D1644895

The Oxford Handbook of Exercise
Psychology

OXFORD LIBRARY OF PSYCHOLOGY

Editor in Chief PETER E. NATHAN

The Oxford Handbook of Exercise Psychology

Edited by

Edmund O. Acevedo

OXFORD
UNIVERSITY PRESS

OXFORD
UNIVERSITY PRESS

Oxford University Press, Inc., publishes works that further
Oxford University's objective of excellence
in research, scholarship, and education.

Oxford   New York
Auckland   Cape Town   Dar es Salaam   Hong Kong   Karachi
Kuala Lumpur   Madrid   Melbourne   Mexico City   Nairobi
New Delhi   Shanghai   Taipei   Toronto

With offices in
Argentina   Austria   Brazil   Chile   Czech Republic   France   Greece
Guatemala   Hungary   Italy   Japan   Poland   Portugal   Singapore
South Korea   Switzerland   Thailand   Turkey   Ukraine   Vietnam

Published by Oxford University Press, Inc.
198 Madison Avenue, New York, New York 10016
www.oup.com

Oxford is a registered trademark of Oxford University Press

Library of Congress Cataloging-in-Publication Data
The Oxford handbook of exercise psychology / edited by Edmund O. Acevedo.
    p. cm. — (Oxford library of psychology)
  ISBN-13: 978-0-19-539431-3 (acid-free paper)
  ISBN-10: 0-19-539431-3 (acid-free paper)
  1. Exercise—Psychological aspects.   2. Physical fitness—Psychological aspects.
  I. Acevedo, Edmund O.
  GV481.2.O94 2012
  613.71—dc23
  2011037048

9 8 7 6 5 4 3 2
Printed in the United States of America
on acid-free paper

CONTENTS

OXFORD LIBRARY OF PSYCHOLOGY

The *Oxford Library of Psychology*, a landmark series of handbooks, is published by Oxford University Press, one of the world's oldest and most highly respected publishers, with a tradition of publishing significant books in psychology. The ambitious goal of the *Oxford Library of Psychology* is nothing less than to span a vibrant, wide-ranging field and, in so doing, to fill a clear market need.

Encompassing a comprehensive set of handbooks, organized hierarchically, the *Library* incorporates volumes at different levels, each designed to meet a distinct need. At one level are a set of handbooks designed broadly to survey the major subfields of psychology; at another are numerous handbooks that cover important current focal research and scholarly areas of psychology in depth and detail. Planned as a reflection of the dynamism of psychology, the *Library* will grow and expand as psychology itself develops, thereby highlighting significant new research that will impact on the field. Adding to its accessibility and ease of use, the *Library* will be published in print and, later on, electronically.

The *Library* surveys psychology's principal subfields with a set of handbooks that capture the current status and future prospects of those major subdisciplines. This initial set includes handbooks of social and personality psychology, clinical psychology, counseling psychology, school psychology, educational psychology, industrial and organizational psychology, cognitive psychology, cognitive neuroscience, methods and measurements, history, neuropsychology, personality assessment, developmental psychology, and more. Each handbook undertakes to review one of psychology's major subdisciplines with breadth, comprehensiveness, and exemplary scholarship. In addition to these broadly conceived volumes, the *Library* includes a large number of handbooks designed to explore in depth more specialized areas of scholarship and research, such as stress, health and coping, anxiety and related disorders, cognitive development, and child and adolescent assessment. In contrast to the broad coverage of the subfield handbooks, each of these latter volumes focuses on an especially productive, more highly focused line of scholarship and research. Whether at the broadest or most specific level, however, all of the *Library* handbooks offer synthetic coverage that reviews and evaluates the relevant past and present research and anticipates research in the future. Each handbook in the *Library* includes an introductory chapter written by its editor to provide a road map to the handbook's table of contents and to offer informed anticipations of significant future developments in that field.

An undertaking of this scope calls for handbook editors and chapter authors who are established scholars in the areas about which they write. Many of the nation's and world's most productive and best-respected psychologists have agreed to edit *Library* handbooks or write authoritative chapters in their areas of expertise.

For whom has the *Oxford Library of Psychology* been written? Because of its breadth, depth, and accessibility, the *Library* serves a diverse audience, including graduate students in psychology and their faculty mentors, scholars, researchers, and practitioners in psychology and related fields. Each will find in the *Library* the information they seek on the subfield or focal area of psychology in which they work or are interested.

Befitting its commitment to accessibility, each handbook includes a comprehensive index, as well as extensive references to help guide research. And because the *Library* was designed from its inception as an online as well as a print resource, its structure and contents will be readily and rationally searchable online. Further, once the *Library* is released online, the handbooks will be regularly and thoroughly updated.

In summary, the *Oxford Library of Psychology* will grow organically to provide a thoroughly informed perspective on the field of psychology, one that reflects both psychology's dynamism and its increasing interdisciplinarity. Once published electronically, the *Library* is also destined to become a uniquely valuable interactive tool, with extended search and browsing capabilities. As you begin to consult this handbook, we sincerely hope you will share our enthusiasm for the more than 500-year tradition of Oxford University Press for excellence, innovation, and quality, as exemplified by the *Oxford Library of Psychology*.

Peter E. Nathan
Editor-in-Chief
Oxford Library of Psychology

ABOUT THE EDITOR

Edmund O. Acevedo

Edmund O. Acevedo, Ph.D., is Professor and Chair in the Department of Health and Human Performance at Virginia Commonwealth University. His primary research focus is on the interaction of mental stress and fitness level on an individual's health. Most recently, he has examined the impact of acute stress on factors that impact the process of cardiovascular disease in obese and lean individuals. The work of his research team suggests an interaction between obesity, psychological stress, and cardiovascular diseases. In summary, his research supports the notion that psychological stress can have deleterious effects on cardiovascular health, and improved fitness may ameliorate these effects. His research has been funded by federal and private sources. He is coauthor with Panteleimon Ekkekakis of an edited text published by Human Kinetics entitled, *"The Psychobiology of Physical Activity"* (2006). He is a Fellow of the American College of Sports Medicine and the American Psychological Association and has served as President of Division 47, which is the Exercise and Sport Psychology division of the American Psychological Association.

Edmund O. Acevedo
Department of Health and Human
   Performance
Virginia Commonwealth University
Richmond, VA

Rebecca L. Bassett
Department of Kinesiology
McMaster University
Hamilton, ON, Canada

Louis Bherer
Department of Psychology
Université du Québec à Montréal
Associate Director for Clinical Research
Institut Universitaire de Gériatrie de
   Montréal
Montréal, Québec, Canada

Christopher D. Black
Department of Health, Exercise Science,
   and Recreation Management
University of Mississippi
Oxford, MS

Robert J. Brustad
School of Sport & Exercise Science
University of Northern Colorado
Greeley, CO

Catherine Conlin
Department of Kinesiology
McMaster University
Hamilton, ON, Canada

Kerry S. Courneya
Faculty of Physical Education and
   Recreation
University of Alberta
Edmonton, AB, Canada

Manolis Dafermos
Department of Psychology
University of Crete
Rethymnon, Crete, Greece

Panteleimon Ekkekakis
Department of Kinesiology
Iowa State University
Ames, IA

Jennifer L. Etnier
Department of Kinesiology
University of North Carolina at Greensboro
Greensboro, NC

Brian C. Focht
Kinesiology
The Ohio State University
Columbus, OH

Karly S. Geller
Cancer Research Center of Hawaii
University of Hawaii at Manoa
Honolulu, HI

Martin S. Hagger
School of Psychology and Speech Pathology
Curtin University
Perth, Australia

Mark Hamer
Department of Epidemiology and Public
   Health
University College London
London, UK

Kate Hefferon
Department of Psychology
University of East London
London, UK

Daniel B. Hollander
Department of Kinesiology and Health
   Studies
Southeastern Louisiana University
Hammond, LA

Chun-Jung Huang
Department of Exercise Science and Health
   Promotion
Florida Atlantic University
Boca Raton, FL

Ian Janssen
School of Kinesiology & Health Studies, and
Department of Community Health &
Epidemiology
Queen's University
Kingston, ON, Canada

Robert R. Kraemer
Department of Kinesiology and Health
Studies
Southeastern Louisiana University
Hammond, LA

Jeffrey D. Labban
Department of Kinesiology
University of North Carolina at Greensboro
Greensboro, NC

Kate Lambourne
Cardiovascular Research Institute
University of Kansas Medical Center
Kansas City, KS

Fuzhong Li
Oregon Research Institute
Eugene, OR

Bess H. Marcus
Department of Family and Preventive
Medicine
University of California, San Diego
La Jolla, CA

Rachel Mark
Behavioural Medicine Laboratory
University of Victoria
Victoria, BC, Canada

Jeffrey J. Martin
Division of Kinesiology, Health, and Sport
Studies
Wayne State University
Detroit, MI

Kathleen A. Martin Ginis
Department of Kinesiology
McMaster University
Hamilton, ON, Canada

Nanette Mutrie
Department of Sport, Culture and the Arts
University of Strathclyde
Glasgow, UK

Jack A. Naglieri
Research Professor
University of Virginia
Charlottesville, VA

Claudio R. Nigg
Department of Public Health Sciences
John A. Burns School of Medicine
University of Hawaii at Manoa
Honolulu, HI

Steven J. Petruzzello
Department of Kinesiology &
Community Health
University of Illinois at Urbana-Champaign
Champaign, IL

Leila A. Pfaeffli
Behavioural Medicine Laboratory
University of Victoria
Victoria, BC, Canada

Ryan E. Rhodes
Behavioural Medicine Laboratory
University of Victoria
Victoria, BC, Canada

Amy E. Speed-Andrews
Faculty of Physical Education and
Recreation
University of Alberta
Edmonton, AB, Canada

Phillip D. Tomporowski
Department of Kinesiology
University of Georgia
Athens, GA

Heather E. Webb
Department of Kinesiology
Mississippi State University
Mississippi State, MS

David M. Williams
Department of Behavioral and Social
Sciences
Program in Public Health
Brown University
Providence, RI

CONTENTS

PART 1

Context, Issues, and Perspectives in Exercise Psychology

Exercise Psychology: Understanding the Mental Health Benefits of Physical Activity and the Public Health Challenges of Inactivity

Edmund O. Acevedo

Abstract

Regular physical activity is important for optimal physical and mental health. Furthermore, physical inactivity has been identified as a leading cause of death (U.S. Department of Health and Human Services, 1996). However, the Centers for Disease Control and Prevention (Barnes, 2007) have reported that fewer than 50% of Americans participate in regular physical activity. This information highlights the public health challenge of increasing participation in physical activity to enhance physical health and to buoy the psychological benefits associated with physical activity.

This chapter presents a brief synopsis of the evidence that compels the study of exercise psychology. In addition, as a basis for assimilating the content of subsequent chapters, this chapter includes explanations for terms often used in exercise psychology, important methodological and conceptual clarifications, and a preface to the topics addressed throughout this text.

Key Words: exercise, mental health, physical activity, motivation, physical activity assessment.

> Lack of activity destroys the good condition of every human being, while movement and methodical physical exercise save it and preserve it.
> —*Plato*

Throughout most of history the physical requirements of survival have been a defining element of human existence. However, within the last 150 years, industrial and technological advancements have made survival no longer intricately dependent on physical demands. With little need for physical activity to perform important work for society, ease of transportation, and almost effortless access to information, most of the population must make a conscious effort to incorporate physical activity into their lifestyles. The challenge to self-regulate exercise behavior has had unexpected, negative health consequences. This challenge, along with the documented psychological benefits associated with participating in physical activity, is central to the arguments supporting the study of exercise psychology.

This chapter provides a brief presentation of the evidence that compels the study of exercise psychology. In addition, it presents explanations for terms that are used in the field of exercise psychology. Together these will serve to define the broad scope of this interdisciplinary field. The cross-fertilization of knowledge has had a tremendously positive effect on the development of exercise psychology. In addition, this chapter clarifies important methodological and conceptual issues that will provide a platform from which to assimilate the content presented in subsequent chapters. In particular, a number of issues relevant to the combined investigation of physical activity and behavior are included—for example, the challenge of assessing physical activity, the relationship of physical health outcomes to mental health outcomes within the context of standard exercise prescription guidelines for physical health outcomes, and, although minimal and far outweighed by the benefits, the health risks associated with exercise. This chapter also includes a preface to the topics addressed in this text.

In 1996 the Surgeon General's Report identified physical inactivity as a leading cause of death. Since the publication of that report, physical inactivity has contributed to the deaths of approximately 200,000 Americans per year (Danaei et al., 2009). Even with the common understanding of the importance of physical activity to health (Bouchard, Blair, & Haskell, 2007), the Centers for Disease Control and Prevention has reported that fewer than 50% of Americans participate in regular physical activity (Barnes, 2007). Furthermore, evidence supports the benefits of physical activity to mental health, including improvements in depression, anxiety, self-concept, quality of life, and cognitive function (see Faulkner & Taylor, 2005). Promoting physical activity has clear relevance to improving physical and mental health. This text provides in-depth analyses of the literature that examines the behavioral, affective, cognitive, and psychobiological antecedents and consequences of physical activity, with a focus on the adoption and maintenance of physical activity and its effects on psychological well-being.

Regular physical activity can help in controlling weight; reducing the risk of cardiovascular disease, type 2 diabetes, metabolic syndrome, and some cancers; improving bone strength; and improving the ability to do daily activities and preventing falls in older adults (USDHHS, 1996). The financial cost of the physical health consequences of inactivity is approximately $250 billion (Chenoweth & Leutzinger, 2006). In addition, the benefits of physical activity include alleviating depression, decreasing anxiety, enhancing self-concept and cognitive function, attenuating the stress response, and improving general mood states (Faulkner & Taylor, 2005). These mental health benefits are important when one considers that at least one in five people in the United States has a diagnosed mental disorder, and the estimated direct cost of mental health services is now more than $99 billion (U.S. Department of Health and Human Service, 1999). These physical and mental health benefits, along with the potential reduction of the dramatic financial costs of poor health, provide great impetus for the promotion of physical activity as a public health goal.

An understanding of the mental health benefits of exercise has developed from an appreciation of the value of interdisciplinary investigation into the psychobiological nature of the physical activity experience. The study of exercise psychology provides an excellent model for examining the link between the mind-brain and the body. This age-old concept is highlighted in the quote that begins this chapter. An even more compelling consideration is that physical fitness is necessary for optimal physical and mental health, including cognitive function (Kramer, Erickson, & Colcombe, 2006), and "to make normal life more fulfilling" (Seligman & Csikszentmihalyi, 2000). This is a central proposition of the conceptualization of positive psychology by Seligman and Csikszentmihalyi.

Terminology

The terms *physical activity* and *exercise* are often used interchangeably; however, there are subtle differences. **Physical activity** is defined as "*any* bodily movement produced by skeletal muscles that results in energy expenditure" (Caspersen, Powell, and Christenson, 1985). In the literature examples of physical activity include activities of daily living, participation in sports, exercise, and leisure-time activity. However, the literature goes further in defining **exercise** as a form of structured physical activity with the specific objective of improving or maintaining physical fitness or health. The psychological study of emotions, thoughts, and behaviors of physical activity versus exercise also maintains this subtle distinction between structured physical activity and physical activity encompassing all types of movement. It is important to appreciate that, as Gill (2009) has noted, "Physical activity is the key to positive health and quality of life, and, thus, lifetime physical activity is the base for healthy lives" (p. 691). However, the primary focus of this text is the development of empirical evidence in support of physical activity programs that promote health. A major challenge in developing such knowledge is assessing physical activity as a stimulus for improvements in health. The necessity or desire to efficiently and effectively quantify, prescribe, and promote physical activity to increase the likelihood of a positive health outcome is the rationale for the use of "exercise psychology" in the title of this text. Nonetheless, throughout this text and in parallel with the literature, "physical activity" and "exercise" are often used interchangeably.

The historical development of exercise psychology has been fueled by a broad range of disciplines and interdisciplinary approaches. In 1986, the research journal *Journal of Sport Psychology* changed its name to the *Journal of Sport and Exercise Psychology* to include this promising area of investigation. Since then a number of new journals addressing exercise psychology have included "exercise" or "physical activity" in their titles, including *Psychology of Sport and Exercise, International Journal of Sport and Exercise Psychology, Mental Health and Physical Activity*, and *International Journal of Behavioral Nutrition and Physical Activity*. Today inquiries into the behavioral aspects of exercise and physical activity originate from health psychology, rehabilitation psychology, positive psychology, psychobiology, neuroscience, behavioral epidemiology, behavioral medicine, and exercise science. Furthermore, scientific journals from these disciplines and subdisciplines frequently publish articles on research that uses physical activity as an independent variable. The plethora of work parallels the demand for knowledge in this area. Comprehensive historical accounts of the field of exercise psychology have been presented by Rejeski and Thompson (1993) and Buckworth and Dishman (2002).

The exercise psychology literature most often examines exercise or physical activity as an independent variable. A clear understanding of the benefits of this stimulus (physical activity or exercise) requires an operational definition. When interpreting the exercise literature one must recognize that the exercise stimulus can be either acute—a single relatively short bout of exercise—or chronic—exercise that is carried out repeatedly over time, usually for a number of weeks. To further describe the physical challenge of an exercise program the duration of the activity, intensity of the activity, the type of activity, and the frequency (per week) must be identified. In 2007 the American College of Sports Medicine (ACSM) and the American Heart Association (AHA) provided updates to their physical activity guidelines based on the most relevant science that links physical activity to enhanced health and quality of life (Haskell et al., 2007). ACSM/AHA guidelines recommend a minimum of 30 minutes of moderate-intensity aerobic physical activity five days a week. Alternatively, individuals can accumulate 30 minutes over the course of a day with shorter bouts that total 30 minutes. These guidelines are considered minimal recommended

amounts. Finally, the exercise stimulus does not have to be aerobic. It can also be anaerobic, which includes resistance exercise (weight training), and it can be a combination of activities. These types of exercise have received little attention in the exercise psychology literature. The parameters of the physical stimulus (exercise) to be studied must be clearly defined so that one is able to compare "apples to apples" or be able to identify differences in the stimulus to compare "apples to oranges."

Key Methodological and Conceptual Clarifications

While the ACSM/AHA guidelines address the activity requirements for physical health, these guidelines do not address the exercise stimulus necessary for mental health benefits. Furthermore, the mechanisms that explain the physiological adaptations to exercise that impact physical health have received much attention, whereas the psychobiological mechanisms that explain the mental health benefits have only recently been investigated. It is intriguing to consider the exercise stimuli that are necessary to elicit positive mental health outcomes, and which mechanisms explain these adaptations. Interestingly, while the mental health benefits of aerobic exercise have begun to be explored, the psychological responses and mental health benefits of anaerobic exercise, resistance exercise (weight lifting), and combinations of activities have received little attention in the literature. Thus, although aerobic physical activity is associated with significant mental health benefits, the challenge still exists to define a specific exercise prescription for a specific mental health benefit. It may be that the mental health outcomes are not contingent on changes in the physiological parameters that have supported the ACSM/AHA guidelines.

In addition, the exercise psychology literature has understandably struggled in its attempt to measure physical activity as a perception and as an objective physical stimulus. Valid and reliable assessment of physical activity is important in the investigation of the direct relationship between physical activity and mental health; in the study of physical activity patterns, determinants, and barriers in different populations; and in evaluating the effectiveness of physical activity interventions (Pols, Peeters, Kemper, & Grobbee, 1998; Washburn, Heath, & Jackson, 2000). Furthermore, addressing the dose–response relationship with psychological outcomes necessitates the accurate measurement of physical activity.

The literature has included subjective (self-report questionnaires, diaries) and objective measures (heart rate monitors, pedometers, accelerometers, doubly labeled water), with the inherent advantages and disadvantages of both. More specifically, self-report measures are relatively inexpensive, are easy to administer, and can be used with large samples. Conversely, objective measures, although they are not subject to recall error and are generally unobtrusive, can often fail to assess specific types of activities (water sports, arm exercise, walking or running on an incline) and can be very expensive. In addition, the use of a specific technique may be limited by the ability of the participant to follow instructions. Thus the age and any special needs or characteristics of the participants must be considered. Welk, Blair, Wood, Jones, and Thompson (2000) have proposed that accelerometers, which measure movement based on acceleration and deceleration of the body, provide the most reliable and valid measure of physical activity for research purposes. However, an objective measure of physical activity does not preclude the importance of assessing individuals' perceptions of the amount of their physical activity participation. Depending on the research question, the perception of activity may be more critical to the research question or outcome of interest than the actual or objective assessment of physical activity. Tudor-Locke and Meyers (2001) in their review have suggested that the use of multiple measures will likely increase the accuracy of the assessment. Our understanding of exercise psychology will continue to progress in parallel with the improvements in the tools for assessing physical activity.

An aspect of exercise that must be considered prior to embarking on an examination of its benefits is the potential health risks associated with physical activity participation. While the benefits clearly outweigh the risks (USDHHS, 1996), understanding the risks provides insight that can be used to minimize the possibility of an adverse event or response to physical activity. The two most discussed risks are myocardial infarction and musculoskeletal injuries. Individuals with underlying heart disease are at increased risk of a cardiac event during physical activity because of the additional stress it places on the heart and circulatory system. However, this stress also serves as a stimulus for improved cardiovascular function. Ultimately, physical activity reduces the risk of cardiovascular disease by at least half (Kohl, Powell, Gordon, Blair, & Paffenbager,

1992). Cardiac patients can experience considerable improvements, but must take appropriate clinical precautions when participating in physical activity (ACSM, 2010).

Most physical activity–related injuries can be categorized as overuse injuries. These musculoskeletal injuries are associated with the frequency, intensity, and duration of exercise (Pate & Macera, 1994). Thus the risk of these injuries can be minimized by a reduction in the frequency, intensity, or the duration of the activity. The recommendations for health-related physical activity by the ACSM (2010) are moderate enough to limit the incidence of overuse injuries for most people (Pate et al., 1995). At very high levels of activity health problems can include dehydration, hyperthermia and hypothermia from exercise in extreme environmental conditions, amenorrhea, anemia, and suppression of immune function. In general, these conditions, when monitored, can be improved with an appropriate decrease in the level of physical exertion or limitation of physical activity participation.

Several mental health problems related to exercise have received some attention in the literature. Exercise dependence—a combination of high levels of physical activity participation and a strong perceived need to exercise despite all obstacles (Davis, Brewer, & Ratusny, 1993)—can interfere with social and work activities and lead to or exacerbate injuries. In addition, in habitual exercisers withdrawal from exercise can elicit depressive symptoms, anxiety, and symptoms of emotional distress (Mondin et al., 1996). Current understanding of the extent and severity of exercise dependency across the population is very limited. Interestingly, Coen and Ogles (1993) have found that participants who rated high on exercise dependency had less psychopathology and less body image distortion than individuals with anorexia nervosa. This distinction suggests that although exercise dependency and anorexia share some similar characteristics, the severity of the potential medical and psychological consequences is much greater for anorexic individuals. Finally, Morgan, Brown, Raglin, O'Connor, and Ellickson (1987) have reported that athletes, as a result of overtraining (when the volume and intensity of exercise exceeds an individual's recovery capacity and performance is compromised), can experience symptoms of chronic fatigue, muscle soreness, insomnia, and disturbed mood. Although substantial evidence supports the detrimental psychological consequences of excessive physical activity, this evidence must be considered in light of the plethora of data demonstrating the beneficial physical and mental health effects of appropriate levels of exercise and the fact that fewer than 15% of U.S. adults, a relatively small portion of the population, regularly participate in vigorous exercise (USDHHS, 1996). Thus the challenge of increasing physical activity is pertinent to enhancing physical and mental health and addressing the tremendous cost to society of inactivity.

The contents of this authoritative and comprehensive text present the breadth and depth of empirical contributions using state-of-the-science theories and approaches in exercise psychology. The authors are leading investigators who have made significant scientific contributions to the literature examining the behavioral aspects of physical activity, and each chapter presents a summary of scientific advances in the topic area as a foundation for future investigation. To provide a context for interpreting the contents of this text, the second chapter of this introductory section addresses the epidemiology of physical activity. Subsequent sections address the effects of physical activity on mental health; knowledge gathered using psychobiological perspectives; behavioral factors that affect exercise motivation; the benefits of physical activity in special populations, including individuals with physical disabilities, older adults, and cancer patients; and promising areas for additional investigation.

References

American College of Sports Medicine. (2010). *ACSM's guidelines for exercise testing and prescription* (8th ed.). Philadelphia, PA: Lippincott Williams & Wilkins.

Barnes P. (2007). *Physical activity among adults: United States, 2000 and 2005*. Hyattsville, MD: U.S. Department of Health and Human Services, Centers for Disease Control and Prevention.

Bouchard, C., Blair, S. N., & Haskell, W. L. E. (2007). *Physical activity and health*. Champaign, IL: Human Kinetics.

Buckworth, J., & Dishman, R. K. (2002). *Exercise psychology*. Champaign, IL: Human Kinetics.

Caspersen, C. J., Powell, K. E., & Christenson, G. M. (1985). Physical activity, exercise, and physical fitness: Definitions and distinctions for health-related research. *Public Health Reports, 100*(2), 126–131.

Chenoweth, D., & Leutzinger, J. (2006). The economic cost of physical inactivity and excess weight in American adults. *Journal of Physical Activity and Health, 3*, 148–163.

Coen, S., & Ogles, B. (1993). Psychological characteristics of the obligatory runner. *Journal of Sport and Exercise Psychology, 15*, 338–354.

Danaei, G., Ding, E. L., Mozaffarian, D., Taylor, B., Rehm, J., Murray, C. J. L., & Ezzati, M. (2009). The preventable causes of death in the United States: Comparative risk assessment of dietary, lifestyle, and metabolic risk factors. *PLoS Medicine 6*(4):e1000058. doi:10.1371/journal.pmed.1000058

Davis, C., Brewer, H., & Ratusny, D. (1993). Behavioral frequency and psychological commitment: Necessary concepts in the study of excessive exercising. *Journal of Behavioral Medicine, 16*, 611–628.

Faulkner, G. E. J., & Taylor, A. H. (2005). *Exercise, health and mental health: Emerging relationships*. New York: Routledge.

Gill, D. L. (2009). Social psychology and physical activity: Back to the future. *Research Quarterly for Exercise and Sport, 80*, 685–695.

Haskell, W. L., Lee, I. M., Pate, R. R., Powell, K. E., Blair, S. N., Franklin, B. A., . . . Bauman, A. (2007). Physical activity and public health. Updated recommendation for adults from the American College of Sports Medicine and the American Heart Association. *Circulation, 116*, 1081–1093.

Kohl, H. W., Powell, K. E., Gordon, N. F., Blair, S. N., & Paffenbarger, R. S., Jr. (1992). Physical activity, physical fitness, and cardiac death. *Epidemiologic Reviews, 14*, 37–57.

Kramer, A. F., Erickson, K. I., & Colcombe, J. (2006). Exercise, cognition, and the aging brain. *Journal of Applied Physiology, 101*, 1237–1242.

Mondin, G. W., Morgan, W. P., Piering, P. N., Stegner, A. J., Stotesbery, C. L., Trine, M. R., & Wu, M. (1996). Psychological consequences of exercise deprivation in habitual exercisers. *Medicine and Science in Sports and Exercise, 28*, 1199–1203.

Morgan, W. P., Brown, D. R., Raglin J. S., O'Connor, P. J., & Ellickson, K. A. (1987). Psychological monitoring of overtraining and staleness. *British Journal of Sports Medicine, 21*, 107–114.

Pate, R. R., & Macera, C. A. (1994). Risks of exercising: Musculoskeletal injuries. In C. Bouchard, R. J. Shephard, & T. Stephens (Eds). *Physical activity, fitness and health* (pp. 1008–1018). Champaign, IL: Human Kinetics.

Pate, R. R., Pratt, M., Blair, S. N., Haskell, W. L., Macera, C. A., Bouchard, C., . . . King, A.C. (1995). Physical activity and public health. A recommendation from the Centers for Disease Control and Prevention and the American College of Sports Medicine. *JAMA, 273*(5), 402–407.

Pols, M. A., Peeters, P. H. M., Kemper, H. C. G., & Grobbee, D. E. (1998). Methodological aspects of physical activity assessment in epidemiological studies. *European Journal of Epidemiology, 14*, 63–70.

Rejeski, W. J., & Thompson, A. (1993). Historical and conceptual roots of exercise psychology. In P. Seraganian (Ed.), *Exercise psychology: The influence of physical exercise on psychological processes* (pp. 3–35). New York: John Wiley & Sons.

Seligman, M. E. P., & Csikszentmihalyi, M. (2000). Positive psychology: An introduction. *American Psychologist, 55*, 5–14.

Tudor-Locke, C. E., & Myers, A. M. (2001). Challenges and opportunities for measuring physical activity in sedentary adults. *Sports Medicine, 31*, 91–100.

U.S. Department of Health and Human Services. (1996). *Physical activity and health: A report of the Surgeon General*. Atlanta, GA: U.S. Dept of Health and Human Services, Centers for Disease Control and Prevention, National Center for Chronic Disease Prevention and Health Promotion.

U.S. Department of Health and Human Services. (1999). *Mental health: A report of the Surgeon General—executive summary*. Rockville, MD: U.S. Department of Health and Human Services, Substance Abuse and Mental Health Services Administration, Center for Mental Health Services, National Institutes of Health, National Institute of Mental Health.

Washburn, R. A., Heath, G. W., & Jackson, A. W. (2000). Reliability and validity issues concerning large scale surveillance of physical activity. *Research Quarterly for Exercise and Sport, 71*, 104–113.

Welk, G. J., Blair, S. N., Wood, K., Jones, S., & Thompson, R. W. (2000) A comparative evaluation of three accelerometry-based physical activity monitors. *Medicine and Science in Sports and Exercise, 32*, S489–S497.

Physical Activity Epidemiology

Ian Janssen

Abstract

The main purpose of the research discipline of physical activity epidemiology is to study the causal relationship between physical activity, or a lack of physical activity, and health. This chapter begins by explaining the importance of studying this relationship. The chapter then provides some information on the methods used to study and interpret the relations between physical activity and health. The next section of the chapter provides an overview of the scientific evidence on the relationship between physical activity and several health outcomes, including mortality, cardiovascular disease, cancer, diabetes, obesity, osteoporosis, mental health, and functional health. Examples from historical and contemporary studies are used to highlight key relationships. The chapter concludes by discussing how the research findings are translated into public health recommendations on the appropriate volume, intensity, and type of physical activity required for good health.

Key Words: epidemiology, physical activity, surveillance, population health, sedentary behavior.

What Is Physical Activity Epidemiology?

Epidemiology is a research field that is concerned with the occurrence of disease and health problems in human populations. Unlike clinical medicine, which typically focuses on individual patients who are already sick, epidemiology focuses on large groups of people and includes among its concerns the prevention of chronic disease and illness in individuals who are not sick. The field of physical activity epidemiology studies the relationship between physical activity, or a lack of physical activity, and health. Physical activity epidemiology also studies the distribution of physical activity and inactivity within the population and the determinants of physical activity and inactivity.

Physical activity epidemiology has traditionally focused on chronic diseases, which can be defined as diseases that are long-lasting or recurrent, such as diabetes, heart disease, and arthritis. The three leading causes of death in North America (diseases of the heart, cancer, and cerebrovascular diseases), which combined account for approximately 6 in 10 deaths, are all chronic diseases (Mokdad, Marks, Stroup, & Gerberding, 2004). A lack of physical activity contributes to all three of these leading causes of death. It has been estimated that 14.2% of breast cancers, 18.0% of colon cancers, 19.4% of coronary artery diseases, and 24.3% of strokes in Canada could be avoided if everyone in the population engaged in an appropriate amount of physical activity (Katzmarzyk & Janssen, 2004). In addition to the leading causes of death, physical inactivity is associated with a host of other chronic diseases and conditions, including but not limited to type 2 diabetes, osteoporosis, physical disability, depression, and dementia (Bouchard, Blair, & Haskell, 2007; Katzmarzyk, Gledhill, & Shephard, 2000; Physical Activity Guidelines Advisory Committee, 2008).

Importance of Studying the Influence of Physical Activity on Health

Participation in vigorous physical activity was a major factor in the evolution of the human species. Hunting, gathering of food and other necessities, and escaping animal predators were necessary parts of daily life for our ancient ancestors. The most physically fit and best performers had an advantage in these activities and were more likely to survive and pass on their genes to the next generation. Thus survival and reproductive success of humanity over tens of thousands of years required high levels of physical activity and performance.

The necessity for the majority of the population to engage in challenging physical activity on a habitual basis for survival persisted until the Industrial Revolution in the latter half of the 18th century. The Industrial Revolution underpinned dramatic increases in production capacity and people became heavily reliant on a variety of power sources such as the internal combustion engine and electrical power generation. By the end of the Industrial Revolution human survival was no longer contingent on the majority of the population performing demanding muscular work.

In the past hundred years technology has continued to develop at an accelerated pace. Personal computers, fiber optics, communication satellites, the World Wide Web, and a host of other inventions have changed the way we work and get from one location to another. Today, jobs in the workplace and home and transportation from one place to another rely even less on muscle power and motor skills than they did just two decades ago. We have reached a point where the reduction in the amount of habitual physical activity required in our daily lives has gone too far, at least as our health is concerned. Unless people make a conscious effort to engage in physical activity and devote a proportion of their leisure time to doing so, it is unlikely that they will accumulate enough physical activity for health benefits.

Surveillance of Physical Activity

This section of the chapter discusses physical activity levels in the population, as well as how they vary across age, sex, ethnicity, socioeconomic status, and nationality. Although physical activity levels in the population are on a continuum, ranging from extremely sedentary (e.g., bedridden individuals) to incredibly active (e.g., elite marathon runners), for surveillance purposes people are usually placed into "physically active" or "physically inactive" groups. In many instances, the cut point used to distinguish between these two groups is based on whether the individual does or does not meet current public health recommendations for physical activity. For example, the U.S. Behavioral Risk Factor Surveillance System (BRFSS) classifies adults as physically active if they meet recommendations of 30 minutes of moderate physical activity on at least five days of the week or 20 minutes of vigorous physical activity on at least three days of the week (National Center for Chronic Disease Prevention and Health Promotion, 2005).

Table 2.1 illustrates age, sex, ethnic, and socioeconomic variations in physical activity in adults using results from the 2005 BRFSS (National Center for Chronic Disease Prevention and Health Promotion, 2005). The 2005 BRFSS is a nationally representative telephone survey that was administered to over 330,000 American adults from across the country. According to the BRFSS, 48.1% of the adult population are physically active (i.e., meet recommendations), 37.7% of the adult population engage in some physical activity but not enough to meet the recommendations, and 14.2% of the adult population engage in no physical activity whatsoever. The percentage of the adult population who are physically active decreases across age, from a high of 57.4% in 18- to 24-year-olds to a low of 39.8% in those aged 65 or older. Men are slightly more likely to be physically active than women (49.9% vs. 46.4%). Whites are more likely to be physically active than blacks and Hispanics (50.3% vs. 41.1% vs. 42.7%). Finally, there is a socioeconomic gradient such that the prevalence of those who are physically active is greatest in the highest-income group and lowest in the lowest-income group.

Results from the 2005/06 Health Behaviour in School-Aged Children Survey (HBSC; see Table 2.2) illustrate sociodemographic differences in physical activity within American youth as well as across countries (Currie et al., 2008). The 2005/06 HBSC studied 41 countries and regions, including the United States, Canada, and several European countries. The study is based on a questionnaire completed in the classroom in 11-, 13-, and 15-year-olds. Youth were classified as physically active if they reported engaging in at least 60 minutes of moderate-to-vigorous activity every day of the week, which aligns with public health recommendations for physical activity in this age group. Within the U.S. sample of the HBSC, boys were more active than girls. For example, 35% of 13-year-old boys were physically active, while only 21% of

Table 2.1. Prevalence of Physically Active and Inactive Adults (≥18 Years) from the United States According to Age, Sex, Ethnicity, and Income

Population group	% Physically active (meets recommendations)	% Not enough physical activity	% No physical activity
All adults	48.1	37.7	14.2
Age			
18–24 years	57.4	32.3	10.3
25–44 years	50.3	38.7	11.0
45–64 years	46.0	39.8	14.2
≥65 years	39.8	35.7	24.6
Sex			
Men	49.9	36.7	13.4
Women	46.4	38.7	14.9
Ethnicity			
White, non-Hispanic	50.3	37.8	11.9
Black, non-Hispanic	41.1	38.2	20.7
Hispanic	42.7	37.1	20.3
Other race	42.5	38.9	16.0
Multiracial	52.1	35.0	12.9
Income			
<$15,000	37.7	35.2	27.2
$15,000–$24,999	42.2	37.3	20.5
$25,000–$34,999	46.1	39.4	14.4
$35,000–$49,999	49.0	39.7	11.4
≥$50,000	54.4	38.2	7.4

Note. Data taken from *Behavioral Risk Factor Surveillance System,* National Center for Chronic Disease Prevention and Health Promotion, 2005; retrieved March 4, 2010, from http://www.cdc.gov/brfss/2005

13-year-old girls were physically active. There was also a noticeable age gradient in girls, such that the 11-year-old girls were more physically active than 13-year-old girls, who were in turn more physically active than 15-year-olds (26% vs. 21% vs. 14%). This age trend was not observed in boys: 33% of 11-year-olds vs. 35% of 13-year-olds vs. 34% of 15-year-olds were physically active. On average, 27% of the boys and girls in the U.S. HBSC sample were physically active. The physical activity statistics for the U.S. youth compared favorably with those for youth from the other 40 HBSC countries: American youth were the fourth most active. Across all countries, the prevalence of physically active youth varied from a low of 13.2% in Switzerland to a high of 42.5% in Slovakia.

It is important to recognize that the vast majority of surveillance studies on physical activity levels in the population are based on subjective measures of physical activity obtained by questionnaires or interview. There is now strong and convincing evidence that, on average, both children and adults

Table 2.2. Prevalence of Physically Active Youth (Meeting Guidelines) within the 41 Participating Countries of the 2005/2006 Health Behavior in School-Aged Children Study

Country	11-year-old girls (%)	11-year-old boys (%)	13-year-old girls (%)	13-year-old boys (%)	15-year-old girls (%)	15-year-old boys (%)	Average	Ranking
Austria	23	29	14	27	10	13	19.3	21
Belgium (Flemish)	15	20	10	21	11	17	15.7	34
Belgium (French)	23	31	20	27	21	24	24.3	8
Bulgaria	26	39	19	32	16	24	26.0	5
Canada	26	36	16	31	13	27	24.8	6
Croatia	26	36	15	31	10	20	23.0	10
Czech Republic	19	25	17	28	16	27	22.0	15
Denmark	26	31	18	23	16	20	22.3	14
England	18	27	14	23	9	18	18.2	25
Estonia	21	24	13	22	9	18	17.8	26
Finland	37	48	15	24	9	15	24.7	7
France	12	24	5	20	5	14	13.3	39
Germany	20	25	13	19	10	16	17.2	29
Greece	16	25	12	21	7	16	16.2	33
Greenland	27	43	23	28	22	30	28.8	3
Hungary	19	28	13	29	11	19	19.8	19
Iceland	23	29	14	24	9	16	19.2	22
Ireland	38	51	23	39	13	27	31.8	2
Israel	15	30	12	24	6	13	16.7	31
Italy	13	23	9	23	7	16	15.2	36
Latvia	23	30	17	27	16	26	23.2	9
Lithuania	20	27	13	22	13	19	19.0	23
Luxembourg	13	18	11	19	11	19	15.2	37
Malta	18	27	14	20	13	19	18.5	24
Netherlands	20	30	20	24	15	18	21.2	16
Norway	17	27	14	15	7	13	15.5	35
Poland	19	24	12	21	10	21	17.8	27
Portugal	12	30	8	21	5	15	15.2	38
Romania	16	29	11	24	6	16	17.0	30

Table 2.2. (Continued)

Country	11-year-old girls (%)	11-year-old boys (%)	13-year-old girls (%)	13-year-old boys (%)	15-year-old girls (%)	15-year-old boys (%)	Average	Ranking
Russia	12	20	10	18	7	12	13.2	40
Scotland	25	40	15	28	9	21	23.0	11
Slovakia	43	51	35	51	29	46	42.5	1
Slovenia	21	25	10	22	9	19	17.7	28
Spain	24	32	14	21	12	19	20.3	18
Sweden	20	23	14	21	10	11	16.5	32
Switzerland	11	19	10	16	10	13	13.2	41
Macedonia	26	29	18	30	11	21	22.5	12
Turkey	21	29	17	22	12	16	19.5	20
Ukraine	22	33	16	32	11	21	22.5	13
United States	*26*	*33*	*21*	*35*	*14*	*34*	*27.2*	*4*
Wales	21	35	12	27	9	21	20.8	17

Note. Data taken from *Inequalities in Young People's Health: HBSC International Report from the 2005/2006 Survey*, edited by C. Currie, S. Nic Gabhainn, N. Godeau, C. Roberts, R. Smith, D. Currie,...V. Barnekow, 2008, Copenhagen: World Health Organization Regional Office for Europe.

substantively overreport their physical activity using these subjective measures (Adamo, Prince, Tricco, Connor-Gorber, & Tremblay, 2009; Prince et al., 2008). Thus the proportion of the population who are physically active is likely much lower than what most surveillance studies suggest, including the BRFSS and HBSC surveys mentioned above. The discrepancy between subjective and objective measures is highlighted by findings from the 2003–2004 U.S. National Health and Nutrition Examination Survey (NHANES; Troiano et al., 2008). In addition to questionnaires, this survey used objective measures of physical activity. These objective measures were obtained over a one-week period using accelerometers, tiny motion sensors worn on the hip. Within the NHANES study adherence to physical activity recommendations in adults was less than 5% according to accelerometer-measured activity, while adherence to physical activity recommendations based on the questionnaire measures was 51% (Troiano et al., 2008). This enormous difference may be attributable to several factors. A leading argument is that accelerometers provide estimates of physical activity that are close to the actual amounts and that research participants

greatly overestimate their moderate and vigorous physical activity levels on questionnaire measures.

Evaluating the Relations between Physical Activity and Health

This section of the chapter starts with a brief explanation of the study methodologies that are used to assess the effects of physical activity on health in epidemiology. This is followed by an explanation of how the relationships between physical activity and health outcomes are evaluated and interpreted. The section ends with a discussion of the criteria that epidemiologists use to determine the strength of the scientific evidence for a causal association between physical activity and a given health outcome.

Study Designs

Studies of relationships between physical activity and health outcomes fall into two broad categories: observational studies and experimental studies. In *observational studies* the researchers collect, record, and analyze data on study participants as they naturally divide themselves. The researchers do not control or manipulate the physical activity level of the subjects in any way. For example, the participants may be asked to fill out a questionnaire about their physical activity habits and medical history, and the researchers see if their reported level of physical activity is related to the presence of a specific health outcome. Conversely, *experimental studies* involve some type of intervention or control of the participants' physical activity levels by the researchers. For example, the participants may be invited into a laboratory three times a week over several months to engage in an exercise program that is prescribed and monitored by the researchers. The researchers see if this exercise program has an effect on one or more health outcomes.

OBSERVATIONAL STUDIES

Three types of observational studies are commonly used in physical activity epidemiology: cross-sectional studies, case-control studies, and prospective cohort studies. In cross-sectional studies the physical activity and health variables are measured at the same point in time. Consider the following cross-sectional study as an example. Liu et al. (2006) sought to examine the relationship between cardiorespiratory fitness level, in this case a measure of maximal oxygen uptake (VO_2max) during a cycling test, and the metabolic syndrome. The metabolic syndrome is a clustering of risk factors for cardiovascular disease (e.g., high blood pressure, high triglycerides, and high blood glucose). Liu et al. found that in a group of 360 Oji-Cree Aboriginals from Sandy Lake, Ontario, for each 10 ml·kg^{-1}·min^{-1} increase in VO_2max, there was a 70% reduction in the likelihood of the metabolic syndrome. Because the temporal sequence in which the low fitness and metabolic syndrome variables occurred was not clear, Liu et al. could not infer that the low fitness *caused* the metabolic syndrome. They were able to say only that these variables were related. In this situation it was plausible, albeit unlikely, that the metabolic syndrome led to low physical activity and low fitness. For physical activity to be considered a cause of the health outcome, there must be evidence that it precedes the outcome. The lack of temporal sequence is a main limitation of all cross-sectional studies.

Case-control studies begin by classifying participants according to their health outcome. Typically, individuals with the health outcome or disease in question are selected (they represent the cases) along with a group of controls who do not have that health outcome or disease. The controls are usually selected based on similarities in age and gender to the cases. The cases and controls are then queried about their physical activity level in the past (e.g.,

"How active were you 20 years ago?"). An association between physical activity and the health outcome exists when the proportion of cases who were physically active is significantly different from the proportion of controls who were physically active. Consider the study by Mao, Pan, Wen, and Johnson (2003). The researchers interviewed 2,128 patients from the Canadian Cancer Registry with lung disease (cases) and 3,106 individuals from the general population without lung disease (controls). All of the study participants completed a questionnaire in which they were asked to report the duration and frequency with which they engaged in moderate- and vigorous-intensity physical activities in previous years. The cases with lung disease reported that they were less active in previous years than did the controls, implying that an association exists between physical activity and lung disease.

Prospective cohort studies begin by measuring the physical activity or fitness level in a group of subjects at the start of the study (baseline). None of these subjects have the health outcome of interest at that time. The subjects, known as the cohort, are followed over time, usually several years, to see who develops the health outcome. A finding that a greater percentage of the inactive subjects develop the outcome during the follow-up period implies that physical inactivity precedes the health outcome. Consider a prospective cohort study that examined the relation between walking and the risk of developing type 2 diabetes. Krishnan, Rosenberg, and Palmer (2009) assessed physical activity in 45,668 African American women, none of whom had been diagnosed with diabetes. These women completed a detailed physical activity questionnaire and were then followed for 10 years. During the follow-up, 2,928 of the 45,668 women in the cohort developed diabetes. The women who reported walking briskly for five hours or more a week at the start of the study were two-thirds as likely to develop type 2 diabetes over the follow-up period as the women who indicated at the start of the study that they did no brisk walking.

EXPERIMENTAL STUDIES

There are two major types of experimental studies: randomized controlled trials and community trials. In randomized controlled trials the participants are randomly allocated into a control group and one or more experimental groups. The health outcome is measured at baseline in all participants. After randomization, the experimental group(s) undergoes the physical activity intervention, while those in the control group are not provided with an intervention and are asked to maintain their previous activity level. After the intervention is completed, the health outcome is measured again to see if improvements have occurred in the experimental group(s) relative to the control group. To illustrate this study design, consider a recent study that examined whether aerobic exercise, resistance exercise, or a combination of both exercise modalities resulted in the greatest improvement in physical function (Davidson et al., 2009). A group of 136 previously inactive older adults were randomly assigned to one of four groups: resistance exercise, aerobic exercise, resistance + aerobic exercise, or control. All exercise interventions, as prescribed and monitored by the researcher team, were conducted over six months. In response to the six-month intervention, physical function improved significantly in all groups compared with the control group. Improvement in the resistance + aerobic exercise group was greater than in the aerobic exercise group but not the resistance exercise group.

Unlike randomized controlled trials, community trials assign interventions to entire communities or groups of people (e.g., schools) rather than at the individual level. Otherwise, the design of community and randomized trials is similar. A classic example of a community trial in the physical activity epidemiology literature is the Minnesota Heart Health Program (Luepker et al., 1994). This program was initiated in 1980 and involved approximately 400,000 persons from six communities. Three of the six communities received the five- to six-year intervention program; the remaining three communities acted as the controls. The community-based intervention advocated blood pressure and blood cholesterol control, healthy eating, not smoking, and regular physical activity. The intervention program alerted people in the community to health issues, informed them of behavioral alternatives that promote good health, provided incentives for new healthy behaviors, and provided reinforcements for such behaviors. A sample of 7,097 adults from the six communities was studied at different times to test the effectiveness of the intervention. At the end of the intervention, the physical activity levels and cardiovascular disease risk factors were not different in the sample of participants in the intervention communities and the sample of participants from the control communities. Thus this behavioral based community intervention was unable to favorably impact physical activity and cardiovascular disease risk factors.

Evaluating the Statistical Associations between Physical Activity and Health

Many of the statistical associations that are commonly used and reported in exercise psychology studies are also used in physical activity epidemiology research. Hopefully you will already be familiar with the simple statistical tests that are used to determine correlations and to compare group means. Those tests will not be discussed here. Rather, we will consider some of the measures of association that are more specific to physical activity epidemiology, particularly for population-based studies that use the observational and experimental designs covered above.

A simple way to compare chronic disease rates according to the level of physical activity in a cross-sectional study is to look at the *prevalence* of the disease in different physical activity groups (e.g., inactive, moderately active, or active). The prevalence rate refers to the proportion (or percentage) of people in a defined group with the disease at a specific time. In prospective cohort studies this measure would be replaced with incidence rates. *Incidence* refers to new cases of the disease or health outcome during a follow-up period. For example, if 10 out of 100 people developed the outcome in a 10-year follow-up, the cumulative incidence rate over the 10 years would be 10%. A second type of incidence rate commonly used in prospective cohort studies is the *person-time incidence rate*. It is calculated as the total number of new cases during the follow-up period divided by the total person-time units at risk, where the total person-time units is a combined measure of the number of persons at risk of a specific health outcome and the time for which they were at risk. Take for instance a 10-year follow-up for coronary heart disease in three participants. If the first participant developed coronary heart disease after one year, the second participant developed coronary heart disease after five years, and the third participant did not develop coronary heart disease during the follow-up period, the total person-time units for these three participants would be 16 years (1 + 5 + 10 = 16). In prospective cohort studies, which often follow thousands of participants over years or even decades, total person-time units are typically expressed relative to 10,000 or 100,000 person-years (e.g., 100 incident cases per 10,000 person-years or 1,000 incident cases per 100,000 person-years).

It is easy to compare the prevalence and incidence rates of chronic disease in groups with different physical activity or fitness levels to get a sense of the association between physical activity and the health outcome of interest. Another way to measure associations is to compare rates in different groups using ratios. A common ratio score used in cross-sectional, case-control, and prospective cohort studies is the *odds ratio*, which is similar to a *relative risk* or *risk ratio*. It is calculated as the prevalence (or incidence) rate in one group divided by the prevalence (or incidence) rate in another, referent group. For example, if the prevalence of hypertension was 10% in the active group and 20% in the inactive group, the odds ratio for hypertension would be 0.5 in the active group relative to the inactive group. The odds ratio is always 1.0 in the referent group. An odds ratio greater than 1.0 in the comparison group, in this case the active group, would indicate a higher risk than in the referent group, while an odds ratio of less than 1.0 in the comparison group would indicate a lower risk. Thus in this example the odds ratio of 0.5 would suggest that active individuals have a 50% lower risk of hypertension than inactive individuals. If the referent group were switched in this example, such that the active group was the referent group and the inactive group was the comparison group, the relative risk of 2.0 (20% ÷ 10%) in the inactive group relative to the active group would indicate a doubling of the risk with inactivity. The inversion of the ratio score, depending on whether the active or inactive group serves as the referent group, has created some confusion in the physical activity epidemiology literature, particularly when the ratio scores from different studies are being compared.

In the scientific literature most ratio scores are presented with a corresponding *95% confidence interval*. Confidence intervals are used to indicate the reliability of the ratio scores, with wider confidence intervals indicating less reliability. The 95% confidence interval indicates with 95% certainty that the true ratio score would fall within that interval. Confidence intervals are closely related to statistical significance. If both the lower and upper confidence intervals are lower than 1.0, or both the lower and upper confidence intervals are higher than 1.0, it indicates the ratio scores are statistically different in the comparison and referent groups. For instance, an odds ratio of 2.26 with a 95% confidence interval of 1.15–4.43 would indicate that we are 95% certain the true odds ratio falls between 1.15 and 4.43 (i.e., if the study were repeated 100 times the odds ratio would fall in this range 95% of the time). Because both the lower and upper confidence intervals are above 1.0, the odds ratio of 2.26 in the comparison group is significantly different from the odds ratio of 1.0 in the referent group.

A ratio score that is interpreted in a similar manner to the odds ratio or relative risk, and that can be used exclusively in prospective cohort studies, is the *hazard ratio*. The hazard ratio calculation is very complex and takes into consideration both the incidence of cases of the chronic disease and the differences in the length of the follow-up period prior to disease development for different research participants.

The limitation of the rates and association measures discussed thus far is that they are crude rates. While these crude rates are easy to calculate and compare, they cannot be compared without fear of distortion due to confounding by differences in other variables in the different physical activity groups such as age, sex, ethnicity, and lifestyle habits such as smoking. A confounding variable in physical activity epidemiology is a variable that is related both to physical activity and the health outcome, and that may in part or in whole explain why physical activity is related to the health outcome. Consider, for instance, a 17-year prospective cohort study that reported a relative risk of 0.58 for coronary heart disease in the most physically active group relative to the inactive group (Wannamethee, Shaper, & Alberti, 2000). In that study 29% of the participants in the most physically active group were smokers, while 54% of the participants in the inactive group were smokers. Thus part of the reason why the physically active group had a lower coronary heart disease risk than the inactive group is because fewer of them smoked. It is possible to control statistically for the confounding effects of smoking and other variables in odds ratio, relative risk, and hazard ratio calculations using a multivariate analysis. Contemporary studies in physical activity epidemiology typically control for several confounding variables in the statistical analyses. With these statistical controls it is hoped that the independent effects of physical activity on the health outcome of interest can be determined. In the example noted earlier on in this paragraph, the hazard ratio for coronary heart disease in the most active group changed from 0.58 to 0.89 after the confounding effects of smoking and several other covariates, such as obesity and social class, were controlled for statistically in the multivariate analysis. Thus, the effect of physical activity on coronary heart disease risk weakened when the confounds were considered.

Evaluating the Strength of Evidence for Causation

A goal in physical activity epidemiology is to establish the existence of a causal association between physical activity and specified health outcomes. Many of the associations that are observed in the literature may have occurred by chance alone, may reflect measurement errors in the studies, may reflect biases of the researchers, or are noncausal (i.e., influenced by confounding variables). Causal associations are those in which the researcher is confident that a change in physical activity would result in a change in the health outcome. Experimental studies, at least when well designed and conducted, come much closer to establishing causation than do observational studies. Within observational studies, prospective cohort studies provide more evidence of causation than do cross-sectional and case-control studies, all else being equal.

In addition to temporal sequence, a number of other criteria are used to determine whether associations are likely to be causal:

- *Strength of the association.* The stronger the association, the more likely it is to be causal. Positive ratio scores (e.g., odds or hazard ratios) below 1.5 and negative ratio scores above 0.70 indicate weak associations. Positive ratio scores above 3.0 and negative ratio scores below 0.40 indicate strong associations.
- *Consistency of the association.* When different researchers obtain similar findings, despite the fact that they studied different research participants at different times using different methodologies, it is more likely that the associations are causal.
- *Dose–response relationship.* In general, if an increase in physical activity along a continuum leads to an increasingly greater change in the health outcome, this is suggestive of a dose–response and causal relationship.
- *Biological plausibility.* Does the association make sense based on possible biological mechanisms? For example, it is biologically plausible that physical activity is negatively associated with obesity because participation in physical activity results in an increase in fat oxidation and energy expenditure.

The information provided in this section on study designs and measures of association should provide you with the background you need to appreciate the research studies discussed in the remainder of this chapter. This information should also give you a basic understanding of how to read and interpret research papers in physical activity epidemiology if you are interested in exploring the relations between physical activity and health in more depth than this chapter provides.

Historical Perspectives on Physical Activity and Health

The history of physical activity epidemiology research began in the 1950s with the pioneering work of Dr. Jeremy Morris. Morris began to study the incidence of heart disease in civil service workers in England using a prospective cohort design (Morris, Heady, Raffle, Roberts, & Parks, 1953). Specifically, he found that a group of highly active conductors who worked on double-decker buses, who spent the majority of their day on their feet and climbed the stairs on the bus numerous times, had a lower risk of having a myocardial infarction during a two-year follow-up than a group of sedentary bus drivers who worked on the same buses. The incidence rates of myocardial infarction in these two groups were 19 and 27 cases per 10,000 person-years, respectively. Morris later reported that postmen had a lower incidence of coronary heart disease than sedentary office clerks and telephone operators (Morris & Crawford, 1958).

Evidence of the health benefits of physical activity continued to build in the latter half of the 20th century. Dr. Ralph Paffenbarger made a number of important contributions. Most notable among Paffenbarger's studies were those based on the alumni of Harvard University, most of whom had very sedentary occupations. The more than 15,000 men who were part of these studies filled in comprehensive physical activity questionnaires and were followed using a prospective cohort study design for coronary artery disease. In a seminal paper published in 1978, Paffenbarger noted that the amount of stairs climbed, blocks walked, strenuous sports played, and a composite physical activity value all opposed risk (Paffenbarger, Wing, & Hyde, 1978). Compared with men with a composite physical activity value above 2,000 kcal/week, men with a physical activity index below 2,000 kcal/week had a relative risk for coronary artery disease of 1.64. This study provided some of the first evidence that leisure-time physical activity—physical activity performed outside of the work environment—has beneficial effects on chronic disease risk.

In the 1980s important developments in the discipline took place with the research of Dr. Steven Blair and colleagues from the Cooper Institute in Dallas, Texas. They assembled the Aerobics Center

Longitudinal Study, a prospective cohort of over 13,000 adults. Rather than measuring physical activity, this research team had their study participants complete a maximal treadmill test to measure their cardiorespiratory fitness (Blair et al., 1989). Physical activity is an important determinant of fitness, so to a certain extent, fitness is an objective measure of physical activity. Prior studies had relied on subjective measures of physical activity obtained by questionnaire, and measures of fitness therefore provided additional insight into the contribution of physical activity to good health. The initial findings from the Blair et al. (1989) prospective cohort study were quite striking. Moderately fit men (40–59th percentile) had a relative risk for mortality from all causes of 1.46 compared with men in the highest fitness quintile (80th percentile and above), whereas men in the lowest fitness quintile (19th percentile and below) had a relative risk of 3.44. The corresponding relative risks in women were 1.43 and 4.65, respectively. Note how strong these associations for fitness (measured objectively) are in comparison with those for physical activity (measured subjectively) observed by Paffenbarger et al. (1978) in the Harvard Alumni Study. One of the consequences of using imprecise measurement techniques, which is typical of physical activity questionnaires, is a diluted association between the physical activity exposure and health outcome.

From these early beginnings, there has been a huge growth spurt in physical activity epidemiology in the past two decades, with an exponential increase in the number of studies. While most of the early studies employed prospective cohort designs, there has also been an infusion of experimental studies. These experimental studies have typically been relatively small (<100 participants), have focused on risk factors (e.g., blood pressure, cholesterol, or bone mineral density) and not disease outcomes (e.g., coronary heart disease or osteoporosis), and have not been as rigorously conducted as in many other disciplines (e.g., pharmacology). Thus the strength of the experimental studies in physical activity epidemiology has traditionally been less than in clinical medicine and other substantive epidemiology disciplines. However, in the past decade or so two large, well-controlled, randomized lifestyle-based interventions have been conducted that meet the most rigorous design standards (Diabetes Prevention Program Research Group, 2002; Tuomilehto et al., 2001). Both of these trials focused on the prevention of diabetes in high-risk patients—specifically,

patients who were obese and had poor glucose tolerance. Consider the Finnish Diabetes Prevention Study (Tuomilehto et al., 2001). The 552 participants were randomly assigned to an intervention group or a control group. The intervention group received individual counseling aimed at reducing weight, increasing physical activity, and improving diet (low fat, high fiber). The cumulative incidence of type 2 diabetes after 4 years was 11% in the intervention group vs. 23% in the control group. Among the participants in the intervention group, the odds ratio for type 2 diabetes in those who achieved the modest physical activity goal was 0.2 (95% confidence interval: 0.1–0.6) compared with those in the intervention group who maintained a sedentary lifestyle.

Relations between Physical Activity and Health

The next section of this chapter discusses the relationship of physical activity to premature mortality and several chronic diseases. Before moving on, it is important to point out that there is an extensive body of scientific literature supporting the beneficial role of physical activity for each of these health outcomes. There have been entire chapters, and in some cases books, that cover each of the relationships that will be discussed here in a few paragraphs. Physical activity is also related to several health outcomes and determinants that are not covered here. The goal in this chapter is to summarize the relationships for several key health outcomes. To do so, example studies from the literature have been selected to highlight some of the key findings and issues. For each of the health outcomes discussed, Table 2.3 shows a summary of the evidence for a causal role of physical activity, based on the criteria described earlier in this chapter.

Physical Activity and All-Cause Mortality

A large body of scientific evidence, all from prospective cohort studies, has examined the association of physical activity with all-cause mortality rates. The data consistently show an inverse relation, with the most active individuals experiencing about a 30% reduction in the risk of dying during follow-up compared with the least active individuals (Physical Activity Guidelines Advisory Committee, 2008). The protective effects of physical activity extend to both sexes, adults of different ages, and different racial and ethic groups (Physical Activity Guidelines Advisory Committee, 2008). Findings in the Harvard Alumni

Table 2.3. Summary of the Causal Evidence That Physical Activity Prevents Mortality, the Development of Chronic Disease, and a Poor Quality of Life

Health outcome	Demonstrated temporal sequence of relationship with physical activity		Strength of association with physical activity	Consistency of association across studies	Evidence of a dose–response relation with physical activity	Biologically plausible relationship with physical activity
	Observational studies	Experimental studies				
All-cause mortality	Yes	No	Weak to modest	Consistent	Yes	Yes
Cardiovascular disease	Yes	No (yes for risk factors)	Modest	Consistent	Yes	Yes
Cancer (colon and breast)	Yes	No	Weak	Somewhat consistent	Yes	Yes
Type 2 diabetes	Yes	Yes	Modest to strong	Consistent	Yes	Yes
Obesity	Yes	Yes	Weak to strong	Somewhat consistent	Yes	Yes
Osteoporosis	No (yes for fractures)	No (yes for bone density)	Modest	Consistent (weight bearing exercise)	Yes	Yes
Mental health	Yes	Yes	Weak	Somewhat consistent	Yes	Yes
Functional health and disability	Yes	Yes	Weak to moderate	Consistent	Yes	Yes

Study indicated that 16% of deaths in the cohort were directly attributable to an inactive lifestyle, and that physically active men lived, on average, over two years longer than physically inactive men (Paffenbarger, Brand, Sholtz, & Jung, 1986).

Research has consistently demonstrated an inverse dose–response relation between the total volume of physical activity and mortality risk, supporting the message that some activity is good, but more is better. The dose–response curve is curvilinear, with moderate differences in mortality risk between sedentary and modestly active individuals and subtle differences in mortality risk between modestly active and highly active individuals. Figure 2.1 shows a typical dose–response curve for the relationship between physical activity and all-cause mortality risk. This figure was created from

the findings of a 5-year prospective cohort study of 27,734 Swedish women (Carlsson, Andersson, Wolk, & Ahlbom, 2006).

Physical activities of different types and intensities have been investigated in a number of studies. Walking, the most common physical activity among adults (Siegel, Brackbill, & Heath, 1995), has been the most extensively studied activity. The data suggest that walking for at least 2 hours per week is associated with significantly reduced all-cause mortality rates (Physical Activity Guidelines Advisory Committee, 2008). Some data also suggest that vigorous-intensity physical activity is associated with additional risk reduction beyond lower-intensity activities, even after accounting for the total energy expenditure. Consider findings from the Copenhagen City Heart Study, a prospective

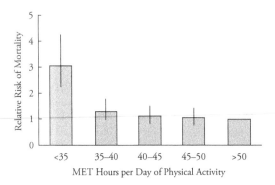

Figure 2.1. Dose–response relation between physical activity level and all-cause mortality in middle-aged and older Swedish women. The error bars represent the 95% confidence intervals for the relative risk estimates. One MET is the energy expenditure at rest, two METs is the energy expenditure for a physical activity that requires twice the expenditure as rest, three METs is the expenditure for a moderate-intensity activity that requires three times the expenditure as rest, and so on. Engaging in a 2-MET physical activity for 1 hour equals 2 MET-hours, engaging in a 3-MET physical activity for 1 hour would equals 3 MET-hours, and so on. Figure created from data presented in "Low Physical Activity and Mortality in Women: Baseline Lifestyle and Health as Alternative Explanations," by S. Carlsson, T. Andersson, A. Wolk, and A. Ahlbom, 2006, *Scandinavian Journal of Public Health, 34*(5), pp. 480–487.

cohort of 7,308 healthy men and women followed over 12 years (Schnohr, Scharling, & Jensen, 2007). Compared with men who walked less than a half hour per day and who tended to walk at a slow pace (hazard ratio = 1.0), men who walked less than a half hour per day but walked at a fast pace had a hazard ratio for all-cause mortality of 0.38 (95% confidence interval: 0.18–0.79), and men who walked at a slow pace but for more than 2 hours a day had a hazard ratio for all-cause mortality of 0.43 (95% confidence interval: 0.22–0.82). These findings demonstrate that low-intensity activities, such as walking at a slow pace, have an effect on mortality risk. They also demonstrate that higher-intensity activities have a greater impact than lower-intensity activities.

In addition to physical activity, there is strong and consistent evidence that cardiorespiratory fitness is inversely related to all-cause mortality risk. One study examining the relation between cardiorespiratory fitness and mortality was based on a follow-up of the 1981 Canada Fitness Survey (Villeneuve, Morrison, Craig, & Schaubel, 1998). In this representative sample of 7,916 Canadian adults, an undesirable fitness level, as measured using the Canadian Aerobic Fitness Test, was associated with a 52% increased risk of all-cause mortality compared with those who had desirable fitness levels.

Physical Activity and Cardiovascular Disease

A vast scientific literature has examined the role that leisure-time physical activity, occupational physical activity, and cardiorespiratory fitness play in the risk of cardiovascular disease. From these studies it can be concluded that physical inactivity and low cardiorespiratory fitness are causally linked to an increased risk of several forms of cardiovascular disease, including coronary artery disease, stroke, and peripheral vascular disease (Kohl, 2001). Both occupational and leisure-time physical activity levels have an effect on cardiovascular disease risk (Kohl, 2001).

There is a dose–response relationship between physical activity level and cardiovascular disease risk (Kohl, 2001). The left panel of Figure 2.2 shows a typical example of the shape of this dose–response relationship for coronary artery disease. This figure shows an inverse, curvilinear association between total weekly physical activity energy expenditure—whether it be strenuous sports or other, nonvigorous activities—and the relative risk of having a myocardial infarction. This figure is based on results from the Harvard Alumni Study (Paffenbarger, Wing, & Hyde, 1978) that were discussed earlier in this chapter.

As with coronary artery disease, physical inactivity and low fitness are causally linked to an increased risk of stroke. A meta-analysis that summarized the evidence from all published studies indicated that, by comparison with inactive persons, moderately active individuals have a 17% reduction in stroke risk and highly active individuals have a 25% reduction in stroke risk (C. D. Lee, Folsom, & Blair, 2003).

As summarized in Table 2.3, there is strong causal evidence that physical activity offers protection against the development of different forms of cardiovascular disease. It is also clear that engaging in physical activity is important in the management of poor health and the prevention of mortality in individuals with cardiovascular disease (Jolliffe et al., 2001; Thompson et al., 2003). A prospective cohort study of 1,045 elderly men and women with coronary artery disease indicated that baseline physical activity was related to all-cause mortality risk over 9 years in a curvilinear, dose–response manner (Janssen & Jolliffe, 2006). Interestingly, the shape of the dose–response relation between physical activity and cardiovascular disease risk in healthy adults (left panel in Figure 2.2) is similar to the shape of

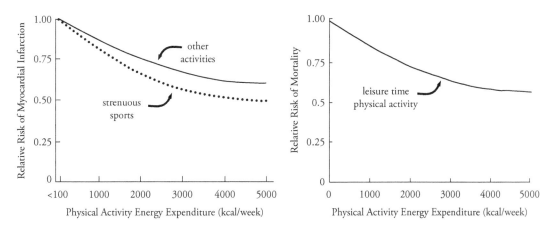

Figure 2.2. *Left panel.* Dose–response relation between physical activity level and risk of coronary heart disease in men without cardiovascular disease. Adapted from "Physical Activity as an Index of Heart Attack Risk in College Alumni," by R. S. Paffenbarger, Jr., A. L. Wing, and R. T. Hyde, 1978, *American Journal of Epidemiology, 108*(3), pp. 161–175. *Right panel.* Dose–response relation between leisure-time physical activity level and all-cause mortality risk in older adults with cardiovascular disease. Adapted with permission from "Influence of Physical Activity on Mortality in Elderly with Coronary Artery Disease," by I. Janssen and C. J. Jolliffe, 2006, *Medicine & Science in Sports & Exercise, 38*(3), pp. 418–427.

the dose–response relation between physical activity and mortality risk in adults with cardiovascular disease (right panel in Figure 2.2).

Physical Activity and Cancer

Cancer can occur at any site on the body, although the risk factors vary by site. Some risk factors, such as physical inactivity, are associated with more than one form of cancer.

Studies of both occupational and leisure-time physical activity have shown significant protection against colon cancer (I.-M. Lee, 2007). Also, results from the Aerobics Center Longitudinal Study indicate that risks for cancer deaths decrease with increasing levels of cardiorespiratory fitness (Farrell, Cortese, LaMonte, & Blair, 2007). Specifically, when moving from the least fit to most fit quintiles, the hazard ratios for cancer mortality in 38,410 men followed for 17 years were 1.0, 0.70, 0.67, 0.70, and 0.49.

There is consistent evidence that routine participation in moderate-to-vigorous physical activity provides some protection against breast cancer, particularly within postmenopausal women. Consider the findings from the American Association of Retired Persons Diet and Health Study (Peters et al., 2009). This prospective cohort design followed 182,862 postmenopausal women over 7 years, during which time 6,609 incident cases of breast cancer occurred. The relative risks of breast cancer were 1.0 (reference group) in women who

were completely inactive, 0.99 in women who were physically active less than once per week on average, 0.94 in women who were active 1–2 times per week, 0.93 in women who were active 3–4 times per week, and 0.87 in women who were active 5 or more times per week.

Next to skin cancer, prostate cancer is the most common type of cancer in men. While there is evidence of a relation between physical activity and prostate cancer, the findings from the more than 40 published studies are mixed, with only about half reporting a significant association (I.-M. Lee, 2007). The mean relative risk across all studies for the most active group compared with the least active group is 0.90, implying that if there are any benefits of physical activity, they are quite subtle (I.-M. Lee, 2007).

A number of recent studies have examined the relationship between physical activity and lung cancer (I.-M. Lee, 2007). Many of these studies have reported that physical activity offers some protection. There have been concerns that the findings in these studies may be attributable, at least in part, to the confounding effects of smoking, because physically active people are less likely to smoke. However, a study of nonsmokers from the Harvard Alumni Study found a clear dose–response relation between physical activity energy expenditure and the relative risk of lung cancer (I. M. Lee, Sesso, & Paffenbarger, 1999). The most active men had a risk reduction of 39% compared with the least active men.

The association between physical activity and cancer has been examined in several sites in addition to those discussed above. Unfortunately, the data for these other cancer sites are too sparse and inconsistent to permit any conclusions (I.-M. Lee, 2007).

In recent years researchers have started to consider whether physical activity provides health benefits for individuals who are diagnosed with cancer (Newton & Galvao, 2008). The results from both observational and intervention studies indicate that participation in physical activity following cancer diagnosis can reduce cancer symptoms, benefit surgical outcomes, help manage the side effects and outcomes of cancer treatment (surgery, radiation, and chemotherapy), improve psychological health, maintain physical function, and reduce fat gain and muscle and bone loss (Newton & Galvao, 2008). Furthermore, the results from prospective cohort studies indicate that regular physical activity post diagnosis increases survivorship by about 50%, with the strongest evidence for breast and colorectal cancers (Newton & Galvao, 2008).

Physical Activity and Type 2 Diabetes

There is a large and consistent body of evidence that low physical activity and a low cardiorespiratory fitness are modest-to-strong risk factors for the development of type 2 diabetes in both men and women (see summary in Table 2.3). Results from the Nurses' Health Study (Hu et al., 1999) highlight these associations. In an 8-year follow-up of 70,102 participants with no history of diabetes at baseline, the relative risks of developing type 2 diabetes from the least to the most physically active quintiles were 1.0, 0.77, 0.75, 0.62, and 0.54. Interestingly, among women who did not perform vigorous activity, relative risks for type 2 diabetes across were 1.0, 0.90, 0.73, 0.69, and 0.58 from the quintile who did the least walking to the quintile who walked the most (Figure 2.3, left panel). These results suggest that physical activity, including physical activity of modest intensity and duration, is associated with a substantial reduction in the risk of type 2 diabetes.

Type 2 diabetes is a major risk factor for other chronic diseases such as renal disease, cardiovascular disease, and cancer. Additional results from the Nurses' Health Study suggest that physical activity provides some protection against the development of these diseases in adults with diabetes (Hu et al., 2001). Hu et al. (2001) examined a subset of 5,125 women from the Nurses' Health Study who had diabetes at baseline. Over a 14-year follow-up period, the relative risk of cardiovascular disease was 0.52 (95% confidence interval: 0.25–1.09) in the most active quartile compared with the least active quartile. Similarly, within those who did not perform any vigorous physical activity, the relative risk of cardiovascular disease was 0.56 (95% confidence interval: 0.31–1.00) in the quartile who walked the most compared with the least quartile who walked the least. The shape of this dose–response relation (Figure 2.3, right panel) is similar to that observed in women without diabetes (Figure 2.3, left panel).

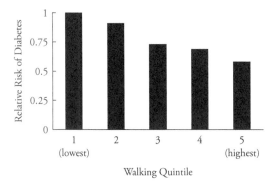 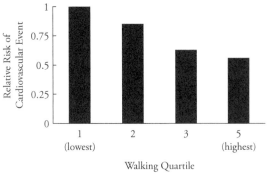

Figure 2.3. *Left panel.* Dose–response relation between walking and the risk of developing type 2 diabetes in women who did not perform vigorous exercise. Figure created from data presented in "Walking Compared with Vigorous Physical Activity and Risk of Type 2 Diabetes in Women: A Prospective Study," by F. B. Hu, R. J. Sigal, J. W. Rich-Edwards, G. A. Colditz, C. G. Solomon, W. C. Willett, F. E. Speizer, and J. E. Manson, 1999, *JAMA, 282*(15), pp. 1433–1439. *Right panel.* Dose–response relation between walking and the risk of developing cardiovascular disease in women with diabetes who did not perform vigorous exercise. Figure created from data presented in "Physical Activity and Risk for Cardiovascular Events in Diabetic Women," by F. B. Hu, M. J. Stampfer, C. Solomon, S. Liu, G. A. Colditz, F. E. Speizer, W. C. Willett, and J. E. Manson, 2001, *Annals of Internal Medicine, 134*(2), pp. 96–105.

Physical Activity and Obesity

Obesity results from a chronic energy imbalance whereby intake exceeds expenditure; physical inactivity therefore plays an important role in the development and treatment of obesity. Results from cross-sectional and prospective cohort studies have shown, in general, that physical activity is inversely related to obesity (Ross & Janssen, 2007). That is, physically active and fit individuals are considerably less likely to have and develop obesity than inactive and unfit individuals. There has been considerable debate in the scientific community about the amount of physical activity required to prevent weight gain throughout adulthood. In 2003, the Institute of Medicine recommended that adults should accumulate 60–90 minutes of physical activity daily to prevent weight gain (Food and Nutrition Board (Institute of Medicine), 2003). Also in 2003, a consensus statement from the International Association for the Study of Obesity suggested that 45–60 minutes of moderate-intensity physical activity per day would be sufficient to achieve weight maintenance for most adults (Saris et al., 2003). The 2008 Physical Activity Guidelines for Americans report, which included a comprehensive and systematic literature review, concluded that a dose of physical activity in the range of 13–26 metabolic equivalent (MET)-hours per week was needed for weight stability over time (Physical Activity Guidelines Advisory Committee, 2008). Thirteen MET-hours per week is equivalent to walking at a 4-mph pace for 150 minutes or jogging at a 6-mph pace for 75 minutes. The wide range from 13 to 26 MET-hours per week of physical activity needed for weight stability probably reflects individual variation in the inherent (nonstructured) level of physical activity, genetic variation, and the degree to which caloric intake is increased with participation in physical activity.

The role of physical activity as a treatment strategy for obese individuals has received considerable attention. Early literature reviews suggested that increasing physical activity in the absence of caloric restriction was associated with only a modest weight loss, in the magnitude of 1–2 kg, in overweight and obese individuals (National Institutes of Health National Heart, Lung, and Blood Institute, 1998). However, few of the earlier weight loss studies prescribed a volume of physical activity that would have resulted in a meaningful energy expenditure (Ross & Janssen, 2001). For example, Mourier et al. (1997) conducted an 8-week randomized controlled exercise trial in a group of 21 overweight patients with diabetes. Participants in the intervention group were asked to complete three aerobic exercise sessions per week, each lasting 45 minutes at 75% of VO_2 peak. This exercise program would have resulted in a total energy expenditure of ~840 kcal/week. Given that 1 kg of fat contains 7,700 kcal of energy, the expected weight loss from this physical activity intervention would have been slightly less than 1 kg over the 8-week intervention period. Thus the fact that participants in the intervention group lost an average of only 1.5 kg in this study should not be surprising given the modest volume of exercise prescribed. In other words, while 135 min/week of moderate-intensity aerobic exercise can have a significant impact on many of the other health outcomes discussed in this chapter, based on the laws of thermodynamics, this volume of exercise would have only a minimal effect on body fat and weight.

Within the past 10 years the results from some experimental studies have indicated that exercise in the absence of a calorie-restricted diet can be associated with significant weight loss in overweight and obese individuals if the volume of physical activity is sufficient. In two randomized controlled trials, Ross et al. (2000, 2004) demonstrated that moderately obese men and women lost about 7% of their body weight over a three- to four-month period by engaging in approximately 60 minutes of moderate-intensity aerobic exercise on a daily basis, primarily in the form of brisk walking, in the absence of changes in caloric intake. Furthermore, results from these two studies indicated that regular aerobic exercise in the absence of weight loss can, over the course of a few months, lead to an impressive reduction in total and abdominal fat. The reduction in abdominal fat is particularly relevant given that obesity-related health risks are in large measure determined by the amount of abdominal fat an individual has (Janssen, Katzmarzyk, & Ross, 2004).

Physical Activity and Osteoporosis

Early understanding about the beneficial effects of physical activity on the risk of osteoporosis was generated from cross-sectional studies (Borer, 2005). The results from these studies suggested that athletes in sports that include running, jumping, and other weight-bearing activities, such as soccer, basketball, and weight lifting, have higher bone mineral density values than nonathlete controls. Conversely, athletes in sports that do not involve running and jumping, such as swimming, speed skating, and cross-country skiing, have bone mineral density values comparable to those of nonathlete controls.

Evidence from several randomized controlled trials has demonstrated that prolonged exercise interventions that involved either ground reaction forces (e.g., running or jumping) or joint reaction forces (e.g., weight training) can improve bone mineral density in young adults (Borer, 2005). For example, one study prescribed 8 months of weight training or running to healthy college-aged women (Snow-Harter, Bouxsein, Lewis, Carter, & Marcus, 1992). The weight training consisted of three sessions per week of three sets of 10 exercises. Participants in the running group were asked to run 7–17 km/week at 75% of their maximal heart rate. Bone mineral density in the lumbar spine region improved in both the weight trainers (+1.2%) and runners (+1.3%) in response to the 8-month exercise interventions. These may seem like trivial changes in bone density, but since bone loss during this time of life is less than 0.5% per year, these 8-month exercise programs reversed approximately three years' worth of bone loss in these young women.

After the fifth decade of life, bone loss is accelerated, particularly in women. Postmenopausal women tend to lose between 1% and 2% of their bone mass per year. Exercise involving ground reaction or joint reaction forces is an effective strategy for reducing and even reversing age-related loss in bone mineral content in this age group (Borer, 2005). In one 11-month-long experimental study of 39 women aged 65–66 years, a ground-reaction-force exercise program consisting of jogging, walking, and stair climbing resulted in a 2.0% increase in total body bone mineral density (Kohrt, Ehsani, & Birge, 1997). Similarly, a joint-reaction-force exercise program consisting of weight training and rowing resulted in 1.6% increase in bone mineral density (Kohrt et al., 1997). The authors of this study concluded that these two exercise programs, which introduced stress to the skeleton through difference forces, both led to significant increases in bone mineral density at clinically important sites.

The research examining the relation between physical activity and bone mineral density, measured on a continuous scale, has been extensive. Limited research has considered whether engagement in physical activity helps prevent the transition into a diseased state of osteoporosis. The few published studies have focused on the occurrence of osteoporotic fractures. Consider two examples. First, in a 20-year prospective cohort study of men aged 50 years and older (Kujala, Kaprio, Kannus, Sarna, & Koskenvuo, 2000), men who participated in vigorous exercise were one-third as likely to have a hip fracture during the follow-up period compared with men who did not participate in vigorous exercise (hazard ratio = 0.38, 95% confidence interval: 0.16–0.91). Second, in a 4-year prospective cohort study (Cummings et al., 1995), elderly women who walked for exercise had a significantly lower risk of hip fracture compared with women who did not walk for exercise (hazard ratio = 0.70, 95% confidence interval: 0.5–0.9). The results from these studies confirm that physical activity, particularly when vigorous, provides some protection against the risk of osteoporosis and related fractures.

Physical Activity and Mental Health

Physical activity is associated with several measures of mental health, including depression, anxiety, distress, cognitive function, and dementia. Cross-sectional and prospective cohort studies provide evidence, albeit somewhat inconsistent, that regular physical activity protects against the onset of depression and its symptoms. In the published prospective cohort studies, the average odds of elevated depression symptoms, after controlling for important confounding variables, was 15–25% lower among active adults than in inactive adults (Physical Activity Guidelines Advisory Committee, 2008).

Although the minimal amount, optimal amount, and type of physical activity needed to help protect against the development of depression and its symptoms is not known, it is clear that the volume of physical activity is related to depression in a dose–response manner. In one study of 1,947 community-dwelling adults aged 50 and older, the odds ratio for depression over the 5 years of follow-up was 1.0 in the highly active group, 2.64 (95% confidence interval: 1.04–6.73) in the moderately active group, and 4.95 (95% confidence interval: 1.95–12.5) in the inactive group (Strawbridge, Deleger, Roberts, & Kaplan, 2002). The effect of a low activity level on the risk of depression in this study was greater than that of any of the other risk factors for depression considered in the analysis, including age, gender, financial status, neighborhood problems, education, and disability status.

The relation between physical activity and reduced feelings of distress or enhanced well-being was virtually unknown until about 15 years ago. Since that time, several observational studies, mostly cross-sectional in design, have provided findings indicating that active people have about 30% lower odds of having feelings of distress and about 30% higher odds of having feelings of enhanced well-being than inactive people (Physical Activity Guidelines Advisory Committee, 2008).

The weight of the available evidence from prospective cohort studies indicates that physical activity delays the onset of cognitive decline and the incidence of dementia, particularly Alzheimer's disease, associated with advancing age. It is encouraging that light- to modest-intensity activities that most older adults are capable of performing, such as walking, have a protective effect. In one prospective cohort study of 2,257 physically capable men aged 71–93 years (Abbott et al., 2004), men who walked less than 0.25 miles/day had a 1.8-fold higher risk of developing dementia than men who walked more than 2 miles/day (17.8 vs. 10.3 events per 1,000 person-years).

In addition to being an effective preventive measure, physical activity is a useful treatment strategy for individuals with mental health problems. A meta-analysis of 14 randomized controlled trials conducted in people diagnosed with depression reported that the mean reduction in depression symptoms across the 14 studies was equivalent to 1 standard deviation of the mean score for those measures (Lawlor & Hopker, 2001). It is also encouraging that the effects of routine physical activity on symptoms within depressed individuals are equivalent to those of drug therapy (Blumenthal et al., 2007). As with depression, a meta-analysis of 10 randomized controlled trials of older adults with cognitive impairments (Heyn, Abreu, & Ottenbacher, 2004) concluded that physical activity interventions provided clinically meaningful benefits.

Physical Activity and Functional Health

This section reviews evidence related to the effects of physical activity on functional health and disability in middle-aged and older adults. Functional activities considered include the ability to walk at a normal speed on a flat surface, to climb a flight of stairs, to perform basic activities of daily living (e.g., bathing, dressing, and grooming), and to perform activities that enable one to live independently (e.g., shopping, traveling in the community, and light housework).

Observational studies have consistently shown that middle-aged and older adults who participate in regular physical activity, particularly aerobic activity, have a reduction on the order of 30% in the risk of developing functional limitations and disability (Physical Activity Guidelines Advisory Committee, 2008). There is a dose–response effect, as higher amounts of physical activity are associated with

lower risks of limitations and disability than modest amounts of physical activity (Physical Activity Guidelines Advisory Committee, 2008). A recent prospective cohort study of 549 older adults who were examined annually from 1984 to 2000 also provides evidence that changes in physical activity influence subsequent disability risk (Berk, Hubert, & Fries, 2006). Four groups were formed based on participants' physical activity levels during the baseline and annual follow-up visits: Sedentary (low activity at baseline and during follow-up), Exercise Increasers (low activity at baseline and high activity during follow-up), Exercise Decreasers (high activity at baseline and low activity during follow-up), and Exercisers (high activity at baseline and during follow-up). Over the 16-year follow-up, the increase in a disability index score was far greater in the Sedentary group (+0.37) and Exercise Decreasers (+0.27) than in the Exercise Increasers (+0.17) and Exercisers (+0.11). These encouraging findings indicate that physical activity, even when begun later in life, can help postpone the onset of physical disability.

There is also evidence that regular physical activity improves functional ability in older adults with existing functional limitations. The majority of the published experimental studies have included both aerobic and muscle-strengthening activities (Physical Activity Guidelines Advisory Committee, 2008). For this reason, exercise programs aimed at improving functional health in older adults with functional limitations involve 30–90 minutes of moderate-to-vigorous physical activity three to five days per week, in which most of this time is devoted to aerobic and muscle-strengthening activity, with a shorter amount of time spent on forms of activity that address issues such as flexibility and balance (Physical Activity Guidelines Advisory Committee, 2008).

Resistance Exercise, Muscular Fitness, and Health

The relations of physical activity and fitness to health that have been covered so far in this chapter are, for the most part, based on aerobic- and cardio-respiratory-based measures of physical activity and fitness. The effects of strength-based physical activities and musculoskeletal fitness on most of the health outcomes considered in this chapter have not been studied as extensively. Nonetheless, the available information suggests that resistive-type activities protect against many chronic diseases and mortality risk. For instance, in the Health Professional's

Follow-up Study of over 40,000 American men, those who reported participating in 30 minutes or more of weight training a week had a 23% reduction in coronary heart disease risk compared with those who performed no weight training (Tanasescu et al., 2002). A 19-year follow-up of 8,677 men from the Aerobics Center Longitudinal Study indicated that men in the highest-muscular-strength tertile had a lower risk of cancer mortality than men in the lowest-muscular-strength tertile (hazard ratio = 0.61, 95% confidence interval: 0.44–0.85) (Ruiz et al., 2009). A 13-year follow-up of 8,116 adults from the 1981 Canada Fitness Survey suggests that musculoskeletal fitness provides some protection against mortality risk (Katzmarzyk & Craig, 2002). Take for example muscular endurance as evaluated using a sit-ups test (maximal number of sit-ups performed in 60 seconds). In comparison to the best performers (e.g., top quartile), men and women in the lowest sit-ups quartiles had relative risks of all-cause mortality of 2.72 (95% confidence interval: 1.56–4.64) and 2.26 (95% confidence interval: 1.15–4.43), respectively (Katzmarzyk & Craig, 2002).

Physical Activity and Health in Children and Adolescents

A considerable amount is known about the health benefits of physical activity in children and adolescents, although not as much as in adults or supported by the same degree of causal evidence. A systematic evaluation of over 850 published studies linking physical activity to several health and behavioral outcomes in school-aged children and adolescents was published in 2005 (Strong et al., 2005). The panel of 13 experts in the field reached the following conclusions: (1) There is *strong* evidence that physical activity has beneficial effects on adiposity within overweight and obese youth, on musculoskeletal health and fitness, and on several components of cardiovascular health. (2) There is *adequate* evidence that physical activity has beneficial effects on adiposity levels in those with a normal body weight, on blood pressure in normotensive youth, on plasma lipid and lipoprotein levels, on nontraditional cardiovascular risk factors (e.g., inflammatory markers, endothelial function, and heart rate variability), and on several components of mental health (e.g., anxiety and depression). Based on the evidence, the expert panel recommended that school-aged children and adolescents accumulate 60 minutes of physical activity on a daily basis. They also recommended that the activity be developmentally appropriate, be enjoyable, and involve a variety of activities.

Sedentary Behaviors and Health

Traditionally, research in physical activity epidemiology has focused on the health benefits of engaging in physical activity of moderate-to-vigorous intensity. However, even very active persons, such as a person who runs for an hour each day, spend less than 10% of their waking hours in moderate-to-vigorous activity. Recent research has started to examine whether the level of low-intensity and incidental activity (e.g., moving around the house vs. sitting) in the remaining 90% or more of waking hours influences health. Sedentary behavior research represents an exciting avenue for future research in physical activity epidemiology (Salmon et al., 2008; Spanier et al., 2006).

Several studies, primarily cross-sectional in design, have demonstrated that the amount of time children and adults spend in sedentary behaviors is related to obesity and other cardiovascular and diabetes risk factors (Healy, Dunstan, et al., 2008; Healy, Wijndaele, et al., 2008; Janssen, Katzmarzyk, Boyce, King, & Pickett, 2004; Janssen et al., 2005; Mark & Janssen, 2008b; Must & Tybor, 2005; Rey-Lopez, Vicente-Rodriguez, Biosca, & Moreno, 2008; Salmon, Dunstan, & Owen, 2008; Spanier, Marshall, & Faulkner, 2006). In fact, these associations are independent of the volume of moderate-to-vigorous activity. Most of this research has focused on screen-time sedentary behaviors such as watching television, using the computer, and playing video games. For instance, a recent cross-sectional study of 1,808 American adolescents reported that the prevalences of the metabolic syndrome across groups with ≤1 hr/day, 2 hr/day, 3 hr/day, 4 hr/day, and 5 hr/day of screen time were 3.7%, 4.6%, 6.6%, 6.7%, and 8.4%, respectively (Mark & Janssen, 2008b). There is also evidence that some sedentary behaviors have a greater impact on health than others. For example, a cross-sectional study conducted on a representative sample of Canadian adults found that obesity was associated with the amount of screen time but not with the amount of time spent reading (Shields & Tremblay, 2008). Finally, although limited, there is emerging evidence that the pattern in which sedentary behaviors are accumulated impacts health. One recent cross-sectional study in 168 adults found that after controlling for the overall volume of sedentary behavior, a greater frequency of breaks in sedentary time (e.g., walking around the house during a TV commercial) was associated with a better cardiovascular risk factor profile (Healy, Dunstan, et al., 2008).

Dose–Response Issues in Physical Activity and Health
Components of Physical Activity Dose

The primary components used to determine physical activity dose are intensity and duration. The intensity of an activity can be characterized in both absolute and relative terms. Absolute intensity refers to the increase in energy required to perform the activity for aerobic-based activities (e.g., VO_2 in liters or METs) or the force produced by the skeletal muscle for resistance-based activities (e.g., amount of weight lifted). Relative intensity refers to the intensity of the activity in relation to the capacity of the person (e.g., percentage of VO_2max, percentage of maximal heart rate, or percentage of one-repetition maximum). In most observational studies activity intensity has been measured in absolute terms. Conversely, in most experimental studies activity intensity has been prescribed in relative terms. Aside from its impact on the total dose of physical activity, the intensity of physical activity is important to consider because higher intensities appear to have a beneficial effect on some health outcomes independent of the total volume or dose of physical activity (Hu et al., 1999; Manson et al., 2002; Paffenbarger, Brand, Sholtz, & Jung, 1978).

Duration is the second main component of physical activity dose. It is a function of the session duration and frequency of participation in activity. Results of numerous experimental studies indicate that when participants performed physical activity several days a week, three or four shorter bouts of activity per day produced changes in fitness and cardiometabolic risk factors that are quite similar to those produced by a single longer bout (Hardman, 2001). There is little data for bouts shorter than 10 minutes; however, the concept that one can achieve health benefits by accumulating physical activity throughout the day in shorter bouts appears to be valid.

Another question to ask is whether one needs to accumulate the suggested weekly dose of physical activity over several days of the week, or whether longer sessions performed on one or two days are acceptable (as in the case of "weekend warriors" who compress all of their weekly activity into the weekend). The rationale for recommending activity on most days of the week comes from experimental studies that have tended to prescribe training in this manner. The results from the only available study of the weekend warrior pattern of physical activity in relation to health outcomes suggest that while it may postpone mortality, particularly in relatively healthy individuals, this pattern of activity may not be as beneficial as a more traditional pattern of regular physical activity throughout the week (I. M. Lee, Sesso, Oguma, & Paffenbarger, 2004).

Minimal and Optimal Amounts of Physical Activity for Health Benefits

Many people in the population are more concerned about knowing the *minimal* amount of physical activity needed to produce meaningful health benefits and not the *optimal* amount of physical activity needed to produce the best health benefits. The minimal amount of activity needed likely depends on a person's current physical activity level. A person who has been at complete bed rest may benefit just from getting out of bed for a few minutes each day. Some of the research presented earlier in this chapter suggests that a small amount of walking, even at a light pace, can reduce mortality risk in very inactive individuals with a chronic disease such as diabetes. Unfortunately, there are few data on the minimal amount of physical activity needed for good health in the general public. The minimal amount of activity may also vary depending on the health outcome. Nonetheless, the dose–response curves for physical activity, such as those presented in Figures 2.1–2.3, indicate that only a modest amount of moderate-intensity activity (i.e., 150 min/week) is required to bring about meaningful benefits for many health outcomes.

Similar to the above conundrum, it is unclear as to what point an increase in physical activity provides no further health benefits. The plateau in physical activity benefit may also vary by health outcome—it may be quite low for some outcomes and quite high for others. For instance, there is a linear dose–response relation between miles run and the likelihood of having high-risk HDL cholesterol levels, even up to 80 miles run per week (Williams, 1997). This would suggest that at least for some health variables, continued health benefits can be achieved even after running 10 hours a week at a vigorous pace. Most dose–response curves suggest that health benefits do not completely level off at high activity levels, although there are certainly diminishing returns once a moderate level of physical activity is reached.

Translation of Research Findings into Public Health Recommendations
Background on Recommendations for Fitness and Health

Scientific understanding of the health benefits of physical activity is of little relevance if this information cannot be translated to the general public so that they can apply it to improve their health. In recent decades there have been increasing efforts to generate public health messages about the appropriate amount, intensity, frequency, and type of physical activity needed for good health. These physical activity recommendations and guidelines have been developed by experts tasked with synthesizing the findings from the scientific literature and applying the resulting information to create messages that can be clearly communicated to the public.

The first endorsed recommendations for physical activity were those of the American College of Sports Medicine. In its 1975 exercise guidelines book (American College of Sports Medicine, 1975) and 1978 position statement (American College of Sports Medicine, 1978), this group recommended that people engage in exercise three to five days a week for 15–60 minutes at an intensity of 50–85% VO$_2$max. These recommendations were geared toward the appropriate exercise for developing and maintaining fitness in healthy adults. They were not geared toward health outcomes. For two decades after these guidelines were developed, physical activity guidelines continued to focus on the appropriate exercise for fitness. This changed in 1995 with the publication of the U.S. Centers for Disease Control and Prevention and the American College of Sports Medicine recommendation on physical activity and public health (Pate et al., 1995). This recommendation was intended to communicate to the American public how much and what types of physical activity are needed to maintain good health. The panel recommended that "every U.S. adult should accumulate 30 minutes or more of moderate-intensity physical activity on most, preferably all, days of the week." Since these initial public health recommendations for physical activity and health, several other organizations and countries have developed their own recommendations. America's most recent physical activity recommendations and guidelines were released in 2008; copies of these guidelines and the scientific basis for their development can be found and downloaded for free at http://www.health.gov/paguidelines/.

America's Physical Activity Guidelines for Adults

The key recommendations within America's physical activity guidelines for adults are as follows:

• All adults should avoid inactivity. Some physical activity is better than none, and adults who participate in any amount of physical activity gain some health benefits.

• For substantial health benefits, adults should do at least 150 minutes a week of moderate-intensity or 75 minutes a week of vigorous-intensity aerobic physical activity, or an equivalent combination of moderate- and vigorous-intensity aerobic activity. Aerobic activity should be performed in episodes of at least 10 minutes, and preferably it should be spread throughout the week.

• For additional and more extensive health benefits, adults should increase their aerobic physical activity to 300 minutes a week of moderate-intensity, or 150 minutes a week of vigorous-intensity aerobic physical activity, or an equivalent combination of moderate- and vigorous-intensity activity. Additional health benefits are gained by engaging in physical activity beyond this amount.

• Adults should also do muscle-strengthening activities that are moderate or high intensity and involve all major muscle groups on 2 or more days a week, as these activities provide additional health benefits.

America's Physical Activity Guidelines for Older Adults

The older adult guidelines were tailored to those aged 65 years and older and contain eight recommendations. The first four recommendations are identical to those listed above for adults. The four recommendations specifically for older adults are as follows:

• When older adults cannot do 150 minutes of moderate-intensity aerobic activity a week because of chronic conditions, they should be as physically active as their abilities and conditions allow.

• Older adults should do exercises that maintain or improve balance if they are at risk of falling.

• Older adults should determine their level of effort for physical activity relative to their level of fitness.

• Older adults with chronic conditions should understand whether and how their conditions affect their ability to do regular physical activity safely.

America's Physical Activity Guidelines for Children and Adolescents

The key recommendations within the child and adolescent physical activity guidelines are as follows:

• Children and adolescents should do 60 minutes or more of physical activity daily.

• Most of the 60 or more minutes a day should involve moderate- or vigorous-intensity aerobic physical activity and should include vigorous-intensity physical activity at least three days a week.

• As part of their 60 or more minutes of daily physical activity, children and adolescents should include muscle-strengthening physical activity on at least three days of the week.

• As part of their 60 or more minutes of daily physical activity, children and adolescents should include bone-strengthening physical activity on at least three days of the week.

• It is important to encourage young people to participate in physical activities that are appropriate for their age, that are enjoyable, and that offer variety.

Future Directions for Research

Most of the available literature linking physical activity and health, as well as the physical activity guidelines derived from the literature, are based on relatively healthy, middle- to upper-class Caucasians. There are limited data for specific subpopulations, including non-Caucasians, persons of low socioeconomic status, obese persons, and people with specific chronic illnesses (e.g., cancer survivors and disabled persons). That is not to say that there is no evidence of a relationship between physical activity and health in such groups; to the contrary, the positive impact of physical activity on health has been demonstrated in numerous subpopulations. The issue is whether the inflection points and slopes of the dose–response curves relating physical activity and health are comparable in different subpopulations.

Consider the following analogous situation in the obesity field. Although obesity as measured by the body mass index (BMI) is associated with several chronic diseases and premature mortality in several ethnic groups (Health Canada, 2003; WHO Expert Committee, 1994), the health risks associated with a given BMI vary considerably by ethnicity. Thus, while a BMI of ≥30 kg/m^2 is used to define obesity in Caucasian, African American, and Hispanic populations (World Health Organization, 1998), a BMI of ≥27 kg/m^2 is used to define obesity in Asian populations, to reflect a different slope and inflection point on the dose–response curve between BMI and health outcomes (WHO Expert Consultation, 2004). One can envision a similar scenario for physical activity, where the volume of activity needed for a meaningful health impact could vary by ethnicity, health status, socioeconomic status, etc. To address this issue, future studies need to include different subpopulations and, more importantly, need to carefully examine whether the relationship between physical activity and health is modified in different subpopulations.

In 2001 an evidence-based symposium was held to address the dose–response relationship between physical activity and health (Kesaniemi et al., 2001). An important outcome of that symposium was the recognition of the need for more dose–response studies in physical activity epidemiology, which led to considerable research efforts and increased knowledge in the last decade. Despite this, there is still much to be learned. Specifically, studies are needed to define the dose of activity that provides the maximal benefit for various health outcomes. Studies are also needed to address the nature of the benefits and characteristics of lower doses (volumes and intensities) of physical activity.

The intensity of physical activity may have particular relevance at low doses. Although this issue has not been addressed directly, anecdotal evidence is offered by the European Youth Heart Survey of approximately 5,000 youth (Andersen et al., 2006) and the US National Health and Nutrition Examination Survey of approximately 1,200 youth (LeBlanc & Janssen, 2009; Mark & Janssen, 2008a). Both studies measured physical activity using accelerometers; however, the European study included low-intensity activity while the US study was restricted to moderate-to-vigorous intensity. Both studies found a dose–response relation between physical activity and cardiovascular risk factors. However, the patterns were different at the low-dose end of the activity spectrum. The European study observed minimal health benefits at the low end of the spectrum, while the US study observed large health benefits. It is possible that the inclusion of low-intensity activity in the European study impacted the findings, implying that a low dose of activity may only have an impact if it is performed at a higher intensity. Clearly this issue needs to be addressed in future studies.

A third area that needs to be addressed in future studies is the relevance of physical activity patterns. Is the pattern by which physical activity is accumulated over a day or week is important? If the total weekly dose of physical activity is constant, does it matter on how many days the activity is accumulated? Within a given day, does it matter whether the activity occurs in a single longer bout or is accumulated in multiple short bouts?

Initial physical activity guidelines in the United States, which were published in 1995, contained a "days per week" recommendation (Pate et al., 1995). More specifically, the guidelines recommended that adults accumulate ≥150 min/week of moderate-to-vigorous activity, but noted that it was important to spread out the activity over most or all days of the week. The recent systematic reviews conducted for the U.S. physical activity guidelines project noted that there is in fact very little evidence to support the days-per-week recommendation (Physical Activity Guidelines Advisory Committee, 2008). This recommendation was therefore removed from the 2008 guidelines.

Extremely limited information is available comparing the health benefits of multiple days of weekly activity to those of one or two days, when the dose of activity is controlled for. One of the only studies to examine this issue is a prospective cohort study of 8,421 older men who were followed for mortality over 9 years (I. M. Lee, Sesso, Oguma, & Paffenbarger, 2004). Within that study physically active men (≥ 1,000 kcal/week) were classified as "weekend warriors" (active 1–2 days/week) or "regularly active" (active 3–7 days/week). Compared with sedentary men, mortality risk was reduced by 15% in weekend warriors and 36% in regularly active men. Although the risk reductions were not statistically different in regularly active men and weekend warriors, the twofold greater reduction in the former group suggests that the days-per-week message may have health relevance.

The concept of accumulating physical activity throughout the day by performing multiple short bouts of at least 10 minutes was introduced in 1995 in the U.S. Centers for Disease Control guidelines (Pate et al., 1995). This recommendation was based on a handful of small experimental studies that compared the effects of a single longer bout of daily exercise (e.g., 40 minutes) with those of multiple short bouts of daily exercise (e.g., four 10-minute

sessions) on cardiorespiratory fitness (VO_2max) and body weight (Hardman, 2001; Pate et al., 1995). For example, in a group of 50 overweight women, Jakicic, Wing, Butler, and Robertson (1995) found that 30 minutes of brisk walking performed in a single session 5 days a week resulted in a 14% increase in VO_2max and a 7% loss in weight. Similarly, in that study 30 minutes of brisk walking accumulated in three sessions 5 days a week resulted in a 16% increase in VO_2max and a 9% loss in weight.

Although accumulating physical activity in multiple short bouts appears to be effective for improving fitness and body weight, the influence of short bouts of physical activity on other health outcomes (e.g., mental health and chronic disease) has not been addressed. In addition, only a single study has addressed the relevance of bouts of less than 10 minutes (Mark & Janssen, 2009). That study is also the only study that has considered the importance of bouts of activity in children and youth, a particularly important issue in this age group given that two-thirds of their total activity is accumulated in brief bursts lasting less than 4 minutes (Mark & Janssen, 2009). The authors of that study demonstrated that after controlling for the total volume of moderate-to-vigorous activity, youth who tended to accumulate their daily activity in bouts of at least 5 minutes were only half as likely to be overweight or obese as youth who tended to accumulate their activity in a more sporadic manner. In addition, longer bouts (≥10 minutes) had a greater impact on obesity than shorter bouts (5–9 minutes). This evidence suggests that bouts of activity is an important factor to consider. Additional studies examining a range of bout lengths on a variety of health outcomes in different subpopulations are warranted.

Research on sedentary behavior is an area of physical activity epidemiology that is still in its infancy. First, it is important to understand the volume of sedentary behavior that is harmful to health in people of different ages. The American and Canadian pediatric associations recommend 2 or fewer hours per day of screen time for school-aged children and youth (American Academy of Pediatrics, 2001; Canadian Paediatric Society, 2003). However, their position statements do offer a scientific justification for this threshold, and recent findings suggest that the 2-hr/day cut point may be overly restrictive (Janssen, Katzmarzyk, Boyce, et al., 2004; Mark & Janssen, 2008b). Second, it is important to understand whether different sedentary behaviors impact health in different ways (Rey-Lopez et al., 2008). The vast majority of research has focused on screen-time behaviors; other common sedentary behaviors such as reading, homework, and time spent driving may impact health in a different manner. Third, it is important to understand whether the pattern in which sedentary behaviors are accumulated impacts health.

Summary and Conclusions

In our technologically driven society it is possible for the majority of the population to be extremely sedentary throughout most or all of their lifespan. Unfortunately, there is now clear and strong scientific evidence that this sedentary and inactive lifestyle is causally related with increased risks of mortality, several chronic diseases, and a reduced quality of life. This is true for people of all ages, sexes, and ethnicities. Adults should be encouraged to accumulate at least 150 minutes of moderate-to vigorous-intensity physical activity on a weekly basis to achieve substantive health benefits, with the understanding that more activity will be associated with even greater health benefits. Current evidence indicates that children and youth require even more physical activity for health purposes—at least an hour every day.

References

Abbott, R. D., White, L. R., Ross, G. W., Masaki, K. H., Curb, J. D., & Petrovitch, H. (2004). Walking and dementia in physically capable elderly men. *JAMA, 292*(12), 1447–1453.

Adamo, K. B., Prince, S. A., Tricco, A. C., Connor-Gorber, S., & Tremblay, M. (2009). A comparison of indirect versus direct measures for assessing physical activity in the pediatric population: A systematic review. *International Journal of Pediatric Obesity, 4*(1), 2–27.

American Academy of Pediatrics. (2001). Children, adolescents, and television. *Pediatrics, 107*(2), 423–426.

American College of Sports Medicine. (1975). *Guidelines for graded exercise testing and prescription*. Philadelphia, PA: Lea & Febiger.

American College of Sports Medicine. (1978). Position statement—the recommended quantity and quality of exercise for developing and maintaining fitness in healthy adults. *Medicine & Science in Sport & Exercise, 10*, vii–x.

Andersen, L. B., Harro, M., Sardinha, L. B., Froberg, K., Ekelund, U., Brage, S.,...Anderssen, S. A. (2006). Physical activity and clustered cardiovascular risk in children: A cross-sectional study (the European Youth Heart Study). *Lancet, 368*(9532), 299–304.

Berk, D. R., Hubert, H. B., & Fries, J. F. (2006). Associations of changes in exercise level with subsequent disability among seniors: A 16-year longitudinal study. *Journals of Gerontology. Series A, Biological Sciences and Medical Sciences, 61*(1), 97–102.

Blair, S. N., Kohl, H. W., 3rd, Paffenbarger, R. S., Jr., Clark, D. G., Cooper, K. H., & Gibbons, L. W. (1989). Physical fitness and all-cause mortality. A prospective study of healthy men and women. *JAMA, 262*(17), 2395–2401.

Blumenthal, J. A., Babyak, M. A., Doraiswamy, P. M., Watkins, L., Hoffman, B. M., Barbour, K. A.,...Sherwood, A. (2007). Exercise and pharmacotherapy in the treatment of major depressive disorder. *Psychosomatic Medicine, 69*(7), 587–596.

Borer, K. T. (2005). Physical activity in the prevention and amelioration of osteoporosis in women: Interaction of mechanical, hormonal and dietary factors. *Sports Medicine, 35*(9), 779–830.

Bouchard, C., Blair, S. N., & Haskell, W. L. E. (2007). *Physical activity and health*. Champaign, IL: Human Kinetics.

Canadian Paediatric Society. (2003). Impact of media use on children and youth. *Paediatrics & Child Health, 8*(5), 301–306.

Carlsson, S., Andersson, T., Wolk, A., & Ahlbom, A. (2006). Low physical activity and mortality in women: Baseline lifestyle and health as alternative explanations. *Scandinavian Journal of Public Health, 34*(5), 480–487.

Cummings, S. R., Nevitt, M. C., Browner, W. S., Stone, K., Fox, K. M., Ensrud, K. E.,...Vogt, T. M. (1995). Risk factors for hip fracture in white women. Study of Osteoporotic Fractures Research Group. *New England Journal of Medicine, 332*(12), 767–773.

Currie, C., Nic Gabhainn, S., Godeau, N., Roberts, C., Smith, R., Currie, D.,...Barnekow, V. (Eds.) (2008). *Inequalities in young people's health: HBSC international report from the 2005/2006 survey*. Copenhagen: World Health Organization Regional Office for Europe.

Davidson, L. E., Hudson, R., Kilpatrick, K., Kuk, J. L., McMillan, K., Janiszewski, P. M.,...ross, R. (2009). Effects of exercise modality on insulin resistance and functional limitation in older adults: A randomized controlled trial. *Archives of Internal Medicine, 169*(2), 122–131.

Diabetes Prevention Program Research Group. (2002). Reduction in the incidence of type 2 diabetes with lifestyle intervention or metformin. *New England Journal of Medicine, 346*(6), 393–403.

Farrell, S. W., Cortese, G. M., LaMonte, M. J., & Blair, S. N. (2007). Cardiorespiratory fitness, different measures of adiposity, and cancer mortality in men. *Obesity (Silver Spring), 15*(12), 3140–3149.

Food and Nutrition Board (Institute of Medicine). (2003). *Dietary reference intakes for energy, carbohydrate, fiber, fat, fatty acids, cholesterol, protein, and amino acids (macronutrients)*. Washington, DC: National Academies Press.

Hardman, A. E. (2001). Issues of fractionization of exercise (short vs long bouts). *Medicine & Science in Sports & Exercise, 33*(6 Suppl.), S421–S427; discussion S452–S423.

Health Canada. (2003). *Canadian guidelines for body weight classification in adults* (Cat. no.: H49–179/2003E). Ottawa, ON: Health Canada Publications Centre.

Healy, G. N., Dunstan, D. W., Salmon, J., Cerin, E., Shaw, J. E., Zimmet, P. Z.,...Owen, N. (2008). Breaks in sedentary time: Beneficial associations with metabolic risk. *Diabetes Care, 31*(4), 661–666.

Healy, G. N., Wijndaele, K., Dunstan, D. W., Shaw, J. E., Salmon, J., Zimmet, P. Z.,...Owen, N. (2008). Objectively measured sedentary time, physical activity, and metabolic risk: The Australian Diabetes, Obesity and Lifestyle Study (AusDiab). *Diabetes Care, 31*(2), 369–371.

Heyn, P., Abreu, B. C., & Ottenbacher, K. J. (2004). The effects of exercise training on elderly persons with cognitive impairment and dementia: A meta-analysis. *Archives of Physical Medicine and Rehabilitation, 85*(10), 1694–1704.

Hu, F. B., Sigal, R. J., Rich-Edwards, J. W., Colditz, G. A., Solomon, C. G., Willett, W. C., ... Manson, J. E. (1999). Walking compared with vigorous physical activity and risk of type 2 diabetes in women: A prospective study. *JAMA, 282*(15), 1433–1439.

Hu, F. B., Stampfer, M. J., Solomon, C., Liu, S., Colditz, G. A., Speizer, F. E., ... Manson, J. E. (2001). Physical activity and risk for cardiovascular events in diabetic women. *Annals of Internal Medicine, 134*(2), 96–105.

Jakicic, J. M., Wing, R. R., Butler, B. A., & Robertson, R. J. (1995). Prescribing exercise in multiple short bouts versus one continuous bout: Effects on adherence, cardiorespiratory fitness, and weight loss in overweight women. *International Journal of Obesity and Related Metabolic Disorders, 19*(12), 893–901.

Janssen, I., & Jolliffe, C. J. (2006). Influence of physical activity on mortality in elderly with coronary artery disease. *Medicine & Science in Sports & Exercise, 38*(3), 418–427.

Janssen, I., Katzmarzyk, P. T., Boyce, W. F., King, M. A., & Pickett, W. (2004). Overweight and obesity in Canadian adolescents and their associations with dietary habits and physical activity patterns. *Journal of Adolescent Health, 35*(5), 360–367.

Janssen, I., Katzmarzyk, P. T., Boyce, W. F., Vereecken, C., Mulvihill, C., Roberts, C., ... pickett, W. (2005). Comparison of overweight and obesity prevalence in school-aged youth from 34 countries and their relationships with physical activity and dietary patterns. *Obesity Reviews, 6*(2), 123–132.

Janssen, I., Katzmarzyk, P. T., & Ross, R. (2004). Waist circumference and not body mass index explains obesity-related health risk. *American Journal of Clinical Nutrition, 79*(3), 379–384.

Jolliffe, J. A., Rees, K., Taylor, R. S., Thompson, D., Oldridge, N., & Ebrahim, S. (2001). Exercise-based rehabilitation for coronary heart disease. *Cochrane Database of Systematic Reviews,* (1), CD001800.

Katzmarzyk, P. T., & Craig, C. L. (2002). Musculoskeletal fitness and risk of mortality. *Medicine & Science in Sports & Exercise, 34*(5), 740–744.

Katzmarzyk, P. T., Gledhill, N., & Shephard, R. J. (2000). The economic burden of physical inactivity in Canada. *CMAJ, 163*(11), 1435–1440.

Katzmarzyk, P. T., & Janssen, I. (2004). The economic costs associated with physical inactivity and obesity in Canada: An update. *Canadian Journal of Applied Physiology, 29*(1), 90–115.

Kesaniemi, Y. K., Danforth, E., Jr., Jensen, M. D., Kopelman, P. G., Lefebvre, P., & Reeder, B. A. (2001). Dose–response issues concerning physical activity and health: An evidence-based symposium. *Medicine & Science in Sports & Exercise, 33*(6 Suppl.), S351–S358.

Kohl, H. W., 3rd. (2001). Physical activity and cardiovascular disease: Evidence for a dose response. *Medicine & Science in Sports & Exercise, 33*(6 Suppl.), S472–S483; discussion S493–S474.

Kohrt, W. M., Ehsani, A. A., & Birge, S. J., Jr. (1997). Effects of exercise involving predominantly either joint-reaction or ground-reaction forces on bone mineral density in older women. *Journal of Bone and Mineral Research, 12*(8), 1253–1261.

Krishnan, S., Rosenberg, L., & Palmer, J. R. (2009). Physical activity and television watching in relation to risk of type 2 diabetes: The Black Women's Health Study. *American Journal of Epidemiology, 169*(4), 428–434.

Kujala, U. M., Kaprio, J., Kannus, P., Sarna, S., & Koskenvuo, M. (2000). Physical activity and osteoporotic hip fracture risk in men. *Archives of Internal Medicine, 160*(5), 705–708.

Lawlor, D. A., & Hopker, S. W. (2001). The effectiveness of exercise as an intervention in the management of depression: Systematic review and meta-regression analysis of randomised controlled trials. *BMJ, 322*(7289), 763–767.

LeBlanc, A. G., & Janssen, I. (2009). Dose–response relation between physical activity and dyslipidemia in youth. *Canadian Journal of Cardiology, 26*(6), e201–e205.

Lee, C. D., Folsom, A. R., & Blair, S. N. (2003). Physical activity and stroke risk: A meta-analysis. *Stroke, 34*(10), 2475–2481.

Lee, I.-M. (2007). Physical activity, fitness, and cancer. In C. Bouchard, S. N. Blair & W. L. Haskell (Eds.), *Physical activity and health* (pp. 205–218). Champaign, IL: Human Kinetics.

Lee, I. M., Sesso, H. D., Oguma, Y., & Paffenbarger, R. S., Jr. (2004). The "weekend warrior" and risk of mortality. *American Journal of Epidemiology, 160*(7), 636–641.

Lee, I. M., Sesso, H. D., & Paffenbarger, R. S., Jr. (1999). Physical activity and risk of lung cancer. *International Journal of Epidemiology, 28*(4), 620–625.

Liu, J., Young, T. K., Zinman, B., Harris, S. B., Connelly, P. W., & Hanley, A. J. (2006). Lifestyle variables, non-traditional cardiovascular risk factors, and the metabolic syndrome in an Aboriginal Canadian population. *Obesity (Silver Spring), 14*(3), 500–508.

Luepker, R. V., Murray, D. M., Jacobs, D. R., Jr., Mittelmark, M. B., Bracht, N., Carlaw, R., ... Folsom, A. R. (1994). Community education for cardiovascular disease prevention: Risk factor changes in the Minnesota Heart Health Program. *American Journal of Public Health, 84*(9), 1383–1393.

Manson, J. E., Greenland, P., LaCroix, A. Z., Stefanick, M. L., Mouton, C. P., Oberman, A., ... Siscovick, D. S. (2002). Walking compared with vigorous exercise for the prevention of cardiovascular events in women. *New England Journal of Medicine, 347*(10), 716–725.

Mao, Y., Pan, S., Wen, S. W., & Johnson, K. C. (2003). Physical activity and the risk of lung cancer in Canada. *American Journal of Epidemiology, 158*(6), 564–575.

Mark, A. E., & Janssen, I. (2008a). Dose–response relation between physical activity and blood pressure in youth. *Medicine & Science in Sports & Exercise, 40*(6), 1007–1012.

Mark, A. E., & Janssen, I. (2008b). Relationship between screen time and metabolic syndrome in adolescents. *Journal of Public Health (Oxford), 30*(2), 153–160.

Mark, A. E., & Janssen, I. (2009). Does physical activity accrued in bouts predict overweight and obesity beyond the total volume of physical activity in youth? *American Journal of Preventive Medicine, 36,* 416–421.

Mokdad, A. H., Marks, J. S., Stroup, D. F., & Gerberding, J. L. (2004). Actual causes of death in the United States, 2000. *JAMA, 291*(10), 1238–1245.

Morris, J. N., & Crawford, M. D. (1958). Coronary heart disease and physical activity of work: Evidence of a national necropsy survey. *BMJ, 30,* 1485–1496.

Morris, J. N., Heady, J. A., Raffle, P. A., Roberts, C. G., & Parks, J. W. (1953). Coronary heart-disease and physical activity of work. *Lancet, 265,* 1053–1057, 1111–1120.

Mourier, A., Gautier, J. F., De Kerviler, E., Bigard, A. X., Villette, J. M., Garnier, J. P., . . . Cathelineau, G. (1997). Mobilization of visceral adipose tissue related to the improvement in insulin sensitivity in response to physical training in NIDDM. Effects of branched-chain amino acid supplements. *Diabetes Care, 20*(3), 385–391.

Must, A., & Tybor, D. J. (2005). Physical activity and sedentary behavior: A review of longitudinal studies of weight and adiposity in youth. *International Journal of Obesity (London), 29*(Suppl. 2), S84–S96.

National Center for Chronic Disease Prevention and Health Promotion. (2005). *Behavioral Risk Factor Surveillance System.* Retrieved March 4, 2010, from http://www.cdc.gov/brfss/

National Institutes of Health National Heart, Lung, and Blood Institute. (1998). Clinical guidelines on the identification, evaluation, and treatment of overweight and obesity in adults: The evidence report. *Obesity Research, 6*(Suppl. 2), S51–S210.

Newton, R. U., & Galvao, D. A. (2008). Exercise in prevention and management of cancer. *Current Treatment Options in Oncology, 9*(2–3), 135–146.

Paffenbarger, R. S., Jr., Brand, R. J., Sholtz, R. I., & Jung, D. L. (1978). Energy expenditure, cigarette smoking, and blood pressure level as related to death from specific diseases. *American Journal of Epidemiology, 108*(1), 12–18.

Paffenbarger, R. S., Jr., Hyde, R. T., Wing, A. L., & Hsieh, C. C. (1986). Physical activity, all-cause mortality, and longevity of college alumni. *New England Journal of Medicine, 314*(10), 605–613.

Paffenbarger, R. S., Jr., Wing, A. L., & Hyde, R. T. (1978). Physical activity as an index of heart attack risk in college alumni. *American Journal of Epidemiology, 108*(3), 161–175.

Pate, R. R., Pratt, M., Blair, S. N., Haskell, W. L., Macera, C. A., Bouchard, C., . . . King, A. C. (1995). Physical activity and public health. A recommendation from the Centers for Disease Control and Prevention and the American College of Sports Medicine. *JAMA, 273*(5), 402–407.

Peters, T. M., Schatzkin, A., Gierach, G. L., Moore, S. C., Lacey, J. V., Jr., Wareham, N. J., . . . Leitzmann, M. F. (2009). Physical activity and postmenopausal breast cancer risk in the NIH–AARP diet and health study. *Cancer Epidemiology, Biomarkers & Prevention, 18*(1), 289–296.

Physical Activity Guidelines Advisory Committee. (2008). *Physical Activity Guidelines Advisory Committee Report, 2008.* Washington, DC: U.S. Department of Health and Human Services.

Prince, S. A., Adamo, K. B., Hamel, M. E., Hardt, J., Gorber, S. C., & Tremblay, M. (2008). A comparison of direct versus self-report measures for assessing physical activity in adults: A systematic review. *International Journal of Behavioral Nutrition and Physical Activity, 5*, 56.

Rey-Lopez, J. P., Vicente-Rodriguez, G., Biosca, M., & Moreno, L. A. (2008). Sedentary behaviour and obesity development in children and adolescents. *Nutrition, Metabolism, and Cardiovascular Diseases: NMCD, 18*(3), 242–251.

Ross, R., Dagnone, D., Jones, P. J., Smith, H., Paddags, A., Hudson, R., . . . Janssen, I. (2000). Reduction in obesity and related comorbid conditions after diet-induced weight loss or exercise-induced weight loss in men. A randomized, controlled trial. *Annals of Internal Medicine, 133*(2), 92–103.

Ross, R., & Janssen, I. (2001). Physical activity, total and regional obesity: Dose–response considerations. *Medicine &* *Science in Sports & Exercise, 33*(6 Suppl.), S521–S527; discussion S528–S529.

Ross, R., & Janssen, I. (2007). Physical activity, fitness, and obesity. In C. Bouchard, S. N. Blair & W. L. Haskell (Eds.), *Physical activity, fitness, and health* (pp. 173–189). Champaign, IL: Human Kinetics.

Ross, R., Janssen, I., Dawson, J., Kungl, A. M., Kuk, J. L., Wong, S. L., . . . Hudson, R. (2004). Exercise-induced reduction in obesity and insulin resistance in women: A randomized controlled trial. *Obesity Research, 12*(5), 789–798.

Ruiz, J. R., Sui, X., Lobelo, F., Lee, D. C., Morrow, J. R., Jr., Jackson, A. W., . . . Blair, S. N. (2009). Muscular strength and adiposity as predictors of adulthood cancer mortality in men. *Cancer Epidemiology, Biomarkers & Prevention, 18*(5), 1468–1476.

Salmon, J., Dunstan, D., & Owen, N. (2008). Should we be concerned about children spending extended periods of time in sedentary pursuits even among the highly active? *International Journal of Pediatric Obesity, 3*(2), 66–68.

Saris, W. H., Blair, S. N., van Baak, M. A., Eaton, S. B., Davies, P. S., Di Pietro, L., . . . Wyatt, H. (2003). How much physical activity is enough to prevent unhealthy weight gain? Outcome of the IASO 1st Stock Conference and consensus statement. *Obesity Reviews, 4*(2), 101–114.

Schnohr, P., Scharling, H., & Jensen, J. S. (2007). Intensity versus duration of walking, impact on mortality: The Copenhagen City Heart Study. *European Journal of Cardiovascular Prevention and Rehabilitation, 14*(1), 72–78.

Shields, M., & Tremblay, M. S. (2008). Sedentary behaviour and obesity. *Health Reports, 19*(2), 19–30.

Siegel, P. Z., Brackbill, R. M., & Heath, G. W. (1995). The epidemiology of walking for exercise: Implications for promoting activity among sedentary groups. *American Journal of Public Health, 85*(5), 706–710.

Snow-Harter, C., Bouxsein, M. L., Lewis, B. T., Carter, D. R., & Marcus, R. (1992). Effects of resistance and endurance exercise on bone mineral status of young women: A randomized exercise intervention trial. *Journal of Bone and Mineral Research, 7*(7), 761–769.

Spanier, P. A., Marshall, S. J., & Faulkner, G. E. (2006). Tackling the obesity pandemic: A call for sedentary behaviour research. *Canadian Journal of Public Health, 97*(3), 255–257.

Strawbridge, W. J., Deleger, S., Roberts, R. E., & Kaplan, G. A. (2002). Physical activity reduces the risk of subsequent depression for older adults. *American Journal of Epidemiology, 156*(4), 328–334.

Strong, W. B., Malina, R. M., Blimkie, C. J., Daniels, S. R., Dishman, R. K., Gutin, B., . . . Trudeau, F. (2005). Evidence based physical activity for school-age youth. *Journal of Pediatrics, 146*(6), 732–737.

Tanasescu, M., Leitzmann, M. F., Rimm, E. B., Willett, W. C., Stampfer, M. J., & Hu, F. B. (2002). Exercise type and intensity in relation to coronary heart disease in men. *JAMA, 288*(16), 1994–2000.

Thompson, P. D., Buchner, D., Pina, I. L., Balady, G. J., Williams, M. A., Marcus, B. H., . . . Wenger, N. K. (2003). Exercise and physical activity in the prevention and treatment of atherosclerotic cardiovascular disease: A statement from the Council on Clinical Cardiology (Subcommittee on Exercise, Rehabilitation, and Prevention) and the Council on Nutrition, Physical Activity, and Metabolism (Subcommittee on Physical Activity). *Circulation, 107*(24), 3109–3116.

Troiano, R. P., Berrigan, D., Dodd, K. W., Masse, L. C., Tilert, T., & McDowell, M. (2008). Physical activity in the United States measured by accelerometer. *Medicine & Science in Sports & Exercise, 40*(1), 181–188.

Tuomilehto, J., Lindstrom, J., Eriksson, J. G., Valle, T. T., Hamalainen, H., Ilanne-Parikka, P., ... Uusitupa, M. (2001). Prevention of type 2 diabetes mellitus by changes in lifestyle among subjects with impaired glucose tolerance. *New England Journal of Medicine, 344*(18), 1343–1350.

Villeneuve, P. J., Morrison, H. I., Craig, C. L., & Schaubel, D. E. (1998). Physical activity, physical fitness, and risk of dying. *Epidemiology, 9*(6), 626–631.

Wannamethee, S. G., Shaper, A. G., & Alberti, K. G. (2000). Physical activity, metabolic factors, and the incidence of coronary heart disease and type 2 diabetes. *Archives of Internal Medicine, 160*(14), 2108–2116.

WHO Expert Committee. (1994). *World Health Organization (WHO) 1994 assessment of fracture risk and its application to screening for postmenopausal osteoporosis: Reports of a WHO study group.* Geneva: World Health Organization.

WHO Expert Consultation. (2004). Appropriate body-mass index for Asian populations and its implications for policy and intervention strategies. *Lancet, 363*(9403), 157–163.

Williams, P. T. (1997). Relationship of distance run per week to coronary heart disease risk factors in 8283 male runners. The National Runners' Health Study. *Archives of Internal Medicine, 157*(2), 191–198.

World Health Organization. (1998). *Obesity: Preventing and managing the global epidemic.* Report of a WHO Consultation on Obesity (WHO/NUT/NCD/98.1.1998). Geneva: World Health Organization.

PART 2

Exercise Psychology and Mental Health

3

The Ultimate Tranquilizer? Exercise and Its Influence on Anxiety

Steven J. Petruzzello

Abstract

One of the most popular research topics in exercise psychology has been the effect of exercise on anxiety. Exercise has been examined as a potential tool for preventing and treating anxiety and anxiety disorders for several decades. Indeed, an extensive literature examining the relationship between exercise and anxiety has accumulated over the last 40 years. The topic was important enough for a National Institute of Mental Health "state-of-the-art workshop" in 1984, out of which came the understanding that the anxiety-reducing effect of exercise was an important topic requiring further investigation. While much has been accomplished since the publication of the Morgan and Goldston (1987) text which resulted from the NIMH workshop, much remains unknown regarding the relationship between exercise and anxiety. This chapter summarizes what is known, what isn't yet known, and what remains to be done to make good on the "potential efficacy of exercise" (Morgan & Goldston, 1987, p. 5).

Key Words: exercise, anxiolysis, anxiety sensitivity, state anxiety, trait anxiety, panic disorder, tranquilizer effect, biological challenge, dose response.

> Exercise has the effect of defusing anger and rage, fear and anxiety. Like music, it soothes the savage in us that lies so close to the surface. It is the ultimate tranquilizer.
> —*George Sheehan*, How to Feel Great 24 Hours a Day

Defining Anxiety

Stress, particularly chronic stress, can lead to mental health problems, including anxiety and anxiety disorders. Chronic stress can come from many things, including lack of sleep, poor dietary habits, juggling busy schedules, deadlines, work pressures, and dealing with employment and economic uncertainties, to name but a few. When such chronic stress leads to a feeling of always being "on guard," anxiety is the resultant experience. This is a feeling that goes beyond normal feelings of worry and fear. In fact, the Surgeon General's Report on Mental Health refers to anxiety as the "pathological counterpart of normal fear, manifest by disturbances of mood, as well as of thinking, behavior, and physiological activity" (U.S. Department of Health and Human Services [USDHHS], 1999, p. 233). Because of the increasingly stressful nature of life in modern society, anxiety and anxiety disorders have become increasingly prevalent. Indeed, the anxiety disorders are the most prevalent of the mental illnesses, resulting in significant distress and impairment of function (Hollander & Simeon, 2003).

The traditional view holds that a stimulus perceived as a threat results in an acute stress response. This response is often characterized by increased arousal (through a complex set of interactions between the central and sympathetic nervous systems, along with the secretion of hormones, namely epinephrine and cortisol), but this increased arousal is not automatically manifested as anxiety. Although stress and anxiety are often viewed synonymously, anxiety goes beyond increased arousal in that (a) the perception and concern over the threat are disproportionate to the actual threat, (b) cognitive and behavioral actions are often undertaken to avoid the symptoms of an anxiety attack, (c) the anxiety is usually experienced even after the arousal has subsided, and (d) the anxiety can occur even in the absence of an actual threat—that is, a perceived threat can result in anxiety (USDHHS, 1999).

Symptomatology

Anxiety can be manifested both psychologically and physiologically. Often, one or more of the following are useful in characterizing anxiety: (a) unpleasant feelings (e.g., uncertainty regarding what to do, or feeling weighed down or overwhelmed), (b) physical symptoms caused by activation of the autonomic nervous system (e.g., increased muscle tension, elevated heart rate, or autonomic hyperactivity), (c) altered cognitive processes (e.g., compulsions; persistent obsessions; or unsubstantiated uncertainties regarding objects, activities, or situations), (d) altered behavior (e.g., avoidance of situations), and (e) vigilance (being constantly on guard for danger or a problem). "Normal" anxiety becomes clinical anxiety when the number and intensity of the aforementioned symptoms increases and the degree of suffering and ensuing dysfunction becomes disruptive of usual activities. Anxiety does not have to manifest itself to the extent that it becomes clinical to cause disruption. When a situation is perceived as exceeding an individual's capacity for effective coping or results in feelings of uncertainty or lack of control over the situation, that person experiences stress. When the person's appraisal of that stress becomes negative, anxiety is the result. This is a state characterized by worry, self-doubt, nervousness, and tension, but it also disrupts thought processes and behavior and alters physiological functioning. When the anxiety affects these processes to the extent that normal behavior is disrupted, it becomes clinical. Table 3.1 lists the

Table 3.1. Characteristics of Main Anxiety Disorders

Panic disorder

- Intense fear and discomfort associated with physical and mental symptoms, including:
  - Sweating, trembling, shortness of breath, chest pain, nausea
  - Fear of dying or loss of control of emotions

- Induces urge to escape or run away and often results in seeking emergency help (e.g., hospital)

- Frequently accompanied by major depressive disorder

- Twice as common in women as in men

Generalized anxiety disorder

- Defined by worry lasting more than six months, along with multiple symptoms (e.g., muscle tension, poor concentration, insomnia, irritability)

- Anxiety and worry not attributable to other conditions (e.g., panic disorder, phobias)

- Disorder has fluctuating course, including periods of increased symptoms, usually linked with life stressors

- Twice as common in women as in men

Posttraumatic stress disorder

- Anxiety and behavioral disturbances following exposure to extreme trauma (e.g., combat, physical assault), which persist for more than one month

- Dissociation, a symptom involving perceived detachment from emotional state or body, is a critical feature

- Symptoms also include generalized anxiety, hyperarousal, avoidance of situations that trigger memories of trauma, recurrent thoughts

- Occurs in about 9% of those exposed to extreme trauma

Agoraphobia

- Severe, pervasive anxiety when in situations perceived to be difficult to escape from, or complete avoidance of certain situations (e.g., crowded areas, alone outside of home, travel in bus or plane)

- Often seen after onset of panic disorder

- Twice as common in women as in men

Table 3.1. (Continued)

Social phobia (social anxiety disorder)

- Marked, persistent anxiety in social situations (e.g., public speaking)
  - Possibility of embarrassment or ridicule is a crucial factor
  - Individual is preoccupied with concern that others will notice the anxiety symptoms (e.g., trembling, sweating, halting or rapid speech)

- Accompanied by anticipatory anxiety days or weeks prior to feared event

- More common in women than in men

Obsessive–compulsive disorder

- Obsessions, such as recurrent thoughts or images that are perceived as inappropriate or forbidden, elicit anxiety

- Individual perceives loss of control, thus acts on impulses or thoughts

- Compulsions, including behaviors or thoughts, reduce anxiety associated with obsessions
  - Include overt behaviors (e.g., hand washing) and mental acts (e.g., counting, praying)
  - Take long periods of time to complete

- Disorder has fluctuating course, including periods of increased symptoms, usually linked with life stressors

- Equally common in women and men

Note. Adapted from *Mental Health: A Report of the Surgeon General* (p. 234–237), By U.S. Department of Health and Human Services, 1999, Rockville, MD: U.S. Department of Health and Human Services, Substance Abuse and Mental Health Services Administration, Center for Mental Health Services, National Institutes of Health, National Institute of Mental Health.

characteristics of the major anxiety disorders (i.e., panic disorder, generalized anxiety disorder, posttraumatic stress disorder, agoraphobia, social anxiety disorder, and obsessive–compulsive disorder).

Prevalence

As noted in the Surgeon General's Report (USDHHS, 1999), anxiety disorders are the most prevalent of the mental disorders (Regier et al., 1990). Anxiety disorders, in order of decreasing lifetime population prevalence, include social phobia (13–16%), specific phobias (10%), posttraumatic stress disorder (7–9%), generalized anxiety disorder (5–7%), agoraphobia (6%), panic disorder (2–4%), and obsessive–compulsive disorder (2–3%) (Hollander & Simeon, 2003). The anxiety disorders contribute significantly to the disease and disability burden of the nation.

Two nationwide probability surveys published in the mid-1990s further highlight the prevalence of such disabling mental conditions. The 23.4% one-year prevalence rate for any mental disorder in the National Comorbidity Survey (Kessler et al., 1994) included an 18.7% one-year prevalence rate for any anxiety disorder, meaning that within a given year, 18.7% of the U.S. adult population will have a diagnosable anxiety disorder. The more recent National Comorbidity Survey Replication study indicated an 18.1% one-year prevalence rate for any anxiety disorder (Kessler, Chiu, Demler, & Walters, 2005). The Epidemiological Catchment Area Study (Regier et al., 1993) estimated a 19.5% one-year prevalence rate for any mental disorder, including 13.1% for any anxiety disorder. From these studies, the best estimate of the one-year prevalence rates has been calculated to be 16.4% for any anxiety disorder (USDHHS, 1999). Of all cases of anxiety disorder, roughly 22.8% were deemed serious in severity, 33.7% were moderate, and 43.5% were mild (Kessler et al., 2005). Although Kessler et al. (2005) caution against interpreting temporal trends, anxiety disorders continue to be the most prevalent of the mental disorders.

Beyond the human suffering that cannot be measured, the prevalence of the anxiety disorders creates an economic burden in terms of both treatment and lost productivity (DuPont, Rice, Miller, Shiraki, Rowland, & Harwood, 1996). Estimated annual national costs associated with anxiety disorders approximated $42 billion in the United States in 1990 ($63 billion in 1998 dollars; Greenberg et al., 1999). Greenberg et al. (1999) estimated this cost at $1,542 per year for each person afflicted (in 1990 dollars). An analysis by Marciniak et al. (2005) estimated the total medical cost, using data from 1996 to 1998, for a patient with any anxiety disorder at approximately $6,500. Using an analysis to assess the effects of various characteristics (e.g., age, sex) and conditions (e.g., generalized anxiety disorder, asthma) on the total medical cost, type of anxiety disorder (e.g., generalized anxiety disorder, panic disorder) contributed ~$1,600-$4,000 to the total medical costs. Of the roughly 42 billion 1990 dollars, psychiatric treatment (e.g., counseling and hospitalization) accounted for 31% of the total, nonpsychiatric medical treatment (e.g., emergency room treatment) for 54%, indirect workplace costs for 10%, and prescription costs and mortality (i.e., anxiety-induced suicide) for approximately 5%. Notably, the vast majority (88%) of workplace costs were derived from lost productivity rather than absenteeism. Anxiety is also a predisposing factor in drug and substance abuse, which further adds to the cost of the disorder.

Treatment

Traditional treatment protocols for anxiety (e.g., medication and psychotherapy) are often expensive and time-consuming, albeit readily available and generally effective. Pharmacotherapies (i.e., medications) are often used to treat anxiety. Benzodiazepines (e.g., diazepam), which inhibit neurotransmitter systems, have sedative effects. Antidepressants (e.g., clomipramine, a tricyclic antidepressant, or specific serotonin reuptake inhibitors such as sertraline and fluoxetine) are also used in the treatment of anxiety because of their antianxiety properties. While efficacious as a treatment, medication usually requires extended periods of use, often lasting up to six months. Additionally, pharmacological treatments often have side effects (e.g., withdrawal symptoms when medication is stopped). Psychotherapy, while also having demonstrated treatment efficacy, can likewise be problematic, primarily in terms of the length of the treatment and the greater financial cost associated with it. Cognitive behavioral therapies can often assist in determining the cause-and-effect relationships among the person's thoughts, feelings, and behaviors and developing strategies for attenuating anxiety symptoms and reducing dysfunctional behaviors (USDHHS, 1999). Time-limited therapies (therapy conducted within a finite time frame, e.g., 12 weeks) are often used to assist the individual in directly coping with the anxiety and its symptoms.

For quite some time, physical activity (e.g., exercise) has been examined as a potential tool in both the prevention and the treatment of anxiety (Martinsen & Raglin, 2007). The National Institute of Mental Health identified examination of the *anxiolytic* (anxiety-reducing) effects of exercise as an important topic (Morgan & Goldston, 1987). Although some of the anxiety disorders (e.g., phobias) are thought to be unaffected by exercise, because they are linked to specific situations or objects (Dunn, Trivedi, & O'Neal, 2001), this is not a uniformly accepted viewpoint (Johnsgard, 1989, 2004). The remainder of this chapter presents the major findings of research on the effects of physical activity on both normal anxiety and anxiety sufficient to be considered clinical. Before examining this work, however, we will examine the ways in which anxiety is assessed.

Measurement

Distinguishing between state and trait forms of anxiety is a necessary backdrop to discussing the ways in which anxiety is measured. State anxiety is a noticeable but *transient* emotional state characterized by feelings of worry and apprehension and by heightened autonomic nervous system activity (e.g., increased heart rate, sweaty palms, increased respiration, and increased muscle tension). Thus state anxiety is an assessment of how the individual feels "right now, at this moment." For example, a self-report measure of state anxiety will ask the extent to which individuals "feel calm," "feel relaxed," or are "presently worrying over possible misfortunes."

Conversely, trait anxiety reflects a more general predisposition to respond across many situations with apprehension, worry, and nervousness. For example, high-trait-anxious individuals would most often respond with increased restlessness, lack of confidence, difficulty in making decisions, and a feeling of inadequacy regardless of the situation. Thus trait anxiety is an assessment of how the individual "generally feels." A self-report measure of trait anxiety will ask the extent to which individuals "generally feel this way, that is, how [you] feel on average" for items like "I feel satisfied with myself," "I feel like a failure," "I wish I could be as happy as others seem to be," and "I take disappointments so keenly that I can't put them out of my mind." Measures of trait anxiety are conceptually analogous to the personality construct of neuroticism. As such, some studies have used measures of neuroticism or emotionality as an assessment of this construct. Because trait anxiety reflects a general predisposition, it makes sense conceptually to assess trait anxiety before and after chronic exercise programs (i.e., exercise programs lasting several weeks or months) rather than before and after single bouts of exercise. In studies examining acute exercise effects (i.e., single bouts of exercise), because the goal is to assess the currently experienced level of anxiety, state anxiety measures are often used pre- and post exercise.

Psychological Measures

Because anxiety can be manifested both psychologically and physiologically, it can be assessed in several ways. The most common method for the psychological assessment of anxiety in exercise studies is through the use of self-report inventories or questionnaires. Of the myriad anxiety questionnaire measures available, the most commonly used has been the Spielberger State–Trait Anxiety Inventory (STAI; Spielberger, 1979, 1983), followed by the Tension subscale of the Profile of Mood States (POMS; McNair, Droppleman, & Lorr, 1981), and the Anxiety subscale of the Multiple Affect Adjective Check List (MAACL; Zuckerman & Lubin, 1965).

Physiological Measures

Numerous measures of physiological activation or arousal (e.g., increased heart rate, muscle tension, or sensations of being jittery or shaky) have been used as physiological indices of anxiety. Using a single physiological measure implicitly assumes that anxiety and physiological activation are linked in a one-to-one relationship. Although this is a questionable assumption, most studies that have used physiological measures have relied on a single measure. It may be more appropriate to use a battery of physiological measures to account for individual response stereotypy (Stern, Ray, & Quigley, 2001), but this goes beyond the scope of the present discussion.

Because anxiety is often manifested as increased activity in skeletal muscle, measures of muscle tension (via electromyography [EMG]), have been used as an index of anxiety. Notable research in this regard was done by Herbert deVries (e.g., deVries, 1981; deVries & Adams, 1972; for an example of this research see the section "Exercise versus Other Anxiety-Reducing Treatments" later in this chapter). Anxiety can also be manifested in the cardiovascular system (e.g., measures of blood pressure or heart rate), the electrodermal system (skin responses such as galvanic skin response, palmar sweating, and skin temperature), and the central nervous system (e.g., electroencephalography [EEG] measure of electrical activity in the brain). Although anxiety responses are likely to have neurochemical components (e.g., increases in catecholamines and cortisol), not many studies in the human exercise–anxiety literature have examined such measures. This is in part due to the expense involved in the collection and analysis of such data. However, a growing research literature using both human and animal models continues to make considerable progress toward understanding the neurochemistry of anxiety and examining how exercise influences such pathways (e.g., Dishman, 1997; O'Connor, Raglin, & Martinsen, 2000).

Research on Exercise and Anxiety

As mentioned in the previous section, exercise can be classified as either *acute* or *chronic*. Acute exercise involves single bouts of exercise at a specified level of intensity and for a specified duration. Chronic exercise, on the other hand, typically involves a bout of acute exercise repeated several times a week for weeks, months, or years. A program of chronic exercise is often designed with the aim of improving aerobic capacity, if the exercise is aerobic, or improving muscular strength, endurance, or both, if the exercise involves resistance training. Popular or folk wisdom posits that physical activity or exercise is a useful tool in alleviating anxiety and anxiety disorders (De Moor, Boomsma, Stubbe, Willemsen, & De Geus, 2008). Physicians, at least to some extent, do prescribe exercise for this purpose. A survey in the *Physician and Sportsmedicine* found that 60% of the 1,750 physicians surveyed prescribed exercise for patients suffering from anxiety (Ryan, 1983), although this is likely a liberal estimate given the sample (i.e., physicians reading a journal that regularly contains information about the physical and mental benefits of exercise).

What is currently known regarding the effects of exercise on anxiety? This question can be answered in several different ways with different sources of data. In what follows, evidence for the effects of exercise on preventing anxiety symptoms or disorders from developing is drawn from epidemiological or prospective studies. Evidence for the relationship between acute vs. chronic exercise and state vs. trait anxiety is drawn from empirical studies and from reviews. The vast majority of studies have not used clinically anxious samples, even though it has been suggested that the greatest impact of exercise may be in such samples (Salmon, 2001). Here, where possible, research is presented that examined the utility of exercise in the treatment of anxiety symptoms or disorders in clinically anxious samples.

The most comprehensive quantitative review of the exercise–anxiety literature was by Petruzzello, Landers, Hatfield, Kubitz, and Salazar (1991) and involved three meta-analyses (one for state anxiety, one for trait anxiety, and one for psychophysiological indices of anxiety) of more than 120 studies that had examined the exercise–anxiety relationship. Several less comprehensive reviews of the literature have since appeared (Landers & Petruzzello, 1994; Long & van Stavel, 1995; Martinsen & Raglin, 2007; McDonald & Hodgdon, 1991; Physical Activity Guidelines Advisory Committee [PAGAC], 2008; Raglin, 1997; Schlicht, 1994; Wipfli, Rethorst, &

Landers, 2008), but none has shown any striking differences from the Petruzzello et al. review.

Evidence for Preventive Effects

Various studies have indicated that exercise may be an important lifestyle factor in the prevention of anxiety symptoms and disorders. Stephens (1988) conducted a cross-sectional epidemiological study examining four large Canadian adult samples (ranging in size from 3,025 to 23,791). It was found that greater self-reported physical activity was associated with better mental health, which included fewer symptoms of anxiety (and fewer symptoms of depression). More recently, De Moor, Beem, Stubbe, Boomsma and De Geus (2006) conducted another population-based study in the Netherlands with over 19,000 adolescent and adult twins and their families. The findings indicated that individuals who exercised had lower trait anxiety scores than sedentary individuals.

A similar study by Goodwin (2003), using data from the National Comorbidity Survey, examined the relationship between regular physical activity (defined as "How often do you get physical exercise—either on your job or in a recreational activity?") and mental disorders, including a variety of anxiety disorders (e.g., generalized anxiety disorder, panic attack, and agoraphobia). From the large sample (N = 5,877 adults, 15–54 years old), 63% (3,707) responded that they exercised regularly, with the remainder (2,170) reporting that they exercised occasionally, rarely, or never. Goodwin's analysis showed regular physical activity to be associated with reduced risk of having generalized anxiety disorder, agoraphobia, panic attack, specific phobias, and social phobia. These relationships remained even after controlling for a variety of demographic and self-reported illness variables. There was also a dose–response effect. Specifically, frequency of reported anxiety disorders increased as the level of physical activity decreased. For example, panic attacks occurred in 3.32% of those reporting regular exercise, 4.85% of those reporting occasional exercise, 7.33% of those who exercised rarely, and 8.52% of those who never exercised. Generalized anxiety disorder showed a similar dose effect, occurring in 2.26% of those who exercised regularly, 2.97% of occasional exercisers, 5.93% of those who rarely exercised, and 6.49% of those who never exercised. Goodwin concluded that such findings provide evidence of a potential link between regular exercise and a reduced likelihood of a variety of anxiety disorders.

Taylor, Pietrobon, Pan, Huff, and Higgins (2004) used another large database of almost 42,000 US adults (the 2001 Behavioral Risk Factor Surveillance System) to examine the potential links between mental health and physical activity. Using the Healthy People 2010 guidelines for physical activity, they found that those who were completely inactive were at significantly greater risk of having reported anxiety symptoms on at least 14 of the 30 days prior to when they responded to the survey. Somewhat surprisingly, among individuals over the age of 40 years, those who were physically active, but at a level below the Healthy People 2010 recommendation, were at less risk of experiencing anxiety symptoms than those who met or exceeded the recommendation. Taylor et al. concluded that some physical activity was better than none when it came to protecting against anxiety symptoms, but more physical activity was not necessarily better. Clearly this relationship needs further examination.

In addition, studies have consistently shown that individuals who are physically fit typically have less anxiety than unfit individuals (Landers and Petruzzello, 1994). This could be the result of healthier lifestyles; that is, more fit individuals may be more active and perhaps have better nutrition. When examining the effects of exercise training programs (which often have the aim of improving cardiovascular fitness), Landers and Petruzzello (1994) concluded that in addition to increasing fitness, trait (i.e., more general) levels of anxiety decrease following such chronic activity protocols. Studies examining levels of neuroticism, a conceptual analogue to trait anxiety, have found neuroticism to decline over the length of a training program, with greater reductions seen with more weeks of training (Petruzzello et al., 1991). Other explanations for this relationship, independent of fitness changes, are possible. However, the overall evidence supports the hypothesis that regular participation in a program of physical activity buffers against anxiety symptoms and anxiety disorders (PAGAC, 2008).

Exercise and Anxiety

The Petruzzello et al. (1991) review concluded that anxiety reduction occurred following a single bout of exercise or following exercise training, but only when the exercise was aerobic. The type of aerobic exercise (e.g., walking, jogging, running, swimming, or cycling) did not influence the anxiety-reducing effects. Anaerobic forms of exercise (e.g., resistance exercise), by contrast, either did not change anxiety or actually resulted in slight increases in anxiety (see the section "Anaerobic Exercise and Anxiety" below). The anxiolytic effects of aerobic activity occurred for state anxiety following acute exercise and for trait anxiety following chronic exercise. These reductions were independent of how the anxiety was operationalized, whether by self-report measures (questionnaires), measures of muscular tension (EMG), cardiovascular measures (heart rate and blood pressure), or alterations in central nervous system measures (e.g., EEG alpha activity)—though effects on the last of these are not always found (e.g., Motl, O'Connor, & Dishman, 2004).

In the acute exercise studies, the anxiolytic effect following exercise was transient. Several studies examining the anxiolytic effect for an extended period following exercise have shown that the reduction in anxiety does not last indefinitely, but instead returns to pre-exercise levels within about 2–4 hours (Martinsen & Raglin, 2007; Petruzzello et al., 1991). Of note, this anxiolytic effect parallels some physiological changes that occur following exercise, such as postexercise hypotension (reduced blood pressure). Many studies have shown the postexercise hypotension response, and numerous studies have shown reductions in anxiety, leading to speculation that the two might be linked. However, such a linkage has yet to be definitively shown.

Given that participants in chronic exercise programs show reductions in trait anxiety at program's end relative to preprogram levels, it is possible that over time pre-exercise levels of state anxiety become reduced (i.e., a new baseline is achieved). Anxiety reduction, however, continues to take place following a single bout of aerobic activity. As an example, a pre-exercise state anxiety baseline might be a score of 35 on the State Anxiety Inventory (SAI, where possible scores range from 20 to 80; Spielberger, 1983). Following a single exercise bout, state anxiety might be reduced to a score of 28. The next day, or prior to the next exercise session, this state anxiety score might again be at 35. Over 12 to 16 weeks of a consistent chronic exercise program, the pre-exercise state anxiety baseline might drop to a value of 30. With this reduction in baseline anxiety, a single exercise bout would still be associated with an anxiolytic effect (e.g., state anxiety might fall to 25), but it would again return to the pre-exercise level of 30 before the next exercise session.

To date, there is no evidence that the anxiolytic effect is greater for one sex than the other. There is also no consistent evidence for any effects of age on the anxiolytic effect with either acute or chronic exercise (Petruzzello et al., 1991).

Exercise versus Other Anxiety-Reducing Treatments

It is important to know the extent to which exercise reduces anxiety compared with other treatment options. Findings in the exercise–anxiety literature have shown exercise to have stronger anxiolytic effects than not doing anything and to be as effective as known anxiety-reducing treatments such as meditation, relaxation, or quiet rest (Petruzzello et al., 1991). A now classic study conducted by Bahrke and Morgan (1978) randomly assigned 75 men to 20 minutes of either treadmill exercise, noncultic meditation, or sitting quietly in a sound-dampened chamber reading a *Reader's Digest* magazine (a condition now known as the "quiet rest" condition). State anxiety was assessed (via the SAI) pretreatment, immediately post treatment, and 10 minutes post treatment. State anxiety was significantly reduced following all three conditions; there were no differences in the magnitude of the reduction among the three (see Figure 3.1). Such a finding can obviously be interpreted as evidence that exercise is not necessary for anxiety reduction. However, while exercise is perhaps no better at reducing anxiety than other known anxiety-reducing treatments, results from studies like the Bahrke and Morgan work show it is just as good. Additionally, the physiological benefits that result from exercise would not accrue from other, nonexercise treatments.

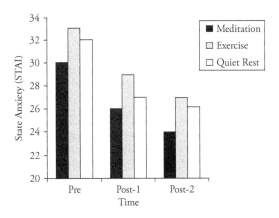

Figure 3.1. State anxiety responses before and after several manipulations known to reduce state anxiety. Adapted with permission from "Anxiety Reduction following Exercise and Meditation," by M. S. Bahrke and W. P. Morgan, 1978, *Cognitive Therapy and Research, 4,* pp. 323–333. Copyright 1978 by Springer Science+Business Media.,

Exercise has the further advantage that the anxiolytic effects seem to last for a longer time. For example, Raglin and Morgan (1987) showed that anxiety was still reduced below pretreatment levels 3 hours following exercise but not quiet rest.

Surprisingly little research has been done comparing exercise with another common treatment for anxiety, namely pharmacotherapy (medication). The available evidence shows, however, that exercise may be as or even more effective than anxiety-reducing drugs (e.g., diazepam). In another classic study, deVries and Adams (1972) recruited 10 older adults (52–70 years old) suffering from anxiety/tension problems (e.g., difficulty concentrating, excessive muscle tension, or nervousness). Each of these individuals was tested three times in each of five treatment conditions: (a) a 400-mg capsule containing meprobamate, a commonly used anxiolytic drug at the time; (b) a 400-mg placebo capsule containing lactose (a sugar pill); (c) 15 min of walking at a moderate intensity designed to elicit a heart rate (HR) of 100 beats per minute (bpm) (~67% of the individual's maximal HR); (d) 15 min of walking at a moderate-hard to vigorous intensity designed to elicit a HR of 120 bpm (~80% of the individual's maximal HR); and (e) a control condition where the participant sat quietly and read. As is often done in pharmacological studies, conditions (a) and (b) were done in double-blind fashion (i.e., neither the participants nor the experimenters interacting with the participants knew whether the participants were receiving the actual drug or the placebo) to reduce expectancy effects. DeVries and Adams assessed anxiety through EMG measures from the biceps taken before each treatment condition and 30 and 60 minutes after each condition. Of the five conditions, only the exercise at moderate intensity elicited significant reductions in muscle tension (although effect in the higher-intensity exercise condition approached significance). The control, drug, and placebo conditions did not reduce muscle tension and were not different from one another.

The deVries and Adams results suggest that exercise may be more effective than anxiolytic medication. Indeed, deVries (1981) consistently referred to the "tranquilizer effect of exercise." Given the widespread use of antianxiety (i.e., tranquilizer) medications for individuals suffering from anxiety disorders, more research in this area is warranted (see Martinsen & Stanghelle, 1997). Only a few other studies examining the effectiveness of exercise relative to anxiety medication have been done. These will be presented in a subsequent section, as they were done with clinical samples of participants.

Anaerobic Exercise and Anxiety

The Petruzzello et al. (1991) meta-analysis indicated that unlike aerobic forms of exercise, anaerobic (e.g., resistance) exercise seems to result in slight *increases* in anxiety. Raglin (1997), in a review of more recent studies involving resistance exercise, concluded that reductions in state anxiety are not consistently seen following such exercise, and in some cases anxiety is even increased. Thus the picture has not really changed. Possible explanations for the lack of change in anxiety include subject (in)experience with the activity and exercise intensity. The intensity explanation has been supported in some studies. Raglin, Turner, and Eksten (1993) found that resistance exercise for 30 min at 70–80% of the individual's one-repetition maximum (1-RM), resulted in brief increases in anxiety, with anxiety returning to baseline levels within 20 min post exercise. Bartholomew and Linder (1998) found that 20 min of self-rated light–intensity weight training resulted in reductions in state anxiety in males but not females; anxiety was increased, however, following self-rated moderate and high-intensity activity. Again, these increased levels of anxiety were brief, dissipating within 5–15 min following completion of the exercise. In a second study using intensity based on estimated 1-RMs, Bartholomew and Linder (1998) found that low-intensity (40–50% 1-RM) resistance exercise led to decreased anxiety 15 and 30 min post exercise, but high-intensity (75–85% 1-RM) exercise led to significant increases in anxiety for up to 15 min following the exercise.

Arent, Landers, Matt, and Etnier (2005) adopted a dose–response approach to examining anxiety responses to resistance exercise. College students performed, on separate days, a no-exercise control session and three resistance exercise sessions each consisting of three sets (10 repetitions) of six upper-body exercises performed at either 40%, 70%, or 100% of the individual's predetermined 10-repetition maximum (10-RM; conditions were counterbalanced). The largest reductions in anxiety occurred with the 70% 10-RM session, but an increase in anxiety of comparable magnitude occurred with the 100% 10-RM session. Unfortunately, although anxiety was assessed 0–5, 15, 30, 45, and 60 min post session, Arent et al. mention no specific time effects, so it is unclear whether this was an immediate postexercise effect or whether it was more persistent. Arent, Alderman, Short, and Landers (2007) found that increased state anxiety persisted up to 15 min following approximately 30 min of resistance exercise (12–20 repetitions each of bench press, shoulder press, lat pull-down, leg press, and dead lift performed at 50% of the participant's 1-RM); anxiety returned to pre-exercise levels within 30 min post exercise and stayed at that level for up to 120 min post exercise, but at no point was there a significant reduction in anxiety.

Bibeau, Moore, Mitchell, Vargas-Tonsing, and Bartholomew (2010) conducted another study examining resistance exercise of varying intensities and rest periods. Participants ($N = 104$, M_{age} = 20.5 years, 58 males) in a university weight training class were randomly assigned to one of five treatment conditions: a no-exercise control; low intensity, short rest; low intensity, long rest; high intensity, short rest; high intensity, long rest. Each of the exercise conditions involved three sets each of chest press, seated row, leg press, and hamstring curl. Low-intensity conditions consisted of 10–11 repetitions of each exercise performed at 50–55% of the individual's 1-RM, whereas high-intensity conditions consisted of 6–7 repetitions performed at 80–85% of the individual's 1-RM; short-rest conditions had 30 s of rest between repetitions, whereas long-rest conditions had 90 s of rest between repetitions. State anxiety was assessed before and within 5 min following exercise as well as 20 and 40 min following exercise completion. Results indicated an elevation in anxiety immediately following the high-intensity, short-rest condition; significant reductions in anxiety were seen at 20 and 40 min post exercise in all exercise conditions.

The PAGAC (2008) concluded, based on six randomized controlled trials published after 1995, that the magnitude of anxiety reduction does not differ based on exercise mode: Resistance exercise and aerobic exercise result in similar reductions in anxiety. Based on studies of resistance exercise like those cited above, it does seem that light- to moderate-intensity resistance exercise may result in reduced anxiety. However, more vigorous intensities seem either to increase anxiety, at least for some brief period post exercise, or to result in no change (e.g., Cassilhas et al., 2007).

It is also entirely possible that the findings of unchanged or increased anxiety result from measurement problems. As articulated by Rejeski, Hardy, and Shaw (1991) and Ekkekakis, Hall, and Petruzzello (1999), such a problem could arise from using the State–Trait Anxiety Inventory (STAI) to measure anxiety (as has been done in the vast majority of exercise studies). Specifically, results taken as indicative of increased anxiety may actually reflect little more than increased activation or arousal (e.g., increased heart rate). Numerous items in the STAI were designed to reflect perceived activation, based on the notion that changes in such perceptions of activation (e.g., jitteriness) would be related to changes in anxiety. However, such altered perceptions with exercise may be more reflective of changes in physiological activity consistent with the demands of the exercise. Thus *immediately* following exercise, particularly resistance exercise, an individual who is breathing hard and senses his or her chest pounding might respond to an STAI item like "jittery" with "somewhat," "moderately so," or "very much so." Although this is a normal and expected outcome of the exertion coincident with the activity, it is reflected as increased anxiety on a measure like the STAI.

Evidence for the Use of Exercise as a Treatment

Much of the research on exercise-associated anxiety reduction has been done on samples that do not have unusually elevated levels of anxiety to begin with. For example, it is not unusual for participants to have pre-exercise levels of anxiety near the floor of the scale being used to assess anxiety. In fact, as demonstrated by Petruzzello (1995), it is quite likely that many participants in laboratory-based studies are actually less anxious on reporting to the laboratory for the study than they are in their "normal" environments. This obviously leaves little room for a decrease in anxiety, but it also speaks to the issue of whether exercise is influencing anxiety at all. That is, if the participants are not anxious to begin with (based on low scores on a measure of anxiety), does a lower score post exercise reflect a reduction in anxiety? One obvious way to study the anxiolytic effect of exercise is to use clinically anxious samples, which has been done, albeit relatively infrequently. Another approach is to use a "biological challenge" model to generate anxiety or anxiety symptoms and examine the effects of exercise in such a scenario.

Biological Challenge Models

An alternative approach to relying on participants who are not suffering from elevated anxiety is to induce anxiety symptoms and then examine the effect of exercise on emotional reactivity. Several such biological challenge models have been used.

Motl and Dishman (2004) experimentally induced anxiety symptoms by having subjects ingest capsules containing either a large dose of caffeine (10 mg per kilogram of body weight) or a placebo and then compared the effects of moderate exercise (60% of the aerobic capacity obtained during graded exercise testing, i.e., VO_{2peak}) and quiet rest on self-reported state anxiety. The caffeine was quite effective for increasing self-reported anxiety symptoms, with an effect size of 1 standard deviation, and state anxiety was reduced to a significantly greater extent after the exercise compared with quiet rest; there was no effect of exercise on anxiety in the placebo condition.

Another biological challenge involves a single vital-capacity inhalation of a gas mixture containing 35% CO_2 and 65% O_2. Several studies have now used this protocol to examine the effectiveness of exercise on subsequent anxiety (more specifically, panic) symptoms. In the initial study, Esquivel, Schruers, Kuipers, and Griez (2002) randomly assigned 20 healthy volunteers to either an exercise or a very light-exercise control condition. In the exercise condition, participants did approximately 12 min of cycling at 70 rpm; the initial workload was 100 W for women and 125 W for men, increasing to 175 W (women) and 200 W (men) for 9 min or until blood lactate level exceeded 6 mM. After 9 min the workload was increased 25 W for an additional 3 min until either blood lactate reached the 6-mM level or the participant was exhausted. In the control condition participants did 12 min of cycling at 70 rpm at a continuous workload of 1 W per kilogram of body weight minus 20. Blood samples were drawn from an indwelling catheter every 3 min. Immediately following both conditions, participants completed a panic symptom list and a visual analog anxiety scale, were then given the CO_2 challenge, and then again completed the panic symptom list and visual analog anxiety scale. Panic symptoms and anxiety increased following the challenge, but the increase for the panic symptoms was significantly less following the exercise condition than the control condition.

Esquivel et al. (2008) performed essentially the same study with patients suffering from panic disorder. Ten patients were assigned to the same exercise protocol as in Esquivel et al. (2002), with the exception that the target end point was 80–90% of predicted maximal heart rate; eight patients were assigned to the control condition. As with the previous study, the CO_2 challenge involved a vital-capacity inhalation of the 35% CO_2/65% O_2 mixture.

Panic symptoms were assessed and a visual analog anxiety scale was completed before and immediately following the CO_2 challenge. Similar to the previous study, the CO_2 challenge evoked a smaller panic reaction in the exercise group (panic symptoms decreased, self-reported anxiety increased minimally) than in the control group (panic symptoms increased, self-reported anxiety increased markedly).

A CO_2 challenge study by Smits, Meuret, Zvolensky, Rosenfield, and Seidel (2009) yielded similar results. After participants (M_{age} = 19.4 ± 2.4 years) were randomly assigned to either 20 min of exercise or quiet rest, they completed several measures, including the Acute Panic Inventory (API; Dillon, Gorman, Liebowitz, Fyer, & Klein, 1987) and a measure of self-reported fear. Those in the exercise condition then walked or ran on a treadmill for 20 min at 70% of their maximal heart rate after a 3 min warm-up, while the control group participants sat quietly for an equivalent length of time. Participants in both groups completed a second API, rested for 3 min, then did the CO_2 challenge and completed the API within 30 seconds afterward. Results revealed that the participants who did moderate-intensity exercise had significantly less reactivity to the CO_2 challenge than did the rest participants. Smits et al. speculated that the reduction in reactivity may have been due in part to a reduced fear of the somatic sensations, with the exercise mediating the interoceptive sensations that accompany panic attacks.

Another biological challenge model involves the injection of cholecystokinin tetrapeptide (CCK_4) to induce panic attacks. Strohle and colleagues (Strohle et al., 2005, 2009; Strohle, Feller, Strasburger, Heinz, & Dimeo, 2006) have shown across several studies that exercise prior to CCK_4 injection results in a significantly lower increase in panic (as assessed via the API) than in control conditions. In one of the studies (Strohle et al., 2009) patients with panic disorder showed elevated somatic symptoms (e.g., palpitations, breathing, and nausea) but not anxiety (e.g., fear of dying and general fear) following exercise; for both measures, exercise resulted in significantly fewer somatic and cognitive anxiety symptoms than in a quiet rest control condition.

Short of working directly with clinically anxious samples, such biological challenge models offer a viable alternative to examining the efficacy of exercise in reducing anxiety. Most of these challenge models appear to have more relevance to panic disorder, but the findings may be applicable to other anxiety disorders as well.

Clinically Anxious Samples

The preventive effects of exercise on anxiety are clearly important, but it is also important to determine the extent to which exercise can be useful as a treatment for anxiety problems once they have manifested themselves. Although the literature using clinical samples is very scant, some evidence does suggest that exercise can be useful in the treatment of mental disorders, and several calls have been made for using exercise for that purpose (Callahan, 2004; Chung & Baird, 1999). Johnsgard (1989) cites numerous case study examples of how he has successfully used exercise in the treatment of both anxiety and mood disorders in his patients. More carefully controlled studies conducted with clinically anxious samples highlight the utility of such an "exercise prescription"—what deVries (1981) referred to as the "ultimate tranquilizer." A summary of these studies is presented below.

Breus and O'Connor (1998) randomly assigned 14 high-trait-anxious women (using trait version of STAI; unless otherwise stated, all references to trait anxiety scores are from the trait version of the STAI) to four conditions: 20 min of low- to moderate-intensity cycling (40% VO_{2peak}) immediately followed by 20 min of recovery (Exercise Only condition); sitting on the bicycle ergometer for 40 min while studying (Study Only); 20 min of low- to moderate-intensity cycling (40% VO_{2peak}) immediately followed by 20 min of studying while seated on the bicycle (Exercise/Study); and 40 min of seated rest on the bicycle (Control). Assessments before and after each condition revealed that state anxiety was significantly reduced following the Exercise Only condition (effect size = -0.52), but not following any of the other three conditions.

Motl et al. (2004) examined the effects of 20 min of either low- to moderate-intensity (40% VO_{2peak}) or high-intensity (70% VO_{2peak}) exercise or 20 min of quiet rest on state anxiety in 40 college-aged men, 20 of whom were selected because they had low trait anxiety scores (mean trait anxiety = 26.4) and the other 20 of whom were selected for high trait anxiety (mean trait anxiety = 51.2). Both exercise intensities resulted in significant reductions in state anxiety for the high-trait-anxious men (effect size = -0.31); much smaller reductions were seen in the low-trait-anxious group (effect size = -0.14), and no change was seen following quiet rest.

Steptoe, Edwards, Moses, and Mathews (1989) examined the effects of a 10-week program of moderate-intensity exercise (20 min of walking or jogging at 60–65% of maximal heart rate (HR_{max})) compared with an attention-placebo condition (20 min of strength, flexibility, and mobility exercises at <50% HR_{max}). Both conditions involved one supervised and three unsupervised sessions per week and included 5–10 min of warm-up and cool-down exercises. Participants were selected based on Hospital Anxiety and Depression (HAD) scale scores that would classify them as having "borderline" or "clinical" anxiety and were matched across the two conditions for age, sex, weight, habitual activity, and baseline anxiety (mean trait anxiety = 49.7, 51.3 and HAD anxiety = 10.4, 10.8 for the exercise and attention-placebo conditions, respectively). The moderate-exercise condition resulted in significant improvements on several psychological outcomes, with significantly greater reductions in anxiety/tension (as assessed via the POMS) compared with the attention-placebo group. Steptoe et al. also performed follow-up assessments on a subsample of the original participants three months after the treatments ended. Using the baseline scores as a covariate, there were significantly greater reductions in trait anxiety and POMS anxiety/tension for the exercise group.

In a sample of 79 inpatients with diagnosed anxiety disorders, Martinsen, Hoffart, and Solberg (1989) found that both aerobic (walking and jogging) and nonaerobic (muscular strength and flexibility) exercise resulted in significant psychological improvements. The exercise treatment protocol involved 8 weeks of 60 min of exercise done three times per week. Martinsen, Sandvik, and Kolbjornsrud (1989) conducted another intervention study with a sample of 92 nonpsychotic inpatients. The intervention again lasted 8 weeks, with at least 60 min of aerobic exercise five times per week. Physical fitness was significantly increased in all patients, as indexed by an increase in physical work capacity. Patients diagnosed with alcohol abuse or substance dependence showed the largest reductions in number of anxiety symptoms. Importantly for the present discussion, patients with unipolar depressive and anxiety disorders (generalized anxiety disorder and agoraphobia) also showed significant symptom reduction. In those patients who responded to a one-year follow-up (84%), those who had established regular exercise habits tended to have lower symptom scores.

Sexton, Maere, and Dahl (1989) examined in a sample of 52 symptomatic neurotics the effects of an 8-week exercise program (walking or jogging) with a follow-up 6 months post program. Patients had nonpsychotic diagnoses as determined by the DSM–III (American Psychiatric Association, 1980). Anxiety and depression were both significantly reduced regardless of whether patients walked or jogged; changes were maintained at follow-up. Indeed, at follow-up Sexton et al. noted a significant relationship between aerobic capacity and anxiety levels, with greater fitness levels associated with lower anxiety. Although not all studies have found such a relationship, this result provides evidence that anxiety reduction is associated with an increase in actual fitness and not just in physical activity. Sexton et al. also highlighted the fact that vigorous exercise was not required for psychological improvements; the effects were comparable for both walking and running. The study further reinforces the point made earlier that moderate-intensity exercise is sufficient to decrease anxiety even in clinical populations. Sexton et al. noted as well that the patients rated exercise as more important than medication and psychotherapy in their improvement.

Meyer, Broocks, Bandelow, Hillmer-Vogel, and Ruther (1998) examined, in a sample of inpatients diagnosed with DSM–III-Revised (American Psychiatric Association, 1987) panic disorder (with or without agoraphobia), the influence of a 10-week exercise program (45–60 min of running three times per week) compared with pharmacotherapy (clomipramine) or a no-treatment control. At the end of the 10 weeks of treatment, the exercise group had significant clinical improvement in their anxiety relative to the control condition. The improvement in anxiety was similar to the improvement seen in the clomipramine group (i.e., exercise was as effective as antianxiety medication).

Broocks et al. (1998), in a randomized, placebo-controlled clinical trial, assigned 46 outpatients diagnosed with DSM–III-Revised moderate to severe panic disorder (with or without agoraphobia) to either a 10-week exercise treatment ($n = 16$; walking progressing to running 3 times per week along a 4-mile outdoor course, with emphasis on completing the course at least 3 times per week), pharmacotherapy ($n = 15$; 112.5 mg/day of clomipramine), or placebo treatment. Results revealed that exercise was as effective as the drug treatment in reducing self-reported anxiety, with both being superior to the placebo. The drug treatment resulted in an earlier improvement in anxiety symptoms (after 4 weeks),

but the exercise treatment had an equivalent effect by the end of the 10-week trial (see Figure 3.2). The drug treatment improved both patient- and observer-rated panic, along with agoraphobia intensity and frequency of attacks, to a greater extent than did exercise, but exercise was superior to placebo in reducing the frequency and intensity of those conditions.

Studies like those by Broocks et al. are particularly salient given the call by Salmon (2001) for more studies examining the usefulness of exercise in dealing with panic disorder. Some researchers have proposed that exercise might actually induce panic attacks in panic-prone individuals, but this is based more on flawed logic than on experimental evidence. O'Connor, Smith, and Morgan (2000) point out that exercise, both acute and chronic, is safe for panic disorder patients and that generally, panic patients show anxiety reductions following exercise similar to those seen in nonanxious individuals. O'Connor et al. (2000) do note, however, that more work is needed to examine the effect of exercise on generalized anxiety disorder. Goodwin's (2003) analysis of the National Comorbidity Survey data indicates that exercise should be helpful with generalized anxiety disorder, but clearly empirical research is needed.

A recent study by Merom et al. (2008) provided group cognitive behavioral therapy (GCBT) to individuals with diagnosed panic disorder, social phobia, or generalized anxiety disorder through an outpatient clinic. A home-based walking program (exercise intervention) or educational sessions were

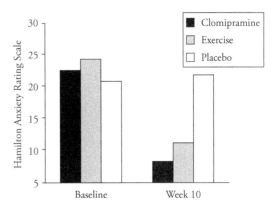

Figure 3.2. Hamilton Anxiety Rating Scale responses at baseline and after 10 weeks of treatment. Adapted with permission from "Comparison of Aerobic Exercise, Clomipramine, and Placebo in the Treatment of Panic Disorder," by A. Broocks, B. Bandelow, G. Pekrun, A. George, T. Meyer, U. Bartmann, U. Hillmer-Vogel, and E. Ruther, 1998, *American Journal of Psychiatry, 155,* pp. 603–609.

added to the GCBT, and self-reported anxiety, stress, and depression were assessed before and after the 8- to 10-week intervention. The exercise intervention consisted of a gradually increasing number of 30-min sessions of moderate-intensity exercise (e.g., brisk walking); the ultimate goal was 150 min of accumulated exercise per week. Participants in the group who completed the exercise intervention showed a significant reduction in anxiety, stress, and depression scores after controlling for several potential confounding factors, compared with the education group. Merom et al. noted that the exercise intervention might have yielded even larger effects had the program lasted longer than 8–10 weeks.

Noting that many cognitive behavioral therapy protocols involve exposure to anxiety-related arousal symptoms, Broman-Fulks and Storey (2008) conducted a follow-up to an earlier study by Broman-Fulks, Berman, Rabian, and Webster (2004) to examine whether acute exercise sessions could reduce anxiety sensitivity (i.e., fear of anxiety and anxiety-related sensations). They noted that anxiety sensitivity is crucial in the etiology of panic disorder and other anxiety disorders, and as such, reducing fears related to somatic symptoms of anxiety may be crucial in preventing and treating such disorders. The Broman-Fulks et al. (2004) study showed that six 20-min bouts of both low-intensity (60% of age-adjusted predicted HR_{max}) and high-intensity (90% of age-adjusted predicted HR_{max}) exercise over a 2-week period were effective at reducing anxiety sensitivity. They noted that the high-intensity exercise resulted in quicker decreases in anxiety sensitivity and produced a greater number of treatment responders (52% of participants) than did the lower-intensity exercise treatment (20%) immediately following the treatment; by a one-week follow-up, responders had increased to 62% and 28% for the high- and low-intensity exercise groups, respectively. These results led Broman-Fulks et al. to conclude that higher-intensity exercise could be particularly effective in reducing the fear associated with physiological activation in high-anxiety-sensitive individuals.

The follow-up work (Broman-Fulks & Storey, 2008) randomly assigned 24 individuals with high scores on an anxiety sensitivity index to either an exercise group or a no-exercise control group. The exercise group again completed six 20-min bouts of aerobic exercise (this time at an intensity resulting in heart rates between 60–90% of age-adjusted predicted HR_{max}) over a 2-week period. The no-exercise control participants reported to the laboratory six times over a 2-week period, but only to complete the anxiety sensitivity measure. Results showed a significant reduction in anxiety sensitivity following the initial session only for the exercise group. This reduction in anxiety sensitivity was maintained throughout the remainder of the exercise sessions and at a 1-week follow-up assessment. This led Broman-Fulks and Storey to suggest that exercise may be an effective intervention for individuals with high levels of anxiety sensitivity, especially if a rapid reduction in that sensitivity is required.

Smits et al. (2008) conducted a study that randomly assigned individuals with high anxiety sensitivity to an exercise group (Ex; $n = 19$), an exercise + cognitive restructuring group (Ex+C; $n = 21$), or a wait-list control group (WL; $n = 20$). The exercise interventions were patterned after the Broman–Fulks studies: Participants completed six 20-min sessions of aerobic exercise over 2 weeks at an intensity of 70% of age-predicted HR_{max}. In addition, participants viewed a 15-min video that presented a rationale for the study along with study procedures. The video provided to the participants in the Ex+C group also included a description of the usefulness of cognitive restructuring. Assessments were made preintervention, after the first week, and then 1 week and 3 weeks following the intervention. Both interventions involving exercise (Ex and Ex+C) showed large and clinically significant reductions in anxiety sensitivity, which Smits et al. stated were comparable to reductions produced by existing protocols for modifying anxiety sensitivity.

It should be noted, however, that no research has directly compared the effects of exercise on anxiety sensitivity with those of other forms of treatment, notably cognitive behavioral therapy, nor has there been research on the effects of exercise in individuals with clinical conditions involving high levels of anxiety sensitivity (e.g., panic disorder and posttraumatic stress disorder). Exercise does offer promise as a possible treatment intervention for conditions like panic disorder and PTSD, either by itself or in combination with other traditional treatments.

It is worth pointing out that the question of causality is not clear-cut. De Moor et al. (2008, p. 898) note: "The evidence from these prospective and experimental studies makes it tempting to interpret the association at the population level as reflecting a causal effect of exercise on the symptoms of anxiety and depression. This explanation fits folk wisdom." Specifically examining the causal effects of exercise on anxiety and depressive symptoms in nearly 6,000 twins, approximately 1,500 of their siblings, and nearly 1,300 parents, De Moor et al. found that in identical twins, fewer anxiety symptoms were not seen in the twin who exercised more frequently, nor did longitudinal analyses indicate that increased exercise resulted in decreased anxiety. Distinguishing between voluntary leisure-time exercise and exercise that is prescribed and supervised in specific groups (e.g., the clinically anxious), De Moor et al. (2008) note that the absence of a causal effect of voluntary exercise doesn't mean exercise can't be useful in alleviating anxiety symptoms. It does mean that the association so often noted on a population level should not be used to justify using exercise as a treatment for clinical anxiety (or depression). Randomized controlled trials are a first necessary step in making such recommendations. In spite of the claim by Wipfli et al. (2008), based on their meta-analytic findings, that solid evidence (i.e., randomized controlled trials) is available for using exercise as a treatment for anxiety, precious little data is available with clinically anxious samples to warrant such a conclusion at present. As clearly articulated by De Geus and De Moor (2008), incorporating "genetic sensitivity" into our research models would also help in better understanding the mental health benefits of exercise.

What Isn't Known: Dose Response

Although we have learned a great deal regarding exercise and anxiety reduction, much, unfortunately, remains unknown. This is particularly true with respect to the relation between dose (i.e., intensity and duration) and response. It has been suggested that thresholds exist for the achievement of anxiety reduction. For example, Dishman (1986) proposed that exercise at at least 70% of aerobic capacity sustained for at least 20 minutes would yield anxiety reduction. Raglin and Morgan (1987) suggested that a more moderate intensity (greater than 60% of maximum aerobic capacity) was sufficient. The minimum intensity needed for anxiety reduction, however, has been poorly investigated. Ekkekakis and Petruzzello (1999), summarizing studies that specifically examined dose–response issues, concluded that evidence shows state anxiety and tension (measured via POMS) are sensitive to exercise intensity effects. They found that higher intensities led to increases in anxiety/tension and lower intensities resulted in no change or decreases (but remember the caveat raised earlier regarding the potential problems with measuring anxiety in the exercise context). Clearly more work is needed

before any firm conclusions can be drawn and certainly before any recommendations about minimal exercise intensity levels can be made.

As for the issue of the minimum duration of exercise needed to achieve anxiety-reducing effects, the meta-analysis by Petruzzello et al. (1991) noted that exercise durations of less than 20 minutes were as effective as durations of greater than 20 minutes for reducing anxiety. Thus research at this point shows that the anxiety-reducing effect that is achieved by exercise is present regardless of the duration of that exercise. Recommendations like those made by Dishman (1986) for a minimum duration of 20 minutes are thus sufficient but not necessarily accurate. The PAGAC report (2008) essentially concluded the same thing as Petruzzello et al. (1991)—minimal and optimal exercise durations or intensities for anxiety reduction are still unknown. More research is clearly needed for a definitive answer, but reductions in anxiety can apparently be realized simply by exercising aerobically.

Another problematic issue is the extent to which anxiety reduction occurs for individuals suffering from clinical levels of anxiety. The vast majority of the research on the relationship between exercise and anxiety has examined the reduction of anxiety symptoms (usually via self-report) in people who are not clinically anxious. The PAGAC report (2008) details that approximately 60% of the randomized controlled trials conducted since 1995 have used individuals, usually patients, with some medical condition (e.g., cancer or cardiovascular disease), but these were not necessarily individuals suffering from clinical anxiety. The Wipfli et al. (2008) meta-analysis, despite claiming that exercise could be used as a treatment for anxiety, does not justify this claim. Wipfli et al. were correct to recommend that future research be conducted with clinical samples, especially considering that fewer than 7.5% (3 of 49) of the studies they reviewed used such samples (a point echoed by Ekkekakis, 2008). Clearly, more such work needs to be done before clear recommendations can be made regarding exercise as a treatment for clinically anxious individuals.

Mechanisms of Change

We do not yet have a definitive picture of the mechanisms responsible for the anxiety-reducing effect of exercise. Many of the mechanisms that have been proposed to explain the anxiolytic effect are the same as those proposed to explain depression reduction. Two additional mechanisms, the thermogenic and the distraction/time-out hypotheses, have been proposed as explanations for anxiety reduction with exercise.

Thermogenic Hypothesis

Derived from research showing that treatments that elevate body temperature (e.g., sauna bathing and warm showers) produce therapeutic benefits (e.g., reduced muscle tension), the *thermogenic hypothesis* states that the elevated body temperature resulting from exercise may also lead to observed psychological changes, such as reduced anxiety. In essence, exercise is thought to result in elevated body temperature. The brain senses this temperature increase, a muscular relaxation response is triggered, and this sensation is fed back to the brain and interpreted psychologically as relaxation or reduced anxiety.

The thermogenic hypothesis is probably the most systematically studied of the proposed mechanisms for the anxiolytic effect of exercise. At present, research seems to indicate that elevated body temperature is probably not directly responsible for the psychological changes (Koltyn, Shake, & Morgan, 1993; Petruzzello, Landers, & Salazar, 1993; Youngstedt, Dishman, Cureton, & Peacock, 1993). The thermogenic hypothesis remains tenable, however, in part because it could very well be that brain temperature and not body temperature is what drives the affective response and decrease in anxiety. Some evidence shows that the temperature of the brain is regulated independently from the body, although this independence is not completely accepted, and researchers have not yet been able to directly measure exercise-related increases in brain temperature in humans. Thus more work is needed to determine the effects of exercise on brain temperature before the thermogenic hypothesis can be accepted or ruled out.

Distraction/Time-out Hypothesis

The *distraction/time-out hypothesis* grew out of the findings from the Bahrke and Morgan (1978) study described earlier, which showed essentially no differences between 20 minutes of treadmill exercise, noncultic meditation, or sitting quietly in a sound-dampened chamber reading a *Reader's Digest* magazine. This particular hypothesis, stated simply, says that the anxiety-reducing effects seen with exercise are due to the distraction it provides from the normal routine. It allows the stressed, anxious, or depressed person to "leave behind" or take a time-out from cares and worries. Other distraction "therapies" have also been shown to reduce anxiety and depression (e.g., meditation, relaxation, and quiet rest). As noted earlier, however, the effect of exercise may be qualitatively different from other cognitively based therapies because the exercise effect lasts longer. The distraction hypothesis remains a possible explanation for anxiety and depression reduction; however, the evidence available indicates that the exercise-related reduction in anxiety and depression is the consequence of more than simply taking time away from one's daily routine.

Practical Recommendations

As is the case with depression, the minimal level of exercise activity needed to alleviate anxiety is currently unknown, but it seems clear that exercise or physical activity done on a regular basis can be useful not only for this purpose but for protecting against the anxiety that we might ordinarily succumb to as a result of our busy, stressful lives if we remained sedentary. The *type* of exercise does seem to matter, as only aerobic forms of exercise appear to be effective in reducing anxiety, although this conclusion may change as more studies examine other types of exercise (e.g., resistance exercise). Individuals suffering from more severe forms of anxiety may also find relief in exercise therapies, but these individuals should certainly consult with a mental health care provider before beginning an exercise program.

Conclusion and Future Directions

As with exercise and depression, it seems reasonable to propose that exercise can be helpful in reducing anxiety in the short term and in reducing general tension, nervousness, and worry, thus increasing emotional stability over the longer term. Exercise can also be successful in treating clinical manifestations of anxiety, such as panic disorder, phobias, and generalized anxiety disorder, although more research with clinically anxious populations is needed. The current state of research is summarized in Table 3.2. Much remains to be done, however, not the least of which is determining what causes this reduced level of anxiety and determining what "doses" of exercise reliably yield such effects. Another important avenue for future research is to continue to examine the effects of exercise as a potential treatment for individuals suffering from clinical levels of anxiety. Related to this will be the important task of determining whether exercise can be a useful treatment for all forms of anxiety disorders or whether certain types are less likely to be positively influenced

Table 3.2. Consensus Statements regarding Exercise and Anxiety

1. Exercise can be associated with reduced state anxiety.

2. Long-term exercise is usually associated with reductions in neuroticism and trait anxiety.

3. Exercise can result in the reduction of various stress indices.

4. Exercise can have beneficial emotional effects across all ages and both genders.

Note. Adapted from *Exercise and Mental Health* (p. 156), by W. P. Morgan and S. E. Goldston (Eds.), 1987, Washington, DC: Hemisphere.

by exercise protocols. The coin of the realm in this regard would be randomized controlled trials, but given the paucity of research with clinical samples all well-designed studies would be warranted at this point.

References

American Psychiatric Association (APA). (1980). *Diagnostic and statistical manual of mental disorders* (3rd ed.).Washington, DC: American Psychiatric Association.

American Psychiatric Association (APA). (1987). *Diagnostic and statistical manual of mental disorders, Third Edition, Revised (DSM-III-R).* Washington, DC: American Psychiatric Association.

Arent, S. M., Alderman, B. L., Short, E. J., & Landers, D. M. (2007). The impact of the testing environment on affective changes following acute resistance exercise. *Journal of Applied Sport Psychology, 19,* 364–378.

Arent, S. M., Landers, D. M., Matt, K. S., & Etnier, J. L. (2005). Dose–response and mechanistic issues in the resistance training and affect relationship. *Journal of Sport and Exercise Psychology, 27,* 92–110.

Bahrke, M. S., & Morgan, W. P. (1978). Anxiety reduction following exercise and meditation. *Cognitive Therapy and Research, 4,* 323–333.

Bartholomew, J. B., & Linder, D. E. (1998). State anxiety following resistance exercise: The role of gender and exercise intensity. *Journal of Behavioral Medicine, 21,* 205–219.

Bibeau, W. S., Moore, J. B., Mitchell, N. G., Vargas-Tonsing, T., & Bartholomew, J. B. (2010). Effects of acute resistance training of different intensities and rest periods on anxiety and affect. *Journal of Strength & Conditioning Research, 24*(8), 2184–2191.

Breus, M. J., & O'Connor, P. J. (1998). Exercise-induced anxiolysis: A test of the "time out" hypothesis in high anxious females. *Medicine & Science in Sports & Exercise, 30*(7), 1107–1112.

Broman-Fulks, J. J., Berman, M. E., Rabian, B. A., & Webster, M. J. (2004). Effects of aerobic exercise on anxiety sensitivity. *Behaviour Research & Therapy, 42,* 125–136.

Broman-Fulks, J. J., & Storey, K. M. (2008). Evaluation of a brief aerobic intervention for high anxiety sensitivity. *Anxiety, Stress & Coping, 21,* 117–128.

Broocks, A., Bandelow, B., Pekrun, G., George, A., Meyer, T., Bartmann, U.,...Ruther, E. (1998). Comparison of aerobic exercise, chloripramine, and placebo in the treatment of panic disorder. *American Journal of Psychiatry, 155,* 603–609.

Callahan, P. (2004). Exercise: A neglected intervention in mental health care? *Journal of Psychiatric & Mental Health Nursing, 11,* 476–483.

Cassilhas, R. C., Viana, V. A. R., Grassmann, V., Santos, R. T., Santos, R. F., Tufik, S., & Mello, M. T. (2007). The impact of resistance exercise on the cognitive function of the elderly. *Medicine & Science in Sports & Exercise, 39,* 1401–1407.

Chung, Y. B., & Baird, M. K. (1999). Physical exercise as a counseling intervention. *Journal of Mental Health Counseling, 21,* 124–135.

De Geus, E. J. C., & De Moor, M. H. M. (2008). A genetic perspective on the association between exercise and mental health. *Mental Health & Physical Activity, 1,* 53–61.

De Moor, M. H. M., Beem, A. L., Stubbe, J. H., Boomsma, D. I., & De Geus, E. J. C. (2006). Regular exercise, anxiety, depression and personality: A population-based study. *Preventive Medicine, 42,* 273–279.

De Moor, M. H. M., Boomsma, D. I., Stubbe, J. H., Willemsen, G., & De Geus, E. J. C. (2008). Testing causality in the association between regular exercise and symptoms of anxiety and depression. *Archives of General Psychiatry, 65,* 897–905.

deVries, H. A. (1981). Tranquilizer effect of exercise: A critical review. *Physician and Sportsmedicine, 9*(11), 47–54.

deVries, H. A., & Adams, G. M. (1972). Electromyographic comparison of single doses of exercise and meprobamate as to effects on muscular relaxation. *American Journal of Physical Medicine, 51,* 130–141.

Dillon, D.J., Gorman, J.M., Liebowitz, M.R., Fyer, A.J., & Klein, D.F. (1987). Measurement of lactate-induced panic and anxiety. *Psychiatry Research, 20,* 97–105.

Dishman, R. K. (1986). Mental health. In V. Seefeldt (Ed.), *Physical activity and well-being* (pp. 303–341). Reston, VA: American Association for Health, Physical Education, Recreation and Dance.

Dishman, R. K. (1997). The norepinephrine hypothesis. In W. P. Morgan (Ed.), *Physical activity & mental health* (pp. 199–212). Washington, DC: Taylor & Francis.

Dunn, A. L., Trivedi, M. H., & O'Neal, H. A. (2001). Physical activity dose–response effects on outcomes of depression and anxiety. *Medicine & Science in Sports & Exercise, 33*(Suppl.), S587–S597.

DuPont, R. L., Rice, D. P., Miller, L. S., Shiraki, S. S., Rowland, C. R., & Harwood, H. J. (1996). Economic cost of anxiety disorders. *Anxiety, 2,* 167–172.

Ekkekakis, P. (2008). The genetic tidal wave finally reached our shores: Will it be a catalyst for a critical overhaul of the way we think and do science? *Mental Health & Physical Activity, 1,* 47–52.

Ekkekakis, P., Hall, E. E., & Petruzzello, S. J. (1999). Measuring state anxiety in the context of acute exercise using the State Anxiety Inventory: An attempt to resolve the brouhaha. *Journal of Sport and Exercise Psychology, 21,* 205–229.

Ekkekakis, P., & Petruzzello, S. J. (1999). Acute aerobic exercise and affect: Current status, problems and prospects regarding dose-response. *Sports Medicine, 28,* 337–374.

Esquivel, G., Diaz-Galvis, J., Schruers, K., Berlanga, C., Lara-Munoz, C., & Griez, E. (2008). Acute exercise reduces the effects of a 35% CO_2 challenge in patients with panic disorder. *Journal of Affective Disorders, 107,* 217–220.

Esquivel, G., Schruers, K., Kuipers, H., & Griez, E. (2002). The effects of acute exercise and high lactate levels on 35% CO_2 challenge in healthy volunteers. *Acta Psychiatrica Scandinavica, 106,* 394–397.

Goodwin, R. D. (2003). Association between physical activity and mental disorders among adults in the United States. *Preventive Medicine, 36,* 698–703.

Greenberg, P. E., Sisitsky, T., Kessler, R. C., Finkelstein, S. N., Berndt, E. R., Davidson, . . . Fyer, A. J. (1999). The economic burden of anxiety disorders in the 1990s. *Journal of Clinical Psychiatry, 60,* 427–435.

Hollander, E., & Simeon, D. (2003). *Concise guide to anxiety disorders.* Washington, DC: American Psychiatric Publishing.

Johnsgard, K. W. (1989). *The exercise prescription for depression and anxiety.* New York: Plenum.

Johnsgard, K. W. (2004). *Conquering depression and anxiety through exercise.* Amherst, NY: Prometheus Books.

Kessler, R. C., Chiu, W. T., Demler, O., & Walters, E. E. (2005). Prevalence, severity, and comorbidity of 12-month DSM-IV disorders in the National Comorbidity Survey Replication. *Archives of General Psychiatry, 62,* 617–627.

Kessler, R. C., McGonagle, K. A., Zhao, S., Nelson, C. B., Hughes, M., Eshleman, S., . . . Kendler, K. S. (1994). Lifetime and 12-month prevalence of DSM-III-R psychiatric disorders in the United States: Results from the National Comorbidity Survey. *Archives of General Psychiatry, 51,* 8–18.

Koltyn, K. F., Shake, C. L., & Morgan, W. P. (1993). Interaction of exercise, water temperature and protective apparel on body awareness and anxiety. *International Journal of Sport Psychology, 24,* 297–305.

Landers, D. M., & Petruzzello, S. J. (1994). Physical activity, fitness, and anxiety. In C. Bouchard, R. J. Shephard, & T. Stephens (Eds.), *Physical activity, fitness, and health: International proceedings and consensus statement* (pp. 868–882). Champaign, IL: Human Kinetics.

Long, B. C., & van Stavel, R. (1995). Effects of exercise training on anxiety: A meta-analysis. *Journal of Applied Sport Psychology, 7,* 167–189.

Marciniak, M. D., Lage, M. J., Dunayevich, E., Russell, J. M., Bowman, L., Landbloom, R. P., & Levine, L. R. (2005). The cost of treating anxiety: The medical and demographic correlates that impact total medical costs. *Depression & Anxiety, 21,* 178–184.

Martinsen, E. W., Hoffart, A., & Solberg, O. Y. (1989). Aerobic and non-aerobic forms of exercise in the treatment of anxiety disorders. *Stress Medicine, 5,* 115–120.

Martinsen, E. W., & Raglin, J. S. (2007). Anxiety/depression: Lifestyle medicine approaches. *American Journal of Lifestyle Medicine, 1,* 159–166.

Martinsen, E. W., Sandvik, L., & Kolbjornsrud, O. B. (1989). Aerobic exercise in the treatment of nonpsychotic mental disorders: An exploratory study. *Nordic Journal of Psychiatry, 43,* 521–529.

Martinsen, E. W., & Stanghelle, J. K. (1997). Drug therapy and physical activity. In W. P. Morgan (Ed.), *Physical activity and mental health* (pp. 81–90). Washington, DC: Taylor & Francis.

McDonald, D. G., & Hodgdon, J. A. (1991). *Psychological effects of aerobic fitness training: Research and theory.* New York: Springer-Verlag.

McNair, D. M., Droppleman, L. F., & Lorr, M. (1981). *Manual for the Profile of Mood States.* San Diego, CA: Educational and Industrial Testing Service.

Merom, D., Phongsavan, P., Wagner, R., Chey, T., Marnane, C., Steel, Z., . . . Bauman, A. (2008). Promoting walking as an adjunct intervention to group cognitive behavioral therapy for anxiety disorders: A pilot group randomized trial. *Journal of Anxiety Disorders, 22,* 959–968

Meyer, T., Broocks, A., Bandelow, B., Hillmer-Vogel, U., & Ruther, E. (1998). Endurance training in panic patients: Spiroergometric and clinical effects. *International Journal of Sports Medicine, 19,* 496–502.

Morgan, W. P., & Goldston, S. E. (Eds.). (1987). *Exercise and mental health.* Washington, DC: Hemisphere.

Motl, R.W., & Dishman, R.K. (2004). Effects of acute exercise on the soleus H-reflex and self-reported anxiety after caffeine ingestion. *Physiology & Behavior, 80,* 577–585.

Motl, R. W., O'Connor, P. J., & Dishman, R. K. (2004). Effects of cycling exercise on the soleus H-reflex and state anxiety among men with low or high trait anxiety. *Psychophysiology, 41,* 96–105.

O'Connor, P. J., Raglin, J. S., & Martinsen, E. W. (2000). Physical activity, anxiety and anxiety disorders. *International Journal of Sport Psychology, 31*(2), 136–155.

O'Connor, P. J., Smith, J. C., & Morgan, W. P. (2000). Physical activity does not provoke panic attacks in patients with panic disorder: A review of the evidence. *Anxiety, Stress and Coping, 13,* 333–353.

Petruzzello, S.J. (1995). Anxiety reduction following exercise: Methodological artifact or "real" phenomenon? *Journal of Sport & Exercise Psychology, 17,* 105–111.

Petruzzello, S. J., Landers, D. M., Hatfield, B. D., Kubitz, K. A., & Salazar, W. (1991). A meta-analysis on the anxiety-reducing effects of acute and chronic exercise: Outcomes and mechanisms. *Sports Medicine, 11,* 143–182.

Petruzzello, S. J., Landers, D. M., & Salazar, W. (1993). Exercise and anxiety reduction: Examination of temperature as an explanation for affective change. *Journal of Sport and Exercise Psychology, 15,* 63–76.

Physical Activity Guidelines Advisory Committee (2008). *Physical Activity Guidelines Advisory Committee Report, 2008.* Washington, DC: U.S. Department of Health and Human Services.

Raglin, J. S. (1997). Anxiolytic effects of physical activity. In W. P. Morgan (Ed.), *Physical activity and mental health* (pp. 107–126). Washington, DC: Taylor & Francis.

Raglin, J. S., & Morgan, W. P. (1987). Influence of exercise and quiet rest on state anxiety and blood pressure. *Medicine & Science in Sports & Exercise, 19,* 456–463.

Raglin, J. S., Turner, P. E., & Eksten, F. (1993). State anxiety and blood pressure following 30 min of leg ergometry or weight training. *Medicine & Science in Sports & Exercise, 25,* 1044–1048.

Regier, D. A., Farmer, M. E., Rae, D. S., Locke, B. Z., Keith, S. J., Judd, L. L., & Goodwin, F. K. (1990). Comorbidity of mental disorders with alcohol and other drug abuse: Results from the Epidemiologic Catchment Area (ECA) Study. *Journal of the American Medical Association, 264,* 2511–2518.

Regier, D. A., Narrow, W. E., Rae, D. S., Manderscheid, R. W., Locke, B. Z., & Goodwin, F. K. (1993). The de facto U.S. mental and addictive disorders service system: Epidemiologic Catchment Area prospective 1-year prevalence rates of disorders and services. *Archives of General Psychiatry, 50,* 85–94.

Rejeski, W. J., Hardy, C. J., & Shaw, J. (1991). Psychometric confounds of assessing state anxiety in conjunction with acute bouts of vigorous exercise. *Journal of Sport and Exercise Psychology, 13,* 65–74.

Ryan, A. J. (1983). Exercise is medicine. *Physician and Sportsmedicine, 11,* 10.

Salmon, P. (2001). Effects of physical exercise on anxiety, depression, and sensitivity to stress: A unifying theory. *Clinical Psychology Review, 21*(1), 33–61.

Schlicht, W. (1994). Does physical exercise reduce anxious emotions? A meta-analysis. *Anxiety, Stress and Coping, 6,* 275–288.

Sexton, H., Maere, A., & Dahl, N. H. (1989). Exercise intensity and reduction in neurotic symptoms. *Acta Psychiatrica Scandinavica, 80,* 231–235.

Sheehan, G. (1983). *How to feel great 24 hours a day.* New York: Simon & Schuster.

Smits, J. A. J., Berry, A. C., Rosenfield, D., Powers, M. B., Behar, E., & Otto, M. W. (2008). Reducing anxiety sensitivity with exercise. *Depression & Anxiety, 25,* 689–699.

Smits, J. A. J., Meuret, A. E., Zvolensky, M. J., Rosenfield, D., & Seidel, A. (2009). The effects of acute exercise on CO_2 challenge reactivity. *Journal of Psychiatric Research, 43,* 446–454.

Spielberger, C. D. (1979). *Preliminary manual for the State–Trait Personality Inventory (STPI).* Unpublished manuscript.

Spielberger, C. D. (1983). *Manual for the State–Trait Anxiety Inventory (Form Y).* Palo Alto, CA: Consulting Psychologists Press.

Stephens, T. (1988). Physical activity and mental health in the United States and Canada: Evidence from four population surveys. *Preventive Medicine, 17,* 35–47.

Steptoe, A., Edwards, S., Moses, J., & Mathews, A. (1989). The effects of exercise training on mood and perceived coping ability in anxious adults from the general population. *Journal of Psychosomatic Research, 33,* 537–547.

Stern, R. M., Ray, W. J., & Quigley, K. S. (2001). *Psychophysiological recording* (2nd ed.). New York: Oxford University Press.

Strohle, A., Feller, C., Onken, M., Godemann, F., Heinz, A., & Dimeo, F. (2005). The acute antipanic activity of aerobic exercise. *American Journal of Psychiatry, 162,* 2376–2378.

Strohle, A., Feller, C., Strasburger, C. J., Heinz, A., & Dimeo, F. (2006). Anxiety modulation by the heart? Aerobic exercise and atrial natriuretic peptide. *Psychoneuroendocrinology, 31,* 1127–1130.

Strohle, A., Graetz, B., Scheel, M., Wittmann, A., Feller, C., Heinz, A., & Dimeo, F. (2009). The acute antipanic and anxiolytic activity of aerobic exercise in patients with panic disorder and healthy control subjects. *Journal of Psychiatric Research, 43,* 1013–1017.

Taylor, M. K., Pietrobon, R., Pan, D., Huff, M., & Higgins, L. D. (2004). Healthy People 2010 physical activity guidelines and psychological symptoms: Evidence from a large nationwide database. *Journal of Physical Activity & Health, 1,* 114–130.

U.S. Department of Health and Human Services. (1999). *Mental health: A report of the Surgeon General.* Rockville, MD: U.S. Department of Health and Human Services, Substance Abuse and Mental Health Services Administration, Center for Mental Health Services, National Institutes of Health, National Institute of Mental Health.

Wipfli, B. M., Rethorst, C. D., & Landers, D. M. (2008). The anxiolytic effects of exercise: A meta-analysis of randomized trials and dose–response analysis. *Journal of Sport & Exercise Psychology, 30,* 392–410.

Youngstedt, S. D., Dishman, R. K., Cureton, K. J., & Peacock, L. J. (1993). Does body temperature mediate anxiolytic effect of acute exercise? *Journal of Applied Physiology, 74,* 825–831.

Zuckerman, M., & Lubin, B. (1965). *Manual for the Multiple Affect Adjective Checklist.* San Diego, CA: Educational and Industrial Testing Service.

Body Image and Exercise

Kathleen A. Martin Ginis, Rebecca L. Bassett-Gunter, *and* Catherine Conlin

Abstract

Exercise has been shown to be an effective intervention for improving body image among both women and men. This chapter begins with a review of the meta-analytic evidence regarding the effects of exercise on body image. We then provide a comprehensive assessment of potential mechanisms underlying the effects of exercise on body image. Three mechanisms are discussed: objective changes in physical fitness, perceived changes in physical fitness, and changes in self-efficacy. An analysis of potential moderators of the exercise–body image relationship follows. Finally, we present a review of emerging topics in the exercise intervention and body image literature and provide recommendations for body image research within the field of exercise psychology.

Key Words: body satisfaction, self-perception, self-efficacy, physical activity, social physique anxiety.

Introduction

Evidence of society's obsession with body image is ubiquitous. Weekly reality TV programs deliver makeovers, surgical interventions, and extreme weight loss regimens to people desperate to change their physical appearance. Countless men's and women's magazines are devoted to providing information that will help readers feel better about their bodies. Typing "body image" into Google yields over 12 million hits. As these examples attest, body image has enormous significance within contemporary society.

What Is Body Image?

Body image is "the multifaceted psychological experience of embodiment, especially but not exclusively one's physical appearance" (Cash, 2004, p. 1), encompassing how people see, feel, think and act toward their bodies. The *perceptual dimension* of body image captures how the body is pictured in one's own mind—that is, how people see themselves when they look in a mirror, and how they imagine

their bodies to look. The *affective dimension* reflects feelings about the body's appearance and function. These feelings may be positive—such as pride and happiness—or negative, such as anxiety and shame. The *cognitive dimension* refers to attitudes, thoughts, and beliefs about one's body. Examples of these cognitions include the value placed on body image and the extent to which people are invested in their appearance. The *behavioral dimension* captures behavioral representations of body image. For instance, wearing revealing clothing and participating in physique-exposing activities (e.g., swimming or sunbathing) can provide indications of how people perceive, think, and feel about their bodies. Finally, the *subjective satisfaction dimension* reflects people's satisfaction with their bodies—individual body parts as well as overall (Stewart & Williamson, 2004; Thompson, Heinberg, Altabe, & Tantleff-Dunn, 1999).

Several large-scale surveys have yielded data indicating that a substantial proportion of men and women have a negative body image (for a review, see Cash, 2002). Negative body image has typically been defined as dissatisfaction with one's physical appearance. For instance, a national study of 4,000 American adults revealed that 43% of men and 56% of women were dissatisfied with their overall appearance (Garner, 1997). Such results have frequently been used as evidence of the prevalence of negative body image (Cash, 2002). However, operationalizing and measuring negative body image solely in terms of body dissatisfaction does not take into account the other four dimensions of body image. This approach also fails to consider the psychological significance and consequences of negative body image evaluations. Indeed, many people may be dissatisfied with their appearance, but their dissatisfaction does not necessarily affect their emotional well-being or daily functioning. The term *body image disorder* has been used to refer to situations where body image concerns are persistent and result in some degree of impairment in social relations, social activities, or occupational functioning (Thompson, 1999).

Very few studies in exercise psychology have examined the impact of body image concerns on emotional and social functioning (i.e., body image disorders), but many have measured aspects of body image other than body satisfaction/dissatisfaction. For example, social physique anxiety (SPA), the anxiety that people experience in response to other's real or imagined evaluations of their bodies (Hart, Leary, & Rejeski, 1989), taps into the affective dimension of body image and has been very well studied in the field of exercise psychology (for reviews see Hausenblas, Brewer, & Van Raalte, 2004; Martin Ginis, Lindwall, & Prapavessis, 2007). Given these trends in the exercise psychology literature, in addition to using the term negative body image, we interchangeably employ the terms *poor body image* and *body image disturbance* throughout this chapter to recognize the multidimensional manifestations of a "negative body image."

The Importance of Body Image Treatments

The health implications of a negative body image and body image disorders cannot be overstated. From a mental health perspective, poor body image has been linked to low self-esteem (Miller & Downey, 1999), is believed to be a cause of depression and anxiety (Stice & Whitenton, 2002), and plays a significant role in the etiology of eating disorders such as anorexia nervosa and bulimia nervosa (Polivy & Herman, 2002). From a physical health perspective, body image concerns have been shown

to influence health risk behaviors such as smoking, alcohol and drug use, and pathological weight loss behaviors (e.g., extreme dieting and use of diet pills; French, Story, Downes, Resnick, & Blum, 1995). Some investigators have even blamed body image concerns for girls' avoidance of physical education classes (e.g., Ennis, 1999). Because the implications can be so severe, efforts have been directed toward developing interventions to improve body image.

Exercise is one intervention that has attracted increasing interest over the past two decades. We begin our chapter by presenting a summary of results from three meta-analyses of these intervention studies. The meta-analytic evidence is used as the basis for a comprehensive discussion of potential mediators and moderators of the effects of exercise on body image. We then examine emerging topics in the exercise intervention and body image literature and conclude with recommendations for the further study of body image within exercise psychology.

The Effects of Exercise Interventions on Body Image

Three meta-analyses have examined the effects of exercise interventions on body image (Campbell & Hausenblas, 2009; Hausenblas & Fallon, 2006; Reel et al., 2007). Two of the meta-analyses (Hausenblas & Fallon, 2006; Reel et al., 2007) also included separate meta-analyses of correlational studies, whereas the third (Campbell & Hausenblas, 2009) included only controlled experiments. Given that the focus of this chapter is on exercise as a treatment for poor body image, our discussion is limited to meta-analytic findings for studies that included an exercise intervention.

Hausenblas and Fallon (2006) conducted the first meta-analysis of the literature on exercise and body image. Their meta-analysis consisted of 121 published and unpublished studies. Studies with an exercise intervention component consisted of both pretest–posttest single-group designs and studies with both an experimental and control group. All of the studies included at least one measure of body image. In the single-group studies, the average effect size was 0.24. For studies with a control group, the overall mean effect size was 0.28. These results provided evidence of small albeit statistically significant effects of exercise on body image.

Reel and colleagues (2007) conducted a meta-analysis of 35 published studies that examined the association between exercise and body concerns. The authors conceptualized "body concerns" as an umbrella category that captured body image as well as related constructs such as body esteem and physical self-concept. Medium-sized effects emerged for both controlled experiments (ES = 0.47) and pretest–posttest studies (ES = 0.45). Based on these findings, the authors concluded that exercise has a significant, positive effect on body concerns.

Most recently, Campbell and Hausenblas (2009) conducted a meta-analysis of 57 published and unpublished exercise intervention studies. All of the studies had a body image variable as a dependent measure, a group that received an exercise intervention, and a control group. The interventions varied widely in terms of the body image outcome measures employed, the types of exercise prescribed, and the populations sampled. Despite such a mix of study features, the authors still found a significant effect of exercise on body image. Overall, there was an average effect size of 0.29 when comparing pre- to postintervention changes in body image for treatment versus control groups.

The results across the three meta-analyses provide a clear indication that exercise has significant positive effects on body image. What is not clear, however, is *how* exercise improves body image. Investigation of the mechanisms underlying the exercise–body image relationship is crucial if researchers are to better understand how these positive effects occur and if interventionists are to develop exercise programs that maximize improvements in body image. In the next section, we examine potential mediators of the effects of exercise interventions on body image.

Mechanisms Underlying the Effects of Exercise Interventions on Body Image

Mechanisms are variables that account for or explain the effects of an intervention on an outcome measure. One way to test for mechanisms is to examine whether change in a proposed mechanism mediates the effects of the intervention. This can be done by calculating a series of regression equations or using structural equation modeling.

Within the exercise and body image literature, three broad categories of variables have been identified as potential mechanisms underlying the effects of exercise interventions: objective improvements in physical fitness, perceived improvements in physical fitness, and increases in self-efficacy (Lox, Martin Ginis, & Petruzzello, 2006). For the purposes of the present chapter, we conducted a review of published exercise interventions that tested these (and other variables) as mediators of the effects of exercise on body image.

We began by retrieving articles referenced in the three exercise and body image meta-analyses and then conducted additional searches through electronic databases (PubMed, PsycINFO, Sociological Abstracts, and SPORTdiscus). For consistency, publications that were deemed "body image studies" in the meta-analyses were included in our review, even if the authors of a publication did not identify their paper as a body image study per se. In particular, studies that used the Physical Self subscale of the Tennessee Self Concept Scale (Fitts, 1965) and the Body Attractiveness subscale of the Physical Self-Perception Profile (Fox & Corbin, 1989) were frequently conceptualized as "self-concept studies" by their respective authors rather than body image studies. However, these subscales could arguably be considered body image measures and were treated as such in the Campbell and Hausenblas (2009) meta-analysis (personal communication, October 12, 2009). To remain consistent, our review included studies with these outcome measures.

Our searches identified only one study that conducted a proper statistical test of mediation (Anderson, Murphy, Murtagh, & Nevill, 2006). Consequently, we expanded our search to include exercise intervention studies that measured change in a potential mechanism over time, and then tested this change as either a predictor or correlate of body image change. In total, 13 relevant studies were identified. Table 4.1 presents characteristics of those studies. The studies included single-group interventions and both randomized and nonrandomized controlled trials. The majority of studies (7) had only female participants, and the remainder had mixed-sex samples. Two studies were of adolescents, one involved university-age participants, and the remainder consisted of participants over the age of 35. Average sample size was $N = 82$ (range of 14–174). Each study demonstrated significant improvements in body image among participants assigned to an exercise training condition.

All of the tested mechanisms could be classified as objective fitness, perceived fitness, or self-efficacy variables. Table 4.2 presents information about the mechanisms and the relationships between changes in the mechanisms and changes in body image. Many of the studies included measures in addition to those presented in Table 4.2. The table shows only those variables that were assessed for change over time and in relation to change in body image.

Table 4.1. Characteristics of Studies Examining Mechanisms Underlying the Effects of Exercise Interventions on Body Image

Study	Baseline N	Sex	Sample characteristics (M_{age}, years)	Exercise intervention
1. Anderson et al. (2006)	37	Women	Sedentary (38.1)	12 weeks of brisk walking or walking + abdominal electric muscle stimulation, moderate intensity, 3/week for 30 min
2. Annesi (2000)	48	Women	Sedentary, obese (36.5)	12 weeks of aerobic training, at 40–50% VO_2max, 2/week for 15–20 min plus weight training 1/week
3. Ben-Shlomo & Short (1986)	14	Women	Sedentary, 23–41 years	6 weeks of arm or leg ergometry at 60–80% max heart rate (HR), 3/week for 20 min
4. Lindwall & Lindgren (2005)	62	Women	Sedentary (16.4)	6 months of exercise, moderate intensity, 2/week for 45 min
5. Martin Ginis et al. (2005)	44	Men = 28 Women = 16	Sedentary (21.6)	12 weeks of high-intensity strength training, 5/week
6. McAuley, Bane, Rudolph, & Lox (1995)	114	Men = 56 Women = 58	Sedentary, middle-aged (54.5)	20 weeks of brisk walking at 65–70% max HR, 3/week for 15–40 min
7. McAuley, Bane, & Mihalko (1995)	114	Men = 56 Women = 58	Sedentary, middle-aged (54.5)	20 weeks of brisk walking at 65–70% max HR, 3/week for 15–40 min
8. McAuley et al. (2000)	174	Men = 49 Women = 125	Older adults (65.5)	6 months of strength and flexibility training or walking at 65–70% VO_2max, 3/week for 40 min
9. McAuley et al. (2002)	174	Men = 49 Women = 125	Older adults (65.5)	6 months of strength and flexibility training or walking at 65–70% VO_2max, 3/week for 40 min
10. Ransdell, Detling, Taylor, Reel, & Shultz (2004)	40	Women	Sedentary mother–daughter pairs (45.2, 15.4)	12 weeks of aerobic and resistance training, 3/week for 60–75 min
11. Shaw et al. (2000)	37	Women	Postmenopausal (54.6)	9 months of strength training, 3/week
12. Taylor & Fox (2005)	142	Men = 53 Women = 89	Individuals at (54) for risk for heart disease	10 weeks of moderate intensity aerobic activity, 2/week 30–40 min
13. Tucker & Mortell (1993)	65	Women	Sedentary (42.5)	12 weeks of resistance training or walking at 65–80% max for 1–4 miles, 3/week

Table 4.2. Mediators, Outcome Measures, and Results in Studies of Mechanisms Underlying the Effects of Exercise on Body Image

Study (see Table 4.1)	Mediator type	Mediator measures	Body image measures	Effect of exercise on body image?	Results
1	Body composition	Weight, BMI, % body fat, body circumference	Body attractiveness, clothes fit, body dissatisfaction, stomach appearance	Yes	Δ in weight, BMI, and thigh circumference mediated Δ in clothes fit; no other significant associations
2	Body composition	Waist-to-hip ratio, weight	Multiple Body-Self Relations Questionnaire	Yes	No significant correlations
3	Aerobic fitness	Submaximal heart rate, maximal workload	Physical self-concept	Yes	No significant correlations
4	Body composition	Weight, BMI	Social physique anxiety, body attractiveness	Yes	No significant correlations
	Aerobic fitness	VO$_2$submax			
5	Body composition	% body fat, muscle mass	Social physique anxiety, body areas satisfaction, muscularity attitudes	Yes	In general, for women, Δ in body image was correlated with Δ in both actual strength and perceived body fat, strength, and muscularity; for men, Δ in body image was correlated only with Δ in perceived fat, strength, and muscularity
	Strength	Leg, shoulder, chest, arm one-repetition maximum			
	Perceived fitness	Body fat, strength, muscularity			
6	Body composition	Body circumference	Social physique anxiety	Yes	In a regression model, Δ in hip circumference predicted Δ in social physique anxiety
7	Body composition	Weight, % body fat, body circumference	Social physique anxiety	Yes	In a regression model, Δ in hip circumference and walking self-efficacy predicted Δ in social physique anxiety
	Self-efficacy	Biking efficacy, walking efficacy, physical efficacy			
8	Body composition	% body fat	Body attractiveness	Yes	In a structural equation model, Δ in physical self-efficacy and body fat predicted Δ in body attractiveness
	Aerobic fitness	VO$_2$ peak			
	Self-efficacy	Physical efficacy			

(Continued)

Table 4.2. (Continued)

Study (see Table 4.1)	Mediator type	Mediator measures	Body image measures	Effect of exercise on body image?	Results
9	Body composition	% body fat	Social physique anxiety	Yes	In a structural equation model, Δ in VO$_2$ peak and physical self-efficacy predicted Δ in social physique anxiety
	Aerobic fitness	VO$_2$ peak			
	Self-efficacy	Physical efficacy			
10	Body composition	Weight	Body attractiveness	Yes	No significant correlations
	Strength	No. of push-ups			
	Aerobic fitness	Estimated VO$_2$max			
	Flexibility	Sit-and-reach			
11	Body composition	Fat mass, lean mass	Body attractiveness	Yes	Δ in leg fat mass correlated with Δ in body attractiveness
	Strength	Strength, peak power			
12	Body composition	BMI, skinfolds, body circumference	Body attractiveness	Yes	Δ in BMI, skinfolds, waist and hip circumference, and BMI correlated with Δ in body attractiveness
	Aerobic fitness	Submaximal heart rate			
13	Strength	Leg, chest, shoulder, biceps one-repetition maximum	Body cathexis	Yes	In a regression model, within the strength training condition, Δ in strength predicted Δ in body cathexis

The following discussion is organized around the three categories of mechanisms.

Objective Improvements in Physical Fitness

Objective measures of change in physical fitness have been the most frequently studied mechanism in the exercise and body image literature. Physical fitness encompasses body composition, cardiorespiratory endurance (aerobic fitness), muscular strength and endurance, flexibility, and the ability to perform functional activities such as those associated with activities of daily living. All 13 studies in our review examined at least one measure of physical fitness as a potential mechanism.

The most frequently examined fitness components were body composition (11 studies), followed by aerobic fitness (6 studies) and muscular strength (4 studies).

Of the 11 interventions that included measures of body composition change, six showed a significant association with body image change. When statistically significant, body composition change accounted for less than 15% of the variance in body image change scores. There was no discernible pattern across the studies in the types of body composition measures that were most frequently associated with body image change. For example, measures of body fatness, body weight, body mass index (BMI), and body circumference each emerged as a significant correlate in some studies but not in others. Of note, in the only study to include a proper statistical test of mediation, changes in weight, BMI, and thigh circumference were shown to mediate the effects of the exercise intervention on women's perceptions of how well an article of clothing fit them (Anderson et al., 2006). However, none of the body composition measures mediated or were even correlated with changes in any of the other three measures of body image in that study.

Together, these findings suggest that changes in body composition play a relatively minor role in exercise-related body image improvements. This conclusion is somewhat surprising given that cross-sectional studies have consistently shown body composition to be a significant correlate of body image. Among women, it is well-established that body weight and BMI are negatively correlated with body image such that smaller women have better body images than larger women. Among men, there is evidence of a curvilinear, inverted-U relationship between body image and BMI (Muth & Cash, 1997), indicating that the thinnest *and* the heaviest men have the poorest body images.

Likewise, changes in strength and cardiovascular fitness variables are not consistently related to change in body image. Changes in body image were significantly correlated with changes in aerobic fitness in just one out of six studies (McAuley, Marquez, Jerome, Blissmer, & Katula, 2002). Using structural equation modeling, McAuley and colleagues found that aerobic fitness change coupled with self-efficacy change explained 19% of the variance in changes in SPA. Self-efficacy was the stronger of the two predictors. Only two of four studies found an association between changes in muscular strength and body image change (Martin Ginis, Eng, Arbour, Hartman, & Phillips, 2005; Tucker & Mortell, 1993). In particular, Tucker and Mortell (1993) found that changes in strength explained 12% of the variance in body image change among women in a strength training program. Subsequently, Martin Ginis and colleagues (2005) found that among female study participants, changes in some strength measures were associated with changes in SPA and body satisfaction. However, the pattern of correlations was not consistent across the body image measures. The significant correlations were quite strong (rs = .48–.70), but some correlations were nonsignificant.

Taken together, these findings suggest that the magnitude of change in body composition and other physical fitness variables does not determine the extent to which an exercise intervention improves body image. Although this conclusion may seem counterintuitive, there are several possible explanations. First, physical fitness may not be a particularly valued component of body image; thus changes in fitness have little impact on body image. While this could be true for the aerobic and strength components of fitness, it seems unlikely that the body composition component would not be valued, given the value that westernized societies place on the possession of a lean physique.

A more likely possibility is that the objective fitness measures employed in most studies do not provide useful or meaningful information to participants. For instance, McAuley and colleagues (2002) suggested that it is not change in a person's VO_2 peak per se that drives changes in body image, but rather the impact of improved VO_2 peak on physical functioning. Most people do not know how to interpret the results of a VO_2 peak test, but they do recognize improvements in their abilities to carry out activities of daily living. Perhaps if functional improvements were assessed (e.g., the ability to climb stairs or carry heavy bags of groceries), people would be able to make better use of fitness test information and thus stronger and more consistent relationships with body image change would emerge.

Another possibility is that changes in some objective measures of fitness (such as VO_2 peak, amount of weight that one can lift, and skinfold measures) may be imperceptible to outside observers. This may be particularly relevant for explaining the lack of association between changes in physical fitness and changes in SPA. SPA is an affective measure of body image that reflects anxiety about *others'* evaluations of one's body (Hart et al., 1989). If other people cannot see changes in the exerciser's aerobic fitness, muscular strength, or skinfold thickness, then the exerciser's SPA may not decrease (McAuley et al., 2002).

We suspect that the most likely reason for the absence of fitness–body image relationships is that the absolute amount of fitness change is not as important as the exerciser's interpretation of that change. For example, some women may experience large improvements in body image after losing relatively small amounts of weight, while other women may remain dissatisfied with their bodies despite losing quite large amounts of weight. Responses to the weight loss will depend on whether the exerciser perceives that she has moved closer to her body ideal. As such, people's *perceptions* of fitness change likely play a more important role in the exercise–body image relationship than does the actual amount of change.

Perceived Improvements in Physical Fitness

Only one study has examined the relationship between perceived changes in physical fitness and changes in body image following an exercise intervention. Martin Ginis and colleagues (2005) looked at changes in perceived muscularity, strength, and body fat after 12 weeks of strength training. Among male participants, changes in all three types of perceptions were significantly associated with changes in body satisfaction, SPA, and muscularity attitudes, with the most consistent relationships emerging for SPA (i.e., change in SPA was significantly correlated with change in all three perception measures, $rs \geq -.33$). In contrast, none of the body image variables correlated significantly with *objective* measures of change in muscularity, strength, and body fat. These results suggest that among men involved in a strength training program, perceived fitness improvements are more important to body image change than actual fitness improvements.

Among female study participants, changes in perceived muscularity, strength, and body fat were significantly associated with changes in body satisfaction and SPA, with the most consistent relationships emerging for body satisfaction (i.e., change in body satisfaction was correlated with change in all three perception measures, $rs \geq .46$). Although changes in body image were not significantly correlated with objective changes in muscularity or body fat, there were some significant relationships between body image and objective strength change. Unfortunately, the study lacked adequate power to examine the relative impact of objective versus perceived changes in strength, so it is not clear which played the more important role in women's body image improvements. Nevertheless, it is clear that perceived body composition changes (i.e., perceived increased muscularity and decreased body fat) were more important to women's body images than were actual body composition changes.

Presumably, the measurement of changes in perceived fitness overcomes some of the limitations identified with regard to measuring changes in actual fitness. In particular, assessment of perceived change indicates whether the exerciser recognizes a meaningful transformation in his or her body. When an individual perceives meaningful change, we would expect improvements in body image to follow.

Improvements in Self-efficacy

Self-efficacy refers to beliefs in one's capabilities to organize and execute the activities required to produce a given outcome (Bandura, 1997). Three studies have examined the relationship between changes in self-efficacy and changes in body image (McAuley, Bane & Mihalko, 1995; McAuley, Blissmer, Katula, Duncan, & Mihalko, 2000; McAuley et al., 2002). All three found significant associations after controlling for objective changes in physical fitness. Specifically, at the end of a walking intervention for middle-aged adults, walking self-efficacy and physical self-efficacy combined to account for 12% of the change in SPA (McAuley et al., 1995). In structural equation models, changes in physical self-efficacy were significant predictors of both body attractiveness (McAuley et al., 2000) and SPA (McAuley et al., 2002) among older adults in either a strength-and-flexibility program or a walking program. In all three of these studies, the predictive strength of self-efficacy was greater than the predictive strength of various objective measures of physical fitness such as body fat (McAuley et al., 1995; McAuley et al., 2002) and aerobic fitness (McAuley et al., 2000).

As with measures of perceived fitness change, measures of self-efficacy capture people's interpretations of their exercise-related improvements. Changes in self-efficacy reflect the sense of personal control and mastery over one's body that is gained from exercise participation. McAuley and colleagues' studies suggest that an enhanced sense of physical mastery plays an important role in body image change. Self-efficacy gains may also reflect feelings of empowerment; that is, the sense of being able to meet one's own needs and solve one's own problems. An enhanced sense of empowerment could also play a mechanistic role in the exercise–body image relationship (Lindwall & Lindgren, 2005).

Conclusions and Recommendations

The exercise and body image literature is characterized by a lack of research on mechanisms. When the mechanisms underlying change are unknown, it is difficult to develop interventions that will maximize that change (Baranowski, Anderson, & Carmack, 1998). Of the studies that have examined potential mechanisms, only one performed a proper test of statistical mediation (Anderson et al., 2006). Thus our conclusions are based primarily on the observed relationships between changes in the potential mechanisms and changes in the measures of body image. Such designs and analyses do not allow for any causal interpretations. Further research using prospective designs and mediational analyses is needed to establish firm conclusions about the mechanistic role of these variables.

Based on the reviewed studies, objective improvements in physical fitness account for minimal variance in body image change. Nevertheless, we do not recommend that researchers remove fitness measures altogether from their designs. It is important to measure and statistically control for objective fitness changes because they sometimes can account for explained variance and they may influence other potential mechanisms such as functional fitness (McAuley et al., 2002). It should also be noted that most of the studies included in our review involved relatively older participants. The relationship between changes in physical fitness and changes in body image among children, adolescents, and young adults is not yet known. These points notwithstanding, it is time for investigators to move past physical fitness variables as the primary mechanisms of interest. As our review indicates, perceived changes in physical fitness and self-efficacy are two viable mechanisms that warrant greater attention.

We also encourage researchers to explore other variables that have been hypothesized to mediate the effects of exercise. For instance, Fox (2000a, 2000b) has suggested that exercise elicits an undetermined psychophysiological mechanism that enhances mood and positive self-regard. In a similar vein, the extent to which people experience enjoyment during exercise has been identified as a potential determinant of body image change (Tucker & Mortell, 1993). Fox has also posited that participation in group exercise programs can lead to an increased sense of belonging that indirectly improves thoughts and feelings about the self. We recommend that investigators test these potential mechanisms in studies of the effects of exercise on body image.

Moderators of the Effects of Exercise Interventions on Body Image

In addition to understanding *how* exercise enhances body image, it is important to understand the conditions under which exercise is most effective for enhancing body image. Addressing this issue requires an examination of moderators. Moderators are variables that alter the direction or strength of an intervention effect (Baron & Kenny, 1986). From a treatment perspective, information on moderators is useful for indicating who will derive the greatest benefit from an exercise intervention and the types of interventions that will yield the largest improvements. From a research perspective, failure to control for moderators during study design and data analysis can result in null or tempered effects if the benefits of exercise vary depending on participant characteristics (e.g., sex or age) or characteristics of the exercise prescription itself (e.g., the type of exercise performed or its frequency). In this section, we examine characteristics of both exercisers and exercise interventions that can moderate the effects of exercise on body image.

Exerciser Characteristics

BASELINE BODY IMAGE AND EXERCISE EXPERIENCE

In general, people with the poorest body images reap the largest gains from exercise interventions (Fox, 2000a, 2000b; Martin Ginis & Bassett, 2011; McAuley, Bane, Rudolph, & Lox, 1995; Tucker & Maxwell, 1992; Tucker & Mortell, 1993)—probably because these people have the most room for improvement in body image measures. Likewise, study participants with less exercise experience may see greater body image improvements than those with more exercise experience; improvements in mechanism variables—fitness, physical self-perceptions, and self-efficacy—can be quite drastic for out-of-shape novice exercisers who lack favorable perceptions of and confidence in their physical abilities.

Meta-analytic data provide support for these proposals. Campbell & Hausenblas (2009) reported greater improvements in body image ($p = .07$) for overweight and obese exercise participants (ES = 0.34) compared with normal-weight participants (ES = 0.18). It is possible that overweight and obese people enter exercise interventions with poorer body image, fitness, physical self-perceptions, and self-efficacy than their normal-weight counterparts. Greater improvements in the mechanism variables can in turn lead to greater improvements in body image.

SEX AND GENDER ROLE ORIENTATION

Historically, men and women have shown differences across all five body image dimensions. For instance, women are generally less satisfied with their bodies than men (e.g., Demarest & Allen, 2000;

Feingold & Mazzella, 1998; Furnham, Badmin, & Sneade, 2002; Smith, Thompson, Raczynski, & Hilner, 1999), report greater SPA (e.g., Davidson & McCabe, 2005), and engage in more body-focused behaviors than men (e.g., restrictive dieting; Neumark-Sztainer, Sherwood, French, & Jeffery, 1999). These types of findings have led to the generally accepted conclusion that women have worse body images than men (Feingold & Mazzella, 1998). However, this assumption is now being challenged, because it is based largely on studies that focused on only one type of body image concern—body fatness. Whereas female body dissatisfaction typically stems from concerns about being overweight, male body dissatisfaction can stem from concerns about being too fat, too thin, insufficiently muscular, or a combination of these (McCabe & Ricciardelli, 2004; Muth & Cash, 1997). When the range of potential male body image concerns are properly measured, poor body image and body image disturbance are probably just as common among men as among women (McCabe & Ricciardelli, 2004).

Few exercise training studies have included both male and female participants and examined sex differences in body image change. Meta-analyses comparing the effect sizes for exercise-related change in male and female body image have produced contradictory findings. The Reel et al. (2007) and Campbell and Hausenblas (2009) meta-analyses indicated no significant sex differences in the magnitude of body image change following participation in an exercise intervention, although in the latter review, the effect for women (ES = 0.32) tended to be larger than that for men (ES = 0.19). Conversely, Hausenblas and Fallon (2006) found a larger effect for women than men in experimental (ES$_{women}$ = 0.43, ES$_{men}$ = 0.39) and single-group studies (ES$_{women}$ = 0.45, ES$_{men}$ = 0.26).

One possible explanation for the conflicting meta-analytic results is that sex moderates the effectiveness of different *types* of exercise interventions. That is, the effectiveness of a particular regimen may depend on whether it brings people closer to the body ideal for their sex. The sociocultural body image ideal for women is an ultrathin, curvy, and toned physique. For men, the sociocultural ideal is a V-shaped physique with broad, muscular shoulders, prominent abdominal muscles, a narrow waist, and muscular legs. Thus an exercise regimen designed solely to maximize fat loss, with no strength training component to increase muscle mass, could have greater body image benefits for women than men, because it would bring women closer to the

ultrathin female body image ideal. Conversely, this regimen would not help the many men who are in pursuit of the muscular male ideal (McCreary & Sasse, 2000).

Another possibility is that gender role orientation, and not biological sex, is the true moderator of the effects of exercise on body image. Gender role orientation refers to the extent to which people identify with stereotypically masculine (e.g., strong and assertive) versus feminine (e.g., gentle and affectionate) traits. The effects of an exercise intervention on body image may depend more on whether the type of exercise promotes the body ideal for the participants' gender role orientation than on the body ideal for their biological sex. The male sociocultural body ideal is associated with the possession of typically masculine traits, whereas a smaller, thinner male body is associated with stereotypically feminine traits. Not surprisingly, men who score high on measures of masculinity are more likely to endorse and pursue the muscular ideal, while men scoring high on measures of femininity are more likely to be concerned with weight loss and attaining a thinner ideal (McCabe & Ricciardelli, 2004). Similarly, women who score high on measures of masculinity may be less concerned with weight loss and thinness than women scoring high on measures of femininity. These tendencies suggest that moderator analyses and intervention decisions based on biological sex (i.e., whether one is male or female) may be overly simplistic, because they assume that all women will have the same body image response to a particular exercise intervention, as will all men.

AGE

The relationship between body image and age is not well understood. Studies have found evidence of a positive (e.g., Demarest & Langer, 1996), negative (Demarest & Allen, 2000; Hetherington & Burnett, 1994), and no relationship (Cash & Henry, 1995; Davis & Cowles, 1991) between body image and age. The meta-analyses have also produced equivocal findings. In both experimental and single-group studies, Hausenblas and Fallon (2006) found larger exercise-related improvements in body image for adolescents (ES = 0.71, 0.98, respectively) than for university students (ES= 0.25, 0.17) and adults (ES = 0.46, 0.40). Likewise, Reel and colleagues (2007) found a larger effect for younger (ES = 0.51) than older adults (ES = 0.41). Yet Campbell and Hausenblas (2009) found a larger effect for studies of adults (ES = 0.44) and older adults (ES = 0.33) than studies of youth (ES = 0.16) and university students (ES = 0.22).

Inconsistent findings for older adults could reflect individual differences in people's responses to the aging process. On the one hand, some people may become increasingly dissatisfied with their bodies as they age and their bodies become further from cultural ideals (Whitborne & Skultety, 2002). These individuals would likely have the most to gain from an exercise intervention. On the other hand, for some people, aging may bring a more relaxed and accepting view of physical appearance (Whitborne & Skultety, 2002), resulting in more positive thoughts and feelings about the body. These individuals could have less to gain from exercise. In short, the magnitude of body image change in studies of middle-aged and older adults may depend on participants' attitudes toward aging.

Another possibility is that age moderates the effects of different types of exercise. For example, there is some evidence to suggest that with age, adults begin to place greater value on physical function than physical appearance (Reboussin et al., 2000). Thus exercise interventions designed to maximize improvements in older adults' physical function may yield greater improvements in body image than interventions focused on weight loss and muscle sculpting. The latter may be most likely to yield body image change in younger adults.

ETHNICITY

Body-related values and norms differ by culture. Accordingly, there are variations in body image across ethnic and cultural groups. For instance, Caucasian women report greater body dissatisfaction than Black (Altabe, 1998; Roberts, Cash, Feingold, & Johnson, 2006; Smith et al., 1999), Asian (Altabe, 1998; Sampei, Sigulem, Novo, Juliano, & Colugnati, 2009), and Hispanic American women (Altabe, 1998). A literature review reported variations in body image among men from differing ethnic backgrounds (Ricciardelli, McCabe, Williams, & Thompson, 2007). Perhaps most interesting was the finding in that review that disturbances in behavioral body image (e.g., extreme body-changing strategies and binge eating) were more prevalent among males from American ethnic minorities (e.g., Blacks, Hispanic Americans, Asian, Middle Eastern) than Whites.

There is very little research on ethnicity as a moderator of the exercise–body image relationship. Campbell and Hausenblas (2009) found that among the few exercise studies that examined or

reported ethnic differences, there was no moderating effect of the percentage of White participants in the sample. Yet presumably if an exercise intervention is conducted among members of an ethnic group that has a lower baseline body image, participants could experience greater improvements in body image than those who are more satisfied at baseline. This effect could be tempered, however, by whether the exercise intervention brings participants' bodies closer to or further from their ethnic group's body ideal.

Exercise Intervention Characteristics

In addition to characteristics of study participants, characteristics of exercise interventions could also moderate body image effects. Excrcise prescriptions generally consist of four components: frequency, intensity, time, and type (commonly referred to as the "FITT principles" of exercise). Frequency refers to the number of exercise sessions prescribed over a given period (e.g., five sessions per week). Intensity refers to the level of effort required during the exercise (e.g., moderate or heavy intensity). Time is the prescribed duration of a given exercise session (e.g., 30 minutes), and type refers to the specific mode of exercise (e.g., aerobic exercise such as jogging or swimming versus resistance exercise such as lifting weights). Well-designed exercise interventions specify all four components of an exercise training program (see Table 4.1 for examples).

Virtually all that is known about the moderating effects of exercise program characteristics has been derived from meta-analyses that have statistically compared effect sizes across studies with different FITT characteristics. Very few studies have directly compared the effects of exercise programs with different characteristics on body image change.

With regard to weekly exercise frequency, one meta-analysis (Hausenblas & Fallon, 2006) found no moderating effect. Another (Campbell & Hausenblas, 2009) found a larger effect for studies with a higher number of weekly exercise sessions. The third meta-analysis (Reel et al., 2007) found a negative correlation between the frequency of exercise sessions and the effect size. Based on these results, it is impossible to draw any firm conclusions about the importance of exercise frequency.

Regarding exercise intensity, meta-analytic findings of experimental and single-group studies show that the effects on body image of strenuous exercise (ES = 0.45, 0.33, respectively) and moderate-intensity exercise (ES = 0.36, 0.31) are larger than that of mild-intensity exercise (ES = -0.04, 0.06)

(Hausenblas & Fallon, 2006). The meta-analyses by Campbell and Hausenblas (2009) and Reel and colleagues (2007) compared only studies involving moderate-intensity and strenuous exercise. While Campbell and Hausenblas found no significant differences, Reel et al. found a larger effect for strenuous (ES = 0.58) than moderate-intensity exercise (ES = 0.35). Based on these results, exercise must be performed at least at a moderate intensity to elicit improvements in body image.

With regard to exercise duration (or time), the results are very consistent. Across all three meta-analyses, the number of minutes of exercise per session did not moderate the effects of exercise on body image (Campbell & Hausenblas, 2009; Hausenblas & Fallon, 2006; Reel et al., 2007). Exercise bouts of longer and shorter duration result in similar changes in body image.

Exercise type is the one FITT component that has been directly examined as a moderator in individual body image studies (e.g., McAuley et al., 2000; Tucker & Mortell, 1993). Tucker and Mortell (1993) showed that resistance training was superior to a walking program for generating improvements in body image among middle-aged women. Conversely, McAuley et al. (2000) found no difference in improvements in body image between older adults who participated in a walking program and those who did a "stretch and strength" exercise program. The meta-analytic data are equally conflicted. Hausenblas and Fallon's (2006) meta-analyses of experimental and single-group studies indicated that a combination of aerobic (e.g., jogging or swimming) and anaerobic (e.g., weight lifting or certain sports) exercise is superior (ES = 0.45 and 0.39 for experimental and single-group studies, respectively) to either mode independently ($ES_{aerobic\ only}$ = 0.25, 0.34; $ES_{anaerobic\ only}$ = 0.27, 0.36). Reel et al.'s (2007) meta-analysis indicated that studies involving anaerobic exercise (ES = 0.64) had a larger effect than studies involving only aerobic exercise (ES = 0.40). Most recently, Campbell and Hausenblas's (2009) meta-analysis found no evidence to support the hypothesis that exercise type moderates the effects of exercise on body image ($ES_{aerobic\ only}$ = 0.30, 0.34; $ES_{resistance}$ = 0.37, $ES_{aerobic+resistance}$ = 0.26). Given these conflicting findings, it is premature to draw any conclusions about the role of exercise type as a moderator of body image effects.

Conclusions and Recommendations

Although some individual exercise intervention studies have tested for moderators (e.g., age and sex,

McAuley, Bane, Rudolph et al., 1995; exercise type, Tucker & Mortell, 1993), most of what is known about the effects of participant and exercise intervention characteristics on body image has been derived from meta-analyses. Meta-analysis allows for the examination of potential moderators across a pooled set of studies. It is a valuable data synthesis technique, particularly when individual studies are too small and underpowered to detect between-group differences. Nevertheless, meta-analysis also has its limitations.

In particular, moderator analyses involve the comparison of effect sizes from studies that are grouped and compared according to a particular moderator characteristic (e.g., sex, ethnicity, or exercise type). There can be tremendous variability in study design features such as how body image was measured, participant inclusion/exclusion criteria, and overall study quality. These differences in design and quality can ultimately confound the results of moderator analyses. In fact, these types of between-study differences might even explain the inconsistent findings reported across the meta-analyses for moderators such as age and sex. To address this limitation, it is important that whenever possible, moderator analyses be conducted and reported within individual studies. This strategy would allow for examination of moderators across participants drawn from the same sampling pool, administered the same measures of body image, and exposed to exercise interventions implemented by the same research team. We also urge investigators to account for baseline body image in their analyses, and use data analytic strategies (such as multilevel modeling) to address the possibility that there are different trajectories of change for individuals with different baseline body image scores.

Another limitation of the existing literature is that neither the individual studies nor the meta-analyses have examined higher-order interactions. As discussed throughout this section, it is likely that participant and intervention characteristics interact. For instance, gender role orientation and exercise type could interact such that masculine-oriented individuals derive greater benefits from strength training and feminine-oriented individuals derive greater benefits from aerobic training interventions. In addition to interacting with one another, moderators may also interact with the proposed mediators. For instance, Martin Ginis et al. (2005) found evidence that different mechanisms drive exercise-related body image change in men versus women. We certainly recognize the challenges and resource demands associated with conducting exercise training studies that are adequately powered to examine multiple moderators and two-way and three-way interactions. Nevertheless, such studies are important next steps toward developing a better understanding of factors that moderate the effects of exercise on body image.

Emerging Topics in Exercise Intervention and Body Image Research

Much of the research on exercise intervention and body image has focused simply on whether exercise is a viable treatment modality for improving body image. But as favorable evidence has accumulated, investigators have begun to examine topics beyond the simple cause-and-effect association between these variables. In this section, we examine three developing areas within the exercise intervention and body image literature: the acute effects of exercise on body image, the effects of exercise on the body image of people drawn from at-risk populations, and the exercise–body image dose–response relationship.

The Effects of Acute Exercise on State Body Image

In most exercise and body image research, body image has been conceptualized as a relatively enduring, cross-situational trait that is amenable to change over a sustained intervention period. However, it is well documented that body image can also be conceptualized as a state variable, with body image experiences varying temporally and across situational contexts (e.g., Haimovitz, Lansky, & Reilly, 1993; Kruisselbrink, Dodge, Swanburg, & MacLeod, 2004; Tiggemann, 2001). This raises the possibility that interventions consisting of single, acute bouts of exercise can positively influence state body image.

A handful of studies have examined this hypothesis, and in general, acute bouts of exercise do seem to have a positive impact on body image. For instance, one experiment showed that a single, 60-minute bout of aerobic dance led to significant increases in women's body satisfaction (McInman & Berger, 1993). Another experiment found that 30 minutes of walking or jogging reduced body dissatisfaction among women who exercised regularly and scored high on a measure of drive for thinness (Fallon & Hausenblas, 2005). In a particularly innovative study, researchers used ecological momentary assessment to examine the effects of exercise on state body dissatisfaction among women who exercised regularly (LePage & Crowther, 2010). Study participants were given electronic pagers and received signals at random times, four times per day, over a 10-day period. They completed measures of state body dissatisfaction on receipt of each random pager signal as well as on completion of each bout of exercise. Analyses indicated that state body dissatisfaction was lower after exercise than after the random pager signals, providing further evidence that acute bouts of exercise can result in acute improvements in body image.

There is evidence, however, that characteristics of the exercise environment and the participant can moderate the acute effects of exercise. For example, studies have shown that women experience higher state SPA when they exercise in mixed-sex than in single-sex environments (Martin Ginis, Murru, Conlin, & Strong, 2011), when they feel less physically attractive than the exercise instructor (Martin Ginis, Prapavessis, & Haase, 2008), and when led by a male than by a female instructor (Bray, Bassett, & Amirthavasar, 2011). Preliminary data also suggest that for women who do not exercise on a regular basis, an acute bout of exercise can have a negative effect on body image. Martin Ginis, Jung, and Gauvin (2003) found that following an acute bout of stationary cycling, women with poor trait body image had increases in state anxiety about their physical appearance. Among women who do not exercise regularly, a single bout of exercise could increase body awareness or elicit negative self-perceptions regarding physical fitness, thus exacerbating preexisting body image concerns. Women unaccustomed to exercise may need to participate in multiple exercise sessions before the acute negative reactions are attenuated or even reversed.

In summary, acute bouts of exercise can provide a transitory "body image boost" to women who are regularly active. Additional research is needed to determine if similar acute effects occur among men who are active. Research is also needed to determine how long the effects of acute exercise persist. Fallon and Hausenblas (2005) found that the positive effects of an exercise bout on body image were immediately wiped out after study participants viewed a slide show consisting of images of "ideal" female bodies. Although these results suggest that acute gains are quickly lost, it is possible that accumulated bouts that enhance state body image contribute to long-term gains in dispositional body image.

At-Risk Populations

We use the term *at-risk populations* to refer to sub-populations at elevated risk for health problems and health complications. At one time, exercise training was often considered to be contraindicated for people with health risk factors. Now exercise is recognized as having significant physical, psychological, and quality-of-life benefits for people with a variety of health conditions (e.g., Martin Ginis and Hicks, 2007; Rimmer, Braddock, & Pitetti, 1996). With growing recognition of these benefits, researchers have begun to investigate the potential for exercise to also improve body image in at-risk populations. Three such populations have received the greatest attention in the exercise and body image literature: people with chronic disease and disability, pregnant women, and patients with eating disorders.

PEOPLE WITH CHRONIC DISEASE AND DISABILITY

Chronic diseases and disabilities that result in disfigurement, altered physical appearance, or body composition changes can compromise body image (Taleporos & McCabe, 2001; Yuen & Hanson, 2002). For instance, after undergoing treatment for breast cancer (e.g., mastectomy or chemotherapy), women often report an increase in body anxiety and dissatisfaction due to the impact of the treatment on their physical appearance (e.g., hair loss, weight gain, or loss of a breast; DeFrank, Bahn Mehta, Stein, & Baker, 2007). In a similar vein, conditions that affect physical function—such as spinal cord injury, multiple sclerosis, or amputation—can result in body dissatisfaction subsequent to the associated functional losses—paralysis, muscle atrophy, or the loss of a limb (Pruzinsky, 2004).

Emerging data indicate that exercise can improve body image among people with different types of diseases and disabilities. For instance, correlational research has shown a positive relationship between exercise and body image among people with various mobility impairments (Wise, 2000; Yuen & Hanson, 2002). Furthermore, exercise training studies have demonstrated significant improvements in body image in people with spinal cord injury (Hicks et al., 2003; Martin Ginis et al., 2003), women with breast cancer (Friedenreich & Courneya, 1996; Pinto, Clark, Maruyama, & Feder, 2003; Pinto, Frierson, Rabin, Trunzo, & Marcus, 2005), people with other types of cancer (for a review see Courneya, 2001), people with arthritis (Chia-Ling Chang et al., 2009), and women with obesity (Foster, Wadden, & Vogt, 1997). Taylor and

Fox's (2005) study of adults with coronary heart disease risk factors is the only intervention we are aware of that has examined potential mechanisms of exercise-induced change in an at-risk population. They found that changes in body composition, but not changes in aerobic fitness, were correlated with changes in body image. However, in cross-sectional research comparing objective with perceived measures of physical fitness, perceptions have been shown to be superior predictors of body image. For instance, in a sample of men enrolled in a cardiac rehabilitation program, perceived physical function explained 37% of the variance in body satisfaction, whereas objective measures of aerobic fitness did not account for any explained variance (Lichtenberger, Martin Ginis, MacKenzie & McCartney, 2003). Thus, paralleling effects observed in the general population, we suspect that among people with disease and disability, exercise-induced improvements in perceived fitness and self-efficacy are more likely to drive body image change than improvements in actual fitness.

PREGNANT WOMEN

The female body undergoes tremendous change during pregnancy. There are mixed findings regarding the effects of these changes on body image. On the one hand, consistent with the idea that changes in body composition—such as weight gain—are related to changes in body image, some research has found that many women experience decreased body satisfaction during pregnancy (Lacey & Smith, 1987; Stein & Fairburn, 1996; Walker, 1998). On the other hand, some research shows no change, or even improvements to body image, during pregnancy (Abraham, King, & Llewellyn, 1994).

Given that roughly 70% of women are inactive during pregnancy, it is quite difficult to conduct research on exercise and body image within this population (Symons Downs, Dinallo, & Kirner, 2008). Nevertheless, preliminary research suggests that women who are more physically active during pregnancy report greater body image satisfaction than those who are less active (Boscaglia, Skouteris, & Wertheim, 2003; Goodwin, Astbury, & McMeeken, 2000; Symons Downs et al., 2008). In terms of mechanisms, exercise likely helps to control changes in body fat and body weight that, in turn, could influence body image. Exercise could also reduce anxiety about bodily changes that are expected during pregnancy. Finally, exercise may help to sustain a woman's perceptions of her physical competence and self-efficacy when fatigue, nausea, and discomfort undermine positive self-beliefs.

PATIENTS WITH EATING DISORDERS

Body image disturbance is a risk factor for the development of eating disorders such as anorexia nervosa (characterized by the refusal to maintain a minimally normal body weight and an intense fear of gaining weight) and bulimia nervosa (characterized by binge eating and excessive compensatory behaviors) (Polivy & Herman, 2002). Indeed, women diagnosed with eating disorders report greater body image dissatisfaction and more distorted body image perceptions than the general population (Cash & Deagle, 1997). Eating disorders might even be considered the ultimate behavioral manifestation of a disturbed body image, as patients engage in dangerous and idiosyncratic activities in response to their negative body images.

Among young women with bulimia nervosa, exercise has been shown to be more effective in reducing negative body image than cognitive behavioral therapy and nutritional counseling (Sundgot-Borgen, Rosenvinge, Bahr, & Sundgot Schneider, 2002). Improvements in eating disorder symptoms have also been found after participation in an exercise intervention. Indeed, a review of exercise interventions in populations with eating disorders suggests that exercise may have positive effects on several psychosocial variables, including body image (Hausenblas, Cook, & Chittester, 2008). For example, among obese women with binge eating disorder, participants in an exercise program had significantly greater reductions in binge eating days than non-exercisers (Pendleton, Goodrick, Poston, Reeves, & Foreyt, 2002). Among inpatient women being treated for anorexia nervosa, bulimia nervosa, and unspecified eating disorders, participants in an exercise program experienced a reduction in obligatory attitudes toward exercise and improved body weight relative to controls (Calogero & Pedrotty, 2004). Structured exercise is believed to alleviate anxiety and increase comfort with weight gain among women being treated for eating disorders, resulting in reduced exercise abuse (i.e., excessive exercise) and improved adherence to meal plans (Calogero & Pedrotty, 2004).

However, caution must be employed in examining exercise as a treatment for body image disturbance among individuals with eating disorders. Exercise abuse is a risk factor for development of eating disorders (Bulik et al. 2006) and is a compensatory behavior for some people with these disorders

(Stice & Agras, 1998). Given these risks, a clinician should provide assistance with the planning and implementation of exercise interventions to treat eating disorder patients.

The Exercise Dose–Response Relationship

The exercise dose–response concept refers to whether increasing amounts of exercise are associated with concomitant changes in the variable of interest (here, body image). Establishment of a dose–response relationship between exercise and body image is an important step toward establishing causality and for developing recommendations regarding the types and amounts of exercise that are most beneficial (cf., Dishman, Washburn, & Heath, 2004). As discussed in the section on moderators, the dose–response relationship for exercise and body image has been assessed primarily through meta-analysis. Of the four components of the exercise prescription (frequency, intensity, type, and time), only intensity has shown a consistent relationship with body image change. However, we also noted the downfalls of relying exclusively on meta-analysis to determine how elements of the exercise prescription are related to changes in body image. Stronger evidence can be provided by examining the dose–response relationship in individual studies.

One of the seminal exercise training studies included a dose–response analysis of the relationship between exercise and body image change. Tucker & Mortell (1993) showed that among women in a strength training condition, higher-intensity workouts (where intensity was measured as average heart rate during the workout) were associated with greater improvements in body image. Despite these encouraging findings, there was little interest in the dose response over the subsequent decade, with the exception of the studies of McAuley et al. (2000, 2002), which found that exercise frequency was unrelated to changes in body image.

Recent years have shown some signs of renewed interest in the dose response. For instance, Taylor and Fox (2005) examined the dose–response relationship in their study of adults at risk for heart disease. They found that adherence to the exercise intervention (operationalized as number of visits to a fitness center) was associated with greater improvements in body image. In addition, Arbour and Martin Ginis (2008) conducted a proper test of statistical mediation, and showed that the number of steps walked over an 11-week exercise intervention mediated the effects on body image change and accounted for a significant 41% of the variance in those changes. Together, these studies provide support for the existence of a dose–response relationship. However, much more research is needed to determine the relationship between the specific elements of the exercise prescription and changes in body image.

Looking to the Future: Recommendations

In this chapter we have provided a comprehensive review of research examining mediators and moderators of the effects of exercise interventions on body image. We have also presented an overview of emerging topics in the exercise and body image literature. In this final section, we provide a series of specific recommendations for future research, followed by some general recommendations to help with the design and implementation of future studies.

Specific Recommendations

Based on our review, we recommend three specific areas of focus in future exercise intervention studies:

1. Greater effort must be directed toward studying the mechanisms underlying the effects of exercise on body image. Having firmly established that exercise has significant effects on body image, investigators must now focus their attention on identifying the mechanisms that account for these effects. Without an understanding of the causes of intervention successes, it is very difficult for interventionists to reliably implement exercise programs to improve body image.

2. More attention needs to be paid to moderators within individual studies. Whenever possible, investigators should report subgroup data (e.g., effect sizes for participants with different demographic characteristics) and carefully monitor adherence to all aspects of the exercise prescription so that dose–response analyses can be undertaken. This information is vital for determining who will benefit most from exercise interventions and under what conditions.

3. Further study is needed of the effects of acute bouts of exercise on state body image. Just as the study of the effects of individual exercise bouts on acute affect is important for understanding the long-term effects of exercise on psychological well-being, studies of acute exercise-related changes in body image states can contribute to a better understanding of how exercise improves body image over the long haul. Acute changes in body image may also be an important determinant of long-term adherence to exercise.

General Recommendations

Exercise training studies are incredibly resource intensive. For instance, considerable effort must be devoted to participant recruitment and retention to ensure that analyses are adequately powered. The provision of exercise equipment and supervision to study participants can also be costly. Given these realities, it is important for researchers to maximize the information that can be obtained from an intervention study. We provide three recommendations to researchers in this regard.

USE THEORY TO GUIDE STUDY DESIGN

Much has been written about the importance of using theory to design and implement studies within exercise psychology (e.g., Brawley, 1993; Lox et al., 2006). In intervention research, theories provide valuable blueprints that identify key sets of variables that can be targeted for change and are susceptible to change. Good theories also elucidate the mediating variables by which an intervention exerts its effects (cf. Baranowski et al., 1998). By using theory to guide the design of body image studies, exercise researchers can maximize the likelihood of targeting and measuring key processes of change.

To date, most research examining the effects of exercise on body image has been atheoretical. For example, of the 13 studies listed in Table 4.1, only six employed a guiding theoretical framework. Three studies (Lindwall & Lindgren, 2005; McAuley et al., 2000; Shaw, Ebbeck, & Snow, 2000) were couched in elements of the Exercise and Self-Esteem Model (EXSEM; Sonstroem & Morgan, 1989), two studies (McAuley, Bane & Mihalko, 1995, 2002) used Bandura's (1997) social cognitive theory, and one study (Martin Ginis et al., 2005) employed Cash's (2002) cognitive–behavioral model of body image. Although none of those frameworks were explicitly designed to explain the effects of exercise on body image, they helped the researchers formulate theoretically tenable hypotheses regarding changes in self-efficacy (social cognitive theory) and in perceived and actual physical fitness (EXSEM and the cognitive–behavioral model of body image) as potential mediators.

We believe that the lack of an explicit model or framework to guide exercise and body image research has been a hindrance to the study of mechanisms. Without a blueprint, investigators have had little direction for selecting and measuring mediators within their experiments. As a step to addressing this shortcoming, we have provided a very basic model, based on our own literature review, to help investigators design exercise intervention studies. As shown in Figure 4.1, our model provides a preliminary list of mechanisms to be assessed. We wish to emphasize that this is not an exhaustive list. Other, unstudied factors such as exercise enjoyment (Tucker & Mortell, 1993), feelings of belonging, and psychophysiological mechanisms (Fox, 2000a, 2000b) may also serve as mediators. Our model also highlights the importance of examining the effects of moderators on changes in the mechanism and outcome measures, and the propensity for interactions between moderator variables. We urge investigators to consider this model when designing their studies and to incorporate tests of potential mediators and moderators within theory-based interventions. Such tests will play a key role in the development of a theory to account for the effects of exercise on body image.

LOOK BEYOND APPEARANCE

At the start of our chapter, body image was defined as "the multifaceted psychological experience of embodiment, especially but not exclusively one's physical appearance" (Cash, 2004, p. 1). Inherent in that definition is the recognition that body image is about more than just appearance. Indeed, satisfaction with physical appearance and satisfaction with physical function have been shown to be independent aspects of body image (Reboussin et al., 2000). Nevertheless, the vast majority of exercise studies have focused only on measuring changes in appearance-related aspects of body image. Given the changes in physical function that can result from exercise participation, researchers may be missing

out on an important element of body image change if satisfaction with function is not assessed.

Assessment of exercise-induced changes in function-related aspects of body image could be particularly relevant in studies involving people who place greater value on function than appearance (Bassett & Martin Ginis, 2010). For instance, it has been suggested that some older adults (Reboussin et al., 2000) and people with chronic diseases (Lichtenberger et al., 2003) and physical disabilities (Bassett, Martin Ginis, & The SHAPE-SCI Research Group, 2009) are more concerned with function than appearance, given their physical challenges and limitations. For these individuals, the "experience of embodiment" may be more about thoughts and feelings regarding what the body can do than about how the body looks.

MEASURE MULTIPLE DIMENSIONS OF BODY IMAGE

Body image consists of evaluative (i.e., subjective satisfaction), affective, cognitive, behavioral, and perceptual components. Currently, it is not known if exercise is effective at improving all of the body image components. In fact, very few exercise intervention studies have included measures other than the subjective satisfaction dimension of body image. In their meta-analysis of experimental exercise studies, Hausenblas and Fallon (2006) noted that 96% of the body image measures employed in these studies assessed subjective satisfaction. About 3% assessed body image affect and less than 1% assessed the perceptual and behavioral domains.

Consistent with Hausenblas and Fallon's (2006) observations, most of the studies cited in Tables 4.1 and 4.2 used measures of subjective

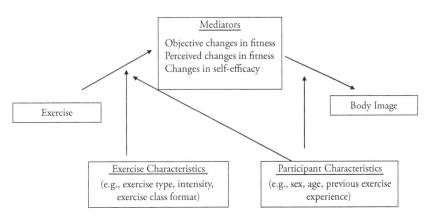

Figure 4.1. Preliminary model to guide research examining the effects of exercise interventions on body image.

satisfaction (e.g., the Body Areas Satisfaction Scale) and affect (e.g., the Social Physique Anxiety Scale). We also note that several of the studies included measures of multiple dimensions of body image. This is a methodological strength: By measuring multiple dimensions, information can be gleaned regarding which body image dimensions are most responsive to exercise interventions. Such information may also provide clues as to the mechanisms underlying body image changes.

For instance, based on the results of intent-to-treat analyses, the exercise intervention employed by Lindwall and Lindgren (2005) led to improvements in SPA but not in perceived body attractiveness. From this pattern of results, one could hypothesize that the exercise intervention primarily alleviated sources of SPA—perhaps by making participants feel less evaluated or by giving them a sense of comfort and belonging (Leary & Kowalski, 1995). Conversely, the intervention may not have been effective for eliciting changes in the variables postulated to underlie improvements in perceived attractiveness (i.e., perceptions of fitness and self-efficacy; Sonstroem & Morgan, 1989).

The use of multiple measures also helps to mitigate the possibility of drawing misleading or inaccurate conclusions about the effects of exercise on body image (Thompson, 2004). For instance, if an exercise study employs just one scale, and that scale captures only a very specific dimension of body image, finding nonsignificant changes may lead to the conclusion that the intervention has no effect on body image. A more accurate conclusion would be that exercise has no effect on that particular body image dimension. Of course, we are not encouraging the strategy of "throwing 'everything body image' at the wall to see what sticks" (Thompson, 2004, p. 9). Rather, we recommend the thoughtful inclusion of multiple theoretically based measures of body image so as to maximize what can be learned from a single study. Given the logistical challenges and resource demands associated with conducting exercise interventions, this recommendation also makes good practical sense.

Conclusions

Based on the findings of three meta-analytic reviews, it is clear that exercise is an effective strategy for improving body image. It is now time for investigators to move beyond simple cause-and-effect studies and begin elucidating the mediators and moderators underlying these effects. A better understanding of these intermediary variables is key to the development of body image theory that leads to successful body image treatments.

Acknowledgment

The preparation of this chapter was supported by a CIHR New Investigator Award (K. A. Martin Ginis) and a SSHRC Doctoral Fellowship (R. L. Bassett).

References

*References marked with an asterisk are included in Tables 4.1 and 4.2.

Abraham, S., King, W., Llewellyn-Jones, D. (1994). Attitudes to body weight, weight gain and eating behavior in pregnancy. *Journal of Psychosomatic Obstetrics and Gynecology, 15,* 189–195.

Altabe, M. (1998). Ethnicity and body image: Quantitative and qualitative analysis. *International Journal of Eating Disorders, 23,* 153–159.

*Anderson, A. G., Murphy, M. H., Murtagh, E., & Nevill, A. (2006). An 8-week randomized controlled trial on the effects of brisk walking with abdominal electrical muscle stimulation on anthropometric, body composition, and self-perception measures in sedentary adult women. *Psychology of Sport and Exercise, 7,* 437–451.

*Annesi, J. J. (2000). Effects of minimal exercise and cognitive behavior modification on adherence, emotion change, self-image, and physical change in obese women. *Perceptual and Motor Skills, 91,* 322–336.

Arbour, K. P., & Martin Ginis, K. A. (2008). Improving body image one step at a time: Greater pedometer step counts produce greater body image improvements. *Body Image, 5,* 331–336.

Bandura, A. (1997). *Self-efficacy: The exercise of control.* New York: W. H. Freeman.

Baranowski, T., Anderson, C., & Carmack, C. (1998). Mediating variable framework in physical activity interventions. How are we doing? How might we do better? *American Journal of Preventive Medicine, 15,* 266–297.

Baron, R. M., & Kenny, D. A. (1986). The moderator–mediator distinction in social psychological research. *Journal of Personality and Social Psychology, 51,* 1173–1182.

Bassett, R. L., & Martin Ginis, K. A. (2011). Issues pertaining to body image measurement in exercise research. In S. B. Greene (Ed.), Body image: perceptions, interpretations and attitudes (pp. 245–254). NY: Nova Science.

Bassett, R. L., Martin Ginis, K. A., & The SHAPE-SCI Research Group. (2009). More than looking good: Impact on quality of life moderates the relationship between functional body image and physical activity in men with SCI. *Spinal Cord, 47,* 252–256.

*Ben-Shlomo, L. S., & Short, M. A. (1986). The effects of physical conditioning on selected dimensions of self concept in sedentary females. *Occupational Therapy in Mental Health, 5,* 27–46.

Boscaglia, N., Skouteris, H., & Wertheim, E. H. (2003). Changes in body image satisfaction during pregnancy: A comparison of high exercising and low exercising women. *Australian and New Zealand Journal of Obstetrics and Gynaecology, 43,* 41–45.

Brawley, L. R. (1993). The practicality of using social psychological theories for exercise and health research and intervention. *Journal of Applied Social Psychology, 5,* 99–115.

Bray, S. R., Bassett, R. L., & Amirthavasar, G. (2011). Self-monitoring and women's self-presentational reactions to gender variations in exercise class composition. *Journal of Applied Biobehavioral Research, 26,* 1–5.

Bulik, C. M., Sullivan, P. F., Tozzi, F., Furberg, H., Lichtenstein, P., & Pederson, N. L. (2006). Prevalence, heritability, and prospective risk factors for anorexia nervosa. *Archives of General Psychiatry, 63,* 305–312.

Calogero, R. M., & Pedrotty, K. N. (2004). The practice and process of healthy exercise: An investigation of the treatment of exercise abuse in women with eating disorders. *Eating Disorders, 12,* 273–291.

Campbell, A., & Hausenblas, H. A. (2009). Effects of exercise interventions on body image: A meta-analysis. *Journal of Health Psychology, 14,* 780–793.

Cash, T. F. (2002). A "negative body image" evaluating epidemiological evidence. In T. F. Cash & T. Pruzinsky (Eds.) *Body Image: A handbook of theory, research, and clinical practice* (pp. 269–276). New York: The Guilford Press.

Cash, T. F. (2004). Body image: Past, present, and future. *Body Image, 1,* 1–5.

Cash, T. F., & Deagle, E. A. (1997). The nature and extent of body-image disturbances in anorexia nervosa and bulimia nervosa: A meta-analysis. *International Journal of Eating Disorders, 22,* 107–125.

Cash, T. F., & Henry, P. E. (1995). Women's body images: The results of a national survey in the U.S.A. *Sex Roles, 33,* 19–28.

Courneya, K. (2001). Exercise interventions during cancer treatment: Biopyschosocial outcomes. *Exercise and Sport Sciences Reviews, 29,* 60–64.

Davidson, T. E., & McCabe, M. P. (2005). Relationships between men's and women's body image and their psychological, social, and sexual functioning. *Sex Roles, 52,* 463–475.

Davis, C., & Cowles, M. (1991). Body image and exercise: A study of relationships and comparisons between physically active men and women. *Sex Roles, 25,* 33–44.

DeFrank, J. T., Bahn Mehta, C., Stein, K. D., & Baker, F. (2007). Body image dissatisfaction in cancer survivors. *Oncology Nursing Forum, 34,* E36–E41.

Demarest, J., & Allen, R. (2000). Body image: Gender, ethnic, and age differences. *Journal of Social Psychology, 140,* 465–472.

Demarest, J., & Langer, E. (1996). Perception of body shape by underweight, average, and overweight men and women. *Perceptual and Motor Skills, 83,* 569–570.

Dishman, R. K., Washburn, R. A., & Heath, G. W. (2004). *Physical activity epidemiology.* Champaign, IL: Human Kinetics.

Ennis, C. (1999). Creating a culturally relevant curriculum for disengaged girls. *Sport, Education and Society, 4,* 31–49.

Fallon, E. A., & Hausenblas, H. A. (2005). Media images of the "ideal" female body: Can acute exercise moderate their psychological impact? *Body Image, 2,* 62–73.

Feingold, A., & Mazzella, R. (1998). Gender differences in body image are increasing. *Psychological Science, 9,* 190–195.

Foster, G. D., Wadden, T. A., & Vogt, R. A. (1997). Body image in obese women before, during, and after weight loss treatment. *Health Psychology, 16,* 226–229.

Fitts, W. H. (1965). *The Tennessee Self-Concept Scale (Manual).* Nashville, TN: Counselor Recordings and Tests.

Fox, K. R. (2000a). The effects of exercise on self-perceptions and self-esteem. In S. J. H. Biddle, K. R. Fox, & S. H. Boutcher (Eds.), *Physical activity and psychological well-being* (pp. 88–118). London: Routledge & Kegan Paul.

Fox, K. R. (2000b). Self-esteem, self-perceptions, and exercise. *International Journal of Sport and Exercise Psychology, 31,* 228–240.

Fox, K. R., & Corbin, C. B. (1989). The physical self-perception profile: Development and preliminary validation. *Journal of Sport and Exercise Psychology, 11*(4), 408–430.

French, S.A., Story, M., Downes, B., Resnick, M. D., & Blum, R. W. (1995). Frequent dieting among adolescents: Psychosocial and health behavior correlates. *American Journal of Public Health, 85,* 695–701

Friedenreich, C. M., & Courneya, K. S. (1996). Exercise as rehabilitation for cancer patients. *Clinical Journal of Sport Medicine, 6,* 237–244.

Furnham, A., Badmin, N., & Sneade, I. (2002). Body image dissatisfaction: Gender differences in eating attitudes, self-esteem, and reasons for exercise. *Journal of Social Psychology, 136,* 581–596.

Garner, D. M. (1997). The 1997 body image survey results. *Psychology Today, 30,* 30–44, 75–80, 84.

Goodwin, A., Astbury, J., & McMeeken, J. (2000). Body image and psychological well-being in pregnancy. *Australia and New Zealand Journal of Obstetrics and Gynaecology, 40,* 442–447.

Haimovitz, D., Lansky, L., & Reilly, P. (1993). Fluctuation in body satisfaction across situations. *International Journal of Eating Disorders, 13,* 77–83.

Hart, E. A., Leary, M. R., & Rejeski, W. J. (1989). The measurement of social physique anxiety. *Journal of Sport and Exercise Psychology, 11,* 94–104.

Hausenblas, H. A., Brewer, B. W., & Van Raalte, J. L. (2004). Self-presentation and exercise. *Journal of Applied Sport Psychology, 16,* 3–18.

Hausenblas, H. A., Cook, B. J., & Chittester, N. I. (2008). Can exercise treat eating disorders? *Exercise and Sport Sciences Reviews, 36,* 43–47.

Hausenblas H. A., & Fallon, E. A. (2006). Exercise and body image: A meta-analysis. *Psychology and Health, 21,* 33–47.

Hetherington, M. M., & Burnett, L. (1994). Ageing and the pursuit of slimness: Dietary restraint and weight satisfaction in elderly women. *British Journal of Clinical Psychology, 33,* 391–400.

Hicks, A. L., Martin, K. A., Ditor, D. S., Latimer, A. E., Craven, C., Bugaresti, J., McCartney, N. (2003). Long-term exercise training in persons with spinal cord injury: Effects on strength, arm-ergometry performance and psychological well-being. *Spinal Cord, 41,* 34–43.

Kruisselbrink, L. D., Dodge, A. M., Swanburg, S. L., & MacLeod, A. L. (2004). Influence of same-sex and mixed-sex exercise settings on the social physique anxiety and exercise intentions of males and females. *Journal of Sport & Exercise Psychology, 26,* 616–622.

Lacey, J. H., & Smith, G. (1987). Bulimia nervosa. The impact of pregnancy on mother and baby. *British Journal of Psychology, 150,* 777–781.

Leary, M. R., & Kowalski, R. M. (1995). *Social anxiety.* New York: Guilford Press.

LePage, M. L., & Crowther, J. H. (2010). The effects of exercise on body dissatisfaction and affect. *Body Image, 7*(2), 124–130.

Lichtenberger, C. M., Martin Ginis, K. A., MacKenzie, C. L., & McCartney, N. (2003). Body image and depressive symptoms as correlates of self-reported versus clinician-reported physiologic function. *Journal of Cardiopulmonary Rehabilitation, 23,* 53–59.

*Lindwall, M., & Lindgren, E. C. (2005). The effects of a 6-month exercise intervention programme on physical self-perceptions and social physique anxiety in non-physically active adolescent Swedish girls. *Psychology of Sport and Exercise, 6,* 643–658.

Lox, C., Martin Ginis, K. A., & Petruzello, S. (2006). *The psychology of exercise: Integrating theory and practice* (2nd ed.). Scottsdale, AZ: Holcomb Hathaway.

Martin Ginis, K. A., & Bassett, R. L. (2011). Exercise and changes in body image. In T. F. Cash, & L. Smolak (Eds.), Body image: A handbook of science, practice, and prevention (2nd ed., pp. 378–386). NY: Guilford Press.

*Martin Ginis, K. A., Eng, J. J., Arbour, K. P., Hartman, J. W., & Phillips, S. M. (2005). Mind over muscle? Sex differences in the relationship between body image change and subjective and objective physical changes following a 12-week strength-training program. *Body Image, 2,* 363–372.

Martin Ginis, K. A., & Hicks, A. L. (2007). Considerations for the development of a physical activity guide for Canadians with physical disabilities. *Canadian Journal of Public Health, 98*(Suppl. 2), S135–S147.

Martin Ginis, K. A., Jung, M. E., & Gauvin, L. (2003). To see or not to see: Effects of exercising in mirrored environments on sedentary women's feeling states and self-efficacy. *Health Psychology, 22,* 354–361.

Martin Ginis, K. A., Latimer, A. E., McKechnie, K., Ditor, D. S., McCartney, N., Hicks, L.,...Craven, C. (2003). Using exercise to enhance subjective well-being among people with spinal cord injury: The mediating influences of stress and pain. *Rehabilitation Psychology, 48,* 157–164.

Martin Ginis, K. A., Lindwall, M., & Prapavessis, H. (2007). Who cares what other people think? Self-presentation in sport and exercise. In G. Tenenbaum & R. Eklund (Eds.), *Handbook of Sport Psychology* (3rd ed., pp. 136–157). New York: Wiley.

Martin Ginis, K. A., Murru, E. C., Conlin, C., & Strong, H. (2011). Construct validation of a state version of the Social Physique Anxiety Scale. *Body Image, 8,* 52–57.

Martin Ginis, K. A., Prapavessis, H., & Haase, A. M. (2008). The effects of physique-salient and physique non-salient exercise videos on women's body image, self-presentational concerns, and exercise motivation. *Body Image, 5,* 164–172.

*McAuley, E., Bane, S. M., & Mihalko, S. (1995). Exercise in middle-aged adults: Self-efficacy and self-presentational outcomes. *Preventive Medicine, 24,* 319–328.

*McAuley, E., Bane, S. M., Rudolph, D. L., & Lox, C. L. (1995). Physique anxiety and exercise in middle-aged adults. *Journal of Gerontology, 50,* 229–235.

*McAuley, E., Blissmer, B., Katula, J., Duncan, T. E., & Mihalko, S. L. (2000). Physical activity, self-esteem, and self-efficacy relationships in older adults: A randomized controlled trial. *Annals of Behavioral Medicine, 22,* 131–139.

*McAuley, E., Marquez, D. X., Jerome, G. J., Blissmer, B., & Katula, J. (2002). Physical activity and physique anxiety in older adults: Fitness and efficacy influences. *Aging and Mental Health, 6,* 222–230.

McCabe, M. P., & Ricciardelli, L. A. (2004). Body image dissatisfaction among males across the lifespan: A review of past literature. *Journal of Psychosomatic Research, 56,* 675–685.

McCreary, D. R., & Sasse, D. K. (2000). An exploration of the drive for muscularity in adolescent boys and girls. *Journal of American College Health, 48,* 297–304.

McInman, A. D., & Berger, B. G. (1993). Self-concept and mood changes associated with aerobic dance. *Australian Journal of Psychology, 45,* 134–140.

Miller, C. T., & Downey, K. T. (1999). A meta-analysis of heavyweight and self-esteem. *Personality and Social Psychology Review, 31,* 68–84.

Muth, J. L., & Cash, T. F. (1997). Body-image attitudes: What difference does gender make? *Journal of Applied Social Psychology, 21,* 1438–1452.

Neumark-Sztainer, D., Sherwood, N. E., French, S. A., & Jeffery, R. W. (1999). Weight loss behaviors among adult men and women: Cause for concern? *Obesity Research, 7,* 179–188.

Pendleton, V. R., Goodrick, G. K., Poston, W. S. C., Reeves, R. S., & Foreyt, J. P. (2002). Exercise augments the effects of cognitive-behavioral therapy in the treatment of binge eating. *International Journal of Eating Disorders, 31,* 172–184.

Pinto, B. M., Clark, M. M., Maruyama, N. C., & Feder, S. I. (2003). Psychological and fitness changes associated with exercise participation among women with breast cancer. *Psycho-Oncology, 12,* 118–126.

Pinto, B. M., Frierson, G. M., Rabin, C., Trunzo, J. J., & Marcus, B. H. (2005). Home-based physical activity intervention for breast cancer patients. *Journal of Clinical Oncology, 23,* 3577–3587.

Polivy, J., & Herman, C. P. (2002). Causes of eating disorders. *Annual Review of Psychology, 53,* 187–213.

Pruzinsky, T. (2004). Enhancing quality of life in medical populations: A vision for body image assessment and rehabilitation as standards of care. *Body Image, 1,* 71–81.

*Ransdell, L. B., Detling, N. J., Taylor, A., Reel, J., & Shultz, B. (2004). Effects of home- and university-based programs on physical self-perception in mothers and daughters. *Women and Health, 39,* 63–81.

Reboussin, B. A., Rejeski, W. J., Martin, K. A., Callahan, K., Dunn, A. L., King, A. C., Sallis, J. F. (2000). Correlates of satisfaction with body function and body appearance in middle and older aged adults: The activity counseling trial (ACT). *Psychology and Health, 15,* 239–254.

Reel, J., Greenleaf, C., Baker, W. K., Aragon, S., Bishop, D., Cachaper, Handwerk, P.,...Hattie, J. (2007). Relations of body concerns and exercise behavior: A meta-analysis. *Psychological Reports, 101,* 927–942.

Ricciardelli, L. A., McCabe, M. P., Williams, R. J., & Thompson, J. K. (2007). The role of ethnicity and culture in body image and disordered eating among males. *Clinical Psychology Review, 27,* 582–606.

Rimmer, J. H., Braddock, D., & Pitetti, K. H. (1996). Research on physical activity and disability: An emerging national priority. *Medicine & Science in Sports & Exercise, 28,* 1366–1372.

Roberts, A., Cash, T. F., Feingold, A., & Johnson, B. T. (2006). Are Black–White differences in females' body dissatisfaction decreasing? A meta-analytic review. *Journal of Consulting and Clinical Psychology, 74,* 1121–1131.

Sampei, M. A., Sigulem, D. M., Novo, N. F., Juliano, Y., & Colugnati, F. A. B. (2009). Eating attitudes and body image in ethnic Japanese and Caucasian adolescent girls in the city of São Paulo, Brazil. *Journal de Pediatria, 85,* 122–128.

*Shaw, J. M., Ebbeck, V., & Snow, C. M. (2000). Body composition and physical self concept in older women. *Journal of Women and Aging, 12,* 59–75.

Smith, D. E., Thompson, J. K., Raczynski, J. M., & Hilner, J. E. (1999). Body image among men and women in a biracial cohort: The CARDIA study. *International Journal of Eating Disorders, 25,* 71–82.

Sonstroem, R. J., & Morgan, W. P. (1989). Exercise and self-esteem: Rationale and model. *Medicine & Science in Sports & Exercise, 21,* 329–337.

Stein, A. & Fairburn, C.G. (1996). Eating habits and attitudes in the post-partum period. *Psychosomatic Medicine, 58,* 321–325.

Stewart, T. M., & Williamson, D. A. (2004). Assessment of body image disturbances. In J. K. Thompson (Ed.), *Handbook of eating disorders and obesity* (pp. 495–514). New York: Wiley.

Stice, W., & Agras, W. S. (1998). Predicting onset and cessation of bulimic behaviors during adolescence: A longitudinal group analysis. *Behavior Therapy, 29,* 257–276.

Stice, E., & Whitenton, K. (2002). Risk factors for body dissatisfaction in adolescent girls: A longitudinal investigation. *Developmental Psychology, 38,* 669–678.

Sundgot-Borgen, J., Rosenvinge, J. H., Bahr, R., & Sundgot Schneider, L. (2002). The effect of exercise, cognitive therapy, and nutritional counseling in treating bulimia nervosa. *Medicine & Science in Sports & Exercise, 34,* 190–195.

Symons Downs, D., Dinallo, J. M., & Kirner, T. L. (2008). Determinants of pregnancy and postpartum depression: Prospective influences of depressive symptoms, body image satisfaction, and exercise behaviour. *Annals of Behavioral Medicine, 36,* 54–63.

Taleporos, G., & McCabe, M. P. (2001). The impact of physical disability on body esteem. *Sexuality and Disability, 19,* 293–307.

*Taylor, A. H., & Fox, K. R. (2005). Effectiveness of a primary care exercise referral intervention for changing physical self-perceptions over 9 months. *Health Psychology, 24,* 11–21.

Thompson, J. K., Heinberg, L., Altabe, M., & Tantleff-Dunn, S. (1999). *Exacting beauty: Theory, assessment and treatment of body image disturbance.* Washington, DC: American Psychological Association.

Thompson, J. K. (2004). The (mis)measurement of body image: Ten strategies to improve assessment for applied and research purposes. *Body Image, 1,* 7–14.

Tiggemann, M. (2001). Person × situation interactions in body dissatisfaction. *International Journal of Eating Disorders, 29,* 65–70.

*Tucker, L. A., & Maxwell, K. (1992). Effects of weight training on the emotional well being and body image of females: Predictors of greatest benefit. *American Journal of Health Promotion, 6,* 338–344, 371.

*Tucker, L. A., & Mortell, R. (1993). Comparison of the effects of walking and weight training programs on body image in middle-aged women: An experimental study. *American Journal of Health Promotion, 8,* 34–42.

Walker, L. (1998). Weight-related distress in the early months after childbirth. *Western Journal of Nursing Research, 20,* 30–44.

Whitborne, S. K., & Skultety, K. M. (2002). Body image development: Adulthood and aging. In T. F. Cash & T. Pruzinsky (Eds.), *Body images: A handbook of theory, research, and clinical practice* (pp. 83–90). New York: Guilford Press.

Wise, J. B. (2000). Benefits derived from weight training by men with cervical spinal cord injuries. *Journal of Strength and Conditioning Research, 14,* 493–495.

Yuen, H. K., & Hanson, C. (2002). Body image and exercise in people with and without acquired mobility disability. *Disability and Rehabilitation, 24,* 289–296.

Physical Activity and Cognitive Function: Theoretical Bases, Mechanisms, and Moderators

Jennifer L. Etnier *and* Jeffrey D. Labban

Abstract

Since Spirduso's seminal study (1975), research examining the relationship between physical activity and cognitive function has burgeoned. Studies examining the effects of a single session of exercise on cognition have demonstrated small effects, with the size of the effect dependent on the particular cognitive task being assessed. Researchers are exploring cerebral blood flow and catecholamines as potential mechanisms of this effect. Studies examining the effects of chronic physical activity on cognitive performance generally report small to moderate effects, with the size of the effect varying based on age, gender, and cognitive task type. Evidence supports changes in cerebral structure and function, reductions in oxidative stress, and increases in cerebral blood flow as potential mechanisms of these effects. Future research is encouraged to further our understanding of mechanisms, of dose–response relationships, and of moderators so that we will be able to prescribe exercise as a means of improving or protecting cognitive performance.

Key Words: cognition, aging, exercise, physical activity, cardiovascular fitness, aerobic fitness.

Introduction

It has long been recognized that physical activity has the potential to benefit both physical and mental health. However, the first empirical evidence of the effects of physical activity on neurocognitive function was not available until the publication of Spirduso's (1975) seminal study, indicating that older men who regularly participated in racket sports had quicker reaction times than older men who were not physically active. Although the conclusions that could be drawn from this study were clearly limited by the cross-sectional nature of the research, this study was important because it paved the way for future interest in exploring the potential benefits of physical activity for neurocognitive function.

Since 1975, well over 200 studies have been conducted to further our understanding of this potential relationship. Reviewing the literature in this area is challenging because of the variety of ways in which the relationship has been explored, the myriad measures of neurocognitive function that have been used, the complexity of the relationship, and the number of potential underlying mechanisms.

At its broadest level, research testing the effects of physical activity on neurocognitive function can be identified as focusing either on the effects of a single bout of exercise (acute exercise) or on the long-term effects of regular participation in physical activity (chronic exercise). The theoretical frameworks, mechanisms, study designs, and targeted populations differ between the acute exercise literature and the chronic exercise literature; hence reviewing this research requires considering these two broad areas separately. In the acute exercise literature, studies can be further identified as focusing on the effects of exercise on cognitive performance measured either concurrently with or following completion of the exercise bout. In the chronic exercise literature, study designs also vary, with researchers using cross-sectional, prospective, and experimental designs to enhance our understanding of how regular participation in physical activity affects cognitive performance.

This area of research is also challenging to synthesize because of the multitude of measures of neurocognitive function that have been used. These include both behavioral measures and measures of cerebral structure and function. Over 450 behavioral measures of cognitive performance have been used in the broader field of neuropsychology (Lezak, Howieson, & Loring, 2004), and at least 100 measures have been used to test the effects of physical activity on cognitive performance (Etnier et al., 1997). With regard to cerebral structure, both studies of nonhuman animals using invasive methods or neuroimaging and human studies using neuroimaging have been used to assess the effects of physical activity. Human studies using neuroimaging techniques have also been conducted to ascertain the effects of physical activity on cerebral function.

The challenges of synthesizing this literature are also related to the complex relationship between physical activity and cognitive performance. The complexity of the relationship is exemplified by considerations of dose–response issues, age-related differences in the magnitude of the effects, and task specificity of the effects. With regard to dose–response issues, researchers must consider the intensity, duration, and mode of the exercise and, for chronic exercise, the number of sessions per week and the length of the exercise program. Our understanding of dose–response relationships for chronic exercise is not well developed, and future research will be necessary to clarify issues relevant to the prescription of physical activity to benefit cognitive performance (Etnier, 2009b). Further adding to the complexity of the dose–response relationship is the fact that age-related differences in the magnitude of the effects for chronic exercise have been reported (Etnier et al., 1997), with larger effects observed for children and older adults. Although research aimed at understanding the effects of regular physical activity on the cognitive performance of children has been increasing, research with chronic exercise is dominated by studies with older adults. It is also interesting to consider whether there might be "windows" of time during which physical activity is particularly important for cognitive performance (e.g., during childhood, when the frontal lobe is developing) and whether physical activity performed during young adulthood and physical activity performed in older age differ in the protection they offer against cognitive decline and dementia with advancing age. Lastly, evidence from meta-analytic reviews (Angevaren, Aufdemkampe, Verhaar, Aleman, & Vanhees, 2008; Colcombe & Kramer, 2003) suggests that the effects of regular physical activity on cognitive performance depend on the type of cognitive task. These findings suggest that cognitive tasks for research must be selected carefully, and these task-specific effects contribute to the difficulty in clearly describing the physical activity–cognition relationship.

To further complicate our ability to synthesize the literature on the effects of physical activity on cognitive performance, a number of mechanisms have been proposed to explain the relationship. These mechanisms differ depending on whether the interest is in the acute or the chronic effects of physical activity on cognitive performance. In the acute literature, recent research is focused on the potential role of cerebral blood flow and catecholamines (epinephrine and norepinephrine). Recent research on mechanisms of the effects of chronic exercise on cognition has focused on cerebral structure, cerebral function, cerebral blood flow, neurotrophic factors, and oxidative stress. It is likely that more than one (or even all) of these mechanisms are involved in explaining the link between physical activity and cognitive performance (Etnier, 2008; McMorris, 2009). Obtaining a better understanding of the relevant mechanisms will likely enhance our understanding of dose–response relationships and will help to elucidate behavioral and pharmacological interventions that might be used in conjunction with physical activity to garner even greater benefits for cognitive performance.

Acute Exercise

The body of research examining the links between acute exercise and cognitive performance is fairly well developed, and this literature has been narratively reviewed on several occasions (Brisswalter, Collardeau, & Rene, 2002; McMorris & Graydon, 2000; Tomporowski, 2003; Tomporowski & Ellis, 1986). The first review of this literature was written by Tomporowski and Ellis (1986), who considered both aerobic and anaerobic exercise. Based on their synthesis of the literature, they concluded that consistent facilitative effects on cognitive performance were evident for anaerobic resistance protocols when cognition was tested during exercise and for aerobic protocols when physically fit individuals were tested either during or following exercise.

Brisswalter and colleagues (2002) examined the acute exercise literature with particular attention to the manner in which the characteristics of the exercise bout (i.e., intensity and duration) affected cognitive outcomes. They concluded that moderate- to high-intensity (40–80% VO$_2$max) and moderate-duration (20–60 minutes) exercise consistently resulted in improvements in decision making. Decrements in cognitive performance were observed in longer-duration (> 60 minutes) exercise protocols, a finding that Brisswalter et al. attributed to the effects of fatigue and dehydration.

A more recent review by Tomporowski (2003) also reported a facilitative effect of exercise on information processing for protocols up to 60 minutes in duration, while decrements in cognitive function were consistently observed for protocols that led to fatigue and dehydration. In both reviews, facilitation of performance on tasks such as visual detection, decisionmaking, and problem solving was observed during periods of submaximal aerobic exercise of durations between 20 and 60 minutes. Also, longer and more intense exercise protocols that stressed physiological resources more severely tended to result in cognitive performance decrements.

Meta-analyses can help overcome one of the shortcomings of narrative reviews, namely, the difficulty of interpreting mixed results in empirical studies. In a meta-analytic review of over 50 studies that used acute protocols, Etnier et al. (1997) reported a small positive effect size ($M=$ 0.16, $SD=$ 0.60, $p<$ 0.05) for the effect of acute exercise on cognitive performance. Thus both narrative and meta-analytic reviews indicate that acute bouts of exercise positively affect cognitive performance. More recently, Lambourne and Tomporowski (2010) meta-analytically reviewed 40 studies assessing the effects of acute exercise on cognitive performance by healthy young adults and concluded that during exercise the effects were small and negative ($d = -0.14$), but after exercise the effects were small and positive ($d = 0.20$).

Theoretical Basis

Multiple theoretical explanations have been proposed for the possible links between acute exercise and cognitive performance. Whereas theories related to chronic exercise paradigms typically focus on changes accrued over time, theories within the acute exercise paradigm focus on alterations in homeostasis that occur during exercise and persist for only a short time following exercise. Four hypotheses of note in the acute exercise literature are the inverted-U hypothesis (Davey, 1973; Easterbrook, 1959; Yerkes & Dodson, 1908), the central fatigue hypothesis (Douchamps-Riboux, Heinz, & Douchamps, 1989), the transient hypofrontality hypothesis (Dietrich, 2003), and the cognitive-energetic hypothesis (Audiffren, 2009).

INVERTED-U HYPOTHESIS

The inverted-U hypothesis was originally proposed by Yerkes and Dodson (1908) to explain the relationship between physiological arousal and performance efficiency. The original assumption was that as arousal increased, performance would be affected in a curvilinear fashion. Davey (1973) applied this approach to exercise-induced arousal and cognitive performance to suggest that cognitive performance during or directly following exercise should benefit from increasing arousal up to a point, after which higher arousal levels should hinder performance. Though there is some empirical evidence to support this curvilinear relationship (Arent & Landers, 2003; Brisswalter, Durand, Delignieres, & Legros, 1995; Chmura, Nazar, & Kaciuba-Uscilko, 1994; Levitt & Gutin, 1971; Martens & Landers, 1970; Reilly & Smith, 1986; Salmela & Ndoye, 1986; Sonstroem & Bernardo, 1982), there is enough contradictory evidence (Cote, Salmela, & Papathanasopoulu, 1992; McMorris & Graydon, 2000; Sjoberg, 1980) to deem overall results equivocal at best. Multiple narrative reviews (Brisswalter et al., 2002; McMorris & Graydon, 2000; Tomporowski, 2003) have come to a similar conclusion and point out that the efficacy of the inverted-U hypothesis to predict cognitive performance may be dependent on characteristics of the task and of the individual. Recent empirical research examining cognitive performance following resistance exercise has lent support to the idea that the relationship may be task specific. Chang and Etnier (2009) observed linear relationships between exercise intensity and performance on tasks that tested simple attention and information processing, but curvilinear relationships for executive function and complex attentional tasks.

Recently, researchers have used electrophysiological measures to further our understanding of how exercise intensity relates to cognitive performance. Specifically, researchers have begun to investigate the P300 component of event-related brain potentials (ERPs). ERPs are measures of cerebral activation that are time-locked to a stimulus. A paradigm that is often used in this literature is to assess the P300 components of ERPs during performance of a flankers task. Researchers use the latency and amplitude of the P300 (a positive-going electrical wave observed approximately 300 ms after stimulus presentation) to make judgments about attention and speed of processing. Specifically, when the P300 occurs after a shorter latency, speed of processing is deemed to be quicker and when the P300 has higher amplitude, the allocation of attentional resources is deemed to be greater. A flankers task requires participants to respond to a stimulus that is presented in the center of "flanking" stimuli. These flankers can either be consistent with (congruent) or in contrast to (incongruent) the central stimulus. Performance of the task when the flankers are incongruent is thought to be indicative of executive function.

Magnie and colleagues (2000) compared P300 amplitude and latency before and after maximal aerobic exercise. Counter to what might be predicted by the inverted-U hypothesis, results indicated a beneficial effect of maximal exercise for both P300 amplitude and latency. However, their design did not directly test the inverted-U hypothesis in that it did not include exercise intensity manipulations. A later study by Kamijo, Nishihira, Higashiura, and Kuroiwa (2007) measured P300 amplitude and latency relative to three different intensities of exercise. Participants were asked to perform a flankers task at baseline and after cycling at intensities rated at 11, 13, and 15 on the Borg Ratings of Perceived Exertion scale. Results showed that reaction time and P300 latency were reduced following exercise compared with baseline levels, again not supporting the inverted-U prediction. Interestingly, though, P300 amplitudes increased above baseline levels following exercise at light and moderate intensities, but not after the highest-intensity exercise. This last result would seem to provide some support for the inverted-U hypothesis.

Taken together, the research does provide evidence that certain cognitive tasks, such as speeded tasks, and certain indices of neurological processes, such as P300 amplitude, are related to arousal level in a curvilinear fashion, but plausible mechanisms that might explain this relationship have yet to be identified. Thus it remains unclear whether the inverted-U relationship is appropriate for explaining the relationship between acute exercise and certain types of cognitive task performance.

CENTRAL FATIGUE

One of the criticisms of the inverted-U hypothesis is that it considers arousal to be a unidimensional construct. One alternate view is the central fatigue hypothesis, which breaks arousal into three dimensions: energetical, emotional, and computational (Douchamps-Riboux et al., 1989). According to this hypothesis, as physical demands are increased above what the individual can readily meet, energetical processing (which is described as the strategic allocation of attentional resources for multiple functions) becomes favored system-wide over computational processing (which is described as multiple structures working collaboratively) (Sanders, 1983). Thus as resources in the central nervous system are taxed by higher physiological demands, cognitive performance that relies on computational processing (i.e., memory, response selection, and stimulus encoding) is predicted to suffer (Hogervorst, Riedel, Jeukendrup, & Jolles, 1996). Research guided by this hypothesis has typically focused on the effects of dehydration, heat stress, and hypoglycemia that result from exhaustive exercise. Though there is some empirical evidence that exercise leading to dehydration and heat stress can result in cognitive impairment (Cian, Barraud, Melin, & Raphel, 2001; Cian et al., 2000; Gopinathan, Pichan, & Sharma, 1988), some of that same research reports that ingestion of carbohydrates and fluids can reduce or eliminate cognitive decrements resulting from exhaustive exercise (Cian et al., 2000, 2001). When Brisswalter and colleagues (2002) reviewed this entire literature, they concluded that exhaustive exercise usually resulted in improvements in cognitive function, arguing against the central fatigue hypothesis.

TRANSIENT HYPOFRONTALITY

The transient hypofrontality hypothesis was developed by Dietrich (2003, 2006), and is based on the suppositions of limited cognitive resources and task-dependent resource distribution. According to this hypothesis, as demand increases beyond the point at which a person is readily able to cope, cognitive resources are redistributed to better support the body's immediate needs. The term hypofrontality refers to the redirection of cognitive resources away from the frontal, more sophisticated processing and output areas of the brain and toward the systems necessary for more basic functions (Dietrich, 2009). Shortly after demand has abated, cognitive resources are presumed to be redistributed back to homeostatic levels (assuming a new demand has not arisen).

As hypofrontality relates to exercise, Dietrich posits that with sufficiently demanding exercise, cognitive resources are redistributed to those regions of the brain most pertinent to carrying out the corresponding physical functions and away from those regions less necessary to meet the physical demands. Thus during strenuous exercise, resources are predicted to be pulled first from regions of the brain involved in higher-order functions (i.e., prefrontal areas) and redirected to regions involved in more basic cognitive processes necessary to maintain and regulate the physical activity. The expected result is a decrement in prefrontal-dependent cognitive tasks. Dietrich points out that this hypofrontality is also dependent on characteristics of the physical activity being performed. Dietrich predicts that hypofrontality during novel forms of physical activity, physical activity that involves high decision-making expectations, or physical activity at a low intensity would be less than would be observed during automatic types of physical activity performed at sufficient intensity to tax cognitive demands (Dietrich, 2003, 2009).

Though direct support for the neuropsychological component of this hypothesis is unavailable in human research, indirect measurement via prefrontal-reliant cognitive tasks can be used to assess its viability. For example, Dietrich and Sparling (2004) assessed performance on two tasks that differed in their dependence on prefrontal activation, comparing two exercise groups with sedentary controls. The tasks were a prefrontal-dependent task—the Wisconsin Card Sorting Task—and a task that was not expected to be dependent on prefrontal activation—the Brief Kaufman Intelligence Test). Cognitive testing for the exercise groups was initiated following 20 minutes of steady-state aerobic exercise and continued during the last 25 minutes of exercise. While no differences in performance were observed on the intelligence test as a function of treatment condition, exercisers exhibited significantly worse performance on the Wisconsin Card Sorting Task than did controls. This result has been interpreted as providing indirect support for the transient hypofrontality hypothesis. Further research testing the viability of this hypothesis using both indirect (Dietrich & Sparling, 2004) and direct (Ekkekakis, 2009) approaches is necessary.

COGNITIVE-ENERGETIC MODEL

The cognitive-energetic model arises from cognitive psychological and energetic approaches to understanding relationships between exercise and cognitive performance (Audiffren, 2009). Though multiple models exist that can be described as "cognitive-energetic," the approach is rooted in the interplay between multiple levels of cognitive operations and multiple dimensions of arousal (Sanders, 1983). Pribram and McGuinness (1975) identified three dimensions of arousal, which can be partitioned into a voluntary subdivision—effort—and involuntary subdivisions—activation and arousal—with effort playing a role in the maintenance and regulation of activation and arousal (Audiffren, Tomporowski, & Zagrodnik, 2008; Tomporowski, 2003). Pribram and McGuinness (1975) define activation as a situational readiness to respond and arousal as a response to stimulus input. Differences between cognitive-energetic models typically revolve around the model of information processing employed and the specific manner of its interaction with the separate components of arousal. Audiffren (2009) explains that the suitability of each model as an explanation of the effects of acute exercise on cognitive performance depends heavily on the characteristics of the exercise session and the time of cognitive assessment relative to exercise.

Sanders (1983) introduced one such model that seeks to describe the manner in which an individual's state with respect to arousal, activation, and effort influences cognitive computational processing speed. Within his model, Sanders identified four computational stages of cognitive processing: stimulus preprocessing, feature extraction, response selection, and motor adjustment. The notion is that arousal has its greatest impact at the feature extraction stage, and activation has its greatest effect at the motor adjustment stage. Effort is thought to play a role both in the response selection stage and in maintaining both arousal and activation at appropriate levels. Further, the entire process is thought to be regulated by an evaluation mechanism that directs effort and receives feedback concerning arousal, activation, and physical response.

A second model, proposed by Humphreys and Revelle (1984), relies on the assumption that cognitive performance increases with increased availability of cognitive resources and, that the availability of cognitive resources can be augmented by increases in motivation. In this model, motivation is broken down into two contributory components: effort and arousal. Effort is described as the level of engagement in a particular task; whereas, arousal is described as a state of alertness or activation, brought about by the sum total of stimulation acting upon the organism. Humphreys and Revelle posit that availability of cognitive resources can only increase cognitive performance up to a point, after which further resources are of no benefit. Moreover, these benefits are not thought to extend similarly to all cognitive functions. Humphreys and Revelle suggest that tasks involving the transfer of information (e.g., reaction time tasks and simple math) benefit most from increases in arousal and effort, while tasks involving information retrieval may benefit from effort but may also be prone to decrements from high levels of arousal. This model also includes predictions about the impact of certain personality traits (impulsivity, anxiety, and achievement motivation) on the impact of arousal and effort on cognitive performance. For example, it may be that higher levels of trait anxiety interact with level of task difficulty to discourage motivation through an avoidance coping style, whereas higher levels of achievement motivation may interact with task difficulty to increase motivation by encouraging an approach coping style.

The last cognitive-energetic model we will discuss was put forth by Hockey (1997). Here again, the allocation of cognitive resources is thought to be important for predicting performance. This model differs from the previous two in that increases in arousal due to exercise are not expected to increase the availability of cognitive resources for cognitive functions. Rather, a "supervisory controller" is thought to determine the division of resources among the present demands. This aspect of the model would suggest that unless either the cognitive or physical task fell within the range of automatic or simple behaviors, performing two tasks simultaneously would result in a decrement in performance on one task or the other. Specifically, resources would be allocated preferentially to the task deemed a higher priority in an effort to keep performance levels on this task in the acceptable range. Performance of the task viewed as less important would suffer until resource demand for the primary task decreased enough to allow adequate reallocation of resources back to the secondary task.

These models share a commonality with respect to the relationship between acute exercise and cognition. They all predict that exercise impacts the availability of attentional and cognitive resources through an increase in arousal and activation. The difference lies in how those resources are predicted to be distributed in response to an acute bout of exercise. Sanders's (1983) and Humphreys and Revelle's (1984) models predict that exercise will increase resource availability and positively affect performance, but Hockey's (1997) model predicts that exercise will decrease resource availability and

negatively affect performance. Though recent literature has continued to examine the cognitive-energetic approach (Audiffren, 2009; Audiffren et al., 2008; Tomporowski, 2003), further research is needed to clarify the cognitive-energetic approach and refine it into a parsimonious model that may be applied generally to predict the effects of acute exercise on cognitive performance.

Underlying Mechanisms

Various mechanisms have been suggested to explain the relationship between acute exercise and cognitive performance. The two that will be discussed here are exercise-induced increases in cerebral blood flow and in catecholamines. While other mechanisms have been suggested, these are the most common within the acute exercise literature.

CEREBRAL BLOOD FLOW

It has been suggested that one manner by which acute exercise might affect cognition is through regional or global increases of cerebral blood flow (CBF). Increases in regional CBF occur during cognitive processing and are thought to reflect adaptations made to provide additional resources to areas of the brain that are activated. However, there is less certainty concerning alterations in blood flow as a function of exercise. Research employing the Kety-Schmidt method of CBF measurement (Kety & Schmidt, 1945, 1948) has consistently reported no increases in global CBF as a function of a single session of exercise (Ide & Secher, 2000). However, several studies have reported that a main weakness of the Kety-Schmidt method is that it relies on the assumption that the two jugular veins drain equally (Querido & Sheel, 2007). Multiple studies point out that the internal jugular, which is typically the larger of the two, drains from the cortical areas of the brain, while the smaller jugular drains from the subcortical areas (Ide & Secher, 2000; Querido & Sheel, 2007; Secher, Seifert, & Van Lieshout, 2008). Given, this asymmetry, conclusions drawn from studies using the Kety-Schmidt method are flawed. Recently, Querido and Sheel (2007) reviewed the literature on CBF changes during exercise and reported that newer measurement methods, such as transcranial Doppler ultrasound (TCD), have shown consistent evidence of a positive, intensity-dependent relationship between acute exercise and CBF. Specifically, Querido and Sheel report that CBF is increased up to approximately 60% VO_2max, after which CBF begins to fall back toward baseline.

Despite consistent evidence for increased CBF (Ide & Secher, 2000; Querido & Sheel, 2007; Secher et al., 2008) and increased cognitive function resulting from acute exercise (Etnier et al., 1997; Lambourne & Tomporowski, 2010), there is no direct evidence that exercise-related increases in CBF are the causal mechanism for improved cognitive performance. Studies using appropriate designs and tests of statistical mediation are required to test the validity of this mechanistic proposal (Etnier, 2008).

CATECHOLAMINES

Finally, a recently reemerging mechanistic possibility is that acute exercise impacts cognitive performance via neuroendocrinological changes. Specifically, it is thought that acute exercise may increase neurotransmitters such as the catecholamine norepinephrine and 5-hydroxytryptamine (serotonin) (Cooper, 1973). Serotonin and norepinephrine are understood to be important to proper cognitive function, and there is consistent evidence that an acute bout of exercise increases serum catecholamine levels (Chmura et al., 1994; McMorris et al., 1999; Zouhal, Jacob, Delamarche, & Gratas-Delamarche, 2008). However, it is still not clear whether or not or to what degree these changes reflect catecholamine and serotonin levels in the brain, as current techniques for measuring those levels are too invasive for human research.

Research with nonhuman animals has been fairly consistent in demonstrating that acute exercise increases cerebral catecholamines and serotonin (Ahmadiasl, Alaei, & Hanninen, 2003; Meeusen, Piacentini, & De Meirleir, 2001). One such study (Pagliari & Peyrin, 1995) found that cerebral norepinephrine and catecholamine metabolite levels increased significantly during treadmill exercise and lasted for approximately one hour following exercise cessation. Ahmadiasl and colleagues (2003) extended this literature by demonstrating a relationship between the amount of increase in cerebral norepinephrine and the amount of improvement in performance on a common learning and memory task (the Morris water maze). Thus these animal studies generally suggest that acute exercise results in increases in catecholamines and serotonin and that these changes are related to cognitive performance.

However, it is unclear whether exercise-induced increases in serotonin and catecholamines have a beneficial effect on cognitive performance in humans. Several empirical studies illustrate the equivocal state of the human literature. McMorris,

Collard, Corbett, Dicks, and Swain (2008) measured plasma metabolites of norepinephrine and dopamine following a rest condition or an acute bout of cycling at either 40% or 80% maximum power output. Though metabolites increased as a function of exercise intensity, cognitive performance did not improve as a function of exercise. A later study (McMorris et al., 2009) with a similar design showed increases in catecholamine and cortisol and decrements in cognitive performance on reaction time and flankers tasks during strenuous aerobic exercise. Though this later study suggests a role for exercise-induced catecholamines in cognitive performance, it seems to predict a deleterious effect. The results of both of these studies contrast with earlier research (Chmura et al., 1994; McMorris et al., 1999) that showed positive effects for cognition as a result of exercise at or above the adrenaline and noradrenaline thresholds. Finally, a study by Winter and colleagues (2007) compared participants' ability to learn and retain lists of words following rest, moderate aerobic running, and intense anaerobic running. Winter et al. found that not only did the participants who did intense anaerobic running exhibit improved list learning over the other two groups, but they also experienced the steepest increases in plasma catecholamine and dopamine levels.

In sum, though there is evidence from nonhuman animal studies that increases in cerebral levels of norepinephrine and serotonin occur as a function of acute exercise and that these increases are related to improvements in cognitive performance, the evidence from human studies is much less clear.

Chronic Exercise

The chronic exercise literature has been summarized meta-analytically on several occasions. The first meta-analysis in this area (Etnier et al., 1997) was comprehensive, in that it included studies using both cross-sectional and experimental designs, acute and chronic exercise paradigms, and all age groups. Results for the chronic exercise paradigms indicated that across age groups, chronic physical activity had a small effect on cognitive performance (effect size[ES] = 0.33). When randomized controlled trials (RCTs) were examined separately, the average ES across age groups was 0.18. Meta-analyses that have been conducted subsequently have been designed to further identify the potential role of physical activity in children and older adults. Sibley and Etnier (2003) summarized the results from 44 studies testing the effects with children and found an average

ES of 0.32. Several meta-analytic reviews have limited their focus to RCTs with older adults. Colcombe and Kramer (2003) reported an average ES of 0.48 from 18 studies with older adults that were identified as using experimental designs. Angevaren et al. (2008) reported on 11 RCTs with older adults without cognitive impairment and reported small effects for certain cognitive functions when compared with other types of interventions (cognitive speed ES=0.26; visual attention ES=0.26) and moderate-to-large effects when compared with no-treatment controls (auditory attention ES=0.52; motor function ES=1.17). However, for nine other cognitive functions Angevaren et al. reported effect sizes that were not significantly different from zero for both comparison groups (i.e., other types of interventions and no-treatment controls). Heyn, Abreu, and Ottenbacher (2004) summarized results for studies that they identified as being RCTs with older adults with cognitive impairment and reported a moderate effect (ES=0.57). Based on the findings of these meta-analyses, the extant literature shows that participation in a chronic exercise intervention is associated with improvements in cognitive performance, that the magnitude of the effect is in the small-to-moderate range, and that there is evidence with older adults that this is a causal relationship.

A number of prospective studies have also been conducted to examine the relationship between current levels of physical activity and subsequent changes in cognitive performance. In these studies, physical activity and cognitive performance have been measured at baseline and then cognitive performance has been measured again 3–21 years later. Some of these studies have focused on clinical outcomes (e.g., Alzheimer's disease, vascular dementia, and other forms of dementia), while others have used performance on standardized tests of general cognition (e.g., Mini Mental Status Exam, Telephone Interview for Cognitive Status) or on batteries of cognitive tests. These studies have been conducted exclusively with older adults (>59 years). The results from prospective studies are mixed. Fourteen studies support a protective effect of physical activity participation on cognitive performance (Abbott et al., 2004; Albert et al., 1995; Barnes, Yaffe, Satariano, & Tager, 2003; Karp et al., 2006; Larson et al., 2006; Laurin, Verreault, Lindsay, MacPherson, & Rockwood, 2001; Lindsay et al., 2002; Lytle, Vander Bilt, Pandav, Dodge, & Ganguli, 2004; Podewils et al., 2005; Rovio et al., 2005; van Gelder et al., 2004; Weuve et al., 2004; Yaffe, Barnes, Nevitt, Lui, & Covinsky, 2001; Yoshitake et al., 1995).

Six studies fail to support this relationship (Broe et al., 1998; Dik, Deeg, Visser, & Jonker, 2003; Sturman et al., 2005; Verghese et al., 2003; Wilson et al., 2002; Yamada et al., 2003). With the exception of Barnes et al. (2003), the prospective studies all suffer from the limitation that they relied on self-report measures of physical activity. Although many self-report measures of physical activity have been shown to provide valid estimates of physical activity behavior (Pereira et al., 1997; Sallis et al., 1985; Sirard & Pate, 2001), the use of self-report measures clearly increases the error inherent in the estimate of the independent variable. Additionally, most of the prospective studies have used self-report measures of physical activity without established psychometrics, potentially further decreasing the accuracy of the measurement of the independent variable. Despite this serious limitation, prospective studies with larger sample sizes have tended to support the role of physical activity as protective against age-related cognitive decline (Etnier, 2009a), and higher levels of aerobic fitness have also been shown to protect against cognitive decline (Barnes et al., 2003).

In general, the evidence regarding the effects of chronic physical activity on cognitive performance is supportive of a beneficial effect. However, the bulk of the research has focused on older adults. Although there is also a body of literature with children, this literature is not nearly as well developed in quantity, design, or interest in mechanisms. For example, Sibley and Etnier (2003) reviewed 44 studies in this area and reported that only nine were published articles that used experimental designs. Since that time, we are aware of only one additional RCT in which the effects of physical activity on cognitive performance were tested in children (Davis et al., 2007). Given that a statistically reliable effect of physical activity on cognitive performance has been reported (Sibley & Etnier, 2003) and that improving the cognitive performance of school-aged children is of great interest, this area of research is deserving of attention.

Theoretical Basis

Several theories have been proposed to explain the potential beneficial effects of chronic physical activity on cognitive performance. The frontal lobe hypothesis and the cognitive reserve hypothesis can be logically applied to explain the benefits of chronic physical activity on cognitive performance. Other theories are more mechanistic and focus on potential physiological mediators of the effects of physical activity on cognitive performance.

FRONTAL LOBE HYPOTHESES

Evidence that physical activity is more benefi-cial to the cognitive performance of children and of older adults than it is for younger adults is con-sistent with frontal lobe hypotheses of development and of aging. With respect to development, there is evidence that the frontal lobe and the ability to perform frontal lobe–dependent tasks develop relatively late during adolescence (Giedd, 2008; Jurado & Rosselli, 2007). With respect to aging, the frontal-aging hypothesis suggests that advanc-ing age results in selective deterioration of cerebral regions that include frontal and prefrontal areas of the brain (Dempster, 1992; West, 1996). As applied to the beneficial effects of physical activity on cog-nitive performance, the implication is that physi-cal activity should be particularly beneficial to the performance of executive control tasks that depend on frontal and prefrontal brain regions (Kramer et al., 1999). Empirical evidence (Davis et al., 2007; Kramer et al., 1999) showing that participation in a chronic physical activity program by children and older adults results in significant improvements in executive function measures, but not in perfor-mance of nonexecutive tasks, supports the viability of the frontal-aging hypothesis, as does the meta-analytic finding that effects are significantly larger for executive processes than for other cognitive pro-cesses (Colcombe & Kramer, 2003).

COGNITIVE RESERVE HYPOTHESIS

The cognitive reserve hypothesis was originally proposed to explain age-related declines in cogni-tive performance. This hypothesis suggests that individuals with greater cognitive reserves will expe-rience less age-related cognitive decline and have less risk of dementia (Fratiglioni, Paillard-Borg, & Winblad, 2004; Scarmeas & Stern, 2003; Whalley, Deary, Appleton, & Starr, 2004). The application to physical activity derives from the further suppo-sition that cognitive reserves are enhanced by life-style factors that include physical activity (Whalley et al., 2004). Thus individuals who are more physi-cally active are expected to have greater cognitive reserves, which then enable them to perform well cognitively even in the face of advancing age or other variables (e.g., chronic illness or a genetic pre-disposition to Alzheimer's disease) that are expected to reduce cognitive reserves. Evidence supporting this hypothesis comes from studies demonstrating that the largest effects of physical activity on cogni-tion are evident in those persons expected to have the greatest demands on their cognitive reserves.

For example, research showing that persons who are at genetic risk for Alzheimer's disease benefit more from physical activity or aerobic fitness than those without such risk factors (Deeny et al., 2008; Etnier et al., 2007; Rovio et al., 2005; Schuit, Feskens, Launer, & Kromhout, 2001) supports this hypoth-esis. Although the cognitive reserves themselves have not been clearly operationalized, it has been proposed that a person's cognitive reserves are deter-mined by cerebral morphology, cerebral function, or both (Stern et al., 2005; Whalley et al., 2004).

Underlying Mechanisms

Recent research has focused on the physiological mechanisms that may explain precisely how chronic physical activity serves to benefit cognitive perfor-mance. Much of this research has been conducted using nonhuman animal models, which allows for tight control of experimental conditions and for the use of invasive measurement procedures to directly assess proposed mechanisms. Research with humans is limited by our dependence on noninvasive tech-niques, but indirect evidence and evidence from neuroimaging techniques are available for each mechanism. The mechanisms that are currently con-sidered the most plausible involve cerebral structure, cerebral function, cerebral blood flow, neurotrophic factors, and oxidative stress.

CEREBRAL STRUCTURE

One mechanism by which exercise is thought to affect cognition is through its impact on cerebral structure. Humans experience decreases in cerebral gray and white matter as they age (Bartzokis et al., 2001; Good et al., 2001; Guttmann et al., 1998; Lim, Zipursky, Watts, & Pfefferbaum, 1992; Sowell et al., 2003). Further, this age-related cerebral tissue loss begins in humans as early as when they are in their 30s (Jernigan et al., 2001; Raz, 2000), and the rate of loss increases with advancing age (Resnick, Pham, Kraut, Zonderman, & Davatzikos, 2003). However, age-related cerebral tissue loss does not appear to occur at the same rate across all regions of the brain. Some brain regions have been identified as particularly susceptible to aging effects, with losses appearing most prominently in prefrontal regions, temporal cortices, and anterior tracts (Colcombe et al., 2003; Gunning-Dixon, Brickman, Cheng, & Alexopoulos, 2009). These losses in cerebral tis-sue largely parallel the observation of age-related declines in particular types of cognitive performance (Colcombe et al., 2003), and multiple studies have reported associations between the rate or amount of gray and white matter loss in specific cerebral regions and age-related declines in memory, executive function, and information processing speed (Gunning-Dixon et al., 2009; Oosterman et al., 2008a, 2008b; Rabbitt et al., 2008). Additionally, decrements in brain volume that threaten the integrity of white matter tracts can result in losses of connectivity in the corpus callosum (Gunning-Dixon et al., 2009), which is responsible for much of the crosstalk between brain hemispheres.

Though it was once thought that cerebral structure development ceased after a certain age, the central nervous system is now thought to be more dynamic, with evidence that new neuronal cells can develop even into advanced age (Galvan & Bredesen, 2007). In particular, evidence suggests that regular participation in physical activity has a beneficial effect on cerebral structure. For example, recent research using nonhuman animal models has demonstrated effects of physical activity on neuronal birth and development. Van Praag and colleagues have shown that adult rodents who are given access to running wheels experience increased neurogenesis as compared with rodents who are not given this access (van Praag, Christie, Sejnowski, & Gage, 1999; van Praag, Kempermann, & Gage, 1999) and that cell survival also is greater for rodents in the running condition (van Praag, Christie, et al., 1999). Van Praag, Shubert, Zhao, and Gage (2005) found that exercise increased the number of new cells in both young and old rodents. Though older mice in the exercise group did not develop as many new cells as younger mice in the exercise group, they developed similar numbers of neurons as did younger mice in a no-activity control condition.

Other researchers have been interested in the effects of "enriched" environments on cognitive performance and cerebral structure. In studies exploring this question, animals are randomly assigned to a variety of conditions, including an enriched environment that allows for physical activity and includes opportunities for exploration. Results from these studies demonstrate that animals raised in an enriched environment that includes physical activity exhibit better learning (Milgram et al., 2005) and develop more new synapses than those in control conditions (Black, Isaacs, Anderson, Alcantara, & Greenough, 1990; Isaacs, Anderson, Alcantara, Black, & Greenough, 1992; Kleim, Lussnig, Schwarz, Comery, & Greenough, 1996; Kleim et al., 1998; Kleim, Vij, Ballard, & Greenough, 1997). This area of inquiry is receiving increasing attention as researchers become interested in applying the idea of an enriched environment to studies with humans. In fact, this notion is supported by the finding from the meta-analysis by Colcombe and Kramer (2003) that studies combining aerobic exercise with resistance exercise demonstrate significantly larger effects than studies using only aerobic exercise.

Research with humans using neuroimaging techniques has also shown that aerobic fitness and physical activity may attenuate age-related cerebral tissue loss and cognitive decline (Colcombe et al., 2003, 2006; Gordon et al., 2008; Marks et al., 2007). In cross-sectional studies with older adults, Colcombe and colleagues (2003) found that greater gray matter tissue density was associated with higher levels of aerobic fitness, Gordon et al. (2008) demonstrated significant preservation of cerebral volume as a function of aerobic fitness, and Marks and colleagues (2007) reported that higher aerobic fitness was associated with greater integrity of white matter tracts. In an experimental study, Colcombe et al. (2006) compared the effects of a six-month aerobic training intervention and a stretching-and-toning program on cerebral volume in older adults. Results showed significant increases in both gray and white matter volume in the aerobic training group but not in the stretching and toning group. Lastly, Rovio and colleagues (2010) found that midlife physical activity levels were negatively associated with gray matter loss in later life. Together, the research consistently shows a beneficial impact of physical activity and fitness on cerebral structure, with some studies simultaneously demonstrating these effects on behavioral measures of cognitive performance.

CEREBRAL FUNCTION

Another mechanism that has been proposed to explain the benefits of physical activity for cognitive performance is improved cerebral function. Much of the research in this area has employed neuroelectric indices of cognitive functioning, such as ERPs.

Themanson and Hillman (2006) compared ERPs between high- and low-fit adults performing a flankers task prior to and following an acute bout of exercise. Results were interpreted as showing that high-fit individuals exhibited better attentional allocation and control, especially following an error, than did low-fit individuals. McDowell, Kerick, Santa Maria, and Hatfield (2003) compared the P300 components of young and old low-fit and high-fit participants during an oddball task. An oddball task is one in which participants are shown a series of frequent stimuli that do not require an action, occasionally interrupted by a stimulus that requires an action. McDowell et al. found that the older high-fit group exhibited a P300 profile similar to those of the younger groups, which did not differ based on fitness. Thus their results support a conclusion that the relationship between aerobic fitness and neurocognitive measures is moderated by age, such that there is a relationship for older adults but not younger adults. When these effects are tested in children, however, there is also evidence for benefits of aerobic fitness on cognitive function. Hillman, Buck, Themanson, Pontifex, and Castelli (2009) reported that high-fit children exhibited greater P300 amplitude (indicative of the allocation of greater attentional resources) during a flankers task than did low-fit children. In general, these studies and others (Prakash et al., 2007; Stroth et al., 2009) have been fairly consistent in reporting positive associations between aerobic fitness and measures of cerebral function, thus supporting this as a potential mechanism of the relationship between chronic physical activity and cognitive performance.

CEREBRAL BLOOD FLOW

Altered cerebral blood flow is another mechanism that has been proposed to explain the effects of chronic physical activity on cognitive performance. It is hypothesized that regular participation in physical activity improves cognitive function by increasing delivery of nutrients and oxygen to the relevant regions of the brain. Using xenon clearance techniques, researchers have shown that acute bouts of exercise result in increases in regional cerebral blood flow (Herholz et al., 1987; Jorgensen, Perko, & Secher, 1992; Thomas, Schroeder, Secher, & Mitchell, 1989). However, evidence for the effects of chronic physical activity on cerebral blood flow is much less well developed.

Studies with nonhuman animals have typically shown that voluntary exercise results in changes to the structure of the brain that would be expected to positively affect cerebral blood flow. Black et al. (1990) found that rats that received chronic physical exercise because of access to a running wheel developed a greater density of cerebral blood vessels than rats assigned to inactive, forced exercise, or acrobatic (obstacle course) conditions. Van Praag and colleagues (2005) reported increased vascular quality in young mice assigned to a running condition as compared with those in a no-exercise control condition. Additionally, increases in vascular surface area and in blood vessel perimeter were observed in the active mice. It therefore appears that exercise results

in greater angiogenesis, which would be expected to benefit cerebral blood flow.

Only one study has been conducted with humans that demonstrates differences in cerebral blood flow as a function of physical activity participation. In a cross-sectional design, Rogers, Meyer, and Mortel (1990) reported that retired older adults who were not physically active experienced significant declines in cerebral blood flow that were not evident in older adults who continued to work or who were retired but physically active. Future research is necessary to further develop our understanding of the role of cerebral blood flow in explaining the effects of physical activity on cognitive performance.

NEUROTROPHIC FACTORS

Neurotrophic factors offer another possible mechanism for the effects of physical activity on cognitive performance. The best-developed empirical evidence for such a mechanism relates to brain-derived neurotrophic factor (BDNF). BDNF plays a critical role in neuronal development and cell survival (Cotman & Engesser-Cesar, 2002), and research supports the impact of BDNF on both regional and global brain volume (Lipsky & Marini, 2007; Toro et al., 2009). It is also believed that BDNF is critical for proper cognitive function, especially in learning and memory tasks (Lipsky & Marini, 2007).

Animal studies have shown that exercise increases BDNF levels in the brain, specifically in the hippocampus (Cotman & Berchtold, 2002; Vaynman & Gomez-Pinilla, 2006), an area heavily involved in learning and memory. Additionally, studies have shown that exercise-induced increases in BDNF are associated with improvements in learning and spatial memory in rats performing cognitively demanding tasks such as the Morris water maze (Vaynman & Gomez-Pinilla, 2005). Lastly, blockage of BDNF activity in animal models has been shown to eliminate the positive effects of exercise on learning and memory (Ang & Gomez-Pinilla, 2007; Gomez-Pinilla, 2008; Vaynman & Gomez-Pinilla, 2006).

Human research has also provided evidence of the relationship between BDNF and cognitive performance and of the effects of physical activity on BDNF. Specifically, humans with BDNF dysfunction exhibit reduced learning abilities, and decreased BDNF levels are commonly found in persons with age-related dementia (Vaynman & Gomez-Pinilla, 2005). Additionally, there is evidence that single bouts of exercise increase serum BDNF levels in humans (Ferris, Williams, & Shen, 2007; Gold et al., 2003; Gustafsson et al., 2009;

Rojas Vega et al., 2006; Tang, Chu, Hui, Helmeste, & Law, 2008) and that well-trained athletes have higher levels of serum BDNF than do untrained participants (Zoladz et al., 2008).

Although evidence regarding the importance of BDNF for cognitive performance is compelling and animal evidence regarding the effects of physical activity on BDNF levels is promising, research testing the effects of regular physical activity on BDNF in humans is in its infancy. Further, the evidence from human studies is limited by our inability to assess cerebral levels of BDNF. The lack of a clear understanding of the relationship between serum levels and cerebral levels of BDNF is a major limitation of this line of research.

OXIDATIVE STRESS

A final proposed mechanism for the effect of chronic physical activity on cognitive performance is based on the free radical theory of aging. The free radical theory of aging (Harman, 1956, 1969, 1972, 1994) predicts that with advancing age comes an increase in the production of free radicals, a decrease in the quantity or quality of antioxidants, or both. The result is an increase in overall level of oxidative stress. The brain is particularly vulnerable to oxidative insults (Fukui et al., 2002), and the free radical theory posits that the damage caused by increased oxidative stress plays a role in age-related cognitive decline and the risk of dementia (Berr, 2000; Butterfield, Howard, Yatin, Allen, & Carney, 1997; Clausen, Doctrow, & Baudry, 2010; Hasnis & Reznick, 2003; Joseph et al., 1998; Liu & Ames, 2005; Meydani, 1999).

Although the results are not unequivocal, the free radical theory of aging has generally been supported by studies that have observed an age-related shift in the prooxidant–antioxidant balance (redox status) toward greater oxidative stress (Berr, 2000; Droge & Schipper, 2007; Hasnis & Reznick, 2003; Junqueira et al., 2004; Meydani, 2001; Polidori, 2003; Sohal & Weindruch, 1996). Additionally, studies in which oxidative stress was induced in younger mice have consistently demonstrated decrements in cognitive function such as are typically observed in older animals (Fukui et al., 2002; Joseph, Shukitt-Hale, Casadesus, & Fisher, 2005). Human studies employing chronic exercise programs have produced consistent evidence for a direct, protective effect of exercise against oxidative stress (Ji, 2001, 2002). For example, Fatouros and colleagues (2004) found that older men participating in a 16-week aerobic exercise program showed significant increases in protective factors against oxidative stress and reductions in several oxidative stress markers. However, on program completion, individuals who returned to baseline levels of physical activity also returned to baseline levels of oxidative stress.

SUMMARY

Overall, the mechanisms underlying the relationship between chronic exercise and cognition remain unclear. It is likely that no one proposed mechanism acts in isolation, but rather that multiple systems interact and influence one another (Etnier, 2008). Future research will benefit from considering more than one mechanism and from using statistical techniques that allow for the assessment of these potential mechanisms as mediators of the relationship.

Moderators

Several variables have been identified as potentially moderating the effects of chronic physical activity on cognitive performance. The identification of moderators is important because it can provide insights into dose–response questions and enable the identification of subgroups that could particularly benefit from physical activity participation. The variables that have been identified thus far as moderators include age, apolipoprotein E, gender, and hormone replacement therapy.

AGE

Age has been mentioned throughout this chapter as important in the relationship between chronic physical activity and cognitive performance. As discussed with regard to the frontal lobe hypotheses, physical activity is predicted to have greater benefits for children because their frontal lobes are developing and for older adults because of age-related structural decline in frontal lobe. In their meta-analytic review, Etnier et al. (1997) found that age was a significant moderator of the relationship between chronic physical activity participation and cognitive performance. Both "older adults" (45–60 years) and "younger adults" (18–30 years) showed significantly larger effects than the oldest adults (60–90 years); older adults also showed significantly greater effects than "adults" (30–45 years). Although these findings appear not to be consistent with the expectation that younger and older adults would experience the greatest benefits, Etnier et al. interpreted them in light of the cognitive reserve hypothesis and suggested that physical activity might be most beneficial to those who are slightly resource limited (i.e., older and younger adults) as compared with those who have no resource limitations (i.e., adults) or those who have substantial resource limitations (oldest adults and children). Among older adults, Colcombe and Kramer (2003) reported a further significant moderating effect of age group, such that studies with participants who were "mid-old" (66–70 years) had significantly larger effects than studies with "old-old" (71–80 years) or "young-old" (55–65 years) participants. Given the importance of nurturing cognitive development in children and the value of maintaining cognitive performance in older adults, additional research with these age groups is of obvious importance. However, it is important to point out that physical activity by young adults may not affect cognitive performance in an observable way, but may increase cognitive reserves, thus protecting young adults against future age-,stress-, or health-related cognitive insults. Empirical studies designed to test the effects of physical activity on various age groups will be necessary to further our understanding of the potential moderating role of age on the physical activity–cognition relationship.

APOLIPOPROTEIN E

The apolipoprotein E epsilon 4 allele (*APOE* ε4) is a major risk factor for the development of Alzheimer's disease (Corder et al., 1993; Farrer et al., 1997; Gomez-Isla et al., 1996; Mayeux et al., 1993; Myers et al., 1996; Poirier et al., 1993; Saunders et al., 1993). In nondemented individuals, *APOE* ε4 carrier status has also been associated with poorer cognitive performance, as well as earlier onset and a greater rate of age-related cognitive decline in carriers versus non-carriers (Blazer, Fillenbaum, & Burchett, 2001; Dik et al., 2001; Jonker, Schmand, Lindeboom, Havekes, & Launer, 1998; Gonzalez McNeal et al., 2001; O'Hara et al., 1998; Riley et al., 2000; Yaffe, Cauley, Sands, & Browner, 1997).

Given this relationship, several researchers have tested the potentially differential effects of physical activity for individuals carrying the *APOE* ε4 allele as compared with noncarriers. In a prospective study, Schuit et al. (2001) tested 390 nondemented men aged 65–84 years at baseline and three years later. Participation in physical activity for more than 1 hour per day was associated with a decrease in the risk of cognitive decline for the ApoE ε4 carriers (odds ratio [*OR*]=1.0 for active participants, *OR*=3.7 for inactive participants) but did not significantly affect the risk of decline for noncarriers (*OR*=1.0 for active, *OR*=0.8 for inactive). Similar findings were reported in a prospective study by

Rovio et al. (2005), who assessed physical activity during "midlife" (39–64 years) and then diagnosed participants for dementia and Alzheimer's disease approximately 21 years later (65–79 years). Participants who reported leisure-time physical activity had a reduced risk of dementia (*OR*=0.47) and Alzheimer's disease (*OR*=0.35) as compared with sedentary individuals. However, physical activity was significantly protective only for the *APOE* ε4 carriers. As compared with sedentary *APOE* ε4 carriers, physically active *APOE* ε4 carriers had less risk of dementia (*OR*=0.38) and of AD (*OR*=0.18).

Using a cross-sectional design, Etnier and colleagues (2007) demonstrated that the relationship between aerobic fitness and cognitive performance in older women (51–81 years) was also moderated by *APOE* genotype. Positive associations between aerobic fitness and cognitive performance were found for the *APOE* ε4 homozygotes (persons with two copies of the ε4 allele), but no significant relationship was found for the *APOE* ε4 heterozygotes (persons with one copy of the ε4 allele) or the *APOE* ε4 noncarriers. Deeny and colleagues (2008) also used a cross-sectional design to test the interactive effects of *APOE* genotype and physical activity level on working memory and cerebral activation in older adults (50–70 years). Results showed that physical activity was predictive of better working memory performance and cerebral activation patterns for the *APOE* ε4 carriers but not for the noncarriers. Specifically, active carriers exhibited decreased reaction times, as well as higher cortical activation in the right temporal lobe, when completing more difficult portions of a working memory task.

In contrast to these four studies, Podewils et al. (2005) found that beneficial effects of physical activity were evident only for *APOE* ε4 noncarriers. They examined the relationship between baseline physical activity and the development of dementia over 5.4 years in adults over 65 years old. Compared with the noncarriers with the lowest energy expenditures and who engaged in the fewest physical activities, the noncarriers who had the highest energy expenditures or performed the most physical activities had significantly lower hazard ratios (0.68 and 0.44, respectively). However, for *APOE* ε4 carriers, the hazard ratios were not significantly different from 1.0 as a function of either measure of physical activity.

Thus the evidence suggests that physical activity interacts with *APOE* genotype to predict cognitive performance and the risk of Alzheimer's disease. In particular, several studies suggest that physical activity and aerobic fitness are most beneficial for older adults who are at genetic risk for Alzheimer's disease. However, the conflicting findings reported by Podewils et al. (2005) emphasize the need for future research in this area and the importance of understanding the mechanisms through which physical activity influences cognition.

GENDER

There is some evidence that physical activity is more important for the maintenance of cognitive function in older women than in older men. Laurin et al. (2001) conducted a prospective study in which they tested 6,434 community-dwelling, cognitively normal men and women over 65 years of age at baseline and then again five years later. Results indicated that women who participated in the most physical activity had less risk of cognitive impairment (50% less risk), dementia (50% less risk), and Alzheimer's disease (60% less risk) than women who were sedentary. No significant effect of physical activity on cognitive performance was observed for the men in the study. Findings from the meta-analysis by Colcombe and Kramer (2003) also support the role of gender as a moderator of the relationship between physical activity and cognitive performance. Their results indicated that studies in which the sample was more than 50% female yielded significantly larger effects than did studies in which the sample was predominantly male (≥50%).

The research demonstrating differential effects of physical activity on cognitive performance as a function of gender has been conducted only with older adults. The role of gender as a moderator with younger samples has not been established.

HORMONE REPLACEMENT THERAPY

In older adults, the moderating role of gender on the effects of chronic physical activity on cognitive performance may be linked to estrogen. Many researchers have suggested that the decrease in estrogen that accompanies menopause has a deleterious effect on the cognitive functioning of older women (Drake et al., 2000; Kampen & Sherwin, 1994; Phillips & Sherwin, 1992; Sherwin, 1994). Relatedly, it has been suggested that physical activity might be more important for older women than for older men because of the potential importance of estrogen in cognitive function. Estrogen may be neuroprotective in women, and there may be a critical window of time during which providing exogenous estrogen is beneficial to women experiencing menopause. Animal research has shown that the

provision of estrogen to rodents that have had their ovaries surgically removed (surgicallyinduced menopause) benefits memory performance (Gibbs, 2000). Kampen and Sherwin (1994) demonstrated that postmenopausal women who were taking estrogen performed better on paragraph recall tests than did women who were not taking estrogen. Phillips and Sherwin (1992) tested cognitive performance in women prior to and following surgery to remove the uterus and both ovaries. Those women who were treated with estrogen after surgery maintained their level of performance on a memory test, while women who received a placebo experienced declines in memory from pretest to posttest.

Most germane to this chapter, researchers have examined the potential interactive effects of physical activity and hormone replacement therapy (HRT) on cognitive performance in postmenopausal women. Etnier and Sibley (2004) found that self-reported physical activity was predictive of better performance on a digit–symbol substitution task and the Trail Making Test, but did not observe any interactive effects with the use of HRT. However, Etnier and Sibley operationalized HRT use by dividing participants into those currently using HRT and those currently not using HRT. Thus they were not able to examine potential differences in the relationship as a function of the duration of use of HRT. Erickson et al. (2007) categorized postmenopausal women as "never" users, short-term users (up to 10 years), medium-term users (11–15 years), and long-term users (16 or more years). These four categories of women were not significantly different in age. Thus, the significant interactive effect of HRT use and aerobic fitness on the number of perseverative errors in the Wisconsin Card Sorting Task was not confounded by age effects. Therefore, the authors concluded that their results demonstrated that aerobic fitness had a larger effect on cognitive performance as the duration of use of HRT increased. These authors also used magnetic resonance imaging (MRI) to obtain measures of cortical volume. The cerebral structure data closely resembled the performance data: Cerebral volume decreased with increasing length of use of HRT, but the effects of aerobic fitness ameliorated these decreases.

Berchtold et al. (2001) conducted a study with ovariectomized rats that also supported an interactive relationship between physical activity and estrogen. Their results showed that exercise increased BDNF levels in rats that had been without estrogen for only a short time, but that exercise had no effect on BDNF in rats that had been without estrogen for a longer time. However, rats that exercised and that received estrogen replacement for a long time experienced the greatest gains in BDNF.

Evidence suggesting that estrogen is predictive of cognitive performance and that chronic physical activity and HRT use have an interactive effect on cognitive performance in postmenopausal women clearly suggests that this area of research is worth pursuing. Given that women are at greater risk of Alzheimer's disease than men (Aronson et al., 1990; Farrer et al., 1997; Gorelick & Bozzola, 1991) and that the population of older women is increasing rapidly, the public health implications are evident.

Summary and Conclusions

Since Spirduso's seminal study in 1975, our knowledge regarding the potential effects of physical activity on cognitive performance has increased greatly. Evidence clearly suggests that both acute bouts of exercise and regular participation in physical activity result in enhanced performance on a variety of cognitive tasks.

In the acute exercise literature, this effect is generally small, but larger effects may be evident when exercise intensity is appropriate for the particular type of cognitive task to be performed. In particular, evidence suggests that high-intensity exercise results in performance gains on relatively simple cognitive tasks, while moderate-intensity exercise is more beneficial for complex cognitive tasks. Further research in this area is necessary to enhance our understanding of mechanisms responsible for the effects, of dose–response issues (especially with regard to exercise duration), of the temporal durability of the effects postexercise, and of variables that may moderate the effects, such as cognitive task type, participant fitness, and time of day. However, it is certainly reasonable to suggest that participation in physical activity has the potential to positively affect cognitive performance on the same day as the activity. The implications are clear for those interested in using physical activity to enhance cognition and are relevant to the promotion of physical activity in a variety of settings, including schools, the workplace, and retirement communities.

In the chronic exercise literature, the effect of physical activity on cognitive performance clearly seems to be moderated by age, with moderate-to-large effects evident for young and older adults and with small effects evident for children. Empirical results suggest that effects of chronic physical activity are also task dependent and are moderated by additional variables including gender, ApoE genotype, and HRT use. Studies testing underlying mechanisms generally support the potential role of changes in cerebral structure and changes in cerebral blood flow and suggest that oxidative stress may also be important in the relationship between physical activity and cognition. Future research in this area will likely focus on identifying ways to further enhance the effect of physical activity by looking at combined interventions (e.g., interventions that include both physical activity and cognitive challenges, or interventions that include both physical activity and a diet that is high in antioxidants). Clearly, we need to improve our understanding of dose–response issues so that we will one day be able to prescribe a physical activity regimen designed to protect or improve cognitive performance. However, the evidence clearly suggests that regular participation in physical activity can benefit cognitive performance in persons of all ages, but that the amount of benefit is likely to be greater for those who would be predicted to benefit the most according to the cognitive reserve hypothesis—children, older adults, older adults at genetic risk for Alzheimer's disease, and older postmenopausal women who are on HRT.

References

Abbott, R. D., White, L. R., Ross, G. W., Masaki, K. H., Curb, J. D., & Petrovitch, H. (2004). Walking and dementia in physically capable elderly men. *JAMA, 292*(12), 1447–1453.

Ahmadiasl, N., Alaei, H., & Hanninen, O. (2003). Effect of exercise on learning, memory and levels of epinephrine in rats' hippocampus. *Journal of Sports Science and Medicine, 2*, 106–109.

Albert, M. S., Jones, K., Savage, C. R., Berkman, L., Seeman, T., Blazer, D., & Rowe, J. W. (1995). Predictors of cognitive change in older persons: MacArthur studies of successful aging. *Psychology and Aging, 10*(4), 578–589.

Ang, E. T., & Gomez-Pinilla, F. (2007). Potential therapeutic effects of exercise to the brain. *Current Medical Chemistry, 14*, 2564–2571.

Angevaren, M., Aufdemkampe, G., Verhaar, H. J., Aleman, A., & Vanhees, L. (2008). Physical activity and enhanced fitness to improve cognitive function in older people without known cognitive impairment. *Cochrane Database of Systematic Reviews, (3)*, CD005381.

Arent, S. M., & Landers, D. M. (2003). Arousal, anxiety, and performance: A reexamination of the inverted-U hypothesis. *Research Quarterly for Exercise & Sport, 74*(4), 436–444.

Aronson, M. K., Ooi, W. L., Morgenstern, H., Hafner, A., Masur, D., Crystal, H.,...Katzman, R. (1990). Women, myocardial infarction, and dementia in the very old. *Neurology, 40*(7), 1102–1106.

Audiffren, M. (2009). Acute exercise and psychological functions: A cognitive-energetic approach. In T. McMorris, P. D. Tomporowski, & M. Audiffren (Eds.), *Exercise and cognitive function* (pp. 1–40). Hoboken, NJ: Wiley-Blackwell.

Audiffren, M., Tomporowski, P. D., & Zagrodnik, J. (2008). Acute aerobic exercise and information processing: Energizing motor processes during a choice reaction time task. *Acta Psychologica (Amsterdam), 129*(3), 410–419.

Barnes, D. E., Yaffe, K., Satariano, W. A., & Tager, I. B. (2003). A longitudinal study of cardiorespiratory fitness and cognitive function in healthy older adults. *Journal of the American Geriatrics Society, 51*(4), 459–465.

Bartzokis, G., Beckson, M., Lu, P. H., Nuechterlein, K. H., Edwards, N., & Mintz, J. (2001). Age-related changes in frontal and temporal lobe volumes in men. *Archives of General Psychiatry, 58*, 461–465.

Berchtold, N. C., Kesslak, J. P., Pike, C. J., Adlard, P. A., & Cotman, C. W. (2001). Estrogen and exercise interact to regulate brain-derived neurotrophic factor mRNA and protein expression in the hippocampus. *European Journal of Neuroscience, 14*(12), 1992–2002.

Berr, C. (2000). Cognitive impairment and oxidative stress in the elderly: Results of epidemiological studies. *Biofactors, 13*(1–4), 205–209.

Black, J. E., Isaacs, K. R., Anderson, B. J., Alcantara, A. A., & Greenough, W. T. (1990). Learning causes synaptogenesis, whereas motor activity causes angiogenesis, in cerebellar cortex of adult rats. *Proceedings of the National Academy of Sciences of the United States of America, 87*(14), 5568–5572.

Blazer, D. G., Fillenbaum, G., & Burchett, B. (2001). The APOE-E4 allele and the risk of functional decline in a community sample of African American and White older adults. *Journals of Gerontology, Series A: Biological Sciences and Medical Sciences, 56*(12), M785–M789.

Brisswalter, J., Collardeau, M., & Rene, A. (2002). Effects of acute physical exercise characteristics on cognitive performance. *Sports Medicine, 32*(9), 555–566.

Brisswalter, J., Durand, M., Delignieres, D., & Legros, P. (1995). Optimal and non-optimal demand in a dual-task of pedaling and simple reaction time: Effects on energy expenditure and cognitive performance. *Journal of Human Movement Studies, 29*, 15–34.

Broe, G. A., Creasey, H., Jorm, A. F., Bennett, H. P., Casey, B., Waite, L. M.,...Cullen, J. (1998). Health habits and risk of cognitive impairment and dementia in old age: A prospective study on the effects of exercise, smoking and alcohol consumption. *Australian and New Zealand Journal of Public Health, 22*(5), 621–623.

Butterfield, D. A., Howard, B. J., Yatin, S., Allen, K. L., & Carney, J. M. (1997). Free radical oxidation of brain proteins in accelerated senescence and its modulation by *N*-tert-butyl-α-phenylnitrone. *Proceedings of the National Academy of Sciences of the United States of America, 94*(2), 674–678.

Chang, Y. K., & Etnier, J. L. (2009). Effects of an acute bout of localized resistance exercise on cognitive performance in middle-aged adults: A randomized controlled trial study. *Psychology of Sport and Exercise, 10*(1), 19–24.

Chmura, J., Nazar, K., & Kaciuba-Uscilko, H. (1994). Choice reaction time during graded exercise in relation to blood lactate and plasma catecholamine thresholds. *International Journal of Sports Medicine, 15*(4), 172–176.

Cian, C., Barraud, P. A., Melin, B., & Raphel, C. (2001). Effects of fluid ingestion on cognitive function after heat stress or exercise-induced dehydration. *International Journal of Psychophysiology, 42*(3), 243–251.

Cian, C., Koulmann, N., Barraud, P. A., Raphel, C., Jimenez, C., & Melin, B. (2000). Influence of variations in body hydration on cognitive function: Effect of hyperhydration, heat stress, and exercise-induced dehydration. *Journal of Psychophysiology, 14*, 29–36.

Clausen, A., Doctrow, S., & Baudry, M. (2010). Prevention of cognitive deficits and brain oxidative stress with superoxide dismutase/catalase mimetics in aged mice. *Neurobiology of Aging, 31*,425–433.

Colcombe, S., & Kramer, A. F. (2003). Fitness effects on the cognitive function of older adults: A meta-analytic study. *Psychological Science, 14*(2), 125–130.

Colcombe, S. J., Erickson, K. I., Raz, N., Webb, A. G., Cohen, N. J., McAuley, E., & Kramer, A. F.(2003). Aerobic fitness reduces brain tissue loss in aging humans. *Journals of Gerontology, Series A: Biological Sciences and Medical Sciences, 58*(2), 176–180.

Colcombe, S. J., Erickson, K. I., Scalf, P. E., Kim, J. S., Prakash, R., McAuley, E.,...Kramer, A. F. (2006). Aerobic exercise training increases brain volume in aging humans. *Journals of Gerontology, Series A: Biological Sciences and Medical Sciences, 61*(11), 1166–1170.

Cooper, C. J. (1973). Anatomical and physiological mechanisms of arousal, with special reference to the effects of exercise. *Ergonomics, 16*(5), 601–609.

Corder, E. H., Saunders, A. M., Strittmatter, W. J., Schmechel, D. E., Gaskell, P. C., Small, G. W.,...Pericak-Vance, M. A. (1993). Gene dose of apolipoprotein E type 4 allele and the risk of Alzheimer's disease in late onset families. *Science, 261*(5123), 921–923.

Cote, J., Salmela, J., & Papathanasopoulu, K. P. (1992). Effects of progressive exercise on attentional focus. *Perceptual and Motor Skills, 75*(2), 351–354.

Cotman, C. W., & Berchtold, N. C. (2002). Exercise: A behavioral intervention to enhance brain health and plasticity. *Trends in Neurosciences, 25*(6), 295–301.

Cotman, C. W., & Engesser-Cesar, C. (2002). Exercise enhances and protects brain function. *Exercise and Sport Sciences Reviews, 30*(2), 75–79.

Davey, C. P. (1973). Physical exertion and mental performance. *Ergonomics, 16*(5), 595–599.

Davis, C. L., Tomporowski, P. D., Boyle, C. A., Waller, J. L., Miller, P. H., Naglieri, J. A., & Gregoski, M.(2007). Effects of aerobic exercise on overweight children's cognitive functioning: A randomized controlled trial. *Research Quarterly for Exercise & Sport, 78*(5), 510–519.

Deeny, S. P., Poeppel, D., Zimmerman, J. B., Roth, S. M., Brandauer, J., Witkowski, S.,...Hatfield, B. D. (2008). Exercise, APOE, and working memory: MEG and behavioral evidence for benefit of exercise in epsilon4 carriers. *BiologicalPsychology, 78*(2), 179–187.

Dempster, F. N. (1992). The rise and fall of the inhibitory mechanism: Toward a unified theory of cognitive development and aging. *Developmental Review, 12*, 45–75.

Dietrich, A. (2003). Functional neuroanatomy of altered states of consciousness: The transient hypofrontality hypothesis. *Consciousness and Cognition, 12*(2), 231–256.

Dietrich, A. (2006). Transient hypofrontality as a mechanism for the psychological effects of exercise. *Psychiatry Research, 145*(1), 79–83.

Dietrich, A. (2009). The transient hypofrontality theory and its implications for emotion and cognition. In T. McMorris, P. D. Tomporowski, & M. Audiffren (Eds.), *Exercise and cognitive function* (pp. 69–90). Hoboken, NJ: Wiley-Blackwell.

Dietrich, A., & Sparling, P. B. (2004). Endurance exercise selectively impairs prefrontal-dependent cognition. *Brain and Cognition, 55*(3), 516–524.

Dik, M., Deeg, D. J., Visser, M., & Jonker, C. (2003). Early life physical activity and cognition at old age. *Journal of Clinical and Experimental Neuropsychology, 25*(5), 643–653.

Dik, M. G., Jonker, C., Comijs, H. C., Bouter, L. M., Twisk, J. W., van Kamp, G. J., & Deeg, D. J. (2001). Memory complaints and APOE-epsilon4 accelerate cognitive decline in cognitively normal elderly. *Neurology, 57*(12), 2217–2222.

Douchamps-Riboux, F., Heinz, J.-K., & Douchamps, J. (1989). Arousal as a tridimensional variable: An exploratory study of behavioural changes in rowers following a marathon race. *International Journal of Sport Psychology, 20*, 31–41.

Drake, E. B., Henderson, V. W., Stanczyk, F. Z., McCleary, C. A., Brown, W. S., Smith, C. A.,...Buckwalter, J. G. (2000). Associations between circulating sex steroid hormones and cognition in normal elderly women. *Neurology, 54*(3), 599–603.

Droge, W., & Schipper, H. M. (2007). Oxidative stress and aberrant signaling in aging and cognitive decline. *Aging Cell, 6*(3), 361–370.

Easterbrook, J. A. (1959). The effect of emotion on cue utilization and the organization of behavior. *Psychological Review, 66*(3), 183–201.

Ekkekakis, P. (2009). Illuminating the black box: Investigating prefrontal cortical hemodynamics during exercise with near-infrared spectroscopy. *Journal of Sport & Exercise Psychology, 31*(4), 505–553.

Erickson, K. I., Colcombe, S. J., Elavsky, S., McAuley, E., Korol, D. L., Scalf, P. E., & Kramer, A. F.(2007). Interactive effects of fitness and hormone treatment on brain health in postmenopausal women. *Neurobiology of Aging, 28*(2), 179–185.

Etnier, J. L. (2008). Mediators of the exercise and cognition relationship. In W. W. Spirduso, L. W. Poon, & W. J. Chodzko-Zajko (Eds.), *Aging, Exercise, and Cognition Series: Exercise and its mediating effects on cognition* (pp. 13–32). Urbana-Champaign, IL: Human Kinetics.

Etnier, J. L. (2009a). Chronic exercise and cognition in older adults. In T. McMorris, P. D. Tomporowski, & M. Audiffren (Eds.), *Exercise and cognitive function* (pp. 227–248). Chichester, West Sussex, UK: Wiley & Sons.

Etnier, J. L. (2009b). Physical activity programming to promote cognitive function: Are we ready for prescription? In W. W. Spirduso, W. Chodzko-Zajko, & L. W. Poon, (Eds.), *Aging, Exercise, and Cognition Series, Vol. 3: Enhancing cognitive functioning and brain plasticity* (pp. 159–176). Urbana-Champaign, IL: Human Kinetics.

Etnier, J. L., Caselli, R. J., Reiman, E. M., Alexander, G. E., Sibley, B. A., Tessier, D., & McLemore, E. C.(2007). Cognitive performance in older women relative to ApoE-epsilon4 genotype and aerobic fitness. *Medicine & Science in Sports & Exercise, 39*(1), 199–207.

Etnier, J. L., Salazar, W., Landers, D. M., Petruzzello, S. J., Han, M., & Nowell, P. (1997). The influence of physical fitness and exercise upon cognitive functioning: A meta-analysis. *Journal of Sport and Exercise Psychology, 19*, 249–277.

Etnier, J. L., & Sibley, B. L. (2004). Physical activity and hormone-replacement therapy: Interactive effects on cognition? *Journal of Aging and Physical Activity, 12*(4), 554–567.

Farrer, L. A., Cupples, L. A., Haines, J. L., Hyman, B., Kukull, W. A., Mayeux, R.,...van Duijn, C. M. (1997). Effects of age, sex, and ethnicity on the association between apolipoprotein E genotype and Alzheimer disease: A meta-analysis. *JAMA, 278*(16), 1349–1356.

Fatouros, I. G., Jamurtas, A. Z., Villiotou, V., Pouliopoulou, S., Fotinakis, P., Taxildaris, K., & Deliconstantinos, G.(2004). Oxidative stress responses in older men during endurance training and detraining. *Medicine & Science in Sports & Exercise, 36*(12), 2065–2072.

Ferris, L. T., Williams, J. S., & Shen, C. L. (2007). The effect of acute exercise on serum brain-derived neurotrophic factor levels and cognitive function. *Medicine & Science in Sports & Exercise, 39*(4), 728–734.

Fratiglioni, L., Paillard-Borg, S., & Winblad, B. (2004). An active and socially integrated lifestyle in late life might protect against dementia. *Lancet Neurology, 3*(6), 343–353.

Fukui, K., Omoi, N.-O., Hayasaka, T., Shinnkai, T., Suzuki, S., Abe, K., & Urano, S.(2002). Cognitive impairments of rats caused by oxidative stress and aging, and its prevention by vitamin E. *Annals of the New York Academy of Sciences, 959*, 275–284.

Galvan, V., & Bredesen, D. E. (2007). Neurogenesis in the adult brain: Implications for Alzheimer's disease. *CNS & Neurological Disorders—Drug Targets, 6*, 303–310.

Gibbs, R. B. (2000). Oestrogen and the cholinergic hypothesis: Implications for oestrogen replacement therapy in postmenopausal women. *Novartis Foundation Symposium, 230*, 94–107; discussion 107–111.

Giedd, J. N. (2008). The teen brain: Insights from neuroimaging. *Journal of Adolescent Health, 42*(4), 335–343.

Gold, S. M., Schulz, K. H., Hartmann, S., Mladek, M., Lang, U. E., Hellweg, R.,...Heesen, C. (2003). Basal serum levels and reactivity of nerve growth factor and brain-derived neurotrophic factor to standardized acute exercise in multiple sclerosis and controls. *Journal of Neuroimmunology, 138*(1–2), 99–105.

Gomez-Isla, T., West, H. L., Rebeck, G. W., Harr, S. D., Growdon, J. H., Locascio, J. J.,...Hyman, B.T. (1996). Clinical and pathological correlates of apolipoprotein E epsilon 4 in Alzheimer's disease. *Annals of Neurology, 39*(1), 62–70.

Gomez-Pinilla, F. (2008). The influences of diet and exercise on mental health through hormesis. *Aging Research Reviews, 7*, 49–62.

Gonzales McNeal, M., Zareparsi, S., Camicioli, R., Dame, A., Howieson, D., Quinn, J.,...Payami, H. (2001). Predictors of healthy brain aging. *Journal of Gerontology, 56A*, B294–B301.

Good, C. D., Johnsrude, I. S., Ashburner, J., Henson, R. N. A., Friston, K. J., & Frackowiak, R. S. J. (2001). A voxel-based morphometric study of aging in 465 normal adult human brains. *Neuroimage, 14*, 21–36.

Gopinathan, P. M., Pichan, G., & Sharma, V. M. (1988). Role of dehydration in heat stress–induced variations in mental performance. *Archives of Environmental Health, 43*(1), 15–17.

Gordon, B. A., Rykhlevskaia, E. I., Brumback, C. R., Lee, Y., Elavsky, S., Konopack, J. F.,...Fabiani, M. (2008). Neuroanatomical correlates of aging, cardiopulmonary fitness level, and education. *Psychophysiology, 45*, 825–838.

Gorelick, P. B., & Bozzola, F. G. (1991). Alzheimer's disease: Clues to the cause. *Postgraduate Medicine, 89*(4), 231–232, 237–238, 240.

Gunning-Dixon, F. M., Brickman, A. M., Cheng, J. C., & Alexopoulos, G. S. (2009). Aging of cerebral white matter: A review of MRI findings. *International Journal of Geriatric Psychiatry, 24*(2), 109–117.

Gustafsson, G., Lira, C. M., Johansson, J., Wisen, A., Wohlfart, B., Ekman, R., & Westrin, A.(2009). The acute response of plasma brain-derived neurotrophic factor as a result of exercise in major depressive disorder. *Psychiatry Research, 169*(3), 244–248.

Guttmann, C. R. G., Jolesz, F. A., Kikinis, R., Killiany, R. J., Moss, M. B., Sandor, T., & Albert, M. S.(1998). White matter changes with normal aging. *Neurology, 50*, 972–978.

Harman, D. (1956). Aging: A theory based on free radical and radiation chemistry. *Journal of Gerontology, 11*, 298–300.

Harman, D. (1969). Prolongation of life: Role of free radical reactions in aging. *Journal of theAmerican Geriatrics Society, 17*(8), 721–735.

Harman, D. (1972). The biologic clock: The mitochondria? *Journal of the American Geriatrics Society, 20*(4), 145–147.

Harman, D. (1994). Free-radical theory of aging. Increasing the functional life span. *Annals of the New York Academy of Sciences, 717*, 1–15.

Hasnis, E., & Reznick, A. Z. (2003). Antioxidants and healthy aging. *Israel Medical Association Journal, 5*(5), 368–370.

Herholz, K., Buskies, W., Rist, M., Pawlik, G., Hollmann, W., & Heiss, W. D. (1987). Regional cerebral blood flow in man at rest and during exercise.*Journal of Neurology, 234*(1), 9–13.

Heyn, P., Abreu, B. C., & Ottenbacher, K. J. (2004). The effects of exercise training on elderly persons with cognitive impairment and dementia: A meta-analysis. *Archives of Physical Medicine and Rehabilitation, 85*(10), 1694–1704.

Hillman, C. H., Buck, S. M., Themanson, J. R., Pontifex, M. B., & Castelli, D. M. (2009). Aerobic fitness and cognitive development: Event-related brain potential and task performance indices of executive control in preadolescent children. *Developmental Psychology, 45*(1), 114–129.

Hockey, G. R. (1997). Compensatory control in the regulation of human performance under stress and high workload: A cognitive-energetical framework. *BiologicalPsychology, 45*(1–3), 73–93.

Hogervorst, E., Riedel, W., Jeukendrup, A., & Jolles, J. (1996). Cognitive performance after strenuous physical exercise. *Perceptual and Motor Skills, 83*(2), 479–488.

Humphreys, M. S., & Revelle, W. (1984). Personality, motivation, and performance: A theory of the relationship between individual differences and information processing. *Psychological Review, 91*(2), 153–184.

Ide, K., & Secher, N. H. (2000). Cerebral blood flow and metabolism during exercise. *Progress in Neurobiology, 61*(4), 397–414.

Isaacs, K. R., Anderson, B. J., Alcantara, A. A., Black, J. E., & Greenough, W. T. (1992). Exercise and the brain: Angiogenesis in the adult rat cerebellum after vigorous physical activity and motor skill learning. *Journal of Cerebral Blood Flow and Metabolism, 12*, 110–119.

Jernigan, T. L., Archibald, S. L., Fennema-Notestine, C., Gamst, A. C., Stout, J. C., Bonner, J., & Hesselink, J. R.(2001). Effects of age on tissues and regions of the cerebrum and cerebellum. *Neurobiology of Aging, 22*(4), 581–594.

Ji, L. L. (2001). Exercise at old age: Does it increase or alleviate oxidative stress? *Annals of the New York Academy of Sciences, 928*, 236–247.

Ji, L. L. (2002). Exercise-induced modulation of antioxidant defense. *Annals of the New York Academy of Sciences, 959*, 82–92.

Jonker, C., Schmand, B., Lindeboom, J., Havekes, L. M., & Launer, L. J. (1998). Association between apolipoprotein E epsilon4 and the rate of cognitive decline in community-dwelling elderly individuals with and without dementia. *Archives of Neurology, 55*(8), 1065–1069.

Jorgensen, L. G., Perko, G., & Secher, N. H. (1992). Regional cerebral artery mean flow velocity and blood flow during dynamic exercise in humans. *Journal of Applied Physiology, 73*(5), 1825–1830.

Joseph, J. A., Shukitt-Hale, B., Casadesus, G., & Fisher, D. (2005). Oxidative stress and inflammation in brain aging: Nutritional considerations. *Neurochemical Research, 30*, 927–935.

Joseph, J. A., Shukitt-Hale, B., Denisova, N. A., Prior, R. L., Cao, G., Martin, A.,...Bickford, P. C. (1998). Long-term dietary strawberry, spinach, or vitamin E supplementation retards the onset of age-related neuronal signal-transduction and cognitive behavioral deficits. *Journal of Neuroscience, 18*(19), 8047–8055.

Junqueira, V. B., Barros, S. B., Chan, S. S., Rodrigues, L., Giavarotti, L., Abud, R. L., & Deucher, G.P. (2004). Aging and oxidative stress. *Molecular Aspects ofMedicine, 25*(1–2), 5–16.

Jurado, M. B., & Rosselli, M. (2007). The elusive nature of executive functions: A review of our current understanding. *Neuropsychology Review, 17*(3), 213–233.

Kamijo, K., Nishihira, Y., Higashiura, T., & Kuroiwa, K. (2007). The interactive effect of exercise intensity and task difficulty on human cognitive processing.*International Journal of Psychophysiology, 65*(2), 114–121.

Kampen, D. L., & Sherwin, B. B. (1994). Estrogen use and verbal memory in healthy postmenopausal women. *Obstetrics & Gynecology, 83*(6), 979–983.

Karp, A., Paillard-Borg, S., Wang, H. X., Silverstein, M., Winblad, B., & Fratiglioni, L. (2006). Mental, physical, and social components in leisure activities equally contribute to decrease dementia risk. *Dementia and Geriatric Cognitive Disorders, 21*(2), 65–73.

Kety, S. S., & Schmidt, C. F. (1945). The determination of cerebral blood flow in man by the use of nitrous oxide in low concentrations. *American Journal of Physiology, 143*, 53–66.

Kety, S. S., & Schmidt, C. F. (1948). The nitrous oxide method for the quantitative determination of cerebral blood flow in man: Theory, procedure, and normal values. *The Journal of Clinical Investigation, 27*, 476–483.

Kleim, J. A., Lussnig, E., Schwarz, E. R., Comery, T. A., & Greenough, W. T. (1996). Synaptogenesis and FOS expression in the motor cortex of the adult rat after motor skill learning. *Journal of Neuroscience, 16*(14), 4529–4535.

Kleim, J. A., Swain, R. A., Armstrong, K. A., Napper, R. M. A., Jones, T. A., & Greenough, W. T. (1998). Selective synaptic plasticity within the cerebellar cortex following complex motor skill learning. *Neurobiology of Learning and Memory, 69*, 274–289.

Kleim, J. A., Vij, K., Ballard, D. H., & Greenough, W. T. (1997). Learning-dependent synaptic modifications in the cerebellar cortex of the adult rat persist for at least four weeks. *Journal of Neuroscience, 17*(2), 717–721.

Kramer, A. F., Hahn, S., Cohen, N. J., Banich, M. T., McAuley, E., Harrison, C. R.,...Colcombe, A. (1999). Ageing, fitness and neurocognitive function. *Nature, 400*(6743), 418–419.

Lambourne, K., &Tomporowski, P. (2010). The effect of exercise-induced arousal on cognitive task performance: A meta-regression analysis. *Brain Research, 1341*, 12–24.

Larson, E. B., Wang, L., Bowen, J. D., McCormick, W. C., Teri, L., Crane, P., & Kukull, W. (2006). Exercise is associated with reduced risk for incident dementia among persons 65 years of age and older. *Annals of Internal Medicine, 144*(2), 73–81.

Laurin, D., Verreault, R., Lindsay, J., MacPherson, K., & Rockwood, K. (2001). Physical activity and risk of cognitive impairment and dementia in elderly persons. *Archives of Neurology, 58*(3), 498–504.

Levitt, S., & Gutin, B. (1971). Multiple choice reaction time and movement time during physical exertion. *Research Quarterly, 42*(4), 405–410.

Lezak, M. D., Howieson, D. B., & Loring, D. W. (2004). *Neuropsychological assessment*(4th ed.). New York: Oxford University Press.

Lim, K. O., Zipursky, R. B., Watts, M. C., & Pfefferbaum, A. (1992). Decreased gray matter in normal aging: An in vivo magnetic resonance study. *Journal of Gerontology, 47*(1), B26–B30.

Lindsay, J., Laurin, D., Verreault, R., Hebert, R., Helliwell, B., Hill, G. B., & McDowell, I.(2002). Risk factors for Alzheimer's disease: A prospective analysis from the Canadian Study of Health and Aging. *American Journal of Epidemiology, 156*(5), 445–453.

Lipsky, R. H., & Marini, A. (2007). Brain-derived neurotrophic factor in neuronal survival and behavior-related plasticity. *Annals of the New York Academy of Sciences, 1122*, 130–143.

Liu, J., & Ames, B. N. (2005). Reducing mitochondrial decay with mitochondrial nutrients to delay and treat cognitive dysfunction, Alzheimer's disease, and Parkinson's disease. *NutritionalNeuroscience, 8*(2), 67–89.

Lytle, M. E., Vander Bilt, J., Pandav, R. S., Dodge, H. H., & Ganguli, M. (2004). Exercise level and cognitive decline: The MoVIES project. *Alzheimer Disease and Associated Disorders, 18*(2), 57–64.

Magnie, M. N., Bermon, S., Martin, F., Madany-Lounis, M., Suisse, G., Muhammad, W., & Dolisi, C.(2000). P300, N400, aerobic fitness, and maximal aerobic exercise. *Psychophysiology, 37*(3), 369–377.

Marks, B. L., Madden, D. J., Bucur, B., Provenzale, J. M., White, L. E., Cabeza, R., & Huettel, S. A.(2007). Role of aerobic fitness and aging on cerebral white matter integrity. *Annals of the New York Academy of Sciences, 1097*, 171–174.

Martens, R., & Landers, D. M. (1970). Motor performance under stress: A test of the inverted-U hypothesis. *Journal of Personality and SocialPsychology, 16*(1), 29–37.

Mayeux, R., Stern, Y., Ottman, R., Tatemichi, T. K., Tang, M. X., Maestre, G.,...Ginsberg, H. (1993). The apolipoprotein epsilon 4 allele in patients with Alzheimer's disease. *Annals of Neurology, 34*(5), 752–754.

McDowell, K., Kerick, S. E., Santa Maria, D. L., & Hatfield, B. D. (2003). Aging, physical activity, and cognitive processing: An examination of P300. *Neurobiology of Aging, 24*, 597–606.

McMorris, T. (2009). Exercise and cognitive function: A neuroendocrinological explanation. In T. McMorris, P. D. Tomporowski, & M. Audiffren (Eds.), *Exercise and cognitive function* (pp. 41–68). Chichester, West Sussex, UK: Wiley & Sons.

McMorris, T., Collard, K., Corbett, J., Dicks, M., & Swain, J. P. (2008). A test of the catecholamines hypothesis for an acute exercise–cognition interaction. *Pharmacology Biochemistry and Behavior, 89*(1), 106–115.

McMorris, T., Davranche, K., Jones, G., Hall, B., Corbett, J., & Minter, C. (2009). Acute incremental exercise, performance of a central executive task, and sympathoadrenal system and hypothalamic-pituitary-adrenal axis activity.*International Journal of Psychophysiology, 73*(3), 334–340.

McMorris, T., & Graydon, J. (2000). The effects of incremental exercise on cognitive performance. *International Journal of Sport Psychology, 31*, 66–81.

McMorris, T., Myers, S., MacGillivary, W. W., Sexsmith, J. R., Fallowfield, J., Graydon, J., & Forster, D.(1999). Exercise, plasma catecholamine concentrations and decision-making performance of soccer players on a soccer-specific test.*Journal of Sports Science, 17*(8), 667–676.

Meeusen, R., Piacentini, M. F., & De Meirleir, K. (2001). Brain microdialysis in exercise research. *Sports Medicine, 31*(14), 965–983.

Meydani, M. (1999). Dietary antioxidants modulation of aging and immune–endothelial cell interaction. *Mechanisms of Ageing and Development, 111*(2–3), 123–132.

Meydani, M. (2001). Nutrition interventions in aging and age-associated disease. *Annals of the New York Academy of Sciences, 928*, 226–235.

Milgram, N. W., Head, E., Zicker, S. C., Ikeda-Douglas, C. J., Murphey, H., Muggenburg, B.,...Cotman, C. W. (2005). Learning ability in aged beagle dogs is preserved by behavioral enrichment and dietary fortification: A two-year longitudinal study. *Neurobiology of Aging, 26*(1), 77–90.

Myers, R. H., Schaefer, E. J., Wilson, P. W., D'Agostino, R., Ordovas, J. M., Espino, A.,...Wolf, P. A. (1996). Apolipoprotein E epsilon4 association with dementia in a population-based study: The Framingham study. *Neurology, 46*(3), 673–677.

O'Hara, R., Yesavage, J. A., Kraemer, H. C., Mauricio, M., Friedman, L. F., & Murphy, G. M., Jr. (1998). The APOE epsilon4 allele is associated with decline on delayed recall performance in community-dwelling older adults. *Journal of the American Geriatrics Society, 46*(12), 1493–1498.

Oosterman, J. M., Van Harten, B., Weinstein, H. C., Scheltens, P., Sergeant, J. A., & Scherder, E. J. (2008a). White matter hyperintensities and working memory: An explorative study. *Neuropsychology, Development, and Cognition. Section B, Aging, Neuropsychology and Cognition, 15*(3), 384–399.

Oosterman, J. M., Vogels, R. L., van Harten, B., Gouw, A. A., Scheltens, P., Poggesi, A.,...Scherder, E. J. A. (2008b). The role of white matter hyperintensities and medial temporal lobe atrophy in age-related executive dysfunctioning. *Brain and Cognition, 68*(2), 128–133.

Pagliari, R., & Peyrin, L. (1995). Norepinephrine release in the rat frontal cortex under treadmill exercise: A study with microdialysis. *Journal of Applied Physiology, 78*(6), 2121–2130.

Pereira, M. A., FitzerGerald, S. J., Gregg, E. W., Joswiak, M. L., Ryan, W. J., Suminski, R. R.,...Zmuda, J. M. (1997). A collection of physical activity questionnaires for health-related research.*Medicine & Science in Sports & Exercise, 29*(6 Suppl.), S1–S205.

Phillips, S. M., & Sherwin, B. B. (1992). Effects of estrogen on memory function in surgically menopausal women. *Psychoneuroendocrinology, 17*(5), 485–495.

Podewils, L. J., Guallar, E., Kuller, L. H., Fried, L. P., Lopez, O. L., Carlson, M., & Lyketsos, C. G.(2005). Physical activity, APOE genotype, and dementia risk: Findings from the Cardiovascular Health Cognition Study. *American Journal of Epidemiology, 161*(7), 639–651.

Poirier, J., Davignon, J., Bouthillier, D., Kogan, S., Bertrand, P., & Gauthier, S. (1993). Apolipoprotein E polymorphism and Alzheimer's disease. *Lancet, 342*(8873), 697–699.

Polidori, M. C. (2003). Antioxidant micronutrients in the prevention of age-related diseases. *Journal of PostgraduateMedicine, 49*(3), 229–235.

Prakash, R. S., Snook, E. M., Erickson, K. I., Colcombe, S. J., Voss, M. W., Motl, R. W., & Kramer, A. F.(2007). Cardiorespiratory fitness: A predictor of cortical plasticity in multiple sclerosis. *Neuroimage, 34,* 1238–1244.

Pribram, K. H., & McGuinness, D. (1975). Arousal, activation, and effort in the control of attention. *Psychological Review, 82*(2), 116–149.

Querido, J. S., & Sheel, A. W. (2007). Regulation of cerebral blood flow during exercise. *Sports Medicine, 37*(9), 765–782.

Rabbitt, P., Ibrahim, S., Lunn, M., Scott, M., Thacker, N., Hutchinson, C.,...Jackson, A. (2008). Age-associated losses of brain volume predict longitudinal cognitive declines over 8 to 20 years. *Neuropsychology, 22*(1), 3–9.

Raz, N. (2000). Aging of the brain and its impact on cognitive performance: Integration of structural and functional findings. In F. I. M. Craik & T. A. Salthouse (Eds.), *The handbook of aging and cognition* (pp. 1–90). Mahwah, NJ: Lawrence Erlbaum.

Reilly, T., & Smith, D. (1986). Effect of work intensity on performance in a psychomotor task during exercise. *Ergonomics, 29*(4), 601–606.

Resnick, S. M., Pham, D. L., Kraut, M. A., Zonderman, A. B., & Davatzikos, C. (2003). Longitudinal magnetic resonance imaging studies of older adults: A shrinking brain. *Journal of Neuroscience, 23*(8), 3295–3301.

Riley, K. P., Snowdon, D. A., Saunders, A. M., Roses, A. D., Mortimer, J. A., & Nanayakkara, N. (2000). Cognitive function and apolipoprotein E in very old adults: Findings from the Nun Study. *Journals of Gerontology, Series B: Psychological Sciences and Social Sciences, 55*(2), S69–S75.

Rogers, R. L., Meyer, J. S., & Mortel, K. F. (1990). After reaching retirement age physical activity sustains cerebral perfusion and cognition. *Journal of the American Geriatrics Society, 38*(2), 123–128.

Rojas Vega, S., Struder, H. K., Vera Wahrmann, B., Schmidt, A., Bloch, W., & Hollmann, W. (2006). Acute BDNF and cortisol response to low intensity exercise and following ramp incremental exercise to exhaustion in humans. *Brain Research, 1121*(1), 59–65.

Rovio, S., Kareholt, I., Helkala, E. L., Viitanen, M., Winblad, B., Tuomilehto, J.,...Kivipelto, M. (2005). Leisure-time physical activity at midlife and the risk of dementia and Alzheimer's disease. *Lancet Neurology, 4*(11), 705–711.

Rovio, S., Spulber, G., Nieminen, L. J., Niskanen, E., Winblad, B., Tuomilehto, J.,...Kivipelto, M. (2010). The effect of midlife physical activity on structural brain changes in the elderly. *Neurobiology of Aging, 31,* 1927–1936.

Sallis, J. F., Haskell, W. L., Wood, P. D., Fortmann, S. P., Rogers, T., Blair, S. N.,...Paffenbarger, R. S. Jr. (1985). Physical activity assessment methodology in the Five-City Project. *American Journal of Epidemiology, 121*(1), 91–106.

Salmela, J., & Ndoye, O. D. (1986). Cognitive distortions during progressive exercise. *Perceptual and Motor Skills, 63,* 1067–1072.

Sanders, A. F. (1983). Towards a model of stress and human performance. *Acta Psychologica (Amsterdam), 53*(1), 61–97.

Saunders, A. M., Strittmatter, W. J., Schmechel, D., George-Hyslop, P. H., Pericak-Vance, M. A., Joo, S. H.,...Roses, A. D. (1993). Association of apolipoprotein E allele epsilon 4 with late-onset familial and sporadic Alzheimer's disease. *Neurology, 43*(8), 1467–1472.

Scarmeas, N., & Stern, Y. (2003). Cognitive reserve and lifestyle. *Journal of Clinical and Experimental Neuropsychology, 25*(5), 625–633.

Schuit, A. J., Feskens, E. J., Launer, L. J., & Kromhout, D. (2001). Physical activity and cognitive decline, the role of the apolipoprotein e4 allele. *Medicine & Science in Sports & Exercise, 33*(5), 772–777.

Secher, N. H., Seifert, T., & Van Lieshout, J. J. (2008). Cerebral blood flow and metabolism during exercise: Implications for fatigue. *Journal of Applied Physiology, 104*(1), 306–314.

Sherwin, B. B. (1994). Sex hormones and psychological functioning in postmenopausal women. *Experimental Gerontology, 29*(3–4), 423–430.

Sibley, B. A., & Etnier, J. L. (2003). The relationship between physical activity and cognition in children: A meta-analysis. *Pediatric Exercise Science, 15*(3), 243–256.

Sirard, J. R., & Pate, R. R. (2001). Physical activity assessment in children and adolescents. *Sports Medicine, 31*(6), 439–454.

Sjoberg, H. (1980). Physical fitness and mental performance during and after work. *Ergonomics, 23*(10), 977–985.

Sohal, R. S., & Weindruch, R. (1996). Oxidative stress, caloric restriction, and aging. *Science, 273*(5271), 59–63.

Sonstroem, R. J., & Bernardo, P. B. (1982). Intraindividual pregame state anxiety and basketball performance: A re-examination of the inverted-U curve. *Journal of Sport Psychology, 4,* 235–245.

Sowell, E. R., Peterson, B. S., Thompson, P. M., Welcome, S. E., Henkenius, A. L., & Toga, A. W. (2003). Mapping cortical change across the human life span. *Nature Neuroscience, 6*(3), 309–315.

Spirduso, W. W. (1975). Reaction and movement time as a function of age and physical activity level. *Journal of Gerontology, 30*(4), 435–440.

Stern, Y., Habeck, C., Moeller, J., Scarmeas, N., Anderson, K. E., Hilton, H. J.,...van Heertum, R. (2005). Brain networks associated with cognitive reserve in healthy young and old adults. *Cerebral Cortex, 15*(4), 394–402.

Stroth, S., Kubesch, S., Dieterle, K., Ruchsow, M., Heim, R., & Kiefer, M. (2009). Physical fitness, but not acute exercise modulates event-related potential indices for executive control in healthy adolescents. *Brain Research, 1269,* 114–124.

Sturman, M. T., Morris, M. C., Mendes de Leon, C. F., Bienias, J. L., Wilson, R. S., & Evans, D. A. (2005). Physical activity, cognitive activity, and cognitive decline in a biracial community population. *Archives of Neurology, 62*(11), 1750–1754.

Tang, S. W., Chu, E., Hui, T., Helmeste, D., & Law, C. (2008). Influence of exercise on serum brain-derived neurotrophic factor concentrations in healthy human subjects. *Neuroscience Letters, 431*(1), 62–65.

Themanson, J. R., & Hillman, C. H. (2006). Cardiorespiratory fitness and acute aerobic exercise effects on neuroelectric and behavioral measures of action monitoring. *Neuroscience, 141,* 757–767.

Thomas, S. N., Schroeder, T., Secher, N. H., & Mitchell, J. H. (1989). Cerebral blood flow during submaximal and maximal dynamic exercise in humans. *Journal of Applied Physiology, 67*(2), 744–748.

Tomporowski, P. D. (2003). Effects of acute bouts of exercise on cognition. *Acta Psychologica (Amsterdam), 112*(3), 297–324.

Tomporowski, P. D., & Ellis, N. R. (1986). Effects of exercise on cognitive processes: A review. *Psychological Bulletin, 3*, 338–346.

Toro, R., Chupin, M., Garnero, L., Leonard, G., Perron, M., Pike, B.,...Paus, T. (2009). Brain volume and Val66Met polymorphism of the BDNF gene: Local or global effects? *Human Brain Structure: Structure, Function & Behavior, 213*, 501–509.

van Gelder, B. M., Tijhuis, M. A., Kalmijn, S., Giampaoli, S., Nissinen, A., & Kromhout, D. (2004). Physical activity in relation to cognitive decline in elderly men: The FINE Study. *Neurology, 63*(12), 2316–2321.

vanPraag, H., Christie, B. R., Sejnowski, T. J., & Gage, F. H. (1999a). Running enhances neurogenesis, learning, and long-term potentiation in mice. *Proceedings of the National Academy of Sciences of the United States of America, 96*(23), 13427–13431.

van Praag, H., Kempermann, G., & Gage, F. H. (1999b). Running increases cell proliferation and neurogenesis in the adult mouse dentate gyrus. *NatureNeuroscience, 2*(3), 266–270.

van Praag, H., Shubert, T., Zhao, C., & Gage, F. H. (2005). Exercise enhances learning and hippocampal neurogenesis in aged mice. *Journal of Neuroscience, 25*(38), 8680–8685.

Vaynman, S., & Gomez-Pinilla, F. (2005). License to run: Exercise impacts functional plasticity in the intact and injured central nervous system by using neurotrophins. *Neurorehabilitation and Neural Repair, 19*, 283–295.

Vaynman, S., & Gomez-Pinilla, F. (2006). Revenge of the "sit": How lifestyle impacts neuronal and cognitive health through molecular systems that interface energy metabolism with neuronal plasticity. *Journal of Neuroscience Research, 84*, 699–715.

Verghese, J., Lipton, R. B., Katz, M. J., Hall, C. B., Derby, C. A., Kuslansky, G.,...Buschke, H. (2003). Leisure activities and the risk of dementia in the elderly. *New England Journal of Medicine, 348*(25), 2508–2516.

West, R. L. (1996). An application of prefrontal cortex function theory to cognitive aging. *Psychological Bulletin, 120*(2), 272–292.

Weuve, J., Kang, J. H., Manson, J. E., Breteler, M. M., Ware, J. H., & Grodstein, F. (2004). Physical activity, including walking, and cognitive function in older women. *JAMA*, 1454–1461.

Whalley, L. J., Deary, I. J., Appleton, C. L., & Starr, J. M. (2004). Cognitive reserve and the neurobiology of cognitive aging. *Ageing Research Reviews, 3*(4), 369–382.

Wilson, R. S., Bennett, D. A., Bienias, J. L., Aggarwal, N. T., Mendes De Leon, C. F., Morris, M. C.,...Evans, D. A. (2002). Cognitive activity and incident AD in a population-based sample of older persons. *Neurology, 59*(12), 1910–1914.

Winter, B., Breitenstein, C., Mooren, F. C., Voelker, K., Fobker, M., Lechtermann, A.,...Knecht, S. (2007). High impact running improves learning. *Neurobiology of Learning and Memory, 87*(4), 597–609.

Yaffe, K., Barnes, D., Nevitt, M., Lui, L. Y., & Covinsky, K. (2001). A prospective study of physical activity and cognitive decline in elderly women:Women who walk. *Archives of Internal Medicine, 161*(14), 1703–1708.

Yaffe, K., Cauley, J., Sands, L., & Browner, W. (1997). Apolipoprotein E phenotype and cognitive decline in a prospective study of elderly community women. *Archives of Neurology, 54*(9), 1110–1114.

Yamada, M., Kasagi, F., Sasaki, H., Masunari, N., Mimori, Y., & Suzuki, G. (2003). Association between dementia and midlife risk factors: The Radiation Effects Research Foundation Adult Health Study. *Journal of the American Geriatrics Society, 51*(3), 410–414.

Yerkes, R. M., & Dodson, J. D. (1908). The relation of strength of stimulus to the rapidity of habit formation. *Journal of Comparative Neurology and Psychology, 18*, 459–482.

Yoshitake, T., Kiyohara, Y., Kato, I., Ohmura, T., Iwamoto, H., Nakayama, K.,...Fujishima, M. (1995). Incidence and risk factors of vascular dementia and Alzheimer's disease in a defined elderly Japanese population: The Hisayama Study. *Neurology, 45*(6), 1161–1168.

Zoladz, J. A., Pilc, A., Majerczak, J., Grandys, M., Zapart-Bukowska, J., & Duda, K. (2008). Endurance training increases plasma brain-derived neurotrophic factor concentration in young healthy men. *Journal of Physiology and Pharmacology, 59*(Suppl. 7), 119–132.

Zouhal, H., Jacob, C., Delamarche, P., & Gratas-Delamarche, A. (2008). Catecholamines and the effects of exercise, training and gender. *Sports Medicine, 38*(5), 401–423.

Exercise and Health-Related Quality of Life

Brian C. Focht

Abstract

Health-related quality of life (HRQL) is a multidimensional subcomponent of quality of life involving subjective appraisal of various dimensions of one's life that can be affected by health or health-related interventions. There is a growing consensus that HRQL is an integral indicant of treatment efficacy across a wide variety of therapeutic interventions. Consistent with this position, interest in delineating the effects of exercise on HRQL has increased considerably in the past 20 years. Results from studies in the physical activity, psychology, medical, and behavioral medicine literatures demonstrate that exercise results in meaningful improvements in an array of HRQL outcomes. The primary objectives of the present chapter are to summarize the empirical evidence addressing the effects of exercise on HRQL, address issues in the conceptualization and measurement of HRQL outcomes, and underscore persisting research considerations that will aid in developing a more comprehensive understanding of the exercise–HRQL relationship.

Key Words: exercise, physical activity, quality of life, subjective well-being, life satisfaction, behavioral medicine, intervention, psychological well-being.

It is well established that regular exercise results in numerous health benefits. Compelling evidence has emerged in the contemporary physical activity literature clearly linking sedentary behavior with increased risk for mortality and morbidity (Blair, LaMonte, & Nichamon, 2004). Across the past 30 years, accumulating epidemiological evidence has demonstrated that regular physical activity participation is inversely related to all-cause mortality (Pate et al., 1995) and to risk for developing a variety of the most prevalent forms of chronic disease, including cardiovascular disease, type 2 diabetes, hypertension, obesity, stroke, and select forms of cancer (Haskell et al., 2007). In light of this evidence, the beneficial role of physical activity in the prevention of and rehabilitation from many prevalent chronic diseases is now widely recognized.

Medical research has traditionally focused on the effects of clinical interventions on objective outcomes such as mortality and morbidity. However, health involves far more than simply the absence of disease or extension of longevity. Contemporary conceptualizations of health directly address the inherent complexity of this construct by acknowledging that health represents a complete state of positive physical, mental, and social well-being (World Health Organization Group, 1995). Assessing quality of life has been proposed to be instrumental in obtaining a comprehensive understanding of both the disease process as well as the efficacy of clinical interventions to prevent or treat chronic disease (Rejeski, Brawley, & Shumaker, 1996; Rejeski & Mihalko, 2001). Consistent with this position, measures of quality of life are now advocated as important indicants of treatment efficacy, and the National Institutes of Health and the Federal Drug Administration in the United States mandate the inclusion of indices of quality of life in most clinical studies examining the efficacy of therapeutic interventions (Kaplan & Bush, 1982; Pavot & Diener, 1993; Shumaker, Anderson, & Czajkowski, 1990). Accordingly, there is a growing consensus among clinicians and researchers that subjective, patient-based evaluations of functional status and well-being are integral to developing a comprehensive understanding of chronic disease processes and treatment efficacy (Ware, Kosinski, & Keller, 1997).

The benefits of a physically active lifestyle for promoting health and preventing disease are of clear public health importance. However, as exercise becomes increasingly advocated in efforts to prevent and treat chronic disease, there is growing interest in the delineating the role of physical activity and exercise behavior in enhancing quality of life. Evidence from the physical activity literature suggests that exercise results in meaningful improvements in quality-of-life outcomes when implemented in the treatment of a variety of populations with or at risk for disease and disability. Notably, there is empirical evidence that physical activity is associated with improvements in select dimensions of quality of life among cancer survivors (Courneya, Campbell, Karvinen, & Ladha, 2006; Winters-Stone & Schwartz, 2006); patients with cardiovascular disease (Tai, Meininger, & Frazier, 2008), osteoarthritis (Focht, 2006; Rejeski et al., 1996), chronic obstructive pulmonary disease (Berry, 2007), and multiple sclerosis (Motl & Gosney, 2008); older adults (McAuley & Katula, 1998; Rejeski & Mihalko, 2001); and overweight or obese individuals (Bouchard, 2001; Wing, 1999). Despite the increased attention devoted to investigation of the effects of exercise on quality of life in recent years, knowledge pertaining to several key research issues remains limited.

First, considerable confusion regarding the conceptualization and measurement of quality-of-life outcomes remains pervasive in the exercise literature. A consensus regarding the meaning of the terms "quality of life" and "health-related quality of life" and the core dimensions that make up these constructs remains absent. Inconsistency in the interpretation and measurement of quality of life has limited what can be concluded about the effects of exercise on quality-of-life outcomes. Second, although exercise has been consistently associated with improvements in select indices of quality of life, the factors that may moderate or mediate the exercise–quality of life relationship have yet to be adequately delineated. Finally, the programmatic,

prescriptive, and behavioral characteristics of exercise interventions that promote the most favorable changes in quality of life have not been well defined. The dearth of knowledge regarding these important research issues has significantly impeded progress toward a more comprehensive understanding of the benefits of exercise for promoting enhanced quality of life (Rejeski & Mihalko, 2001).

As recognition of the value of physical activity as a viable public health intervention for preventing and treating chronic disease accumulates, the importance of advancing knowledge of the effects of exercise on quality-of-life outcomes becomes of added significance. Accordingly, this chapter provides a summary of the effects of exercise on health-related quality of life. The present review has the following objectives:

• to address conceptual considerations concerning the meaning and measurement of quality of life and health-related quality of life
• to summarize the existing literature investigating the effects of exercise on health-related quality of life, with particular emphasis on select patient populations that have been focuses of physical activity and exercise interventions
• to examine what factors may influence the relationship between exercise and health-related quality of life, with a focus on the role of psychological variables that may serve as mediators underlying the beneficial effects of exercise on health-related quality-of-life outcomes
• to address several research considerations that, if adequately addressed in future inquiry, will aid in providing integration and progress in delineating the effects of exercise on quality-of-life outcomes

Conceptual and Measurement Issues in Health-Related Quality of Life

Over the years, numerous definitions of quality of life have been proposed. However, an overall consensus about the meaning of the terms "quality of life" and "health-related quality of life" and the specific dimensions that make up each construct remains lacking. In the absence of a widely accepted conceptualization of the terms, discipline-specific definitions of the constructs have emerged. For example, within the mainstream psychology literature, quality of life is often conceptualized and measured as an index of overall life satisfaction (Diener, 2000; Pavot & Diener, 1993; Rejeski & Mihalko, 2001). Indeed, there is a well-established literature that uses global measures of quality of life to conduct cross-cultural examinations of differences in life satisfaction and its determinants (Diener, Oishi, & Lucas, 2003).

In contrast to the conceptualization of quality of life as an index of overall life satisfaction in the psychology literature, other social, medical, and behavioral science disciplines have espoused a multidimensional perspective on quality-of-life outcomes (Mayou & Bryant, 1993). The World Health Organization Group (1995) defines quality of life as a multidimensional construct reflecting an individual's perception of his or her position in life based on an appraisal of key life components such as physical health, psychological well-being, social relationships, and level of independence. In this context, quality of life has frequently been viewed as being synonymous with constructs such as subjective well-being, life satisfaction, or satisfaction with functional domains that influence one's evaluation of their lives (Berger & Tobar, 2007).

In the aging and medical literature, the term "quality of life" has frequently been replaced with the terms "health status" or "health-related quality of life" (HRQL). This conceptualization views HRQL as a multidimensional, umbrella concept that constitutes broad categories of well-being and functioning (Stewart & King, 1991) and more discrete, specific aspects reflecting core dimensions of those generic categories (Rejeski & Mihalko, 2001; Lox, Martin Ginis, & Petruzzello, 2006). Thus quality of life and HRQL represent related but not isomorphic constructs (Motl & McAuley, 2010). Emerging evidence from the behavioral medicine literature also suggests that quality-of-life and HRQL outcomes are hierarchically organized, with change in proximal HRQL constructs predicting change in distal, global quality-of-life outcomes (Elavsky et al., 2005; Motl & McAuley, 2010). Collectively, it is clear that there remains considerable heterogeneity in the conceptualization and definition of quality-of-life outcomes across medical, social, and behavioral science disciplines.

Similar variability is evident in the methods used to measure HRQL. Measures used to assess quality-of-life and HRQL outcomes can be generally classified into two broad categories: objective and subjective. Objective measures of quality of life or HRQL involve a quantitative rating made by an external observer rather than the individual person or patient. These measures, such as quality-adjusted life years, are frequently used by health economists to determine the cost-effectiveness of treatments (Kaplan & Bush, 1982). Because these measures fail to account for individuals' perceptions of health, function, and well-being, this assessment approach has been viewed as controversial (Lox et al., 2006).

By contrast, subjective measures of quality of life and HRQL involve patient-defined evaluations of life satisfaction and functioning in core dimensions of well-being. As noted, provided that quality of life is viewed as a cognitive evaluation of one's overall life satisfaction in this context, it is assessed using global life satisfaction measures such as the Satisfaction with Life Scale (Diener, 2000 Pavot & Diener, 1993 or Cantril's Life Ladder (Cantril, 1965). Generic measures of HRQL tap broad dimensions of HRQL that are posited to be relevant across populations. The Short-Form 36 (SF-36) from the Medical Outcomes Study is one of the scales most widely employed to assess generic HRQL (Ware et al., 1997). Conversely, targeted HRQL instruments are designed to tap HRQL information specific to a particular disease or population (or both) that may not be adequately captured by broad, generic measures. For example, the Functional Assessment of Cancer Therapy has both a general version and disease-specific versions that are designed to assess concerns that may be specific to particular subgroups of cancer patients and survivors (Courneya et al., 2006).

In summary, quality of life is now well established as an important indicant of treatment efficacy across a wide variety of therapeutic interventions and populations. The divergence in the conceptualization and definition of quality-of-life and HRQL terms across disciplines, as well as the breadth of measures used to assess these outcomes, presents a considerable challenge to effectively synthesizing knowledge of the effects of exercise on quality-of-life outcomes. For the purposes of the present chapter, HRQL will be operationally defined as a subcomponent of quality of life that involves the subjective appraisal of various dimensions of one's life that can be affected by health or health-related interventions. Within this context, HRQL is an umbrella construct representing both broad domains of functioning and well-being and more specific core dimensions of HRQL including, but not limited to, perceptions of physical function, emotional well-being, social functioning, health states, and physical symptoms and states. Given the heterogeneity in perspectives that persists regarding the conceptualization of quality-of-life outcomes, it is unlikely that all researchers interested in the effects of exercise on quality of life would agree with each aspect of this operational definition of HRQL. Nonetheless this definition is similar to, if not synonymous with, accepted definitions proposed and used in prior reviews (Lox et al., 2006; Rejeski et al., 1996) and provides a basis for the synthesis of findings in the extant exercise–HRQL literature.

Effects of Exercise on HRQL

Exercise is increasingly applied as an adjuvant approach in the prevention and treatment of disease. Accordingly, several population subgroups with or at high risk for disease and disability have been the target of focal research addressing the efficacy of exercise for enhancing or maintaining HRQL. Given that HRQL is a multidimensional construct that has been assessed in numerous healthy and chronic disease samples, summarizing all outcomes in all populations that have been focuses of exercise research is clearly beyond the scope of any single review. Thus in the following section of this chapter, I will provide a general overview of the exercise–HRQL relationship in select chronic disease populations that have been focuses of study in the contemporary exercise and behavioral medicine literatures. These populations include individuals with knee osteoarthritis, cancer patients and survivors, patients with chronic obstructive pulmonary disease, individuals with or at risk for cardiovascular disease, and overweight or obese individuals.

For each population, I will provide a brief summary of the research literature emphasizing select examples of seminal studies, recent investigations, or both. Several comprehensive reviews of the effects of exercise on overall quality of life and HRQL (Berger & Tobar, 2007; Courneya et al., 2006; Gillison, Skevington, Sato, Standage, & Evangelidou, 2009; Schmitz, Holzman, et al., 2005; Speed-Andrews & Courneya, 2009) and specific dimensions of HRQL in select chronic disease populations (Focht, 2006; Lawlor & Hopker, 2001; Linden, Stossel, & Maurice, 1996; Winters-Stone & Schwartz, 2006) have been conducted previously. To limit redundancy with these prior narrative or meta-analytic syntheses of the literature, I will summarize their overall conclusions and present more focused discussion of select findings and of investigations that have been emerged since those reviews were published.

Other populations have been targets of important, systematic exercise–HRQL research, such as older adults at risk for functional decline or disability and individuals with multiple sclerosis. These subgroups that have yielded meaningful findings

that are pertinent to the present review. However, the effects of exercise on HRQL in these samples have been ably reviewed previously (McAuley & Katula, 1998; Motl & Gosney, 2008; Rejeski et al., 1996; Rejeski & Mihalko, 2001), and many of the findings from this line of inquiry will be covered in the present chapter, both within the overviews of specific subgroups and in a later segment of the chapter addressing potential mediators of the effects of exercise on HRQL outcomes.

Exercise and HRQL in Knee Osteoarthritis

Knee osteoarthritis (OA) is a progressive, degenerative disease characterized by joint damage associated with the degradation of articular cartilage, joint space narrowing, and development of osteophytes. Pain, stiffness, and fatigue are the principal adverse symptoms accompanying the progression of knee OA. The deleterious effects of knee OA on physical function and quality of life are well established (Focht, 2007). There is considerable evidence for the benefits of exercise for improving physical function, pain symptoms, and fatigue among individuals burdened with knee OA. Consequently, exercise is now advocated in the medical management of knee OA (Roddy et al., 2005).

Several narrative and meta-analytic reviews have addressed the benefits of exercise in the treatment of knee OA (Baker & McAlindon, 2000; Focht, 2006; Lange, Vanwanseele, & Fiatarone Singh, 2008; Minor, 2004; Petrella, 2000). Additionally, there have been at least 32 randomized controlled trials examining the benefits of aerobic exercise, resistance exercise, or physical therapy--based exercises for knee OA patients (Fransen & McConnell, 2008). Overall, findings in prior randomized trials and reviews of the exercise–knee OA literature demonstrate that exercise is consistently associated with improvements in multiple HRQL outcomes. The majority of studies focused on the effects of aerobic exercise, resistance exercise, or both on disease-specific indices of HRQL or symptoms. For example, many studies have used the Western Ontario McMaster Arthritis Scale (WOMAC) and Arthritis Impact Measurement Scale (AIMS) inventories, which are targeted measures designed to tap OA-related symptoms (pain, stiffness, and fatigue) and core dimensions of HRQL particularly affected by the disease and its treatments, such as physical function and ability to complete activities of daily living.

Collectively, the effects of exercise on HRQL outcomes have been found to be similar in magnitude to those observed with the use of nonsteriodal anti-inflammatory drugs (NSAIDs) Fransen & McConnell, 2008). Select randomized trials have also demonstrated that exercise elicits significant improvements in generic indices of HRQL (Rejeski, Focht, et al., 2002). Findings from the exercise–knee OA literature also reveal differential effects of exercise across core dimensions of HRQL. For example, whereas the effects of exercise on HRQL are generally characterized as being small to moderate in magnitude, the HRQL constructs most favorably influenced by exercise vary considerably across studies. Some studies indicated that the exercise produced the greatest change in physical function (Messier et al., 2004), whereas other investigations observed the most pronounced improvements in relevant disease symptoms such as pain (O'Reilly, Muir, & Doherty, 1999). By contrast, other large trials suggested that exercise resulted in comparable improvements in various assessments of core dimensions of HRQL (Ettinger et al., 1997). Consistent with this position, recent meta-analyses observed meaningful, comparable effects of exercise on pain (Cohen's d = 0.40) and physical function (d = 0.37) outcomes (Fransen & McConnell, 2008). Differences in the HRQL measures employed across studies likely play a role in the inconsistent results. However, these findings also underscore the unique effects that exercise can have on select dimensions of HRQL in arthritic populations.

One of the seminal randomized controlled trials of exercise for knee OA patients was the Fitness and Arthritis in Seniors Trial (FAST; Ettinger et al., 1997). The FAST study was an 18-month, multicenter, single-blind trial that compared the effects of aerobic exercise, resistance exercise, and a health education control intervention in 459 older knee OA patients. Results from FAST demonstrated that both aerobic exercise and resistance exercise produced significantly greater improvements in self-reported disability and knee pain symptoms than in the health education control group. Ancillary analyses from FAST also revealed dose-dependent improvements in select HRQL outcomes. Participants with greater attendance at prescribed center-based exercise sessions reported superior improvement in pain and self-reported physical function (Rejeski, Brawley, Ettinger, Morgan, & Thompson, 1997).

The Arthritis, Diet, and Activity Promotion Trial (ADAPT) was a recent randomized controlled trial examining the efficacy of exercise in the treatment of 316 older overweight or obese individuals burdened with knee OA (Messier et al., 2004). ADAPT was a single-blind 18-month trial comparing the effects of exercise and dietary weight loss interventions, separately and in combination, on weight loss, physical function, and HRQL. Findings from ADAPT demonstrated that compared with a health education control group, the group receiving the combination of exercise and diet showed significantly greater improvements in generic indices of HRQL (SF-36) as well as self-reported and performance measures of physical function at the 18-month follow-up assessment (Messier et al., 2004; Rejeski, Focht, et al., 2002). Exercise alone was also associated with more favorable changes in select performance measures of physical function than was the control treatment arm. The results from ADAPT demonstrate that dietary interventions can augment the benefits of exercise alone in the treatment of overweight and obese knee OA patients.

Ancillary meditational analyses from both FAST and ADAPT also provided meaningful data addressing the pathways through which exercise may lead to improvements in HRQL. These findings will be summarized in a later section of the chapter focusing on the mediators and moderators of the effects of exercise on HRQL.

Overall, findings from randomized trials in the exercise–knee OA literature demonstrate that aerobic exercise and resistance exercise interventions result in statistically significant and clinically meaningful improvements in various measures of HRQL. The magnitude of the change in commonly assessed dimensions of HRQL is similar to that observed with NSAID treatment (Fransen & McConnell, 2008; Focht, 2006). The benefits of exercise do not appear to systematically vary as a function of demographic or exercise program characteristics (i.e., length of intervention; mode, intensity, frequency, or duration of exercise; or whether the intervention was home based or center based). There was considerable variability in the prescriptive components of the exercise interventions that yielded comparable benefits in the same HRQL outcomes. Consequently, from a prescription perspective, the characteristics of exercise interventions that facilitate improvements in HRQL remain unclear.

Exercise and HRQL in Cancer Treatment and Survivorship

Improvements in detection and treatment strategies have resulted in dramatic increases in survival rates across a variety of different cancer sites. It is well established, however, that many cancer treatments are accompanied by negative side effects such as fatigue, pain, unfavorable changes in body weight and body composition, and reduced physical functioning. These adverse effects have a deleterious effect on quality of life and can persist for a considerable amount of time following the cessation of treatment. As survival rates improve, identifying behavioral interventions that can alleviate adverse treatment symptoms and enhance quality of life is becoming a primary consideration during both the active treatment and survivorship phases of the cancer continuum (Courneya, 2009). Additionally, emerging evidence suggests that cancer survivors are at increased risk for developing chronic diseases such as heart disease, diabetes, and osteoporosis compared with individuals with no history of cancer (Newton & Galvao, 2008). In light of these findings, developing effective strategies to prevent and manage these diseases in cancer survivors is an important clinical and public health consideration.

There is mounting empirical evidence that exercise is an efficacious lifestyle intervention that can offset the adverse effects of traditional cancer therapies and ameliorate a variety of quality-of-life outcomes both during and following cancer treatment (Courneya, 2009; Galvao & Newton, 2008; Schmitz, Holtzman, et al., 2005). Accordingly, the American Cancer Society now recommends regular exercise for cancer patients and survivors (American Cancer Society, 2008). The accumulating evidence that exercise can elicit significant improvements in HRQL has been particularly influential in calls advocating the integration of exercise as an adjuvant supportive care intervention across the cancer continuum.

The majority of exercise–cancer research conducted to date has focused on the effects of aerobic exercise during active treatment in women with early-stage breast cancer (Conn, Hafdahl, Porock, McDaniel, & Neilson, 2006; Courneya et al., 2006; Galvao & Newton, 2005; Schmitz, Holtzman, et al., 2005; Schwartz, 2008). However, a growing number of investigations are focusing on the benefits of exercise for breast cancer survivors in the period following the cessation of active treatment (Courneya, 2009; Speed-Andrews & Courneya, 2009). Focal study of the HRQL benefits in single-site cancers other than breast cancer is also beginning to emerge, as underscored by recent reviews of the efficacy of exercise interventions in prostate cancer (Thorsen, Courneya, Stevinson, & Fossa, 2008) and hematological cancer (Liu, Chinapow, Huijgens, & Mechelen, 2008).

A variety of HRQL and quality-of-life outcomes have been assessed in the exercise–cancer literature. Generic indices of HRQL, targeted measures of disease-specific symptoms, measures of core dimensions of physical functioning and well-being, and global ratings of life satisfaction have all been implemented in exercise intervention trials (Courneya, 2009; Courneya et al., 2006; Schmitz, Holtzman, et al., 2005; Schwartz, 2008; Speed-Andrews & Courneya, 2009). Exercise interventions implemented during and following cancer treatment were heterogeneous in exercise mode, intervention length, and duration and intensity of exercise. Studies have examined both aerobic and resistance exercise as well as both supervised center-based and home-based exercise interventions. A wide range of exercise characteristics were employed across studies, with interventions lasting from 10 weeks to six months, using frequencies ranging from three to five sessions per week. Prescriptions for aerobic exercise ranged from 50% to 85% of aerobic capacity and from 15 to 60 minutes in duration. Prescriptions for resistance exercise interventions consisted of six to nine exercises for the major muscle groups. Participants in resistance exercise interventions completed a range of one to three sets of 8–20 repetitions per set at loads ranging from 60% to 70% of an individual's one-repetition maximum (1RM).

Overall, the findings from the extant exercise–cancer research revealed that exercise consistently results in significant, clinically meaningful improvements in multiple HRQL outcomes. Specifically, exercise was associated with increases in global satisfaction with life, generic dimensions of HRQL, physical function, and specific disease- or treatment-related symptoms such as pain and fatigue (Courneya et al., 2006; Schwartz, 2008; Winters-Stone & Schwartz, 2006). Exercise is generally associated with small-to-moderate improvements in the quality-of-life outcomes that have been assessed, though substantial variability in the magnitude of the effects of exercise has been observed across studies and measures of HRQL.

In addition to the findings evident in prior exercise–cancer reviews, several recent randomized controlled trials have examined the effects of exercise on HRQL during active cancer treatment. For example, Courneya et al. (2007) conducted the Supervised Trial of Aerobic and Resistance Training (START), the largest multicenter randomized controlled trial conducted in breast cancer patients undergoing chemotherapy to date. The START trial compared the effects of aerobic and resistance exercise with those of usual-care treatment approaches across a 6-month intervention period. Findings from START revealed that both aerobic and resistance exercise yielded superior changes in select HRQL outcomes relative to usual care. However, each mode of exercise elicited unique benefits. Specifically, aerobic exercise was associated with superior improvements in self-esteem, whereas resistance exercise was associated with the most favorable change in a cancer-specific measure of HRQL, particularly among breast cancer patients who preferred resistance exercise to aerobic exercise. Results from the START trial demonstrated that women randomized to receive resistance exercise reported the best chemotherapy completion rate. This is the first study to document this exceptionally meaningful benefit of exercise.

In a large, single-blind randomized controlled trial, Segal and colleagues (2009) recently compared the effects of 6 months of resistance exercise, aerobic exercise, and usual-care interventions in 121 prostate cancer patients receiving adjuvant radiation and hormone therapy. Results of intention-to-treat analyses revealed that both resistance exercise and aerobic exercise resulted in significant, comparable improvements in fatigue relative to usual care at 12 weeks of each respective intervention. Resistance exercise yielded greater improvements in fatigue and disease-specific HRQL than the usual-care condition at the 24-week follow-up assessment.

Recent findings focusing on the effects of exercise on HRQL following cancer treatment have also been reported. Vallance, Courneya, Plotnikoff, Yasui, and Mackey (2007) compared the effects of pedometer, print-based physical activity promotion materials, and a combination of the two interventions in 377 breast cancer survivors. Results revealed that combining breast cancer–specific print materials and pedometers produced superior changes in global HRQL and fatigue relative to a usual-care treatment approach. Additionally, Schmitz and colleagues have recently convincingly extended the quality-of-life benefits of exercise for breast cancer survivors to include resistance exercise: Results from the Weight Training and Breast Cancer Trial (Ohira, Schmitz, Ahmed, & Yee, 2006; Schmitz, Ahmed, Hannan, & Yee, 2005) and the Physical Activity and Lymphedema trial (Schmitz et al., 2009) demonstrate that resistance exercise is a safe, well-tolerated exercise intervention that elicits meaningful improvements in generic and disease-specific indices of HRQL among breast cancer survivors. Contrary to common clinical observation, resistance exercise did not exacerbate lymphedema symptoms or increase risk of onset of lymphedema.

The majority of studies examining the effects of exercise on HRQL outcomes during and following cancer treatment have focused on breast cancer patients or survivors. However, the quality-of-life benefits of exercise and physical activity are rapidly being investigated and documented in numerous subgroups of cancer patients. Emerging evidence from observational studies suggests that physical activity participation is associated with superior HRQL in such diverse cancer populations as patients with ovarian, colorectal, and endometrial cancer, multiple myeloma, and non-Hodgkin's lymphoma (Speed-Andrews & Courneya, 2009).

Taken collectively, evidence from the exercise–cancer literature demonstrates that exercise results in significant improvements in multiple HRQL outcomes both during and following cancer treatment in a variety of cancer patient groups. Aerobic forms of exercise have been the most frequently studied mode of exercise. However, mounting evidence underscores the ability of resistance exercise to elicit beneficial effects on HRQL in cancer patients. Indeed, resistance exercise is associated with unique improvements in generic and disease-specific HRQL measures in recent research involving breast cancer survivors, breast cancer patients undergoing chemotherapy, and prostate cancer patients on hormone and radiation therapy (Courneya et al., 2007; Ohira et al., 2006; Segal et al., 2009; Schmitz, Holtzman, et al., 2005; Schmitz et al., 2009). Comparable, clinically meaningful improvements in HRQL have been observed during and following treatment in multiple randomized controlled trials. The HRQL benefits accompanying exercise do not appear to be limited to any cancer population subgroup, stage in the cancer continuum, or specific exercise characteristic (mode, duration, intensity, etc.). However, much of the research has focused on the periods during or soon after active treatment. The extent to which exercise may result in similar improvements in quality-of-life outcomes at other stages of the cancer experience, such as the buffering or palliative stages of the cancer continuum, has yet to be determined. Additionally, the pathways through which exercise may elicit improvements in HRQL are not well understood. Clearly, addressing these important research considerations will help to advance knowledge pertaining to the HRQL benefits accompanying exercise across the cancer continuum.

Exercise and HRQL in Chronic Obstructive Pulmonary Disease

Chronic obstructive pulmonary (COPD) is one of the leading causes of mortality and disease burden in the United States. Exercise intolerance and dyspnea (perceived breathlessness) are primary adverse symptoms accompanying COPD. The symptoms of COPD are linked with reductions in physical function, quality of life, and the ability to perform common activities of daily living. Exercise training is now well established as an integral component of treatment and rehabilitation of patients with COPD (Berry, 2007; Berry et al., 2003). There have been several prior narrative and meta-analytic reviews of the effects of exercise on HRQL in COPD patients (CambachWagenaar, Koelman, VanKeimpema, & Kemper,1999; Lacasse et al., 1996; Lacasse, Martin, Lasserson, & Goldstein, 2007). Within the literature summarized in those prior reports, in the past 30 years there have been over 30 randomized controlled trials examining the benefits of exercise therapy, often within the context of respiratory rehabilitation programs, on HRQL among individuals burdened with COPD. Eight different disease-targeted indices were used to examine changes in HRQL in the 13 trials that included such indices (Lacasse et al., 2007). The effects of exercise on global quality of life or generic measures of HRQL have not been systematically investigated among COPD patients.

Findings from the extant literature suggest that exercise results in significant, clinically meaningful improvements in several dimensions of disease-specific HRQL. Notably, exercise is associated with moderate improvements in dyspnea, fatigue, and psychological well-being (Berry, 2007; Lacasse et al., 2007). Exercise also produced significant yet smaller improvements in exercise tolerance and select performance measures of physical function. However, exercise–induced improvements in HRQL are not strongly related to increases in objective measures of exercise capacity or physical functioning in COPD patients.

The majority of studies examining the effects of exercise on HRQL in COPD patients have focused on short-term exercise training interventions lasting 4 to 12 weeks. There is strong evidence that the benefits of exercise on several dimensions of HRQL diminish markedly following the cessation of exercise therapy (Berry, 2007). In light of this limitation, several recent randomized trials have examined the efficacy of long-term exercise training in producing improved HRQL outcomes.

The Reconditioning and Chronic Obstructive Pulmonary Disease Trial (REACT) was a single-blind randomized controlled trial designed to examine the effects of short-term (3 months) and long-term (18 months) exercise interventions in 140 COPD patients. Findings from REACT revealed that the long-term exercise intervention yielded significantly more favorable improvements in select HRQL outcomes, including symptoms of dyspnea and fatigue, psychological functioning and well-being, and self-reported physical function (Berry et al., 2003; Foy, Rejeski, Berry, Zaccarro, & Woodard, 2001). In contrast to changes in HRQL outcomes observed in numerous other exercise trials, gender was found to moderate the effect of exercise on HRQL in the REACT study. With short-term exercise therapy, men and women reported comparable, significant improvements in HRQL. However, men in long-term exercise therapy reported superior changes in select dimensions of HRQL compared with women.

Maltais and colleagues (2008) recently compared the effects of home-based and center-based exercise, within the context of comprehensive pulmonary rehabilitation programs, on HRQL in 252 patients with COPD. Results from this trial revealed that the two programs produced comparable improvements in disease-specific indices of HRQL. These benefits were maintained, irrespective of location of training, at a one-year follow-up assessment.

The findings of studies addressing the effects of exercise in COPD patients demonstrate that exercise consistently produces significant improvements in a variety of dimensions of disease-specific HRQL. Consistent with findings for other clinical populations, the effects of exercise do not appear to systematically vary as a function of various individual differences or program characteristics. Some findings suggest that men may benefit more than women and that long-term exercise therapy may be associated with added benefit for some patients (Berry et al., 2003; Foy et al., 2001). However, the effects of exercise on generic HRQL or global measures of quality of life have not been evaluated. Additionally, there is still little evidence of the minimal amount of exercise that produces significant improvements in HRQL for COPD patients, and knowledge of the pathways underlying the favorable effect of exercise on HRQL in this population is limited.

Exercise and HRQL in Cardiovascular Disease

Cardiac rehabilitation is a complex, multicomponent intervention that comprises a variety of therapeutic strategies including risk factor education, psychological and behavioral counseling, and pharmacotherapy. In addition to these strategies, exercise remains a central component of the rehabilitation programs designed for people with or at high risk for cardiovascular disease. Primary goals of cardiac rehabilitation–based exercise therapy are to restore optimal physical function, prevent or reverse the progression of cardiovascular disease risk factors, reduce disease-related morbidity, and extend longevity. Promoting enhanced HRQL in the added years of life associated with therapy is now widely recognized as an integral objective of multicomponent cardiac rehabilitation programs.

It is well established that cardiac rehabilitation programs that use exercise therapy as a cornerstone of treatment result in significant improvements in total and cardiac mortality, total cholesterol, trigylcerides, and systolic blood pressure (Taylor et al., 2004). Although quality of life is an important outcome of exercise therapy for cardiovascular disease patients, close inspection of systematic reviews of the cardiac rehabilitation literature shows that measures of HRQL outcomes have not been consistently incorporated in randomized controlled trials investigating the efficacy of rehabilitation programs. For example, in a recent meta-analysis of 48 randomized trials comparing exercise-based cardiac rehabilitation with usual-care interventions, measures of HRQL were included in only 12 of the studies (Taylor et al., 2004). Other narrative and meta-analytic reviews of the exercise therapy literature find that HRQL outcomes are assessed in a similar proportion of reviewed trials (Eshah & Bond, 2009; Tai et al., 2008). Thus while enhancing and maintaining quality of life is an inherently important consideration in rehabilitation programs targeting recovery from cardiovascular disease, a relatively small proportion of randomized trials have examined the effects of exercise therapy on HRQL outcomes.

Existing evidence supporting the HRQL benefits of exercise-based cardiac rehabilitation is surprisingly equivocal. Studies documenting improvements in HRQL following exercise therapy suggest these changes are relatively modest. For example, Taylor et al. (2004) reported that moderate improvements in HRQL relative to baseline levels were consistently observed across the 12 randomized controlled trials mentioned above. However, when compared with usual-care treatments, superior improvements in HRQL were documented in only two of the 12 trials.

The inconsistent evidence addressing the effects of exercise on HRQL in cardiovascular disease patients is possibly attributable to several factors. As noted for other population subgroups included in the present review, there is considerable heterogeneity in the HRQL assessments used across studies in the cardiac rehabilitation literature (Tai et al., 2008; Taylor et al., 2004). Many trials are also characterized by relatively small sample sizes. Thus while these investigations allow for the assessment of within-treatment effects that have been frequently observed across studies, they may not have sample sizes that provide adequate statistical power to detect meaningful differences between exercise therapy and usual-care treatment conditions. Finally, an emphasis on the use of global quality-of-life or generic HRQL measures that may lack sensitivity to detect changes in dimensions of HRQL that are of relevance to cardiac rehabilitation patients may also contribute to the relatively modest effect observed for exercise (Taylor et al., 2004). Thus whereas exercise therapy clearly results in meaningful improvements in a wide array of indicants of cardiovascular disease, a relatively limited number of studies demonstrate that exercise therapy is associated with improvements in HRQL.

Although findings addressing the effects of exercise on HRQL in cardiovascular disease remain surprisingly sparse and equivocal, Rejeski and colleagues (2003) demonstrated that exercise therapy can elicit meaningful changes in HRQL among patients undergoing cardiac rehabilitation in the Cardiovascular Health and Physical Activity Maintenance Program (CHAMP) trial. CHAMP was a single-blind randomized controlled trial comparing the effects of a theoretically driven, group-mediated cognitive behavioral (GMCB) exercise therapy intervention with those of traditional cardiac rehabilitation–based exercise therapy in 147 older adults with or at high risk for cardiovascular disease. Findings from the CHAMP trial revealed significant improvements in a generic measure of HRQL (SF-36) and perceived physical function (Focht, Brawley, Rejeski, & Ambrosius, 2004; Rejeski, Foy, et al., 2002). Results indicated that improvements in HRQL were influenced by initial HRQL levels, gender, and treatment group assignment. More specifically, men in both exercise interventions and women assigned to the GMCB intervention exhibiting the lowest baseline levels of HRQL demonstrated the most favorable changes in the Mental Health summary scale and Vitality subscale of the SF-36 at 12-month follow-up (Focht et al., 2004). Additionally, participants reporting the greatest difficulty in performing activities of daily living prior to initiating therapy who were assigned to the GMCB intervention experienced the most favorable change in self-reported physical function at follow-up (Rejeski, Foy, et al., 2002).

Consistent with the results of prior meta-analytic reviews (Jolly, Taylor, Lip, & Stevens, 2006), finding from the CHAMP trial suggest that exercise results in modest yet meaningful improvements in generic measures of HRQL. The results from this study also extend these benefits to specific dimensions of HRQL that are of importance to individuals burdened with cardiovascular disease, such as perceptions of physical function. The CHAMP findings also demonstrate that baseline HRQL values are independent predictors of improvement in HRQL following exercise interventions. It appears that those who have the least favorable levels of HRQL prior to exercise accrue the most benefit through exercise training. Results from CHAMP also revealed that the effects of exercise therapy on HRQL in cardiovascular disease patients may be augmented through the integration of a component involving self-regulatory skills counseling. Finally, similar to results observed in the REACT trial among COPD patients (Foy et al., 2001), the benefits of exercise therapy on HRQL for cardiac rehabilitation patients may vary as a function of gender.

Careful review of the cardiac rehabilitation literature reveals that few studies have systematically addressed the effects of exercise on HRQL. Consequently, evidence of individual differences in treatment effects or of the amount of exercise that yields the best improvements in HRQL remains lacking. Given that exercise is an integral component of treatment in cardiac rehabilitation, the question of what factors may strengthen the beneficial effect of exercise on HRQL in this population should be examined further.

Exercise and HRQL in Obesity

The prevalence of overweight and obesity in the United States has increased dramatically in the past 25 years, and more than a third of adult Americans are now classified as obese (Ogden et al., 2006). Overweight and obesity are associated with increased risk of all-cause mortality and the onset of a variety of chronic diseases, including cardiovascular disease, select forms of cancer, diabetes, and arthritis. In the United States alone, estimates of the annual health care costs of obesity exceed $100 billion (Harrington, Gibson, & Cottrell, 2009; Jakicic, 2009).

Successful weight management interventions are associated with meaningful improvements in health and disease outcomes among overweight and obese individuals (Williamson et al., 2009), and the promotion of regular participation in physical activity at moderate or greater intensities represents an integral component of behavioral weight management efforts (National Task Force on the Prevention and Treatment of Obesity, 2000). Increased physical activity and exercise participation is associated with superior maintenance of weight loss and improvements in various chronic disease risk factors among obese individuals (Jakicic, 2009). In addition to these valuable health outcomes, physical activity is independently associated with enhanced HRQL in overweight adults. The 2005 Behavioral Risk Factor Surveillance Study survey found that overweight and obese adults who attained recommended daily levels of physical activity reported significantly higher HRQL than sedentary adults with a similar obesity status (Heath & Brown, 2009).

In spite of the well-established health benefits of exercise for overweight or obese individuals and the priority of promoting physical activity in this population, empirical evidence demonstrating the efficacy of exercise for enhancing HRQL among this group remains surprisingly limited (Fontaine & Barofsky, 2001). Furthermore, randomized trials addressing the HRQL benefits of behavioral weight loss interventions in samples of obese participants have yielded mixed findings. For example, Maciejewski, Patrick, and Williamson (2005) conducted a meta-analytic review of 34 randomized controlled trials assessing change in HRQL following weight loss interventions targeting overweight or obese adults. Twenty-two of the trials used behavioral intervention approaches, with 10 of these studies specifically incorporating exercise as a component of the behavioral treatment. Findings from the review suggested that the effect of weight loss on HRQL outcomes was inconsistent and varied across the dimensions of HRQL assessed. It should be acknowledged, however, that interpretation of the HRQL benefits of exercise or weight loss observed following interventions that included an exercise component is complicated by the fact that the majority of studies in this meta-analysis used multicomponent interventions that incorporated approaches including but not limited to dietary modification, cognitive behavioral therapy, social support, and surgical and pharmacologic treatment.

Although the effects of exercise on HRQL in the obese have yet to be systematically investigated, findings from several recent randomized controlled trials provide compelling evidence of links between exercise, weight management, and HRQL among overweight and obese individuals. For example, the Action for Health in Diabetes Trial, also known as the Look AHEAD trial (Ryan et al., 2003), is a multicenter, randomized trial designed to compare the effects of an intensive lifestyle intervention involving modification of exercise and dietary behavior with those of a usual-care diabetes education and support treatment in 5,145 overweight or obese adults with type 2 diabetes. Baseline results from Look AHEAD demonstrated that less favorable scores on the Physical Component summary scale of the SF-36 were associated with higher body mass index (BMI) and lower MET capacity (Rejeski et al., 2006). Additionally, interactions between obesity category and MET capacity revealed that while greater BMI was associated with lower HRQL in individuals with lower MET capacities, this relationship was not observed among higher-obesity individuals with greater MET capacities. Thus cross-sectional analysis of baseline data from Look AHEAD suggests that higher aerobic fitness levels may attenuate the adverse effect of BMI on select dimensions of HRQL.

Longitudinal analysis of changes in HRQL in the Look AHEAD trial also yielded promising results. The lifestyle exercise and dietary intervention resulted in significantly greater improvement in both the Physical Component summary scale of the SF-36 and depressive symptoms relative to the usual-care treatment arm (Williamson et al., 2009). Consistent with prior research (Rejeski et al., 1996), individuals reporting the lowest baseline HRQL status exhibited the greatest improvement in HRQL following participation the lifestyle intervention. Additionally, the beneficial effects of lifestyle intervention on HRQL were mediated by change in body weight, aerobic fitness, and physical symptoms. Recent ancillary analyses of a subsample of Look AHEAD participants reporting knee pain at baseline also revealed that the lifestyle exercise and dietary intervention produced significantly greater improvement in self-reported physical function than did usual-care diabetes treatment (Foy et al., 2010).

Evidence from the Lifestyle Interventions for the Elderly Pilot (LIFE-P) study also suggests that obesity classification may be an important determinant of change in select dimensions of HRQL. LIFE-P is a randomized controlled trial examining the effects of a moderate-intensity exercise intervention with those of a successful aging education program across 12 months of treatment in 424 older adults. Findings from LIFE-P revealed that mobility performance improved following exercise in nonobese participants (Manini et al., 2010). Conversely, mobility performance decreased irrespective of treatment arm assignment in obese participants. Consequently, one's obesity status may attenuate the effects of exercise on the physical functioning dimension of HRQL.

Overall, a relatively limited number of studies have addressed the effects of exercise on HRQL in overweight or obese individuals. Effectively summarizing the exercise–HRQL relationship in the obese is further complicated by the challenge of disentangling the effects of exercise from those of complementary treatment approaches, such as diet, counseling, or medical interventions, that are frequently employed in conjunction with efforts promoting physical activity in the treatment of obesity. Therefore, it is difficult at present to discriminate the independent effects of exercise on HRQL from the potentially synergistic effects of multicomponent lifestyle interventions on HRQL outcomes. These challenges notwithstanding, emerging evidence from several contemporary randomized controlled trials provides support for the position that behavioral interventions involving exercise result in significant, clinically meaningful improvements in select HRQL outcomes. Although there is considerable variability across studies in both the dimensions of HRQL that are most affected and the observed magnitude of change in these outcomes, it is reasonable to conclude from the present findings that exercise is a promising intervention for enhancing HRQL outcomes in overweight or obese individuals. Much additional research is necessary to adequately define both the relationship between obesity and HRQL and the efficacy of exercise in enhancing HRQL in the obese and overweight populations.

Taken collectively, it is evident from the summary of the exercise–HRQL relationship in the select population subgroups addressed in this review that exercise consistently results in small-to-moderate, yet meaningful, improvements in multiple HRQL outcomes, ranging from global indices of life satisfaction to disease-specific measures of core HRQL dimensions and symptoms. In light of the strong empirical evidence supporting the beneficial effect of exercise on HRQL, there is growing interest in identifying the factors that may influence the strength of the exercise–HRQL relationship or serve as intermediate variables that account for the favorable effect of exercise on HRQL outcomes. In this regard, potential moderating and mediating variables have become a focal area of research in the contemporary exercise psychology and behavioral medicine literature. The following section of the chapter will address emerging evidence of the variables that serve as effect modifiers of the exercise–HRQL relationship.

Pathways from Exercise to Enhanced HRQL

In the context of the exercise–HRQL relationship, a *moderator* is a variable that influences the strength of the effect of exercise on HRQL outcomes. A *mediator* is an intermediate variable that serves as an underlying mechanism for the effect of exercise on HRQL outcomes. A mediator variable essentially represents a proximal outcome that, when positively affected by exercise, subsequently contributes to improvements on more distal HRQL outcomes.

One of the most frequently observed moderators of the exercise–HRQL relationship is initial level of HRQL. Baseline HRQL values have consistently been found to serve as independent predictors of subsequent change in HRQL outcomes (Focht et al., 2004; Gillison et al., 2009; Rejeski et al., 1996; Rejeski, Focht et al., 2002; Rejeski & Mihalko, 2001). This effect has been documented across population subgroups (both healthy and various chronic disease samples) and for multiple HRQL outcomes, including global ratings of life satisfaction, generic HRQL, and disease- or population-specific measures of perceived physical function and psychological well-being (Berger & Tobar, 2007; Focht, 2006; Focht et al., 2004; Gillison et al., 2009; Rejeski et al., 1996; Rejeski & Mihalko, 2001). Consequently, there is strong empirical support for the position that, from a quality-of-life perspective, those who have the most to gain at the outset of exercise interventions derive the greatest benefit across an array of HRQL outcomes.

Although less compelling than the evidence supporting the influence of initial HRQL status, there are some recent findings from randomized controlled trials that suggest gender may moderate the effects of exercise on select HRQL outcomes. For example, findings from the REACT trial demonstrated that while men exhibited significant improvements in multiple aspects of disease-specific HRQL following long-term exercise training, women did not obtain similar added benefits beyond those conferred by a short-term exercise intervention (Foy et al., 2001). Furthermore, in the CHAMP trial, men reported more favorable improvements than women in a generic index of HRQL and in perceived physical functioning (Focht et al., 2004; Rejeski et al., 2003; Rejeski, Foy, et al., 2002). In interpreting these results, it should be recognized that gender differences have not been observed in the majority of studies addressing changes in HRQL accompanying exercise interventions. However, it is equally important to acknowledge that many randomized trials examining exercise have not been stratified by gender and have lacked the statistical power to detect potentially meaningful gender differences in treatment responsivity (Focht et al., 2004). In light of the equivocal findings, it seems prudent to propose that gender may be an important individual difference that moderates exercise-induced changes in select HRQL outcomes among targeted chronic disease samples (i.e., patients with COPD and cardiovascular disease). Accordingly, the role of gender in influencing responses to exercise therapy should be considered in future investigations of the efficacy of exercise interventions.

The importance or value one places on a particular dimension of functioning has also been proposed to impact the strength of the exercise–HRQL relationship. Importance or value appears to be particularly relevant when HRQL is assessed as an index of satisfaction with life or satisfaction with a specific HRQL domain. For example, Rejeski and colleagues found that knee OA and COPD patients who had the greatest difficulty completing valued functional tasks reported the least satisfaction with their physical function (Katula, Rejeski, Wickley, & Berry, 2004; Rejeski, Martin, Miller, Ettinger, & Rapp, 1998). Individuals who appear to adapt to disease and compromised levels of functioning by cognitively devaluing physical function have also been found to report less physical activity participation, placing them at greater risk for the onset of functional limitations and subsequent progression toward disability (Martin et al., 1999; Rejeski & Focht, 2002). Together, these findings suggest that value one places on particular dimensions of HRQL may affect satisfaction with one's function, well-being, and capabilities related to that domain. Thus, when assessed as an index of satisfaction, overall or domain-specific aspects of HRQL may be influenced by the importance ascribed to this aspect of quality of life. These evaluations also appear to have meaningful consequences for the perception of and participation in exercise behavior.

Findings from several recent randomized controlled trials have also expanded knowledge pertaining to potential mediators of the effects of exercise on HRQL. Within the context of the exercise–HRQL relationship, mediation is observed when each of the following criteria is satisfied: (1) Exercise has a significant effect on HRQL; (2) exercise significantly influences a targeted potential mediator variable; (3) change in the potential mediator variable is significantly related to change in the HRQL outcome; and (4) the effects of exercise on the HRQL outcome become nonsignificant after the effects of the mediator have been controlled for in a composite model.

Ancillary analyses from the FAST trial provided some of the first evidence that self-related psychological variables can serve as mediators of the effects of exercise on HRQL (Rejeski, Ettinger, Martin, & Morgan, 1998). Within a large sample of knee OA patients, self-efficacy beliefs relating to mobility (e.g., confidence in one's ability to complete incrementally more challenging amounts of a stair climb task) and knee pain symptoms were found to mediate the beneficial effect of exercise on a measure of functional performance. Additionally, knee pain mediated the effects of exercise on a generic index of HRQL. More recently evidence of similar meditational pathways was observed in the ADAPT trial (Rejeski, Focht, et al., 2002). Satisfaction with physical function and pain ratings were shown to be independent mediators of the effect of the lifestyle intervention involving exercise and dietary weight loss on the Physical Health summary scale of the SF-36. Mobility-related self-efficacy and knee pain were also shown to be significant, independent partial mediators of the effect of the combined exercise and diet intervention on select performance measures of physical function (Focht, Rejeski, Katula, Ambrosius, & Messier, 2005).

Both FAST and ADAPT addressed the effects of exercise in older adults burdened with knee OA. Consistent with the abovementioned findings from those studies, select psychological constructs such as self-efficacy beliefs, satisfaction with physical function, perceptions of physical symptoms, and affective responses have been observed to act as mediators of the effects of exercise on HRQL in other population subgroups. Notably, self-efficacy and satisfaction with physical function and appearance served as independent mediators of the effects of exercise on life satisfaction in the Activity Counseling Trial (Rejeski et al., 2001). Recent evidence has also demonstrated that the effects of exercise on global quality of life were mediated by changes in intermediate psychological constructs within samples of community-dwelling older adults. More specifically, improvements in ratings of overall life satisfaction were mediated in part by the positive effects of exercise on affective responses, self-efficacy, and perceptions of social support among older adults at risk for functional decline (Elavsky et al., 2005; McAuley et al., 2006).

Similarly, recent findings of research addressing the effects of exercise training in individuals diagnosed with multiple sclerosis provides support for the assertion that the effects of exercise on global quality-of-life and generic HRQL constructs are mediated by its influence on intermediate psychological variables. Results of path analyses demonstrated that exercise positively influenced self-efficacy, disease symptoms, and select indicants of psychological well-being. In turn, changes in these intermediate outcomes were linked with more favorable ratings of global quality of life (Motl & McAuley, 2009; Motl, McAuley, Snook, & Gliottoni, 2009; Motl & Snook, 2008).

These emerging findings suggest that the effects of exercise on generic indices of HRQL and global ratings of life satisfaction are consistently mediated in part by changes in intermediate psychological outcomes. The recent evidence demonstrating the indirect effect of exercise on HRQL and quality of life suggests that these potential mediators should be targeted and assessed in future exercise intervention trials. These findings also have important implications for the conceptualization of quality-of-life outcomes. The results indicate a hierarchical organization of quality-of-life outcomes in which change in proximal HRQL constructs predicts change in more distal, global indices of quality of life. Thus exercise may influence proximal HRQL dimensions assessed by measures of generic core dimensions of HRQL and disease- or population-specific symptoms. In turn, favorable changes in these proximal intermediate HRQL outcomes subsequently contribute to improvements in overall ratings of life satisfaction. Clearly, these findings have important implications for the design and delivery of exercise interventions as well as for the way in which HRQL and quality of life should be measured in future exercise trials.

Exercise and HRQL: Overall Summary

As noted in prior systematic reviews of the exercise–quality of life relationship (Berger & Tobar, 2007; Rejeski et al., 1996; Rejeski & Mihalko, 2001), heterogeneity in the conceptualization and measurement of salient quality-of-life constructs makes attempts to synthesize the effects of exercise on HRQL particularly challenging. The exercise–quality of life relationship is unquestionably complex. Nonetheless, findings from the contemporary exercise psychology, medical, and behavioral medicine literature clearly demonstrate that exercise consistently results in statistically significant, clinically meaningful improvements in a variety of quality-of-life outcomes, including global measures of overall life satisfaction, generic domains of HRQL, and targeted measures of specific HRQL dimensions and physical symptoms relevant to particular diseases or populations.

Although the wide array of HRQL benefits can be generally characterized as small to moderate in magnitude, not all dimensions of HRQL are equally responsive to exercise. There is sufficient evidence to conclude that certain dimensions of HRQL, such as perceptions of physical function and select physical symptoms and aspects of psychological well-being, are more sensitive to change with exercise interventions than others that are not as readily tied to the stimulus properties of exercise (e.g., social function). Current findings also suggest that improvements in HRQL do not appear to be limited to any particular population subgroup. Both healthy individuals and those with or at increased risk for chronic disease exhibit favorable changes in HRQL outcomes following exercise training interventions (Focht, 2006; Gillison et al., 2009; Lacasse et al., 2008; Rejeski et al., 1996). However, initial perceptions of health status are consistently independent predictors of the magnitude of improvement observed. Those individuals with the worst level of or the least satisfaction with a particular quality-of-life outcome at baseline report the most favorable improvement following exercise. This effect has been observed across numerous HRQL outcomes and population subgroups (Focht et al., 2004; Rejeski et al., 1996; Rejeski, Focht, et al., 2002). Additionally, the development and application of targeted measures of HRQL has led some to conclude that individuals with disease benefit more from exercise training than do healthy individuals (Gillison et al., 2009). Nonetheless, whereas the magnitude of the benefit may differ based on one's initial HRQL status, improvements in HRQL do not appear to systematically vary as a function of demographic variables or exercise intervention characteristics such as exercise mode, duration, intensity, or frequency.

With regard to exercise characteristics, it is particularly important to acknowledge that the effects of different amounts or "doses" of exercise on quality of life remain poorly understood. Accordingly, the minimum amount of exercise training required to produce improvements in various HRQL outcomes is not known. This dearth of information detracts from the ability to develop accurate guidelines for the recommended amount of exercise for enhancing and maintaining HRQL. There is emerging evidence that individuals meeting or exceeding public health recommendations for physical activity participation report superior HRQL relative to those failing to accrue this amount of activity (Blanchard, Stein, & Courneya, 2009). Accordingly, adhering to public health recommendations for physical activity and exercise may hasten improvements in HRQL (Speed-Andrews & Courneya, 2009). It has also been proposed that moderate-intensity exercise can facilitate superior changes in select dimensions of HRQL compared with more demanding or less demanding amounts of activity (Berger & Tobar, 2007).

There is certainly sufficient empirical evidence to warrant advancing such intuitively appealing proposals. However, current recommendations for physical activity and exercise prescription are largely based on the amounts of activity associated with physical health promotion and disease prevention benefits. Compelling arguments have been forwarded that these recommendations are based on a passive stimulus–response paradigm that erroneously assumes that any prescribed dose of activity will yield a uniform response across both physiological and psychological domains (Rejeski, 1994; Rejeski & Focht, 2002). Although accruing recommended amounts of physical activity and exercise may elicit a specific physiological adaptation, participants' tolerance for and perception of a given exercise prescription is shaped in part by the cognitive appraisals of and affective responses to that prescription that they experience directly or that they perceive to be related to the prescription. Given that HRQL inherently involves an individual's perception of a variety of dimensions of function and well-being, any single dose of exercise is unlikely to affect all valued aspects of HRQL equally. Additionally, improvements in HRQL outcomes are influenced by perceptions of initial health status and functional value. Hence while it seems prudent to suggest that achieving current public health recommendations for exercise participation will be sufficient to enhance HRQL, this amount of activity may not be appropriate for all people or elicit favorable changes in all relevant HRQL outcomes. As such, when a primary objective of the exercise prescription is to enhance HRQL, flexible prescriptions tailored to individuals' deficits, values, and preferences with respect to function and well-being would be preferable to advocating any single dose.

Directions for Future Research

Recognition of the value of exercise for improving and maintaining HRQL has increased dramatically in the past two decades. Although there is now a considerable body of empirical evidence supporting the position that exercise represents a viable public health intervention for enhancing HRQL, relatively modest advances in knowledge in this area of inquiry have been realized since one of the seminal reviews of the exercise–HRQL relationship was published nearly 15 years ago (Rejeski et al., 1996). Rejeski et al. (1996) offered several proposals that have yet to be consistently integrated into investigations of the effects of exercise on HRQL outcomes. To conclude the present chapter, I will present a brief overview of the most pressing issues identified by Rejeski et al. over a decade ago that have yet to be systematically addressed in contemporary exercise–HRQL literature. Future investigations that target the following issues will aid in developing a more comprehensive understanding of the complex exercise–HRQL relationship. Furthermore, expanded knowledge of these issues will also provide important information regarding how to more effectively design and implement exercise interventions to improve HRQL outcomes.

Consistency in the Conceptualization and Measurement of HRQL

Rejeski and colleagues (Rejeski et al., 1996; Rejeski & Mihalko, 2001) convincingly argued that one of the primary barriers to synthesizing and advancing knowledge of the effects of exercise on quality-of-life outcomes is inconsistency in the definition and measurement of quality-of-life and HRQL constructs (Berger & Tobar, 2007; Lox et al., 2006; Rejeski et al., 1996; Rejeski & Mihalko, 2001). There is little evidence to suggest that this and other calls for progress toward a unifying conceptualization of quality-of-life outcomes have been heeded. However, advances in this area have

recently emerged. Recent findings from the physical activity literature provide strong support for the assertion that quality of life and HRQL are related yet conceptually distinct constructs (Elavsky et al., 2005; McAuley et al., 2006; Motl & Snook, 2008; Motl et al., 2009). Perhaps more importantly, there is compelling evidence that quality-of-life outcomes may be hierarchically organized. Within the proposed hierarchical model of quality of life, exercise is purported to influence global quality of life (life satisfaction) indirectly through its effect on both generic domains and specific indices of HRQL as well as self-related psychological constructs such as self-efficacy beliefs, satisfaction with select aspects of function and well-being, affect, and social support (Elavsky et al., 2005; McAuley et al., 2006; Motl et al., 2009).

Both the proposed hierarchical structure of quality of life and findings indicating that exercise positively influences higher-order quality-of-life and HRQL outcomes indirectly have important implications for the design of future exercise interventions intended to improve HRQL. Notably, it suggests that quality of life and HRQL should be viewed and measured as distinct constructs. The consistent integration of a multilevel assessment approach that includes global indices of life satisfaction, generic measures of HRQL, and targeted measures of disease- or population-specific assessments of HRQL will be critical to advancing toward a more comprehensive understanding of the effects of exercise on quality-of-life outcomes. Additionally, measurement of select, conceptually relevant intermediate psychological constructs that may serve as mediator variables of the effect of exercise on quality of life and HRQL will aid in elucidating the mechanisms underlying the beneficial effect of exercise on HRQL. Recognition of the conceptual distinction between quality-of-life and HRQL outcomes and inclusion of multilevel measures of these outcomes is integral to achieving meaningful advances in knowledge of the effects of exercise on HRQL.

Appropriate Interpretation of Exercise-Related Changes in HRQL

Adoption of a hierarchical model of quality of life and inclusion of a multilevel measurement strategy will also aid in addressing other important research issues. Rejeski et al. (1996) proposed that many researchers mistakenly equate change in a core dimension of HRQL with improvements in more broad indices of function and well-being or overall quality of life. Given that quality of life and

HRQL are not isomorphic constructs, it is erroneous to assume that improvements in a core dimension of HRQL, such as physical function, will also produce concomitant improvements in perceived physical health status or overall life satisfaction. The effects of exercise on HRQL are not consistent across all outcomes. Consequently, change in one particular index of HRQL cannot be used to infer change in separate measures of HRQL. Provided that HRQL is seen as an umbrella construct comprising numerous core dimensions and disease- or population-specific symptoms, acknowledging that exercise may have unique influences on those outcomes is both practically and conceptually relevant for future inquiry.

Consideration of the Influence of Individual Differences in Initial Status and Perceived Importance of HRQL

Improvements in HRQL are also not consistent for all individuals. Individuals with normative levels of perceived function or well-being will not demonstrate as much improvement as those who exhibit compromised levels of these outcomes prior to exercise. Thus initial values are salient predictors of HRQL responses to exercise and must be carefully considered when interpreting the efficacy of any exercise intervention. Individuals vary considerably in the importance they place on various aspects of HRQL. The beneficence of exercise for HRQL is partially determined by the extent to which an individual values a particular aspect of HRQL. Furthermore, the extent to which change in a lower-order HRQL outcome will facilitate improvements in global ratings of quality of life would be expected to be influenced by the value ascribed to that dimension of HRQL. That is, exercise-related improvements in highly valued aspects of functioning and well-being should have more pronounced effects on global quality of life, as these personally meaningful aspects of HRQL are most likely to be to be sufficiently relevant to alter perceptions of overall life satisfaction. Because few investigations have directly addressed the role of perceptions of initial health status or of the importance and value attached to particular domains of HRQL, evidence supporting these relationships remains sparse.

Recognition of the Importance of Social and Behavioral Characteristics of Exercise Interventions

To develop appropriate exercise recommendations for enhancing HRQL, it is obviously critical to more fully explicate the range of exercise program characteristics that facilitate favorable changes in HRQL. The heterogeneity of exercise program factors (exercise mode, intervention length, intensity, frequency, and duration) that have been used in investigations of the exercise–HRQL relationship considerably restricts the ability to synthesize exercise recommendations for optimizing HRQL benefits. As noted above, efforts to determine a single optimal prescription reflect a passive stimulus–response paradigm that ultimately lacks utility or generalizability (Rejeski, 1994; Rejeski & Focht, 2002). No single exercise prescription will be equally efficacious in producing improvements in all facets of HRQL for all participants. In progressing toward the development of appropriate exercise guidelines it must be recognized that the impact of exercise on HRQL outcomes is due not only to the physiological dynamics of the exercise stimulus but also to the social and behavioral characteristics of the exercise intervention.

Findings from the CHAMP trial illustrated that exercise combined with a cognitive behavioral intervention produced superior changes in HRQL compared with exercise alone (Focht et al., 2004). Determining the "dose" of exercise that facilitates the most favorable changes in HRQL involves more than simply quantifying the exercise stimulus characteristics. Consequently, while identifying more precise ranges of exercise characteristics through the implementation of flexible, individually tailored prescriptive approaches seems prudent, the social, environmental, and behavioral factors that influence perceptions of health status are also critical considerations in enhancing treatment efficacy. The emerging evidence that exercise influences higher-order quality-of-life constructs through improvements in intermediate, self-related psychological variables underscores the potential importance of integrating behavioral intervention components that enhance self-efficacy beliefs, tolerance for and affective responses to exercise, and perceptions of social support. Expanding the conceptualization of the aspects of exercise interventions that comprise a given dose of exercise is a necessary step in facilitating meaningful advances in understanding the psychosocial mechanisms through which exercise results in HRQL benefits.

In summary, there is sufficient evidence to conclude that exercise is an efficacious intervention for promoting enhanced HRQL. Exercise has been linked with small-to-moderate improvements in numerous HRQL outcomes. Although exercise does not influence all HRQL outcomes equally, these benefits do not at present appear to systematically vary as a function of population subgroup or exercise intervention characteristics. However, the initial levels of HRQL prior to exposure to the exercise intervention and the amount of importance one places on a particular dimension of HRQL have been shown to influence the magnitude of the exercise effect. Individuals with compromised perceptions of function and well-being will demonstrate more pronounced changes in those specific aspects of HRQL than will individuals exhibiting higher levels of function.

Exercise also has great potential to positively influence value dimensions of HRQL that change in response to exercise participation. In turn, within the context of a hierarchical model of quality of life, exercise-related improvements in aspects of HRQL that are personally important have the greatest potential to contribute to enhancing subjective evaluations of generic HRQL domains and appraisals of overall satisfaction with life. This suggests that the beneficial effect of exercise on quality of life may be indirect, operating through its favorable influence on intermediate psychological and HRQL constructs. Given the clear value of exercise as a public health intervention and the relevance of HRQL as an indicant of treatment efficacy, further inquiry designed to provide a more comprehensive understanding of the complex exercise–HRQL relationship is warranted. In conclusion, as more consistent conceptualizations of HRQL are adopted, the likelihood of meaningful progress toward designing and delivering exercise interventions that are effective in enhancing HRQL is likely to be realized.

Acknowledgment

Dr. Focht was supported by grants R21 AR054595 from the National Institutes of Health and by the Lance Armstrong Foundation Survivorship Center of Excellence.

References

American Cancer Society (2008). *Cancer facts and figures—2008.* Atlanta, GA: American Cancer Society.

Baker, K., & McAlindon, T. (2000). Exercise for knee osteoarthritis. *Current Opinion in Rheumatology, 12,* 456–463.

Berger, B. G., & Tobar, D. A. (2007). Physical activity and quality of life: Key considerations. In G. Tennenbaum & R. C. Eklund (Eds.), *Handbook of sport psychology* (pp. 598–620). Hoboken, NJ: John Wiley & Sons.

Berry, M. J. (2007). The relationship between exercise tolerance and other outcomes in COPD. *Journal of Chronic Obstructive Pulmonary Disease, 4,* 205–216.

Berry, M. J., Rejeski, W. J., Adair, N. E., Ettinger, W. H., Zacarro, D. J., & Sevick, M. A. (2003). A randomized controlled trial comparing long-term and short-term exercise in patients with chronic obstructive pulmonary disease. *Journal of Cardiopulmonary Rehabilitation, 23,* 60–68.

Blair, S. N., LaMonte, M. J., & Nichamon, M. Z. (2004). The evolution of physical activity recommendations: How much is enough? *American Journal of Clinical Nutrition, 79,* 913S–920S.

Blanchard, C. M., Stein, K., & Courneya, K. S. (2010). BMI, physical activity, and health-related quality of life in cancer survivors. *Medicine & Science in Sports & Exercise, 42,* 665–671.

Bouchard, C. (2001). *Physical activity and obesity.* Champaign, IL: Human Kinetics.

Cambach, W., Wangenaar, R. C., Koelman, T. W., VanKeimpema, A. R., & Kemper, H. C. (1999). The long-term effects of pulmonary rehabilitation in patients with asthma and chronic obstructive pulmonary disease: A research synthesis. *Archives of Physical Medicine and Rehabilitation, 80,* 103–111.

Cantril, H. (1965). *The pattern of human concerns.* New Brunswick, NJ: Rutgers University Press.

Conn, V. S., Hafdahl, A. R., Porock, D. C., McDaniel, R., & Neilson, P. J. (2006). A meta-analysis of exercise interventions among people treated for cancer. *Supportive Care in Cancer, 14,* 699–712.

Courneya, K. S. (2009). Physical activity in cancer survivors: A field in motion. *Psychooncology, 18,* 337–342.

Courneya, K. S., Campbell, K. L., Karvinen, K. H., & Ladha, A. B. (2006). Exercise and quality of life in survivors of cancer other than breast. In A. McTiernan (Ed.), *Cancer prevention and management through exercise and weight control* (pp. 367–386). New York, NY: Taylor & Francis.

Courneya, K. S., Segal, R. J., Mackey, J. R., Gelmon, K., Reid, R. D., Friedenreich, C. M.,…McKenzie, D. C. (2007). Effects of aerobic and resistance exercise in breast cancer patients receiving adjuvant chemotherapy: A multi-center randomized controlled trial. *Journal of Clinical Oncology, 25,* 4396–4404.

Diener, E. (2000). Subjective well-being: The science of happiness and a proposal for a national index. *American Psychologist, 55,* 34–43.

Diener, E., Oishi, S., & Lucas, R. E. (2003). Personality, culture, and subjective well-being: Emotional and cognitive evaluations of life. *Annual Review of Psychology, 54,* 403–425.

Elavsky, S., McAuley, E., Motl, R. W., Konopack, J. F., Marquez, D. X., Hu, L.,…Diener, E. (2005). Physical activity enhances long-term quality of life in older adults: Efficacy, esteem, and affective influences. *Annals of Behavioral Medicine, 30,* 138–145.

Eshah, N. F., & Bond, A. E. (2009). Cardiac rehabilitation programme for coronary heart disease patients: An integrative review. *International Journal of Nursing Practice, 15,* 131–139.

Ettinger, W. H., Burns, R., Messier, S. P., Applegate, W., Rejeski, W. J., Morgan, T.,…Craven, T. (1997). A randomized clinical trial comparing aerobic exercise and resistance exercise with a health education program in older adults with knee osteoarthritis. *JAMA, 277,* 25–31.

Focht, B. C. (2006). Effectiveness of exercise interventions in reducing pain symptoms among older adults with knee osteoarthritis: A review. *Journal of Aging and Physical Activity, 14,* 212–235.

Focht, B. C. (2007). Obesity and knee osteoarthritis: Behavioral considerations in weight management. *International Journal of Advances in Rheumatology, 4*, 128–132.

Focht, B. C., Brawley, L., Rejeski, W. J., & Ambrosius, W. T. (2004). Effects of lifetime physical activity and traditional exercise therapy programs upon health-related quality of life among older adults in cardiac rehabilitation. *Annals of Behavioral Medicine, 28*, 52–61.

Focht, B. C., Rejeski, W. J., Katula, J. A., Ambrosius, W., & Messier, S. P. (2005). Exercise, self-efficacy, and mobility performance in overweight and obese older adults with knee osteoarthritis. *Arthritis and Rheumatism, 53*, 659–665.

Fontaine, K. R., & Barofsky, I. (2001). Obesity and health-related quality of life. *Obesity Reviews, 2*, 173–182.

Foy, C. G., Lewis, C. E., Hairston, K. G., Miller, G. D., Lang, W., Jakicic, J. M.,...Wagenknecht, L. E. (2011). Intensive lifestyle intervention improves physical function among obese adults with knee pain: Findings from the Look AHEAD Trial. *Obesity, 19*, 83-93.

Foy, C. G., Rejeski, W. J., Berry, M. J., Zaccaro, D, & Woodard, C. M. (2001). Gender moderates the effects of exercise therapy on health-related quality of life among COPD patients. *Chest, 119*, 70–76.

Fransen, M., & McConnell, S. (2008). Exercise for osteoarthritis of the knee. *Cochrane Database of Systematic Reviews, (4)*, CD004376.

Galvao, D. A., & Newton, R. U. (2005). Review of exercise intervention studies in cancer patients. *Journal of Clinical Oncology, 23*, 899–909.

Gillison, F. B., Skevington, S. M., Sato, A., Standage, M., & Evangelidou, S. (2009). The effects of exercise interventions in clinical and healthy populations: A meta-analysis. *Social Science and Medicine, 68*, 1700–1710.

Harrington, M., Gibson, S., & Cottrell, R. C. (2009). A review and meta-analysis of the effect of weight loss on all-cause mortality. *Nutrition Research Reviews, 22*, 93–108.

Haskell, W. L., Lee, I. M., Pate, R. R., Powell, K. E., Blair, S. N., Franklin, B. A.,...Bauman, A. (2007). Physical activity and public health: Updated recommendations for adults from the American College of Sports Medicine and the American Heart Association. *Circulation, 116*, 1081–1093.

Heath, G. W., & Brown, D. W. (2009). Recommended levels of physical activity and health-related quality of life among overweight and obese adults in the United States. *Journal of Physical Activity and Health, 6*, 403–411.

Jakicic, J. M. (2009). The effect of physical activity on body weight. *Obesity, 17(3)*, S34–S38.

Jolly, K., Taylor, R. S., Lip, G. Y. H., & Stevens, A. (2006). Home-based cardiac rehabilitation compared with center-based rehabilitation and usual care: A systematic review and meta-analysis. *International Journal of Cardiology, 111*, 343–351.

Katula, J. A., Rejeski, W. J., Wickley, K. L., & Berry, M. J. (2004). Perceived difficulty, importance, and satisfaction with physical function in COPD patients. *Health and Quality of Life Outcomes, 2*, 18.

Kaplan, R. M., & Bush, J. W. (1982). Health-related quality of life measurement for evaluation research and policy analysis. *Health Psychology, 1*, 61.

Lacasse, Y., Martin, S., Lasserson, T. J., & Goldstein, R. S. (2007). Meta-analysis of respiratory rehabilitation in chronic obstructive pulmonary disease: A Cochrane systematic review. *Europa Medicophysica, 43*, 475–485.

Lacasse, Y., Wong, E., Guyatt, G. H., King, D., Cook, D. J., & Goldstein, R. S. (1996). Meta-analysis of respiratory rehabilitation in chronic obstructive pulmonary disease. *Lancet, 348*, 1115–1119.

Lange, A. K., Vanwanseele, B., & Fiatarone Singh, M. A. (2008). Strength training for treatment of osteoarthritis of the knee: A systematic review. *Arthritis and Rheumatism, 59*, 1488–1494.

Lawlor, D. A., & Hopker, S. W. (2001). The effectiveness of exercise as an intervention in the management of depression: A systematic review and meta-regression analysis of randomized controlled trials. *British Medical Journal, 322*, 1–8.

Linden, W., Stossel, C., & Maurice, J. (1996). Psychosocial interventions for patients with coronary heart disease: A meta-analysis. *Archives of Internal Medicine, 156*, 745–752.

Liu, D. K. S, Chinapow, M. J. M., Huijgens, P. C., & Mechelen, W. V. (2008). Physical exercise interventions in haematological cancer patients, feasible to conduct but effectiveness to be established: A systematic review. *Cancer Treatment Reviews, 35*, 185–192.

Lox, C. L., Martin Ginis, K. A., & Petruzzello, S. J. (2006). *Psychology of exercise: Integrating theory and practice.* Scottsdale, AZ: Holcomb Hathaway.

Maciejewski, M. L., Patrick, D. L., & Williamson, D. F. (2005). A structured review of randomized controlled trials of weight loss showed little improvement in health-related quality of life. *Journal of Clinical Epidemiology, 58*, 568–578.

Maltais, F., Bourbeau, J., Shapiro, S., Lacasse, Y., Perrault, H., & Baltzan, M. (2008). Effects of home-based pulmonary rehabilitation in patients with chronic obstructive pulmonary disease. *Annals of Internal Medicine, 149*, 869–878.

Manini, T. D., Newman, A. B., Fielding, R., Fielding, R., Blair, S. N., Perri M. G.,...Pahor M; LIFE Research Group.(2010. Effects of exercise on mobility in obese and non-obese adults. *Obesity, 18*, 1168–1175.

Martin, K. A., Rejeski, W. J., Miller, M. E., James, M. K., Ettinger, W. H., & Messier, S. P. (1999). Validation of the PASE in older adults with knee pain and physical disability. *Medicine & Science in Sports & Exercise, 31*, 627–633.

Mayou, R., & Bryant, B. (1993). Quality of life in cardiovascular disease. *British Heart Journal, 69*, 460–466.

McAuley, E., & Katula, J. A. (1998). Physical activity interventions in the elderly: Influence on physical health and psychological function. In R. Schulz, G. Maddox, & M. P. Lawton (Eds.), *Annual review of gerontology and geriatrics* (pp. 111–154). New York: Springer-Verlag.

McAuley, E., Konopack, J. F., Motl, R. W., Morris, K. S., Doerksen, S. E., & Rosengren, K. R. (2006). Physical activity and quality of life in older adults: Influence of health status and self-efficacy. *Annals of Behavioral Medicine, 31*, 99–103.

Messier, S. P., Loeser, R. F., Miller, G. D., Morgan, T. M., Rejeski, W. J., & Sevick, M. A. (2004). Exercise and dietary weight loss in overweight and obese older adults with knee osteoarthritis. *Arthritis and Rheumatism, 50*, 1501–1510.

Minor, M. (2004). Impact of exercise on osteoarthritis outcomes. *Journal of Rheumatology, 31*, 81–85.

Motl, R. W., & Gosney, J. L. (2008). Effect of exercise training on quality of life in multiple sclerosis: A meta-analysis. *Multiple Sclerosis, 14*, 129–135.

Motl, R. W., & McAuley, E. (2009). Pathways between physical activity and quality of life in adults with multiple sclerosis. *Health Psychology, 28*, 682–689.

Motl, R. W., & McAuley, E. (2010). Physical activity, disability, and quality of life in older adults. *Physical Medicine and Rehabilitation Clinics of North America, 21*, 299–308.

Motl, R. W., McAuley, E., Snook, E. M., & Gliottoni, R. C. (2009). Physical activity and quality of life in multiple sclerosis: Intermediary roles of disability, fatigue, mood, pain, self-efficacy, and social support. *Psychology, Health, & Medicine, 14*, 111–124.

Motl, R. W., & Snook, E. M. (2008). Physical activity, self-efficacy, and quality of life in multiple sclerosis. *Annals of Behavioral Medicine, 35*, 111–115.

National Task Force on the Prevention and Treatment of Obesity. (2000). Overweight, obesity, and health risk. *Archives of Internal Medicine, 160*(7), 898–904.

Newton, R. U., & Galvao, D. A. (2008). Exercise in the prevention and management of cancer. *Current Treatment Options in Oncology, 9*, 135-146.

Ogden, C. L., Carroll, M. D., Curtin, L. R., McDowell, M. A., Tabak, C. J., & Flegal, K. M. (2006). The prevalence of overweight and obesity in the United States: 1999–2004. *JAMA, 295*, 1549–1555.

Ohira, T., Schmitz, K. H., Ahmed, R. L., & Yee, D. (2006). Effects of weight training on quality of life in recent breast cancer survivors: The Weight Training for Breast Cancer Survivors study. *Cancer, 106*, 2076–2083.

O'Reilly, S. C., Muir, K. R., & Doherty, M. (1999). Effectiveness of home exercise on pain and disability from osteoarthritis of the knee: A randomized controlled trial. *Annals of Rheumatic Disease, 58*, 15–19.

Pate, R. R., Pratt, M., Blair, S. N., Haskell, W. L., Macera, C. A., Bouchard, C.,...Wilmore, J. H. (1995). Physical activity and public health: A recommendation from the Centers for Disease Control and Prevention and the American College of Sports Medicine. *JAMA, 273*, 402–407.

Pavot, W., & Diener, E. (1993). Review of the Satisfaction with Life Scale. *Psychological Assessment, 5*, 164–172.

Petrella, R. J. (2000). Is exercise an effective treatment for osteoarthritis of the knee? *British Journal of Sports Medicine, 34*, 326–331.

Rejeski, W. J. (1994). Dose–response issues from a psychosocial perspective. In C. Bouchard, R. J. Shepard, & T. Stephens (Eds.), *Physical activity, fitness, and health: International proceedings and consensus statement* (pp. 1040–1053). Champaign, IL: Human Kinetics.

Rejeski, W. J., Brawley, L., Ambrosius, W. T., Brubaker, P. H., Focht, B. C., Foy, C. G., & Fox, L. (2003). Older adults with chronic disease: The benefits of group-mediated counseling in the promotion of physically active lifestyles. *Health Psychology, 22*, 414–423.

Rejeski, W. J., Brawley, L. R., Ettinger, W. H., Morgan, T., & Thompson, C. (1997). Compliance to exercise therapy in older participants with knee osteoarthritis: Implications for treating disability. *Medicine & Science in Sports & Exercise, 29*, 977–985.

Rejeski, W. J, Brawley, L. R., & Shumaker, S. A. (1996). Physical activity and health-related quality of life. *Exercise and Sport Science Reviews, 24*, 71–108.

Rejeski, W. J., Ettinger, W. H., Martin, K. A., & Morgan, T. (1998). Treating disability in knee osteoarthritis: A central role for self-efficacy and pain. *Arthritis Care and Research, 11*, 94–101.

Rejeski, W. J., & Focht, B. C. (2002). Aging and physical disability: On integrating group and individual counseling in the promotion of physical activity. *Exercise and Sport Science Reviews, 30*, 166–171.

Rejeski, W. J., Focht, B. C., Messier, S. P., Morgan, T., Pahor, M., & Penninx, B. (2002). Obese older adults with knee osteoarthritis: Weight loss, exercise, and quality of life. *Health Psychology, 21*, 419–426.

Rejeski, W. J., Foy, C. G., Brawley, L., Brubaker, P., Focht, B. C., Norris, J. L., & Smith, M. (2002). Lifestyle physical activity and traditional exercise therapy: Effects upon physical functioning among older men and women in cardiac rehabilitation. *Medicine & Science in Sports & Exercise, 34*, 1705–1713.

Rejeski, W. J., Lang, W., Neiberg, R. H., VanDoresten, B., Foster, G. D., Maciejewski, M. L.,...Williamson, D. F. (2006). Correlates of health-related quality of life in overweight and obese adults with type 2 diabetes. *Obesity, 14*, 870–883.

Rejeski, W. J., Martin, K. A., Miller, M. E., Ettinger, W. H., & Rapp, S. (1998). Perceived importance and satisfaction with physical function in patients with knee osteoarthritis. *Annals of Behavioral Medicine, 20*, 141–148.

Rejeski, W. J., & Mihalko, S. L. (2001). Physical activity and quality of life in older adults. *Journals of Gerontology, 56A*, 23–35.

Rejeski, W. J., Shelton, B., Miller, M., Dunn, A. L., King, A. C.,...Sallis, J. F. (2001). Mediators of increased physical activity and change in subjective well-being: Results from the Activity Counseling Trial. *Journal of Health Psychology, 6*, 159–168.

Roddy, E., Zhang, W., Doherty, M., Arden, N. K., Barlow, J., Birrell, F.,...Richards, S. (2005). Evidence-based recommendations for the role of exercise in the management of osteoarthritis of the hip or knee: The MOVE consensus. *Rheumatology, 44*, 67–73.

Ryan, D. H., Espeland, M. A. Foster, G. D., Haffner S. M., Hubbard, V. S., Johnson, K. C.,...Yanovski, S. Z.; Look AHEAD Research Grooup. (2003). Look AHEAD (Action for Health in Diabetes): Design and methods for a clinical trial of weight loss for the prevention of cardiovascular disease in type 2 diabetes. *Controlled Clinical Trials, 24*, 610–628.

Schmitz, K. H., Ahmed, R. L., Hannan, P. J., & Yee, D. (2005). Safety and efficacy of weight training in recent breast cancer survivors to alter body composition, insulin, and insulin-like growth factor axis proteins. *Cancer Epidemiology, Biomarkers, and Prevention, 14*, 1672–1680.

Schmitz, K. H., Ahmed, R. L., Troxel, A., Checille, A., Smith, R., Lewis-Grant, L.,...Greene, Q. P. (2009). Weight lifting in women with breast cancer-related lymphedema. *New England Journal of Medicine, 361*, 664–673.

Schmitz, K. H., Holtzman, J., Courneya, K. S., Masse, L. C., Duval, S., & Kane, R. (2005). Controlled physical activity trials in cancer survivors: A systematic review and meta-analysis. *Cancer Epidemiology, Biomarkers, and Prevention, 14*, 1588–1595.

Schwartz, A. L. (2008). Physical activity. *Seminars in Oncology Nursing, 24*, 164–170.

Segal, R. J., Reid, R. J., Courneya, K. S., Sigal, R. J., Kenny, G. P., Prud'Homme, D. G.,...DeAngelo, M. E. (2009). Randomized controlled trial of resistance exercise and aerobic exercise in men receiving radiation therapy for prostate cancer. *Journal of Clinical Oncology, 27*, 344–351.

Shumaker, S. A., Anderson, R. T., & Czajkowski, S. M. (1990). Psychological tests and scales. In B. Spiker (Ed.), *Quality* of life assessment in clinical trials (pp. 95–113). New York: Raven Press.

Speed-Andrews, A. E., & Courneya, K. S. (2009). Effects of exercise on quality of life and prognosis in cancer survivors. Current Sports Medicine Reports, 8, 176–181.

Stewart, A. L., & King, A. C. (1991). Evaluating the efficacy of physical activity for influencing quality of life outcomes in older adults. Annals of Behavioral Medicine, 13, 108–116.

Tai, M. E., Meininger, J. C., & Frazier, L. Q. (2008). A systematic review of exercise interventions in patients with heart failure. Biological Research for Nursing, 10, 156–182.

Taylor, R. S., Brown, A., Ebrahim, S., Jolliffe, J., Noorani, H., Rees, K., . . . Oldridge, N. (2004). Exercise-based rehabilitation for patients with coronary heart disease: Systematic review and meta-analysis of randomized controlled trials. American Journal of Medicine, 116, 682–692.

Thorsen, L., Courneya, K. S., Stevinson, C., & Fossa, S. D. (2008). A systematic review of physical activity in prostate cancer survivors: Outcomes, prevalence, and determinants. Supportive Care in Cancer, 16, 987–991.

Vallance, J. K., Courneya, K. S., Plotnikoff, R. C., Yasui, Y., & Mackey, J. R. (2007). Randomized controlled trial of the effects of print materials and step pedometers on physical activity and quality of life in breast cancer survivors. Journal of Clinical Oncology, 25, 2352–2359.

Ware, J. E., Kosinski, M., & Keller, S. D. (1997). SF-36 Physical and Mental Health summary scales: A user's manual. Boston: Health Institute New England Medical Center.

Williamson, D. A., Rejeski, W. J., Lang, W., Van Dorsten, B., Fabricatore, A. N., Toledo, K.; Look AHEAD Research Group. (2009). Impact of a weight management program on health-related quality of life in overweight adults with type 2 diabetes. Archives of Internal Medicine, 169(2), 163–171.

Wing, R. R. (1999). Physical activity in the treatment of adulthood overweight and obesity: Current evidence and research issues. Medicine & Science in Sports & Exercise, 31, S547–S552.

Winters-Stone, K., & Schwartz, A. L. (2006). Quality of life and fatigue in breast cancer. In A. McTiernan (Ed.), Cancer prevention and management through exercise and weight control (pp. 357–366). New York: Taylor & Francis.

World Health Organization Group (1995). The World Health Organization Quality of Life Group (WHOQOL): Position paper from the World Health Organization. Social Science and Medicine, 41, 1403–1409.

Physical Activity as a "Stellar" Positive Psychology Intervention

Kate Hefferon *and* Nanette Mutrie

Abstract

This chapter discusses the origins of the positive psychology movement; the main theoretical areas within positive psychology, such as positive emotions, resilience, and psychological well-being; and how physical activity provides a stellar medium for application of these concepts. Furthermore, the chapter discusses the links between the disciplines of positive psychology and physical activity in relation to interventions for well-being. The chapter concludes with a critical reflection and suggestions for future research.

Key Words: positive psychology, physical activity, psychological well-being, positive emotions, resilience, positive psychology interventions.

Introduction

For centuries, humans have been searching for the answer to "What makes us happy?" In 2010, we now have a psychological science that is dedicated to uncovering the response to that "million dollar question." That science is *positive psychology* (Peterson, 2006; Seligman, 2002). Positive psychology is defined as the science of optimal functioning It is as concerned with strength as with weakness and as interested in building the best things in life as in repairing the worst (Peterson, 2006; Seligman, 2002). The key concepts of interest in the discipline of positive psychology include optimism, resilience, goal setting, and strengths, which have been found to enable the psychologically healthy population to flourish.

Studying happiness and well-being is not a fruitless endeavor. There are a lot of benefits derived from being happy; it's not just an end in itself. Happier people tend to be more creative, persist at tasks longer, be more optimistic, live longer, be less vulnerable to illness, and be more socially giving, less hostile, and less self-centered (Argyle, 2001; Biswas-Diener & Diener, 2008; Myers, 2000). Thus

enhancing flourishing and well-being within the normal population produces benefits not only at a micro (individual) level but at a macro (community and society) level.

Although the positive psychology movement has gained rapid momentum over the past decade, its lack of acknowledgment of the role of the physical self is a common criticism (Resnick, Warmoth, & Serlin, 2001), with even the founder of positive psychology proclaiming that it has become a "neck-up"-focused discipline (Seligman, 2008). In 2004, Mutrie and Faulkner wrote a concise, groundbreaking chapter highlighting the absence of any focus on the body and its impact on well-being within the positive psychology literature. In particular, they argued that positive psychology should be looking at the benefits to well-being that are available from regular physical activity, and they suggested that the ability to build psychological and emotional strength via the building of physical strength be referred to as the *somatopsychic principle*. Both current authors support this perspective, which underpins the content of this chapter.

The aim of this chapter is to provide an overview of the major theories within positive psychology and to describe how they connect to exercise and physical activity.[1] The chapter commences with a brief overview of positive psychology, followed by a detailed consideration of the relation of positive emotions, resilience, psychological well-being, motivation, and individual strengths to physical activity. The chapter concludes with a critical reflection on the positive psychology movement, its inclusion of the body, and suggestions for future research and applications.

Overview of Positive Psychology

The following section will focus on the conception of the positive psychology movement and definitions of well-being. Positive psychology is the scientific study of optimal human functioning that "aims to discover and promote the factors that allow individuals and communities to thrive" (Seligman, 1998). It is concerned with enhancing flourishing and well-being at three levels (Seligman, 1998):

1) the *subjective node* (positive experiences and states across past, present, and future, e.g., happiness, optimism, and well-being)
2) the *individual node* (characteristics of the "good person," e.g., talent, wisdom, love, courage, and creativity)
3) the *group node* (positive institutions, citizenship, and communities, e.g., altruism, tolerance, and work ethic)

This trifold perspective has many implications for its usefulness and application in physical activity settings. As exercise psychologists know, participation in exercise can have copious benefits for the individual's physical, psychological, and emotional well-being (subjective node) as well as foster a sense of purpose, personal growth, self-determination, and citizenship (individual node). Furthermore, communities and organizations (group node) that support local participation in physical activities have the potential to flourish via reduction in social exclusion, reduction in crime, and an increased sense of community involvement (Coalter, 2005).

At this point, it is important to take a step back and look at the reasons surrounding the positive psychology movement's profound shift in thinking to the "positive side" of life. Prior to World War II, psychology had three main tasks: (1) to cure mental illness, (2) to enhance the well-being of the normal population, and (3) to study geniuses

(Seligman & Csikszentmihalyi, 2000). As a result of the terrible atrocities of the war, posttraumatic stress disorder and mental illness flew to the forefront of psychology's priorities. This remained so for over 50 years. Due to this intense focus of funding, psychologists can now say that at least 14 disorders can be cured or considerably relieved (Seligman & Csikszentmihalyi, 2000). However, the downside of this achievement is that for decades, psychology was focused on healing a small fraction of the population suffering from mental health problems rather than on giving the larger fraction a chance and the knowledge to enhance their life and flourish.

This imbalance was addressed at the American Psychological Association in 1998 by Professor Martin Seligman, who shifted the trajectory of psychology to focus on building strengths and living "the good life." In 2000, a special issue of the *American Psychologist* focused on this area and stated a clear and forceful message: The positive psychology movement was here to stay.

What Is Well-Being?

There are several ways to characterize well-being, and there is no firm consensus on the best one (Snyder & Lopez, 2002). Terms used interchangeably with well-being include *happiness, self-actualization, contentment, adjustment, economic prosperity, quality of life, positive mental health, positive mental well-being, positive health, mental well-being,* and *flourishing.* Although there is still confusion outside and within the discipline of positive psychology, two terms help separate the theories into two camps: *hedonic* and *eudaimonic* well-being.

Hedonic theorists define happiness as a direct result of *subjective well-being* (SWB) (Diener 1984; Diener, Emmons, Larsen, & Griffin, 1985). SWB encompasses how people evaluate their own lives in terms of affective and cognitive explanations (Diener, Suh, Lucas, & Smith, 1999). The formula for SWB, according to these theorists, is "satisfaction with life + high positive affect + low negative affect.") (Diener 1984; Diener, Emmons, Larsen, & Griffin, 1985). *Satisfaction with life* represents the cognitive component and refers to the discrepancy between the person's present situation and their ideal standard (Veenhoven, 1991). *Affect* represents the emotional side of well-being and refers to both moods and emotions associated with experiencing momentary events (Diener et al., 1999). There are multiple SWB scales, with the most widely used and best validated being the Satisfaction with Life Scale (Diener et al., 1985).

Eudaimonic theorists view well-being as a combination of happiness and meaning (Snyder & Lopez, 2007). Researchers became disgruntled with the focus on well-being as simply "feeling good" and argued that the discipline was failing to answer the question of what it means to be well psychologically (Ryff & Keyes, 1995). Most importantly, they said, meaning and purpose were ignored (King & Napa, 1998; McGregor & Little, 1998). Thus the eudaimonic perspective within positive psychology focuses on self-actualization, purpose, meaning and growth as being important for well-being along with feeling good.

Together, these two camps are reflected in Seligman's (2002) three routes to happiness, or authentic happiness model:

1) the pleasant life (includes positive emotions, gratification)

2) the good life (includes absorption, engagement, "flow")

3) the meaningful life (includes using your strengths in the service of something greater than yourself)

Within this chapter, we discuss both hedonic and eudaimonic theories of well-being in relation to physical activity. As there are numerous topic areas within the umbrella term of positive psychology, this chapter is not an exhaustive review (see Hefferon & Boniwell, 2011, for further reading). The next section will review the rationale for physical activity as a part of positive psychology. We will then address major theories such as positive emotions, resilience, psychological well-being, motivation, interventions, and strengths.

Physical Activity and Well-Being

Why should we focus on physical activity as important for well-being? For optimal human functioning, we need to function at our optimum physiological level. Activity participation is influential on both physical and psychological functioning. Specifically, activity participation has been found to reduce the risks of developing obesity, cardiovascular disease, coronary heart disease, stroke, diabetes (type 2), osteoporosis, sleep disorders, high blood pressure, certain cancers (colon, breast, rectal, lung, prostate, and endometrial), and even premature death (Department of Health, 2004; Paffenbarger, Hyde, Wing, & Hsieh, 1986; Salonen et al, 1983). In addition, physical activity has been reported to reduce the risk of developing depression, dementia, and cognitive impairment (Fox & Mutrie, under

review). Having a healthy mind within a healthy body is not a new idea, but the increased knowledge we now have of the integration between physiological and psychological processes has provided several potential mechanisms for enhanced well-being with enhanced physiological function. Possible mechanisms include:

• changes associated with an increase in core body temperature with exercise—the thermogenic hypothesis (Koltyn, 1997)

• increase in endorphin production following exercise—the endorphin hypothesis (Hoffmann, 1997)

• changes in central serotonergic systems due to exercise—the serotonin hypothesis (Chaouloff, 1997)

• effects of exercise on neurotransmitters, as in the norepinephrine/noradrenaline hypothesis (Dishman, 1997)

• changes in physical self-worth and self-esteem due to mastering new tasks, having a greater sense of personal control, or getting time away from negative or more stressful aspects of one's life (Fox, 2000)

Exercise scientists are investigating which of these mechanisms remain plausible or if all of them work in a simultaneous and synergistic way to provide enhanced well-being following physical activity participation.

Ironically, positive psychology has traditionally focused on passive leisure activities to enhance well-being. Interventions such as "expressing gratitude" and visualizing a "best possible self" focus on changing perceptions of the self via cognitive reframing and not holistically engaging the person. Research has shown that choosing to participate in active leisure activities can have significant positive effects on one's well-being and satisfaction with life (Holder, Coleman, & Sehn, 2009). Thus if we are not using or developing our bodies to their optimal levels of functioning, how are we going to ensure that our cognitive and affective functioning is at its best? It seems remiss to focus on the cognitive side of well-being without including the physical side of well-being in tandem.

Is Physical Activity a Positive Psychology Intervention?

Although the first representation of sport and exercise psychologists in positive psychology was evident at the International Positive Psychology Association world congress in Philadelphia in June

2009, the connection between activity and well-being is still often ignored in the field. Indeed, the major textbooks in positive psychology have limited references to the benefits of exercise on flourishing.[2]

Sin and Lyubomirsky (2009) conducted a meta-analysis of 52 positive psychology interventions (PPIs). However, their explicit exclusion of physical activity from this meta-analysis raises several questions regarding positive psychology's reluctance to fully embrace physical activity as a PPI. They defined PPIs as

> treatment methods or intentional activities that aim to cultivate positive feelings, behaviours or cognitions.... Programs, interventions, or treatments aimed at fixing, remedying, or healing something that is pathological or deficient—as opposed to building strengths—do not fit the definition of a PPI.
>
> (*Sin & Lyubormirsky,* 2009, p. 468)

Given this definition, we see no reason to exclude physical activity, which is often used as a therapeutic tool precisely (and very literally) to build strength. Well-being is not simply the absence of depression and anxiety, but the presence of subjective and psychological well-being. We see physical activity as a stellar (by which we mean exceptionally good) method of intervening to promote well-being. The research on the enhancement of positive emotions following activity participation has focused on *producing* positive psychological emotions rather than solely *reducing* negative ones. Positive psychology offers exercise psychology access to a battery of well-being measurement tools that are easy to administer and well validated, including the following:

1) Positive and Negative Affect Schedule (PANAS) (Watson, Clark, & Tellegen, 1988)
2) Scale of Positive and Negative Experiences (SPANE) (Diener et al., 2009)
3) Satisfaction with Life Scale (SWLS) (Diener et al., 1985)
4) Subjective Happiness Scale (Lyubomirsky, 2008)
5) Flourishing Scale (Diener et al., 2009)
6) Subjective Vitality (Ryan & Frederick, 1997)

Ultimately, these tools, and many more, can give exercise psychology researchers a broader picture of the positive effects of activity. The next section will review the main theories in positive psychology, commencing with positive emotions (i.e., affect or mood) at the individual level (subjective node).

Positive Psychology Theories and Links to Well-Being
Positive Emotions

One of the most influential and empirically supported theories in positive psychology is the importance of positive emotions for well-being. Early research into the purpose of positive emotions demonstrated novel evidence that positive emotions have evolutionary value (Fredrickson, 2009). While negative emotions allow us to narrow in on danger and alert us to risk, positive emotions have been shown to help broaden our thought-action repertoires, allowing humans to "think outside the box" and become more creative, open, and tolerant. These emotions include joy, gratitude, serenity, interest, hope pride, amusement, inspiration, awe, and love (Fredrickson, 2009). The proposed optimal ratio of positive to negative emotions is three positive for every one negative emotion felt (Fredrickson & Losada, 2005).

Even more notably, positive emotions appear to have a protective effect, meaning that the accumulation of positive emotions can build resilient psychological tendencies. Studies have shown that individuals who are manipulated to feel positive emotions are able to bounce back physiologically and psychologically from adverse conditions (Fredrickson, 2009). The "broadening" features of positive emotions paired with the "building" of psychological resources has been coined the *broaden-and-build theory* of positive emotions (Fredrickson, Tugade, Waugh, & Larkin, 2003). More on the effects of positive emotions and resilience is reviewed in the next section.

The link between positive emotions and physical activity can be illustrated with the literature on the "feel good" effects of activity participation. At the extreme positive end of the feel-good effect is the "runner's high," which is anecdotally recognized throughout the exercise world as a euphoric state that can be reached through distance running. Recent research in this area has explored a number of themes. For example, it now seems clear that there is a complex relationship between the intensity of exercise or physical activity and the affective responses to that activity (Ekkekakis, Hall, & Petruzzello, 2005). Biddle and Mutrie, in their overview of this area (2008, Chapter 8), concluded that exercise and physical activity participation is consistently associated with positive mood and affect and that experimental trials support the effect of moderate exercise on psychological well-being.

Thus if most positive psychology interventions are focused on inducing and prolonging positive emotions within individuals, and physical activity participation has been shown to have this result, then we would argue that such activity is a PPI in its purest form.

Flow, or optimal experience, is one of the leading states in which individuals can actively engage and increase their positive-emotion ratio. The majority of research on flow stems from the sports discipline, where the engagement in activity provides a perfect environment for flow experiences (Hefferon & Ollis, 2006). Flow is defined as

> the intense experiential involvement in moment-to-moment activity, which can be either physical or mental. Attention is fully invested in the task at hand and the person functions at her or his fullest capacity. (*Csikszentmihalyi*, 2009, p. 394)

Originally termed an "autotelic experience," flow entails a common set of structural characteristics that distinguish patterns of action that produce flow from the rest of everyday life (Csikszentmihalyi, 1998, p. 8). Csikszentmihalyi (1998) proposed nine elements required for the flow experience:

1) structured activity
2) balance of challenges vs. skills
3) clear goals and immediate feedback
4) complete concentration
5) merging of action and awareness
6) loss of awareness of oneself and self-consciousness
7) sense of control
8) transformation of time
9) activity for the sake of activity

Once these have been satisfied, a person in able to enter into the flow state, feeling immense joy, pleasure, and positive emotions as well as performance success. Interestingly, 10–15% of the US and European populations have never experienced flow, and yet another 10–15% of the same population report experiencing flow every day (Csikszentmihalyi, 2009). Participation in physical activity, whether in competitive, team, or individual sport environments or in everyday activities such as walking or gardening, can potentially facilitate the flow experience.

Resilience

We now turn to how physical activity participation can build both physiological and psychological resilience. Like well-being, *resilience* is a commonly used term with many definitions used interchangeably. A clear, all-encompassing definition of resilience is "the flexibility in response to changing situational demands, and the ability to bounce back from negative emotional experiences" (Tugade, Fredrickson, & Barrett, 2004, p. 1169). Resilience has been further subdivided into three dimensions: recovery, resistance and reconfiguration (Lepore & Revenson, 2006). *Recovery* is said to occur when someone simply "bounces back" from an adverse situation and returns to normal levels of functioning. Some researchers hold that it is the time line over which you recover (the faster, the better) that determines whether or not you have exhibited resilient tendencies (Bonanno, 2004). *Resistance* occurs when someone exhibits no signs of disturbance or low distress while in the midst of an adverse situation. *Reconfiguration* refers to the ability to be changed (or reconfigured) by adversity into someone stronger than before the adverse event occurred. This definition is related to the theory of posttraumatic growth, which states that people can derive positive benefits following a traumatic event, (Lepore & Revenson, 2006; Tedeschi, Park & Calhoun, 1998).

Resilience has been suggested to be a key process in buffering individuals from depression and inoculating them against future stressors (Carver, 1998). Exercise psychologists have established that buffering and inoculation occur as a result of physical activity involvement (Biddle & Mutrie, 2008; Salmon, 2001). Some researchers take a more biological stance than others; suggesting that by training individuals either psychological or physically to adapt to stressors, one can build stronger, more resilient individuals. Physical activity can therefore be seen as one of the ways in which to inoculate individuals against psychological dysfunction. Engaging in physical activity can potentially reduce depression (in intensity, duration, and likelihood of relapse), emotional and generalized stress, and anxiety (Babyak et al., 2000; Camacho, Roberts, Lazarus, Kaplan, & Cohen, 1991; Hassmen, Koivula, & Utela, 2000; Kritz-Silverstein, Barrett-Connor, & Corbeau, 2001; McDonald & Hodgdon, 1991; Steptoe & Butler, 1996).

Psychological Well-Being

As discussed above, psychological well-being (PWB) differs from mainstream SWB (Diener et al., 1999), which is the cognitive appraisal of satisfaction with life and more closely linked to hedonic well-being (which involves the pleasant life and positive emotions). PWB theory falls under the umbrella of eudaimonic well-being, which is a deeper level of happiness in which one has developed a connection to one's meaningful, true self.

Ryff and Singer's (1996; 2006) model of PWB is one of the models that come closest to explaining why physical activity can facilitate well-being. This model proposes that there are six major components for PWB. We next review each of these six components and how they may apply to physical activity.

SELF-ACCEPTANCE

The *self-acceptance* component of Ryff and Singer's (1996) model focuses on the need for individuals to accept and be at peace with themselves. Enhanced self-acceptance and self-esteem is imperative for PWB (Mutrie & Faulkner, 2004). Research on activity participation has repeatedly demonstrated the significant positive effects on people's body image, self-perceptions, and global self-esteem (Fox, 2000; Moses, Steptoe, Mathews, & Edwards, 1989). Therefore physical activity participation can enable this component to thrive.

Fox and Corbin (1989) developed the Physical Self-Perception Profile (PSPP)) as a measure of physical self-worth. They suggested that physical self-worth is a component of global self-esteem and proposed four subdomains of physical self-worth: sport competence, body attractiveness, perceived strength, and physical condition. The PSPP enables the investigation of exercise's effects on different aspects of self-perception and of their impact on self-esteem. For example, participation in exercise may improve one's perception of one's physical condition, which may in turn increase one's overall physical self-worth and global self-esteem.

AUTONOMY

According to the well-researched area of self-determination theory, *autonomy* is regarded as essential for well-being and self-development (Ryan & Deci, 2000). Autonomy refers to the ability to feel independent and believe that one has choice over one's life decisions. People need to feel that they have influence over what happens to them and that they are not controlled by external forces. Participation in exercise can help foster a person's sense of autonomy in several ways, which we can illustrate using weight loss as an example. First, individuals can create their own exercise plans to lose weight around their own lives, thereby exerting control over their environments. Second, as they engage in their individual programs, lose weight, and increase their self-esteem, they will revel in the fact that they alone achieved these feats and derive a deep sense of autonomous pleasure.

ENVIRONMENTAL MASTERY

Environmental mastery refers to a person's belief and confidence in their ability to negotiate their environmental surroundings. Environmental mastery has two applications for exercise. First, exercise allows a person to gain a sense of mastery or control over his or her own body. This phenomenon has been documented throughout the literature in normal populations and especially within clinical populations (e.g., individuals with cancer, HIV, and multiple sclerosis; see Hefferon, Grealy, & Mutrie, 2008, 2009, 2010). For individuals who perceive their bodies as declining in physical functioning (e.g., elderly adults and cancer and HIV patients), participation in exercise can allow them to gain a sense of mastery and control over their bodies and to develop positive physical self-perceptions. This is especially true for those who viewed themselves as having an athletic identity and derived satisfaction from their physical self (Netz, Wu, Becker, & Tenenbaum, 2005). There is evidence supporting the fact that mastering a sense of environmental efficacy enables the production and maintenance of positive emotions (Netz et al., 2005).

The second application involves the development of environmental mastery in special populations: people who are suffering from any type of mild-to-severe mental illness (e.g., depression, anxiety, and schizophrenia). Specifically, exercise interventions have been developed for people who are in remission from mental illness, to help them integrate them back into society and gain confidence and environmental mastery over their own lives (e.g., by arranging training sessions, traveling to the gym, exercising in normal surroundings, and identifying as a gym-goer, not a person with mental illness). As an adjunct to therapy, exercise participation can enhance self-esteem, give a person the confidence to leave his or her "inner world," and reintegrate the individual into society (Biddle & Mutrie, 2008).

POSITIVE RELATIONSHIPS

Social connections and the development of positive relationships are among the most important components of well-being. Again, the literature is rich with documentation of group-based exercise interventions and the bonds that are created via working with, and sweating with, a team (Emslie,

2005; Emslie et al., 2007; Sabiston, McDonough, & Crocker, 2007; Stevinson & Fox, 2006). The majority of the research involves groups of cancer patients, who have participated in activities such as dragon boat racing (Sabiston et al., 2007) and controlled aerobic trials (Mutrie et al., 2007).

PURPOSE IN LIFE

The *purpose in life* component of PWB touches upon the "meaningful life" that Seligman named as important for authentic happiness. Although the connection between purpose and exercise may not appear evident at first, there are many circumstances in which this link rings true. Holahan, Holahan, and Suzuki (2008), for example, found a significant relationship between maintaining purpose in life, a sense of personal growth, and physical activity among cardiac patients. Those patients who reported higher levels of purposefulness were more likely to adopt and adhere to healthy exercise behaviors. As a second example, a person may have a "teachable moment" when a diagnosis of illness highlights the importance of healthy living, with the result that staying healthy and exercising in an attempt to prevent any further disease becomes a huge focus (purpose) of that person's life (Demark-Wahnefried, Aziz, Rowland, & Pinto, 2005; Demark-Wahnefried, Peterson, McBride, Lipkus, & Clipp, 2000). Third, for isolated and socially excluded individuals (e.g., the elderly and those with mental health issues), exercise participation may provide a reason to get up in the morning. Taking part in an exercise group enables people to feel part of something; they are responsible to a group of people, a team, and the team doesn't work without all of them. Research continually finds that people develop a sense of camaraderie when they have something to do and somewhere to be and people are counting on them.

PERSONAL GROWTH

Humanistic psychologists believed that personal growth or self-actualization was the ultimate goal for all human beings. Thus it is appropriate that this concept fits within the eudaimonic perspective or model of PWB. Merleau-Ponty (1945/2005) argued that all humans are embodied creatures, that our experiences are not just physical but also phenomenological, and that our bodies ultimately affect our emotions, feelings, and experiences. Thus the body and what we do to it will inevitably affect our experience of growth. Hefferon et al. (2008) found that exercise participation was a key contributor to the attainment of personal and psychological growth among women with breast cancer.

In conclusion, the combination of the first five components of PWB (Ryff & Singer, 2006)—self-acceptance, autonomy, environmental mastery, positive relationship, and purpose in life—appears to inevitably influence the sixth component- a personal sense of achievement and growth.

Adapting Positive Psychology Interventions for Exercise Adoption and Adherence

Theories of and interventions used in positive psychology can be used to promote adoption of and adherence to physical activity participation. In the past several years the number of interventions created and tested in the realm of positive psychology has exploded. Within the discipline, the theory of *hedonic adaptation,* or *set point theory,* is the foundation for research into well-being interventions. This theory posits that we each have our own individual set points for happiness. Thus after a positive or negative event, we will eventually return to our previous levels of happiness. Lyubomirsky (2008) goes further into this theory and has proposed the "happiness pie," or *40% solution.* According to this idea, after the contributions of genes (50%) and circumstances (10%), we are left with 40% of our happiness to play with. This is the fundamental argument for PPIs and the continued research into enhancing human flourishing.

The next section will adapt approaches and interventions based on the concepts of self-determination theory, "best possible self," and individual strengths to an exercise context. Activity consultants, practitioners, trainers, and those in similar occupations can use the ideas presented to enhance activity participation by their clients.

Self-Determination Theory

Self-determination theory is a theory of motivation that posits that humans strive to be self-governed, a situation in which their behavior is "volitional, intentional and self-caused or self-initiated" (Wehmeyer & Little, 2009, p. 869). According to this notion, *intrinsic motivation* is key for a healthy, fulfilling, and meaningful life. Over the decades, researchers have proposed that the social environment has a powerful influence in promoting intrinsically healthy, self- determined development. In particular, there are three proposed psychological components individuals require for well-being: *autonomy, competence* and *relatedness* (Deci & Ryan, 2008; Ryan & Deci, 2000). The most important of these three is autonomy, which is the need to feel that one is in charge of one's own life and own choices. Competence relates to people's need to feel that they have the skills to complete what is asked of them. When one feels incompetent, anxiety increases and it becomes less and less possible to achieve well-being. Finally, relatedness has to do with the need for humans, who are social creatures, to have social networks and connections. People need to feel part of something and that they have people they trust and rely on.

When these three needs are met, it is thought that the person is moving toward becoming self-determined, or acting intrinsically. Exercise environments have the ability to foster the satisfaction of these needs and thereby increase intrinsic motivation and well-being. By giving people choice in developing exercise routines (autonomy), starting slowly and building on already developed exercises (competence), and getting people to participate in groups or buddy systems (relatedness), one can enable them to feel more intrinsic motivation to continue and thus psychologically benefit from their participation.

"Best Possible Self"

Individual interventions aimed at the adoption of an activity can focus on the importance of goals for well-being and persistence For example, one can adapt positive psychology's validated goal-setting tool, the *best possible self* intervention (Lyubomirsky, 2008), to have clients create visualizations or images of their best possible selves as they relate to activity participation. One might, for instance, ask clients to write, for 15 minutes for three consecutive days, about their best possible selves in terms of what they will feel, think, and look like after they have adopted and adhered to their goals with regard to exercise. One could further ask the clients to write out exactly how they could achieve their best possible selves and what they need to do, step by step, goal by goal, to reach their potential. This exercise allows people to gain insight into and organize their thoughts, values, and goals and enables them to recognize where they are in their lives and where they would like to be in the future.

Pedometers are one excellent, simple, cheap way for individuals to keep track of their goals and set realistic, gradual targets with clear and immediate feedback. Research has shown that by simply making people aware of their activity level via monitoring and feedback, one can promote an increase in walking of up to 30% (Biddle & Mutrie, 2008;

Baker, Mutrie & Lowry, 2008). While the recommended goal for walking has been 10,000 steps or the equivalent of 333 kcal/day, interventions with pedometers of course need to be individualized and set relative to baseline statistics (Bravata et al., 2007). Small goals set frequently will give the exerciser the commitment and sense of achievement to continue (in accord with self-determination theory).

Strengths

We propose here for the first time an approach to physical activity predicated on the *strengths movement* within positive psychology. The discipline has developed several assessment tools, underpinned by different theories, to assess individuals' inner strengths and talents. The Values in Action (VIA) and the Gallup Strengths Finder are the two most widely used tools, supported with data on over 100,000 users. The VIA is a tool that anyone can use for free online (www.authentichappiness.org). The Strengths Finder test is purchasable via Gallup's books (Rath, 2007). Both tools give a report detailing one's top five *signature strengths*. Research suggests that by using these "top five" in our daily lives one can significantly increase one's well-being and reduce depression (Seligman, Steen, Park, & Peterson, 2005).

There are fundamental differences between the two approaches, however. The VIA was created by two of the "founding fathers" of positive psychology (Peterson & Seligman, 2004). Based on a global search for values and virtues that appear in every society, they came up with 24 strengths that are valued in their own right and that, when used, do not hurt or hinder anyone. These strengths can be cultivated with attention and effort. When individuals use their strengths, it is believed that they are acting in their most authentic way. The Strengths Finder, however, comes from a slightly more corporate perspective and concentrates not on virtues but on talents that are innate (i.e., that one cannot cultivate). The Strengths Finder has 34 strengths and focuses on their use for performance achievement.

To incorporate strengths into physical activity, we suggest that individuals build an exercise program around using their VIA top five signature strengths in new and challenging ways. There are several ways of fusing a person's natural strengths with a bespoke exercise program. For example, say a client had the top five signature strengths of "love and be loved," curiosity, self-regulation, playfulness and humor, and spirituality. This person's top strength is their ability to love and be loved—to connect to others, to build friendships and keep them. This immediately suggests that the client should join a group class or get an exercise buddy to nourish the client's strength in and desire for connection. The client's strengths of curiosity and playfulness and humor suggest a taste for fun and adventure. A trainer could thus suggest dance classes such as Zumba, salsa, or tango; hula-hooping; hill walking; hiking; mountain biking; or rock climbing. Again, some of these activities can be done in groups to reinforce the client's top signature strength. The report also suggests that this person seems able to regulate his or her life very well and draws strength from this regulation. Thus incorporating continuity and structure would be important for a successful exercise program. Finally, the client's focus on spirituality may lead the trainer to arrange activity sessions in outdoor settings or natural environments, where the person may be able to connect to his or her spiritual side. Ultimately, programs that tap into the strengths of individuals will resonate far deeper than ones that don't.

Risks of Activity to Positive Well-Being

We have presented more evidence for the psychological benefit of physical activity or exercise than for detrimental effects. However, a person reading this chapter who has had negative experiences such as being ridiculed for lack of skill by schoolmates might tell a different story. Novice exercisers who judge themselves to be failures because they give up their exercise plans may also have trouble accepting that exercise is good for mental health. There is an acknowledged "dark side" to physical activity in which poor experiences may damage self-esteem or create physique anxiety, but much less literature exists on that topic than on the beneficial effects.

Recent evidence has suggested that some people approach exercise in a way that many would see as mentally unhealthy. Some can become dependent on or addicted to exercise and exhibit very high levels of activity on a daily or twice-daily basis. The term *exercise dependence* was first used by Veale (1987) to describe a state in which exercise has become a compulsive behavior. However, it is difficult to say how harmful exercise dependence really is. If the person continues to exercise against medical advice, then the risk of chronic injury is clear. It may also be economically harmful to neglect work responsibilities in favor of exercise. Damage to personal and social relationships due to exercise dependence may be psychologically harmful. It is clear in these cases that the exercise-dependent individual needs to regain a balance between their need to exercise and other important life issues. Veale (1987) noted that cases of primary exercise dependence appear to be rare. What is more common is dependence on exercise secondary to underlying problems such as eating disorders or muscle dysmorphia (Choi, Pope, & Olivardia, 2002).

We propose that the potential benefits of a physically active life outweigh the risk of negative consequences, but teachers, exercise leaders, and coaches should be aware of the potential for exercise to engender harmful psychological consequences.

Conclusion

Positive psychology is the science of well-being and, as argued here, should therefore include the role of the body and physical activity in the facilitation of well-being. As we have described, activity participation is an exceptionally effective strategy for facilitating psychological well-being within individuals and societies.

The original vision of the positive psychology movement was to integrate the ideas into mainstream psychology and not fragment from it. However, it appears that this separate discipline is here to stay, for a little while longer at least. Furthermore, criticisms of positive psychology as a fad or as based on unstable theoretical bases have been raised (Lazarus, 2003). One in particular is that the movement will create a "tyranny of positive thinking" that promotes constant happiness and makes people feel bad about feeling blue. In response to these criticisms, we would say that positive psychology is not about negating negative feelings, nor does it want to suppress such feelings to create a false sense of well-being. Negative emotions are important, natural, subjective, and contextual. Positive psychology's mission is simply to redress the imbalance supported for the past 60 years.

In conclusion, we have several visions of the future of positive psychology:

1) Positive psychology will move toward becoming a more holistic discipline, starting with the inclusion of the body (including notions of embodiment, sexual pleasure, nutrition, and human touch) and physical activity.

2) Positive psychology will become even more integrated with other disciplines. Recognizing that some theories overlap strongly with domains such as sport and performance psychology will give positive psychologists a better footing within academia. People need to know what has come before them to understand where they are going.

3) Positive psychology will start to validate more physically based PPIs alongside its more cognitively based interventions.

4) Physical activity will be seen as a stellar intervention in the science of positive psychology.

Notes

1. Although there is a distinction between exercise (which is planned and structured with a focus on fitness progression) and physical activity (which simply entails movement and energy expenditure), we will use these terms interchangeably throughout the chapter unless otherwise noted.

2. Carr (2004) has 387 pages and only two general paragraphs (with no references) on physical activity. The *Handbook of Positive Psychology* (Snyder & Lopez, 2002) has 829 pages and only seven references to activity. Finally, none of the assessment handbooks (e.g., Ong & Dulmen, 2006)) contain any reference to the benefits of exercise for well-being.

References

Argyle, M. (2001). *The psychology of happiness*. London: Routledge.

Babyak, M., Blumenthal, J. A., Herman, S., Khatri, P., Doraiswamy, M., Moore, K.,…Krishnan, K. R. (2000). Exercise treatment for major depression: Maintenance of therapeutic benefit at 10 months. *Psychosomatic Medicine, 62*(5), 633–638.

Baker, G., Mutrie, N., & Lowry, R. (2008). Using pedometers as motivational tools: Are goals set in steps more effective than goals set in minutes for increasing walking? *International Journal of Health Promotion, 46,* 21–26.

Biddle, S. J. H. & Mutrie, N. (2008). *Psychology of physical activity: Determinants, well-being, and interventions* (2nd ed.). London: Routledge.

Blumenthal, J. A., Babyak, M. A., Moore, K. A., Craighead, E., Herman, S., Khatri, P.,…Krishnan, K. R (1999). Effects of exercise training on older patients with major depression. *Archives of Internal Medicine, 159*(19), 2349–2356.

Bonanno, G. A. (2004). Loss, trauma, and human resilience—have we underestimated the human capacity to thrive after extremely aversive events? *American Psychologist, 59*(1), 20–28.

Bravata, D. M., Smith-Spangler, C., Sundaram, V., Gienger, A. L., Lin, N., Lewis, R.,…Sirard, J. R. (2007). Using pedometers to increase physical activity and improve health: A systematic review. *JAMA, 298,* 2296–2304.

Camacho, T. C., Roberts, R. E., Lazarus, N. B., Kaplan, G. A., & Cohen, R. D. (1991). Physical activity and depression: Evidence from the Alameda County Study. *American Journal of Epidemiology, 134*(2), 220–231.

Carr, A. (2004). *Positive psychology: The science of happiness and human strengths*. Sussex: Routledge.

Carver, C. S. (1998). Resilience and thriving: Issues, models, and linkages. *Journal of Social Issues, 54,* 245–266.

Chaouloff, F. (1997). The serotonin hypothesis. In W. P. Morgan (Ed.), *Physical activity and mental health* (pp. 179–198). Washington, DC: Taylor & Francis.

Choi, P. Y. L., Pope, H. G., & Olivardia, R. (2002). Muscle dysmorphia: A new syndrome in weightlifters. *British Journal of Sports Medicine, 36*(5), 375–376.

Coalter, F. (2005). *Social benefits of sport: An overview to inform the community planning process*. Edinburgh: Sportscotland.

Csikszentmihalyi, M. (2009). Flow. In S. Lopez (Ed), *The Encyclopedia of positive psychology* (pp. 394–400). Chichester: Blackwell Publishing Ltd.

Csikszentmihalyi, M. (1998). *Finding flow: The psychology of engagement with everyday life*. New York: Basic Books.

Deci, E. L., & Ryan, R. M. (2008). Self-determination theory: A macrotheory of human motivation, development, and health. *Canadian Psychology—Psychologie Canadienne, 49*(3), 182–185.

Demark-Wahnefried, W., Aziz, N. M., Rowland, J. H., & Pinto, B. M. (2005). Riding the crest of the teachable moment: Promoting long-term health after the diagnosis of cancer. *Journal of Clinical Oncology, 23*(24), 5814–5830.

Demark-Wahnefried, W., Peterson, B., McBride, C., Lipkus, I., & Clipp, E. C. (2000). Current health behaviours and readiness to pursue lifestyle change among men and women diagnosed with early-stage prostate and breast cancer. *Cancer, 88,* 674–684.

Department of Health. (2004). *At least five a week: Evidence on the impact of physical activity and its relationship to health. A report from the Chief Medical Officer* (No. 2389). London.

Diener, E. (1984). Subjective well-being. *Psychological Bulletin, 95,* 542–575.

Diener, E., Emmons, R. A., Larsen, R. J., & Griffin, S. (1985). The Satisfaction with Life Scale. *Journal of Personality Assessment, 49,* 71–75.

Diener, E., Suh, E. M., Lucas, R. E., & Smith, H. L. (1999). Subjective well-being: Three decades of progress. *Psychological Bulletin, 125,* 276–302.

Diener, E., Wirtz, D., Tov, W., Kim-Prieto, C., Choi. D., Oishi, S., & Biswas-Diener, R. (2009). New measures of well-being: Flourishing and positive and negative feelings. *Social Indicators Research, 39,* 247–266.

Dishman, R. K. (1997). The norepinephrine hypothesis. In W. P. Morgan (Ed.), *Physical activity and mental health* (pp. 199–212). Washington, DC: Taylor & Francis.

Ekkekakis, P., Hall, E. E., & Petruzzello, S. J. (2005). Variation and homogeneity in affective responses to physical activity of varying intensities: An alternative perspective on dose-response based on evolutionary considerations. *Journal of Sports Sciences, 23*(5), 477–500.

Emslie, C. (2005). Women, men and coronary heart disease: A review of the qualitative literature. *Journal of Advanced Nursing, 51*(4), 382–395.

Emslie, C., Whyte, F., Campbell, A., Mutrie, N., Lee, L., Ritchie, D., & Kearney, N. (2007). 'I wouldn't have been interested in just sitting round a table talking about cancer'; exploring the experiences of women with breast cancer in a group exercise trial. *Health Education Research, 22,* 827–838.

Fox, K. R. (2000). Self-esteem, self-perceptions and exercise. *International Journal of Sport Psychology, 31*(2), 228–240.

Fox, K. R., & Corbin, C. B. (1989). The Physical Self-Perception Profile: Development and preliminary validation. *Journal of Sport and Exercise Psychology, 11,* 408–430.

Fredrickson, B. (2009). *Positivity: Groundbreaking research reveals how to embrace the hidden strength of positive emotions, overcome negativity, and thrive*. New York: Crown.

Fredrickson, B. L., & Losada, M. (2005). Positive affect and the complex dynamics of human flourishing. *American Psychologist, 60*(7), 678–686.

Fredrickson, B., Tugade, M., Waugh, C., & Larkin, G. (2003). What good are positive emotions in crises? A prospective study of resilience and emotions following the terrorist attacks on the United States on September 11th, 2001. *Journal of Personality and Social Psychology, 84*, 365–376.

Hassmen, P., Koivula, N., & Utela, A. (2000). Physical exercise and psychological well-being: A population study in Finland. *Preventive Medicine, 30*(1), 17–25.

Hefferon, K., Grealy, M., & Mutrie, N. (2008). The perceived influence of an exercise class intervention on the process and outcomes of posttraumatic growth. *Journal of Mental Health and Physical Activity, 1*(2), 47–88.

Hefferon, K., Grealy, M., & Mutrie, N. (2009). Posttraumatic growth and life threatening physical illness: A systematic review of the qualitative literature. *British Journal of Health Psychology, 14*(2), 343–378.Hefferon, K., Grealy, M., & Mutrie, N. (2010). Transforming from cocoon to butterfly: The potential role of the body in the process of posttraumatic growth. *Journal of Humanistic Psychology, 50*(2), 224–247.

Hefferon, K., & Ollis, S. (2006). "Just clicks": An interpretive phenomenological analysis of professional dancers' experience of flow. *Research in Dance Education, 7*, 141–159.

Hoffmann, P. (1997). The endorphin hypothesis. In W. P. Morgan (Ed.), *Physical activity and mental health* (pp. 163–177). Washington, DC: Taylor & Francis.

Holahan, C. K., Holahan, C. J., & Suzuki, R. (2008). Purposiveness, physical activity, and perceived health in cardiac patients. *Disability & Rehabilitation, 30*(23), 1772–1778.

Holder, M. D., Coleman, B., & Sehn, Z. L. (2009). The contribution of active and passive leisure to children's well-being. *Journal of Health Psychology, 14*(3), 378–386.

King, L. A., & Napa, C. K. (1998). What makes a life good? *Journal of Personality and Social Psychology, 75*, 156–165.

Koltyn, K. F. (1997). The thermogenic hypothesis. In W. P. Morgan (Ed.), *Physical activity and mental health* (pp. 213–226). Washington, DC: Taylor & Francis.

Kritz-Silverstein, D., Barrett-Connor, E., & Corbeau, C. (2001). Cross-sectional and prospective study of exercise and depressed mood in the elderly: The Rancho Bernardo Study. *American Journal of Epidemiology, 153*(6), 596–603.

Lazarus, R. S. (2003). Does the positive psychology movement have legs? *Psychological Inquiry, 14*(2), 93–109.

Lepore, S., & Revenson, T. (2006). Resilience and posttraumatic growth: Recovery, resistance and reconfiguration. In R. G. Tedeschi & L. G. Calhoun (Eds.), *Handbook of posttraumatic growth* (pp. 24–46). Mahwah, NJ: Lawrence Erlbaum Associates.

Lyubomirsky, S. (2008). *The HOW of happiness.* London: Sphere.

McDonald, D. G., & Hodgdon, J. A. (1991). *The psychological effects of aerobic fitness training: Research and theory.* New York: Springer-Verlag.

McGregor, I., & Little, B. (1998). Personal projects, happiness, and meaning: On doing well and being yourself. *Journal of Personality and Social Psychology, 74*(2), 494–512.

Merleau-Ponty, M. (2005). *Phenomenology of perception.* London: Routledge. (Original work published 1945.)

Moses, J., Steptoe, A., Mathews, A., & Edwards, S. (1989). The effects of exercise training on mental well-being in the normal population: A controlled trial. *Journal of Psychosomatic Research, 33*, 47–61.

Mutrie, N., Campbell, A.,Whyte, F., McConnachie, A., Emslie, C., Lee, L.,…Ritchie, D. (2007). Benefits of supervised group exercise programme for women being treated for early stage breast cancer: pragmatic randomised controlled trial. *British Medical Journal, 334*, 517–520.

Mutrie, N., & Faulkner, G. (2004). Physical activity: Positive psychology in motion. In P. A. Linley & S. Joseph (Eds.), *Positive psychology in practice* (pp. 146–164). Hoboken, NJ: Wiley.

Myers, D. G. (2000). The funds, friends, and faith of happy people. *American Psychologist, 55*, 56–67.

Netz, Y., Wu, M., Becker, B. J., & Tenenbaum, G. (2005). Physical activity and psychological well-being in advanced age: A meta-analysis of intervention studies. *Psychology and Aging, 20*(2), 272–284.

Ong, A. & Dulmen, M. (2006). *Oxford handbook of methods in positive psychology.* Oxford University Press.

Paffenbarger, R. S., Hyde, R. T., Wing, A. L., & Hsieh, C. C. (1986). Physical activity, all-cause mortality, and longevity of college alumni. *New England Journal of Medicine, 314*, 605–613.

Peterson, C. (2006). *A primer in positive psychology.* New York: Oxford University Press.

Peterson, C., & Seligman, M. E. P. (2004). *Character strengths and virtues: A handbook and classification.* Washington, DC: APA Press and Oxford University Press.

Rath, T. (2007). *Strengths Finder 2.0.* New York: Gallup Press.

Resnick, S., Warmoth, A., & Serlin, I. (2001). The humanistic psychology and positive psychology connection: Implications for psychotherapy. *Journal of Humanistic Psychology, 41*, 73–101.

Ryan, R. M., & Deci, E. L. (2000). Self-determination theory and the facilitation of intrinsic motivation, social development, and well-being. *American Psychologist, 55*, 68–78.

Ryan, R. M., & Frederick, C. M. (1997). On energy, personality and health: Subjective vitality as a dynamic reflection of well-being. *Journal of Personality, 65*, 529–565.

Ryff, C. D., & Keyes, C. L. M. (1995). The structure of psychological well-being revisited. *Journal of Personality and Social Psychology, 69*, 719–727.

Ryff, C. D., & Singer, B. (1996). Psychological well-being: Meaning, measurement, and implications for psychotherapy research. *Psychotherapy and Psychosomatics, 65*(1), 14–23.

Ryff, C. D., & Singer, B. H. (2006). Best news yet on the six-factor model of well-being. *Social Science Research, 35*(4), 1103–1119.

Sabiston, C. M., McDonough, M. H., & Crocker, P. R. E. (2007). Psychosocial experiences of breast cancer survivors involved in a dragon boat program: Exploring links to positive psychological growth. *Journal of Sport & Exercise Psychology, 29*(4), 419–438.

Salmon, P. (2001). Effects of physical exercise on anxiety, depression, and sensitivity to stress: A unifying theory. *Clinical Psychology Review, 21*(1), 33–61.

Salonen, J., Puska, P., Nissinen A, & Kottke, T. (1983) Decline in mortality from coronary heart disease in Finland from 1969 to 1979. *British Medical Journal, 286*, 1857–1860.

Seligman, M. (1998). *Positive Psychology Network concept paper.* American Psychological Association.

Seligman, M. E. P. (2002). *Authentic happiness: Using the new positive psychology to realize your potential for lasting fulfillment.* New York: Free Press.

Seligman, M. E. P. (2008). Positive health. *Applied Psychology: An International Review, 57*, 3–18.

Seligman, M. E. P., & Csikszentmihalyi, M. (2000). Positive psychology: An introduction. *American Psychologist, 55*, 5–14.

Seligman, M. E. P., Steen, T. A., Park, N., & Peterson, C. (2005). Positive psychology progress: Empirical validation of interventions. *American Psychologist, 60*, 410–421.

Sin, N. L., & Lyubomirsky, S. (2009). Enhancing well-being and alleviating depressive symptoms with positive psychology interventions: A practice-friendly meta-analysis. *Journal of Clinical Psychology, 65*, 467–487.

Snyder, C. R., & Lopez, S. J. (Eds.). (2002). *Handbook of positive psychology.* London: Oxford University Press.

Snyder, C. R., & Lopez, S. J. (2007). *Positive psychology: The scientific and practical explorations of human strengths.* Thousand Oaks, CA: Sage.

Steptoe, A., & Butler, N. (1996). Sports participation and emotional wellbeing in adolescents. *Lancet, 347*, 1789–1792.

Stevinson, C., & Fox, K. R. (2006). Feasibility of an exercise rehabilitation programme for cancer patients. *European Journal of Cancer Care, 15*, 386–396.

Tedeschi, R. G., Park, C., & Calhoun, L. G. (1998). Posttraumatic growth: Conceptual issues. In R. G. Tedeschi, C. Park, & L. G. Calhoun (Eds.), *Posttraumatic growth* (pp. 1–22). Mahwah, NJ: Lawrence Erlbaum Associates.

Tugade, M., Fredrickson, B., & Barrett, L. (2004). Resilient individuals use positive emotions to bounce back from negative emotional experiences. *Journal of Personality and Social Psychology, 86*, 1161–1190.

Veale, D. M. W. (1987). Exercise dependence. *British Journal of Addiction, 82*, 735–740.

Veenhoven, R. (1991). Is happiness relative? *Social Indicators Research, 24*, 1–34.

Watson, D., Clark, L. A., & Tellegen, A. (1988). Development and validation of brief measures of positive and negative affect: The PANAS scales. *Journal of Personality and Social Psychology, 54*(6), 1063–1070.

Wehmeyer, M., & Little, T. D. (2009). Self-determination. In S. Lopez (Ed.), *The encyclopedia of positive psychology* (pp. 868–873). UK: John Wiley & Sons.

PART 3

Exercise Psychology and Psychobiological Perspectives

Psychoneuroendocrinology and Physical Activity

Mark Hamer

Abstract

Psychoneuroendocrinology is the clinical study of hormone fluctuations and their relationship to human behavior. The hypothalamic-pituitary-adrenal (HPA) axis is central to this area of study. Salivary cortisol is considered to be a reliable indicator of HPA function and can be used as a biomarker of physical and mental stress. Several aspects of psychoneuroendocrinology are relevant to physical activity and exercise. First, regular physical activity can both result in physiological adaptations to the HPA axis that might have implications for health and modify HPA and immune responses to mental stress. Second, cortisol appears to be important in preparing for mental and physical demands and may have an impact on sports performance. Overtraining in athletes provides a model for examining neuroendocrine function and chronic stress.

Key Words: cortisol, catecholamines, exercise, immunity, mental stress, physical activity, psychophysiology, recovery.

Introduction

Psychoneuroendocrinology is the clinical study of hormone fluctuations and their relationship to human behavior. The field of psychoneuroendocrinology covers a number of interrelated disciplines, including psychology, neurobiology, endocrinology, immunology, neurology, and psychiatry. The hypothalamic-pituitary-adrenal (HPA) axis and sympathetic nervous system are central to this area of study. Psychological events initiate an HPA response by activating corticotrophin-releasing factor (CRF) and arginine vasopressin (AVP) neurons in the paraventricular nucleus of the hypothalamus (Chrousos & Kino 2007). This leads to the release of adrenocorticotrophic hormone (ACTH) from the pituitary, which triggers release of glucocorticoids from the adrenal glands (Figure 8.1). In addition, the sympathetic nervous system releases catecholamines (norepinephrine and epinephrine) that are important in regulating cardiovascular functions such as heart rate and blood pressure. The primary physiological role of glucocorticoid secretion is to help mobilize stored energy by allocating glucose to the brain, thus increasing the chances of survival under conditions of enduring stress. Physical and mental stressors elicit similar responses, even though those of a psychological nature are not matched by a need for increased metabolic demand. The interplay between physical and mental stress with regard to neuroendocrinological responses is therefore an intriguing topic.

In this chapter I examine four main areas. First, I discuss how regular physical activity can result in physiological adaptations to the HPA axis that might also modify HPA responses to mental stress. Second, I consider the link between neuroendocrine and immune responses in relation to mental stress and physical activity. Third, I discuss the relevance of HPA responses to chronic stress in both preparing for and coping with competitive environments.

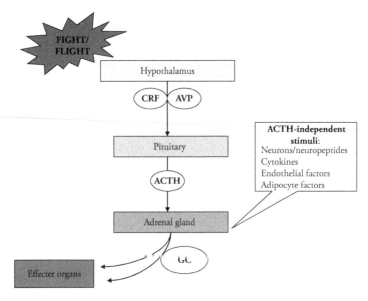

Figure 8.1. The hypothalamic-pituitary-adrenal (HPA) axis. Psychological events initiate an HPA response by activating corticotrophin-releasing factor (CRF) and arginine vasopressin (AVP) neurons in the paraventricular nucleus of the hypothalamus. This leads to the release of adrenocorticotrophic hormone (ACTH) from the pituitary, which triggers release of glucocorticoids (GC) from the adrenal glands. ACTH and GC levels can be influenced by altered sensitivity of the adrenal cortex and other ACTH-independent stimuli.

Last, I explore the use of a variety of hormones, including cortisol, testosterone, and catecholamines, in monitoring training load and recovery in athletes and others exposed to chronic physical and psychological stress.

Individual Differences in HPA Activity

There are large variations in HPA function among individuals as well as across situations. These differences can be largely accounted for by age and gender, although other factors also appear to contribute. One of the most compelling findings is that men show larger cortisol responses to psychological stress tasks than women (Kajantie & Phillips, 2006). Some of these differences may be explained by differences in endogenous and exogenous levels of sex steroids (due to, for example, the menstrual cycle, use of oral contraceptives, and hormone replacement therapy). Health behavior also accounts for individual variability in HPA function. Physical activity is an important determinant of HPA function and will be covered in more detail in later sections. Other factors include obesity, nicotine use, caffeine, alcohol, and dietary intake. Nicotine stimulates the HPA axis through induction of CRF release after binding to cholinergic receptors in the hypothalamus, which can result in chronically elevated cortisol levels and reduced responsiveness of the HPA axis to acute challenge (Kudielka, Hellhammer, & Wüst, 2009). Evidence for the effects of caffeine and alcohol on HPA function is far less consistent, with some studies reporting significant HPA stimulatory effects of caffeine and blunting effects of alcoholism while others report none. Blood glucose level appears to be strongly related to cortisol responses, and participants in a fasted state demonstrate little or no response compared with those receiving glucose. When undertaking standardized laboratory stress testing (a commonly used technique in psychoneuroendocrinology that will be described in detail in later sections), it is therefore desirable to strictly control the use of nicotine, caffeine, and alcohol and dietary intake. Of course, in ambulatory settings it may not always be possible to control for these factors that can limit the interpretation of the findings.

HPA function can also be influenced by a range of other factors, including perinatal environment (Phillips, 2007), early-childhood adversity (Heim et al., 2000), and genetic factors (Bartels, van den Berg, Sluyter, Boomsma, & de Geus, 2003; Wüst et al., 2004). Estimates on the heritability of basal cortisol levels have ranged from 30% to 60%, and the findings generally suggest that cortisol levels soon after waking and early in the day are heritable, while resting cortisol levels later in the day are not (Franz, et al 2010). Studies of the heritability of cortisol reactivity to laboratory-induced stressors have also been inconsistent (Steptoe, van Jaarsveld, Semmler, Plomin, & Wardle, 2009). However, recent evidence has demonstrated a sex-specific association between glucocorticoid receptor gene polymorphisms and cortisol reactivity (Kumsta et al., 2007).

Physical Activity and Psychophysiological Stress Responses
Exercise Adaptations to the HPA Axis and Sympathetic Nervous System

A single bout of acute exercise can result in significant activation of the HPA axis and sympathetic nervous system, causing increases in cortisol, ACTH, and the catecholamines. Significant HPA axis responses are generally observed only with exercise at a moderate or higher intensity (Hill et al., 2008). Norepinephrine increases in a curvilinear fashion with increasing workload, and epinephrine is released with higher-intensity exercise. In addition to hormone release, some changes in receptor sensitivity can also be observed, such as enhanced postexercise beta-adrenergic receptor responsivity (Brownley et al., 2003).

Long-term voluntary exercise in animals causes an increase in mass of the adrenal glands , although no changes in CRF, AVP, or ACTH are generally observed (Droste, Chandramohan, Hill, Linthorst, & Reul, 2007). Exercise training leads to adaptation in HPA responses to acute exercise, including a higher threshold of activation, resulting in blunted responses to exercise at the same absolute intensity but greater responses to maximal exercise. For example, trained rats demonstrate enhanced corticosterone responses to forced swimming in comparison with untrained rats. In humans, physically trained and unfit women demonstrate similar cortisol responses to high-intensity exercise, although during recovery the physically trained have a greater rate of recovery of ACTH levels but higher cortisol (Traustadóttir, Bosch, Cantu, & Matt, 2004). This finding would tend to suggest physical training increases sensitivity of the adrenal glands to ACTH. Other evidence also suggests that trained individuals demonstrate increased tissue sensitivity to glucocorticoids following a bout of acute exercise (Duclos, Gouarne, & Bonnemaison, 2003), which may act as a mechanism to prevent excessive muscle inflammatory responses. Some evidence suggests that after prolonged physical training there are reduced basal levels of cortisol via a reduction in glucocorticoid

receptor sensitivity, which might be beneficial in terms of chronic HPA activation (Silva et al., 2008). However, some studies have not demonstrated reduced corticotropic sensitivity to negative feedback due to chronic exercise stress (Strüder et al., 1999), which might be explained by individual variability (see the section "Individual Differences in HPA Activity" above). In addition, animal data suggest that glucocorticoid receptor adaptation to exercise might be tissue specific, such that glucocorticoid action is decreased in skeletal muscle and increased in the visceral fat (Coutinho, Campbell, Fediuc, & Riddell, 2006). Several adaptations to the sympathetic nervous system are also observed: Classic training effects involve a blunted heart rate response to a standardized workload, which is caused primarily by reduced catecholamine responses. Reduced basal levels of catecholamines following exercise training are also thought to explain reductions in blood pressure via a lowering of peripheral vascular resistance.

Psychophysiological Stress Responses

Psychophysiological stress testing allows individual differences in cardiovascular and biological responses to standardized laboratory stress tasks to be evaluated and related to psychosocial risk factors (Chida & Hamer, 2008) and various health outcomes. It is desirable to select laboratory stress tasks that are novel, so that factors such as intelligence or education do not influence individual responses. Such tasks include mirror tracing (illustrated in Figure 8.2), which has been used to elicit robust and reproducible stress responses (Hamer,

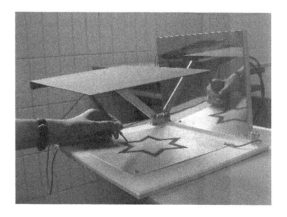

Figure 8.2. The mirror tracing task can be used to elicit robust psychophysiological responses. Participants are asked to trace around the shape using the mirror image, and any deviations from the black line are signaled by a high-pitched noise.

Gibson, Vuononvirta, Williams, & Steptoe, 2006). Heightened cardiovascular and biological stress reactions have been shown to predict future hypertension (Flaa, Eide, Kjeldsen, & Rostrup, 2008), increases in lipid levels and adiposity (Steptoe & Brydon, 2005; Steptoe & Wardle, 2005), and the progression of subclinical cardiovascular disease (Treiber et al., 2003).

Since responses to standardized laboratory stressors appear to be a reliable marker for health outcomes, there has been considerable interest in examining if certain lifestyle factors are associated with more favorable stress response profiles. In particular, physical activity has gained attention. Similarities between central and peripheral responses to exercise and psychological stressors have led to the theory of "cross-stressor adaptation," according to which adaptations resulting from regular exercise lead to improved physiological control not only during exercise but also in response to psychological stressors. Much of the existing psychophysiological work relating to physical activity has focused on cardiovascular responses. In particular, acute exercise and physical fitness have been associated with buffering blood pressure and cardiac responses to standardized behavioral challenges in the laboratory (Hamer, Taylor, & Steptoe, 2006), although there are inconsistencies in the literature (Forcier et al., 2006; Jackson & Dishman 2006).

Far less work has focused on the association between physical activity and HPA stress responses. Acute HPA responses to mental stressors appear to be an important indicator of health. For example, Hamer, O'Donnell, Lahiri, and Steptoe (2010) found that excessive cortisol responses to laboratory-induced mental stress are associated with greater coronary artery calcification in healthy older adults. Other investigators have suggested that psychosocial risk factors such as depressive symptoms are strongly associated with cortisol stress responses (Lopez-Duran, Kovacs, & George, 2009). Since cortisol has a strong diurnal variation that peaks in the morning after awakening and then steadily declines throughout the day, one of the difficulties in this area of work has been in producing consistent cortisol responses to laboratory-induced stress. Reliable cortisol responses can be induced using stressors with a socially evaluative component, such as the Trier Social Stress Test, which generally produces two- to threefold increases in cortisol. Recent studies that have employed appropriate stress tasks have consistently demonstrated blunted HPA responses to mental stressors in physically trained individuals

(Rimmele et al., 2009; Traustadóttir, Bosch, & Matt, 2005). For example, in a sample of elderly women, those defined as physically fit demonstrated plasma cortisol stress responses that were comparable to those of younger, sedentary participants but were blunted in comparison to elderly unfit counterparts (Traustadóttir et al., 2005). Interestingly, physical fitness levels were not associated with cardiovascular responses to mental stress in elderly women. In young men a blunted HPA stress response was apparent only in highly trained athletes; amateur athletes had similar responses to untrained men (Rimmele et al., 2009). This suggests that a certain threshold of exercise training is required to produce adaptations in HPA stress responses. In addition, highly trained participants are more likely to have undertaken exercise prior to stress testing; thus the results may to some extent reflect carryover effects of acute exercise. Alternatively the results could be explained by different psychological profiles. For example, the different psychophysiological responses of highly trained individuals might be partly explained by the fact that they are likely to be more competitive, have higher levels of self-efficacy, and have different coping styles compared with those with less training. Indeed, certain psychological characteristics, such as better adaptive coping styles, have been associated with lower cortisol levels over the day (O'Donnell, Badrick, Kumari, & Steptoe, 2008). The correct interpretation of these findings may only be obtained by performing controlled training studies to examine the direct effect of exercise training on HPA response to mental stressors.

Studies in animals appear to suggest stress-specific effects in relation to exercise training. Trained animals demonstrate exaggerated corticosterone responses to physical stressors such as forced swimming but reduced responses to novel "anxiety-promoting" stressors (Droste et al., 2007). This apparent stress-specific response might be explained by a dissociation of ACTH and glucocorticoids under certain stress conditions (Bornstein, Engeland, Ehrhart-Bornstein, & Herman, 2008). Further data has shown that exercise-trained animals demonstrate better HPA habituation to repeated noise stress (Sasse et al., 2008). This may represent a critical adaptation, because the inability to adequately adapt to ongoing stressors may have long-term consequences for health (McEwen, 2007).

A single acute bout of exercise can also have striking effects on psychophysiological responses. For example, postexercise blood pressure responses to mental stress are blunted (Hamer, Taylor, & Steptoe, 2006), and several studies have demonstrated reduced catecholamine responses following exercise (Brownley et al., 2003; Péronnet, Massicotte, Paquet, Brisson, & de Champlain, 1989). Interestingly, when mental stress is performed during exercise this appears to exacerbate the stress responses, including greater norepinephrine and cortisol, in comparison to exercise alone (Webb et al., 2008). This finding demonstrates that hormonal responses to physical and mental stress are partly independent and that cognitive appraisal and emotional state play an important role in those responses.

Diurnal Neuroendocrine Patterns

As noted above, certain hormones have a strong diurnal variation. Cortisol, for example, peaks in the morning shortly after awakening and then steadily declines throughout the day (see Figure 8.3). The cortisol response to awakening is thought to be a sensitive marker of stress and other psychosocial factors (Chida & Steptoe, 2009). For example, there is a positive association between the cortisol awakening response and general life stress, although a negative association with fatigue, burnout, and exhaustion. Some investigators have employed the cortisol awakening response and daytime cortisol variation as a marker of fatigue induced by strenuous exercise training (see the section "Hormonal Biomarkers of Training Status" below). In addition, disturbed diurnal cortisol patterns have been associated with health risk factors such as hypertension (Wirtz et al., 2007) and atherosclerotic burden (Dekker et al., 2008; Matthews, Schwartz, Cohen, & Seeman, 2006). Recent data also suggest that elevated daytime cortisol partly explains the association

between depression and increased metabolic risk (Muhtz, Zyriax, Klähn, Windler, & Otte, 2009).

Relatively few studies have examined the influence of physical activity on diurnal neuroendocrine patterns. A four-month behavioral change intervention in chronically stressed caregivers showed that an increase in physical activity was associated with a more favorable morning cortisol pattern (Urizar, Garovoy, Castro, & King, 2010). In a randomized controlled trial of overweight hypertensive adults, six months of exercise and weight loss resulted in lower levels of blood pressure measured over the day, especially during periods of emotional distress (Steffen et al., 2001). These effects might be attributed to lower levels of circulating catecholamines that are important in regulating blood pressure. In addition, adiposity levels and weight loss may affect neuroendocrine function. For example, measures of central adiposity have been consistently associated with stress-related daytime cortisol secretion (Rosmond, Dallman, & Björntorp, 1998) and the cortisol awakening response (Steptoe, Kunz-Ebrecht, Brydon, & Wardle, 2004). Therefore, some of the associations between physical activity and neuroendocrine function might be attributable to lower levels of adiposity.

Mood and Mental Health

Physical activity has consistently been associated with better mood and lower levels of depressive symptoms in prospective cohort studies (Brown, Ford, Burton, Marshall, & Dobson, 2005; Hamer, Molloy, de Oliveira, & Demakakos, 2009), although the mechanisms remain poorly understood. Much work in psychoneuroendocrinology

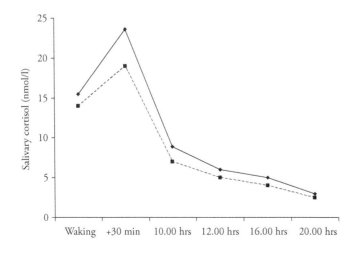

Figure 8.3. The diurnal cortisol profile. The cortisol response to awakening occurs in the first 30 to 45 minutes after waking. Cortisol levels tend to decline steadily throughout the day, reaching a nadir in the evening. The cortisol slope (gradient of decline) can be used as a sensitive marker of stress and health. Diamond symbols with a solid line represent a normal cortisol profile; square symbols with a dashed line represent a hypothesized healthier cortisol profile in habitual exercisers.

has focused on the link between the HPA axis and mental health. For example, dysregulation of the HPA axis is a common feature of major depression (Pariante & Lightman, 2008) that might also be connected with impaired immune responses and low-grade inflammation (Miller, Maletic, & Raison, 2009). Neurodegenerative changes in the hippocampus, prefrontal cortex, and amygdala are frequently linked with changes in the HPA axis and the immune system, providing further evidence in support of these mechanisms. Major depression has been associated with decreased responsiveness to glucocorticoids (glucocorticoid resistance), which is believed to be related in part to impaired functioning of the glucocorticoid receptor. Since exercise is known to affect glucocorticoid sensitivity, this may be an important mechanism in explaining the antidepressant effects of physical activity.

There is, however, a paucity of direct evidence to shed light on the potential mechanisms of the antidepressant effect of exercise. For example, in a randomized controlled trial of mildly depressed women, eight weeks of moderate exercise resulted in lower levels of depressive symptoms and reduced 24-hour cortisol and catecholamine secretion (Nabkasorn et al., 2006). In a population-based prospective study of older men and women, a higher baseline physical activity level was associated with over a 40% reduction in the risk of depressive symptoms at four-year follow-up, after accounting for a range of psychosocial factors and physical health. The physically active participants also displayed lower levels of inflammatory markers, although this factor did not explain a substantial amount of the association between physical activity and risk of depression (Hamer et al., 2009).

Since exercise is thought to alter serotonin metabolism, release endogenous opioids, and increase central noradrenergic neurotransmission, all of these mechanisms might also contribute to antidepressant and anxiolytic effects (Cotman, Berchtold, & Christie, 2007). In particular, brain-derived neurotrophic factor (BDNF) has attracted interest in this area of work. Unlike cortisol, BDNF is known to promote and improve neuronal plasticity, retard neuron cell death, induce neural regeneration, and stimulate neuronal survival (Lewin & Barbe, 1996). Thus not surprisingly, BDNF has been linked with depression and cognitive function. Early studies in animals demonstrated an immediate increase in BDNF concentration after voluntary exercise, and repeated exercise sessions were shown to increase concentrations of BDNF in brain regions including

the hippocampus, cerebellum, cortex, and lumbar spinal cord (van Praag, Kempermann, & Gage, 1999). In addition, after prior exercise exposure, a brief second exercise reexposure insufficient to cause a BDNF change in naïve animals rapidly reinduced BDNF protein, suggesting that exercise primes a molecular memory for BDNF induction (Berchtold, Chinn, Chou, Kesslak, & Cotman, 2005). Exercise-induced increases in BDNF have also been associated with enhanced neurogenesis in the hippocampus in mice (Rhodes et al., 2003). Studies in humans have shown acute increases in BDNF after high-intensity exercise with rapid returns to baseline (Rojas Vega et al., 2006) and elevated resting concentrations of BDNF after five weeks of exercise training (Zoladz et al., 2008). In another study, however, the acute increases in BDNF did not appear to correlate with improvements in postexercise cognitive function (Ferris, Williams, & Shen, 2007). The mechanisms contributing to BDNF expression with exercise remain unclear, although both noradrenaline and the HPA axis have been implicated. For example, in rats the combination of exercise with administration of a selective noradrenaline reuptake inhibitor produced greater increases in BDNF than either treatment alone (Russo-Neustadt, Alejandre, Garcia, Ivy, & Chen, 2004). These findings were not, however, replicated in humans (Goekint et al., 2008). Far more work is therefore required to tease out the neuroendocrinological mechanisms that link physical activity with improved mental health.

It is likely that the association between physical activity and mental health is bidirectional, in that not only does physical activity promote better mental health, but poor mental health negatively affects physical activity behavior. Depression promotes changes in the function of the HPA axis and the immune system. Such changes are thought to promote a sickness-like behavior that favors sedentary activity. Patients with mental illness appear to be significantly less active than the general population (Hamer, Stamatakis, & Steptoe, 2008). Feelings of low confidence and social support towards exercising may partly contribute to this association. In addition, psychiatric symptoms such as poor attention, memory loss, apathy, and amotivation might be barriers to behavioral modification. Thus although exercise can be used in the treatment of depression, some initial improvement in mental health might be required before structured exercise can be initiated. Indeed, combined treatment with antidepressant medication and exercise seems to be a favorable modality (Blumenthal et al., 2007).

Physical Activity and Psychoneuroimmunology
Mental Stress, HPA Responses, and Immune Activation

Psychoneuroimmunology is the study of interactions among behavioral, neural, endocrine, and immune systems. Immune system function can be categorized into innate and adaptive responses. Innate immunity is a barrier to various low-specificity infectious agents and consists of phagocytic cells (macrophages and neutrophils) and natural killer cells (NKC). Adaptive immunity refers to the "memory" aspect of the immune system; it is highly specific in its recognition of antigens consisting of lymphocyte subsets such as T and B cells (including antibodies).

There is a close link between neuroendocrine and immune functioning in the context of mental stress. Acute mental stress has been generally associated with immune stimulation, involving increases in delayed-type hypersensitivity (DTH) response, NKC activity, CD8+ cell number, inflammatory monokines, type 2 (Th2) cytokines, and mucosal immunoglobins (Ig); a reduced lymphocyte proliferation response is an exception to this pattern. Cortisol release during acute stress is thought to shift the immune system balance away from Th1-driven cell-mediated (innate) responses toward Th2-driven antibody-mediated (adaptive) responses, which may increase susceptibility to certain infections. For example, some evidence suggests that high HPA reactivity to acute stress predicts immunosuppression to latent Epstein-Barr virus (Cacioppo et al., 1998). Participants with greater cortisol reactivity to a simulated public speaking task had increased risk of verified upper respiratory tract infection (URTI), but only when they reported a high amount of negative life events (Cohen et al., 2002). In addition, participants with smaller immune responses (NKC activity and CD8+ cell reactivity) to the speech task had increased risk of self-reported URTI during high-stress weeks.

Chronic stress such as family conflict and high life event stress are generally correlated with an increased incidence of serologically confirmed URTIs. However, stressful life events or emotional distress does not consistently predict immune responses in experimental studies where participants were exposed to a cold or influenza virus. Nevertheless, various studies have provided evidence that chronic stress or stressful life events suppress the secondary immune response to vaccination (Vedhara et al., 1999). In summary, upregulation

of the immune system in response to acute stress may be viewed as a normal adaptation to psychological challenge, whereas chronic stress is associated with more serious impairment of immune function, which may have negative implications for health.

Physical Activity and Immune Responses

In many ways exercise stress provokes similar physiological responses to psychological stress and can also be viewed in terms of acute and chronic. Acute exercise results in a number of immune responses (Gleeson, 2007). For example, reductions in lymphocyte proliferation response (on a per-cell basis) are observed after high-intensity exercise; increases in NKC activity of up to 100% are seen during or immediately after exercise (which may be a reflection of changes in circulating cell numbers as opposed to changes in cytotoxic function), followed by a 10–60% suppression of NKC activity during recovery; increases in the phagocytic function of neutrophils are observed that may remain elevated for up to 24 hours. Studies have also shown effects of exercise on various cellular adhesion molecules (CAMs), which are thought to play an important role in the recruitment of immune cells to sites of infection and cell–cell interactions, a process that is critical in host defense. Essentially, CAMs consist of homing receptors found on the lymphocytes (e.g., L-selectin, LFA-1, and VLA-4) and their ligands on endothelial cells (e.g., ICAM-1 and VCAM-1). However, CAM responses vary depending on the intensity and duration of exercise (Hong & Mills, 2006). More recent interest has focused on the role of cytokine responses to exercise. Interleukin-6 (IL-6), for example, is a cytokine that is typically released by the immune cells in response to injury or infection. It has also become evident that exercising muscle produces a number of cytokines, including IL-6, that may have an important influence on the metabolic response to prolonged exercise (Pedersen & Febbraio, 2008). The increases in circulating IL-6 that are consistently observed after exercise are thought to promote an anti-inflammatory environment by increasing synthesis of IL-1 receptor antagonist and IL-10 but inhibiting release of tumor necrosis factor-alpha (TNF-α). The exercise-induced production of IL-6 is thought to partly explain an enhancement in antibody response to vaccination following acute exercise (Edwards, Burns, Carroll, Drayson, & Ring, 2007). The IL-6 response might also explain why a large number of observational studies have confirmed an inverse association between regular physical activity and various proinflammatory markers (Hamer, 2007).

There is a general perception that moderate physical activity promotes immune function although excessive, high-intensity exercise might increase the risk of URTI (for a review, see Gleeson, 2007). Thus a J-shaped association between exercise and immune function has been proposed. The incidence of URTI in runners after a major endurance event such as a marathon is elevated between 2 and 6 times compared with matched nonparticipants, and an impaired DTH response has been observed in endurance athletes following a long triathlon event. Also, a relationship has been observed in athletes between declines in salivary IgA concentration during acute intense exercise and the appearance of URTI. However, there are inconsistencies in the literature. For example, competitive swimmers who were monitored for seven months throughout their training and who exhibited Ig levels in the lowest 10th percentile relative to clinical norms were still able to mount clinically appropriate antibody responses when immunized with a pneumococcal vaccine (Gleeson, 2007). Furthermore, no impairment of antibody response to other vaccines (tetanus and diphtheritis toxoid) was found in triathletes compared with controls. In summary, the literature suggests that in response to high-intensity, acute exercise and intense training periods, athletes suffer mild suppression of the immune system. It is possible that these mild immunosuppressive effects of exercise become detrimental to the athlete's health only if combined with other factors such as psychological stress, poor nutritional status, and inadequate recovery and rest.

Few studies have examined the interaction between physical activity and immune responses to acute mental stress. A higher level of physical fitness was associated with lower inflammatory cytokine (IL-6 and TNF-α) responses to laboratory mental stressors in a sample of middle-aged men and women (Hamer & Steptoe, 2007). These findings were partly replicated by recent work showing less lipopolysaccharide-stimulated IL-6 production in response to the stressor among expert yoga practitioners compared with novices (Kiecolt-Glaser et al., 2010). Other work has shown that regular exercisers had attenuated expression of leukocyte trafficking and adhesion molecules in response to a speech task stressor compared with sedentary participants (Hong, Farag, Nelesen, Ziegler, & Mills, 2004).

The mechanisms linking physical activity to more favorable immune function remain unclear.

Research has indicated an intriguing link between efferent cholinergic activity of the vagus nerve (the parasympathetic arm of the autonomic nervous system) and inhibition of inflammatory processes (Tracey, 2002). In addition, fitter individuals who demonstrated lower inflammatory responses to stress also maintained greater cardiac parasympathetic control during mental stress (Hamer & Steptoe, 2007). The decline in parasympathetic control with aging is attenuated with regular exercise training (Carter, Banister, & Blaber, 2003). Thus fitness-related improvements in parasympathetic activity may play some role in mediating the inhibition of stress-induced inflammatory processes. Other mechanisms might involve increased tissue sensitivity to glucocorticoids (see the section "Exercise Adaptations to the HPA Axis and Sympathetic Nervous System" above), increased high-density lipoprotein, increased adiponectin, and reduced reactive oxygen species, all of which have anti-inflammatory actions and are influenced by regular physical activity. Taken together, these data suggest that regular physical activity might buffer the immunosuppressive effects of mental stress, although further studies are required to fully understand the interaction between physical activity, stress, and immune function.

Psychoneuroendocrinology in Sports Performance
Cortisol, Anxiety, and Performance

An increase in cortisol appears to be important in preparing for mental and physical demands and may have an impact on performance. Cortisol can often increase up to twofold compared with resting values before sports competition; this increase is mostly linked with precompetition anxiety, which might be facilitative or debilitative to performance depending on the athlete's perception (Hanton, Neil, & Mellalieu, 2008). Furthermore, high training intensities and repetitive competition provide a model for examining chronic stress.

Findings about the effects of winning, losing, and performance on hormone levels following a sporting event are contradictory and may vary according to the type of sport. For example, female soccer players on a winning team demonstrated increased levels of testosterone following the game compared with the losers, although there were no differences in cortisol (Oliveira, Gouveia, & Oliveira, 2009). The testosterone response was associated with observed performance and with an increase in self-reported mood. In several other studies of rugby and soccer games in men and women, however, competition outcome was not associated with testosterone responses. The findings are also inconsistent in relation to cortisol responses. For example, among male and female tennis players, losers had significantly higher cortisol levels than winners (Filaire, Alix, Ferrand, & Verger, 2009), while in contact sports such as wrestling and judo the opposite has been found (Suay et al., 1999).

Some of these discrepancies might be partly explained by differences in sampling intervals, the importance of the game, and levels of physical exertion. Individual differences are also important and may be masked when looking at the team as a whole. For example, a series of studies by Mehta and colleagues have used experimental laboratory competition to examine how individual basal testosterone levels can influence cortisol responses and behavior following victory and defeat. In these studies men and women high in basal testosterone demonstrated rises in cortisol following defeat but reductions in cortisol following victory (Mehta, Jones, & Josephs, 2008). Furthermore, participants high in basal testosterone who won chose to repeat the competitive task, while those who lost did not. In contrast, for participants low in basal testosterone the cortisol response was not related to winning or losing, and winners and losers did not differ in their preference to repeat the task. A subsequent study by Mehta and colleagues demonstrated that testosterone responses may also differ according to whether the competition is individual or group based (Mehta, Wuehrmann, & Josephs, 2009). These data might suggest that high-testosterone individuals may be predominantly more motivated by performing in individual competition, whereas low-testosterone individuals may perform better in teams. Indeed, higher testosterone is known to regulate social dominance in a number of species, and thus high-testosterone individuals may be motivated to gain higher status.

Hormonal Biomarkers of Training Status

The HPA axis is thought to play an important role in adaptation to regular exercise. Given that athletes are exposed to increased cortisol levels during and following each bout of acute exercise, several training adaptations have evolved to protect them from excessive exposure to glucocorticoids. The biological effects of cortisol on the target tissues are not fully understood. Intracellular bioavailability depends on tissue-specific enzymes that interconvert active cortisol to inactive cortisone, thereby modulating cortisol action on target cells. This process appears to be important in maintaining equilibrium during regular and intensive exercise training. During nocturnal sleeping the hormone profile is anabolic (increased growth hormone and testosterone) and thus most advantageous for exercise recovery. Higher production of overnight urinary cortisone has been found in endurance athletes compared with untrained controls (Gouarné, Groussard, Gratas-Delamarche, Delamarche, & Duclos, 2005), which might indicate higher tissue inactivation of cortisol. In athletes who have overtrained (characterized by a drop in performance, lethargy, fatigue, loss of appetite, and sleep disturbance) there appears to be lower inactivation of cortisol. Researchers have suggested that an increase in overnight cortisol-to-cortisone ratio above 1 might be a sensitive marker of overtraining or identify individuals at high risk of overtraining. However, further research is required to further understand these data. Some notable effects on neuroendocrine function were demonstrated in young female tennis players followed over seven months with an increasing training volume (Rouveix, Duclos, Gouarne, Beauvieux, & Filaire, 2006). In particular, there appeared to be an increase in cortisol secretion, which was not compensated by a parallel inactivation into cortisone. Increases in cortisol were associated with reduced vigor and increased total mood disturbance, which is consistent with previous evidence implicating cortisol as a marker of overtraining and fatigue. The ratio of epinephrine to norepinephrine also decreased over time, and this decrease was related to fatigue, implicating a role of the sympathetic nervous system.

Several lines of evidence have linked overtraining with exhaustion of the adrenal glands and changes in the ratio of testosterone to cortisol production. These changes are thought to reflect an imbalance in anabolic and catabolic processes that are vital for recovery and performance. In burnout and vital exhaustion, for example, the cortisol response to awakening is diminished. The relevance of the cortisol awakening response to athletes, however, is less clear. For example, seven days of intensified exercise training in soccer players resulted in a heightened cortisol awakening response. However, less lower performance decrement was associated with increased awakening Cortisol response, post-awakening peak cortisol, rate of cortisol increase, and area under the curve (Minetto et al., 2008). In contrast, there were no differences in cortisol awakening responses between highly trained and overtrained endurance athletes over several months

(Gouarne et al., 2005). These discrepancies might reflect differences between chronic overtraining and a short period of voluntary heavy training. Indeed, in rugby players monitored for seven days following intensive competition, the testosterone-to-cortisol ratio was increased compared to baseline, which might suggest an increase in anabolic processes during recovery to encourage muscle repair (Elloumi, Maso, Michaux, Robert, & Lac, 2003). Other data indicate that the first sign of overtraining in athletes is a decreased resting level of free testosterone and a lower maximal exercise-induced increase in free testosterone concentration (Mäestu, Jürimäe, & Jürimäe, 2005). It therefore remains questionable whether simple measures of testosterone-to-cortisol ratio provide useful information on overtraining or chronic stress; provocation of the HPA axis through stress or dexamethasone (a synthetic version of the hormone cortisol that has potent anti-inflammatory properties) may be a more sensitive indicator.

Conclusions

Several aspects of psychoneuroendocrinology are relevant to physical activity. Regular physical activity can result in physiological adaptations to the HPA axis, cardiovascular system, and immune system that have been shown to modify psychophysiological responses. Since heightened stress reactivity has implications for health and well-being, a better understanding of these effects will be important in preventing chronic disease. The HPA axis and brain–immune interactions might also play an important mechanistic role in explaining the mental health benefits of regular physical activity. In relation to sports performance, several hormones appear to be important during preparation for and in coping with competitive environments, although it is not clear how neuroendocrine responses relate to the outcome of winning or losing. Lastly, a variety of hormones, including cortisol, testosterone, and catecholamines, have been used to monitor training load and recovery in athletes. Some evidence suggests that short periods of intense physical training, chronic overtraining, and mental fatigue cause disturbances in these hormones, although further evidence is required before such markers can be used as reliable diagnostic criteria.

Several key questions therefore remain unanswered in the area of physical activity and psychoneuroendocrinology. First, can HPA and immune responses to laboratory-induced stressors be modified by physical exercise training? Second, what is the impact of regular physical activity on the diurnal cortisol profile? Third, can the effects of exercise on glucocorticoid sensitivity and the immune system partly explain the antidepressant effects of physical activity? Lastly, can markers of neuroendocrine function be used as reliable indicators of overtraining in athletes?

References

Bartels, M., van den Berg, M., Sluyter, F., Boomsma, D. I., & de Geus, E. J. (2003). Heritability of cortisol levels: Review and simultaneous analysis of twin studies. *Psychoneuroendocrinology, 28*, 121–137.

Berchtold, N. C., Chinn, G., Chou, M., Kesslak, J. P., & Cotman, C. W. (2005). Exercise primes a molecular memory for brain-derived neurotrophic factor protein induction in the rat hippocampus. *Neuroscience, 133*(3), 853–861.

Blumenthal, J. A., Babyak, M. A., Doraiswamy, P. M., Watkins, L., Hoffman, B. M., Barbour, K. A.,...Sherwood, A. (2007). Exercise and pharmacotherapy in the treatment of major depressive disorder. *Psychosomatic Medicine, 69*(7), 587–596.

Bornstein, S. R., Engeland, W. C., Ehrhart-Bornstein, M., & Herman, J. P. (2008). Dissociation of ACTH and glucocorticoids. *Trends in Endocrinology and Metabolism, 19*(5), 175–180.

Brown, W. J., Ford, J. H., Burton, N. W., Marshall, A. L., & Dobson, A. J. (2005). Prospective study of physical activity and depressive symptoms in middle-aged women. *American Journal of Preventive Medicine, 29*(4), 265–272.

Brownley, K. A., Hinderliter, A. L., West, S. G., Girdler, S. S., Sherwood, A., & Light, K. C. (2003). Sympathoadrenergic mechanisms in reduced hemodynamic stress responses after exercise. *Medicine & Science in Sports & Exercise, 35*(6), 978–986.

Cacioppo, J. T., Berntson, G. G., Malarkey, W. B., Kiecolt-Glaser, J. K., Sheridan, J. F., Poehlmann, K. M.,...Glaser, R. (1998). Autonomic, neuroendocrine, and immune responses to psychological stress: The reactivity hypothesis. *Annals of the New York Academy of Sciences, 840*, 664–673.

Carter, J. B., Banister, E. W., & Blaber, A. P. (2002) Effect of endurance exercise on autonomic control of heart rate. *Sports Medicine, 33*, 33–46.

Chida, Y., & Hamer, M. (2008). Chronic psychosocial factors and acute physiological responses to laboratory-induced stress in healthy populations: A quantitative review of 30 years of investigations. *Psychological Bulletin, 134*(6), 829–885.

Chida, Y., & Steptoe, A. (2009). Cortisol awakening response and psychosocial factors: A systematic review and meta-analysis. *Biological Psychology, 80*(3), 265–278.

Chrousos, G. P., & Kino, T. (2007). Glucocorticoid action networks and complex psychiatric and/or somatic disorders. *Stress, 10*(2), 213–219.

Cohen, S., Hamrick, N., Rodriguez, M. S., Feldman, P. J., Rabin, B. S., & Manuck, S. B. (2002). Reactivity and vulnerability to stress-associated risk for upper respiratory illness. *Psychosomatic Medicine, 64*, 302–310.

Cotman, C. W., Berchtold, N. C., & Christie, L. A. (2007). Exercise builds brain health: Key roles of growth factor cascades and inflammation. *Trends in Neurosciences, 30*(9), 464–472.

Coutinho, A. E., Campbell, J. E., Fediuc, S., & Riddell, M. C. (2006). Effect of voluntary exercise on peripheral tissue glucocorticoid receptor content and the expression and activity of 11beta-HSD1 in the Syrian hamster. *Journal of Applied Physiology*, 100(5), 1483–1488.

Dekker, M. J., Koper, J. W., van Aken, M. O., Pols, H. A., Hofman, A., de Jong, F. H., ... Tiemeier, H. (2008). Salivary cortisol is related to atherosclerosis of carotid arteries. *Journal of Clinical Endocrinology & Metabolism*, 93, 3741–3747.

Droste, S. K., Chandramohan, Y., Hill, L. E., Linthorst, A. C., & Reul, J. M. (2007). Voluntary exercise impacts on the rat hypothalamic-pituitary-adrenocortical axis mainly at the adrenal level. *Neuroendocrinology*, 86(1), 26–37.

Duclos, M., Gouarne, C., & Bonnemaison, D. (2003). Acute and chronic effects of exercise on tissue sensitivity to glucocorticoids. *Journal of Applied Physiology*, 94(3), 869–875.

Edwards, K. M., Burns, V. E., Carroll, D., Drayson, M., & Ring, C. (2007). The acute stress-induced immunoenhancement hypothesis. *Exercise and Sport Sciences Reviews*, 35(3), 150–155.

Elloumi, M., Maso, F., Michaux, O., Robert, A., & Lac, G. (2003). Behaviour of saliva cortisol [C], testosterone [T] and the T/C ratio during a rugby match and during the post-competition recovery days. *European Journal of Applied Physiology*, 90(1–2), 23–28.

Ferris, L. T., Williams, J. S., & Shen, C. L. (2007). The effect of acute exercise on serum brain-derived neurotrophic factor levels and cognitive function. *Medicine & Science in Sports & Exercise*, 39(4), 728–734.

Filaire, E., Alix, D., Ferrand, C., & Verger, M. (2009). Psychophysiological stress in tennis players during the first single match of a tournament. *Psychoneuroendocrinology*, 34(1), 150–157.

Flaa, A., Eide, I. K., Kjeldsen, S. E., & Rostrup, M. (2008). Sympathoadrenal stress reactivity is a predictor of future blood pressure: An 18-year follow-up study. *Hypertension*, 52(2), 336–341.

Forcier, K., Stroud, L. R., Papandonatos, G. D., Hitsman, B., Reiches, M., Krishnamoorthy, J., & Niaura, R. (2006). Links between physical fitness and cardiovascular reactivity and recovery to psychological stressors: A meta-analysis. *Health Psychology*, 25(6), 723–739.

Franz, C. E., York, T. P., Eaves, L. J., Mendoza, S. P., Hauger, R. L., Hellhammer, D. H., ... Kremen, W. S. (2010) Genetic and environmental influences on cortisol regulation across days and contexts in middle-aged men. *Behaviour and Genetics*, 40(4), 467–479.

Gleeson, M. (2007). Immune function in sport and exercise. *Journal of Applied Physiology*, 103(2), 693–699.

Goekint, M., Heyman, E., Roelands, B., Njemini, R., Bautmans, I., Mets, T., & Meeusen, R. (2008). No influence of noradrenaline manipulation on acute exercise-induced increase of brain-derived neurotrophic factor. *Medicine & Science in Sports & Exercise*, 40(11), 1990–1996.

Gouarné, C., Groussard, C., Gratas-Delamarche, A., Delamarche, P., & Duclos, M. (2005). Overnight urinary cortisol and cortisone add new insights into adaptation to training. *Medicine & Science in Sports & Exercise*, 37(7), 1157–1167.

Hamer, M. (2007). The relative influences of fitness and fatness on inflammatory markers. *Preventive Medicine, 44*(1), 3–11.

Hamer, M., Gibson, E. L., Vuononvirta, R., Williams, E., & Steptoe, A. (2006). Inflammatory and hemostatic responses to repeated mental stress: Individual stability and habituation over time. *Brain, Behavior, and Immunity*, 20(5), 456–459.

Hamer, M., Molloy, G. J., de Oliveira, C., & Demakakos, P. (2009). Leisure time physical activity, risk of depressive symptoms, and inflammatory mediators: The English Longitudinal Study of Ageing. *Psychoneuroendocrinology*, 34(7), 1050–1055.

Hamer, M., O'Donnell, K., Lahiri, A., & Steptoe, A. (2010). Salivary cortisol responses to mental stress are associated with coronary artery calcification in healthy men and women. *European Heart Journal, 31*(4), 424–429.

Hamer, M., Stamatakis, E., & Steptoe, A. (2008). Psychiatric hospital admissions, behavioral risk factors, and all-cause mortality: The Scottish health survey. *Archives of Internal Medicine*, 168(22), 2474–2479.

Hamer, M., & Steptoe, A. (2007). Association between physical fitness, parasympathetic control, and proinflammatory responses to mental stress. *Psychosomatic Medicine*, 69(7), 660–666.

Hamer, M., Taylor, A., & Steptoe, A. (2006). The effect of acute aerobic exercise on stress related blood pressure responses: A systematic review and meta-analysis. *Biological Psychology*, 71(2), 183–190.

Hanton, S., Neil, R., & Mellalieu, S. D. (2008). Recent developments in competitive anxiety direction and competition stress research. *International Review of Sport and Exercise Psychology*, 1, 45–47.

Heim, C., Newport, D. J., Heit, S., Graham, Y. P., Wilcox, M., Bonsall, R., ... Nemeroff, C. B. (2000). Pituitary-adrenal and autonomic responses to stress in women after sexual and physical abuse in childhood. *JAMA, 284*, 592–597.

Hill, E. E., Zack, E., Battaglini, C., Viru, M., Viru, A., & Hackney, A. C. (2008). Exercise and circulating cortisol levels: The intensity threshold effect. *Journal of Endocrinological Investigation*, 31(7), 587–591.

Hong, S., Farag, N. H., Nelesen, R. A., Ziegler, M. G., & Mills, P. J. (2004). Effects of regular exercise on lymphocyte subsets and CD62L after psychological vs. physical stress. *Journal of Psychosomatic Research*, 56, 363–370.

Hong, S., & Mills, P. J. (2006). Physical activity and psychoneuroimmunology. In E. O. Acevedo & P. Ekkekakis (Eds.), *Psychobiology of physical activity* (pp. 177–188). Champaign, IL: Human Kinetics.

Jackson, E. M., & Dishman, R. K. (2006). Cardiorespiratory fitness and laboratory stress: A meta-regression analysis. *Psychophysiology*, 43(1), 57–72.

Kajantie, E., & Phillips, D. I. (2006). The effects of sex and hormonal status on the physiological response to acute psychosocial stress. *Psychoneuroendocrinology*, 31(2), 151–178.

Kiecolt-Glaser, J. K., Christian, L., Preston, H., Houts, C. R., Malarkey, W. B., Emery, C. F., & Glaser, R. (2010). Stress, inflammation and yoga practice. *Psychosomatic Medicine, 72*(2), 113–121.

Kudielka, B. M., Hellhammer, D. H., & Wüst, S. (2009). Why do we respond so differently? Reviewing determinants of human salivary cortisol responses to challenge. *Psychoneuroendocrinology*, 34(1), 2–18.

Kumsta, R., Entringer, S., Koper, J. W., van Rossum, E. F., Hellhammer, D. H., & Wüst, S. (2007). Sex specific associations between common glucocorticoid receptor gene variants and hypothalamus-pituitary-adrenal axis responses to psychosocial stress. *Biological Psychiatry*, 62(8), 863–869.

Lewin, G. R., & Barbe, Y. A. (1996). Physiology of neurotrophins. *Annual Review of Neuroscience*, 19, 289–317.

Lopez-Duran, N. L., Kovacs, M., & George, C. J. (2009). Hypothalamic-pituitary-adrenal axis dysregulation in depressed children and adolescents: A meta-analysis. *Psychoneuroendocrinology*, *34*(9), 1272–1283.

Mäestu, J., Jürimäe, J., & Jürimäe, T. (2005). Hormonal response to maximal rowing before and after heavy increase in training volume in highly trained male rowers. *Journal of Sports Medicine and Physical Fitness*, *45*(1), 121–126.

Matthews, K., Schwartz, J., Cohen, S., & Seeman, T. (2006). Diurnal cortisol decline is related to coronary calcification: CARDIA study. *Psychosomatic Medicine*, *68*, 657–661.

McEwen, B. S. (2007). Physiology and neurobiology of stress and adaptation: Central role of the brain. *Physiology Review*, *87*(3), 873–904.

Mehta, P. H., Jones, A. C., & Josephs, R. A. (2008). The social endocrinology of dominance: Basal testosterone predicts cortisol changes and behavior following victory and defeat. *Journal of Personality and Social Psychology*, *94*(6), 1078–1093.

Mehta, P. H. Wuehrmann, E. V., & Josephs, R. A. (2009). When are low testosterone levels advantageous? The moderating role of individual versus intergroup competition. *Hormones and Behavior*, *56*(1), 158–162.

Miller, A. H., Maletic, V., & Raison, C. L. (2009). Inflammation and its discontents: The role of cytokines in the pathophysiology of major depression. *Biological Psychiatry*, *65*(9), 732–741.

Minetto, M. A., Lanfranco, F., Tibaudi, A., Baldi, M., Termine, A., & Ghigo, E. (2008). Changes in awakening cortisol response and midnight salivary cortisol are sensitive markers of strenuous training-induced fatigue. *Journal of Endocrinology Investigation*, *31*(1), 16–24.

Muhtz, C., Zyriax, B. C., Klähn, T., Windler, E., & Otte, C. (2009). Depressive symptoms and metabolic risk: Effects of cortisol and gender. *Psychoneuroendocrinology*, *34*(7), 1004–1011.

Nabkasorn, C., Miyai, N., Sootmongkol, A., Junprasert, S., Yamamoto, H., Arita, M., & Miyashita, K. (2006). Effects of physical exercise on depression, neuroendocrine stress hormones and physiological fitness in adolescent females with depressive symptoms. *European Journal of Public Health*, *16*(2), 179–184.

O'Donnell, K., Badrick, E., Kumari, M., & Steptoe, A. (2008). Psychological coping styles and cortisol over the day in healthy older adults. *Psychoneuroendocrinology*, *33*(5), 601–611.

Oliveira, T., Gouveia, M. J., & Oliveira, R. F. (2009). Testosterone responsiveness to winning and losing experiences in female soccer players. *Psychoneuroendocrinology*, *34*(7), 1056–1064.

Pariante, C. M., & Lightman, S. L. (2008). The HPA axis in major depression: Classical theories and new developments. *Trends in Neurosciences*, *31*(9), 464–468.

Pedersen, B. K., & Febbraio, M. A. (2008). Muscle as an endocrine organ: Focus on muscle-derived interleukin-6. *Physiological Review*, *88*(4), 1379–1406.

Péronnet, F., Massicotte, D., Paquet, J. E., Brisson, G., & de Champlain, J. (1989). Blood pressure and plasma catecholamine responses to various challenges during exercise-recovery in man. *European Journal of Applied Physiology and Occupational Physiology*, *58*(5), 551–555.

Phillips, D. I. (2007). Programming of the stress response: A fundamental mechanism underlying the long-term effects of the fetal environment? *Journal of Internal Medicine*, *261*, 453–460.

Rhodes, J. S., van Praag, H., Jeffrey, S., Girard, I., Mitchell, G. S., Garland, T., Jr., & Gage, F. H. (2003). Exercise increases

hippocampal neurogenesis to high levels but does not improve spatial learning in mice bred for increased voluntary wheel running. *Behavioral Neuroscience*, *117*(5), 1006–1016.

Rimmele, U., Seiler, R., Marti, B., Wirtz, P. H., Ehlert, U., & Heinrichs, M. (2009). The level of physical activity affects adrenal and cardiovascular reactivity to psychosocial stress. *Psychoneuroendocrinology*, *34*(2), 190–198.

Rojas Vega, S., Strüder, H. K., Vera Wahrmann, B., Schmidt, A., Bloch, W., & Hollmann, W. (2006). Acute BDNF and cortisol response to low intensity exercise and following ramp incremental exercise to exhaustion in humans. *Brain Research*, *1121*(1), 59–65.

Rosmond, R., Dallman, M. F., & Björntorp, P. (1998). Stress-related cortisol secretion in men: Relationships with abdominal obesity and endocrine, metabolic and hemodynamic abnormalities. *Journal of Clinical Endocrinology & Metabolism*, *83*(6), 1853–1859.

Rouveix, M., Duclos, M., Gouarne, C., Beauvieux, M. C., & Filaire, E. (2006). The 24 h urinary cortisol/cortisone ratio and epinephrine/norepinephrine ratio for monitoring training in young female tennis players. *International Journal of Sports Medicine*, *27*(11), 856–863.

Russo-Neustadt, A. A., Alejandre, H., Garcia, C., Ivy, A. S., & Chen, M. J. (2004). Hippocampal brain-derived neurotrophic factor expression following treatment with reboxetine, citalopram, and physical exercise. *Neuropsychopharmacology*, *29*(12), 2189–2199.

Sasse, S. K., Greenwood, B. N., Masini, C. V., Nyhuis, T. J., Fleshner, M., Day, H. E. W., & Campeau, S. (2008). Chronic voluntary wheel running facilitates corticosterone response habituation to repeated audiogenic stress exposure in male rats. *Stress*, *11*(6), 425–437.

Silva, T. S., Longui, C. A., Faria, C. D., Rocha, M. N., Melo, M. R., Faria, T. G., . . . Kater, C. E. (2008). Impact of prolonged physical training on the pituitary glucocorticoid sensitivity determined by very low dose intravenous dexamethasone suppression test. *Hormone and Metabolic Research*, *40*(10), 718–721.

Steffen, P. R., Sherwood, A., Gullette, E. C., Georgiades, A., Hinderliter, A., & Blumenthal, J. A. (2001). Effects of exercise and weight loss on blood pressure during daily life. *Medicine & Science in Sports & Exercise*, *33*(10), 1635–1640.

Steptoe, A., & Brydon, L. (2005). Associations between acute lipid stress responses and fasting lipid levels 3 years later. *Health Psychology*, *24*(6), 601–607.

Steptoe, A., Kunz-Ebrecht, S. R., Brydon, L., & Wardle, J. (2004). Central adiposity and cortisol responses to waking in middle-aged men and women. *International Journal of Obesity (London)*, *28*(9), 1168–1173.

Steptoe, A., & Wardle, J. (2005). Cardiovascular stress responsivity, body mass and abdominal adiposity. *International Journal of Obesity (London)*, *29*(11), 1329–1337.

Steptoe, A., van Jaarsveld, C. H., Semmler, C., Plomin, R., & Wardle, J. (2009). Heritability of daytime cortisol levels and cortisol reactivity in children. *Psychoneuroendocrinology*. *34*(2), 273–280.

Strüder, H. K., Hollmann, W., Platen, P., Rost, R., Weicker, H., Kirchhof, O., & Weber, K. (1999). Neuroendocrine system and mental function in sedentary and endurance-trained elderly males. *International Journal of Sports Medicine*, *20*(3), 159–166.

Suay, F., Salvador, A., González-Bono, E., Sanchís, C., Martínez, M., Martínez-Sanchis, S., . . . Montoro, J. B. (1999). Effects of competition and its outcome on serum testosterone, cortisol and prolactin. *Psychoneuroendocrinology, 24*(5), 551–566.

Tracey, K. J. (2002). The inflammatory reflex. *Nature, 420,* 853–859.

Traustadóttir, T., Bosch, P. R., & Matt, K. S. (2005). The HPA axis response to stress in women: Effects of aging and fitness. *Psychoneuroendocrinology, 30*(4), 392–402.

Traustadóttir, T., Bosch, P. R., Cantu, T., & Matt, K. S. (2004). Hypothalamic-pituitary-adrenal axis response and recovery from high-intensity exercise in women: Effects of aging and fitness. *Journal of Clinical Endocrinology & Metabolism, 89*(7), 3248–3254.

Treiber, F. A., Kamarck, T., Schneiderman, N., Sheffield, D., Kapuku, G., & Taylor, T. (2003). Cardiovascular reactivity and development of preclinical and clinical disease states. *Psychosomatic Medicine, 65*(1), 46–62.

Urizar, G. G., Garovoy, N., Castro, C. M., & King, A. C. (2010). Effects of exercise and nutrition on cortisol regulation among older adults. *Psychosomatic Medicine, 72*(3), A-75.

van Praag, H., Kempermann, G., & Gage, F. H. (1999) Running increases cell proliferation and neurogenesis in the adult mouse dentate gyrus. *Nature Neuroscience, 2*(3), 266–270.

Vedhara, K., Cox, N. K., Wilcock, G. K., Perks, P., Hunt, M., Anderson, S., . . . Shanks, N. M. (1999). Chronic stress in elderly carers of dementia patients and antibody response to influenza vaccination. *Lancet, 353*(9153), 627–631.

Webb, H. E., Weldy, M. L., Fabianke-Kadue, E. C., Orndorff, G. R., Kamimori, G. H., & Acevedo, E. O. (2008). Psychological stress during exercise: Cardiorespiratory and hormonal responses. *European Journal of Applied Physiology, 104*(6), 973–981.

Wirtz, P. H., von Känel, R., Emini, L., Ruedisueli, K., Groessbauer, S., Maercker, A., & Ehlert, U. (2007). Evidence for altered hypothalamus-pituitary-adrenal axis functioning in systemic hypertension: Blunted cortisol response to awakening and lower negative feedback sensitivity. *Psychoneuroendocrinology, 32*(5), 430–436.

Wüst, S., Van Rossum, E. F., Federenko, I. S., Koper, J. W., Kumsta, R., & Hellhammer, D. H. (2004). Common polymorphisms in the glucocorticoid receptor gene are associated with adrenocortical responses to psychosocial stress. *Journal of Clinical Endocrinology & Metabolism, 89*, 565–573.

Zoladz, J. A., Pilc, A., Majerczak, J., Grandys, M., Zapart-Bukowska, J., & Duda, K. (2008). Endurance training increases plasma brain-derived neurotrophic factor concentration in young healthy men. *Journal of Physiology and Pharmacology, 59*(Suppl. 7), 119–132.

Muscle Pain During and Following Exercise

Christopher D. Black

Abstract

This chapter discusses the psychobiology of muscle pain during and following exercise. The chapter includes a general discussion of peripheral nociceptive inputs from noxious biochemicals and mechanical pressure as well as a discussion of central nociceptive processing in spinal and supraspinal areas. Descending modulation of pain via endogenous opioids is also discussed. Particular attention is paid to likely mechanisms of muscle pain during exercise and delayed-onset soreness following exercise. A second section of the chapter covers commonly used methods for assessing muscle pain, such as questionnaires and measures of pain threshold, pain tolerance, and pain intensity. The final section discusses individual attributes and treatment modalities that may affect pain perception. Included are specific discussions on the repeated-bout effect, differences in pain perceptions between men and women, analgesia after exercise, and pharmacological and other commonly employed treatments for pain, such as massage, ice, and heat.

Key Words: muscle pain, delayed-onset muscle soreness, exercise, pain threshold, pain tolerance.

Introduction

The International Association for the Study of Pain (ISAP) defines pain as an unpleasant sensory and emotional experience associated with actual or potential tissue damage, or described in the terms of such damage (Merskey & Bogduk, 1994). For the purpose of this chapter, the conscious, perceptual experience of pain or unpleasantness will be referred to as *muscle pain* and as *delayed-onset muscle soreness* (DOMS) when discussing pain that is caused by eccentrically biased exercise (exercise where a muscle is actively lengthened during a contraction), and experienced in the hours and days following a bout of exercise. From a neurobiological perspective, a distinction must be made between the perceptual experience of pain and the reception of signals evoked by specialized sensory receptors in peripheral tissues (e.g., skeletal muscle) and central tissues (spinal and supraspinal neurons). This process is

termed *nociception,* and the individual stimuli are termed *noxious* stimuli. When a noxious stimulus evokes a greater pain response than normal, this is termed *hyperalgesia* (Merskey & Bogduk, 1994). When a stimulus that does not normally evoke pain (e.g., massaging a muscle) does result in pain, this is termed *allodynia* (Merskey & Bogduk, 1994). The scope of this chapter will be limited to the perceptual experience, nociceptive inputs, and processing of pain that are commonly experienced in skeletal muscle(s) during a single bout of exercise or the pain experienced in the muscles in the hours and days following a bout of exercise. It should be noted that an extensive literature exists regarding nociception and skeletal muscle pain during and following exercise. The contents of this chapter are by no means comprehensive, and readers are referred to previous reviews for more detailed discussions (Mense, 2009, Millan, 1999, O'Connor & Cook, 1999)

In a recent study, it was reported that approximately 10% of visits to clinical medical practices in the United States were the consequence of some form of musculoskeletal pain (Caudill-Slosberg et al., 2004). Roughly 50% of the respondents of the Nuprin Pain Report, a survey of Americans in the mid-1980s, reported experiencing some type of muscle pain, with 9% of respondents reporting the loss of at least one working day in the previous year due to muscle pain (Sternbach, 1986). Low back pain affects upward of 70% of all people at some point in their life (Frymoyer et al., 1980) and is thought to be one of the most costly, in direct medical costs and in lost productivity, and most disabling disorders for Americans. While less prevalent, chronic muscle pain is also experienced in other clinical disorders, such as fibromyalgia and arthritis. Treatment strategies for chronic, persistent muscle and musculoskeletal pain, especially drug treatments, are not always effective (Cohen et al., 2004, Curatolo & Bogduk, 2001). Given the number of individuals who suffer from musculoskeletal pain and the profound economic costs associated with chronic pain, a better understanding of the mechanisms that underlie muscle pain could lead to the development of more efficacious treatments and improved diagnosis of these disorders.

Peripheral and Central Nociception and Pain
Skeletal Muscle Nociceptors

The free nerve endings that function as skeletal muscle nociceptors are located in and around the small arteries, arterioles, and venules as well as connective tissue located in and around skeletal muscle (Stacey, 1969). Individual muscle fibers are not thought to be directly innervated by free nerve endings. Nociceptive free nerve endings are unmyelinated axons that have direct access to interstitial fluid and have axonal expansions that contain various neuropeptides and endogenous substances such as substance P, calcitonin gene-related peptide, and a host of others (Messlinger, 1996, Reinert et al., 1998). They synapse primarily on neuronal cell bodies in the dorsal root ganglia in the dorsal horn of the spinal cord (Cervero et al., 1976). Within skeletal muscle, two primary types of afferent nerve fibers transmit nociceptive signals. Type III afferent fibers, also known as A-delta (Aδ) fibers, are thinly myelinated and may end in free nerve endings, paciniform corpuscles, or other types of receptors. Aδ fibers tend to respond preferentially to mechanical pressure and deformation, and their activation

in skeletal muscle results in dull, aching-, or cramping-type pain (Marchettini et al., 1996). Type IV afferent fibers, also known as cutaneous C fibers, are unmyelinated, end exclusively in free nerve endings (Stacey, 1969), respond preferentially to various chemical stimuli, and result in dull, burning, and aching-type pain (Mense, 1993). Molecular receptors for many algesic substances are also thought to be present in muscle tissue (Julius & Basbaum, 2001).

Muscle nociceptors are typically activated by mechanical pressure or chemical or thermal stimuli. Application of a noxious stimulus to a nociceptor results in the generation of an electrical signal. If the stimulus is sufficiently large, then the electrical signal may exceed a threshold value, resulting in the generation of an action potential that is then transmitted along the axon to the dorsal horn; this represents activation of the nociceptor. Additionally, a nociceptor may be "sensitized" by a given stimulus. During sensitization the binding of a noxious agent, often a noxious biochemical, to a receptor lowers the threshold for activation of the nociceptor. Thus after a receptor has been sensitized, less input is required for activation. Receptors that respond to mechanical stimuli are termed *high-threshold mechanosensitive (HTM) muscle receptors* and require high levels of tissue-threatening mechanical pressure to be activated (Kumazawa & Mizumura, 1977). As a consequence, weak mechanical stimuli that are typical of many everyday sensations are often not perceived as painful because the stimuli are not sufficient to activate HTM nociceptors. Aside from mechanical pressure a host of chemical substances directly activate and sensitize muscle nociceptors. These biochemicals include bradykinin, serotonin, histamine, potassium, protons (hydrogen ions), prostaglandin E$_2$ (PGE$_2$), substance P, and adenosine triphosphate (ATP) (Mense, 2009). Not surprisingly, many of these algesic substances are produced or released during a bout of exercise and in response to tissue damage and inflammation that may occur as a result of exercise-induced muscle injury.

Noxious Biochemicals and Exercise
PROTONS/H⁺ IONS

Intense exercise, ischemia, and tissue inflammation often result in a decrease in tissue pH and an increase in proton, or hydrogen ion (H⁺), concentrations (Hood et al., 1988, Issberner et al., 1996). Proton-sensitive nociceptors are likely contributors to exercise-related pain in skeletal muscles. Tonic, low-force contractions can lead to ischemia within the activated muscles and result in a lowering of muscle pH via accumulation of lactic acid that dissociates into lactate and H^+ ions. Moderate- to high-intensity dynamic exercise such as running or cycling can also lead to the production of lactic acid and can thus result in the aching- or cramping-type pain experienced during intense exercise. Intramuscular injection of a buffer solution of pH 5.2--6.0 resulted in moderate-intensity pain that activates more than 50% of mechanosensitive afferent nociceptors and leads to increased sensitivity to mechanical pressure (Hoheisel et al., 2004). H^+ ions signal through acid-sensing ion channels (ASICs), and high densities of ASIC1 and ASIC3 are found on skeletal muscle nociceptors (Hoheisel et al., 2004, Sluka et al., 2003). ASIC3 channels are found in the dorsal root ganglion (Price et al., 2001) and are thought to play an important role in central sensitization to noxious stimuli.

BRADYKININ

Another potent activator of skeletal muscle nociceptors is bradykinin (BKN). BKN is a peptide whose precursors are found in blood plasma. It is synthesized by the enzyme kallikrein in response to ischemia, plasma extravasation, and when certain factors involved in the clotting system are activated. Thus it is formed in response to direct tissue damage and other situations common to exercise, such as ischemia, hypoxia, and tissue acidification. BKN activates both type III and type IV afferent fibers in skeletal muscle, and intramuscular injections of BKN have been shown to be mildly painful (V. Babenko et al., 1999, V. V. Babenko et al., 1999, Kaufman et al., 1982). BKN signals through the bradykinin B1 and B2 receptors. In addition to leading to synthesis and release of BKN, tissue damage and inflammation leads to increased expression of B1 receptors in dorsal root ganglia and in free nerve endings (Perkins & Kelly, 1993). BKN also plays a role in sensitizing nociceptive afferents. Activation of the B1 and B2 receptors alters the resting membrane potential of nociceptors and can enhance their responsiveness to other noxious stimuli, such as serotonin (Hu et al., 2005). Additionally, BKN leads to the production of prostaglandins, which are important inflammatory mediators that also function to sensitize afferent nociceptive fibers and enhance and prolong the effects of BKN (Mense, 1981).

SEROTONIN (5-HT)

Serotonin is a monoamine neurotransmitter with wide-ranging functions throughout the body and nervous system. Much like BKN, serotonin activates both type III and IV nociceptors in skeletal muscle (Mense, 1977). Injection of 5-HT into muscle in sufficiently large doses results in pain, while in lower doses, serotonin functions to sensitize nociceptors to BKN, leading to a greater pain response to a given dose (V. Babenko et al., 1999, V. V. Babenko et al., 1999). 5-HT may also play a role with BKN in sensitizing HTM receptors to mechanical stimulation (V. V. Babenko et al., 1999).

SUBSTANCE P

Substance P is an endogenous neuropeptide present in skeletal muscle nociceptive fibers and in neurons of the dorsal root ganglion (Mense et al., 1996). It is released in response to noxious stimulation and in response to exercise and inflammation (Lind et al., 1996). It is often colocalized with calcitonin gene-related peptide, which increases its action by inhibiting its breakdown (Levine et al., 1993). Substance P signals through the neurokinin-1 receptor and is known to increase the release of other algesic agents, such as PGE_2 and histamine (Levine et al., 1993, O'Connor & Cook, 1999). Depletion of substance P in neurons and afferent nerve endings via stimulation from substances such as capsaicin has been shown to decrease pain perceptions in response to chemical and mechanical stimuli (Hoheisel et al., 2004).

PROSTAGLANDIN E$_2$

PGE_2 is a metabolite of arachidonic acid and is synthesized via the action of enzymes of the cyclooxygenase (COX) family. It plays a role in a range of body functions, such as the control of blood vessel diameter, blood pressure, and the inflammatory response to tissue damage. It exhibits very little activation of muscle nociceptors but plays a key role in sensitizing nociceptors to BKN and other algesic substances (Mense, 1981). Nonsteroidal anti-inflammatory drugs such as aspirin and ibuprofen blunt the action of the COX enzymes (Vane, 1978) and thus may function to limit inflammation and pain following tissue damage.

ADENOSINE AND ATP

Adenosine is a purine that mediates numerous cellular and physiological processes. ATP is a high-energy molecule that is found in all cells throughout the body. In skeletal muscle ATP serves as the primary source of energy for exercise metabolism. ATP is rapidly metabolized into adenosine, and damage to muscle cells may lead to membrane disruption and result in release of adenosine, ATP, or both from the cells. A host of adenosine receptors exist, and A_1 and A_{2a} receptors are thought to play a role in nociception in human pain models (Millan, 1999, Sawynok, 1998, Sawynok & Liu, 2003). Administration of caffeine, a nonspecific adenosine receptor antagonist, has been shown to reduce muscle pain during and following exercise (Maridakis et al., 2007, Motl et al., 2006, Motl et al., 2003, O'Connor et al., 2004).

Nociception and Pain Processing in the Brain and Spinal Cord

SPINAL CORD AND BRAIN PATHWAYS OF PAIN

After peripheral nociceptors in skeletal muscle have been activated by noxious biochemicals, mechanical pressure, or a thermal stimulus, an electrical signal is transmitted through the afferent fibers to the spinal cord. The spinal cord then transmits the signal to the brain, where it is perceived as painful. Early theories regarding pain pathways, which date from Descartes (1644/1972), suggested that nociceptive inputs traveled from the periphery to the brain as if along simple cables. More recently advances in immunohistochemistry and neuroimaging have allowed researchers to look more closely into the spinal cord and brain to gain insight into how stimulation of peripheral nociceptors is processed at the spinal and supraspinal level and is ultimately perceived as pain. Not surprisingly these techniques have demonstrated that the sensation of pain involves much more than a simple connection from a peripheral receptor to the central nervous system. It is a complex and integrative sensation that is greatly processed and modified in multiple areas (Melzack & Wall, 1965).

Afferent fibers enter the dorsal root ganglia and synapse in the dorsal horn primarily in lamina I and II but also in lamina V (Mense, 1993). If the intensity of the stimulation is sufficient it will produce a postsynaptic output that is transmitted to supraspinal regions of the brain along one of several projection nerve tracts. Within the dorsal horn, afferent fibers and projection neurons communicate using a host of amino acid and peptide neurotransmitters such as glutamate and substance P (DeLeo, 2006, Millan, 1999). They also possess receptors for endogenous opioids, which play a role in pain processing and especially hypoalgesia.

Depending on the type of nociceptor activated, a stimulus is transmitted along the spinal cord to various areas within the brain via the contralateral spinothalamic, spinoreticular, spinomesencephalic, spinoparabrachial, spinohypothalamic, and dorsal column tracts (Millan, 1999). The spinothalamic tract is composed of two separate tracts, a lateral (neospinothalamic) tract, which projects through the medulla to the ventroposterolateral areas of the thalamus, and a medial (paleospinothalamic) tract, which projects to the reticular formation in the brain stem, the periaqueductal gray (PAG), hypothalamus, amygdala, and parts of the thalamus (Millan, 1999). Signals from Aδ fibers travel may travel along the neospinothalamic tract and are thought to be responsible for sharp, fast pain, while signals from C fibers travel along the paleospinothalamic tract and result primarily in dull, aching pain. Along the spinoreticular tract, nociceptive inputs travel to the reticular formation and synapse in the medial thalamus and nucleus paragigantocellularis, which inputs to the locus coeruleus (Millan, 1999). The spinomesencephalic tract transmits signals to the PAG, much like the spinothalamic tract, and the PAG provides inputs to limbic system structures such as the amygdala and anterior cingulate cortex (ACC).

This discussion of pain-related inputs is by no means comprehensive, as many different brain regions have been found to be active during pain processing. However, it begins to demonstrate the complex nature of spinal and supraspinal nociceptive inputs and processing. Activation of the primary and secondary somatosensory systems in the cortex via projections from the thalamus can provide information regarding the location and intensity of a painful stimulus. Other areas, such as the ACC, PAG, and amygdala, may provide information regarding the affective and emotional dimension of pain. As illustrated in Figure 9.1, it is overly simple to view pain perception as occurring via transmission of peripheral nociceptive signals to the spinal cord, then to the thalamus, then to the somatosensory cortex, where it is perceived as painful. Parallel signals are sent to multiple brain areas whose functions encompass cognition, emotion, and attention and to the autonomic nervous system; these complex inputs make pain a multifaceted and complex sensation. There are thus numerous mechanisms for modulation of pain (both hyperalgesia and hypoalgesia).

MODULATION OF PAIN

Many people are familiar with anecdotes about a soldier or an athlete who sustains substantial tissue damage but does not immediately appear to find the injury to be painful. Also, people who have

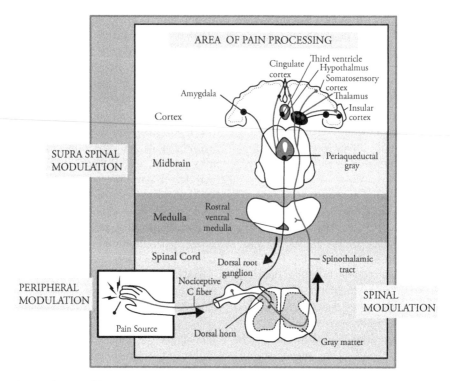

Figure 9.1. Schematic diagram of the primary anatomical pathway by which a nociceptive input would travel from peripheral tissue to spinal and supraspinal areas. Anatomical locations of pain modulation are also shown. Reprinted with permission from "Basic Science of Pain," By J. A. DeLeo, 2006, *Journal of Bone and Joint Surgery, American Volume, 88*(Suppl. 2), pp. 58–62.

been sunburned know that a light touch across the skin that normally would produce no pain can be perceived as quite painful. Hypoalgesia and allodynia are well documented and illustrate how the brain and spinal cord can exert a modulatory effect on how inputs from peripheral nociceptors are perceived. In addition to receiving inputs from peripheral nociceptors (ascending), projection neurons in the dorsal horn of the spinal cord receive input from a host of brain regions (descending) that play an important role in the processing of sensory and nociceptive information. Inputs from non-nociceptive afferent fibers from skeletal muscle as well as cutaneous and visceral sites converge with nociceptive inputs on neurons in the dorsal horn. This complex network of connections allows for the integration of signals from multiple tissues and can exert both excitatory and inhibitory effects on the nociceptive signal and modulate perceptions of a noxious stimulus. Additionally, the release of endogenous opioids in peripheral and central tissue can act to decrease afferent nociceptive input to the dorsal horn (Mense, 1993).

Originally proposed by Melzack and Wall (1965), the *gate-control theory* suggests that input

from non-nociceptive afferent fibers activates interneurons in the dorsal horn that then inhibit the activity of nociceptive neurons, thus blunting nociceptive input from the periphery. This theoretical framework helped to explain a variety of phenomena, such as why a balm that irritates the skin around a painful bruise or cut may provide temporary pain relief. Descending modulation of pain from supraspinal areas also occurs. Stimulation of the PAG has also been shown to result in analgesia without affecting alertness, attention, or motor control in response to non-noxious stimuli (D. J. Mayer & Price, 1976). The PAG integrates ascending noxious stimuli with descending inputs from the hypothalamus, amygdala, insula, and ACC (Brooks & Tracey, 2005). Bidirectional connections also exist between the PAG and the rostral ventromedial medulla (RVM) (Brooks & Tracey, 2005). Electrical stimulation of the PAG, amygdala, or RVM produces analgesia (Hosobuchi et al., 1977, O'Connor & Cook, 1999). Analgesic signals from the PAG are likely transmitted to the spinal cord via the RVM. The RVM is a primary source of serotonin in the spinal cord, and serotonin has been shown to selectively inhibit nociceptive neurons in the dorsal horn (Jordan et al., 1978).

Additionally, the RVM has neurons that synapse on projection neurons in the spinothalamic tract and may reduce nociceptive inputs by activating inhibitory interneurons or inhibiting excitatory interneurons. The PAG, RVM, and amygdala also contain high concentrations of receptors for opioids. Administration of exogenous opioids in the PAG has been shown to induce analgesia. Endogenous opioids such as enkephalins, beta-endorphins, and endomorphins likely play a role in pain modulation in the brain and spinal cord as well as at the afferent nociceptive fibers in the periphery. Opioid administration can lead to hyperpolarization of dorsal horn neurons and inhibition of release of substance P (Meintjes et al., 1995), which could play an antinociceptive role. Levels of endogenous opioids have been shown to increase during exercise, particularly intense exercise (Goldfarb & Jamurtas, 1997), leading to the suggestion that endogenous opioids may play a role in exercise-induced analgesia (Janal et al., 1984, Pertovaara et al., 1984).

In summary, the sensation of pain begins with the activation of peripheral nociceptors, central nociceptors, or both. Skeletal muscle nociceptors are generally located in and around the small arteries, arterioles, and venules as well as connective tissue found in skeletal muscle tissue. These nociceptors signal to the dorsal horn of the spinal cord via type III or IV afferent nerve fibers and respond to a host of noxious biochemicals, thermal stimuli, and mechanical pressure. Afferent nociceptors synapse in the dorsal horn of the spinal cord, typically in lamina I, II, and V, and nociceptive signals are then transmitted to the brain along several tracts that project to numerous regions of the brain, including the thalamus, reticular formation, PAG, ACC, hypothalamus, and amygdala. Nociceptive input is processed at the level of the peripheral receptors, in the dorsal horn, and in higher brain areas, and pain sensations may be modulated in these regions by numerous exogenous and endogenous substances (e.g., opioids and other analgesic drugs) and neural input from other tissue (e.g., afferent input from contracting skeletal muscle). Thus the sensation of pain represents the end product of a complex and multifaceted integration of both excitatory and inhibitory signals.

Pain and Exercise

Pain is a common experience for those who exercise, be it the "burning" of muscles during all-out sprints in a soccer match or the dull ache of muscle soreness that inevitably follows the first bout of resistance training after a long layoff. Two common types of skeletal muscle pain with exercise are (1) pain experienced during active muscle contractions during exercise and (2) delayed pain and tenderness experienced in skeletal muscle in the days following exercise. While both types of pain represent unpleasant sensory experiences, the underlying causes and consequences of each are unique.

Pain following Exercise

Delayed-onset muscle soreness or pain, often referred to as DOMS, is a common experience following unaccustomed exercise. While DOMS can occur following exercise consisting of mainly concentric (shortening) or isometric (static) muscle actions, it most commonly occurs following high-intensity exercise that includes a large eccentric (lengthening) component. Eccentric contractions place greater mechanical stress on the internal structures of skeletal muscles than their concentric and isometric counterparts because fewer muscle fibers are recruited to generate any given level of force (Enoka, 1996). Thus we use a smaller portion of the available muscle fibers in our biceps to lower a 10-kg dumbbell than we would use to curl the same 10-kg dumbbell up. The force per area of recruited or activated muscle is termed *specific force* or *specific tension*. When the specific force of active muscles exceeds the tensile strength of the internal structures of a muscle, damage may occur to the ultrastructure of the muscle fiber (Black et al., 2008, Black & McCully, 2008a). Evidence indicates that lengthening the muscle over a greater distance (Lieber & Friden, 1993) as well as performing contractions at longer (more anatomically extended) initial muscle lengths (Nosaka & Sakamoto, 2001) leads to greater damage.

This damage is characterized by streaming and smearing of the Z disks (the area where one sarcomere connects to another) when observed using electron microscopy (Friden et al., 1983). The damage to the muscle tends to worsen over the several days following the exercise bout and then is gradually repaired within the subsequent two to four weeks (Clarkson & Sayers, 1999). Consequent to the initial mechanical insult to the muscle fibers, damage also occurs to the sarcoplasmic reticulum (Yasuda et al., 1997) and plasma membrane (Clarkson & Sayers, 1999). Disruption of these structures can lead to increased levels of calcium in intracellular spaces and activate calcium-dependent degradation pathways. The calcium-activated protease calpain has been shown to cleave key structural proteins (such as desmin and vimentin) found in the cytoskeleton of muscle fibers and may play a role in the worsening of muscle damage following the initial insult (Belcastro et al., 1998). Muscle damage following eccentric exercise has been shown to lead to acute infiltration of inflammatory cells such as neutrophils and monocytes in the 2 to 24 hours following exercise (MacIntyre et al., 1996), which aids in the removal of damaged tissue and debris and helps to promote repair of the injured tissue. Infiltration by neutrophils and monocytes/macrophages also leads to increases in intramuscular and blood levels of proinflammatory cytokines such as interleukin 1 (IL-1) and 6 (IL-6) and tumor necrosis factor-alpha (TNF-α) in the hours and days following eccentric exercise (Cannon & St Pierre, 1998). Edema or swelling in the exercised musculature is also a common occurrence. Damage to skeletal muscle is also associated with decreased function in the muscle,

characterized by a reduced ability to generate force, stiffness, and decreased joint range of motion as well as increased levels of muscle-specific proteins such as creatine kinase in the blood (Clarkson & Sayers, 1999, Warren et al., 1999). A final consequence of exercise-induced muscle injury is pain and tenderness in the damaged muscle and tendon.

The dull, aching pain and tenderness following muscle injury typically does not occur immediately. It develops in the hours to days after the injurious bout of exercise. While the time course has been shown to vary, it tends to initially develop over the 24 hours after exercise and to reach its peak intensity 24–72 hours post exercise (Clarkson et al., 1992) (Figure 9.2). The intensity of pain is not always strongly associated with other markers of muscle damage, but eccentric exercise performed with a greater percentage of maximal strength (Poudevigne et al., 2002) and an increased number of eccentric

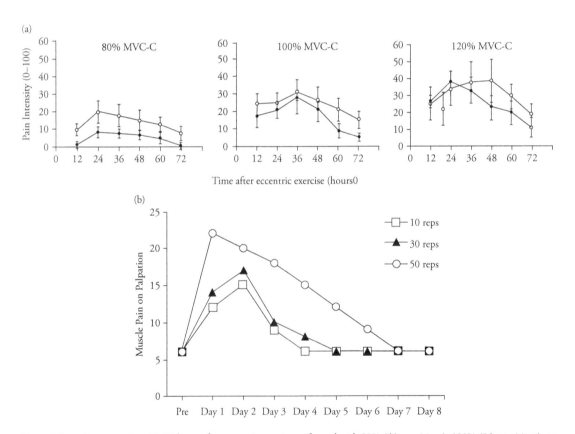

Figure 9.2. *a:* Soreness ratings 12–72 hours after eccentric exercise performed with 80% (45 repetitions), 100% (36 repetitions), or 120% (30 repetitions) of the one-repetition maximum with the elbow flexors. MVC-C, (Maximal Voluntary Contraction). Reprinted from "Lack of Both Sex Differences and Influence of Resting Blood Pressure on Muscle Pain Intensity," by M. S. Poudevigne, P. J. O'Connor, and J. D. Pasley, 2002, *Clinical Journal of Pain, 18*(6), pp. 386–393. *b:* Soreness ratings prior to (Pre) and for 8 days following 10, 30, and 50 repetitions of maximal voluntary isokinetic eccentric exercise of the knee extensors. Based on data from "Exercise-Induced Skeletal Muscle Damage and Adaptation following Repeated Bouts of Eccentric Muscle Contractions," by S. J. Brown, R. B. Child, S. H. Day, and A. E. Donnelly, 1997, *Journal of Sports Science, 15*(2), pp. 215–222.

contractions (Brown et al., 1997) have been shown to increase pain intensity. This pain usually abates within five days post exercise. If ultrastructure damage occurs immediately during a bout of high-intensity eccentric exercise, what then is the cause of DOMS and why is its onset delayed? Accumulation of lactic acid has been proposed as an explanation, since it is known to occur during high-intensity exercise, and the buildup of hydrogen ions produced by the dissociation of lactic acid is known to activate skeletal muscle nociceptors (Mense, 2009). However, evidence exists disproving this hypothesis (Miles & Clarkson, 1994). The most likely explanation, especially given the time course, is that local inflammation induces increased intramuscular pressure due to edema and an increased concentration of biochemicals that both activate and sensitize muscle nociceptors.

DOMS is characterized by muscle tenderness and pain during movements or palpation that would not be painful under "normal" circumstances. This suggests that following muscle damage the HTM muscle nociceptors have been sensitized and the stimulus required to activate them has been reduced. While the exact mechanisms remain unclear, two primary mechanisms of DOMS have been hypothesized. First, noxious biochemicals such as BKN, serotonin, histamine, and PGE_2, which are known to activate or sensitize muscle nociceptors, are associated with tissue inflammation following damage (Mense, 2009). Damage and inflammation are also associated with a decreased tissue pH via accumulation of H^+ ions and a leakage of

adenosine and ATP from damaged muscle fibers into the extracellular space (Mense, 2009, Sawynok, 1998). Intramuscular injection of BKN following administration of either serotonin or PGE_2 has been shown to induce greater pain and lower the pain threshold to mechanical stimuli compared with an injection of BKN alone (V. V. Babenko et al., 1999, Mense, 1981). The accumulation of some combination of these noxious biochemicals following tissue damage, resulting in activation and sensitization of muscle nociceptors, appears to be the most likely explanation for the mechanical hyperalgesia and allodynia observed with DOMS. In addition to chemical stimulation and sensitization, the edema associated with tissue inflammation may play a role in the increased pain and tenderness of DOMS. Swelling of the injured muscle tissue may increase intramuscular pressure, and this pressure may activate the mechanoreceptors.

Pain during Exercise

Pain emanating from the contracting muscles during exercise is also very common. During cycling exercise, pain in the quadriceps muscle group has been shown to increase as a positively accelerating function of relative exercise intensity expressed as either a percentage of peak power output or peak oxygen consumption (Cook et al., 1997) (Figure 9.3). Similarly, pain response during cycling appears to be somewhat dependent on exercise intensity, with cycling at 80% of peak oxygen consumption generally eliciting greater muscle pain than exercise at 60% of peak oxygen consumption (Gliottoni et al.,

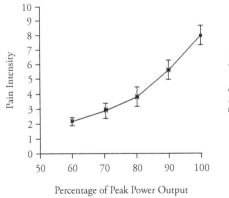
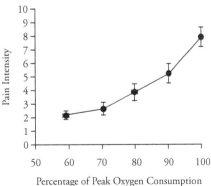

Figure 9.3. Pain ratings during a graded, maximal cycling exercise test as a function of percentage of peak power output and percentage of peak oxygen consumption. Reprinted from "Naturally Occurring Muscle Pain during Exercise: Assessment and Experimental Evidence," by D. B. Cook, P. J. O'Connor, S. A. Eubanks, J. C. Smith, and M. Lee, 1997, *Medicine & Science in Sports & Exercise, 29*(8), pp. 999–1012.

2009, Gliottoni & Motl, 2008, Motl et al., 2006, Motl et al., 2003, O'Connor et al., 2004). Following cessation of exercise, muscle pain does not abate immediately. Rather, it has been shown to decline in an exponential manner over several minutes. This decline very closely mimics the decline in ratings of perceived exertion and oxygen consumption following cessation of exercise (Cook et al., 1997). Pain during high-intensity cycling exercise has been described as exhausting, intense, sharp, burning, tiring, cramping, pulling, and rasping, and it seems plausible that other types of aerobic exercise would elicit similar pain (Cook et al., 1997). This naturally occurring pain that accompanies exercise has been shown to exhibit a reproducible pain threshold of approximately 50% of peak power output or peak oxygen consumption, suggesting that high-intensity exercise or high-force muscle contractions are not necessary to evoke muscle pain (Cook et al., 1997, Weiser et al., 1973). Muscle pain can be evoked during very brief bouts of exercise, as short as 8 seconds (Cook et al., 1997), but tends to be more pronounced during longer exercise bouts.

Muscle pain experienced during exercise tends to show large inter-subject variability when similar modes, relative exercise intensities, and exercise durations are employed. This raises the question of what nociceptive mechanisms are responsible for muscle pain during exercise. As is the case for DOMS, the exact mechanisms of naturally occurring muscle pain remain unclear and may vary based on exercise mode, intensity, and duration. However, it is plausible to group the potential mechanisms into two general categories: (1) accumulation of noxious biochemicals and (2) increases in intramuscular pressure due to muscle contractions. Exercise, especially exercise of high relative intensity, leads to the buildup of metabolic by-productions such as lactic acid. Once produced, lactic acid dissociates into lactate and hydrogen ions. H^+ ions decrease muscle pH and are potent activators of type III and IV afferent nociceptors (Mense, 2009). During typical exercise, even in "untrained" individuals, accumulation of H^+ ions only occurs at moderate-to-high exercise intensities (over 50–60% of peak oxygen consumption). However, muscle pain is commonly associated with work-related situations where repetitive, low-force, tonic muscle contractions are performed (Mense, 2009). In this context, the low-force contractions may generate sufficient force to overcome systolic blood pressure and lead to occlusion of the blood vessels that supply oxygen-rich blood to the working muscle and remove venous blood containing

metabolic by-products such as lactic acid and other noxious biochemicals. Some of those other noxious biochemicals may play a role in pain experienced during exercise. Exercise has been shown to increase interstitial levels of BKN and adenosine in skeletal muscle (Langberg et al., 2002) and has also been shown to increase the release of potassium, histamine, and PGE_2 (Rotto et al., 1990). Increased brain levels of serotonin have been associated with exercise (Caperuto et al., 2009), and exercise has been shown to increase substance P concentrations in the ventral horn of the spinal cord (Lind et al., 1996, Wilson et al., 1993). While none of these findings provides direct evidence that accumulation of these noxious biochemicals underlies the naturally occurring pain experienced during exercise, they at least demonstrate a plausible association. Furthermore, the findings that pain increases with longer durations of exercise and does not abate immediately following cessation of exercise suggest that pain may build up as noxious biochemicals accumulate and abate as the biochemicals are gradually removed during recovery (Cook et al., 1997).

However, some evidence exists that biochemicals are not solely responsible for naturally occurring muscle pain during exercise. Administration of aspirin, which would reduce PGE_2 levels, was not found to reduce muscle pain during cycling exercise (Cook et al., 1997). Furthermore, leg pain has been shown to occur after only 8 seconds of exercise, which would potentially limit the accumulation of biochemicals (Cook et al., 1997). These findings suggest that such accumulation is not a requirement for eliciting muscle pain during exercise. Another plausible mechanism for pain during exercise is increased intramuscular pressure associated with muscle contractions and force production. Exercise requires skeletal muscle to generate force, with higher-intensity exercise typically requiring greater and greater levels of force production. If force levels are high enough, the mechanical deformation of the muscle and the rise in intramuscular pressure could be sufficient to activate the HTM nociceptive fibers. Mechanistically, activation of HTM fibers by high-force muscle contractions could be responsible for the pain experienced during short-term, high-intensity exercise.

It is likely that muscle pain during exercise is the result of a combination of stimulation and sensitization of nociceptors by noxious biochemicals and mechanical pressure. It is easy to envision a situation in which exercise results in an increase in substances such as H^+ ions, BKN, substance P, and PGE_2 during repeated high-force muscle contractions. The biochemicals and contractions may independently activate various nociceptors, and the biochemicals may also function to sensitize receptors for both the noxious biochemicals and the HTM receptors, thus amplifying the response to each.

Measurement of Pain

The perception of pain is a complex, multifaceted experience that is likely unique to each person. Thus the challenge lies in how to assess this perception. While it has been suggested that no single "best" measure of pain during and following exercise exists (O'Connor & Cook, 1999), several commonly used methods have been shown to provide reliable and valid information regarding certain dimensions of pain. These methods include objective measures of pain thresholds and pain tolerance and subjective measures of pain intensity or magnitude.

Pain Threshold

The minimum noxious stimulus required to be perceived as "painful" or "tender" is defined as the *pain threshold*. Thermal, pressure, and electrical stimuli are commonly used to investigate pain thresholds. In a typical experiment, the intensity of noxious stimuli is increased or decreased in a stepwise manner in small increments. During "ascending" trials, intensities below the pain threshold are initially applied and then intensity is gradually increased until the stimulus is perceived as painful, and during "descending" trials the stimulus is initially set above the pain threshold and then gradually lowered until it is no longer perceived as painful. This "method of limits" procedure has its roots in scaling methods and signal detection theory, and readers are referred to Gracely and colleagues (Gracely & Kwilosz, 1988, Gracely et al., 1988) as well as Wall and Melzack (1999) for more complete explanations of the methodology underlying these techniques.

Several factors outside of nociceptive inputs can play a role in determining pain thresholds. Response bias is a measure of a person's willingness to call a stimulus painful and may be influenced by the individual's previous experiences and attitudes toward pain (O'Connor & Cook, 1999). In exercise-related research, the most commonly used method for determining pain tolerance is the use of manually applied force or pressure to various points on a muscle or other anatomical structures (e.g., fingers) during or following exercise. DOMS has repeatedly been shown to lower the pressure pain threshold (Baker et al., 1997, Dannecker et al., 2005, Hedayatpour et al.,

2008, Maridakis et al., 2007). While large interindividual and intraindividual differences can exist in threshold measures, the measures can provide meaningful information regarding peripheral and central sensitization during and following exercise. They can also be useful in determining the effects of various analgesic interventions.

Pain Tolerance

Pain tolerance represents the greatest (largest) noxious stimulus a person is able to endure (O'Connor & Cook, 1999). It is difficult and perhaps unethical to obtain a true measure of pain tolerance in human subjects, given that the applied stimulus could result in substantial tissue damage. Approximations of a true "pain tolerance" could be made by application of mechanical pressure, and application of hot or electrical stimuli. However, given the potential for tissue damage, assessments more often involve examining the length of time a person can or will endure a noxious stimulus (e.g., submersion of the hand in ice water, application of a mechanical stimulus, etc.). Assessing pain tolerance in this manner often imposes maximal exposure times to the noxious stimulus, thus setting a ceiling on the possible length of tolerance times (O'Connor & Cook, 1999).

Pain Intensity Ratings

Subjective ratings of *pain intensity* can be made for any noxious stimulus that exceeds a person's pain threshold. Multiple scales and questionnaires have been developed to aid in the quantification of pain intensity. Visual analog (VA) scales, category scales, and magnitude estimation are all commonly used. VA scales consist of a line (typically 50–100 mm in length) with verbal anchors of "no pain" at the left end and "worst pain imaginable" at the right end. Individuals are instructed to place a vertical mark on the line so that the distance from the left edge represents the pain being experienced at that moment in a given part of the body (Figure 9.4a). The distance in millimeters from the left edge of the line to the mark is used as the pain score. This scale is popular in both clinical and research settings because of its ease of use and ability to obtain a rapid rating. VA scales provide reliable and valid assessments of pain intensity (Revill et al., 1976), possess inherent ratio properties, and have been shown to be sensitive to interventions that provide analgesia. Numerical or verbal category scales (e.g., 0–10, "no pain," "moderate pain," "very strong pain," etc.) are also commonly used, and like the VA scales have been shown to be both reliable and valid measures

(a) **Visual analog pain intensity scale**

No pain at all ————————————————————————— Most intense pain imaginable

(b) **Pain Intensity Scale**

0   No pain at all

1/2 Very faint pain (just noticeable)

1   Weak pain

2   Mild pain

3   Moderate pain

4   Somewhat strong pain

5   Strong pain

6   Very stong pain

7

8

9

10   Extremely intense pain
     (almost unbearable)

•   Unbearable pain

Figure 9.4. Scales for assessing pain intensity. *a:* Visual analog scale. *b:* Category–ratio scale.

of pain intensity (Cook et al., 1997). Despite this fact, the nature of the category scales may introduce some bias and the sensitivity of the scales has been questioned. Because of their fixed end points these scales present difficulties for assessing the effects of treatments on pain conditions. A person who rates the pain during exercise as the highest possible using a category scale will not be able to provide a higher pain rating during subsequent conditions even if he or she experiences greater pain. The category scale shown in Figure 9.4b is designed to possess some ratio properties—it has a "true" zero and is unbounded. This scale allows individuals to choose a number above 10 when necessary and thus overcomes the fixed-end-point problem associated with typical category scales. While not a true ratio scale, this scale has been shown to perform in a similar manner to VA ratio scales (Cook et al., 1997).

Pain intensity can also be assessed using magnitude estimation, in which pain is rated compared with a previous painful stimulus. For example, a participant rating the pain associated with DOMS following eccentric exercise could compare it with the pain experienced during an experimentally

controlled electrical shock applied prior to the exercise. If the pain of the electrical shock was rated as a 50 and the pain from DOMS was judged to be twice as painful, the person would rate the pain from DOMS as a 100. Rating pain in this manner, using an open-ended ratio scale, can reduce the response bias that may be introduced using nonratio scales (O'Connor & Cook, 1999). While potentially less biased, magnitude estimation is often unwieldy for use in clinical settings and prevents comparisons across individuals (O'Connor & Cook, 1999). This highlights the subjective nature and inherent difficulties in quantifying pain among many persons. One individual may rate a noxious stimulus as a 10 while another might rate the same stimulus as a 60. Additionally, an individual's pain report may be altered by numerous factors, including personal experience, anxiety, attention, or perceived expectations of the researchers.

While useful for assessing the intensity of pain, a limitation of the use of a single VA, category, or numerical scale in the assessment of pain is that these scales treat pain as a unidimensional experience lacking qualities besides intensity. The pain experience clearly involves other dimensions, such as unpleasantness and emotional impact. Measurement tools beyond VA pain intensity scales are needed to better capture the totality of the pain experience.

Multidimensional Measures of Pain

In addition to intensity, pain has an affective dimension. Intensity is considered a sensory component, while the affective component can provide information about the location and quality (e.g., dull, sharp, or aching) of the pain and about how bothersome or unpleasant the experienced pain may be. Individual ratings of both the sensory and affective components can be obtained to provide a more complete assessment of the pain a person is experiencing. Scales of this type have not been widely used when evaluating pain during and following exercise, but they could provide more detailed information regarding the efficacy of various treatments for pain. For example, a pharmacological treatment such as ibuprofen could reduce the intensity of DOMS but might not reduce it enough to lessen how bothersome the pain was during a particular movement. Individual VA scales asking subjects to rate pain affect could be used to assess pain domains other than intensity. The McGill Pain Questionnaire (MPQ), another instrument that has been developed to assess pain in a multidimensional manner, classifies pain into three unique dimensions: sensory, affective, and evaluative. It assesses pain intensity and location as well as the sensory and affective quality of pain and the overall experience of the pain. The MPQ has been shown to be both reliable and valid (Reading, 1982, Wilkie et al., 1990) and can provide useful information about the nature of the pain experience during and following exercise.

Attributes and Interventions That Affect Muscle Pain
Gender Differences in Pain

It is well documented that men and women often but not always differ in pain perception (Fillingim et al., 2009). The weight of the experimental evidence indicates that women on average rate identical noxious stimuli as more painful than their male counterparts do. Women also tend to have lower pain thresholds and exhibit a reduced tolerance to pain compared with men. Both physiological and psychological factors have been suggested to influence the differential pain reports by men and women. Although too numerous to comprehensively review here, physiological factors such

as differences in hormones (especially estrogen) and differences in blood pressure have been proposed to play a role in the gender differences in pain. Elevated blood pressure has been shown to lead to decreased sensitivity to painful stimuli (Dworkin et al., 1994, Randich & Maixner, 1984). Given that hypertension is more prevalent in men, it could play a role in men's greater pain tolerance and threshold, and lower perceived pain intensity. Psychologically, cognition surrounding "sex role expectations" may lead to women being more willing to report a stimulus as painful (Fillingim et al., 2009). Clinical conditions such as anxiety and depression, which tend to be more prevalent in women, may also play a role in the increased sensitivity of women to pain (Fillingim et al., 2009).

Given the wealth of evidence regarding other types of experimental pain, one would expect that women would also report experiencing greater pain than men during exercise and greater DOMS following exercise that results in muscle damage. However, this has not been supported by the available research. Very few experiments have sought to examine if there are gender differences in muscle pain perception during a bout of exercise. Cook and colleagues (1998) found that women reported greater leg muscle pain than men at any given absolute work rate during a graded exercise test on a cycle ergometer, but when work rate was normalized to peak power output, women actually reported less leg pain than men. Although not designed to compare pain between men and women, additional insight can be drawn from several studies performed exclusively using men or women as participants but employing identical exercise protocols. Relatively similar levels of quadriceps muscle pain were observed during 30 minutes of cycling at 60% of VO_2 peak in studies examining the effects of caffeine on leg pain in men (O'Connor et al., 2004) and in a follow-up study performed in women (Motl et al., 2006). In separate studies, men and women also reported relatively similar quadriceps pain during 30 minutes of cycling at 80% of VO_2 peak (Gliottoni et al., 2009, Gliottoni & Motl, 2008). It is unclear why the otherwise consistent differences in pain reporting between men and women seem to be ameliorated during exercise. Research is needed in this area to determine the role, if any, of a host of plausible factors, including blood pressure, physical activity history, hormones, endogenous opioids, and other pain-processing mechanisms.

Much like muscle pain during a bout of exercise, the intensity of DOMS reported after eccentric exercise is similar in men and women. The role of estrogen in muscle injury, inflammation, and repair following exercise is a topic of much debate, with evidence on both sides of the argument. DOMS is a symptom and indirect measure of muscle damage that is likely consequent to the inflammation and edema that occur following tissue disruption. In rodent models of muscle injury, estrogen appears to exert a protective effect and has consistently been shown to blunt inflammation and potentially accelerate recovery from damaging exercise (Amelink & Bar, 1986, Enns et al., 2008, Tiidus et al., 2001). These findings have not been repeated in human studies, especially in regard to DOMS. Men and women demonstrate similar magnitudes of injury following eccentric exercise, as indicated by similar decreases in isometric force production (strength), which is considered the best indirect measure of muscle injury (Hubal et al., 2008, Rinard et al., 2000, Sayers & Clarkson, 2001). Similar results have also been found for DOMS. Several relatively large studies (Dannecker et al., 2005 [32 women, 27 men]; (Dannecker et al., 2008)[47 women, 48 men]; Rinard et al., 2000 [83 women, 82 men]; (Sewright et al., 2008); [58 women, 42 men]) that matched men and women on age and activity history (to avoid the confounding effects of the repeated-bout effect on DOMS) have all found no differences between men and women in the intensity of DOMS following eccentric exercise (Figure 9.5). The question remains unanswered as to why men and women report similar pain following eccentric exercise, and the failure to find a sex-related effect may be the result of methods used in the relatively few studies conducted in this area. As with pain during exercise, future research examining the mechanism(s) responsible for these findings is needed.

Exercise as an Analgesic
REPEATED-BOUT EFFECT

As outlined previously, performance of unaccustomed exercise that has an eccentric component very often leads to muscle injury and DOMS. We have all likely experienced this when we begin a new exercise program, start to exercise again after a significant layoff, or perform a physical task to which we are unaccustomed for the first time. If we perform that same task or bout of exercise a second time within a few weeks, very often the magnitude of the DOMS, while still present, will be reduced compared with the initial bout (Figure 9.6). This well-documented phenomenon has been termed the *repeated-bout* or *protective effect* (McHugh et al., 1999). Mechanistically, the reduced DOMS experienced after the second exercise bout is likely the consequence of reduced muscle damage and inflammation, leading to less activation and sensitization of muscle nociceptors. Following the second bout, less swelling and smaller changes in force production and range of motion are commonly observed, indicating that less structural damage has occurred to the muscle (Black & McCully, 2008b, Foley et al., 1999, Hirose et al., 2004, McHugh et al., 1999, Nosaka & Clarkson, 1996). It appears that skeletal muscle rapidly adapts following damaging

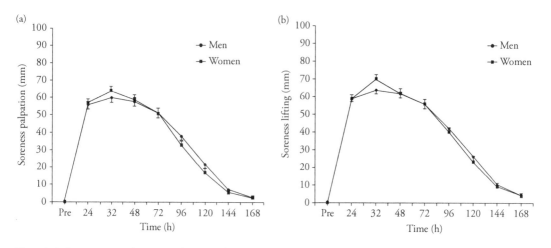

Figure 9.5. Soreness ratings during (a) palpation and (b) lifting for men and women over the 7 days following performance of 70 maximal eccentric contractions of elbow flexors. Reprinted with permission from "Response of Males and Females to High-Force Eccentric Exercise," by J. Rinard, P. M. Clarkson, L. L. Smith, and M. Grossman, 2000, *Journal of Sports Science, 18*(4), pp. 229–236.

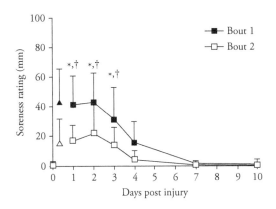

Figure 9.6. Demonstration of the repeated-bout effect. Soreness ratings were made immediately after and over the course of 10 days following performance of 80 eccentric contractions of the knee extensors (using 120% of concentric one-repetition maximum) during an initial bout (bout 1) and an identical bout performed 7 weeks later (bout 2). Reprinted from "Muscle Injury after Repeated Bouts of Voluntary and Electrically Stimulated Exercise," by C. D. Black and K. K. McCully, 2008, *Medicine & Science in Sports & Exercise, 40*(9), pp. 1605–1615.

exercise and this "protects" the muscle from future damage.

Several mechanisms are thought to underlie the reduced damage observed with the repeated-bout effect, including changes in muscle recruitment patterns, longitudinal addition of sarcomeres, increased structural proteins within the muscle, and adaptations in the inflammatory response (McHugh et al., 1999). Irrespective of the mechanism, the repeated-bout effect has been shown to last for six to nine months (Nosaka et al., 2001) following an initial bout of exercise, but is most pronounced during the first two to four weeks. Severe muscle damage and DOMS is not required to confer protection and reduce DOMS in subsequent exercise. Low-volume (two or three contractions), high-intensity eccentric contractions and very light (10% of maximal isometric strength) eccentric exercise have been shown to reduce future muscle damage and DOMS (Lavender & Nosaka, 2008, Paddon-Jones & Abernethy, 2001). Protection seems to be specific to the muscles used in the initial exercise bout. This phenomenon has several important practical applications. First, it may help to explain why many athletes experience less pain following exercise than their untrained counterparts. It may not be that they simply perceive less pain as a result of increased descending modulation and processing of nociceptive inputs. Rather, they likely have adapted to the intense exercise and, in turn, experience less

muscle damage and inflammation. Second, knowledge about the repeated-bout effect could aid in promoting exercise adherence. While it is speculative to say that pain is a barrier to exercise adherence, it is certainly plausible that people who begin an exercise program and experience significant pain and soreness may be reluctant to continue. Since the repeated-bout effect can occur with very low-volume or light exercise that causes little to no soreness following the initial bout, exercise programs that gradually increase volume and intensity could help prevent severe DOMS.

ANALGESIA DURING AND FOLLOWING EXERCISE

While many types of exercise, especially high-intensity exercise, often result in pain in the exercising muscles, certain aspects of pain, such as pain threshold, are altered during and following exercise (Figure 9.7). Several studies have demonstrated reduced sensitivity to noxious electrical stimuli applied to dental pulp (Kemppainen et al., 1986, Kemppainen et al., 1985, Paddon-Jones & Abernethy, 2001, Pertovaara et al., 1984), the forearm (Feine et al., 1990), and finger (Droste et al., 1991) during exercise and that this reduced sensitivity may occur in a dose-dependent manner with exercise intensity (i.e., greater stimulation is required to evoke pain at higher exercise intensities).

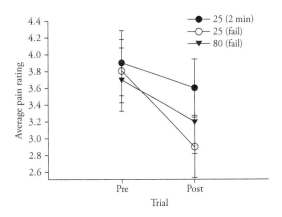

Figure 9.7. Demonstration of the analgesic effects of exercise. Pain ratings in response to pressure applied to a finger prior to (pre) and following (post) isometric contractions performed at 25% of MVC (maximal voluntary contraction) for 2 minutes, 25% of MVC until fatigue, or 80% of MVC until fatigue.. Reprinted from "Dose Response of Isometric Contractions on Pain Perception in Healthy Adults," by M. K. Hoeger Bement, J. Dicapo, R. Rasiarmos, and S. K. Hunter, 2008, *Medicine & Science in Sports & Exercise, 40*(11), pp. 1880–1889.

Additionally, the threshold of mechanical pressure required to evoke muscle pain has been shown to be increased during static, isometric contractions (Kosek & Ekholm, 1995). Reductions in pain following exercise have also been observed. Numerous studies have demonstrated increases in pain thresholds to electrical stimulation of the dental pulp, heat, mechanical pressure, and compression ischemia following exercise (Koltyn, 2000). Exercise has been shown to have little effect on the pain response to the cold-pressure test, indicating that analgesia does not occur for all possible painful stimuli (Janal et al., 1984, Padawer & Levine, 1992). The effects occur more often after high-intensity aerobic exercise, are most pronounced immediately following exercise, and gradually dissipate (Koltyn, 2000, 2002).

While the mechanism(s) of the analgesic effects observed during and following exercise are not completely understood, several explanations have been proposed. Exercise, especially strenuous exercise (> 60% of VO_2 peak) lasting longer than 30 minutes, is known to result in the release of endogenous opioids such as beta-endorphins, which could function to modulate pain at peripheral, spinal, and supraspinal sites. Administration of opioid antagonists such as naloxone have yielded mixed results, with some studies showing prevention or blunting of analgesia during and following exercise (Droste et al., 1988, Haier et al., 1981, Janal et al., 1984) and others finding no effect (Droste et al., 1991, Janal et al., 1984, Olausson et al., 1986). These results indicate that both opioid and nonopioid mechanisms may play a role in exercise-induced reductions in pain. A second possibility is the gate-control theory proposed by Melzack and Wall (1965). This theory states that exercise increases non-nociceptive afferent input (from Golgi tendon organs and muscle spindles) to spinal and supraspinal regions, which reduces pain by inhibiting the activity of nociceptive neurons. Another possibile explanation is suggested by the observation that distraction that focuses attention away from noxious stimuli can lead to reductions in pain during exercise (Fillingim et al., 1989, McCaul & Malott, 1984). Similarly, increases in heart rate and respiration have been suggested to lead to increases in pain thresholds by drawing perceptual attention away from painful stimuli (Fuller & Robinson, 1993).

While the exact mechanism of analgesia remains somewhat unclear and may vary based on the mode, duration, and intensity of exercise, research clearly and consistently demonstrates that intense exercise transiently increases pain thresholds.

Analgesic Interventions
PHARMACOLOGICAL INTERVENTIONS FOR DOMS

Many prescription and over-the-counter drugs have been purported to reduce the pain and soreness associated with muscle damage. However, the weight of the experimental evidence regarding their efficacy is not compelling (Baldwin Lanier, 2003, Connolly et al., 2003). Most over-the-counter pain drugs, such as aspirin, ibuprofen, naproxen, diclofenac, indomethacin, and ketoprofen, are nonsteroidal anti-inflammatory drugs (NSAIDs) designed to inhibit the action of COX-1 and COX-2 enzymes and blunt the production of prostaglandins and the inflammatory response. Reducing levels of PGE_2 would lead to less sensitization of peripheral nociceptors in skeletal muscle and require greater input from noxious biochemicals and mechanical pressure to evoke a pain response. Most studies using NSAIDs employ the maximum recommended daily dose and administer the drugs over the course of several days before a damaging bout of exercise (termed a *prophylactic dose*), following a damaging exercise bout (a *therapeutic dose*), or both.

Comparison between studies using NSAIDs is difficult, because different exercise modes, doses, dosing schedules, subject populations, and measures to quantify pain have been used. For studies where NSAIDs have been given over multiple days, the results have been equivocal, with some studies demonstrating reduced DOMS and other finding no difference (Baldwin Lanier, 2003, Connolly et al., 2003). In the studies that have found reduced pain, the reduction often has occurred at only a single time point following the exercise bout—indicating even in these studies the drugs did not provide consistent pain relief. These findings may indicate that it takes multiple days of drug administration to significantly reduce PGE_2 concentrations and lead to some pain relief. Also, it is possible that the exercise regimes employed in many of the studies result in pronounced DOMS, much more than is typically experienced in daily life, and that the pain is too great to be alleviated by drugs of this type. Far fewer studies have examined the effect of a single dose of medication on the pain experienced in the hours subsequent to an exercise bout. Sayers et al. (2001) demonstrated that both a 25-mg and a 100-mg dose of ketoprofen given 48 hours after eccentric exercise reduced pain in the 8 hours following administration (Figure 9.8). Future research is necessary to better determine whether NSAIDs are more efficacious for treating lower levels of pain and soreness that may be more representative of the DOMS experienced following normal daily activities.

Caffeine, while less studied than NSAIDs, has been shown to reduce DOMS measured during active contraction of the injured muscle approximately one hour after administration of a dose of 5 mg per kilogram of body weight (Maridakis et al., 2007). Caffeine is an adenosine receptor antagonist; thus the mechanism of action differs from that of the NSAIDS. It is unclear whether caffeine exerts its analgesic effects by acting on peripheral, spinal, or supraspinal nerves, and if so, whether it acts separately or concurrently on those tissues.

NUTRITIONAL AND NUTRACEUTICAL INTERVENTIONS FOR DOMS

The use of dietary and nutritional supplements to prevent or limit muscle injury and the consequent DOMS has grown in recent years. Many of these supplements function as antioxidants and limit the production of reactive oxygen species. When a skeletal muscle is damaged with exercise, inflammation and the generation of reactive oxygen species typically occur. Reactive oxygen species may contribute to secondary damage, making the injury more pronounced and potentially increasing the magnitude of the associated DOMS. It is plausible that consumption of an antioxidant could blunt the production of reactive oxygen species, reduce secondary damage and inflammation, and consequently reduce DOMS. Experimental interventions administering an antioxidant, typically vitamin C or vitamin E, have yielded mixed results in studies of humans (Goldfarb, 1999). Supplementation with vitamin E has been shown in several studies to reduce markers of oxidative stress and reduce leakage from the muscle membranes (Meydani et al., 1993, Rokitzki et al., 1994), potentially indicating less secondary damage. Studies assessing the effect of vitamin E on DOMS have failed to find reductions in pain (Avery et al., 2003). Administration of vitamin C has yielded mixed results for DOMS, with several studies demonstrating no effect on pain (Avery et al., 2003, Thompson et al., 2004, Thompson et al., 2003, Thompson, Williams, Kingsley et al., 2001, Thompson, Williams, McGregor et al., 2001) and other studies demonstrating less DOMS compared with a placebo (Bryer & Goldfarb, 2006, Kaminski & Boal, 1992). It is difficult to compare across the studies, because different doses, administration times, and types of exercise were employed to induce muscle damage. The weight of the experimental evidence suggests that antioxidant supplementation with vitamin E or vitamin C is not a particularly effective treatment for DOMS.

Other nutraceuticals, many derived from what would generally be considered culinary spices, have also been proposed as analgesic agents. Many spices have been shown to mimic the anti-inflammatory actions of NSAIDs by inhibiting the action of COX enzymes, binding to the capsaicin receptor, TRPV1, or both. Full discussion of the structure, function, and potential analgesic effects associated with the TRPV1 receptor is beyond the scope of this chapter; interested

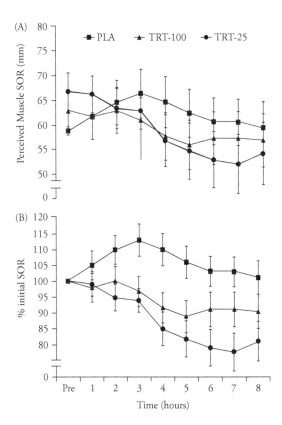

Figure 9.8. Soreness ratings (A) using a visual analog scale (0-100mm) prior to (Pre) and over the 8 hours following administration of placebo (PLA) or a 25-mg (TRT-25) or 100-mg (TRT-100) dose of ketoprofen 36 hours after performing 50 maximal eccentric contractions of the elbow flexors. Panel B shows percentage of initial soreness from pre-dose measurement for PLA, TRT-25, and TRT-100 conditions. Reprinted from "Effect of Ketoprofen on Muscle Function and sEMG Activity after Eccentric Exercise," by S. P. Sayers, C. A. Knight, P. M. Clarkson, E. H. Van Wegen, and G. Kamen, 2001, *Medicine & Science in Sports & Exercise, 33*(5), pp. 702–710.

readers are referred to recent reviews (Palazzo et al., 2008, Wong & Gavva, 2009). A growing number of in vitro experiments and studies using animal models have demonstrated the potential of ginger (Ojewole, 2006), piperine (black pepper) (Bang et al., 2009), and curcumin (Davis et al., 2007) as analgesic agents due to their anti-inflammatory actions. Very few human experiments have been performed, but 11 days of supplementation with a 2-g daily dose of ginger resulted in lower DOMS associated with eccentric exercise of the elbow flexors than was seen with placebo (Black et al., 2010).

OTHER COMMON THERAPEUTIC MODALITIES

Once an injury to skeletal muscle has occurred, several physical therapeutic modalities (agents) are often prescribed by physical therapists, athletic trainers, and other health care providers. The primary goals of these modalities are pain relief; recovery of strength, flexibility, or range of motion; and ultimately a resumption of normal daily activity or athletic competition. Research regarding the efficacy of many such modalities, especially for the treatment of DOMS, is limited. For instance, massage therapy is commonly practiced with athletes and in clinical settings as a treatment for muscle damage and soreness. It has been hypothesized that massage of an injured muscle may increase blood flow to the muscle and thereby promote healing, reduce soreness, and aid recovery of muscle strength and function (Tiidus, 1997). It may also function to reduce DOMS in accordance with the gate-control theory, as massage provides additional sensory input. However, most research examining the effects of massage on DOMS has found either a lack of an effect (Jonhagen et al., 2004, Weber et al., 1994) or relatively small and inconsistent effects occurring at only a single time point following eccentric exercise (Farr et al., 2002, Hilbert et al., 2003, Tiidus & Shoemaker, 1995).

Ultrasound has also been widely used to treat injuries to skeletal muscle. It is thought to increase blood flow via thermal effects on the muscle tissue and also to provide mechanical stimulation to the tissue. As is the case for massage, limited scientific evidence exists regarding the efficacy of ultrasound for treating DOMS. The few studies that have examined the effects of ultrasound on DOMS have employed multiple pulse rates, intensities, and durations of ultrasound application. Although some studies have shown a beneficial effect of ultrasound on DOMS (Hasson et al., 1990), others have shown little to no therapeutic effect (Craig et al.,

1999, Stay et al., 1998, Tiidus et al., 2002), and ultrasound has even been observed to increase pain associated with DOMS (Ciccone et al., 1991). The weight of the experimental evidence appears to indicate ultrasound is not a particularly effective treatment for DOMS.

Application of ice (cryotherapy) and heat to injured muscles experiencing DOMS is also a common clinical practice. Cryotherapy could function to blunt inflammation and swelling following muscle damage via short-term vasoconstriction of the blood vessels within the muscle. Like the other modalities, cryotherapy has not been widely tested, but the available evidence has consistently found it to have little to no effect on DOMS (Gulick et al., 1996, Howatson et al., 2005, Howatson & Van Someren, 2003, Isabell et al., 1992, Sellwood et al., 2007). The application of heat as a treatment for DOMS has yielded mixed results, but very few studies have been performed. J. M. Mayer et al. (2006) demonstrated that a heat pack applied to the lower back was effective at reducing DOMS following eccentric low back exercise, while Jayaraman et al. (2004) found no effect of two weeks of application of moist heat on soreness following eccentric exercise of the knee extensors.

A final treatment modality that is commonly used is transcutaneous electrical nerve stimulation (TENS). TENS is performed by the application of an electrical current that is below the threshold required to elicit a muscle contraction but is sufficient to depolarize smaller, afferent sensory fibers. Much like massage, TENS could provide pain relief by increasing sensory stimulation and thereby interfering with spinal transmission of nociceptive inputs from skeletal muscle. TENS has been widely used and tested in the treatment of many clinical pain conditions (e.g., low back pain and neuropathies). Although it has not been extensively examined for its efficacy in treating soreness following exercise, and the results have been mixed, there is evidence that it may provide some relief from DOMS (Denegar & Perrin, 1992, Denegar et al., 1989).

In conclusion, while many therapeutic modalities are commonly used in clinical practice, there is a paucity of data regarding their efficacy, and the limited evidence often suggests that they have little to no therapeutic effect on DOMS.

PHARMACOLOGICAL INTERVENTIONS
FOR PAIN DURING EXERCISE

Muscle pain is a common experience during moderate- to high-intensity exercise, with pain thresholds in the contracting musculature occurring at approximately 50% of a person's peak power output (Cook et al., 1997). This naturally occurring muscle pain increases as exercise intensity is increased, with exhaustive exercise leading to pain ratings commonly described as very intense. Additionally, muscle pain has been suggested as a limiting factor in exercise and athletic performance. It stands to reason that if muscle pain limits performance, then reducing pain could augment and improve athletic performance. While still poorly understood, there are increases with acute exercise in the levels of known algesic agents such as BKN, potassium, serotonin, histamine, hydrogen ions, adenosine, and substance P centrally in the spinal cord, in muscles, and in the peripheral circulation (Caperuto et al., 2009, Langberg et al., 2002, Lind et al., 1996, Mense et al., 1996, Rotto et al., 1990, Wilson et al., 1993). Muscle contractions, if strong enough, also activate HTM nociceptors. Thus any type of pharmacological intervention that could blunt the accumulation or action of these agents could function to reduce muscle pain experienced during exercise.

Aspirin in a dose of 20 mg per kilogram of body weight (which is approximately twice the suggested over-the-counter dose) given 1 hour prior to an exhaustive cycling exercise bout did not alter the exercise intensity at which muscle pain began, nor did it alter pain ratings at any point during or following the exercise bout or have any effects on exercise performance (Cook et al., 1997). Being a nonselective COX-1 and COX-2 inhibitor, aspirin should blunt the accumulation of PGE_2 during exercise and prevent it from sensitizing skeletal muscle nociceptors. These results suggest that prostaglandins may not play a major role in muscle pain during exercise. A 60-mg dose of the opioid codeine also demonstrated no effects on pain threshold and pain intensity during progressively more intense short-duration hand grip exercise (Cook et al., 2000). These findings call into question the role of the opioid system in the perception of muscle pain during this type of exercise.

Caffeine, especially in moderate-to-high doses, has been repeatedly shown to reduce muscle pain during cycling exercise. Dose-dependent effects have been shown in men, with a dose of 10 mg per kilogram of body weight dose (equivalent to approximately five 8-ounce cups of ground roasted coffee) showing greater hypoalgesia than a 5-mg/kg dose (O'Connor et al., 2004), but not in women (Motl et al., 2006), during exercise at 60% of VO_2 peak (Figure 9.9).

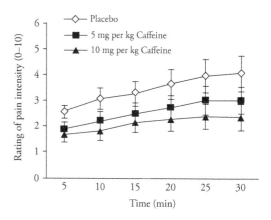

Figure 9.9. Ratings of naturally occurring muscle pain in the quadriceps of males during 30 minutes of cycling exercise at 60% of VO_2 peak 1 hour after administration of a placebo or caffeine doses of 5 or 10 mg per kilogram of body weight. Reprinted with permission from "Dose-Dependent Effect of Caffeine on Reducing Leg Muscle Pain during Cycling Exercise Is Unrelated to Systolic Blood Pressure," by P. J. O'Connor, R. W. Motl, S. P. Broglio, and M. R. Ely, 2004, *Pain, 109*(3), pp. 291–298.

A 5-mg/kg dose has also been shown to reduce ratings of leg muscle pain in response to exercise at 80% of VO_2 peak in both men (Gliottoni et al., 2009) and women (Gliottoni & Motl, 2008) to yield similar hypoalgesic effects in low and high habitual caffeine consumers (Gliottoni et al., 2009). Caffeine is an antagonist to both central and peripheral adenosine A_1 and A_{2a} receptors, which are known to play a role in nociception (Sawynok, 1998). Whether caffeine's analgesic effects during exercise are peripheral or central is unclear, but the robust findings clearly implicate a role for adenosine receptors in naturally occurring muscle pain during exercise.

Pain and Exercise Performance

The concept that muscle pain limits exercise or athletic performance is interesting but experimentally unclear. It seems plausible that experiencing intense pain could reduce motivation to exercise, leading an individual to reduce exercise intensity to reduce pain or prevent further increases in pain perceptions. It has been suggested that pain "sets ultimate limits on the performance of athletes during training and competition" and consequently athletes with the greatest pain tolerances could perform at a higher percentage of their maximal capacities and outperform athletes with lower pain tolerances (O'Connor & Cook, 1999, p. 151). Despite these beliefs, relatively few scientific studies have attempted to elucidate the role of pain in exercise performance.

Many studies examining performance have not measured pain, and many studies measuring and assessing pain during exercise have not measured performance. Pain during exercise is well documented. Cook and colleagues (1997) demonstrated a pain intensity threshold for quadriceps muscle during cycling exercise of approximately 50% of VO_2 peak, and pain increased with exercise intensity until participants reached exhaustion. However, all participants indicated that even though they experienced very strong-to-severe muscle pain during the exercise test, muscle pain did not play a role in their ceasing to exercise. Experimental manipulation of pain during exercise could also yield insight into its role in exercise performance. Caffeine has been consistently shown to enhance exercise performance in the form of both increased exercise time to exhaustion and increased work performed in a fixed period of time (i.e., time trial performance) (Ganio et al., 2009, Keisler & Armsey, 2006). Additionally, multiple studies have demonstrated reduced muscle pain during exercise following caffeine consumption (Gliottoni et al., 2009, Gliottoni & Motl, 2008, Motl et al., 2006, Motl et al., 2003, O'Connor et al., 2004). However, the role of pain in performance is unclear, because most studies examining the effects of caffeine on exercise performance have not measured muscle pain, while the studies examining caffeine's effects on pain have failed to measure exercise performance. A recent study by Jenkins et al. (2008) examined time trial performance in trained cyclists who were administered multiple low doses of caffeine or a placebo and also measured muscle pain during the time trial. The study found that leg pain during exercise did not differ between the caffeine and placebo conditions, but that time trial performance increased with caffeine. While on the surface these findings appear to agree with those of Cook et al. (1997) that muscle pain may not be a primary limiting factor in exercise performance, a second explanation may actually support a role for pain in determining performance. Research has shown that exercise participants can adjust the work rate during cycling exercise such that muscle pain ratings are constant over a period of 20–30 minutes (O'Connor & Cook, 2001). Given this finding, it is possible that the cyclists in the Jenkins et al. (2008) study self-selected a work rate during the time trial that produced a muscle pain intensity that was near the maximal intensity they could tolerate while continuing to exercise. The experimental protocol could have masked the analgesic effects of caffeine. It is possible that the caffeine allowed participants to exercise at higher work rates at near-maximal pain tolerance levels.

Several studies have also attempted to increase pain perception during exercise by administration of the opioid antagonist naloxone. Administration of naloxone should increase pain during exercise, and a concomitant reduction in performance would potentially demonstrate a role for pain in exercise performance. In one experiment administration of naloxone prior to treadmill running to exhaustion led to increased pain as assessed via the McGill Pain Questionnaire (an increase of 30% in overall pain intensity) and reduced exercise time to exhaustion (Surbey et al., 1984). Another study, by Paulev et al. (1989), found increased pain during a 12-minute running test, but performance was not compromised.

Additional evidence examining the role of pain during exercise can be gleaned from studies examining exercise performance in the presence of DOMS from muscle injury. Diminished performance in short-term (20–30 seconds), high-intensity cycling exercise (Byrne & Eston, 2002, Sargeant & Dolan, 1987), in 5-minute cycling (Twist & Eston, 2009), and in 30-minute running time trials (Marcora & Bosio, 2007) has been reported following the induction of DOMS, as has decreased time to exhaustion (Davies et al., 2009). Additionally, pilot data have shown reductions in VO_2 peak of approximately 9% and heightened ratings of muscle pain during 30 minutes of submaximal cycling at 60% of VO_2 peak in the presence of DOMS (Black & Dobson, In Press). While these data present a potential association between the existence of muscle pain and reduced performance, it is difficult to say conclusively that pain per se is the culprit leading to decreased exercise performance in these studies. Muscle damage also leads to decreased joint range of motion and, most significantly, decreased ability of muscles to generate force. It is certainly possible that the reduced force-generating capacity of the muscles rather than muscle pain was the primary factor responsible for the decreased performance. Consequently, while it seems plausible that muscle pain during exercise plays some role in limiting maximal exercise capacity, very few experimental studies have been able determine the individual effects of pain compared with other factors in exercise performance. Given that exercise performance can be influenced by a host of physiological and psychological factors, future research attempting to determine the contribution of pain to performance is necessary.

Summary

Pain in skeletal muscles is a subjective experience that is a manifestation of peripheral and central nociceptive inputs via type III and type IV afferent nerve fibers that undergo complex processing in the dorsal horn of the spinal cord and higher brain areas. Muscle pain is commonly assessed in terms of intensity, threshold (the minimum input required to evoke pain), and tolerance (the amount of time a painful stimulus can be endured).

Pain during exercise is a common experience, and it increases as exercise intensity is increased. While the exact mechanisms of this increase remain somewhat unclear, it is likely the consequence of activation of peripheral nociceptors due to an accumulation of noxious biochemicals and increased intramuscular pressure during muscle contractions. Similarly, DOMS is a common occurrence following novel eccentric muscle contractions that result in muscle damage. The tenderness and pain associated with muscle damage likely results from the sensitization of HTM nociceptors by inflammatory mediators such as PGE_2, BKN, and serotonin. Women generally experience more pain and exhibit lower pain thresholds than men in response to a similar noxious stimulus. This effect does not appear to be the case for muscle pain during a bout of exercise or for DOMS following muscle damage, although studies on the subject are limited.

Exercise has been consistently shown to result in increased pain thresholds both during and following exercise. This effect has been observed with electrical, thermal, and mechanical stimuli. While not completely understood, analgesia of this type may be mediated by the release of endogenous opioids during exercise. Many pharmacological and other therapeutic interventions have been employed to attempt to treat or reduce pain sensations during exercise and once DOMS is present. Little scientific evidence exists supporting many of the commonly used modalities. Varying doses of caffeine have consistently reduced muscle pain during exercise, but NSAIDs such as aspirin have not been effective. Caffeine has also been shown to reduce DOMS, but NSAIDs, while widely studied, have demonstrated inconsistent results as a treatment for soreness. Other modalities, such as massage, ultrasound, ice, heat, and TENS, have shown very little efficacy for the treatment of DOMS, with perhaps the most promising results from TENS. The role pain plays in exercise performance is unclear, because of the difficulty of independently testing and manipulating pain during exercise.

Muscle pain is an extensively studied phenomenon with far-reaching clinical relevance given the prevalence of clinical conditions such as chronic low back pain, fibromyalgia, and arthritis. However, pain during and following exercise has not received as much attention. Exercise presents a unique method for studying pain because it can transiently and reproducibly evoke muscle pain that closely mimics clinical muscle pain in intensity and affect. A better understanding of the causes of muscle pain and how exercise may result in analgesia can help lead to better and more effective treatments for pain in the future.

Future Directions

While much is known about muscle pain during and after exercise, many questions remain unanswered. The interaction among pain, exercise, and physical performance/function is an area where future research is needed. A few potential areas of future study are listed below.

1. Further research into the supraspinal areas activated during exercise and when DOMS is present, using advanced techniques such as electroencephalography (EEG) and functional magnetic resonance imaging (fMRI), could lead to a better understanding of nociceptive inputs and processing and help explain differences in the pain experience between individuals.

2. Future studies should focus on examining the efficacy of both drug and manual therapies for pain management using lower doses of eccentric exercise and consequently lower intensities of DOMS. Studies have traditionally employed very high-intensity exercise and often included only participants who report high levels of soreness that may not be representative of muscle pain experienced in everyday life.

3. Further studies examining the potential influence of estrogen on pain during exercise seem warranted. A clear gender effect is seen in response to most nociceptive inputs and pain measures, but this effect seems to be ameliorated for pain during and following exercise.

4. The role of muscle pain in exercise and athletic performance needs to be more clearly delineated.

5. The role of pain in adherence to and participation in physical activity and exercise programs is also a key area that requires greater study. Physical inactivity is strongly associated with increased risk of a host of chronic diseases (e.g., cardiovascular disease, diabetes, and cancer). Despite this fact, a large

and growing number of people remain inactive. A better understanding of the impact of pain during exercise on exercise adherence could aid in promoting physical activity.

6. Future research should also focus on the effects of chronic disease states or clinical conditions (e.g., obesity, heart disease, hypertension, diabetes, and cancer) on pain perception during exercise. Do individuals suffering from some form of clinical condition experience pain during exercise in an altered manner compared with healthy individuals?

References

Amelink, G. J., & Bar, P. R. (1986). Exercise-induced muscle protein leakage in the rat. Effects of hormonal manipulation. *Journal of the Neurological Sciences, 76*(1), 61–68.

Avery, N. G., Kaiser, J. L., Sharman, M. J., Scheett, T. P., Barnes, D. M., Gomez, A. L., et al. (2003). Effects of vitamin E supplementation on recovery from repeated bouts of resistance exercise. *Journal of Strength and Conditioning Research, 17*(4), 801–809.

Babenko, V., Graven-Nielsen, T., Svensson, P., Drewes, A. M., Jensen, T. S., & Arendt-Nielsen, L. (1999). Experimental human muscle pain and muscular hyperalgesia induced by combinations of serotonin and bradykinin. *Pain, 82*(1), 1–8.

Babenko, V. V., Graven-Nielsen, T., Svensson, P., Drewes, A. M., Jensen, T. S., & Arendt-Nielsen, L. (1999). Experimental human muscle pain induced by intramuscular injections of bradykinin, serotonin, and substance P. *European Journal of Pain, 3*(2), 93–102.

Baker, S. J., Kelly, N. M., & Eston, R. G. (1997). Pressure pain tolerance at different sites on the quadriceps femoris prior to and following eccentric exercise. *European Journal of Pain, 1*(3), 229–233.

Baldwin Lanier, A. (2003). Use of nonsteroidal anti-inflammatory drugs following exercise-induced muscle injury. *Sports Medicine, 33*(3), 177–185.

Bang, J. S., Oh da, H., Choi, H. M., Sur, B. J., Lim, S. J., Kim, J. Y., et al. (2009). Anti-inflammatory and antiarthritic effects of piperine in human interleukin 1beta-stimulated fibroblast-like synoviocytes and in rat arthritis models. *Arthritis Research and Therapy, 11*(2), R49.

Belcastro, A. N., Shewchuk, L. D., & Raj, D. A. (1998). Exercise-induced muscle injury: A calpain hypothesis. *Molecular and Cellular Biochemistry, 179*(1-2), 135–145.

Black, C. D., & Dobson, R. M. (In Press). Prior eccentric exercise reduces VO$_2$ peak and ventilatory threshold, but does not alter movement economy during cycling exercise. *Journal of Strength and Conditioning Research*.

Black, C. D., Elder, C. P., Gorgey, A., & Dudley, G. A. (2008). High specific torque is related to lengthening contraction-induced skeletal muscle injury. *Journal of Applied Physiology, 104*(3), 639–647.

Black, C. D., Herring, M. P., Hurley, D. J., & O'Connor, P. J. (2010). Ginger (Zingiber officinale) Reduces Muscle Pain Caused by Eccentric Exercise. *Journal of Pain*, 11(9), 894–-903.

Black, C. D., & McCully, K. K. (2008a). Force per active area and muscle injury during electrically stimulated contractions. *Medicine & Science in Sports & Exercise, 40*(9), 1596–1604.

Black, C. D., & McCully, K. K. (2008b). Muscle injury after repeated bouts of voluntary and electrically stimulated exercise. *Medicine & Science in Sports & Exercise, 40*(9), 1605–1615.

Brooks, J., & Tracey, I. (2005). From nociception to pain perception: Imaging the spinal and supraspinal pathways. *Journal of Anatomy, 207*(1), 19–33.

Brown, S. J., Child, R. B., Day, S. H., & Donnelly, A. E. (1997). Exercise-induced skeletal muscle damage and adaptation following repeated bouts of eccentric muscle contractions. *Journal of Sports Sciences, 15*(2), 215–222.

Bryer, S. C., & Goldfarb, A. H. (2006). Effect of high dose vitamin C supplementation on muscle soreness, damage, function, and oxidative stress to eccentric exercise. *International Journal of Sport Nutrition and Exercise Metabolism, 16*(3), 270–280.

Byrne, C., & Eston, R. (2002). Maximal-intensity isometric and dynamic exercise performance after eccentric muscle actions. *Journal of Sports Sciences, 20*(12), 951–959.

Cannon, J. G., & St Pierre, B. A. (1998). Cytokines in exertion-induced skeletal muscle injury. *Molecular and Cellular Biochemistry, 179*(1-2), 159–167.

Caperuto, E. C., dos Santos, R. V., Mello, M. T., & Costa Rosa, L. F. (2009). Effect of endurance training on hypothalamic serotonin concentration and performance. *Clinical and Experimental Pharmacology and Physiology, 36*(2), 189–191.

Caudill-Slosberg, M. A., Schwartz, L. M., & Woloshin, S. (2004). Office visits and analgesic prescriptions for musculoskeletal pain in US: 1980 vs. 2000. *Pain, 109*(3), 514–519.

Cervero, F., Iggo, A., & Ogawa, H. (1976). Nociceptor-driven dorsal horn neurones in the lumbar spinal cord of the cat. *Pain, 2*(1), 5–24.

Ciccone, C. D., Leggin, B. G., & Callamaro, J. J. (1991). Effects of ultrasound and trolamine salicylate phonophoresis on delayed-onset muscle soreness. *Physical Therapy, 71*(9), 666–675.

Clarkson, P. M., Nosaka, K., & Braun, B. (1992). Muscle function after exercise-induced muscle damage and rapid adaptation. *Medicine & Science in Sports & Exercise, 24*(5), 512–520.

Clarkson, P. M., & Sayers, S. P. (1999). Etiology of exercise-induced muscle damage. *Canadian Journal of Applied Physiology, 24*(3), 234–248.

Cohen, S. P., Mullings, R., & Abdi, S. (2004). The pharmacologic treatment of muscle pain. *Anesthesiology, 101*(2), 495–526.

Connolly, D. A., Sayers, S. P., & McHugh, M. P. (2003). Treatment and prevention of delayed onset muscle soreness. *Journal of Strength & Conditioning Research, 17*(1), 197–208.

Cook, D. B., O'Connor, P. J., Eubanks, S. A., Smith, J. C., & Lee, M. (1997). Naturally occurring muscle pain during exercise: Assessment and experimental evidence. *Medicine & Science in Sports & Exercise, 29*(8), 999–1012.

Cook, D. B., O'Connor, P. J., & Ray, C. A. (2000). Muscle pain perception and sympathetic nerve activity to exercise during opioid modulation. *American Jornal of Physiology—Regulatory, Integrative and Comparative Physiology, 279*(5), R1565–R1573.

Craig, J. A., Bradley, J., Walsh, D. M., Baxter, G. D., & Allen, J. M. (1999). Delayed onset muscle soreness: Lack of effect of therapeutic ultrasound in humans. *Archives of Physical Medicine and Rehabilitation, 80*(3), 318–323.

Curatolo, M., & Bogduk, N. (2001). Pharmacologic pain treatment of musculoskeletal disorders: Current perspectives and future prospects. *Clinical Journal of Pain, 17*(1), 25–32.

Dannecker, E. A., Hausenblas, H. A., Kaminski, T. W., & Robinson, M. E. (2005). Sex differences in delayed onset muscle pain. *Clinical Journal of Pain, 21*(2), 120–126.

Dannecker, E. A., Knoll, V., & Robinson, M. E. (2008). Sex differences in muscle pain: Self-care behaviors and effects on daily activities. *Journal of Pain, 9*(3), 200–209.

Davies, R. C., Rowlands, A. V., & Eston, R. G. (2009). Effect of exercise-induced muscle damage on ventilatory and perceived exertion responses to moderate and severe intensity cycle exercise. *European Journal of Applied Physiology, 107*(1), 11–19.

Davis, J. M., Murphy, E. A., Carmichael, M. D., Zielinski, M. R., Groschwitz, C. M., Brown, A. S., et al. (2007). Curcumin effects on inflammation and performance recovery following eccentric exercise-induced muscle damage. *American Journal of Physiology - Regulatory, Integrative and Comparative Physiology, 292*(6), R2168–R2173.

DeLeo, J. A. (2006). Basic science of pain. *Journal of Bone and Joint Surgery, American Volume, 88 Suppl 2*, 58–62.

Denegar, C. R., & Perrin, D. H. (1992). Effect of Transcutaneous Electrical Nerve Stimulation, Cold, and a Combination Treatment on Pain, Decreased Range of Motion, and Strength Loss Associated with Delayed Onset Muscle Soreness. *Journal of Athletic Training, 27*(3), 200–206.

Denegar, C. R., Perrin, D. H., Rogol, A. D., & Rutt, R. A. (1989). Influence of transcutaneous electrical nerve stimulation on pain, range of motion, and serum cortisol concentration in females experiencing delayed onset muscle soreness. *Journal of Orthopaedic & Sports Physical Therapy, 11*(3), 100–103.

Droste, C., Greenlee, M. W., Schreck, M., & Roskamm, H. (1991). Experimental pain thresholds and plasma beta-endorphin levels during exercise. *Medicine & Science in Sports & Exercise, 23*(3), 334–342.

Droste, C., Meyer-Blankenburg, H., Greenlee, M. W., & Roskamm, H. (1988). Effect of physical exercise on pain thresholds and plasma beta-endorphins in patients with silent and symptomatic myocardial ischaemia. *European Heart Journal, 9 Suppl N*, 25–33.

Dworkin, B. R., Elbert, T., Rau, H., Birbaumer, N., Pauli, P., Droste, C., et al. (1994). Central effects of baroreceptor activation in humans: Attenuation of skeletal reflexes and pain perception. *Proceedings of the National Academy of Sciences of the United States of America, 91*(14), 6329–6333.

Enns, D. L., Iqbal, S., & Tiidus, P. M. (2008). Oestrogen receptors mediate oestrogen-induced increases in post-exercise rat skeletal muscle satellite cells. *Acta physiologica (Oxford, England), 194*(1), 81–93.

Enoka, R. M. (1996). Eccentric contractions require unique activation strategies by the nervous system. *Journal of Applied Physiology, 81*(6), 2339–2346.

Farr, T., Nottle, C., Nosaka, K., & Sacco, P. (2002). The effects of therapeutic massage on delayed onset muscle soreness and muscle function following downhill walking. *Journal of Sports Science and Medicine, 5*(4), 297–306.

Feine, J. S., Chapman, C. E., Lund, J. P., Duncan, G. H., & Bushnell, M. C. (1990). The perception of painful and nonpainful stimuli during voluntary motor activity in man. *Somatosens Mot Res, 7*(2), 113–124.

Fillingim, R. B., King, C. D., Ribeiro-Dasilva, M. C., Rahim-Williams, B., & Riley, J. L., 3rd. (2009). Sex, gender, and pain: A review of recent clinical and experimental findings. *Journal of Pain, 10*(5), 447–485.

Fillingim, R. B., Roth, D. L., & Haley, W. E. (1989). The effects of distraction on the perception of exercise-induced symptoms. *Journal of Psychosomatic Research, 33*(2), 241–248.

Foley, J. M., Jayaraman, R. C., Prior, B. M., Pivarnik, J. M., & Meyer, R. A. (1999). MR measurements of muscle damage and adaptation after eccentric exercise. *Journal of Applied Physiology, 87*(6), 2311–2318.

Friden, J., Sjostrom, M., & Ekblom, B. (1983). Myofibrillar damage following intense eccentric exercise in man. *International Journal of Sports Medicine, 4*(3), 170–176.

Frymoyer, J. W., Pope, M. H., Costanza, M. C., Rosen, J. C., Goggin, J. E., & Wilder, D. G. (1980). Epidemiologic studies of low-back pain. *Spine (Phila Pa 1976), 5*(5), 419–423.

Fuller, A. K., & Robinson, M. E. (1993). A test of exercise analgesia using signal detection theory and a within-subjects design. *Perceptual & Motor Skills, 76*(3 Pt 2), 1299–1310.

Ganio, M. S., Klau, J. F., Casa, D. J., Armstrong, L. E., & Maresh, C. M. (2009). Effect of caffeine on sport-specific endurance performance: A systematic review. *Journal of Strength & Conditioning Research, 23*(1), 315–324.

Gliottoni, R. C., Meyers, J. R., Arngrimsson, S. A., Broglio, S. P., & Motl, R. W. (2009). Effect of caffeine on quadriceps muscle pain during acute cycling exercise in low versus high caffeine consumers. *International Journal of Sport Nutrition and Exercise Metabolism, 19*(2), 150–161.

Gliottoni, R. C., & Motl, R. W. (2008). Effect of caffeine on leg-muscle pain during intense cycling exercise: Possible role of anxiety sensitivity. *International Journal of Sport Nutrition and Exercise Metabolism, 18*(2), 103–115.

Goldfarb, A. H. (1999). Nutritional antioxidants as therapeutic and preventive modalities in exercise-induced muscle damage. *Can Journal of Applied Physiology, 24*(3), 249–266.

Goldfarb, A. H., & Jamurtas, A. Z. (1997). Beta-endorphin response to exercise. An update. *Sports Medicine, 24*(1), 8–16.

Gracely, R. H., & Kwilosz, D. M. (1988). The Descriptor Differential Scale: Applying psychophysical principles to clinical pain assessment. *Pain, 35*(3), 279–288.

Gracely, R. H., Lota, L., Walter, D. J., & Dubner, R. (1988). A multiple random staircase method of psychophysical pain assessment. *Pain, 32*(1), 55–63.

Gulick, D. T., Kimura, I. F., Sitler, M., Paolone, A., & Kelly, J. D. (1996). Various Treatment Techniques on Signs and Symptoms of Delayed Onset Muscle Soreness. *Journal of Athletic Training, 31*(2), 145–152.

Haier, R. J., Quaid, K., & Mills, J. C. (1981). Naloxone alters pain perception after jogging. *Psychiatry Research, 5*(2), 231–232.

Hasson, S., Mundorf, R., Barnes, W., Williams, J., & Fujii, M. (1990). Effect of pulsed ultrasound versus placebo on muscle soreness perception and muscular performance. *Scandinavian Journal of Rehabilitation Medicine, 22*(4), 199–205.

Hedayatpour, N., Falla, D., Arendt-Nielsen, L., & Farina, D. (2008). Sensory and electromyographic mapping during delayed-onset muscle soreness. *Medicine & Science in Sports & Exercise, 40*(2), 326–334.

Hilbert, J. E., Sforzo, G. A., & Swensen, T. (2003). The effects of massage on delayed onset muscle soreness. *British Journal of Sports Medicine, 37*(1), 72–75.

Hirose, L., Nosaka, K., Newton, M., Laveder, A., Kano, M., Peake, J., et al. (2004). Changes in inflammatory mediators following eccentric exercise of the elbow flexors. *Exercise Immunology Review, 10,* 75–90.

Hoheisel, U., Reinohl, J., Unger, T., & Mense, S. (2004). Acidic pH and capsaicin activate mechanosensitive group IV muscle receptors in the rat. *Pain, 110*(1-2), 149–157.

Hood, V. L., Schubert, C., Keller, U., & Muller, S. (1988). Effect of systemic pH on pHi and lactic acid generation in exhaustive forearm exercise. *American Journal of Physiology, 255*(3 Pt 2), F479–F485.

Hosobuchi, Y., Adams, J. E., & Linchitz, R. (1977). Pain relief by electrical stimulation of the central gray matter in humans and its reversal by naloxone. *Science, 197*(4299), 183–186.

Howatson, G., Gaze, D., & van Someren, K. A. (2005). The efficacy of ice massage in the treatment of exercise-induced muscle damage. *Scandinavia Journal of Medicine and Science in Sports, 15*(6), 416–422.

Howatson, G., & Van Someren, K. A. (2003). Ice massage. Effects on exercise-induced muscle damage. *Journal of Sports Medicine and Physical Fitness, 43*(4), 500–505.

Hu, W. P., Li, X. M., Wu, J. L., Zheng, M., & Li, Z. W. (2005). Bradykinin potentiates 5-HT3 receptor-mediated current in rat trigeminal ganglion neurons. *Acta Pharmacologica Sinica, 26*(4), 428–434.

Hubal, M. J., Rubinstein, S. R., & Clarkson, P. M. (2008). Muscle function in men and women during maximal eccentric exercise. *Journal of Strength & Conditioning Research, 22*(4), 1332–1338.

Isabell, W. K., Durrant, E., Myrer, W., & Anderson, S. (1992). The Effects of Ice Massage, Ice Massage with Exercise, and Exercise on the Prevention and Treatment of Delayed Onset Muscle Soreness. *Journal of Athletic Training, 27*(3), 208–217.

Issberner, U., Reeh, P. W., & Steen, K. H. (1996). Pain due to tissue acidosis: A mechanism for inflammatory and ischemic myalgia? *Neuroscience Letters, 208*(3), 191–194.

Janal, M. N., Colt, E. W., Clark, W. C., & Glusman, M. (1984). Pain sensitivity, mood and plasma endocrine levels in man following long-distance running: Effects of naloxone. *Pain, 19*(1), 13–25.

Jayaraman, R. C., Reid, R. W., Foley, J. M., Prior, B. M., Dudley, G. A., Weingand, K. W., et al. (2004). MRI evaluation of topical heat and static stretching as therapeutic modalities for the treatment of eccentric exercise-induced muscle damage. *European Journal of Applied Physiology, 93*(1-2), 30–38.

Jenkins, N. T., Trilk, J. L., Singhal, A., O'Connor, P. J., & Cureton, K. J. (2008). Ergogenic effects of low doses of caffeine on cycling performance. *Internaltional Journal of Sport Nutrition and Exercise Metabolism, 18*(3), 328–342.

Jonhagen, S., Ackermann, P., Eriksson, T., Saartok, T., & Renstrom, P. A. (2004). Sports massage after eccentric exercise. *American Journal of Sports Medicine, 32*(6), 1499–1503.

Jordan, L. M., Kenshalo, D. R., Jr., Martin, R. F., Haber, L. H., & Willis, W. D. (1978). Depression of primate spinothalamic tract neurons by iontophoretic application of 5-hydroxytryptamine. *Pain, 5*(2), 135–142.

Julius, D., & Basbaum, A. I. (2001). Molecular mechanisms of nociception. *Nature, 413*(6852), 203–210.

Kaminski, M., & Boal, R. (1992). An effect of ascorbic acid on delayed-onset muscle soreness. *Pain, 50*(3), 317–321.

Kaufman, M. P., Iwamoto, G. A., Longhurst, J. C., & Mitchell, J. H. (1982). Effects of capsaicin and bradykinin on afferent fibers with ending in skeletal muscle. *Circulation Research, 50*(1), 133–139.

Keisler, B. D., & Armsey, T. D., 2nd. (2006). Caffeine as an ergogenic aid. *Current Sports Medicine Reports, 5*(4), 215–219.

Kemppainen, P., Pertovaara, A., Huopaniemi, T., & Johansson, G. (1986). Elevation of dental pain threshold induced in man by physical exercise is not reversed by cyproheptadine-mediated suppression of growth hormone release. *Neuroscience Letters, 70*(3), 388–392.

Kemppainen, P., Pertovaara, A., Huopaniemi, T., Johansson, G., & Karonen, S. L. (1985). Modification of dental pain and cutaneous thermal sensitivity by physical exercise in man. *Brain Research, 360*(1-2), 33–40.

Koltyn, K. F. (2000). Analgesia following exercise: A review. *Sports Medicine, 29*(2), 85–98.

Koltyn, K. F. (2002). Exercise-induced hypoalgesia and intensity of exercise. *Sports Medicine, 32*(8), 477–487.

Kosek, E., & Ekholm, J. (1995). Modulation of pressure pain thresholds during and following isometric contraction. *Pain, 61*(3), 481–486.

Kumazawa, T., & Mizumura, K. (1977). Thin-fibre receptors responding to mechanical, chemical, and thermal stimulation in the skeletal muscle of the dog. *Journal of Physiology, 273*(1), 179–194.

Langberg, H., Bjorn, C., Boushel, R., Hellsten, Y., & Kjaer, M. (2002). Exercise-induced increase in interstitial bradykinin and adenosine concentrations in skeletal muscle and peritendinous tissue in humans. *Journal of Physiology, 542*(Pt 3), 977–983.

Lavender, A. P., & Nosaka, K. (2008). A light load eccentric exercise confers protection against a subsequent bout of more demanding eccentric exercise. *Journal of Sports Science and Medicine, 11*(3), 291–298.

Levine, J. D., Fields, H. L., & Basbaum, A. I. (1993). Peptides and the primary afferent nociceptor. *Journal of Neuroscience, 13*(6), 2273–2286.

Lieber, R. L., & Friden, J. (1993). Muscle damage is not a function of muscle force but active muscle strain. *Journal of Applied Physiology, 74*(2), 520–526.

Lind, H., Brudin, L., Lindholm, L., & Edvinsson, L. (1996). Different levels of sensory neuropeptides (calcitonin generelated peptide and substance P) during and after exercise in man. *Clinical Physiology, 16*(1), 73–82.

MacIntyre, D. L., Reid, W. D., Lyster, D. M., Szasz, I. J., & McKenzie, D. C. (1996). Presence of WBC, decreased strength, and delayed soreness in muscle after eccentric exercise. *Journal of Applied Physiology, 80*(3), 1006–1013.

Marchettini, P., Simone, D. A., Caputi, G., & Ochoa, J. L. (1996). Pain from excitation of identified muscle nociceptors in humans. *Brain Research, 740*(1-2), 109–116.

Marcora, S. M., & Bosio, A. (2007). Effect of exercise-induced muscle damage on endurance running performance in humans. *Scandinavia Journal of Medicine and Science in Sports, 17*(6), 662–671.

Maridakis, V., O'Connor, P. J., Dudley, G. A., & McCully, K. K. (2007). Caffeine attenuates delayed-onset muscle pain and force loss following eccentric exercise. *Journal of Pain, 8*(3), 237–243.

Mayer, D. J., & Price, D. D. (1976). Central nervous system mechanisms of analgesia. *Pain, 2*(4), 379–404.

Mayer, J. M., Mooney, V., Matheson, L. N., Erasala, G. N., Verna, J. L., Udermann, B. E., et al. (2006). Continuous low-level heat wrap therapy for the prevention and early phase treatment of delayed-onset muscle soreness of the low back: A randomized controlled trial. *Archives of Physical Medicine and Rehabilitation, 87*(10), 1310–1317.

McCaul, K. D., & Malott, J. M. (1984). Distraction and coping with pain. *Psychological Bulletin, 95*(3), 516–533.

McHugh, M. P., Connolly, D. A., Eston, R. G., & Gleim, G. W. (1999). Exercise-induced muscle damage and potential mechanisms for the repeated bout effect. *Sports Medicine, 27*(3), 157–170.

Meintjes, A. F., Nobrega, A. C., Fuchs, I. E., Ally, A., & Wilson, L. B. (1995). Attenuation of the exercise pressor reflex. Effect of opioid agonist on substance P release in L-7 dorsal horn of cats. *Circulation Research, 77*(2), 326–334.

Melzack, R., & Wall, P. D. (1965). Pain mechanisms: A new theory. *Science, 150*(699), 971–979.

Mense, S. (1977). Nervous outflow from skeletal muscle following chemical noxious stimulation. *Journal of Physiology, 267*(1), 75–88.

Mense, S. (1981). Sensitization of group IV muscle receptors to bradykinin by 5-hydroxytryptamine and prostaglandin E2. *Brain Research, 225*(1), 95–105.

Mense, S. (1993). Nociception from skeletal muscle in relation to clinical muscle pain. *Pain, 54*(3), 241–289.

Mense, S. (2009). Algesic agents exciting muscle nociceptors. *Experimental Brain Research, 196*(1), 89–100.

Mense, S., Hoheisel, U., & Reinert, A. (1996). The possible role of substance P in eliciting and modulating deep somatic pain. *Progress in Brain Research, 110*, 125–135.

Merskey, H., & Bogduk, N. (Eds.). (1994). *Classification of Chronic Pain: Descriptions of chronic pain syndromes and definitions of pain terms.* Seattle: IASP Press.

Messlinger, K. (1996). Functional morphology of nociceptive and other fine sensory endings (free nerve endings) in different tissues. *Progress in Brain Research, 113*, 273–298.

Meydani, M., Evans, W. J., Handelman, G., Biddle, L., Fielding, R. A., Meydani, S. N., et al. (1993). Protective effect of vitamin E on exercise-induced oxidative damage in young and older adults. *American Journal of Physiology, 264*(5 Pt 2), R992–R998.

Miles, M. P., & Clarkson, P. M. (1994). Exercise-induced muscle pain, soreness, and cramps. *Journal of Sports Medicine and Physical Fitness, 34*(3), 203–216.

Millan, M. J. (1999). The induction of pain: An integrative review. *Progress in Neurobiology, 57*(1), 1–164.

Motl, R. W., O'Connor P, J., Tubandt, L., Puetz, T., & Ely, M. R. (2006). Effect of caffeine on leg muscle pain during cycling exercise among females. *Medicine & Science in Sports & Exercise, 38*(3), 598–604.

Motl, R. W., O'Connor, P. J., & Dishman, R. K. (2003). Effect of caffeine on perceptions of leg muscle pain during moderate intensity cycling exercise. *Journal of Pain, 4*(6), 316–321.

Nosaka, K., & Clarkson, P. M. (1996). Changes in indicators of inflammation after eccentric exercise of the elbow flexors. *Medicine & Science in Sports & Exercise, 28*(8), 953–961.

Nosaka, K., & Sakamoto, K. (2001). Effect of elbow joint angle on the magnitude of muscle damage to the elbow flexors. *Medicine & Science in Sports & Exercise, 33*(1), 22–29.

Nosaka, K., Sakamoto, K., Newton, M., & Sacco, P. (2001). How long does the protective effect on eccentric exercise-induced muscle damage last? *Medicine & Science in Sports & Exercise, 33*(9), 1490–1495.

O'Connor, P. J., & Cook, D. B. (1999). Exercise and pain: The neurobiology, measurement, and laboratory study of pain in relation to exercise in humans. *Exercise and Sport Science Review, 27*, 119–166.

O'Connor, P. J., & Cook, D. B. (2001). Moderate-intensity muscle pain can be produced and sustained during cycle ergometry. *Medicine & Science in Sports & Exercise, 33*(6), 1046–1051.

O'Connor, P. J., Motl, R. W., Broglio, S. P., & Ely, M. R. (2004). Dose-dependent effect of caffeine on reducing leg muscle pain during cycling exercise is unrelated to systolic blood pressure. *Pain, 109*(3), 291–298.

Ojewole, J. A. (2006). Analgesic, antiinflammatory and hypoglycaemic effects of ethanol extract of Zingiber officinale (Roscoe) rhizomes (Zingiberaceae) in mice and rats. *Phytotherapy Research, 20*(9), 764–772.

Olausson, B., Eriksson, E., Ellmarker, L., Rydenhag, B., Shyu, B. C., & Andersson, S. A. (1986). Effects of naloxone on dental pain threshold following muscle exercise and low frequency transcutaneous nerve stimulation: A comparative study in man. *Acta Physiologica Scandinavia, 126*(2), 299–305.

Padawer, W. J., & Levine, F. M. (1992). Exercise-induced analgesia: Fact or artifact? *Pain, 48*(2), 131–135.

Paddon-Jones, D., & Abernethy, P. J. (2001). Acute adaptation to low volume eccentric exercise. *Medicine & Science in Sports & Exercise, 33*(7), 1213–1219.

Palazzo, E., Rossi, F., & Maione, S. (2008). Role of TRPV1 receptors in descending modulation of pain. *Molecular and Cellular Endocrinology, 286*(1-2 Suppl 1), S79–83.

Paulev, P. E., Thorboll, J. E., Nielsen, U., Kruse, P., Jordal, R., Bach, F. W., et al. (1989). Opioid involvement in the perception of pain due to endurance exercise in trained man. *Japanese Journal of Physiology, 39*(1), 67–74.

Perkins, M. N., & Kelly, D. (1993). Induction of bradykinin B1 receptors in vivo in a model of ultra-violet irradiation-induced thermal hyperalgesia in the rat. *British Journal of Pharmacology, 110*(4), 1441–1444.

Pertovaara, A., Huopaniemi, T., Virtanen, A., & Johansson, G. (1984). The influence of exercise on dental pain thresholds and the release of stress hormones. *Physiology & Behavior, 33*(6), 923–926.

Poudevigne, M. S., O'Connor, P. J., & Pasley, J. D. (2002). Lack of both sex differences and influence of resting blood pressure on muscle pain intensity. *Clinical Journal of Pain, 18*(6), 386–393.

Price, M. P., McIlwrath, S. L., Xie, J., Cheng, C., Qiao, J., Tarr, D. E., et al. (2001). The DRASIC cation channel contributes to the detection of cutaneous touch and acid stimuli in mice. *Neuron, 32*(6), 1071–1083.

Randich, A., & Maixner, W. (1984). Interactions between cardiovascular and pain regulatory systems. *Neuroscience & Biobehavioral Reviews, 8*(3), 343–367.

Reading, A. E. (1982). A comparison of the McGill Pain Questionnaire in chronic and acute pain. *Pain, 13*(2), 185–192.

Reinert, A., Kaske, A., & Mense, S. (1998). Inflammation-induced increase in the density of neuropeptide-immunoreactive nerve endings in rat skeletal muscle. *Experimental Brain Research, 121*(2), 174–180.

Revill, S. I., Robinson, J. O., Rosen, M., & Hogg, M. I. (1976). The reliability of a linear analogue for evaluating pain. *Anaesthesia, 31*(9), 1191–1198.

Rinard, J., Clarkson, P. M., Smith, L. L., & Grossman, M. (2000). Response of males and females to high-force eccentric exercise. *Journal of Sports Science, 18*(4), 229–236.

Rokitzki, L., Logemann, E., Huber, G., Keck, E., & Keul, J. (1994). alpha-Tocopherol supplementation in racing cyclists during extreme endurance training. *International Journal of Sports Nutrition, 4*(3), 253–264.

Rotto, D. M., Schultz, H. D., Longhurst, J. C., & Kaufman, M. P. (1990). Sensitization of group III muscle afferents to static contraction by arachidonic acid. *Journal of Applied Physiology, 68*(3), 861–867.

Sargeant, A. J., & Dolan, P. (1987). Human muscle function following prolonged eccentric exercise. *European Journal of Applied Physiology and Occupational Physiology, 56*(6), 704–711.

Sawynok, J. (1998). Adenosine receptor activation and nociception. *European Journal of Pharmacology, 347*(1), 1–11.

Sawynok, J., & Liu, X. J. (2003). Adenosine in the spinal cord and periphery: Release and regulation of pain. *Progress in Neurobiology, 69*(5), 313–340.

Sayers, S. P., & Clarkson, P. M. (2001). Force recovery after eccentric exercise in males and females. *European Journal of Applied Physiology, 84*(1-2), 122–126.

Sellwood, K. L., Brukner, P., Williams, D., Nicol, A., & Hinman, R. (2007). Ice-water immersion and delayed-onset muscle soreness: A randomised controlled trial. *British Journal of Sports Medicine, 41*(6), 392–397.

Sewright, K. A., Hubal, M. J., Kearns, A., Holbrook, M. T., & Clarkson, P. M. (2008). Sex differences in response to maximal eccentric exercise. *Medicine & Science in Sports & Exercise, 40*(2), 242–251.

Sluka, K. A., Price, M. P., Breese, N. M., Stucky, C. L., Wemmie, J. A., & Welsh, M. J. (2003). Chronic hyperalgesia induced by repeated acid injections in muscle is abolished by the loss of ASIC3, but not ASIC1. *Pain, 106*(3), 229–239.

Stacey, M. J. (1969). Free nerve endings in skeletal muscle of the cat. *Journal of Anatomy, 105*(Pt 2), 231–254.

Stay, J. C., Richard, M. D., Draper, D. O., Schulthies, S. S., & Durrant, E. (1998). Pulsed Ultrasound Fails To Diminish Delayed-Onset Muscle Soreness Symptoms. *Journal of Athletic Training, 33*(4), 341–346.

Sternbach, R. A. (1986). Pain and 'hassles' in the United States: Findings of the Nuprin pain report. *Pain, 27*(1), 69–80.

Surbey, G. D., Andrew, G. M., Cervenko, F. W., & Hamilton, P. P. (1984). Effects of naloxone on exercise performance. *Journal of Applied Physiology, 57*(3), 674–679.

Thompson, D., Bailey, D. M., Hill, J., Hurst, T., Powell, J. R., & Williams, C. (2004). Prolonged vitamin C supplementation and recovery from eccentric exercise. *European Journal of Applied Physiology, 92*(1-2), 133–138.

Thompson, D., Williams, C., Garcia-Roves, P., McGregor, S. J., McArdle, F., & Jackson, M. J. (2003). Post-exercise vitamin C supplementation and recovery from demanding exercise. *European Journal of Applied Physiology, 89*(3-4), 393–400.

Thompson, D., Williams, C., Kingsley, M., Nicholas, C. W., Lakomy, H. K., McArdle, F., et al. (2001). Muscle soreness and damage parameters after prolonged intermittent

shuttle-running following acute vitamin C supplementation. *International Journal of Sports Medicine, 22*(1), 68–75.

Thompson, D., Williams, C., McGregor, S. J., Nicholas, C. W., McArdle, F., Jackson, M. J., et al. (2001). Prolonged vitamin C supplementation and recovery from demanding exercise. *Internaltional Journal of Sport Nutrition and Exercise Metabolism, 11*(4), 466–481.

Tiidus, P. M. (1997). Manual massage and recovery of muscle function following exercise: A literature review. *Journal of Orthopaedic & Sports Physical Therapy, 25*(2), 107–112.

Tiidus, P. M., Cort, J., Woodruff, S. J., & Bryden, P. (2002). Ultrasound treatment and recovery from eccentric-exercise induced muscle damage. *Journal of Sport Rehabilitation, 11*, 305–314.

Tiidus, P. M., Holden, D., Bombardier, E., Zajchowski, S., Enns, D., & Belcastro, A. (2001). Estrogen effect on post-exercise skeletal muscle neutrophil infiltration and calpain activity. *Canadian Journal of Physiology and Pharmacology, 79*(5), 400–406.

Tiidus, P. M., & Shoemaker, J. K. (1995). Effleurage massage, muscle blood flow and long-term post-exercise strength recovery. *International Journal of Sports Medicine, 16*(7), 478–483.

Twist, C., & Eston, R. G. (2009). The effect of exercise-induced muscle damage on perceived exertion and cycling endurance performance. *European Journal of Applied Physiology, 105*(4), 559–567.

Vane, J. R. (1978). The mode of action of aspirin-like drugs. *Agents & Actions, 8*(4), 430–431.

Warren, G. L., Lowe, D. A., & Armstrong, R. B. (1999). Measurement tools used in the study of eccentric contraction-induced injury. *Sports Medicine, 27*(1), 43–59.

Weber, M. D., Servedio, F. J., & Woodall, W. R. (1994). The effects of three modalities on delayed onset muscle soreness. *Journal of Orthopaedic & Sports Physical Therapy, 20*(5), 236–242.

Weiser, P. C., Kinsman, R. A., & Stamper, D. A. (1973). Task-specific symptomatology changes resulting from prolonged submaximal bicycle riding. *Medicine & Science in Sports, 5*(2), 79–85.

Wilkie, D. J., Savedra, M. C., Holzemer, W. L., Tesler, M. D., & Paul, S. M. (1990). Use of the McGill Pain Questionnaire to measure pain: A meta-analysis. *Nursing Research, 39*(1), 36–41.

Wilson, L. B., Fuchs, I. E., Matsukawa, K., Mitchell, J. H., & Wall, P. T. (1993). Substance P release in the spinal cord during the exercise pressor reflex in anaesthetized cats. *Journal of Physiology, 460*, 79–90.

Wong, G. Y., & Gavva, N. R. (2009). Therapeutic potential of vanilloid receptor TRPV1 agonists and antagonists as analgesics: Recent advances and setbacks. *Brain Research Reviews, 60*(1), 267–277.

Yasuda, T., Sakamoto, K., Nosaka, K., Wada, M., & Katsuta, S. (1997). Loss of sarcoplasmic reticulum membrane integrity after eccentric contractions. *Acta Physiologica Scandinavia, 161*(4), 581–582.

Cardiovascular Health Implications of Combined Mental and Physical Challenge

Edmund O. Acevedo, Heather E. Webb, *and* Chun-Jung Huang

Abstract

Acute physical and psychological stressors individually alter physiological homeostasis, and chronic psychological stress is considered a determinant of cardiovascular diseases including hypertension, stroke, and atherosclerosis. Military personnel, law enforcement officers, firefighters, and rescue workers are examples of individuals subjected to dual-challenge conditions—combinations of physical and psychological stress (i.e., mental stress, physiological exertion, and environmental and physical dangers)—in the course of participating in occupational challenges. These professions have also demonstrated increased rates of ischemic heart disease compared with other population cohorts. The present chapter summarizes the empirical studies that have addressed cardiorespiratory, neuroendocrine, and immunoinflammatory adaptations to dual-challenge conditions. It also explores plausible mechanisms that may help to explain the relationship between exposure to dual stressors and health outcomes, including cardiovascular disease.

Key Words: psychological stress, physical stress, cardiorespiratory, neuroendocrine, immunoinflammatory, cardiovascular disease, occupational challenges, obesity.

Introduction

The impact of psychological stress on health has received much attention in the popular media (e.g., Sapolsky, 1998), and a considerable amount of empirical evidence supports the relationship between psychological stress and clinical depression, cardiovascular disease (CVD), human immunodeficiency virus infection, and cancer (Cohen, Janicki-Deverts, & Miller, 2007). Furthermore, dysregulation of the stress system can hinder production of sex hormones (testosterone, estrogen, and progesterone), hinder the release of stomach acid and emptying of the stomach, directly stimulate the colon, and increase abdominal fat, and is linked to behavioral responses associated with poor mental and physical health (see Chrousos, 2009, for a review). To alleviate the potential for these negative health outcomes, numerous investigators are

examining plausible mechanisms that may help to explain the relationship between stress and health and foster support for potential strategies and interventions. An area of investigation that has received less attention is the impact when a mental stress or challenge occurs simultaneously with physical stress (e.g., physical exertion, heat, cold, or pain). This chapter focuses on the combination of mental stress and the stress of physical activity or exertion. This combination of stressors provides an ecologically valid model when you consider the mental and physical challenges associated with occupations such as firefighting, law enforcement, and engaging in military operations.

Psychological stress occurs "when an individual perceives that environmental demands tax or exceed his or her adaptive capacity" (Cohen, Kessler, & Gordon, 1995). This perception leads to an activation of the physiological stress response (stress system) in an attempt to prepare the body to adapt to the stress. Conversely, physiological stress activates the stress response by perturbing or challenging homeostasis (Chrousos & Gold, 1992). The body's response is to activate the system to adapt to the physical stress and reestablish homeostasis. This response is coupled with behavioral coping responses. Physical stimuli that can trigger a stress response include physical trauma, exposure to cold, physical activity or exertion, infection, shock, decreased oxygen supply, and sleep deprivation.

The stress response, as an evolutionary adaptation to stressful stimuli, serves individuals very effectively when they are confronted with the need for an immediate response. Charmandari, Tsigos, and Chrousos (2005) have provided a comprehensive description of the neuroendocrine response to stress. An immediate response is an elevation of catecholamines (epinephrine and norepinephrine) following sympathetic–adrenal medullary (SAM) axis activation. These catecholamines, released from the adrenal medulla and nerve endings, are responsible for central nervous system activation, cardiovascular activation, enhanced metabolic efficiency, and hemostatic alterations that prepare the system to fight or flee. This response is commonly referred to as the "fight or flight" response. In addition, the catecholamines activate the immune system to prepare for an injury or combat infection.

The neuroendocrine system, in parallel with activation of the SAM axis, activates the hypothalamic-pituitary-adrenocortical (HPA) axis. The result is the release of glucocorticoids (e.g., cortisol) from the adrenal cortex approximately 15–20 minutes following initial exposure to the stimulus. Cortisol is involved in glucose metabolism, regulation of blood pressure, insulin release, and immune function. In addition, cortisol is important in the regulation of the inflammatory response, a series of immune system alterations that (a) protect tissues from infection and (b) are part of the initial response to injury. The aforementioned responses to stress are critical to our survival. However, when we are exposed to very high levels of stress and prolonged stress (chronic stress), the activation of this system can lead to a number of negative health consequences related to the functions of the body regulated by the catecholamines and glucocorticoids (i.e., the central nervous system, cardiovascular system, digestive system, metabolic system, and immune system).

Occupational epidemiology provides ecologically valid support for the study of the cardiovascular health implications of combined stressors. A number of occupations require physical exertion and often expose the worker to mental challenges and stressors. Furthermore, members of a number of these occupations have proportionately high incidences of CVD than the general population. For example, law enforcement officers and firefighters have proportionately higher mortality rates for ischemic heart disease than other cohort population (Baris et al., 2001; Calvert, Merling, & Burnett, 1999; Hessl, 2001). In addition, heart disease is the primary cause of on-duty deaths and nonfatal cardiovascular events in firefighters (Franke et al., 2010; Kales, Soteriades, Christophi, & Christiani, 2007; Soteriades et al., 2002).

Although these professionals are exposed to a broad range of stressful stimuli that may affect the development of CVD, a greater understanding of the body's response to the combination of physical and mental stress may help to explain their proportionately higher incidences of such disease. This chapter presents an overview of the literature that has used a combination of acute laboratory stressors as a paradigm to examine the cardiorespiratory, neuroendocrine, and immune–inflammatory adaptations to physical and mental challenge. A focus will be on the potential cardiovascular health implications.

Cardiorespiratory Adaptations to Physical and Mental Challenge

The potential influence of psychological states on physiological responses during exercise is of meaningful importance to individuals concerned with the efficiency of energy production and human performance, including military personnel, firefighters, law enforcement agents, rescue workers, athletes, and cardiac patients. Several investigators have reviewed the research examining the effects of relaxation techniques, biofeedback, attentional strategies, and hypnosis on cardiorespiratory (CR) and metabolic efficiency (Crews, 1992; Hatfield & Landers, 1987; Lind, Welch, & Ekkekakis, 2009; Morgan, 1985). In summary, these reviews concur that psychological states can raise or lower CR responses and possibly alter metabolic efficiency. Furthermore, an intricate examination of the available data also suggests that the impact of psychological factors may be influenced by gender, fitness levels, and past exposure to the psychological stimulus. The effects of fitness level can be further complicated by considering absolute versus relative changes (e.g., absolute change in heart rate [HR] versus relative change from baseline) and different measures of fitness (e.g., maximal oxygen consumption, percent of maximal oxygen consumption, lactate threshold, or ventilatory threshold).

It would seem metabolically appropriate and efficient for human physiology to have developed mechanisms to assess the body's current physiological and mental status and determine an effective response to combinations of stressors (Dayas, Buller, Crane, Xu, & Day, 2001). To examine this proposition several investigations (Delistraty, Greene, Carlberg, & Raver, 1991, 1992; Turner & Carroll, 1985, Turner, Carroll, Hanson, & Sims, 1988) have used regression equations to predict the change in HR when a mental challenge is added to a physical workload. The calculations from these studies determined that there would be an exacerbation in HR of 10–14 beats per minute with the addition of a psychological challenge. Additionally, studies have been conducted incorporating a mental challenge while participants perform aerobic exercise (Acevedo et al., 2006; Roth, Bachtler, & Fillingim, 1990; Rousselle, Blascovich, & Kelsey, 1995; Szabo, Peronnet, Gauvin, & Furedy, 1994; Webb et al., 2008, 2010). Each of these studies has demonstrated a clear increase in cardiovascular response in response to the combination of stressors. However, with regard to determining whether or not this is an "efficient" response, one could argue that this increase in CR responses may be uneconomical for the athlete and occupational athlete (e.g., firefighter, rescue worker, or military personnel) or unsafe for the cardiac patient and unsuspecting soon-to-be cardiac patient. This has led investigators to examine factors that may affect this cardiovascular adjustment.

Women have demonstrated elevated HR responses to combined mental and physical challenge compared with men (Freedman, Sabharwal, & Desai, 1987; Girdler, Turner, Sherwood, & Light, 1990; Lawler, Wilcox, & Anderson, 1995; Yoon et al., 2009). This could be due to a greater sensitivity in peripheral alpha- and beta-adrenergic receptors in women (Freedman et al., 1987; Girdler et al., 1990). Another proposed mechanism that may account for the greater cardiac response in women is a greater sensitivity, density, or both of adrenergic receptors in the myocardium (Girdler et al., 1990). Furthermore, Lundberg and Frankenhaeuser (1999) have shown that women respond with greater catecholamine secretion than men during an acute psychological stress.

The type of mental challenge is another factor that can affect the cardiac response. Psychological stressors have been classified as cardiac tasks (e.g., mental arithmetic and Stroop color-word tasks) that primarily cause β-adrenergic activation (Iwanaga, Liu, Shimomura, & Katsuura, 2005; Kasprowicz, Manuck, Malkoff, & Krantz, 1990; Sherwood, Dolan, & Light, 1990) and vascular tasks (e.g., cold-pressor and memory recall tasks) that primarily cause α-adrenergic activation (Lawler et al., 2001). If the mental challenges used in the studies exhibiting differences between women and men were classified as cardiac tasks, then one would expect that the β-adrenergic activation was greater because of the greater sensitivity, density, or both of adrenergic receptors in the myocardium of the female subjects (Girdler et al., 1990). Although this hypothesis has not been specifically examined, there is evidence in its support(Girdler, Hinderliter, & Light, 1993).

Fitness Level and Cardiorespiratory Responses

One of the purported benefits associated with aerobic fitness is the attenuation of the cardiovascular response during psychological stress and recovery (Dienstbier, 1989; Sothmann et al., 1996; Spalding, Lyon, Steel, & Hatfield, 2004). Dienstbier (1989) has proposed that this physiologically toughened response is explained by an attenuation of activation of the central nervous system, including the sympathoadrenal axis, in response to a perceived threat. The existence of this response is further supported by the research on the physiological mechanisms responsible for the Cross-Stressor Adaptation Hypothesis, which has been reviewed by Sothmann and colleagues (1996). Dienstbier's model of "physiological toughness" is also supported by the documented attenuation of HR and ventilation response to a combined stress in trained individuals. Acevedo, Dzewaltowski, Kubitz, and Kraemer (1999) have demonstrated that this proposed attenuation can occur during exercise with anticipatory challenge. Using a group of high-fit endurance runners, this study proposed to participants a bogus challenge of running to physical exhaustion. Though this proposed challenge elicited an increase in self-reported state anxiety, CR responses were similar to those in a control exercise-only condition without the proposed challenge.

In the area of cardiovascular reactivity to mental challenge there has been some controversy over the relative versus absolute cardiovascular adjustment from resting baseline to mental challenge in trained versus untrained individuals. However, more recent studies addressing several methodological limitations of initial studies in this area and investigating potential mechanisms of CR responses have clarified that although absolute HR following a cognitive challenge at rest is lower for trained individuals than for untrained individuals, HR increase relative to resting HR is greater for trained individuals (Boutcher & Nugent, 1993; Boutcher, Nugent, McLaren, & Weltman, 1998; Boutcher, Nugent, & Weltman, 1995; Boutcher, Nurhayati, & McLaren, 2001; de Geus, van Doornen, de Visser, & Orlebeke, 1990; Franks & Boutcher, 2003; Spalding et al., 2004; Stein & Boutcher, 1992, van Doornen & de Geus, 1989). These changes seem to occur primarily as a result of an alteration in the balance of sympathetic and parasympathetic activity in response to training (Blumenthal et al., 1990; de Geus, van Doornen, & Orlebeke, 1993; Spalding, Jeffers, Porges, & Hatfield, 2000; Spalding et al., 2004; Szabo, Brown, Gauvin, & Seraganian, 1993). Several adaptations with training, including enhanced parasympathetic tone and increased stroke volume, explain the reduction in resting HR (Boutcher, Meyer, Craig, & Astheimer, 1998; De Meersman, 1993; Kenney, 1985). Mental challenge in aerobically trained individuals with resting bradycardia (reduced HR) has been shown to elicit greater vagal withdrawal (greater decrease in parasympathetic activity than in untrained individuals (Boutcher et al., 1998). In addition, aerobic training adaptations seem to lead to an enhanced sympathetic response in rats (Sothmann & Kastello, 1997). Thus, at rest the enhanced parasympathetic activity seen in trained individuals leads to a reduction in HR; however, when presented with a mental challenge, trained individuals demonstrate greater vagal withdrawal and possibly an enhanced sympathetic response compared with untrained individuals. This explains, at least in part, the relative increase in HR seen in trained individuals.

Acevedo and colleagues (2006) set out to examine the relative HR (resting baseline to mental challenge while exercising) and absolute HR (mental challenge while exercising) in low- fit and high-fit individuals. The expected relative increase in HR in the high-fit group did not occur, although there was a tendency for relative HR increases in this group. In addition, absolute HR did not differ between the two groups. These HR responses suggest that the mechanisms responsible for adaptations to the dual stress of exercise and mental challenge may differ from those responsible for the adaptations in response to a single stressor (mental challenge). More specifically, the balance of parasympathetic

and sympathetic influence is likely altered in the combined-stress condition. In particular, during exercise sympathetic activity is increased and the withdrawal of parasympathetic activity is enhanced; thus these changes may have resulted in a lessening of the fitness-related differences in relative and absolute HR seen during a single stressor (mental challenge without exercise). In addition, the time of HR measurement, following 8 minutes of mental challenge, may have limited a clear understanding of the HR response. It may also be that once the system in activated there is a diminished sensitivity to additional stressors, thus limiting our ability to demonstrate fitness-related differences in HR adaptations. The peripheral adjustment to the exercise may have had an impact on cardiac function that diminished the effects of an additional stressor. A clear interpretation of the observed results may have been further confounded by training-induced cardiovascular adaptations that led to a more rapid steady-state adjustment to acute exercise by fit individuals and by the cardiovascular drift demonstrated by the subjects in this study. Finally, evidence exists that an individual's interpretation of the stressor can influence his or her physiological response to the stressor (Dienstbier, 1989). The body's ability to have specific responses to specific types of stressor (Obrist et al., 1978) would suggest that the stressor in the Acevedo et al. (1999) study may have been interpreted differently from the stressor in the Acevedo et al. (2006) study, resulting in a different CR response.

The mode of physical activity and the assessment of exercise intensity are two important methodological issues to consider in the design of the two studies by Acevedo and colleagues. These studies used different modes of activity: treadmill running (Acevedo, et al., 1999) and stationary cycling (Acevedo, et al., 2006). It is not known whether or not mode of activity and past experience with a mode will alter the physiological response to combined challenges. Fitness levels in the aforementioned studies were assessed using a maximal oxygen consumption test and were quite varied between groups (endurance runners: $VO_2max = 68.46 \pm 1.47$ ml·kg^{-1}·min^{-1}; high fit: $VO_2max = 52.68 \pm 7.67$ ml·kg^{-1}·min^{-1}; low fit: $VO_2max = 35.28 \pm 7.69$ ml·kg^{-1}·min^{-1}). From this assessment, considered the most valid measure for determining fitness, relative exercise intensity (%VO_2max) was calculated. However, this relative intensity does not take into account the physiological challenge associated with the metabolic shift from primarily aerobic to primarily anaerobic metabolism. The concern is that this transition also affects cardiovascular, ventilatory, and endocrine adaptations to the physical workload. Thus using a percentage of maximal oxygen consumption with disregard for the individual's metabolic challenge to his or her system is not a reliable method for standardizing the intensity of exercise across individuals. A more accurate method for standardizing intensity is to select an intensity that is in relation to this metabolic transition e.g., lactate or gas exchange threshold).

A Model for Examining Occupational Stressors

A majority of the studies that have examined combined stress have been limited in scope, in that they have used primarily college-aged individuals and lab-induced psychological stressors such as Stroop color-word and mental arithmetic tasks. A number of investigators have questioned the ecological relevance of the findings in these studies. A compelling area of investigation that has attempted to address this limitation has examined the physical and mental challenges associated with firefighting. Firefighters are of interest for several important reasons: (1) Firefighters have one of the highest rates of on-the-job heart attack deaths among all occupations (Kales et al., 2007; Kales, Soteriades, Christoudias, & Christiani, 2003). (2) Heart disease is the primary cause of line-of-duty deaths in firefighters (Kales et al., 2007; Soteriades et al., 2002). (3) Firefighters have increased mortality rates of ischemic heart disease compared with other cohort populations (Baris et al., 2001; Calvert et al., (1999). (4) Statistics obtained from the United States Fire Administration (2004) demonstrate that for the 10 years prior to 2000, approximately 50% of firefighters' line-of-duty deaths were the result of "stress/exertion" (e.g., myocardial infarctions and cerebrovascular incidents). A more recent study by Kunadharaju, Smith, and DeJoy (2011) presents similar data. Notably, the explanation for the elevated line-of-duty deaths and nonfatal CVD events is unknown.

One occupational characteristic that may help to explain the increased risk of CVD in firefighters is the amount of stress associated with fighting fires. Firefighters are often subjected to combinations of physical and psychological challenges (coping with physical dangers, mental stress, physiological exertion, heat, etc.) in the course of fulfilling occupational responsibilities (Beaton, Murphy, Johnson, Pike, & Corneil, 1998, 1999). Kales and colleagues

(Kales et al., 2003, 2007) found a significantly higher relative risk of CVD death during fire suppression tasks and alarm responses than during nonemergency duties. Numerous unique environmental factors associated with fighting fires likely contribute to these findings (Kales et al., 2007), including the impact of physical workload on cardiovascular responses during firefighting. However, the combination of mental and physical stress has not been investigated extensively, and this combination may further explain the high mortality due to CVD among firefighters.

The effects of firefighting on cardiovascular reactivity and stress hormones has been examined using a pre- and posttest design during fire suppression training (Perroni et al., 2010; Smith, Manning, & Petruzzello, 2001; Smith & Petruzzello, 1998; Smith, Petruzzello, Chludzinski, Reed, & Woods, 2005; Smith, Petruzzello, Kramer, & Misner, 1996). Each of these studies has demonstrated increases in cardiovascular or CR responses to fire suppression drills. However, these studies did not control for physical workload during the fire suppression activities; hence it is difficult to clarify whether the increases were the result of physiological or psychological stressors or a combination of these.

The hazards of fire suppression make it difficult to conduct research during actual or training-related fire suppression activities. Factors such as protective equipment, environmental extremes, and the unpredictability of when and where a fire might occur present researchers with data collection limitations that are difficult to overcome. In addition, although controlled-fire training activities are similar to actual fire scenarios, there are still limitations to using these conditions for investigation. Safety considerations for both researchers and firefighters again limit the ability to obtain measurements during suppression activities. To avoid the dangers of firefighting while facilitating the training of firefighters in the decision-making challenges associated with firefighting, computer-based firefighting scenarios have been developed. The use of computer scenarios has become more prevalent in fire training (Bliss, Tidwell, & Guest, 1997; Lieberman et al., 2006; Tate, Sibert, & King, 1997; Throne, Bartholomew, Craig, & Farrar, 2000). These simulations can predictably require firefighters to respond to challenges similar to those presented at an actual fire, but in an environment that poses less physical risk. These computerized simulations may be beneficial in further examining physiological mechanisms responsible for the increased rate of line-of-duty deaths due to cardiovascular incidents.

Webb et al. (2010), using a controlled workload and a computerized firefighting strategies and tactics drill (FSTD), examined the cardiorespiratory responses (HR, respiration rate [RR], minute ventilation [V_E], oxygen consumption [VO_2], ventilatory efficiency [V_E/VO_2], and respiratory exchange ratio [RER]) to this combined challenge. Results demonstrated that the participants perceived overall workload to be higher in the combined-stress condition than in an exercise-alone condition and showed significantly greater elevations in HR, RR, V_E, and V_E/VO_2; there were was no difference in VO_2 or RER values between the conditions. These investigators concluded that "the increased response of cardiovascular indices demonstrates that a mental challenge, when combined with a physiological challenge seems to exacerbate the cardiorespiratory response" and "the additional cardiorespiratory response may be mediated by central nervous system activation in response to the mental challenge." (p. 380)

The results of the studies provide evidence of an uneconomical increase in CR responses to combined physical activity and mental challenge. It is likely that this response occurs because of an enhanced activation of the sympathoadrenal axis and the subsequent release of epinephrine and norepinephrine. These stress hormones prepare the body, including the CR system, for fight or flight. However, the CR elevations suggest that the response to the psychological stress during exercise is relatively uneconomical and unnecessary for meeting the O_2 demands of the exercise. Furthermore, although some evidence supports the idea of a physiologically toughened response associated with elevated fitness, a clear understanding of "how much" fitness is necessary to exhibit this response is lacking. Finally, although studies are consistent in demonstrating a HR adaptation, findings for respiratory responses are less consistent. It may be that a more stressful stimulus is necessary to elicit respiratory increases, or it could be that the respiratory system is more responsive at higher intensities or intensities closer to the ventilatory threshold.

Stress Hormone Responses to Combined Stress

When psychological and physical stressors are considered independently, the inability to adapt and maintain allostatic balance between the SAM and HPA axes has been linked to numerous disease states (Chrousos, 2009; Ho, Neo, Chua, Cheak, & Mak, 2010; Tsigos & Chrousos, 2002). Pathological responses by the SAM and HPA axes have been linked to hypertension, atherosclerosis, endothelial dysfunction, obesity, depression, and immunosuppression (Charmandari et al., 2005; Chrousos, 2000a, 2000b, 2000c, 2009; Ho et al., 2010). It is plausible that exacerbated adaptations to stress can lead to CVD, immune system suppression, and other cardiometabolic conditions. When considering the occupational health of populations that are often subjected to a combination of physical and psychological stress, such as military personnel, law enforcement officers, rescue workers, and firefighters, it may be informative to investigate the mechanisms that link specific illnesses and the stress response. It is well established that the combination of mental and physical stress results in exacerbated CR responses relative to the unique response from one of these stressors alone (Acevedo et al., 2006; Roth et al., 1990; Rousselle et al., 1995; Szabo et al., 1994; Webb et al., 2008, 2010). Furthermore, our understanding of the stress response and of activation of the SAM axis and the HPA axis would intuitively imply that concurrent stressors (as when a firefighter performs a rescue or military personnel are in a firefight) would elicit an exacerbation of the stress hormone response. An examination of these elevations in stress hormones may lead to a greater understanding of the relationship between occupational stress and stress-related disorders.

Critical to recognizing the impact of concurrent stress on the HPA and SAM axes is a basic understanding of the unique stress hormone responses to physical and mental stress independently. Epinephrine (EPI) and norepinephrine (NE) both demonstrate unique responses to physical activity. EPI increases linearly at workloads greater than 60% VO_2max, whereas NE shows a curvilinear response to increases in workload (Frankenhaeuser, 1991; Kjaer, 1989). In addition, physical activity yields significant increases in cortisol at fairly high exercise intensity levels ($\geq$80% VO_2max) (Hill et al., 2008; Wittert et al., 1991) and following longer durations (>60 min) at moderate intensities (70% VO_2max) (Inder, Hellemans, Swanney, Prickett, & Donald, 1998). The response of these hormones to mental stress has not been delineated relative to the magnitude of the perceived stress because of the interest in human subject protection and idiosyncratic perceptions of distinct stressors. However, investigators have been able to document consistent elevations in EPI and NE in response to mental stressors (Gerra et al., 2001; Schoder et al., 2000). Cortisol has also demonstrated an elevation that occurs 15–20 min following the initiation of a stress (Gerra et al., 2001; Miller et al., 1993; Mutti et al., 1989).

A number of studies have used pretest–posttest designs to examine ecologically valid dual-stress situations in populations including bus drivers (Roohi & Hayee, 2010), firefighters (Perroni et al., 2009; Smith & Petruzzello, 1998; Smith, Manning, & Petruzzello, 2001; Smith et al., 1996, 1998, 2005; Taverniers, Van Ruysseveldt, Smeets, & von Grumbkow, 2010), law enforcement officers (Groer et al., 2010; Piercecchi-Marti et al., 1999; Violanti et al., 2009; Zefferino et al., 2006), medical personnel (Baig et al., 2006; Yang et al., 2001), and military personnel (Nindl et al., 2002; Taverniers et al., 2010; Taylor et al., 2007, 2008). A number of these studies have found increases in activity of the SAM axis (Smith et al., 1996, 2001; Smith & Petruzzello, 1998), the HPA axis (Baig et al., 2006; Groer et al., 2010; Perroni et al., 2009; Smith et al., 2005; Taverniers et al., 2010; Taylor et al., 2007, 2008; Violanti et al., 2009; Wittert et al., 1991; Yang, et al., 2001; Zefferino et al., 2006), or both (Piercecchi-Marti et al., 1999; Roohi & Hayee, 2010). However, all of these studies were either unable to control for or did not measure the physiological workload that occurred during the activities being assessed, thus making it difficult to distinguish whether the neuroendocrine increases reported were the result of physiological or psychological stressors or a combination of the two.

A number of investigations have controlled for physiological workload and have demonstrated an additive effect of mental stress on CR, stress hormone responses, or both (Huang, Webb, Evans, et al., 2010; Huang, Webb, Garten, Kamimori, & Acevedo, 2010; Huang, Webb, Garten, Kamimori, et al., 2010; Webb et al., 2008, 2010;). The results from these studies—the first to measure CR and neuroendocrine responses to the combination of stressors—suggest that the elevations in CR measures seen in response to a dual challenge are the result of greater SAM activation during the concurrent stressor. Furthermore, prolonged or frequent elevations of the catecholamines can result in vasoconstriction in most systemic arteries and veins, leading to allostatic alterations in cardiovascular responses. Thus these alterations provide conditions favorable for the development of hypertension and endothelial dysfunction and can contribute to the development of arteriosclerosis (Seals & Dinenno, 2004). The catecholamine responses include increases in blood pressure and HR, changes in cardiac vagal tone, vasodilation of skeletal muscle

vasculature, the release of hemostatic and inflammatory factors, and stimulation of various immune cells, all of which may be contributing factors to the increased risks of CVD in dual-stress professions (Hamer & Malan, 2010).

The HPA axis functions to maintain processes critical to the survival of an organism during times of stress and to mediate inflammatory events (Black, 2006). The HPA axis hormones are known to have rhythmic and pulsatile secretions (Csernus & Mess, 2003). For example, adrenocorticotrophic hormone (ACTH) is secreted by corticotrophic cells in an episodic fashion with pulsatile bursts and ultradian rhythms (Carnes, Kalin, Lent, Barksdale, & Brownfield, 1988; Carnes, Lent, Erisman, & Feyzi, 1988; Gudmundsson & Carnes, 1997). In contrast, cortisol has not only an intrinsic rhythmicity but also an endogenous pulsatility, which is an alteration in response to a challenge to the system (Young, Abelson, & Lightman, 2004).

Additionally, while it takes 8–10 minutes for cortisol levels to rise significantly in the saliva and 15–20 minutes for the levels to become significant in the blood, cortisol clearance time is 70–90 minutes (Chrousos, 1998c). Cortisol released in response to stress stimulates metabolism and serves as an anti-inflammatory agent. As components of the acute stress response, these adaptations are beneficial. However, chronic increases in cortisol are associated with adverse health consequences, including depression, suppression of the immune system, and enhancement of the inflammatory processes of the body. In addition, a number of investigators have provided evidence in support of a relationship between cortisol and CVD, depression, and other neuroendocrine disorders (Chrousos, 1998a, 1998b, 2009; Ho et al., 2010).

A growing body of scientific literature is showing positive associations between increased cortisol levels and weight gain, enhanced secretion of proinflammatory hormones, and increased levels of adipokine, which are cytokines released by adipose tissues. Chronically elevated cortisol is suggested to contribute to insulin resistance and accumulation of visceral fat, while circulating adipokines can activate the acute-phase reaction and may chronically stimulate the HPA axis, forming a vicious cycle (Kyrou, Chrousos, & Tsigos, 2006; Kyrou & Tsigos, 2007, 2009). The combination of interleukin-6 (IL-6) and cortisol has also been suggested to influence the release rate of acute-phase proteins, including C-reactive protein (CRP), which is released in response to tissue damage. Inflammatory responses are recognized as a key cause of CVD (Ho et al., 2010; Merched, Ko, Gotlinger, Serhan, & Chan, 2008; Serhan, Yacoubian, & Yang, 2008), and CRP and other inflammatory markers have been demonstrated to exert proinflammatory, proatherogenic, and prothrombotic effects (Jain, Mills, von Kanel, Hong, & Dimsdale, 2007; Kereiakes, 2003; Maes et al., 2002; Pearson et al., 2003). It has also been suggested that stress can indirectly contribute to CVD by influencing other CVD risk factors such as lipid profiles, blood pressure, amount of physical activity, and obesity (Franke, Ramey, & Shelley, 2002; Ramey, 2003).

Finally, two studies have investigated cortisol responses to a dual-stress situation (Webb et al., 2008, 2011). These studies have both shown elevated levels of cortisol, indicating greater HPA axis activation, during a dual-stress condition compared with an exercise-alone condition. When considering the occupational health of populations that are often subject to a combination of physical and psychological stress, such as military personnel, law enforcement officers, rescue workers, and firefighters, it may be informative to investigate the mechanisms that link specific illnesses and the stress response.

Overview of Stress and the Immune System

A substantial body of research in psychoneuroimmunology has investigated the effects of psychological and physical stress on immune system responses, both innate and adaptive. Innate immunity is antigen nonspecific and provides immediate defense, including the activation of natural killer (NK) cells, whereas adaptive or acquired immunity specifically responds to a particular foreign antigen, creating immunological memory. Acquired immunity is mediated by T and B lymphocytes. Elevated levels of stress hormones (cortisol and catecholamines) are thought to have detrimental effects on the immune system, leading to an imbalance between innate and adaptive immunity via cytokine release from immune cells (Elenkov & Chrousos, 2002). This imbalance can result in a proinflammatory milieu. A critical area of current interest has been the link between the immune system and CVD. In particular, the inflammatory response has been implicated in mechanisms that explain, at least in part, the development of atherosclerosis (Libby, Ridker, & Maseri, 2002). For example, recent studies have focused on the effects of stress on circulating proinflammatory cytokines such as tumor necrosis factor-alpha (TNF-α), IL-1b, and IL-6, which plays

a critical role in coordinating the body's response to inflammation by recruiting leukocytes to the site of infection or injury (Papanicolaou, Wilder, Manolagas, & Chrousos, 1998; Vassali, 1992). This stress–immune interaction fosters the elimination of invading microorganisms and a proinflammatory response (Black, 2006; Paulose, Bennett, Manning, & Essani, 1998).

Although immune cells perform other critical functions in response to stress, including protection against pathogenic organisms to ensure that the body's immune response is efficient or to elicit an effective immunoprotection, the focus of this chapter will be on the stress-induced proinflammatory response. It is well documented that the stress response includes changes in immune cell distribution (Burleson et al., 1998; Isowa, Ohira, & Murashima, 2004; Mills, Dimsdale, Nelesen, & Dillion, 1996; Willemsen, Carrol, Ring, & Drayson, 2002) linked to proinflammatory responses and that proinflammatory state can negatively impact oxidative stress, which plays a central role in the development of CVD (Sies, 1997). These stress–immune changes have been documented in response to psychological and physical stressors independently (Vincent, Inners, & Vincent, 2007; Wirtz et al., 2007); however, there is limited information on the relationship between inflammation and oxidative stress in response to dual challenge. This section will also discuss the impact of psychological stress on inflammation and CVD in normal-weight populations and in individuals with obesity (a chronic proinflammatory condition). An understanding of the differences between normal-weight and obese individuals can enhance our understanding of the link between obesity, psychological stress, and CVD.

Cytokine Responses and Immune Cell Redistribution to Combined Stress
STRESS-INDUCED INFLAMMATORY CYTOKINE RESPONSES

As previously discussed, acute stress alters physiological homeostasis, and chronic stress is associated with greater incidence of CVDs including hypertension, stroke, and atherosclerosis (Dimsdale, 2008; Olinski et al., 2002). A recent study has suggested that individuals who have a greater laboratory-induced stress response are more likely to experience higher stress in daily life (Wirtz, Ehlert, Emini, & Suter, 2008). Furthermore, an exaggerated cardiovascular response to mental stress is associated with atherosclerosis (Kamarck et al., 1997). Research by Singhai (2005) has indicated that one of the earliest subclinical stages in the atherosclerotic process is an impairment of endothelium-dependent vasodilation, also known as endothelial dysfunction, and Ghiadoni et al. (2000) have demonstrated that acute psychological stress induces transient endothelial dysfunction. Moreover, markers of inflammation, specifically cytokines that serve as signaling proteins of immune cells, have been shown to play important roles in the initiation and propagation of vascular inflammation, a finding that may provide insight into the mechanisms of the inflammatory processes both in health and in stress-related diseases (Black, 2006; Paulose et al., 1998).

One potential mechanism that links acute psychological stress to endothelial dysfunction is the level of circulating proinflammatory cytokines such as TNF-α and IL-6. There is evidence that elevated plasma levels of TNF-α and IL-6 are linked to endothelial dysfunction (Lutzky, 2001) and are associated with increased risk for inflammatory diseases (Niskanen et al., 2004; Ridker et al., 2000; Tosi, 2005). Acute stressors either increase or decrease the production of proinflammatory cytokines through rapid signaling from the SAM system to immune cells (Elenkov & Chrousos, 2002; Elenkov, Wilder, Chrousos, & Vizi, 2000; Nance & Sanders, 2007). More specifically, on immune cells the β-adrenergic receptors have been shown to have an inhibitory effect on TNF-α and IL-6 cytokine release; whereas α-adrenergic receptors mediate stimulation of TNF-α and IL-6 (Elenkov et al., 2000; Hasko & Szabo, 1998; Izeboud, Monshouwer, van Miert, & Witkamp, 1999; Nance & Sanders, 2007). Moreover, stress-induced catecholamines increase activation of nuclear factor-kappa B (NF-κB), which enhances production of proinflammatory cytokines (Barnes & Karin, 1997; Bierhaus et al., 2003).

The effects of acute psychological stress on production of TNF-α and IL-6 have been studied using assays that measure either circulating cytokines or in vitro release of cytokines from blood cells stimulated by an immunogen, such as lipopolysaccharide (LPS). Steptoe, Willemsen, Owen, Flower, and Mohamed-Ali (2001) observed an increase in circulating TNF-α and IL-6 after acute psychological stress. However, investigators examining the effects of acute psychological stress on in vitro production of LPS-stimulated TNF-α and IL-6 cytokines have obtained inconsistent results. For example, Maes et al. (1998) observed an increase and Wirtz et al. (2007) found a decrease in LPS-stimulated TNF-α and IL-6 following acute psychological

stress. Although Goebel, Mills, Irwin, and Ziegler (2000) found that acute stress increases LPS-stimulated IL-6, they found no effects of stress on LPS-stimulated TNF-α. In the same subjects they found that injection of the β-adrenergic agonist isoproterenol decreases LPS stimulation of TNF-α but has no effect on IL-6. A recent review by Steptoe, Hamer, and Chida (2007) concluded that these conflicting results may be due to delayed stress-induced increases in these proinflammatory cytokines. For example, studies have reported that IL-6 increases between 45 and 120 minutes after an acute psychological stress (e.g., Stroop color-word and mirror tracing tasks) (Brydon, Edwards, Mohamed-Ali, & Steptoe, 2004; Kunz-Ebrecht, Mohamed-Ali, Feldman, Kirschbaum, & Steptoe, 2003; Owen & Steptoe, 2003; Steptoe, Owen, Kunz-Ebrecht, & Mohamed-Ali, 2002; Steptoe et al., 2001). Further investigation is needed to clarify the duration and timing of the peak response. In addition to the findings on TNF-α and IL-6, research has shown that exposure to acute psychological stress is associated with increased IL-2 levels (Heinz et al., 2003).

Using a more prolonged stress model, Uchakin, Tobin, Cubbage, Marshall, & Sams (2001) examined several inflammatory cytokines 24 hours following an examination in medical students and found that IL-2 levels were lower than in the control group, but no changes were observed in interferon-gamma (IFN-γ) and IL-10. Kang and Fox (2001) also examined chronic academic stress during examinations and found decreased IL-2 levels (in both peripheral blood mononuclear cells and whole blood measures) and IFN-γ levels (only peripheral blood mononuclear cells), whereas IL-6 levels were elevated (in both peripheral blood mononuclear cells and whole blood measures).

As discussed above, numerous occupations (e.g., firefighting, military operations, and law enforcement) are subject to inherent physical and psychological stresses. The combination of physical and psychological challenge, as in fire suppression activities, can alter hormonal and immunological responses as a consequence of the inability to adapt and maintain allostasis among the HPA and SAM axes (Elenkov, 2004). In turn, this may contribute to high mortality rates (Beaton et al., 1998; Hessl, 2001). Physical and psychological stressors, when induced separately, have been shown to elicit elevated levels of proinflammatory cytokines such as IL-2 and IL-6 depending on the stimulus. The magnitude and direction of the IL-2 and IL-6 cytokine responses to acute exercise vary and are dependent on intensity and duration of physical activity. For example, Akimoto, Akama, Tatsuno, Saito, and Kono (2000) found that plasma IL-12 levels increased significantly after brief anaerobic maximal exercise. IL-12 has been demonstrated to generate the IL-2 response, further enhancing the activity of cytotoxic T cells and NK cells (Kobayashi et al., 1989; Morel & Oriss, 1998; Stern et al., 1990). In addition, Steensberg et al. (2001) found that IL-6 increased following 2.5 hours of aerobic treadmill exercise at 75% of maximal oxygen uptake. Although IL-6 acts as a proinflammatory cytokine, it has also been identified as an anti-inflammatory agent. More specifically, Steensberg, Fischer, Keller, Moller, and Pedersen (2003) infused IL-6 in human subjects to produce intense exercise induced concentrations and observed elevated anti-inflammatory cytokines (e.g., IL-10) after 1 hour of infusion. These findings indicate that an elevation in circulating IL-6 following exercise may initiate a reciprocal anti-inflammatory response that can promote recovery. However, limited information exists on cytokine responses following a combined physical and psychological stress.

In a recent study, Huang and colleagues (Huang, Webb, Garten, Kamimori, et al., 2010) examined stress hormone and immunological responses to a dual challenge in professional firefighters. This study utilized a computerized FSTD as the mental challenge. The dual challenge consisted of 37 minutes of exercise at 60% of VO$_2$max along with 20 minutes of the FSTD. This combination of physical and psychological challenge activated the SAM axis, eliciting the release of catecholamines (NE and EPI) and elevating HR. Furthermore, firefighters demonstrated greater IL-2 levels following the dual challenge, with a significant increase in CD56+ lymphocytes (mostly NK cells) in both conditions, but no change was observed in cytotoxic T cells and IL-6. These findings suggest that the addition of a mental challenge to physical stress can alter hormonal and immunological responses during firefighting activities and, if exacerbated or prolonged, may play a role in the development of stress-related diseases. Using a different protocol, Brenner et al. (1999) found elevations in IL-6 following exercise. Specifically, Brenner et al. used 2 hours of cycle ergometry at 60% VO$_2$max as opposed to the 37 minutes used by Huang et al. It is possible that changes in IL-6 occurred following the last measure, taken at 1 hour of recovery, in the latter study.

To foster a better understanding of the cytokine responses to dual challenges, further studies are needed to investigate extended recovery periods for examining IL-6 responses and to examine the effects of stress on the synthesis of other proinflammatory cytokines. In turn, a greater understanding of cytokine responses will facilitate efforts to address the potential negative impact of the immune system responses associated with professions exposed to dual challenges.

CATECHOLAMINE-INDUCED IMMUNE CELL REDISTRIBUTION

An appropriate distribution of peripheral immune cells enables the performance of the surveillance and effector functions of the immune system (Dhabhar, Miller, McEwen, & Spencer, 1995). It is well established that psychological stress alters immune cell responses, including the numbers and percentages of circulating monocytes and lymphocytes (e.g., NK, T, and B cells) (Burleson et al., 1998; Isowa et al., 2004; Mills et al., 1996; Willemsen et al., 2002). The release of both catecholamines and cortisol in response to psychological or physical stress can mediate changes in the distribution in immune cells (Benschop, Schedlowski, Wienecke, Jacobs, & Schmidt, 1997; Rhind, Shek, & Shephard, 1995). Furthermore, Isowa et al. (2004) have concluded that under acute psychological stress the influence of cortisol on immune function is minimal and the acute immune response is primarily regulated by catecholamines. Stress-induced catecholamines (EPI and NE) from the SAM axis have been shown to alter immune cell numbers and function via β-adrenergic receptor regulation (Graafsma et al., 1989; Sanders & Straub, 2002). More specifically, studies have demonstrated that β$_2$-adrenergic receptors expressed on immune cells respond to psychological stressors (Graafsma et al., 1989) and are important for numerous immune cell functions such as NK-cell cytotoxic activity, antibody production, and cytokine production (Mills et al., 2004; Sanders & Straub, 2002). β$_2$-Adrenergic receptors have been shown to have an inhibitory effect on the release of proinflammatory cytokines, including TNF-α and IL-6, whereas α-adrenergic receptors mediate stimulation of TNF-α and IL-6 (Elenkov et al., 2000; Hasko & Szabo, 1998; Izeboud et al., 1999; Nance & Sanders, 2007). Schedlowski et al. (1993) found that administration of both EPI and NE increased NK cell numbers and activity and decreased total T cells and helper T cells, but they observed no change in cytotoxic T cells. Other studies have demonstrated that administration of a β-adrenergic antagonist inhibited elevation in NK and cytotoxic T cells following psychological and physical stress (Bachen et al., 1995; Murray et al., 1992; Watson et al., 1986). Furthermore, investigators examining the effect of psychological stress on lymphocyte β_2-adrenergic receptor responsiveness (receptor density and sensitivity) found that higher tension/anxiety scores on the Profile of Mood States were correlated with downregulation of β_2-adrenergic receptors (Yu, Dimsdale, & Mills, 1999). Other studies have shown that individuals with high life stress and hostility scores have less lymphocyte β_2-adrenergic sensitivity (Dimsdale, Mills, Patterson, Ziegler & Dillon, 1994; Suarez et al., 1997). These findings indicate that stress-induced β-adrenergic receptor dysregulation may be an important contributing factor to the proinflammatory immune response to stress, although the mechanisms of β_2-adrenergic receptor regulation in immune cells in response to stress have not been fully elucidated.

A number of experimental protocols using laboratory-induced acute psychological stressors have observed a transient immune cell redistribution via β-adrenergic activation through the activation of the sympathetic nervous system (Benschop, Nijkamp, Ballieux, & Heijnen, 1994; Benschop, Rodriguez-Feuerhahn, & Schedlowski,1996; Benschop et al., 1997; Willemsen et al., 2002). Specifically, following acute psychological stress an elevation has been observed in monocytes, NK cells, and cytotoxic T cells (Bosch, Berntson, Cacioppo, Dhabhar, & Marucha, 2003; Mills et al., 1996; Willemsen et al., 2002), whereas helper T cells and B cells have been shown to decrease (Burleson et al., 1998; Isowa et al., 2004; Mills et al., 1996; Willemsen et al., 2002). Furthermore, in the case of physical stress the magnitude of these immune cell responses depends on exercise intensity and duration (Gleeson, Nieman, & Pedersen, 2004). High-intensity exercise has been shown to induce the release of catecholamines, with corresponding alterations in various immune cells (Natale et al., 2003). Typically, following exercise, monocytes and NK cells exhibit the greatest fluctuations, followed by T cells and B cells (Hong & Mills, 2008; Rhind, Shek, Shinkai, & Shephard, 1996). Moyna et al. (1996) demonstrated that following incremental exercise the percentage of CD3+ T cells and CD19+ B cells (adaptive immunity) decreases and the percentage of NK cells (CD3–, CD16+, CD56+) increases (cellular immunity). These findings indicate that acute stress enhances cellular immunity and suppresses adaptive immunity and that these alterations can be enhanced

at higher intensities of psychological and physical stress. The appropriate redistribution of immune cells in response to psychological stress, physical stress, or both is imperative for effective and efficient immune response in preparation for potential invaders (Dhabhar & McEwen,1997, 2001; Dhabhar et al., 1995).

Greater EPI and NE responses to dual-stress conditions have been demonstrated in apparently healthy individuals (Webb et al., 2008) and professional firefighters (Huang, Webb, Garten, et al., 2010b; Webb et al., 2011). These findings suggests that the additional increase in catecholamines compared with exposure to a single stressor may further alter the components of cellular immunity (proinflammatory components) associated with the high mortality rates of the combined mental and physical stress of conducting fire suppression activities (Beaton et al., 1998; Kales et al., 2007). Recently, Huang, Webb, Garten, Kamimori, and Acevedo (2010) examined the associations between catecholamines and immune cell distribution in professional firefighters exposed to a computerized FSTD while participating in moderate-intensity exercise. Firefighters participated in two counterbalanced exercise conditions: 37 min of cycle ergometry at 60% VO_2max (exercise-alone condition) and 37 min of cycle ergometry at 60% VO_2max along with 20 min of FSTD (firefighting strategies condition). As expected, the firefighting strategies condition elicited significantly greater increases in HR, NE, and EPI when compared with exercise alone. Furthermore, both the exercise-alone and firefighting strategies condition elicited increases in CD3–CD56+ NK cells. The percentages of CD3+ T cells, CD3+CD4+ helper T cells, CD19+ B cells, and total lymphocytes, as well as the CD4/CD8 ratio, were lower than pre-test resting values immediately following both conditions. These findings are consistent with previous studies, suggesting that acute dual challenge does not elicit a greater fluctuation in immune cell responses than does a single stressor. Most importantly, these results provide the basis for further examination of the lymphocyte subset redistribution following prolonged or repeated bouts of physical stress, psychological stress, or both. In addition, Huang and colleagues found that following dual challenge, NE area under the curve (AUC) was negatively correlated with percentage of CD19+ B cells immediately post challenge, and HR was negatively associated with the percent change in the CD4/CD8 ratio from pre- to post challenge. The simultaneous elevations in NE and HR in response to the dual challenge suggest greater sympathetic activation, which in turn could explain the alteration in the distribution of lymphocyte subsets, which could lead to an ineffective cell-mediated immune responses (Kimura, Isowa, Ohira, & Murashima, 2005; Kimura, Isowa, Matsunaga, Murashima, & Ohira, 2008). It is important to note that firefighters are advised to engage in fire suppression activities with standard work-to-rest ratios: approximately 15–20 min of work, then rest for approximately 10 min (United States Fire Administration, 2004). The repeated work–rest regimen of firefighting may exacerbate catecholamine and HR responses (Ray, Basu, Roychoudhury, Banik, & Lahiri, 2006; Ronsen, Haug, Pedersen, & Bahr, 2001), further contributing to the perturbation of lymphocyte subsets. Early studies reported reduced NK and cytotoxic cell number and cytotoxicity and suppression of lymphocyte proliferation in humans after exposure to chronic stress (Kiecolt-Glaser, Glaser, Gravenstein, Malarkey, & Sheridan, 1996; Maisel & Michel, 1990).

The examination of the lymphocyte subset redistribution following prolonged or repeated bouts of physical or psychological stress or a combination of the two is warranted. A greater understanding of these responses to stress may assist in finding strategies (e.g., exercise training) to overcome the inherent psychobiological challenges associated with mentally and physically demanding professions.

Oxidative and Inflammatory Responses to Combined Stress

OXIDATIVE RESPONSE TO ACUTE STRESS

Psychological stress has been implicated as a risk factor for CVDs such as atherosclerosis (von Känel, Mills, Fainman, & Dimsdale, 2001). One of the earliest subclinical stages in the atherosclerotic process is an impairment of endothelium-dependent vasodilation, also known as endothelial dysfunction (Singhai, 2005). A mediator of endothelial dysfunction is "shear stress," which is a dragging frictional force generated by blood flow in the vasculature, leading to oxidative stress (Arcaro et al., 1999). Oxidative stress is an imbalance between antioxidants, including nitric oxide (NO), and reactive oxygen species (ROS), including superoxide (O_2^-), hydrogen peroxide (H_2O_2), and hydroxyl radical (OH^-) (Sies, 1997). In healthy vascular cells, ROS are generated during the metabolization of oxygen, with the rate of ROS production being balanced by the rate of oxygen elimination (Vider et al., 2001). Elevated ROS production causes cell damage,

which may facilitate the development of CVD (Ji, Gomez-Cabrera, & Vina, 2006). Furthermore, although the body has adequate antioxidant capacity against ROS, any increase in vascular shear stress from cardiovascular alterations in response to a mental or physical perturbation can influence the balance of oxidative stress. For example, research has shown that psychological stress may contribute to the development of atherosclerosis by eliciting an elevation in ROS, which can induce oxidative DNA damage (Adachi, Kawamura, & Takemoto, 1993; Olinski et al., 2002; Sivonova et al., 2004). In a study on medical students, Sivonova et al. (2004) found greater nuclear DNA damage in lymphocytes on the day of an examination (stress condition) than during the time between two examination periods (nonstress condition).

In the case of physical activity, the magnitude of the oxidative response depends on exercise intensity and duration. Bloomer, Goldfarb, Wideman, McKenzie, and Consitt (2005) observed that both high-intensity aerobic and anaerobic exercise elevated the biomarkers of oxidative stress in blood. Elevated oxidative stress during psychological or physical stress could be the effect of increased circulating levels of catecholamines (Cosentino et al., 2004; McIntosh & Sapolsky, 1996; Sivonova et al., 2004). In support of the role of catecholamines in altering oxidative stress, Baez, Segura-Aguilar, Widersten, Johansson, and Mannervik (1997) found that catecholamine metabolism generates free radicals and other reactive species. This is further supported by research by Flint, Baum, Chambers, and Jenkins (2007), which demonstrated that EPI and NE released during psychological stress could induce DNA damage in mice within 10 minutes.

LINK BETWEEN INFLAMMATION AND OXIDATIVE STRESS DURING DUAL CHALLENGE

Inflammation and its subsequent impact on oxidative stress may also play a crucial role in the pathogenesis of CVD (Nathan, Murray, Wiebe, & Rubin, 1983). The development of vascular inflammation is the result of the activation of endothelial cells (Ross, 1993, 1999). Vascular inflammation can be generated by proinflammatory cytokine production induced by immune cells such as macrophages and T cells. The formation of ROS is associated with elevated levels of proinflammatory cytokines such as TNF-α. TNF-α is a potent activator of nicotinamide adenine dinucleotide phosphate (NADPH) oxidase (an enzyme for synthesis of O_2^-) (Umeki, 1994), and NADPH oxidase shows a strong correlation with endothelial dysfunction in patients with coronary heart diseases (Schachinger, Britten, Dimmeler, & Zeiher, 2001). Furthermore, IL-6 is thought to induce oxidative stress and play a major role in the pathogenesis of atherosclerosis (Wassmann et al., 2004). The formation of ROS is also associated with other proinflammatory cytokines. For example, IL-2 and IFN-γ, both released by type 1 helper T cells, are thought to be the most potent triggers for macrophage-induced ROS production (Nathan et al., 1983). Thus one explanation for increased oxidative stress in response to either psychological or physical stress may be the direct impact of elevated proinflammatory cytokines (e.g. IL-2 and IL-6) that correspond with high concentrations of stress hormones (e.g. catecholamines). However, only limited investigative work has addressed the impact of dual challenge (psychological and physical stress) on the oxidative stress and inflammation responses.

To investigate the impact of combined stress on oxidative stress, Huang, Webb, Evans, et al. (2010) examined the changes in levels of catecholamines (EPI and NE), IL-2, and a biomarker of oxidative stress (8-isoprostane) in healthy individuals who were exposed to a physical and mental challenge. Subjects participated in two experimental conditions: an exercise-alone condition that consisted of cycling at 60% VO_2max for 37 min and a dual-stress condition that included 20 min of a mental challenge (Stroop color-word and mental arithmetic tasks) while cycling at the same intensity. Results revealed that the dual-stress condition elicited greater EPI and 8-isoprostane levels. NE and IL-2 showed significant change across time in both conditions. In addition, following dual stress, EPI AUC demonstrated a positive correlation with NE AUC and peak 8-isoprostane, and peak IL-2 was positively correlated with peak 8-isoprostane. These findings suggest that the addition of a mental challenge to physical stress may exacerbate SAM activation and enhance the inflammatory response, providing a possible explanation for elevated oxidative stress.

An important task for future investigation is to examine the catecholamine response to real-life stressors in occupations such as military operations and law enforcement. In addition, further investigation should examine other forms of oxidative stress and the impact of these changes on cellular function, to facilitate a better understanding of the immunoendocrine and oxidative responses to a combined physical and psychological stress. In turn, an understanding of the interaction between oxidative stress and inflammatory cytokines may explain the link between the stress response, the immune system, and CVD.

The Effect of Acute Stress in a Chronic Stress Condition (Obesity)

INFLAMMATION AS THE LINK BETWEEN OBESITY AND CVD

The epidemic of obesity and overweight has evolved to now include 64.1% of American women and 72.3% of American men (Flegal, Carroll, Ogden, & Curtin, 2010). Along with physical illnesses, obesity is associated with psychosocial disorders such as depression and chronic anxiety (Petry, Barry, Pietrzak, & Wagner, 2008; Stunkard, Faith, & Allison, 2003). Obesity-attributable illnesses are associated with chronic inflammatory responses such as elevated proinflammatory cytokine production and activation of inflammatory signaling pathways (Festa et al., 2000). In obese individuals, the vascular response to shear stress is attenuated (Arcaro et al., 1999). This obesity-induced endothelial dysfunction may be due to the interaction of obesity-induced elevations in leptin and elevations in inflammation. Leptin, an adipocyte-derived hormone, is positively associated with elevated percentage body fat; plays an important role in metabolism, adiposity, and vascular inflammation; and has been implicated in the development of coronary heart disease (Wannamethee et al., 2007).

Obese individuals have serum leptin concentrations up to fourfold greater than those of normal-weight individuals (Considine et al., 1996) and up to threefold increases in both circulating TNF-α levels and TNF-α mRNA expression (Hotamisligil, Arner, Caro, Atkinson, & Spiegelman, 1995). Mechanistic investigations in animals have shown that exogenous leptin regulates the production of proinflammatory cytokines, specifically TNF-α and IL-6 (Loffreda et al., 1998) and that an inflammatory stimulus, such as the administration of TNF-α or IL-1, can increase leptin production (Faggioni et al., 1998; Grunfeld et al., 1996; Sarraf et al., 1997). Zumbach et al. (1997) have also shown elevated serum leptin levels after the infusion of TNF-α in human subjects. These findings are consistent with the findings that leptin activates circulating mononuclear cells (Santos-Alvarez, Goberna, & Sanchez-Margalet, 1999) and that these cells in turn activate adipocytes, resulting in the production of proinflammatory cytokines (Ghanim et al., 2004; Weisberg et al., 2003).

The leptin proinflammatory cytokine relationship is further supported by research by La Cava and Matarese (2004) demonstrating that leptin receptors are expressed in macrophages and T cells. Additionally, studies have shown a positive relationship between plasma leptin and IL-6 levels independent of adiposity (Maachi et al., 2004; Wannamethee et al., 2007). Most importantly, elevated levels of leptin and proinflammatory cytokines have been shown to contribute to the risk of CVD and obesity-related metabolic syndrome (Moon, Kim, & Song, 2004; Singh, Bedi, Singh, Arora, & Khosla, 2009). In addition, obesity-induced elevation in proinflammatory cytokines (e.g., IL-6) may be due to leptin-activated NF-κB (Tang et al., 2007). Normally, NF-κB is bound to inhibitor κB (IκB-α and IκB-β), to prevent its movement into the nucleus (Barnes & Karin, 1997). However, following stress-induced stimulation, IκB is phosphorylated by IκB kinase, resulting in dissociation of IκB from NF-κB. The activated NF-κB is translocated into the nucleus and binds DNA to induce the transcription of proinflammatory cytokines (e.g., TNF-α, IL-1, and IL-6) (McKay & Cidlowski, 1999). NF-κB binding activity has been demonstrated to be associated with obesity and elevated proinflammatory cytokine production (Ghanim et al., 2001). In addition, a study by Sheu et al. (2008) showed that after participants lost 5% of their body weight as a result of 12 weeks of caloric restriction and exercise, leptin levels decreased, with corresponding reductions in NF-κB binding activity and in TNF-α and IL-6 mRNA expression. These studies demonstrate a link between obesity, leptin elevation, NF-κB binding activity, and inflammation, suggesting a mechanism for the connection between obesity and diseases associated with proinflammatory conditions.

PSYCHOLOGICAL STRESS AND OBESITY

Chronic stress has been shown to be associated with disturbances of the HPA and SAM axes and is linked to abdominal adiposity (Bjorntorp, 2001). Furthermore, elevated cortisol responses to mental stress are associated with high central adiposity (Benson et al., 2009; Epel et al., 2000; Rosmond, Dallman, & Bjorntorp, 1998) and with corresponding elevations in pulse pressure and HR (Ljung et al., 2000; Waldstein, Burns, Toth, & Poehlman, 1999). This elevation in cortisol as a result of acute stress, in the presence of catecholamines, may not have a suppressive effect on proinflammatory cytokine responses in obese individuals. More specifically, Wirtz et al. (2008) found that individuals

with a higher body mass index (BMI) demonstrated lower glucocorticoid sensitivity, resulting in less ability to inhibit production of TNF-α following acute psychological stress. This finding suggests that in response to acute psychological stress, individuals with higher BMI exhibit elevations in production of proinflammatory cytokines (e.g., TNF-α) as a consequence of diminished glucocorticoid suppression.

Greater plasma EPI and NE concentrations have been reported in obese individuals (Sowers et al., 1982), and reductions in body weight have shown a correlation with decreased plasma NE levels (Grassi et al., 1998). However, recent studies have shown that obese subjects exhibit higher IL-6 levels than normal-weight subjects in response to acute psychological stress (Benson et al., 2009; Huang et al., 2011). This suggests the possibility that obesity diminishes the inhibitory effect of β_2-adrenergic receptors on the release of proinflammatory cytokines in response to psychological stress. In addition, studies have shown that people who undergo acute psychological stress demonstrate increases in leptin levels and that these increases are positively correlated with waist circumference (Brydon et al., 2008; Otsuka et al., 2006). Furthermore, Wannamethee et al. (2007) found a positive correlation between basal circulating leptin levels and IL-6 responses in response to mental stress. However, the mechanisms contributing to the relationship of the stress response, obesity, and proinflammatory cytokines remain unknown.

Finally, it is important to note that a recent study reported 77% of young emergency responders, in Massachusetts, USA (firefighters and ambulance worker recruits) were overweight and obese (Tsismenakis et al., 2009). Similar rates of overweight and obesity have been reported in professions such as police work and the military (Franke et al., 2002; Hsu, Nevin, Tobler, & Rubertone, 2007). Thus future investigation on the possible interaction, be it additive or synergistic, of obesity and psychological stress in the development of CVD in these professions is warranted and may help in finding practical and perhaps innovative strategies (e.g., weight loss, exercise training, and pharmacological interventions) for the prevention and treatment of stress-related diseases.

Concluding Remarks

Numerous investigators have examined plausible mechanisms that may help explain the relationship between stress and health and foster strategies and interventions. Occupational epidemiology provides ecologically valid support for the study of the cardiovascular health implications of combined stressors. There are a number of occupations that require physical exertion and often expose the worker to mental challenges, including firefighting, law enforcement, rescue work, and participation in military operations. Identifying mechanisms that link specific illnesses and the stress response is warranted when one considers the occupational health of populations that are subject to combinations of physical and psychological stressors, often in occupations responsible for the health and safety of others.

A limited number of studies have used a combination of acute laboratory stressors as a paradigm to examine the CR, neuroendocrine, and immune–inflammatory adaptations to physical and mental challenge. The results of these studies provide evidence in support of an uneconomical increase in CR responses to combined physical activity and mental challenge. This response occurs following an enhanced activation of the SAM axis and the subsequent release of EPI and NE. These stress hormones prepare the body, including the CR system, for the "fight or flight" response.

The CR elevations suggest that the response to psychological stress during exercise is relatively uneconomical and unnecessary for meeting the O_2 demands of the exercise. Although some evidence supports the idea that a physiologically toughened response is associated with elevated fitness, the level of fitness necessary to experience this benefit is not known. In addition, although studies are consistent in demonstrating a HR adaptation, respiratory responses are less consistent. A more stressful stimulus may be necessary to elicit respiratory increases, or it may be that the respiratory system is more responsive at higher exercise intensities or intensities closer to the ventilatory threshold. Thus the assessment of exercise intensity and the mode of physical activity are two important methodological issues to consider in the design of studies on these issues. Finally, the examination of mechanisms that could help to explain the gender differences in physiological stress responses documented in the literature would enhance understanding of the factors that contribute to differences in CVD rates in men and women.

When psychological and physical stressors are considered independently, the inability to adapt and maintain allostatic balance between the SAM and HPA axes has been linked to hypertension, atherosclerosis, endothelial dysfunction, obesity, depression, and immunosuppression (Charmandari et al., 2005; Chrousos, 2000a, 2000b, 2000c, 2009; Ho et al., 2010). It is plausible that exacerbated adaptations to stress can lead to CVD, immune system suppression, and other cardiometabolic conditions. These stress-induced disturbances in stress hormones (cortisol and catecholamines) are thought to also have detrimental effects on the immune system. Immune cells perform critical functions in response to stress, including immunoprotection and a stress-induced proinflammatory response that can negatively affect oxidative stress, further contributing to the development of CVD (Sies, 1997). These stress-related immune changes have been documented in response to psychological and physical stressors independently (Vincent, Inners, & Vincent, 2007; Wirtz et al., 2007); however, there has been only limited investigation of the relationship of inflammation to oxidative stress in response to dual challenge. In addition, the impact of psychological stress on inflammation and CVD in normal-weight populations and individuals with obesity, which is a chronic proinflammatory condition, has received limited attention, even though an understanding of the differences between normal-weight and obese individuals could enhance our understanding of the links among obesity, psychological stress, and CVD. Future investigation of the possible interactions, whether additive or synergistic, of obesity and psychological stress in the development of CVDs in professions where obesity is prevalent, such as recruits for ambulance work, the military, and firefighting, is warranted and may help in finding practical and innovative strategies for the prevention and treatment of stress-related diseases.

References

Acevedo, E. O., Dzewaltowski, D. A., Kubitz, K. A., & Kraemer, R. R. (1999). Effects of proposed challenge on effort sense and cardiorespiratory responses during exercise. *Medicine & Science in Sports & Exercise, 31,* 1460–1465.

Acevedo, E. O., Webb, H. E., Weldy, M. L., Fabianke, E. C., Orndorff, G. R., & Starks, M. A. (2006). Cardiorespiratory response of high fit and low fit subjects to mental challenge during exercise. *International Journal of Sports Medicine, 27,* 1013–1022.

Adachi, S., Kawamura, K., & Takemoto, K. (1993). Oxidative damage of nuclear DNA in liver of rats exposed to psychological stress. *Cancer Research, 53,* 4153–4155.

Akimoto, T., Akama, T., Tatsuno, M., Saito, M., & Kono, I. (2000). Effect of brief maximal exercise on circulating levels of interleukin-12. *European Journal of Applied Physiology, 81,* 510–512.

Arcaro, G., Zamboni, M., Ross, L., Turcato, E., Armellini F., Bosello, O., & Lechi, A. (1999). Body fat distribution predicts the degree of endothelial dysfunction in uncomplicated obesity. *International Journal of Obesity and Related Metabolic Disorders, 23,* 936–942.

Bachen, E. A., Manuck, S. B., Cohen, S., Muldoon, M. F., Raible, R., Herbert, T. B., & Rabin, B. S. (1995). Adrenergic blockade ameliorates cellular immune responses to mental stress in humans. *Psychosomatic Medicine, 57,* 366–372.

Baez, S., Segura-Aguilar, J., Widersten, M., Johansson, A. S., & Mannervik, B. (1997). Glutathione transferases catalyse the detoxication of oxidized metabolites (o-quinones) of catecholamines and may serve as an antioxidant system preventing degenerative cellular processes. *Biochemical Journal, 324,* 25–28.

Baig, A., Siddiqui, I., Naqvi, H., Sabir, S., Jabbar, J., & Shahid, M. (2006). Correlation of serum cortisol levels and stress among medical doctors working in emergency departments. *Journal of the College of Physicians and Surgeons—Pakistan, 16*(9), 576–580.

Baris, D., Garrity, T. J., Telles, J. L., Heineman, E. F., Olshan, A., & Zahm, S. H. (2001). Cohort mortality study of Philadelphia firefighters. *American Journal of Industrial Medicine, 39,* 463–476.

Barnes, P. J., & Karin, M. (1997). Nuclear factor-κB : A pivotal transcription factor in chronic inflammatory diseases. *New England Journal of Medicine, 226,* 1066–1071.

Beaton, R., Murphy, S., Johnson, C., Pike, K., & Corneil, W. (1998). Exposure to duty-related incident stressors in urban firefighters and paramedics. *Journal of Traumatic Stress, 11,* 821–828.

Beaton, R., Murphy, S., Johnson, C., Pike, K., & Corneil, W. (1999). Coping responses and posttraumatic stress symptomatology in urban fire service personnel. *Journal of Traumatic Stress, 12,* 293–308.

Benschop, R. J., Nijkamp, F. P., Ballieux, R. E., & Heijnen, C. J. (1994). The effects of beta-adrenoceptor stimulation on adhesion of human natural killer cells to cultured endothelium. *British Journal of Pharmacology, 113,* 1311–1316.

Benschop, R. J., Rodriguez-Feuerhahn, M., & Schedlowski, M. (1996). Catecholamine-induced leukocytosis: Early observations, current research, and future directions. *Brain, Behavior, and Immunity, 10,* 71–91.

Benschop, R. J., Schedlowski, M., Wienecke, H., Jacobs, R., & Schmidt, R. E. (1997). Adrenergic control of natural killer cell circulation and adhesion. *Brain, Behavior, and Immunity, 11,* 321–332.

Benson, S., Arck, P. C., Tan, S., Mann, K., Hahn, S., Janssen, O. E., ... Elsenbruch, S. (2009). Effects of obesity on neuroendocrine, cardiovascular and immune cell responses to acute psychological stress in premenopausal women. *Psychoneuroendocrinology, 34,* 181–189.

Bierhaus, A., Wolf, J., Andrassy, M., Rohleder, N., Humpert, P. M., Petrov, D., ... Nawroth, P. P. (2003). A mechanism converting psychosocial stress into mononuclear cell activation. *Proceedings of the National Academy of Sciences of the United States of America, 100,* 1920–1925.

Bjorntorp, P. (2001). Do stress reactions cause abdominal obesity and comorbidities? *Obesity Reviews, 2,* 73–86.

Black, P. H. (2006). The inflammatory consequences of psychologic stress: Relationship to insulin resistance, obesity, atherosclerosis and diabetes mellitus, type II. *Medical Hypotheses, 67,* 879–891.

Bliss, J. P., Tidwell, P. D., & Guest, M. A. (1997). The effectiveness of virtual reality for administering spatial navigation training to firefighters. *Presence (Cambridge, Mass.), 6,* 73–86.

Bloomer, R. J., Goldfarb, A. H., Wideman, L., McKenzie, M. J., & Consitt, L. A. (2005). Effects of acute aerobic and anaerobic exercise on blood markers of oxidative stress. *Journal of Strength and Conditioning Research, 19,* 276–286.

Blumenthal, J. A., Fredrikson, M., Kuhn, C. M., Ulmer, R. L., Walsh-Riddle, M., & Applebaum, M. (1990). Aerobic exercise reduces levels of cardiovascular and sympathoadrenal responses to mental stress in subjects without prior evidence of myocardial ischemia. *American Journal of Cardiology, 65,* 93–98.

Bosch, J. A., Berntson, G. B., Cacioppo, J. T., Dhabhar, F. S., & Marucha, P. T. (2003). Acute stress evokes selective mobilization of T cells that differ in chemokine receptor expression: A potential pathway linking immunologic reactivity to cardiovascular disease. *Brain, Behavior, and Immunity, 17,* 251–259.

Boutcher, S. H., Meyer, B. J., Craig, G. A., & Astheimer, L. (1998). Resting autonomic function in aerobically trained and untrained postmenopausal women. *Journal of Aging and Physical Activity, 6,* 310–316.

Boutcher, S. H., & Nugent, F. W. (1993). Cardiac response of trained and untrained males to a repeated psychological stressor. *Behavioral Medicine, 19,* 21–27.

Boutcher, S. H., Nugent, F. W., McLaren, P. F., & Weltman, A. L. (1998). Heart period variability of trained and untrained men at rest and during mental challenge. *Psychophysiology, 35,* 16–22.

Boutcher, S. H., Nugent, F. W., & Weltman, A. L. (1995). Heart rate response to psychological stressors of individuals possessing resting bradycardia. *Behavioral Medicine, 21,* 40–46.

Boutcher, S. H., Nurhayati, Y., & McLaren, P. F. (2001). Cardiovascular responses of trained and untrained old men to mental challenge. *Medicine & Science in Sports & Exercise, 33,* 659–664.

Brenner, I. K., Natale, V. M., Vasiliou, P., Moldoveanu, A. I., Shek, P. N., & Shephard, R. J. (1999). Impact of three different types of exercise on components of the inflammatory response. *European Journal of Applied Physiology and Occupational Physiology, 80,* 452–460.

Brydon, L., Edwards, S., Mohamed-Ali, V., & Steptoe, A. (2004). Socioeconomic status and stress-induced increases in interleukin-6. *Brain, Behavior, and Immunity, 18,* 281–290.

Brydon, L., Wright, C. E., O'Donnell, K., Zachary, I., Wardle, J., & Steptoe, A. (2008). Stress-induced cytokine responses and central adiposity in young women. *International Journal of Obesity, 32,* 443–450.

Burleson, M. H., Malarkey, W. B., Casioppo, J. T., Poehlmann, K. M., Kiecolt-Glaser, J. K., Berntson, G. G., & Glaser, R. (1998). Postmenopausal hormone replacement: Effects on autonomic, neuroendocrine, and immune reactivity to brief psychological stressors. *Psychosomatic Medicine, 60,* 17–25.

Calvert, G. M., Merling, J. W., & Burnett, C. A. (1999). Ischemic heart disease mortality and occupation among 16- to 60-year-old males. *Journal of Occupational and Environmental Medicine, 41,* 960–966.

Carnes, M., Kalin, N. H., Lent, S. J., Barksdale, C. M., & Brownfield, M. S. (1988). Pulsatile ACTH secretion: Variation with time of day and relationship to cortisol. *Peptides, 9*(2), 325–331.

Carnes, M., Lent, S. J., Erisman, S., & Feyzi, J. (1988). Changes in mean plasma ACTH reflect changes in amplitude and frequency of secretory pulses. *Life Sciences, 43*(22), 1785–1790.

Charmandari, E., Tsigos, C., & Chrousos, G. P. (2005). Endocrinology of the stress response. *Annual Review of Physiology, 67,* 259–284.

Chrousos, G. P. (1998a). Stress as a medical and scientific idea and its implications. *Advances in Pharmacology, 42,* 552–556.

Chrousos, G. P. (1998b). Stressors, stress, and neuroendocrine integration of the adaptive response: The 1997 Hans Selye Memorial Lecture. *Annals of the New York Academy of Sciences, 851,* 311–335.

Chrousos, G. P. (1998c). Ultradian, circadian, and stress-related hypothalamic-pituitary-adrenal axis activity—a dynamic digital-to-analog modulation. *Endocrinology, 139*(2), 437–440.

Chrousos, G. P. (2000a). The HPA axis and the stress response. *Endocrine Research, 26*(4), 513–514.

Chrousos, G. P. (2000b). Stress, chronic inflammation, and emotional and physical well-being: Concurrent effects and chronic sequelae. *Journal of Allergy and Clinical Immunology, 106*(5 Suppl.), S275–S291.

Chrousos, G. P. (2000c). The stress response and immune function: Clinical implications. The 1999 Novera H. Spector Lecture. *Annals of the New York Academy of Sciences 917,* 38–67.

Chrousos, G. P. (2009). Stress and disorders of the stress system. *Nature Reviews Endocrinology, 5*(7), 374–381.

Chrousos, G. P., & Gold, P. W. (1992). The concepts of stress and stress system disorders: Overview of physical and behavioral homeostasis. *JAMA, 267,* 1244–1252.

Cohen, S., Janicki-Deverts, D., & Miller, G. E. (2007). Psychological stress and disease. *JAMA, 298,* 1685–1687.

Cohen, S., Kessler, R. C., & Gordon, U. L. (1995). Strategies for measuring stress in studies of psychiatric and physical disorder. In S. Cohen, R. C. Kessler, & U. L. Gordon (Eds.), *Measuring stress: A guide for health and social scientists* (pp. 3–26 XXX–XXX). New York: Oxford University Press.

Considine, R. V., Sinha, M. K., Heiman, M. L., Kriauciunas, A., Stephens, T. W., Nyce, M. R.,... Bauer, T. L. (1996). Serum immunoreactive-leptin concentrations in normal-weight and obese humans. *New England Journal of Medicine, 334,* 292–295.

Cosentino, M., Rasini, E., Colombo, C., Marino, F., Blandini, F., Ferrari, M.,... Frigo, G. (2004). Dopaminergic modulation of oxidative stress and apoptosis in human peripheral blood lymphocytes: Evidence for a D1-like receptor-dependent protective effect. *Free Radical Biology and Medicine, 36,* 1233–1240.

Crews, D. J. (1992). Psychological state and running economy. *Medicine & Science in Sports & Exercise, 24,* 475–482.

Csernus, V., & Mess, B. (2003). Biorhythms and pineal gland. *Neuroendocrinology Letters, 24,* 404–411.

Dayas, C. V., Buller, K. M., Crane, J. W., Xu, Y., & Day, T. A. (2001). Stressor categorization: Acute physical and psychological stressors elicit distinctive recruitment patterns in the amygdala and in medullary noradrenergic cell groups. *European Journal of Neuroscience, 14,* 1143–1152.

de Geus, E. J., van Doornen, L. J., de Visser, D. C., & Orlebeke, J. F. (1990). Existing and training induced differences in aerobic fitness: Their relationship to physiological response pattern during different types of stress. *Psychophysiology, 27,* 457–478.

de Geus, E. J., van Doornen, L. J., & Orlebeke, J. F. (1993). Regular exercise and aerobic fitness in relation to psychological make-up and physiological stress reactivity. *Psychosomatic Medicine, 55,* 347–363.

Delistraty, D. A., Greene, W. A., Carlberg, K. A., & Raver, K. K. (1991). Use of graded exercise to evaluate physiological hyperreactivity to mental stress. *Medicine & Science in Sports & Exercise, 23,* 476–481.

Delistraty, D. A., Greene, W. A., Carlberg, K. A., & Raver, K. K. (1992). Cardiovascular reactivity in Type A and B males to mental arithmetic and aerobic exercise at an equivalent oxygen uptake. *Psychophysiology, 29,* 264–271.

De Meersman, R. E. (1993). Heart rate variability and aerobic fitness. *American Heart Journal, 125,* 726–731.

Dhabhar, F. S., & McEwen, B. S. (1997). Acute stress enhances while chronic stress suppresses cell-mediated immunity in vivo: A potential role for leukocyte trafficking. *Brain, Behavior, and Immunity, 11,* 286–306.

Dhabhar, F. S., & McEwen, B. S. (2001). Bidirectional effects of stress and glucocorticoid hormones on immune function: Possible explanations for paradoxical observations. In R. Ader, D. L. Felten, & N. Cohen (Eds.), *Psychoneuroimmunology* (3rd ed., pp. 301–338). San Diego, CA: Academic Press.

Dhabhar, F. S., Miller, A. H., McEwen, B. S., & Spencer, R. L. (1995). Effects of stress on immune cell distribution: Dynamics and hormonal mechanisms. *Journal of Immunology, 154,* 5511–5527.

Dienstbier, R. A. (1989). Arousal and physiological toughness: Implications for mental and physical health. *Psychological Review, 96,* 84–100.

Dimsdale, J. E. (2008). Psychological stress and cardiovascular disease. *Journal of the American College of Cardiology, 51,* 1237–1246.

Dimsdale, J. E., Mills, P., Patterson, T., Ziegler, M., & Dillon, E. (1994). Effects of chronic stress on beta-adrenergic receptors in the homeless. *Psychosomatic Medicine, 56,* 290–295.

Elenkov, I. J. (2004). Glucocorticoids and the Th1/Th2 balance. *Annals of the New York Academy of Sciences, 1024,* 138–146.

Elenkov, I. J., & Chrousos, G. P. (2002). Stress hormones, proinflammatory and antiinflammatory cytokines, and autoimmunity. *Annals of the New York Academy of Sciences, 966,* 290–303.

Elenkov, I. J., Wilder, R. L., Chrousos, G. P., & Vizi, E. S. (2000). The sympathetic nerve—an integrative interface between two supersystems: The brain and the immune system. *Pharmacological Reviews, 52,* 595–638.

Epel, E. S., McEwen, B., Seeman, T., Mathews, K., Castellazzo, G., Brownell, K. D.,... Ickovics, J. R. (2000). Stress and body shape: Stress-induced cortisol secretion is consistently greater among women with central fat. *Psychosomatic Medicine, 62,* 623–632.

Faggioni, R., Fantuzzi, G., Fuller, J., Dinarello, C. A., Feingold, K. R., & Grunfeld, C. (1998). IL-1b mediates leptin induction during inflammation. *American Journal of Physiology, 274,* R204–R208.

Festa, A., D'Agostino. R., Jr., Howard, G., Mykkanen L., Tracy, R. P., & Haffner, S. M. (2000). Chronic subclinical inflammation as part of the insulin resistance syndrome: The Insulin Resistance Atherosclerosis Study (IRAS). *Circulation, 102,* 42–47.

Flegal, K. M., Carroll, M. D., Ogden, C. L., & Curtin, L. R. (2010). Prevalence and trends in obesity among US adults, 1999–2008. *JAMA, 303,* 235–241.

Flint, M. S., Baum, A., Chambers, W. H., & Jenkins, F. J. (2007). Induction of DNA damage, alteration of DNA repair and transcriptional activation by stress hormones. *Psychoneuroendocrinology, 32,* 470–479.

Franke, W. D., Kohut, M. L., Russell, D. W., Yoo, H. L., Ekkekakis, P., & Ramey, S. P. J. (2010). Is job-related stress the link between cardiovascular disease and the law enforcement profession? *Occupational and Environmental Medicine, 52,* 561–565.

Franke, W. D., Ramey, S. L., & Shelley, M. C., 2nd. (2002). Relationship between cardiovascular disease morbidity, risk factors, and stress in a law enforcement cohort. *Journal of Occupational and Environmental Medicine, 44,* 1182–1189.

Frankenhaeuser, M. (1991). The psychophysiology of workload, stress, and health: Comparison between the sexes. *Annals of Behavioral Medicine, 13*(4), 197–204.

Franks, P. W., & Boutcher, S. H. (2003). Cardiovascular responses of trained preadolescent boys to mental challenge. *Medicine & Science in Sports & Exercise, 35,* 1429–1435.

Freedman, R. R., Sabharwal, S. C., & Desai, N. (1987). Sex differences in peripheral vascular adrenergic receptors. *Circulation Research, 61,* 581–585.

Gerra, G., Zaimovic, A., Mascetti, G. G., Gardini, S., Zambelli, U., Timpano, M.,…Brambilla, F. (2001). Neuroendocrine responses to experimentally-induced psychological stress in healthy humans. *Psychoneuroendocrinology, 26,* 91–107.

Ghanim, H., Aljada, A., Hofmeyer, D., Syed, T., Mohanty, P., & Dandona, P. (2004). Circulating mononuclear cells in the obese are in a proinflammatory state. *Circulation, 110,* 1564–1571.

Ghanim, H., Garg, R., Aljada, A., Mohanty, P., Kumbkarni, Y., Assian, E.,…Dandona, P. (2001). Suppression of nuclear factor-kappa B and stimulation of inhibitor kappa B by troglitazone: Evidence for an anti-inflammatory effect and a potential antiatherosclerotic effect in the obese. *Journal of Clinical Endocrinology and Metabolism, 86,* 1306–1312.

Ghiadoni, L., Donald, A. E., Cropley, M., Mullen, M. J., Oakley, G., Taylor, M.,…Deanfield, J. E. (2000). Mental stress induces transient endothelial dysfunction in humans. *Circulation, 102,* 2473–2478.

Girdler, S. S., Turner, J. R., Sherwood, A., & Light, K. C. (1990). Gender differences in blood pressure control during a variety of behavioral stressors. *Psychosomatic Medicine, 52,* 571–591. Girdler, S. S., Hinderliter, A. L., & Light, K. C. (1993). Peripheral adrenergic receptor contributions to cardiovascular reactivity: Influence of race and gender. *Journal of Psychosomatic Research, 37,* 177–193.

Gleeson, M., Nieman, D. C., & Pedersen, B. K. (2004). Exercise, nutrition, and immune function. *Journal of Sports Science, 22,* 115–125.

Goebel, M. U., Mills, P. J., Irwin, M. R., & Ziegler, M. G. (2000). Interleukin-6 and tumor necrosis factor-alpha production after acute psychological stress, exercise, and infused isoproterenol: Differential effects and pathways. *Psychosomatic Medicine, 62,* 591–598.

Graafsma, S. J., van Tits, L. J., van Heijst, P., Reyenga, J., Lenders, J. W., Rodrigues de Miranda, J. F., & Thien, T. (1989). Adrenoceptors on blood cells in patients with essential hypertension before and after mental stress. *Journal of Hypertension, 7,* 519–524.

Grassi, G., Seravalle, G., Colombo, M., Bolla, G., Cattaneo, B. M., Cavagnini, F., & Mancia, G. (1998). Body weight reduction, sympathetic nerve traffic, and arterial baroreflex in obese normotensive humans. *Circulation, 97,* 2037–2042.

Groer, M., Murphy, R., Bunnell, W., Salomon, K., Van Eepoel, J., Rankin, B.,…Bykowski, C. A. (2010). Salivary measures of stress and immunity in police officers engaged in simulated critical incident scenarios. *Journal of Occupational and Environmental Medicine, 52*(6), 595–602.

Grunfeld, C., Zhao, C., Fuller, J., Pollock, A., Moser, A., Friedman, J., & Feingold, K. R. (1996). Endotoxin and cytokines induce expression of leptin, the *ob* gene product, in hamsters: A role for leptin in the anorexia of infection. *Journal of Clinical Investigation, 97,* 2152–2157.

Gudmundsson, A., & Carnes, M. (1997). Pulsatile adrenocorticotropic hormone: An overview. *Biological Psychiatry, 41,* 342–365.

Hamer, M., & Malan, L. (2010). Psychophysiological risk markers of cardiovascular disease. *Neuroscience and Biobehavioral Reviews, 35,* 76–83.

Hasko, G., & Szabo, C. (1998). Regulation of cytokine and chemokine production by transmitters and co-transmitters of the autonomic nervous system. *Biochemical Pharmacology, 56,* 1079–1087.

Hatfield, B. D., & Landers, D. M. (1987). Psychophysiology in exercise and sport research: An overview. *Exercise and Sport Sciences Reviews, 15,* 351–387.

Heinz, A., Hermann, D., Smolka, M. N., Rieks, M., Graf, K. J., Pohlau, D.,…Bauer, M. (2003). Effects of acute psychological stress on adhesion molecules, interleukins and sex hormones: Implications for coronary heart disease. *Psychopharmacology, 165,* 111–117.

Hessl, S. (2001). Police and corrections. *Occupational Medicine, 16,* 39–49.

Hill, E. E., Zack, E., Battaglini, C., Viru, M., Viru, A., & Hackney, A. C. (2008). Exercise and circulating cortisol levels: The intensity threshold effect. *Journal of Endocrinological Investigation, 31*(7), 587–591.

Ho, R. C., Neo, L. F., Chua, A. N., Cheak, A. A., & Mak, A. (2010). Research on psychoneuroimmunology: Does stress influence immunity and cause coronary artery disease? *Annals of the Academy of Medicine, Singapore, 39*(3), 191–196.

Hong, S., & Mills, P. J., 2008. Effects of an exercise challenge on mobilization and surface marker expression of monocyte subsets in individuals with normal vs. elevated blood pressure. *Brain, Behavior, and Immunity, 22,* 590–599.

Hotamisligil, G. S., Arner, P., Caro, J. F., Atkinson, R. L., & Spiegelman, B. M. (1995). Increased adipose tissue expression of tumor necrosis factor-alpha in human obesity and insulin resistance. *Journal of Clinical Investigation, 95,* 2409–2415.

Hsu, L. L., Nevin, R. L., Tobler, S. K., & Rubertone, M. V. (2007). Trends in overweight and obesity among 18-year-old applicants to the United States military, 1993–2006. *Journal of Adolescent Health, 41,* 610–612.

Huang, C. J., Stewart, J. K., Franco, R. L., Evans, R. K., Lee, Z. P., Cruz, T. D.,…Acevedo, E. O. (2011). LPS-stimulated tumor necrosis factor-alpha and interleukin-6 mRNA and cytokine responses following acute psychological stress. *Psychoneuroendocrinology, 36,* 1553–1561

Huang, C. J., Webb, H. E., Evans, R. K., McCleod, K. A., Tangsilsat, S. E., Kamimori, G. H., & Acevedo, E. O. (2010). Psychological stress during exercise: Immunoendocrine and oxidative responses. *Experimental Biology and Medicine (Maywood), 235,* 1498–1504.

Huang, C. J., Webb, H. E., Garten, R. S., Kamimori, G. H., & Acevedo, E. O. (2010). Psychological stress during exercise:

Lymphocyte subset redistribution in firefighters. *Physiology and Behavior, 101,* 320–326.

Huang, C. J., Webb, H. E., Garten, R. S., Kamimori, G. H., Evans, R. K., & Acevedo, E. O. (2010). Stress hormones and immunological responses to a dual challenge in professional firefighters. *International Journal of Psychophysiology, 75,* 312–318.

Inder, W. J., Hellemans, J., Swanney, M. P., Prickett, T. C., & Donald, R. A. (1998). Prolonged exercise increases peripheral plasma ACTH, CRH, and AVP in male athletes. *Journal of Applied Physiology, 85*(3), 835–841.

Isowa, T., Ohira, H., & Murashima, S. (2004). Reactivity of immune, endocrine and cardiovascular parameters to active and passive acute stress. *Biological Psychology, 65,* 101–120.

Iwanaga, K., Liu, X. X., Shimomura, Y., & Katsuura, T. (2005). Approach to human adaptability to stresses of city life. *Journal of Physiological Anthropology and Applied Human Science, 24,* 357–361.

Izeboud, C. A., Monshouwer, M., van Miert, A. S., & Witkamp, R. F. (1999). The β-adrenoceptor agonist clenbuterol is a potent inhibitor of the LPS-induced production of TNF- α and IL-6 in vitro and in vivo. *Inflammation Research, 48,* 497–502.

Jain, S., Mills, P. J., von Kanel, R., Hong, S., & Dimsdale, J. E. (2007). Effects of perceived stress and uplifts on inflammation and coagulability. *Psychophysiology, 44,* 154–160.

Ji, L. L., Gomez-Cabrera, M. C., & Vina, J. (2006). Exercise and hormesis. *Annals of the New York Academy of Sciences, 1067,* 425–435.

Kales, S. N., Soteriades, E. S., Christophi, C., & Christiani, D. (2007). Emergency duties and deaths from heart disease among firefighters in the United States. *New England Journal of Medicine, 356,* 1207–1215.

Kales, S. N., Soteriades, E. S., Christoudias, S. G., & Christiani, D. C. (2003). Firefighters and on-duty deaths from coronary heart disease: A case control study. *Environmental Health, 2,* 14.

Kamarck, T. W., Everson, S. A., Kaplan, G. A., Manuck, S. B., Jennings, J. R., Salonen, R., & Salonen, J. T. (1997). Exaggerated blood pressure responses during mental stress are associated with enhanced carotid atherosclerosis in middle-aged Finnish men: Findings from the Kuopio Ischemic Heart Disease Study. *Circulation, 96,* 3842–3848.

Kang, D. H., & Fox, C. (2001). Th1 and Th2 cytokine responses to academic stress. *Research in Nursing and Health, 24,* 245–257.

Kasprowicz, A. L., Manuck, S. B., Malkoff, S. B., & Krantz D. S. (1990). Individual differences in behaviorally evoked cardiovascular response: Temporal stability and hemodynamic patterning. *Psychophysiology, 27,* 605–619.

Kenney, W. L. (1985). Parasympathetic control of resting heart rate: Relationship to aerobic power. *Medicine & Science in Sports & Exercise, 17,* 451–455.

Kereiakes, D. J. (2003). The fire that burns within: C-reactive protein. *Circulation, 107*(3), 373–374.

Kiecolt-Glaser, J. K., Glaser, R., Gravenstein, S., Malarkey, W. B., & Sheridan, J. (1996). Chronic stress alters the immune response to influenza virus vaccine in older adults. *Proceedings of the National Academy of Sciences of the United States of America, 93,* 3043–3047.

Kimura, K., Isowa, T., Matsunaga, M., Murashima, S., & Ohira, H. (2008). The temporal redistribution pattern of NK cells under acute stress based on CD62L adhesion

molecule expression. *International Journal of Psychophysiology, 70,* 63–69.

Kimura, K., Isowa, T., Ohira, H., & Murashima, S. (2005). Temporal variation of acute stress response in sympathetic nervous and immune systems. *Biological Psychology, 70,* 131–139.

Kjaer, M. (1989). Epinephrine and some other hormonal responses to exercise in man: With special reference to physical training. *International Journal of Sports Medicine, 10,* 2–15.

Kobayashi, M., Ritz, L., Ryan, M., Hewick, R. M., Clark, S. C., Chan, S., . . . Trinchieri, G. (1989). Identification and purification of natural killer cell stimulatory factor (NKSF), a cytokine with multiple biologic effects on human lymphocytes. *Journal of Experimental Medicine, 170,* 827–845. Kunadharaju, K. Smith, T.D., & DeJoy, D.M. (2011). Line-of-duty deaths among U.S. firefighters: An analysis of fatality investigations. *Accident Analysis & Prevention, 43,* 1171–1180.

Kunz-Ebrecht, S. R., Mohamed-Ali, V., Feldman, P. J., Kirschbaum, C., & Steptoe, A. (2003). Cortisol responses to mild psychological stress are inversely associated with proinflammatory cytokines. *Brain, Behavior, and Immunity, 17,* 373–383.

Kyrou, I., Chrousos, G. P., & Tsigos, C. (2006). Stress, visceral obesity, and metabolic complications. *Annals of the New York Academy of Sciences, 1083,* 77–110.

Kyrou, I., & Tsigos, C. (2007). Stress mechanisms and metabolic complications. *Hormone and Metabolic Research, 39*(6), 430–438.

Kyrou, I., & Tsigos, C. (2009). Stress hormones: Physiological stress and regulation of metabolism. *Current Opinion in Pharmacology, 9*(6), 787–793.

La Cava, A., & Matarese, G. (2004). The weight of leptin in immunity. *Nature Reviews Immunology, 4,* 371–379.

Lawler, K. A., Kline, K. A., Adlin, R. F., Wilcox, Z. C., Craig, F. W., Krishnamoorthy, J. S., & Piferi, R. L. (2001). Psychophysiological correlates of individual differences in patterns of hemodynamic reactivity. *International Journal of Psychophysiology, 40,* 93–107.

Lawler, K. A., Wilcox, Z. C., & Anderson, S. F. (1995). Gender differences in patterns of dynamic cardiovascular regulation. *Psychosomatic Medicine, 57,* 357–365.

Libby, P., Ridker, P. M., & Maseri, A. (2002). Inflammation and atherosclerosis. *Circulation, 105,* 1135–1143.

Lieberman, H. R., Niro, P., Tharion, W. J., Nindl, B. C., Castellani, J. W., & Montain, S. J. (2006). Cognition during sustained operations: Comparison of a laboratory simulation to field studies. *Aviation, Space, and Environmental Medicine, 77,* 929–935.

Lind, E., Welch, A. S., & Ekkekakis, P. (2009). Do "mind over muscle" strategies work? Examining the effects of attentional association and dissociation on exertional, affective, and physiological responses to exercise. *Sports Medicine, 39,* 743–764.

Ljung, T., Holm, G., Friberg, P., Andersson, B., Bengtsson, B., Svensson, J., . . . Bjorntorp, P. (2000). The activity of the hypothalamic-pituitary-adrenal axis and the sympathetic nervous system in relation to waist/hip circumference ratio in men. *Obesity Research, 8,* 487–495.

Loffreda, S., Yang, S. Q., Lin, H. Z., Karp, C. L., Brengman, M. L., Wang, D. J., . . . Diehl, A. M. (1998). Leptin regulates proinflammatory immune responses. *FASEB Journal, 12,* 57–65.

Lundberg, U., & Frankenhaeuser, M. (1999). Stress and workload of men and women in high ranking positions. *Journal of Occupational Health Psychology, 4,* 142–151.

Lutzky, J. (2001). Inflammatory pathways in atherosclerosis and acute coronary syndromes. *American Journal of Cardiology, 88,* 10–15.

Maachi, M., Pieroni, L., Bruckert, E., Jardel, C., Fellahi, S., Hainque, B.,…Bastard, J. P. (2004). Systemic low-grade inflammation is related to both circulating and adipose tissue TNF-alpha, leptin and IL-6 levels in obese women. *International Journal of Obesity and Related Metabolic Disorders, 28,* 993–997.

Maes, M., Song, C., Lin, A., Jongh, R. D., Van Gastel, A., Kenis, G.,…Smith, R. (1998). The effects of psychological stress on humans: Increased cytokines and a Th1-like response in stress induced anxiety. *Cytokine, 10,* 313–318.

Maes, M., Van Gastel, A., Delmeire, L., Kenis, G., Bosmans, E., & Song, C. (2002). Platelet alpha2-adrenoceptor density in humans: Relationships to stress-induced anxiety, psychasthenic constitution, gender and stress-induced changes in the inflammatory response system. *Psychological Medicine, 32*(5), 919–928.

Maisel, A. S., & Michel, M. C. (1990). Beta-adrenoreceptor control of immune function in congestive heart failure. *British Journal of Clinical Pharmacology, 30,* 49S–53S.

McIntosh, L., & Sapolsky, R. (1996). Glucocorticoids increase the accumulation of reactive species and enhance adriamycin-induced toxicity in neuronal culture. *Experimental Neurology, 141,* 201–216.

McKay, L. I., & Cidlowski, J. A. (1999). Molecular control of immune/inflammatory responses: Interactions between nuclear factor- κB and steroid receptor-signaling pathways. *Endocrine Reviews, 20,* 435–459.

Merched, A. J., Ko, K., Gotlinger, K. H., Serhan, C. N., & Chan, L. (2008). Atherosclerosis: Evidence for impairment of resolution of vascular inflammation governed by specific lipid mediators. *FASEB Journal, 22,* 3595–3606.

Miller, P. F., Light, K. C., Bragdon, E. E., Ballenger, M. N., Herbst, M. C., Maixner, W.,…Sheps, D. S. (1993). Beta-endorphin response to exercise and mental stress in patients with ischemic heart disease. *Journal of Psychosomatic Research, 37,* 455–465.

Mills, P. J., Alder, K. A., Dimsdale, J. E., Perez, C. J., Ziegler, M. G., Ancoli-Israel, S.,…Grant, I. (2004). Vulnerable caregivers of Alzheimer disease patients have a deficit in β-adrenergic receptor sensitivity and density. *American Journal of Geriatric Psychiatry, 12,* 281–286.

Mills, P. J., Dimsdale, J. E., Nelesen, R. A., & Dillion, E. (1996). Psychologic characteristics associated with acute stressor-induced leukocyte subset redistribution. *Journal of Psychosomatic Research, 40,* 417–423.

Moon, Y. S., Kim, D. H., & Song, D. K. (2004). Serum tumor necrosis factor-alpha levels and components of metabolic syndrome in obese adolescents. *Metabolism, 53,* 863–867.

Morel, P. A., & Oriss, T. B. (1998). Crossregulation between Th1 and Th2 cells. *Critical Reviews in Immunology, 18,* 275–303.

Morgan, W. P. (1985). Psychogenic factors and exercise metabolism: A review. *Medicine & Science in Sports & Exercise, 17,* 309–316.

Moyna, N. M., Acker, G. R., Fulton, J. R., Weber, K., Goss, F. L., & Robertson, R. J. (1996). Lymphocyte function and cytokine production during incremental exercise in active and sedentary males and females. *International Journal of Sports Medicine, 17,* 585–591.

Murray, D. R., Irwin, M., Rearden, C. A., Ziegler, M., Motulsky, H., & Maisel, A. S. (1992). Sympathetic and immune interactions during dynamic exercise. Mediation via a beta 2-adrenergic-dependent mechanism. *Circulation, 86,* 203–213.

Mutti, A., Ferroni, C., Vescovi, P. P., Bottazzi, R., Selis, L., Gerra, G., & Franchini, I. (1989). Endocrine effects of psychological stress associated with neurobehavioral performance testing. *Life Sciences, 44*(24), 1831–1836.

Nance, D. M., & Sanders, V. M. (2007). Autonomic innervations and regulation of the immune system (1987–2007). *Brain, Behavior, and Immunity, 21,* 736–745.

Natale, V. M., Brenner, I. K., Moldoveanu, A. I., Vasiliou, P., Shek, P., & Shephard, R. J. (2003). Effects of three different types of exercise on blood leukocyte count during and following exercise. *São Paulo Medical Journal, 121,* 9–14.

Nathan, C. F., Murray, H. W., Wiebe, M. E., & Rubin, B. Y. (1983). Identification of interferon-gamma as the lymphokine that activates human macrophage oxidative metabolism and antimicrobial activity. *Journal of Experimental Medicine, 158,* 670–689.

Nindl, B. C., Leone, C. D., Tharion, W. J., Johnson, R. F., Castellani, J. W., Patton, J. F., & Montain, S. J. (2002). Physical performance responses during 72 h of military operational stress. *Medicine & Science in Sports & Exercise, 34,* 1814–1822.

Niskanen, L., Laaksonen, D. E., Nyyssonen, K., Punnonen, K., Valkonen, V. P., Fuentes, R.,…Salonen, J. T. (2004). Inflammation, abdominal obesity, and smoking as predictors of hypertension. *Hypertension, 44,* 859–865.

Obrist, P. A., Gaebelein, C. J., Teller, E. S., Langer, A. W., Grignolo, A., Light, K. C., & McCubbin, J. A. (1978). The relationship among heart rate, dP/dt, and blood pressure in humans as a function of the type of stress. *Psychophysiology, 15,* 102–115.

Olinski, R., Gackowski, D., Foksinski, M., Rozalski R., Roszkowski, K., & Jaruga, P. (2002). Oxidative DNA damage: Assessment of the role in carcinogenesis, atherosclerosis, and acquired immunodeficiency syndrome. *Free Radical Biology and Medicine, 33,* 192–200.

Otsuka, R., Yatsuya, H., Tamakoshil, K., Matsushita, K., Wada, K., & Toyoshima, H. (2006). Perceived psychological stress and serum leptin concentrations in Japanese men. *Obesity (Silver Spring), 14,* 1832–1838.

Owen, N., & Steptoe, A. (2003). Natural killer cell and proinflammatory cytokine responses to mental stress: Associations with heart rate and heart rate variability. *Biological Psychology, 63,* 101–115.

Papanicolaou, D. A., Wilder, R. L., Manolagas, S. C., & Chrousos, G. P. (1998). The pathophysiologic roles of interleukin-6 in human disease. *Annals of Internal Medicine, 128,* 127–137.

Paulose, M., Bennett, B. L., Manning, A. M., & Essani, K. (1998). Selective inhibition of TNF-alpha induced cell adhesion molecule. *Microbial Pathogenesis, 25,* 33–41.

Pearson, T. A., Mensah, G. A., Alexander, R. W., Anderson, J. L., Cannon, R. O., 3rd, Criqui, M.,…Vinicor, F. (2003). Markers of inflammation and cardiovascular disease: Application to clinical and public health practice. A statement for healthcare professionals from the Centers for Disease Control and Prevention and the American Heart Association. *Circulation, 107*(3), 499–511.

Perroni, F., Tessitore, A., Cibelli, G., Lupo, C., D'Artibale, E., Cortis, C., . . . Capranica, L. (2009). Effects of simulated fire-fighting on the responses of salivary cortisol, alpha-amylase and psychological variables. *Ergonomics, 52*(4), 484–491.

Perroni, F., Tessitore, A., Cortis, C., Lupo, C., D'Artibale, E., Cignitti, L., & Capranica, L. (2010). Energy cost and energy sources during a simulated firefighting activity. *Journal of Strength and Conditioning Research, 24,* 3457–3463.

Petry, N. M., Barry, D., Pietrzak, R. H., & Wagner, J. A. (2008). Overweight and obesity are associated with psychiatric disorders: Results from the National Epidemiologic Survey on Alcohol and Related Conditions. *Psychosomatic Medicine, 70,* 288–297.

Piercecchi-Marti, M. D., Leonetti, G., Pelissier, A. L., Conrath, J., Cianfarani, F., & Valli, M. (1999). Evaluation of biological stress markers in police officers. *Medicine and Law, 18*(1), 125–144.

Ramey, S. L. (2003). Cardiovascular disease risk factors and the perception of general health among male law enforcement officers: Encouraging behavioral change. *AAOHN Journal: Official Journal of the American Association of Occupational Health Nurses, 51*(5), 219–226.

Ray, M. R., Basu, C., Roychoudhury, S., Banik, S., & Lahiri, T. (2006). Plasma catecholamine levels and neurobehavioral problems in Indian firefighters. *Journal of Occupational Health, 48,* 210–215.

Rhind, S. G., Shek, P. N., & Shephard, R. J. (1995). The impact of exercise on cytokines and receptor expression. *Exercise Immunology Review, 1,* 97–148.

Rhind, S. G., Shek, P. N., Shinkai, S., & Shephard, R. J. (1996). Effects of moderate endurance exercise and training on in vitro lymphocyte proliferation, interleukin-2 (IL-2) production, and IL-2 receptor expression. *European Journal of Applied Physiology, 74,* 348–360.

Ridker, P. M., Rifai, N., Pfeffer, M., Sacks, F., Lepage, S., & Braunwald, E. (2000). Elevation of tumor necrosis factor-alpha and increased risk of recurrent coronary events after myocardial infarction. *Circulation, 101,* 2149–2153.

Ronsen, O., Haug, E., Pedersen, B. K., & Bahr, R. (2001). Increased neuroendocrine response to a repeated bout of endurance exercise. *Medicine & Science in Sports & Exercise, 33,* 568–575.

Roohi, N., & Hayee, S. (2010). Work stress related physiological responses in professional bus drivers. *Acta Physiologica Hungarica, 97*(4), 408–416.

Rosmond, R., Dallman, M., & Bjorntorp, P. (1998). Stress-related cortisol secretion in men: Relationships with abdominal obesity and endocrine, metabolic, and hemodynamic abnormalities. *Journal of Clinical Endocrinology and Metabolism, 83,* 1853–1859.

Ross, R. (1993). The pathogenesis of atherosclerosis: A perspective for the 1990s. *Nature, 362,* 801–809.

Ross, R. (1999). Atherosclerosis—an inflammatory disease. *New England Journal of Medicine, 340,* 115–126.

Roth, D. L., Bachtler, S. D., & Fillingim, R. B. (1990). Acute emotional and cardiovascular effects of stressful mental work during aerobic exercise. *Psychophysiology, 27,* 694–701.

Rousselle, J. G., Blascovich, J., & Kelsey, R. M. (1995). Cardiorespiratory responses under combined psychological and exercise stress. *International Journal of Psychophysiology, 20,* 49–58.

Sanders, V. M., & Straub, R. H. (2002). Norepinephrine, the β-adrenergic receptor, and immunity. *Brain, Behavior, and Immunity, 16,* 290–332.

Santos-Alvarez, J., Goberna, R., & Sanchez-Margalet, V. (1999). Human leptin stimulates proliferation and activation of human circulating monocytes. *Cellular Immunology, 194,* 6–11.

Sapolsky, R. M. (1998). *Why zebras don't get ulcers.* New York: W. H. Freeman.

Sarraf, P., Frederich, R. C., Turner, E. M., Ma, G., Jaskowiak, N. T., Rivet, D. J., . . . Alexander, H. R. (1997). Multiple cytokines and acute inflammation raise mouse leptin levels: Potential role in inflammatory anorexia. *Journal of Experimental Medicine, 185,* 171–175.

Schachinger, V., Britten, M. B., Dimmeler S., & Zeiher, A. M. (2001). NADH/NADPH oxidase p22 phox gene polymorphism is associated with improved coronary endothelial vasodilator function. *European Heart Journal, 22,* 96–101.

Schedlowski, M., Falk, A., Rohne, A., Wagner, T. O., Jacobs, R., Tewes, U., & Schmidt, R. E. (1993). Catecholamines induce alterations of distribution and activity of human natural killer (NK) cells. *Journal of Clinical Immunology, 13,* 344–351.

Schoder, H., Silverman, D. H., Campisi, R., Sayre, J. W., Phelps, M. E., Schelbert, H. R., & Czernin, J. (2000). Regulation of myocardial blood flow response to mental stress in healthy individuals. *American Journal of Physiology: Heart and Circulatory Physiology, 278*(2), H360–H366.

Seals, D. R., & Dinenno, F. A. (2004). Collateral damage: Cardiovascular consequences of chronic sympathetic activation with human aging. *American Journal of Physiology: Heart and Circulatory Physiology, 287,* H1895–H1905.

Serhan, C. N., Yacoubian, S., & Yang, R. (2008). Anti-inflammatory and proresolving lipid mediators. *Annual Review of Pathology, 3,* 279–312.

Sherwood, A., Dolan, C. A., & Light, K. C. (1990). Hemodynamics of blood pressure response during active and passive coping. *Psychophysiology, 27,* 656–668.

Sheu, W. H., Chang, T. M., Lee, W. J., Ou, H. C., Wu, C. M., Tseng, L. N., . . . Lee, I. T. (2008). Effect of weight loss on pro-inflammatory state of mononuclear cells in obese women. *Obesity (Silver Spring), 16,* 1033–1038.

Sies, H. (1997). Oxidative stress: Oxidants and antioxidants. *Experimental Physiology, 82,* 291–295.

Singh, M., Bedi, U. S., Singh, P. P., Arora, R., & Khosla, S. (2009). Leptin and the clinical cardiovascular risk. *International Journal of Cardiology, 140,* 266–271.

Singhai, A. (2005). Endothelial dysfunction: Role in obesity-related disorders and the early origins of CVD. *Proceedings of the Nutrition Society, 64,* 15–22.

Sivonova, M., Zitnanova, I., Hlincikova, L., Skodacek, I., Trebaticka, J., & Durackova, Z. (2004). Oxidative stress in university students during examinations. *Stress, 7,* 183–188.

Smith, D. L., Manning, T. S., & Petruzzello, S. J. (2001). Effect of strenuous live-fire drills on cardiovascular and psychological responses of recruit firefighters. *Ergonomics, 44,* 244–254.

Smith, D. L., & Petruzzello, S. J. (1998). Selected physiological and psychological responses to live-fire drills in different configurations of firefighting gear. *Ergonomics, 41,* 1141–1154.

Smith, D. L., Petruzzello, S. J., Chludzinski, M. A., Reed, J. J., & Woods, J. A. (2005). Selected hormonal and immunological responses to strenuous live-fire firefighting drills. *Ergonomics, 48,* 55–65.

Smith, D. L., Petruzzello, S. J., Kramer, J. M., & Misner, J. E. (1996). Physiological, psychophysical, and psychological responses of firefighters to firefighting training drills. *Aviation, Space, and Environmental Medicine, 67,* 1063–1068.

Soteriades, E., Kales, S. N., Liarokapis, D., Christoudias, S. G., Tucker, S. A., & Christiani, D. (2002). Lipid profile of firefighters over time: Opportunities for prevention. *Journal of Occupational and Environmental Medicine, 44,* 840–846.

Sothmann, M. S., Buchworth, J., Claytor, R. P., Cox, R. H., White-Welkley, J. E., & Dishman, R. K. (1996). Exercise training and the cross-stressor adaptation hypothesis. *Exercise and Sport Sciences Reviews, 24,* 267–287.

Sothmann, M. S., & Kastello, G. K. (1997). Simulated weightlessness to induce chronic hypoactivity of brain norepinephrine for exercise and stress studies. *Medicine & Science in Sports & Exercise, 29,* 39–44.

Sowers, J. R., Whitfield, L. A., Catania, R. A., Stern, N., Tuck, M. L., Dornfeld, L., & Maxwell, M. (1982). Role of the sympathetic nervous system in blood pressure maintenance in obesity. *Journal of Clinical Endocrinology and Metabolism, 54,* 1181–1186.

Spalding, T. W., Jeffers, L. S., Porges, S. W., & Hatfield, B. D. (2000). Vagal and cardiac reactivity to psychological stressors in trained and untrained men. *Medicine & Science in Sports & Exercise, 32,* 581–591.

Spalding, T. W., Lyon, L. A., Steel, D. H., & Hatfield, B. D. (2004). Aerobic exercise training and cardiovascular reactivity to psychological stress in sedentary young normotensive men and women. *Psychophysiology, 41,* 552–562.

Steensberg, A., Fischer, C. P., Keller, C., Moller, K., & Pedersen, B. K. (2003). IL-6 enhances plasma IL-1ra, IL-10, and cortisol in humans. *American Journal of Physiology: Endocrinology and Metabolism, 285,* E433–E437.

Steensberg, A., Toft, A. D., Bruunsgaard, H., Sandmand, M., Halkjaer-Kristensen, J., & Pedersen, B. K. (2001). Strenuous exercise decreases the percentage of type 1 T cells in the circulation. *Journal of Applied Physiology, 9,* 1708–1712.

Stein, P. K., & Boutcher, S. H. (1992). The effect of participation in an exercise training program on cardiovascular reactivity in sedentary middle-aged males. *International Journal of Psychophysiology, 13,* 215–223.

Steptoe, A., Hamer, M., & Chida, Y. (2007). The effects of acute psychological stress on circulating inflammatory factors in humans: A review and meta-analysis. *Brain, Behavior, and Immunity, 21,* 901–912.

Steptoe, A., Owen, N., Kunz-Ebrecht, S., & Mohamed-Ali, V. (2002). Inflammatory cytokines, socioeconomic status, and acute stress responsivity. *Brain, Behavior, and Immunity, 16,* 774–784.

Steptoe, A., Willemsen, G., Owen, N., Flower, L., & Mohamed-Ali, V. (2001). Acute mental stress elicits delayed increases in circulating inflammatory cytokine levels. *Clinical Science, 101,* 185–192.

Stern, A. S., Podlaski, F. J., Hulmes, J. D., Pan, Y. C., Quinn, P. M., Wolitzky, A. G., . . . Gately, M. K. (1990). Purification to homogeneity and partial characterization of cytoxic lymphocyte maturation factor from human B-lymphoblastoid cells. *Proceedings of the National Academy of Sciences of the United States of America, 87,* 6808–6812.

Stunkard, A. J., Faith, M. S., & Allison, K. C. (2003). Depression and obesity. *Biological Psychiatry, 54,* 330–337.

Suarez, E. C., Shiller, A. D., Kuhn, C. M., Schanberg, S., Williams, R. B., Jr., & Zimmermann, E. A. (1997). The relationship between hostility and beta-adrenergic receptor physiology in healthy young males. *Psychosomatic Medicine, 59,* 481–487.

Szabo, A., Brown, T. G., Gauvin, L., & Seraganian, P. (1993). Aerobic fitness does not influence directly heart rate reactivity to mental stress. *Acta Physiologica Hungarica, 81,* 229–237.

Szabo, A., Peronnet, F., Gauvin, L., & Furedy, J. J. (1994). Mental challenge elicits "additional" increases in heart rate during low and moderate intensity cycling. *International Journal of Psychophysiology, 17,* 197–204.

Tang, C. H., Lu, D. Y., Yang, R. S., Tsai, H. Y., Kao, M. C., Fu, W. M., & Chen, Y. F. (2007). Leptin-induced IL-6 production is mediated by leptin receptor, insulin receptor substrate-1, phosphatidylinositol 3-kinase, Akt, NF-κB, and p300 pathway in microglia. *Journal of Immunology, 179,* 1292–1302.

Tate, D. L., Sibert, L., & King, T. (1997). Using virtual environments to train firefighters. *IEEE Computer Graphics and Applications, 17,* 23–29.

Taverniers, J., Van Ruysseveldt, J., Smeets, T., & von Grumbkow, J. (2010). High-intensity stress elicits robust cortisol increases, and impairs working memory and visuo-spatial declarative memory in Special Forces candidates: A field experiment. *Stress, 13*(4), 323–333.

Taylor, M. K., Reis, J. P., Sausen, K. P., Padilla, G. A., Markham, A. E., Potterat, E. G., Drummond, S. P. A. (2008). Trait anxiety and salivary cortisol during free living and military stress. *Aviation, Space, and Environmental Medicine, 79,* 129–135.

Taylor, M. K., Sausen, K. P., Potterat, E. G., Mujica-Parodi, L. R., Reis, J. P., Markham, A. E., . . . Taylor, D. L. (2007). Stressful military training: Endocrine reactivity, performance, and psychological impact. *Aviation, Space, and Environmental Medicine, 78,* 1143–1149.

Throne, L., Bartholomew, J., Craig, J., & Farrar, R. (2000). Stress reactivity in fire fighters: An exercise intervention. *International Journal of Stress Management, 7,* 235–246.

Tosi, M. F. (2005). Innate immune responses to infection. *Journal of Allergy and Clinical Immunology, 116,* 241–249.

Tsigos, C., & Chrousos, G. (2002). Hypothalamic-pituitary-adrenal axis, neuroendocrine factors and stress. *Journal of Psychosomatic Research, 53,* 865–871.

Tsismenakis, A. J., Christophi, C. A., Burress, J. W., Kinney, A. M., Kim, M., & Kales, S. N. (2009). The obesity epidemic and future emergency responders. *Obesity (Silver Spring), 17,* 1648–1650.

Turner, J. R., & Carroll, D. (1985). Heart rate and oxygen consumption during mental arithmetic, a video game, and graded exercise: Further evidence of metabolically-exaggerated cardiac adjustments? *Psychophysiology, 22,* 261–267.

Turner, J. R., Carroll, D., Hanson, J., & Sims, J. (1988). A comparison of additional heart rates during active psychological challenge calculated from upper body and lower body dynamic exercise. *Psychophysiology, 25,* 209–216.

Uchakin, P. N., Tobin, B., Cubbage, M., Marshall, G. Jr., & Sams, C. (2001). Immune responsiveness following academic stress in first-year medical students. *Journal of Interferon and Cytokine Research, 21,* 687–694.

Umeki, S. (1994). Activation factors of neutrophil NADPH oxidase complex. *Life Science, 55,* 1–13.

United States Fire Administration. (2004). *Health and wellness guide* (Publication No. FA-267). Emmitsburg, MD: Federal Emergency Management Agency.

van Doornen, L. J., & de Geus, E. J. (1989). Aerobic fitness and the cardiovascular response to stress. *Psychophysiology, 26,* 17–28.

Vassali, P. (1992). The pathophysiology of tumor necrosis factor. *Annual Review of Immunology, 10,* 411–452.

Vider, J., Laaksonen, D. E., Kilk, A., Atalay, M., Lehtmaa, J., Zilmer, M., & Sen, C. K. (2001). Physical exercise induces activation of NF-κB in human peripheral blood lymphocytes. *Antioxidants and Redox Signaling, 3,* 1131–1137.

Vincent, H. K., Inners, K. E., & Vincent, K. R. (2007). Oxidative stress and potential interventions to reduce oxidative stress in overweight and obesity. *Diabetes, Obesity, and Metabolism, 9,* 813–839.

Violanti, J. M., Burchfiel, C. M., Fekedulegn, D., Andrew, M. E., Dorn, J., Hartley, T. A.,...Miller, D. B. (2009). Cortisol patterns and brachial artery reactivity in a high stress environment. *Psychiatry Research, 169,* 75–81.

von Känel, R., Mills, P. J., Fainman, C., & Dimsdale, J. E. (2001). Effects of psychological stress and psychiatric disorders on blood coagulation and fibrinolysis: A biobehavioral pathway to coronary artery disease? *Psychosomatic Medicine, 63,* 531–544.

Waldstein, S. R., Burns, H. O., Toth, M. J., & Poehlman, E. T. (1999). Cardiovascular reactivity and central adiposity in older African Americans. *Health Psychology,18,* 221–228.

Wannamethee, S. G., Tchernova, J., Whincup, P., Lowe, G. D., Kelly, A., Rumley, A.,...Sattar, N. (2007). Plasma leptin: Associations with metabolic, inflammatory and haemostatic risk factors for cardiovascular disease. *Atherosclerosis, 191,* 418–426.

Wassmann, S., Stumpf, M., Strehlow, K., Schmid, A., Schieffer, B., Böhm, M., & Nickenig, G. (2004). Interleukin-6 induces oxidative stress and endothelial dysfunction by overexpression of the angiotensin II type 1 receptor. *Circulation Research, 94,* 534–541.

Watson, R. R., Moriguchi, S., Jackson, J. C., Werner, L., Wilmore, J. H., & Freund, B. J. (1986). Modification of cellular immune functions in humans by endurance exercise training during beta-adrenergic blockade with atenolol or propranolol. *Medicine & Science in Sports & Exercise, 18,* 95–100.

Webb, H. E., Garten, R. S., McMinn, D. R., Beckman, J. L., Kamimori, G. H., & Acevedo, E. O. (2011). Stress hormones and vascular function in firefighters during concurrent challenges. *Biological Psychology, 87*(1), 152–160.

Webb, H. E., McMinn, D. R., Garten, R. S., Beckman, J. L., Kamimori, G. H., & Acevedo, E. O. (2010). Cardiorespiratory responses of firefighters to a computerized fire strategies and tactics drill during physical activity. *Applied Ergonomics, 41,* 376–381.

Webb, H. E., Weldy, M. L., Fabianke-Kadue, E. C., Orndorff, G. R., Kamimori, G. H., & Acevedo, E. O.

(2008). Psychological stress during exercise: Cardiorespiratory and hormonal responses. *European Journal of Applied Physiology, 104,* 973–981.

Weisberg, S. P., McCann, D., Desai, M., Rosenbaum, M., Leibel, R. L., & Ferrante, A. W., Jr. (2003). Obesity is associated with macrophage accumulation in adipose tissue. *Journal of Clinical Investigation, 112,* 1796–1808.

Willemsen, G., Carrol, D., Ring, C., & Drayson, M. (2002). Cellular and mucosal immune reactions to mental and cold stress: Associations with gender and cardiovascular reactivity. *Psychophysiology, 39,* 222–228.

Wirtz, P. H., Ehlert, F. U., Emini, L., & Suter, T. (2008). Higher body mass index (BMI) is associated with reduced glucocorticoid inhibition of inflammatory cytokine production following acute psychological stress in men. *Psychoneuroendocrinology, 33,* 1102–1110.

Wirtz, P. H., von Känel, R., Emini, L., Suter, T., Fontana, A., & Ehlert, U. (2007). Variations in anticipatory cognitive stress appraisal and differential proinflammatory cytokine expression in responses to acute stress. *Brain, Behavior, and Immunity, 21,* 851–859.

Wittert, G., Stewart, D. E., Graves, M. P., Ellis, M. J., Evans, M., Wells, J. E.,...Espinar, E. A. (1991). Plasma corticotrophin releasing factor and vasopressin responses to exercise in normal man. *Clinical Endocrinology, 35,* 311–317.

Yang, Y., Koh, D., Ng, V., Lee, F. C., Chan, G., Dong, F., & Chia, S. E. (2001). Salivary cortisol levels and work-related stress among emergency department nurses. *Journal of Occupational and Environmental Medicine, 43,* 1011–1018.

Yoon, T., Keller, M. L., De-Lap, B. S., Harkins, A., Lepers, R., & Hunter, S. K. (2009). Sex differences in response to cognitive stress during a fatiguing contraction. *Journal of Applied Physiology, 107,* 1486–1496.

Young, E. A., Abelson, J., & Lightman, S. L. (2004). Cortisol pulsatility and its role in stress regulation and health. *Frontiers in Neuroendocrinology, 25,* 69–76.

Yu, B. H., Dimsdale, J. E., & Mills, P. J. (1999). Psychological states and lymphocyte beta-adrenergic receptor responsiveness. *Neuropsychopharmacology, 21,* 147–152.

Zefferino, R., Facciorusso, A., Lasalvia, M., Narciso, M., Nuzzaco, A., Lucchini, R., & L'Abbate, N. (2006). Salivary markers of work stress in an emergency team of urban police (1 degree step). *Giornale Italiano di Medicina del Lavoro ed Ergonomia, 28,* 472–477.

Zumbach, M. S., Boehme, M. W., Wahl, P., Stremmel, W., Ziegler, R., & Nawroth, P. P. (1997). Tumor necrosis factor increases serum leptin levels in humans. *Journal of Clinical Endocrinology and Metabolism, 82,* 4080–4082.

PART 4

Psychology of Exercise Motivation

Personality and Physical Activity

Ryan E. Rhodes *and* Leila A. Pfaeffli

Abstract

This chapter updates a prior meta-analysis of the relationship between higher-order personality traits and physical activity with new literature, extends the findings to include an appraisal of personality facet or subtraits, evaluates mechanisms mediating between personality and physical activity, and examines evidence for personality as a moderator of physical activity social cognition. Two literature searches were conducted on five key search engines. The first search yielded 370 hits. Nine studies were included in this review update. The second search for lower-order personality traits yielded 1165 hits. Twenty-nine passed the eligibility criteria. Results showed similar findings to the prior review but with considerable heterogeneity. Evidence showed a link between physical activity and the activity facet trait of extraversion. The mediating capacity of social cognitive variables was generally poor. Evidence for personality moderation came from the conscientiousness trait and its interaction with the physical activity intention–behavior relationship. Overall, some lower-order traits may be better predictors of physical activity than their higher-order structures and may moderate motivation.

Key Words: personality, physical activity, exercise, mediator, moderator, social cognitive.

Introduction
Physical Activity and Health

The health benefits of regular moderate physical activity have been well established (Warburton, Nicol, & Bredin, 2006). By contrast, physical inactivity has been linked to all-cause mortality as well as over 25 chronic disease conditions (Bouchard, Shephard, & Stephens, 1994; Warburton, Katzmarzyk, Rhodes, & Shephard, 2007). These include but are not limited to cardiovascular disease, type 2 diabetes, some cancers, and mental health conditions such as depression and anxiety. The general populace is well versed on the general benefits of regular physical activity, yet participation rates remain very low (Canadian Fitness and Lifestyle Research Institute, 2002; U.S. Department of Health and Human Services,

1996). Thus physical activity promotion beyond simple education is a public health priority.

Correlates of Physical Activity

Understanding the modifiable correlates of physical activity is an important first-stage endeavor in developing intervention efforts to promote physical activity participation (Rhodes & Pfaeffli, 2009). Interventions can then target these critical variables with the expectation that changes in them will result in subsequent changes in physical activity (Baranowski, Anderson, & Carmack, 1998). A large body of research has provided evidence that physical activity participation is related to many factors, spanning policy, environmental, social, and personal categories (Trost, Owen, Bauman, Sallis, & Brown, 2002).

While the appeal of identifying modifiable determinants is obvious, an understanding of less modifiable factors (e.g., age, sex, culture, and socioeconomic status) and their impact on population physical activity also has merit. Nonmodifiable factors may represent "at risk" populations who need additional attention or physical activity promotion initiatives. Knowing the mechanisms mediating and reinforcing nonmodifiable correlates may also be important to fully understanding how nonmodifiable factors affect physical activity behavior. These intermediate factors may be critical in attenuating the relationship between nonmodifiable factors and their impact on behavior. One less modifiable factor that has received continued albeit modest attention in exercise and health psychology across the years is personality.

Personality

Personality trait psychology has a long history, and interest in it has waxed and waned over the years (Digman, 1990; McCrae & Costa, 1995). Over the last 20 years, however, there has been a robust reemergence of personality research, stemming from improved psychometric instrumentation (Funder, 2001) and growing evidence that personality is structured similarly across cultures, is extremely heritable, has high temporal (rank order) stability, and does not relate strongly to parental rearing style (McCrae et al., 2000). Personality has numerous definitions, but most encompass the concept that traits are enduring and consistent individual-level differences in tendencies to show consistent patterns of thoughts, feelings, and actions (McCrae et al., 2000). Many researchers further theorize that personality has a biological/genetic basis (Eysenck, 1970; Funder, 2001; McCrae et al., 2000). Thus personality traits are often considered culturally conditioned responses founded on biological predispositions.

While the accumulation of evidence for the enduring nature of personality is clearly an important source of the resurgence in personality research, the improved conceptual basis of personality has likely contributed the most to the contemporary research process. Mid-20th-century personality trait psychology suffered from an abundance of investigator-created traits and independent research agendas (Digman, 1990); thus it was difficult for research to advance with any common theoretical model. A move toward a common higher-order trait taxonomy has helped bridge the gap between specific subtraits and more general factors (Digman, 1990; Goldberg, 1993). Common taxonomies range from two to seven basic factors, but the most popular personality model is a five-factor taxonomy (Digman, 1990). This model suggests that the basic factors of personality structure are neuroticism (tendency to be emotionally unstable, anxious, self-conscious, vulnerable, etc.), extraversion (tendency to be sociable, be assertive, be energetic, seek excitement, experience positive affect, etc.), openness to experience/intellect (tendency to be perceptive, creative, and reflective; to appreciate fantasy and aesthetics; etc.), agreeableness (tendency to be kind, cooperative, altruistic, trustworthy, generous, etc.), and conscientiousness (tendency to be ordered, dutiful, self-disciplined, achievement oriented, etc.). The second most popular, and more established, model of personality is Eysenck's (1970) three-factor model, which includes extraversion and neuroticism traits similar to those of the five-factor model and a psychoticism trait (e.g., tendency toward risk taking, impulsiveness, irresponsibility, manipulativeness, sensation-seeking, tough-mindedness).

These common factors are thought to represent the basic building blocks of personality and to cause the expression of more specific subtraits. Thus individuals high in extraversion may express this higher-order trait through excitement seeking, sociability, a positive outlook, energetic activity, or other outlets that are feasible within and socially conditioned by their environments. An interaction among higher-order factors may also cause the expression of traits of interest. For example, Type A behavior (Jenkins, 1976) may be a combination of high extraversion, high neuroticism, low agreeableness, and high conscientiousness. While it is important to continue to investigate with a higher-order conceptual understanding of personality and behavior, specific, or facet, traits may help define the relationship between personality and specific behaviors (Costa & McCrae, 1992). The greater specificity provided by these facet traits allows for a more precise understanding of personality relationships with an outcome variable; indeed it is this higher level of specificity and its applied value in understanding traits and behavior that defines the facet approach to instrumentation (Costa & McCrae, 1995).

Personality and Physical Activity

Several pathways for how personality interacts with health have been postulated, but Wiebe and Smith's (1997) health behavior model of personality is the most likely one with respect to physical activity behavior. This model suggests that the principal impact of personality on health behaviors is through the quality of one's health practices. More specifically, personality is hypothesized to affect social cognitions (e.g., perceptions, attitudes, norms, and self-efficacy), habits, or social and environmental access to a behavior, which in turn influences the health behavior itself (Ajzen, 1991; McCrae & Costa, 1995; Rhodes, 2006).

Research on personality and physical activity has spanned over 40 years. While early work considered sport performance and the potential impact of physical activity on personality (Eysenck, Nias, & Cox, 1982), more recent approaches have focused on physical activity and the health behavior model. In 2006, Rhodes and Smith reviewed and systematically appraised the relationship between personality and physical activity. That review, however, focused almost entirely on the higher-order traits of the five- and three-factor personality models. The purpose of this chapter is to (1) highlight the results of that prior review but update them with new research published since that paper, (2) extend the review to include an appraisal of facet or subtraits of personality and physical activity, (3) review the evidence for mediating mechanisms of personality, and (4) examine the evidence for personality as a moderator of relationships between physical activity motivation and behavior. We conclude the chapter by providing suggestions for advancing this field of enquiry and highlighting related research in other health behavior domains that may serve as a template for studies of the relationship between personality and physical activity.

Method

The literature search was completed in July, 2009. Databases searched included Web of Science, PsycINFO, PubMed, and Medline. We also conducted manual cross-referencing of bibliographies.

Updating the Rhodes and Smith (2006) Review

To update the Rhodes and Smith (2006) review, we conducted one literature search yielding 370 potential articles. Search words were based on the prior review and included various combinations of the key words *personality, disposition, extraversion, neuroticism, introversion, openness to experience, agreeableness, conscientiousness, Eysenck, Cattell, psychoticism, individual difference, emotional stability, pessimism, optimism, sociability, hardiness,* and *intellect* with *physical activity, exercise, activity,* and *active living.* Studies were eligible if they were

from peer-reviewed scholarly journals, published in English, from 2005 to 2009. Inclusion criteria included studies with adult samples (age 18 years or older) that included a measure of physical activity behavior and a comprehensive personality model or major trait. Studies that used dependent variables such as physiological markers, preferences of physical activity or related factors, stages of change, or social cognitive constructs rather than physical activity behavior were excluded because these are less direct indicators of actual physical activity. In addition, included studies measured physical activity as a discrete or continuous variable and compared active versus inactive groups. Studies that measured the physical activity of athletes or compared groups of athletes were not included because their baselines did not include the absence of activity.

Thirty-four relevant abstracts were read and reviewed by both authors, resulting in addition of nine studies with major personality traits to the Rhodes and Smith (2006) review (see Table 11.1). Consensus was reached in 100% of the cases.

The Review of Lower-Order Personality Traits

A second literature search was conducted to review studies examining lower-order personality traits, which were excluded in Rhodes and Smith (2006). Search words included combinations of the key words *personality, disposition, extraversion, neuroticism, introversion, openness to experience, agreeableness, conscientiousness, excitement seeking, activity, goal driven, industriousness, Type A, Type D, Eysenck, Cattell, psychoticism, individual difference, emotional stability, pessimism, optimism, sociability, hardiness,* and *intellect* with *physical activity, exercise,* and *active living.* The search yielded 1165 potential studies, from 1969–2009. Studies were eligible if they were from peer-reviewed scholarly journals, published in English, and used adult samples (age 18 years or older). Inclusion criteria included studies with a measure of physical activity behavior and a distinct measure of a lower-order personality trait. Fifty-three relevant abstracts were read and reviewed by both authors. Consensus was reached in 100% of the cases. The lower-order personality trait review included 29 peer-reviewed studies and 42 samples (see Table 11.2). One study (Castaneda, Bigatti, & Cronan, 1998) missed in the Rhodes and Smith (2006) paper was found in this second search and was also included in the major-trait review.

Table 11.1. Higher-Order Personality Traits and Physical Activity Behavior—Studies Used to Update Rhodes and Smith (2006) Review

Study	Participants	Design	Personality measure	PA measure	Findings
Castaneda et al. (1998)	197 (71 male, 126 female) members of a large HMO with symptoms of osteoarthritis (mean age: 69.39)	Cross-sectional	NEO-FFI	Self-report of exercise type, frequency, and duration over last 7 days. Kilocalories estimated	Exercisers scored higher on E ($\eta2 = .022$) and lower on N ($\eta2 = .033$) than nonexercisers. No sig. diff. for O, A, or C. In regression analysis, E accounted for 6.7% of variance in total kilocalories.
T. B. Adams & Mowen (2005)	287 government employees (mean age: 45)	Cross-sectional	Previously developed scales (Mowen, 2000)	Self-report items from Mowen (2000) and Behavioral Risk Factor Surveillance System	Exercise was predicted by emotional instability (negative relationship), A (negative relationship), openness to experience, and C ($R2 = .16$ for total model). No effects were found for E.
Conner et al. (2007)	146 undergraduate students	1-month prospective	IPIP	GLTEQ	No sig. relationship found between C and exercise behavior during regular or unusual week.
Huang et al. (2007)	142 adults belonging to a fitness center	Cross-sectional	NEO-PI-R	Self-report exercise frequency questionnaire	Higher scores on five personality factors (emotional stability, E, O, A, C) associated with higher levels of exercise participation ($R^2 = .524$)
Rhodes et al. (2007)	358 adults (mean age of males: 57; mean age of females: 50.6)	2-month prospective	Goldberg's Unipolar Markers: E, N, C	Variation of GLTEQ	No sig. correlations between walking behavior and E, N, or C.

Study	Sample	Design	Personality measure	Exercise measure	Findings
Saklofske et al. (2007)	497 university students (mean age: 24)	Cross-sectional	Short form EQ-I Mini-Marker Scale	Self-report exercise frequency questionnaire	Positive correlations between exercise behavior and overall Emotional Intelligence ($r = .14$), intrapersonal ($r = .10$), interpersonal ($r = .12$), and general mood ($r = .12$). Positive correlations of regular exercise with E ($r = .12$), A ($r = .11$), and C ($r = .11$); negative correlation with N ($r = -.14$); no correlation with O.
Chatzisarantis & Hagger (2008)	180 university students (mean age: 19.4)	5-week prospective	NEO-FFI	Self-report physical activity questionnaire based on GLTEQ	Personality variables explained 5% of variance in PA participation; only C made sig. contribution to this prediction. A was only trait associated with PA participation ($r = .20$). No sig. correlations for O, N, or E.
Ingledew & Markland (2008)	252 office workers (mean age: 40)	Cross-sectional	Public domain scales from IPIP	Self-report exercise participation questionnaire analogous to GLTEQ	No sig. correlations between personality traits and exercise participation. O and C had indirect positive effects on exercise; N had indirect negative effect on exercise.
J. Adams & Nettle (2009)	423 (mean age: 34.7)	Cross-sectional	IPIP	Self-report questionnaire (frequency of moderate and vigorous PA per week)	C was positively associated with frequency of vigorous PA.

Note. GLTEQ = Godin Leisure Time Exercise Questionnaire; IPIP = International Personality Item Pool; NEO-FFI = NEO Five Factor Inventory; NEO-PI-R = Revised NEO Personality Inventory; PA = physical activity.

Table 11.2 Lower-Order Personality Traits and Physical Activity Behavior

Study	Participants	Design	Lower-order trait	Lower-order trait measure	PA measure	Findings
Adams-Campbell et al. (1990)	192 black college freshman (mean age: 18.5)	Cross-sectional	Type A	Framingham scale (Type A Fram); Bortner scale (Type A Bort)	Harvard Alumni Survey self-report leisure-time PA questionnaire	Type A Bort was associated with leisure-time PA among black women. Neither Type A measurement was associated with leisure-time PA among men.
Adams & Mowen (2005)	287 government employees (mean age: 45)	Cross-sectional	Activity	Previously developed scales (Mowen, 2000)	Self-report items from Mowen (2000) and Behavioral Risk Factor Surveillance System	Activity was sig. correlated with exercise.
Allen et al. (2001)	5,115 adults between 18 and 30 years of age participating in CARDIA study	Cross-sectional	Hostility	Cook and Medley Hostility subscale of MMPI	Checklist of forms of exercise and frequency/duration of participation used to create a total intensity score	Association between high hostility and greater PA found in white women only. No correlations found for white men, black men, or black women.
Bogg (2008)	566 adults (college and community samples; mean age: 26)	Cross-sectional	Conscientiousness (conventionality and industriousness)	Checklist by Roberts et al. (2004)	GLTEQ	Small negative relationship between strenuous exercise and conventionality ($r = -.09$). Positive relationship between exercise that produced sweat and industriousness ($r = .17$) and negative relationship between mild exercise and industriousness ($r = -.11$).
Buchman et al. (1991)	207 first-year medical students (mean age: 23.4)	Cross-sectional	Type A	Bortner Short Rating Scale	Self-report questionnaire	Type A correlated negatively with exercise duration ($r = -.021$) in men. No sig correlations for women. In multiple regression analysis, exercise frequency correlated with Type A ($\beta = .156$).
Chatzisarantis & Hagger (2007)	226 university students (mean age: 19.23)	5-week prospective	Mindfulness	MAAS	Self-report	Mindfulness moderated the intention–behavior relationship.

Study	Design	Sample	Personality construct	Personality measure	PA measure	Results
Chen & Fu (2008)	Cross-sectional	499 Taiwanese older adults (mean age: 70.49)	Sociability	3 question items	Self-report PA scale	Two sociability items correlated with PA: "daily contact" (OR = 1.252) and "wish to make friends through leisure activities" (OR = 1.273).
Davis (1990)	Cross-sectional	86 women in exercise group (mean age: 22.92); 72 women in nonexercising group (mean age: 25.46)	Emotional reactivity of N	EPI Neuroticism–Stability scale	Participants identified themselves as exercisers (at least 30 min, 3*week) or nonexercisers	No differences in N between groups.
DePanfilis et al. (2008)	Group weight loss intervention	92 (80 female, 12 male) obese outpatients (mean age: 41.8)	4 temperament dimensions (novelty seeking, harm avoidance, reward dependence, persistence), 3 character dimensions (self-directedness, cooperativeness, self-transcendence)	TCI	Completers (67.4%)—still attending program 6 months after initial evaluation; noncompleters (32.6%)—dropped out or lost at follow-up	Completers showed higher harm avoidance scores than noncompleters. Treatment attendance predicted by high reward dependence scores (OR = .863). No effect for other TCI dimensions.
Eason et al. (2002)	Cross-sectional	227 African American and Hispanic women (mean age: 49.3)	Type A	10-item Activity Temperament Scale	7-day diary, coded with MET code and value using the Compendium of Physical Activities	Higher scores on Activity Temperament Scale were associated with higher PA scores. Weak associations between TABP and total activity (R^2 = .08), leisure activity (R^2 = .02), and inactivity (R^2 = .04).

(Continued)

Table 11.2. (Continued)

Study	Participants	Design	Lower-order trait	Lower-order trait measure	PA measure	Findings
Geers et al. (2009)	136 psychology undergraduate students	Cross-sectional	Dispositional optimism	Revised Life Orientation Test	Aerobic exercise index (frequency and duration)	Optimism scores did not predict aerobic exercise. However, optimism did mediate relationship between goal value and exercise. Greater goal value predicted greater exercise among participants high in optimism ($\beta = .38$) but was not sig. related to exercise among participants low in optimism.
Hershberger et al. (1999)	49 men entering a cardiac rehabilitation program (mean age: 62.4)	Cross-sectional	20 personality variables, including sociability, dominance, capacity for status, social presence, self-acceptance, independence, empathy, responsibility, socialization, self-control, good impression, and communality	California Psychological Inventory	Adherence: % of exercise appointments kept while patient was enrolled in cardiac rehab program	Participants who withdrew from the program ($n = 10$) had sig. lower socialization and good impression scores than adherers. 18 personality variables were nonsig.
Hoyt et al. (2009)	507 university students (mean age: 21.27)	Cross-sectional	6 facets of each of 5 personality domains (N, E, O, A, C)	NEO-PI-R	GLTEQ	Exercise correlated with E4, activity ($\beta = .19$), and C5, self-discipline ($\beta = .017$). 28 personality variables were nonsig.
Kobasa et al. (1982)	137 male middle- and upper-level management personnel of a large utility company	Cross-sectional	Hardiness	Alienation Test (alienation from self and work, control), California Life Goals Evaluation Schedule (challenge)	4-item questionnaire used to create a composite exercise score	No correlation found between hardiness and exercise ($r = .009$).

Study	Sample	Design	Variable	Measure	PA Measure	Findings
Manning & Fusilier (1999)	192 health insurance and manufacturing employees (mean age: 35.29)	1-year prospective	Hardiness	Alienation Test (alienation from self and work, control), External Locus of Control Scale (control), California Life Goals Evaluation Schedule (challenge)	Checklist of forms of exercise and frequency/duration of participation	No correlation found between hardiness and exercise.
Milam et al. (2004)	886 adults with HIV infection	Cross-sectional	Optimism/pessimism	LOT-R	Single self-report item (weekly level of exercising)	No sig. relationships found between optimism or pessimism and exercise.
Milligan et al. (1997)	1,119 18-year-olds	Cross-sectional	Type A	AATABS	Self-report questionnaire	Type A behavior associated with greater PA in males ($p = .002$) but not females. Inactive females scored higher on the hostility subscale compared with active group ($p = .04$).
Musante et al. (1992)	138 adults participating in Project SCAN (mean age: 35.3)	Cross-sectional	Hostility	Cook and Medley Hostility subscale (total hostility); Braefoot et al. composite hostility scale (cynicism, hostile affect, aggressive responding)	Harvard Alumni Survey self-report PA questionnaire; averaged over all 4 visits during a 2.5-year period.	Total and composite hostility were positively correlated with vigorous PA for men ($r = .24$) and women ($r = .19$).
Palomo et al. (2008)	113–300 in several occupations (age ranged from 14 to 60)	12 Cross-sectional samples examining relationships between PA and various instruments with different populations	Dispositional optimism; impulsiveness; Type A; character	LOT; Barratt's Impulsiveness Scale; Type A scale; TCI	Health questionnaire	Propensity for physical exercise and activity was predicted by character ($\beta = .14$) in study II and by optimism ($\beta = .26$) in study VIII. (Character was tested in 1 study; optimism was tested in 7 studies.) No relationship between PA and Type A or impulsiveness.

(Continued)

Table 11.2. (Continued)

Study	Participants	Design	Lower-order trait	Lower-order trait measure	PA measure	Findings
Poppius et al. (1999)	4405 Finnish working men participating in the Helsinki Heart Study	8-year prospective	Sense of coherence	29-item questionnaire	Leisure-time PA measured with 4-point Gothenburg scale	Leisure-time PA positively related with sense of coherence.
Rhodes & Courneya (2000)	209 undergraduate students (mean age: 19.69)	Experimental	Self-monitoring	Self-Monitoring Scale	GLTEQ	No interaction effect involving exercise status (active vs. inactive) and self-monitoring.
Rhodes, Courneya, & Jones (2002)	301 female undergraduate students	2-week prospective	Three facets of N (anxiety, depression, self-reproach), E (positive affect, sociability, activity), and C (order, dependability, goal striving)	NEO-FFI	Study-created measure	Activity predicted exercise independent of intention and E with a sig. effect (β = .33). All other 8 personality variables were nonsig.
Rhodes & Courneya (2003a)	Sample 1: 303 undergraduate students Mean age: 19.99 Sample 2: 272 cancer survivors Mean age: 60.7	Sample 1: 2-week prospective Sample 2: cross-sectional	Three facets of N (anxiety, depression, self-reproach), E (positive affect, sociability, activity), and C (order, dependability, goal striving)	NEO-FFI	GLTEQ	Activity predicted exercise independent of intention, and self-efficacy/perceived behavioral control had a sig. effect (sample 1: β = .20; sample 2: β = .31). 8 personality variables were nonsig.
Rhodes et al. (2004)	298 undergraduate students	2-week prospective	Activity	Goldberg's Unipolar Markers	GLTEQ	Activity had sig. effect on exercise behavior (χ^2 = 0.23).

Study	Sample	Design	Personality variable	Personality measure	PA measure	Findings
Rhodes et al. (2005)	298 undergraduate students (mean age: 19.97)	2-week prospective	Lower-order facet traits of N (irritability, insecurity, emotionality), E (sociability, assertiveness, activity/adventurousness), C (orderliness, reliability, industriousness/ambition)	Goldberg's Unipolar Markers	GLTEQ	Exercise behavior had sig. relationships with sociability ($r = .26$), assertiveness ($r = .25$), activity ($r = .39$), industriousness/ambition ($r = .25$), and insecurity ($r = -.14$). Other 4 personality variables were nonsig.
Rimmele et al. (2009)	18 elite sportsmen; 50 amateur sportsmen; 24 untrained men	Cross-sectional	Competitiveness	CI Sports Orientation Questionnaire	Self-report of weekly frequency/ duration of PA (this helped determine in which group participants were classified)	Elite sportsmen sig. different from amateur sportsmen and untrained men in general and sport-specific competitiveness.
Rutledge & Linden (2000)	127 adults (mean age: 29.2)	3-year prospective	Defensiveness	BIDR (self-deception and impression management)	Self-report avg. weekly hours of exercise and changes in exercise over 3 years	No correlation between exercise and level of self-deception.
Spano (2001)	210 adults (mean age: 36.54)	Cross-sectional	Narcissism	NPI	Frequency of Physical Activity Form (Davis et al., 1993)	Low, positive correlations between narcissism and PA ($r = .22$), indicating that higher levels of narcissism are associated with higher levels of PA.
Welsh et al. (1991)	26 sedentary women (mean age: 35.7); 26 sedentary women (mean age: 36.4)	RCT, 6-week jogging program with 6-month follow-up	Type A	Type A and Type H (hard-driving) scale of Jenkins Activity Survey	Compliance (20–30 min, 3*week) in daily log book	Relationship between compliance to program and Type A ($r = .59$) and Type H ($r = .49$) scores of Jenkins survey. No sig. relationship between Type A and adherence/frequency of runs each week. Type H correlated with exercise sessions attended ($r = .577$).

Note. AATABS = Adolescent/Adult Type A Behaviour Scale; BIDR = Balanced Inventory of Desirable Responding]; CI = Competitiveness Index; EPI = Eysenck Personality Inventory; GLTEQ = Godin Leisure Time Exercise Questionnaire; LOT = [[Life Orientation Test]; LOT-R = Life Orientation Test - revised]; MAAS = Mindful Attention Awareness Scale; MET = metabolic equivalend; MMPI = Minnesota Multiphasic Personality Inventory; NEO-FFI = NEO Five Factor Inventory; NEO-PI-R = Revised NEO Personality Inventory; NPI = Narcissistic Personality Inventory]]; OR = odds ratio; PA = physical activity; TABP = Type A Behavior Pattern]; TCI = Temperament and Character Inventory

The Review of Mediating and Moderating Mechanisms for Personality and Physical Activity

The nine new major-trait studies, the prior studies identified by Rhodes and Smith (2006), and the 29 lower-order-trait studies were then further examined for mediation and moderator relationships. Seventeen studies examined mediation and are presented in Table 11.3. Eleven studies examined moderators and are presented in Table 11.4.

Analysis and Synthesis

For the update to Rhodes and Smith (2006), we have kept the subtopics outlined in that paper where relevant: extraversion, neuroticism, agreeableness, openness to experience/intellect, conscientiousness, gender, age, cultural differences, physical activity mode, and study design. We outline the findings of the prior review, followed by analyses of our new studies since that time. For the review of lower-order traits, we created subtopics where at least three studies had addressed a given factor.

Finally, we review all relevant mechanisms that mediated the personality–physical activity behavior relationship and all personality traits that moderated physical activity behavior. Moderating traits are organized by each personality trait identified (e.g., conscientiousness) in the review. Only moderators of physical activity behavior are considered, given the search criteria (i.e., the dependent variable must be physical activity). Mediating mechanisms are addressed according to the theory used to predict physical activity behavior (e.g., theory of planned behavior). We discuss these studies in terms of a modified approach used by Cerin, Barnett, & Baranowski (2009) that breaks mediator models into tests of action theory, tests of conceptual theory, and simultaneous tests of both action and conceptual theories (i.e., mediated effect). Specifically, the action theory test examines whether the personality trait is related to the proposed mediator, the conceptual theory test examines whether the mediator is linked to physical activity, and the simultaneous test evaluates the extent to which the trait effect is mediated by the mechanisms hypothesized to affect physical activity. Analyses for all papers were based on the significance criterion within the study and on estimates of effect size, where small $r = .10$, medium $r = .30$, and large $r = .50$ (Cohen, 1992).

Results
Update to Rhodes and Smith (2006)

Of the 35 samples included in the Rhodes and Smith (2006) review, 18 were cross-sectional, and 17 were prospective/longitudinal. The personality instruments used by the included samples were as follows: 10 used the Eysenck Personality Inventory (EPI; Eysenck & Eysenck, 1963) or a variant, 10 used the NEO Five Factor Inventory (NEO-FFI; Costa & McCrae, 1992), 3 used Cattell's 16 Primary Factors, 3 used Goldberg's Unipolar Markers, 2 used the Big Five Inventory, 2 used the Minnesota Multiphasic Personality Inventory, and 1 sample each used the Maudsley Personality Inventory, Karolinska Scale of Personality, 300 Adjective List, and 25 Personality Aspects.

Of the nine studies with which the Rhodes and Smith (2006) review was updated, six were cross-sectional and three used prospective designs (see Table 11.1). The five personality traits (extraversion, neuroticism, agreeableness, openness to experience/intellect, and conscientiousness) were measured with various instruments. Two studies used the NEO-FFI, two studies used the International Personality Item Pool, and one study each used the Revised NEO Personality Inventory (NEO-PI-R), Goldberg's Unipolar Markers, the Five Factor Personality Inventory, the short-form EQ-I Mini Marker Scale, and author-derived scales. Physical activity measures included the Godin Leisure Time Exercise Questionnaire (GLTEQ) (two studies), and various forms of self-report instruments (seven studies). Participant sample sizes in the nine studies ranged from 142 to 497.

NEUROTICISM (N)

Rhodes and Smith (2006) identified twenty-one samples with which to evaluate the neuroticism trait in their review and concluded that it had a small (Cohen, 1992) negative relationship with physical activity. The most common measures of N applied were the EPI and the NEO-FFI, but all scales showed roughly equivalent findings. Our literature update included seven additional samples that appraised the relationship between physical activity and N (T. B. Adams & Mowen, 2005; Castaneda et al., 1998; Chatzisarantis & Hagger, 2008; Huang, Lee, & Chang, 2007; Ingledew & Markland, 2008; Rhodes, Courneya, Blanchard, & Plotnikoff, 2007; Saklofske, Austin, Rohr, & Andrews, 2007). Four of these studies found significant negative associations with physical activity

Table 11.3. Mediators of Personality and Physical Activity Behavior

Study	Participants	Design	Personality—mediators examined (measure)	Mediator variables Antecedent variable; Outcome variable	Mediating effect
T. B. Adams & Mowen (2005)	287 government employees (mean age: 45)	Cross-sectional	Emotional instability, A, O, C (Previously developed scales Mowen, 2000)	Emotional instability AV: health motivation OV: exercise, C, O, A AV: body resource needs OV: exercise	Health motivation fully mediated the effects of emotional instability on exercise. C was mediated by body resource needs. No evidence of mediation for O or A.
Bryan & Rocheleau (2002)	210 university students	3-month follow-up	E (EQ-I Mini-Marker Scale)	TPB for aerobic and strength training	Perceived behavioural control mediated the effect of E on aerobic and strength training exercises.
Chatzisarantis & Hagger (2008)	180 university students (mean age: 19.4)	5-week prospective	C (NEO-FFI)	Continuation intention AV: C, E OV: PA	Continuation intentions did not mediate the effects of C and E on PA.
Conner & Abraham (2001)	123 university students (mean age: 21.8)	2-week prospective	C (BFI + NEO-FFI)	TPB AV: C OV: intention, exercise behavior	Effect of C on intention was totally mediated by TPB variables. Effect of C on behavior was partially mediated by TPB variables.
Conner et al. (2007)	146 undergraduate students	1-month prospective	C (IPIP)	Intention and perceived behavioral control AV: C OV: exercise behavior	No effect of C on behavior.
Courneya et al. (1999)	Sample 1: 300 female university students (mean age: 19.6) Sample 2: 67 females in exercise class (mean age: 25)	Sample 1: cross-sectional Sample 2: 11-week prospective	E, N, C (NEO-FFI)	TPB AV: N, C, E OV: exercise behavior	TPB mediated the relationship between N and C and exercise behavior. It did not mediate the relationship between E and exercise behavior.
Courneya et al. (2002)	51 cancer survivors	10-week prospective	NEO-FFI	TPB and demographics	TPB failed to mediate the effect of E on exercise adherence.

(Continued)

Table 11.3. (Continued)

Study	Participants	Personality—mediators examined (measure)	Design	Mediator variables Antecedent variable; Outcome variable	Mediating effect
Hoyt et al. (2009)	507 university students (mean age: 21.27)	Six facets of each of 5 personality domains (N, E, O, A, C) (NEO-PI-R)	Cross-sectional	Attitude and perceived behavioral control AV: activity facet of E OV: exercise behavior	E's activity facet was mediated through attitude and perceived behavioral control.
Ingledew & Markland (2008)	252 office workers	IPIP	Cross-sectional	Motives and Self Determination Theory	N had a direct effect on appearance motives, which affected external regulation and subsequent exercise (−). O had a direct effect on health motives, which had a direct effect on identified regulation and subsequent exercise (+). C had a direct effect on external regulation (−), which had an effect (−) on exercise.
Rhodes et al. (2002)	301 female undergraduate students (mean age: 19.42)	Activity facet of E (NEO-FFI)	1-month prospective	TPB AV: activity OV: exercise behavior	E's activity facet had a sig. effect on exercise behavior when TPB was controlled for.
Rhodes & Courneya (2003a)	Sample 1: 303 undergraduate students (mean age: 19.99) Sample 2: 272 cancer survivors (mean age: 60.7)	Activity facet of E (NEO-FFI)	Sample 1: 2-week prospective Sample 2: cross-sectional	TPB AV: activity OV: exercise behavior	Activity had a sig. effect on exercise behavior when intention, controllability, and self-efficacy were controlled for. Activity appears to account for prediction of exercise beyond one's planned behavior. TPB did not mediate effect of E on intention.
Rhodes et al. (2004)	298 undergraduate students	Activity facet of E (Goldberg's Unipolar Markers)	2-week prospective	TPB AV: activity OV: intention, exercise behavior	Activity had a sig. effect on intention and exercise behavior when TPB was controlled for. TPB did not mediate the effect of activity on intention or behavior.

Study	Sample	Design	Measures	Variables	Findings
Rhodes et al. (2005)	298 undergraduate students (mean age: 19.97)	2-week prospective	Lower-order facet traits of N (irritability, insecurity, emotionality), E (sociability, assertiveness, activity/adventurousness), C (orderliness, reliability, industriousness/ambition) (Goldberg's Unipolar Markers)	TPB AV: industriousness/ambition, activity OV: exercise behavior	TPB mediated the effects of industriousness/ambition on behavior. TPB did not mediate activity.
Rhodes et al. (2007)	358 adults (mean age of males: 57; mean age of females: 50.6)	2-month prospective	E, N, C (Goldberg's Unipolar Markers)	TPB AV: E, N, C DV: exercise behavior	No effect of personality traits on walking behavior.
Rimmele et al. (2009)	18 elite sportsmen; 50 amateur sportsmen; 24 untrained men	Cross-sectional	Competitiveness (CI Sports Orientation Questionnaire)	Competitiveness AV: exercise (elite sportsmen vs. untrained men) OV: stress response	Competitiveness did not mediate group differences in stress response.
Saklofske et al. (2007)	497 university students (mean age: 24)	Cross-sectional	E, N (Short-form EQ-I Mini-Marker Scale)	Emotional intelligence AV: E, N OV: exercise behavior	Emotional intelligence mediated the relationship between personality and exercise behaviour.
Yeung & Hemsley (1997)	46 women	8-week aerobics program	EPQ	Self-efficacy	Self-efficacy failed to mediate the relationship between E and adherence.

Note. AV = antecedent variable; BFI = Big Five Inventory; CI = Competitiveness Index DV = dependent variable; IPIP = International Personality Item Pool; NEO-FFI = NEO Five Factor Inventory; NEO-PI-R = Revised NEO Personality Inventory; OV = outcome variable; PA = physical activity; TPB = theory of planned behavior.

Table 11.4. Moderators of Personality and Physical Activity Behavior

Study	Participants	Design	Personality moderator (measure)	Moderator Independent variable: Dependent variable:	Moderating effect
Allen et al. (2001)	5,115 adults between 18 and 30 years of age participating in CARDIA study	Cross-sectional	Hostility (Cook and Medley Hostility subscale of MMPI)	Hostility IV: social support DV: exercise behavior	High-hostile men exercised more if they had high support than if they had low support. For women, finding was in the same direction but nonsig.
Chatzisarantis & Hagger (2007)	226 university students (mean age: 19.23)	5-week prospective	Mindfulness (MAAS)	Mindfulness IV: intention DV: exercise behavior	Mindfulness moderated the intention–behavior relationship. Intention predicted PA among mindful individuals but not among less mindful individuals. Habitual binge drinking obstructed PA intention among individuals acting less mindfully.
Chatzisarantis & Hagger (2008)	180 university students (mean age: 19.4)	5-week prospective	C (NEO-FFI)	C IV: continuation intention of failure DV: PA participation	C and perceived achievement moderated effects of continuation intentions of failure on PA participation. Continuation intentions of failure predicted PA participation among conscientious individuals but not among those lower in C. E was also examined but showed no effect.
Conner et al. (2007)	146 undergraduate students	Cross-sectional, surveys completed during a regular week and after an unusual week (reading week)	C (IPIP)	C IV: intention DV: exercise behavior performed in unusual context	Among high intenders, participants high in C were more likely to maintain exercise behaviors during reading week compared with a normal week. High intenders low in C showed sig. drops in exercise during reading week compared with a normal week.

Study	Sample	Design	Personality construct (measure)	Variables	Findings
Geers et al. (2009)	136 psychology undergraduate students	Cross-sectional	Dispositional optimism (Revised Life Orientation Test)	Goal value IV: optimism DV: exercise behavior	Greater goal value predicted greater exercise among participants high in optimism. Goal value was not sig. related to exercise among persons low in optimism
Giacobbi et al. (2006)	48 community-dwelling individuals with physical disabilities (mean age: 27.9)	Repeated-measures, 8 days	N (NEO-FFI)	N IV: exercise DV: affect	N moderated exercise–affect relationship. Participants with high N were more likely to have more positive and less negative affect on days when they exercised more.
Hoyt et al. (2009)	507 university students (mean age: 21.27)	Cross-sectional	Anxiety facet of N (NEO-PI-R)	Anxiety facet trait (N1) IV: intention DV: exercise behavior	N1 anxiety independently moderated intention–behavior relationship, indicating that intention–behavior relationship is smaller under higher levels of anxiety. C and E did not moderation intention–behavior relationship.
Rhodes & Courneya (2000)	209 undergraduate students (mean age: 19.69)	Experimental	Self-monitoring (Self-Monitoring Scale)	Self-monitoring IV: message content DV: exercise status	No interaction effect involving exercise status (active vs. inactive) and self-monitoring.
Rhodes, Courneya, & Hayduk(2002)	300 undergraduate students (mean age: 19.99)	2-week prospective	E, N, C (NEO-FFI)	N, E IV: subjective norm DV: intention E IV: intention DV: exercise behavior C IV: affective attitude DV: intention C IV: intention DV: exercise behavior	Participants high in E and C had stronger intention–behavior relationships than those lower in E and C. Participants lower in N had stronger intention–behavior relationships than those higher in N.

(Continued)

Table 11.4. (Continued)

Study	Participants	Design	Personality moderator (measure)	Moderator Independent variable: Dependent variable:	Moderating effect
Rhodes et al. (2005)	298 undergraduate students (mean age: 19.97)	2-week prospective	Lower-order facet traits of N (irritability, insecurity, emotionality), E (sociability, assertiveness, activity/adventurousness), C (orderliness, reliability, industriousness/ambition) (Goldberg's Unipolar Markers)	Industriousness/ambition IV: intention DV: exercise behavior Irritability IV: affective attitude DV: exercise behavior Insecurity IV: subjective norm DV: exercise behavior Activity/adventurousness IV: perceived control of behavior DV: intention	High levels of industriousness/ambition resulted in a stronger effect of intention on behavior than moderate or low levels of industriousness/ambition. High levels of irritability resulted in stronger effect of affective attitude on behavior than moderate or low levels of irritability. High levels of insecurity resulted in stronger effect of subjective norm on behavior than moderate or low level.. High levels of activity/adventurousness resulted in stronger effect of perceived control of behavior on intention than moderate or low levels.
Rhodes et al. (2007)	358 adults (mean age of males: 57; mean age of females: 50.6)	2-month prospective	C (Goldberg's Unipolar Markers)	C IV: intention DV: walking behavior	C moderated relationship between intention and walking. Participants high and medium in C had a larger effect of intention on walking than those low in C.

Note. DV = dependent variable; IPIP = International Personality Item Pool;IV = independent variable; MAAS = Mindful Attention Awareness Scale MMP = Minnesota Multiphasic Personality Inventory; NEO-FFI = NEO Five Factor Inventory; NEO-PI-R = Revised NEO Personality Inventory; PA = physical activity.

(T. B. Adams & Mowen, 2005; Castaneda et al., 1998; Huang et al., 2007; Saklofske et al., 2007) in the small effect size range. All personality measures followed the five-factor model conceptualization and comprised either adjective markers or the NEO. Thus the findings generally support a small relationship ($r = -.10$) between N and physical activity, and differences across samples do not appear to be based on the instrumentation applied.

EXTRAVERSION (E)

Twenty-three samples were available with which to evaluate the extraversion trait in the Rhodes and Smith (2006) review. The result was a point estimate $r = .23$, suggesting that E is a correlate of physical activity with a small-to-medium effect. Instrumentation differences did not appear to affect the overall results considerably when comparing the NEO-FFI with the EPI. In the literature update, seven additional studies evaluated E and its relationship with physical activity (T. B. Adams & Mowen, 2005; Castaneda et al., 1998; Chatzisarantis & Hagger, 2008; Huang et al., 2007; Ingledew & Markland, 2008; Rhodes et al., 2007; Saklofske et al., 2007). Of these, three showed E as significantly correlated with physical activity, with coefficient rs ranging from .33 to.12. The results point out the heterogeneity of findings with this trait and the potential presence of moderators. Similar to N, E has been measured in physical activity studies over the past four years with either NEO or adjective marker conceptualizations within the five-factor model.

OPENNESS TO EXPERIENCE/INTELLECT (O)

Twelve samples in the Rhodes and Smith (2006) review included the openness to experience/intellect trait of the five-factor model of personality. Of these 12 studies, only two found this trait to be a statistically significant correlate of physical activity (Courneya, Friedenreich, Sela, Quinney, & Rhodes, 2002; Rhodes, Courneya, & Jones, 2003). Rhodes and Smith (2006) concluded that this factor was unrelated to physical activity. This review update includes an additional six studies that evaluated O and physical activity (T. B. Adams & Mowen, 2005; Castaneda et al., 1998; Chatzisarantis & Hagger, 2008; Huang et al., 2007; Ingledew & Markland, 2008; Saklofske et al., 2007). The findings are similar to those of Rhodes and Smith (2006). Specifically, two studies showed support for a correlation (T. B. Adams & Mowen, 2005; Huang et al., 2007), while the remaining four found null effects. Overall, the results suggest O is not related to physical activity.

AGREEABLENESS (A)

Rhodes and Smith (2006) found no evidence for a relationship between the agreeableness trait and physical activity among 11 samples. In the current update six studies appraised this relationship (T. B. Adams & Mowen, 2005; Castaneda et al., 1998; Chatzisarantis & Hagger, 2008; Huang et al., 2007; Ingledew & Markland, 2008; Saklofske et al., 2007). Four of these studies found a significant but small positive relationship with physical activity (T. B. Adams & Mowen, 2005; Chatzisarantis & Hagger, 2008; Huang et al., 2007; Saklofske et al., 2007). When combined with the prior review, the majority (13/17) of studies still identify a null correlation between A and physical activity, yet there appears to be more heterogeneity than previously stated. The possible presence of moderators should be examined.

CONSCIENTIOUSNESS (C)

Of the 12 samples that permitted an evaluation of the relationship between the conscientiousness trait and physical activity in Rhodes and Smith (2006), nine showed significant positive findings, and the point estimate was $r = .20$. Nine additional studies are now available with which to assess the relationship between C and physical activity (J. Adams & Nettle, 2009; T. B. Adams & Mowen, 2005; Castaneda et al., 1998; Chatzisarantis & Hagger, 2008; Conner, Rodgers, & Murray, 2007; Huang et al., 2007; Ingledew & Markland, 2008; Rhodes et al., 2007; Saklofske et al., 2007). Among these studies, five showed a significant association between C and physical activity (J. Adams & Nettle, 2009; T. B. Adams & Mowen, 2005; Castaneda et al., 1998; Huang et al., 2007; Saklofske et al., 2007). Although the small estimated effect size points to some heterogeneity among the findings, the majority of studies (14/21) support a positive relationship between C and physical activity.

GENDER

Rhodes and Smith (2006) identified six studies that directly compared correlations between personality and physical activity by gender. Gender variation for E was mixed, with three studies showing no difference (Arai & Hisamichi, 1998; DeMoor, Beem, Stubbe, Boomsma, & DeGeus, 2006; Szabo, 1992) and three studies indicating a gender difference (Kjelsas & Augestad, 2004; Sale, Guppy, & El-Sayed, 2000; van Loon, Tijhuis, Surtees, & Ormel, 2001). Among the gender-discrepant findings, two studies found significant relations between E and physical activity for females but not males (Kjelsas & Augestad, 2004; Sale et al., 2000), while the other study found the opposite (van Loon et al., 2001). Most important, the two large-scale population assessments of E by gender indicated no gender differences (Arai & Hisamichi, 1998; DeMoor et al., 2006). The findings for N showed less gender discrepancy than was observed for E. Specifically, across four studies, including the two large-scale population surveys, there were no gender differences (Arai & Hisamichi, 1998; DeMoor et al., 2006; Sale et al., 2000; van Loon et al., 2001). No studies had compared males and females on the five-factor traits of A, O, and C.

Our literature update identified one study that allowed for gender comparison of men and women and that used the five-factor taxonomy (Castaneda et al., 1998). That study did not use direct statistical tests for gender comparison, but effect sizes were trivial across the five-factor traits by gender, with the possible exception of O, which had a larger relationship with physical activity for women than for men. As the prior review also concluded, more evidence is needed before conclusions can be drawn about gender as a moderator of personality and physical activity.

AGE

Only one study in Rhodes and Smith (2006) covered a wide enough age spectrum to permit evaluation of young, middle-aged, and older adults (DeMoor et al., 2006). No age-related differences were identified for E or N despite the age-related decline in physical activity. This was also found in the analysis of specific ages across studies. It was noted that the personality and physical activity literature is biased toward young adults but that the results of existing studies generally suggested that age is not a moderator.

Our literature update included samples of young adults (Chatzisarantis & Hagger, 2008; Conner et al., 2007; Saklofske et al., 2007), middle-aged adults (J. Adams & Nettle, 2009; T. B. Adams & Mowen, 2005; Huang et al., 2007; Ingledew & Markland, 2008; Rhodes et al., 2007) and older adults (Castaneda et al., 1998). Similar to the prior review, no discernible difference in personality–physical activity relationships by these age groups was identified. This supports the temporal stability inherent in personality research generally (McCrae et al., 2000) and suggests that personality may be a systematic and continual correlate of activity.

COUNTRY/CULTURE

Eight countries were represented in the prior review: Canada, the United States, the United Kingdom, the Netherlands, Japan, Norway, Germany, and South Africa. Overall, E was positively related to physical activity in 11 of 12 Canadian samples, three of four U.S studies, one of four U.K. studies, both of the Netherlands studies, and the studies from Japan, Germany, and Norway. N and C relationships with physical activity were relatively commensurate by country. Rhodes and Smith (2006) tentatively concluded that a null relationship between E and physical activity in the U.K. might represent a discrepant finding, but they observed that null results could also be due to low sample size and thus limited power.

Our update to this literature featured three samples from Canada (Conner et al., 2007, Rhodes et al., 2007; Saklofske et al., 2007) and the U.S. (J. Adams & Nettle, 2009; T. B. Adams & Mowen, 2005; Castaneda et al., 1998), two samples from the U.K. (Chatzisarantis & Hagger, 2008; Ingledew & Markland, 2008), and one mixed sample (Huang et al., 2007). While the findings showed some heterogeneity within country for Canada and the U.S., both U.K. samples had null findings for the relationship of the five-factor model to physical activity. This is in agreement with the findings of the prior review and suggests there may be cultural factors in the U.K. that affect personality–physical activity relationships compared with other countries. Future analyses by country with matched sample sizes would be helpful in evaluating the effect of culture on these relationships.

PHYSICAL ACTIVITY MODE

Five studies were identified in Rhodes and Smith (2006) as examining personality with respect to a particular mode or modes of physical activity. Overall, E was positively associated with aerobic activity in three of five possible evaluations, and N was negatively associated in one of three possible evaluations. The most detailed evaluation of mode and personality was conducted by Howard, Cunningham, and Rechnitzer (1987). These researchers found that high-E individuals were more likely to engage in swimming, aerobic conditioning, dancing, and tennis. By contrast, lower-E individuals were more inclined to engage in gardening and home improvement. No differences were identified for walking, jogging, golf, and cycling.

The update to the prior review included only one study that did not measure physical activity at a general level without consideration of mode. Rhodes et al. (2007) measured leisure-time walking behavior and found no relationship with N, E, or C. This result complement those of Howard et al. (1987) but also demonstrates the paucity of research investigating personality by physical activity mode. The results of these studies are interesting and may have implications for physical activity prescription and intervention tailoring (Rhodes, 2006). More work is needed on this topic to reach definitive conclusions.

STUDY DESIGN

The Rhodes and Smith (2006) review encompassed studies that ranged from cross-sectional to prospective with a length of 46 years. Overall, 15 studies were cross-sectional and 13 were prospective. For the N factor there was a summary r of $-.15$ for the cross-sectional design and a summary r of $-.10$ for prospective designs. For E, the summary rs were .24 for the cross-sectional design and .21 for prospective designs, suggesting a minimal difference. Similar null differences were observed for C. Thus Rhodes and Smith concluded that personality and physical activity relations are robust to static or prospective designs.

Our updated literature featured six cross-sectional investigations (J. Adams & Nettle, 2009; T. B. Adams & Mowen, 2005; Castaneda et al., 1998; Huang et al., 2007; Ingledew & Markland, 2008; Saklofske et al., 2007) and three short-term prospective studies (Chatzisarantis & Hagger, 2008; Conner et al., 2007; Rhodes et al., 2007). Similar to the prior review, no clearly identifiable differences by design were present. However, personality failed to correlate with physical activity in all of the prospective studies, which had follow-ups of two months or less. Thus longitudinal studies evaluating personality and physical activity across the life span are needed.

Lower-Order Traits and Physical Activity

The review of lower-order traits and physical activity included 29 studies with 42 unique samples. Sample designs were cross-sectional ($N = 30$), prospective/longitudinal ($N = 8$), and experimental ($N = 4$). Sample sizes ranged from 26 to 5,115, and participants included university students ($N = 11$), employed adults ($N = 6$), and clinical populations ($N = 4$). Most samples examined both sexes ($N = 31$), while 5 samples examined women only and 4 samples examined men only.

Lower-order traits were included in the results section if three or more studies examined the trait. These traits were Type A ($N = 6$), optimism ($N = 3$), industriousness ($N = 4$), sociability ($N = 6$), and activity ($N = 6$). The excluded traits included hardiness (Kobasa, Maddi, & Puccetti, 1982; Manning & Fusilier, 1999) and hostility (Allen, Markovitz, Jacobs, & Knox, 2001; Musante, 1992), which were examined in two studies each. Other excluded traits were examined in one study each, including character (Palomo, Beninger, Kostrzewa, & Archer, 2008), pessimism (Milam, Richardson, Marks, Kemper, & McCutchan, 2004), conventionality (Bogg, Voss, Wood, & Roberts, 2008), competitiveness (Rimmele et al., 2009), narcissism (Spano, 2001), self-discipline (Rhodes, Courneya, & Jones, 2005), assertiveness (Rhodes et al., 2005), insecurity (Rhodes et al., 2005), emotional reactivity (Davis, 1990), sense of coherence (Poppius, Tenkanen, Kalimo, & Heinsalmi, 1999), harm avoidance (DePanfilis et al., 2008), reward dependence (DePanfilis et al., 2008), mindfulness (Chatzisarantis & Hagger, 2007), self-monitoring (Rhodes & Courneya, 2000), and defensiveness (Rutledge & Linden, 2000).

Type A was measured with various instruments, including the Activity Temperament Scale ($N = 1$), Adolescent/Adult Type A Behaviour Scale ($N = 1$), Jenkins Activity Survey ($N = 1$), and Bortner Short Rating Scale ($N = 2$). Optimism was measured consistently across studies with the Life Orientation Test ($N = 3$). Industriousness was measured with various instruments, including a checklist, NEO-PI-R, NEO-FFI, and Goldberg's Unipolar Markers, each of which was used in one study. Sociability was measured with various instruments, including the California Psychological Inventory ($N = 1$), author-derived items ($N = 1$), NEO-PI-R ($N = 1$), NEO-FFI ($N = 2$), and Goldberg's Unipolar Markers ($N = 1$). The activity personality trait was assessed using instruments such as NEO-PI-R ($N = 1$), NEO-FFI ($N = 2$), Goldberg's Unipolar Markers ($N = 2$), and author-derived scales ($N = 1$). Across these five lower-order traits, physical activity was measured using self-report (questionnaires or diaries; $N = 9$), GLTEQ ($N = 6$), compliance or adherence to program ($N = 2$), Harvard Alumni Survey ($N = 1$), aerobic exercise index ($N = 1$), health questionnaire ($N = 1$), and the Frequency of Physical Activity Form ($N = 1$).

TYPE A

The concept of Type A personality gained popularity from its association with coronary heart disease (Jenkins, 1976). Type A personality is marked by a blend of competitiveness and hostility with agitated behavior and continual movement patterns; thus physical activity could conceivably be a natural extension of Type A personality. Our review identified six studies that appraised the relationship between Type A and physical activity (Adams-Campbell, Washburn, & Haile, 1990; Buchman, Sallis, Criqui, Dimsdale, & Kaplan, 1990; Eason, Masse, Tortolero, & Kelder, 2002; Milligan et al., 1997; Palomo et al., 2008; Welsh, Labbe, & Delaney, 1991). These studies used a mix of measures and ranged in sample size from 26 to 583. Five of the six studies showed some significant positive association between Type A and physical activity, with effect sizes in the small-to-medium range (Adams-Campbell et al., 1990; Buchman et al., 1990; Eason et al., 2002; Milligan et al., 1997; Welsh et al., 1991). The one discrepant study (Palomo et al., 2008) had an unreported sample size and thus it is difficult to assess its quality in relation to the other studies. Some of the findings suggest heterogeneity. For example, Adams-Campbell et al. (1990) found that Type A was not related to physical activity among men, while Milligan et al. (1997) found the opposite. Eason et al. (2002) also found that Type A was related to total activity and leisure activity but not to household activity or sedentary behavior. Additional and sustained research is needed to evaluate whether Type A individuals engage in certain modes of activity (e.g., competitive sports) more than other modes. Despite limited research, the evidence suggests that Type A personality is positively associated with physical activity.

DISPOSITIONAL OPTIMISM

Dispositional optimism is defined as generalized expectations of positive outcomes. It stands to reason that individuals with high optimism would conceivably hold higher regard for the positive health benefits of physical activity and thus participate more than their more pessimistic (or less optimistic) counterparts. The trait has been evaluated in three studies within the exercise domain (Geers, Wellman, & Lassiter, 2009; Milam et al., 2004; Palomo et al., 2008), with samples of undergraduate students, employed adults, and HIV rehabilitation patients. In all cases, there was no support for optimism as a correlate of physical activity. Thus while the current literature is scant, dispositional optimism seems unlikely to be related to forms of exercise.

ACTIVITY FACET OF EXTRAVERSION

The NEO-PI-R has six underlying facet traits that provide more precision than the five factor

structure and specificity to key personality domains underlying the five-factor model (Costa & McCrae, 1995). These have been applied to physical activity either in their full form (Hoyt, Rhodes, Hausenblas, & Giacobbi, 2009) or an abbreviated form (Rhodes & Courneya, 2003a). Among these facets, the activity facet of extraversion has emerged as the best predictor in multivariate analyses. Individuals high in the activity subtrait are typically "high energy" and fast talking, with a disposition toward a "fast" lifestyle and keeping busy as opposed to a more laissez faire disposition. While the facet is organized under E, it also has been suggested as a subtrait of C due to the goal achievement and organizational properties necessary for this trait to manifest (Costa & McCrae, 1995). The energy, organizational, and self-regulatory demands could conceivably make regular physical activity a behavior of choice for individuals ranked high in the trait.

Our literature review identified six studies that have applied the activity trait to physical activity (T. B. Adams & Mowen, 2005; Hoyt et al., 2009; Rhodes & Courneya, 2003a; Rhodes, Courneya, & Jones, 2002, 2004; Rhodes et al., 2005). In all cases, the trait showed a correlation with behavior, with medium-to-large effect sizes ($r = .24$ to $r = .52$). More compelling, the three tests that directly compared the predictive capacity of activity against E for physical activity showed the superiority of the activity trait (T. B. Adams & Mowen, 2005; Rhodes & Courneya, 2003a; Rhodes, Courneya, & Jones, 2002). The one potential caveat, outlined by Rhodes and colleagues (2004), when using this trait is whether some of its measurement variance is simply a description of physical activity itself. An item that says "I am an active person" could be construed as an assessment of physical activity. A correlation between two measures of physical activity would hardly be informative in any causal sense. The one study to test this concern found no difference when this item was removed from the activity measure, so it appears to not affect the findings (Rhodes et al., 2004). Overall, the results suggest that E's activity facet trait is a reliable and strong predictor of physical activity.

INDUSTRIOUSNESS FACET OF
CONSCIENTIOUSNESS

While multivariate assessments of five-factor trait structures have favored the activity trait of E, the industriousness/ambition facet of conscientiousness has received attention in four studies (Bogg, 2008; Hoyt et al., 2009; Rhodes, Courneya, &

Jones, 2002; Rhodes et al., 2005). The trait comprises aspects of striving for achievement and self-discipline, and a natural extension of this type of disposition could be regular exercise, given its challenge, impact on health and appearance, and self-regulatory demands. Three of the four studies found a significant bivariate relationship between this trait and behavior (Hoyt et al., 2009; Rhodes, Courneya, & Jones, 2002; Rhodes et al., 2005), but only one study found support in a multivariate analysis with other traits (Hoyt et al., 2009). Thus while there is evidence that industriousness/ambition is related to physical activity, it may not be an independent predictor when considered with other personality traits such as E's activity facet trait.

SOCIABILITY

E's sociability facet trait is often considered its cornerstone (Costa & McCrae, 1995). People high in sociability prefer the company of others and gravitate to social situations. The social component that accompanies many physical activities could make for a logical outlet among highly sociable people. Sociability has been assessed for its relationship with physical activity in six studies (Chen & Fu, 2008; Hershberger, Robertson, & Markert, 1999; Hoyt et al., 2009; Rhodes & Courneya, 2003a; Rhodes, Courneya, & Jones, 2002; Rhodes et al., 2005). Only two of these studies supported a relationship between sociability and physical activity (Hershberger et al., 1999; Rhodes et al., 2005). These two studies were discrepant in their samples (undergraduates vs. cardiac rehabilitation patients), the measures employed, and the type of behavior assessed (exercise frequency vs. adherence to a program); thus drawing conclusions is difficult at this time.

Mediators of Personality and Physical Activity

This review also examined mediation of the relationship between personality and physical activity. Seventeen studies looked for mediation variables (see Table 11.3). Most studies used the theory of planned behavior to test for mediation ($N = 15$). Other theories used included self-determination theory ($N = 1$) and self-efficacy ($N = 1$). Of the 17 studies examining mediation, 11 studies came from the Rhodes and Smith (2006) review, and six studies were from the update to that review (see Table 11.1). These studies assessed mediation of the higher-order personality traits. Six studies examined mediation of lower-order personality and physical

activity (see Table 11.2), which included activity ($N = 5$), industriousness/ambition ($N = 1$), and competitiveness ($N = 1$).

THEORY OF PLANNED BEHAVIOR

Personality theorists and social psychologists generally agree that behavioral action is unlikely to arise directly from personality (Ajzen, 1991; Bandura, 1998; Eysenck, 1970; McCrae & Costa, 1995; McCrae et al., 2000; Rhodes, 2006). Instead, personality is thought to influence behavioral perceptions, expectations, and cognitions. The theory of planned behavior (TPB; Ajzen, 1991) has been the leading model to test this assumption in the physical activity domain, with 14 samples (Bryan & Rocheleau, 2002; Chatzisarantis & Hagger, 2008; Conner & Abraham, 2001; Conner et al., 2007; Courneya, Bobick, & Schinke, 1999; Courneya et al., 2002; Hoyt, Rhodes, Hausenblas, & Giacobbi, 2009; Rhodes & Courneya, 2003a; Rhodes et al., 2007; Rhodes, Courneya, & Jones, 2002; Rhodes et al., 2004, 2005).

TPB proposes that the proximal antecedent of behavior is one's intention to act. Intention represents the summary motivation (e.g., willingness to try hard) for that behavior and it is proposed to be influenced by ones' affective (e.g., enjoyment) and instrumental (e.g., utility) evaluations of that behavior, which comprise affective and instrumental attitudes, respectively; one's perceived pressure to act, which is manifest in subjective norms (i.e., perceived pressure from others to perform a behaviour); and the perception of one's capability to enact the behavior independent of behavior motivation (Rhodes & Courneya, 2003b), which is considered perceived behavioral control. The relationship between personality and TPB is specific. According to Ajzen (1991), personality should affect behavior through the constructs of attitude, subjective norm, and perceived behavioral control. Thus, TPB should mediate relations between personality and physical activity.

Using Cerin and colleagues' template for assessing mediation (Cerin & Mackinnon, 2008), the personality traits under consideration were linked to physical activity in 12 of 14 samples (Bryan & Rocheleau, 2002; Chatzisarantis & Hagger, 2008; Conner & Abraham, 2001; Courneya et al., 1999; Courneya et al., 2002; Hoyt et al., 2009; Rhodes & Courneya, 2003a; Rhodes, Courneya, & Jones, 2002; Rhodes et al., 2004, 2005). Among these 12 samples, the action theory test (of whether personality relates to TPB constructs) was supported in all but one of these samples (Chatzisarantis & Hagger, 2008) and the conceptual theory test (of whether TPB relates to behavior) was supported in all samples. The simultaneous mediation test, however, was supported in only two samples (Bryan & Rocheleau, 2002; Hoyt et al., 2009). In these cases extraversion was mediated through perceived behavioral control (Bryan & Rocheleau, 2002), and E's activity facet was mediated through attitude and perceived behavioral control (Hoyt et al., 2009).

The remaining tests showed evidence for only partial mediation of the constructs of E (Courneya et al., 1999; Courneya et al., 2002; Rhodes, Courneya, & Jones, 2002), E's activity trait (Rhodes & Courneya, 2003a; Rhodes, Courneya, & Jones, 2002; Rhodes et al., 2004, 2005), and conscientiousness (Chatzisarantis & Hagger, 2008; Conner & Abraham, 2001). Among the studies that provided evidence for partial mediation, E's activity facet had some of its effect through attitude (Rhodes & Courneya, 2003a; Rhodes, Courneya, & Jones, 2002; Rhodes et al., 2004) and perceived behavioral control (Rhodes & Courneya, 2003a; Rhodes, Courneya, & Jones, 2002). Overall, the results suggest that TPB does not effectively mediate personality.

Personality Moderators of Physical Activity

The final subtopic concerns personality moderators of physical activity. Of the studies examined in this review and in Rhodes and Smith (2006), 11 examined moderation. Three studies came from the update on major traits (see Table 11.1), while seven came from the lower-order-trait review (see Table 11.2). One study came from the Rhodes and Smith (2006) review. Traits assessed in these 11 studies included conscientiousness ($N = 6$), extraversion ($N = 4$), and neuroticism ($N = 3$).

CONSCIENTIOUSNESS

The effect of C on the relationship between intention and physical activity behavior has been evaluated in six studies (Chatzisarantis & Hagger, 2008; Conner et al., 2007; Hoyt et al., 2009; Rhodes et al., 2007; Rhodes, Courneya, & Hayduk, 2002; Rhodes et al., 2005). It has been theorized that people who are more conscientious are more likely to act on their good intentions. Five of these six studies have supported this moderation effect (Chatzisarantis & Hagger, 2008; Conner et al., 2007; Rhodes et al., 2007; Rhodes, Courneya, & Hayduk, 2002; Rhodes et al., 2005). Thus the evidence is fairly robust to suggest that high-C

individuals have stronger intention–behavior relationships than those low in C. Rhodes et al. (2005) also investigated this effect using subtraits of C. In this analysis, industriousness/ambition and not organization or reliability was the significant moderator. This provides some insight into how C may affect intention–behavior relations. It may be that the disposition toward achievement helps high-C individuals keep to their original physical activity plans. However, that the other facet-level analysis of C (Hoyt et al., 2009) yielded null results, so more research is needed to evaluate the reliability of Rhodes et al.'s findings.

EXTRAVERSION

The intention–physical activity relationship has also been investigated with E as a moderator. The theory behind this proposed relationship is that individuals high on E may facilitate their intentions by gravitating more toward active environments than more introverted individuals do. Four studies have evaluated E as a moderator of intention–behavior relations (Chatzisarantis & Hagger, 2008; Hoyt et al., 2009; Rhodes, Courneya, & Hayduk, 2002; Rhodes et al., 2005). Three of these studies found support for moderation (Hoyt et al., 2009; Rhodes, Courneya, & Hayduk, 2002; Rhodes et al., 2005), but of these, two showed that the effect did not hold when other personality traits were considered in a multivariate equation (Hoyt et al., 2009; Rhodes et al., 2005). It appears that E may moderate the intention–behavior relationship but is not the dominant or independent personality trait in this equation.

NEUROTICISM

N represents maladaptive feeling states, and it stands to reason that individuals high on N could have more difficulty holding to good intentions with respect to physical activity than their more emotionally stable counterparts. N has been evaluated as a moderator of the intention–behavior relationship in three studies (Hoyt et al., 2009; Rhodes, Courneya, & Hayduk, 2002; Rhodes et al., 2005). Only one of these, however, has provided evidence for moderation (Hoyt et al., 2009). In this study, N's facets of anxiety, depression, self-consciousness, and vulnerability all showed significant moderator effects. In multivariate analyses, however, anxiety was the critical moderator of all these effects as well as of the possible effects from other personality facets from the five-factor model. Given the limited literature, more research is required before any definitive conclusions about N's moderation capacity can be drawn.

Conclusions

This review was intended to update the findings of Rhodes and Smith (2006), to extend them to personality subtraits and their relationship with physical activity, and to evaluate mechanisms mediating this relationship and the evidence for personality as a moderator of physical activity motivation. For the update of higher-order personality traits, nine studies from 1998 to 2009 met our review criteria. Twenty-nine studies with 42 unique samples from 1982 to 2009 met our review criteria for lower-order traits. Of the studies included in Rhodes and Smith (2006) and our review, 17 studies examined mediators and 11 studies examined moderators of personality and physical activity.

The prior review by Rhodes and Smith (2006) identified E ($r = .23$), N ($r = -.11$) and C ($r = .20$) as correlates of physical activity. Our review update generally complemented these findings, but with some heterogeneity. For example, only three of seven recent studies showed a correlation between E and physical activity, while most of the updated literature showed evidence for a relationship between Agreeableness and physical activity. Part of the heterogeneity may be due to small effect sizes and the differences that can occur around the probability criterion when detecting effects between $r = .10$ and $r = .25$. It seems prudent to conduct a meta-analysis in a few more years to reappraise the findings.

From our updated review, however, it appears that N, E, and C are still the most reliable if small correlates of physical activity. E concerns differences in preferences for social interaction and lively activity (Eysenck, 1970; McCrae & Costa, 1995). The seeking of physical activity behaviors would appear to be a logical extension for people high in this trait, while disinterest in physical activity seems likely for those low in E (Eysenck et al., 1982). High-N individuals have less emotional stability and more distress, anxiety, and depression than those with lower N. Avoidance of physical activity or cancellation of physical activity plans is a logical extension of this trait. A relationship between C and health behaviors more generally has also been established (Booth-Kewley & Vickers, 1994). High scores on C indicate a purposeful, self-disciplined individual (Digman, 1990; McCrae & Costa, 1995), suggesting that this factor may be important in adherence behavior. It seems logical that higher-C individuals would show a greater predisposition to maintain physical activity behavior than their low-C counterparts.

Future Directions

Our results on potential moderators of personality–physical activity relationships, such as gender, age, culture/country, and study design, were inconclusive given the small number of studies. Still, the existing evidence suggested that the personality–physical activity relationship is relatively invariant to these factors. In the U.K., however, unlike other countries, there were continued null effects for personality and physical activity. Future research focusing on personality comparisons by country with some theoretical basis for these discrepancies would be helpful.

Our review of facet or subtraits of personality and physical activity proved more interesting and helps extend the literature on this topic. Type A personality and E's activity facet trait both showed convincing evidence of correlating with physical activity. Indeed, the activity trait showed medium effect sizes and was a better predictor of physical activity than E in three studies. These results advance our understanding of the types of traits that influence regular physical activity and suggest that subtrait approaches may be more valuable to understanding behavior than higher-order approaches (Hoyt et al., 2009). Both Type A and the activity trait are linked with high-energy, fast-paced lifestyles where physical activity seems a logical outlet. It will be interesting to see whether future research can tie this trait to biological/neurological aspects of individual differences.

A review of the processes mediating between personality and physical activity demonstrated that social cognitive constructs generally fail to account for this covariation. Almost all studies applied Ajzen's (1991) theory of planned behavior (TPB), which has shown excellent predictive efficacy within the physical activity domain (Symons Downs & Hausenblas, 2005). No other theory has shown better predictive capability, so while it seems prudent to expand these analyses to different theories, the differences may be minimal.

Personality traits of E, E's activity facet, and C have all demonstrated evidence of direct effects on behavior after controlling for TPB, with some limited partial mediation through attitude and perceived behavioral control. Rhodes and colleagues (Rhodes & Courneya, 2003a; Rhodes et al., 2004) have argued that this direct effect may indicate the temporal stability problems surrounding social cognition when compared with more generalized traits. That is, while intentions and attitudes waver across time, personality remains predictive of behavior. Nevertheless, the findings suggest that understanding "at risk" personalities may be important because interventions targeting social cognitions may underestimate the role of underlying individual trait differences. Interventions that consider one's introversion, for example, and target behaviors accordingly (e.g., by having activity be done at home, solo or with one friend, or at low intensity) may have utility. Research is needed to examine this augmentation or personality-matching strategy.

This review is also the first to systematically appraise personality moderators of social cognition and behavior. Like the mediation papers, most focused on the TPB intention construct and its relationship with behavior. Convincing evidence was found for C and its role in moderating intention–behavior discordance. Individuals high in C were shown to have larger correlations than those low in C, and it seems logical to surmise that this is due to the achievement striving and industrious nature of high-C people. Some evidence was also found for E and N and their potential moderating role in intention–behavior relations, but more research is needed in this domain before any conclusions should be drawn. Intention–behavior discordance is a major problem in the physical activity domain, as nearly half of initial intenders fail to be active (Canadian Fitness and Lifestyle Research Institute, 2004; Rhodes & Plotnikoff, 2006; Rhodes, Plotnikoff, & Courneya, 2008). Indeed, most of the populace has the intention to be active (Canadian Fitness and Lifestyle Research Institute, 2004), suggesting that action control (translating intentions into behavior) is more important than action planning (forming an intention). Current theories such as TPB are ill prepared for an action control approach to intervention because they assume that intention is the proximal antecedent of behavior (Ajzen & Fishbein, 2005). The role that traits like C play in this intention–behavior gap is important to understand so that appropriate interventions can be implemented. It appears that low-C individuals require additional motivational intervention to meet their initial positive physical activity intentions. Research examining intervention augmentation in this group is warranted.

At the same time that this review helps summarize the existing research on personality correlates and behavior, it also paves the way for future directions. Indeed, research on personality and physical activity has remained fairly basic across the last 30 years, focusing largely on bivariate correlations or univariate analyses of variance in cross-sectional or very short prospective designs. Eysenck et al. made this same commentary in 1982. Longitudinal studies across the life span with multivariate designs are needed. These studies would be critical in ascertaining how personality development relates to physical activity as well as how changes in age match with changes in personality. For example, E tends to decline with age (McCrae et al., 2000), and whether this matches declines in physical activity has yet to be investigated. Similarly, C has been able to predict longevity and health behavior from childhood (Friedman et al., 1995). Knowing its association with physical activity across the life span and its mediation via physical activity would add to this interesting finding. Use of socioecological models (Stokols, 1996) that include biological, sociodemographic, social, individual, and environmental variables will also aid in understanding the role of personality within the more complex systems that lead to physical activity behavior.

Experimental and intervention studies are also desperately needed. Personality-matched interventions have great appeal but have never been put to any sort of examination (Rhodes, 2006). Research is needed to evaluate the potentially important roles of personality in message elaboration, physical activity environments, physical activity modes, and responses to exercise. Finally, objective assessment of physical activity will undoubtedly aid the accuracy of personality research. Just as personality assessment has improved over the decades, physical activity assessment is now moving into the age of direct measures (e.g., accelerometry). Thus far, most studies on personality and physical activity behavior have used self-report instrumentation that varies in validity, and studies using more objective means such as program attendance have relied on very small sample sizes.

In summary, the results demonstrate that some lower-order traits, such as extraversion's activity facet, may be better predictors of exercise than their higher-order structures (e.g., extraversion). Personality does not appear to be mediated by social cognition, which suggests that individual traits may serve as markers of personalities at risk for inactivity in intervention. Further, conscientiousness appears to have a consistent moderating effect on the exercise intention–behavior gap. Future research on personality-matched physical activity interventions, longitudinal designs, and ecological models that include interactions between personality and the exercise environment is recommended.

Acknowledgments

Ryan E. Rhodes is supported by a new investigator award from the Canadian Institutes of Health Research and with funds from the Social Sciences and Humanities Research Council of Canada and the Canadian Diabetes Association.

References

Adams, J., & Nettle, D. (2009). Time perspective, personality and smoking, body mass, and physical activity: An empirical study. *British Journal of Health Psychology, 14*, 83–105.

Adams, T. B., & Mowen, J. C. (2005). Identifying the personality characteristics of healthy eaters and exercisers: A hierarchical model approach. *Health Marketing Quarterly, 23*, 22–41.

Adams-Campbell, L. L., Washburn, R. A., & Haile, G. T. (1990). Physical activity, stress, and type A behavior in blacks. *Journal of the National Medical Association, 82*, 701–705.

Ajzen, I. (1991). The theory of planned behavior. *Organizational Behavior and Human Decision Processes, 50*, 179–211.

Ajzen, I., & Fishbein, M. (2005). Theory-based behavior change interventions: Comments on Hobbis and Sutton. *Journal of Health Psychology, 10*, 27–31.

Allen, J., Markovitz, J., Jacobs, D. R., & Knox, S. S. (2001). Social support and health behavior in hostile black and white men and women in CARDIA. *Psychosomatic Medicine, 63*, 609–618.

Arai, Y., & Hisamichi, S. (1998). Self-reported exercise frequency and personality: A population-based study in Japan. *Perceptual and Motor Skills, 87*, 1371–1375.

Bandura, A. (1998). Health promotion from the perspective of social cognitive theory. *Psychology and Health, 13*, 623–649.

Baranowski, T., Anderson, C., & Carmack, C. (1998). Mediating variable framework in physical activity interventions: How are we doing? How might we do better? *American Journal of Preventive Medicine, 15*, 266–297.

Bogg, T. (2008). Conscientiousness, the transtheoretical model of change, and exercise: A neo-socioanalytic integration of trait and social-cognitive frameworks in the prediction of behavior. *Journal of Personality, 76*, 775–801.

Bogg, T., Voss, M. W., Wood, D., & Roberts, B. W. (2008). A hierarchical investigation of personality and behavior: Examining neo-socioanalytic models of health related outcomes. *Journal of Research in Personality, 42*, 183–207.

Booth-Kewley, S., & Vickers, R. R. (1994). Associations between major domains of personality and health behavior. *Journal of Personality, 62*, 281–298.

Bouchard, C., Shephard, R. J., & Stephens, T. (1994). The consensus statement. In C. Bouchard, R. J. Shephard, & T. Stephens (Eds.), *Physical activity fitness and health: International proceedings and consensus statement* (pp. 9–76). Champaign, IL: Human Kinetics.

Bryan, A. D., & Rocheleau, C. A. (2002). Predicting aerobic versus resistance exercise using the theory of planned behavior. *American Journal of Health Behavior, 26*, 83–94.

Buchman, B. P., Sallis, J. F., Criqui, M. H., Dimsdale, J. E., & Kaplan, R. (1991). Physical activity, physical fitness, and psychological characteristics of medical students. *Journal of Psychosomatic Research*, 35,197–208.

Canadian Fitness and Lifestyle Research Institute. (2002). *2002 Physical activity monitor*. Retrieved August, 2004, from http://72.10.49.94/node/595

Canadian Fitness and Lifestyle Research Institute. (2004). *Increasing physical activity: Trends for planning effective communication*. Retrieved February 24, 2006, from http://www.cflri.ca/eng/statistics/surveys/capacity2004.php

Castaneda, D. M., Bigatti, S., & Cronan, T. A. (1998). Gender and exercise behavior among women and men with osteoarthritis. *Women and Health, 27*, 33–53.

Cerin, E., Barnett, A., & Baranowski, T. (2009). Testing theories of dietary behavior change in youth using the mediating variable model with intervention programs. *Journal of Nutrition Education and Behavior, 41*, 309–318.

Cerin, E., & Mackinnon, D. P. (2008). A commentary on current practice in mediating variable analyses in behavioural nutrition and physical activity. *Public Health Nutrition, 12*, 1182–1188.

Chatzisarantis, N. L. D., & Hagger, M. (2007). Mindfulness and the intention–behaviour relationship within the theory of planned behavior. *Personality and Social Psychology Bulletin, 33*, 663–676.

Chatzisarantis, N. L. D., & Hagger, M. (2008). Influences of personality traits and continuation intentions on physical activity participation within the theory of planned behaviour. *Psychology and Health, 23*, 347–367.

Chen, S. Y., & Fu, Y. C. (2008). Leisure participation and enjoyment among the elderly: Individual characteristics and sociability. *Educational Gerontology, 34*, 871–889.

Cohen, J. (1992). A power primer. *Psychological Bulletin, 112*, 155–159.

Conner, M., & Abraham, C. (2001). Conscientiousness and the theory of planned behavior: Toward a more complete model of the antecedents of intentions and behavior. *Personality and Social Psychology Bulletin, 27*, 1547–1561.

Conner, M., Rodgers, W., & Murray, T. (2007). Conscientiousness and the intention–behaviour relationship: Predicting exercise behavior. *Journal of Sport and Exercise Psychology, 29*, 518–533.

Costa, P. T., & McCrae, R. R. (1992). *Revised NEO Personality Inventory (NEO-PI-R) and NEO Five Factor Inventory (NEO-FFI) Professional Manual*. Odessa, FL: Psychological Assessment Resources.

Costa, P. T., & McCrae, R. R. (1995). Domains and facets: Hierarchical personality assessment using the revised NEO Personality Inventory. *Journal of Personality Assessment, 64*, 21–50.

Courneya, K. S., Bobick, T. M., & Schinke, R. J. (1999). Does the theory of planned behavior mediate the relation between personality and exercise behavior? *Basic and Applied Social Psychology, 21*, 317–324.

Courneya, K. S., Friedenreich, C. M., Sela, R., Quinney, H. A., & Rhodes, R. E. (2002). Correlates of adherence and contamination in a randomized controlled trial of exercise in cancer survivors: An application of the theory of planned behavior and the five factor model of personality. *Annals of Behavioral Medicine, 24*, 257–268.

Davis, C. (1990). Body image and weight preoccupation: A comparison between exercising and nonexercising women. *Appetite, 15*, 13–21.

Davis, C., Brewer, H., & Ratusny, D. (1993). Behavioral frequency and psychological commitment: Necessary concepts in the study of excessive exercising. *Journal of Behavioral Medicine, 16*, 611–628.

DeMoor, M. H. M., Beem, A. L., Stubbe, J. H., Boomsma, D. I., & DeGeus, E. J. C. (2006). Regular exercise, anxiety, depression and personality: A population-based study. *Preventive Medicine, 42*, 273–279.

DePanfilis, C. D., Torre, M., Cero, S., Salvatore, P., Aglio, E. D., Marchesi, C., Cabrino, C., … Maggini C. (2008). Personality and attrition from behavioral weight-loss treatment for obesity. *General Hospital Psychiatry, 30*, 515–520.

Digman, J. M. (1990). Personality structure: Emergence of the five-factor model. *Annual Review of Psychology, 41*, 417–440.

Eason, K. E., Masse, L. C., Tortolero, S. R., & Kelder, S. H. (2002). Type A behavior and daily living activity among older minority women. *Journal of Women's Health & Gender-Based Medicine, 11*, 137–146.

Eysenck, H. J. (1970). *The structure of human personality* (3rd ed.). London: Methuen.

Eysenck H. J., & Eysenck, S. B. J. (1963). *Manual for the Eysenck Personality Inventory.* San Diego, CA: Educational and Industrial Testing Service.

Eysenck, H. J., Nias, D. K. B., & Cox, D. N. (1982). Sport and personality. *Advances in Behaviour Research and Therapy, 4*, 1–56.

Friedman, H. S., Tucker, J. S., Tomlinson-Keasey, C., Schwartz, J. E., Wingard, D. L., & Criqui, M. H. (1995). Childhood conscientiousness and longevity: Health behaviors and cause of death. *Journal of Personality and Social Psychology, 65*, 176–185.

Funder, D. C. (2001). Personality. *Annual Review of Psychology, 52*, 197–221.

Geers, A. L., Wellman, J. A., & Lassiter, G. D. (2009). Dispositional optimism and engagement: The moderating role of goal prioritization. *Journal of Personality and Social Psychology, 96*, 913–932.

Giacobbi P. R. Jr., Hardin, B., Frye, N., Hausenblas, H. A., Sears, S., & Stegelin, A. (2006). A multi-level examination of personality, exercise, and daily life events for individuals with physical disabilities. *Adapted Physical Activity Quarterly, 23*, 129–147.

Goldberg, L. R. (1993). The structure of phenotypic personality traits. *American Psychologist, 48*, 26–34.

Hershberger, P. J., Robertson, K. B., & Markert, R. J. (1999). Personality and appointment-keeping adherence in cardiac rehabilitation. *Journal of Cardiopulmonary Rehabilitation, 19*, 106–111.

Howard, J. H., Cunningham, D. A., & Rechnitzer, P. A. (1987). Personality and fitness decline in middle-aged men. *International Journal of Sport Psychology, 18*, 100–111.

Hoyt, A. L., Rhodes, R. E., Hausenblas, H., & Giacobbi, P. R. (2009). Integrating five-factor model facet level traits with the theory of planned behavior and exercise. *Psychology of Sport and Exercise, 10*, 565–572.

Huang, C. H., Lee, L. Y., & Chang, M. L. (2007). The influences of personality and motivation on exercise participation and quality of life. *Social Behavior and Personality, 35*, 1189–1210.

Ingledew, D. K., & Markland, D. (2008). The role of motives in exercise participation. *Psychology and Health, 23*(7), 807–828.

Jenkins, C. D. (1976). Recent evidence supporting psychologic and social risk factors for coronary disease. *New England Journal of Medicine, 294*, 987–1033.

Kjelsas, E., & Augestad, L. B. (2004). Gender, eating behavior, and personality characteristics in physically active students. *Scandinavian Journal of Medicine and Science in Sports, 14*, 258–268.

Kobasa, S. C., Maddi, S. R., & Puccetti, M. C. (1982). Personality and exercise in the stress–illness relationship. *Journal of Behavioral Medicine, 3*, 391–404.

Manning, M. R., & Fusilier, M. R. (1999). The relationship between stress and health care use: An investigation of the buffering roles of personality, social support, and exercise. *Journal of Psychosomatic Research, 47*, 159–173.

McCrae, R. R., & Costa, P. T. (1995). Trait explanations in personality psychology. *European Journal of Personality, 9*, 231–252.

McCrae, R. R., Costa, P. T., Ostendorf, F., Angleitner, A., Hrebickova, M., Avia, M. D., … Smith, P. B. (2000). Nature over nurture: Temperament, personality, and life-span development. *Journal of Personality and Social Psychology, 78*, 173 186.

Milam, J. E., Richardson, J. L., Marks, G. R., Kemper, C. A., & McCutchan, A. J. (2004). The roles of dispositional optimism and pessimism in HIV disease progression. *Psychology and Health, 19*, 167–181.

Milligan, R. A. K., Burke, V., Beilin, L. J., Richards, J., Dunbar, D., Spencer, M., … Gracey, M. P. (1997). Health-related behaviours and psycho-social characteristics of 18 year-old Australians. *Social Science & Medicine, 45*, 1549–1562.

Mowen, J. C. (2000). *The 3M Model of motivation and personality*, Boston: Kluwer Academic Publishers.

Musante, L. Treiber, F. A., Davis, H., Strong, W. B., Levy, M. (1992). Hostility: Relationship to lifestyle behaviors and physical risk factors. *Behavioral Medicine, 18*, 21–26.

Palomo, T., Beninger, R. J., Kostrzewa, R. M., & Archer, T. (2008). Affective status in relation to impulsive, motor and motivational symptoms: Personality, development, and physical exercise. *Neurotoxicity Research, 14*, 151–168.

Poppius, E., Tenkanen, L., Kalimo, R., & Heinsalmi P. (1999). The sense of coherence, occupation and the risk of coronary heart disease in the Helsinki Heart Study. *Social Science & Medicine, 49*, 109–120.

Rhodes, R. E. (2006). The built-in environment: The role of personality with physical activity. *Exercise and Sport Sciences Reviews, 34*, 83–88.

Rhodes, R. E., & Courneya, K. S. (2000). Effects of a health-based versus appearance-based persuasive message on attitudes towards exercise: Testing the moderating role of self-monitoring. *Journal of Social Behavior and Personality, 15*, 321–330.

Rhodes, R. E., & Courneya, K. S. (2003a). Relationships between personality, an extended theory of planned behaviour model, and exercise behaviour. *British Journal of Health Psychology, 8*, 19–36.

Rhodes, R. E., & Courneya, K. S. (2003b). Self-efficacy, controllability, and intention in the theory of planned behavior: Measurement redundancy or causal independence? *Psychology and Health, 18*, 79–91.

Rhodes, R. E., Courneya, K. S., Blanchard, C. M., & Plotnikoff, R. C. (2007). Prediction of leisure-time walking: An integration of social cognitive, perceived environmental, and personality factors. *International Journal of Behavioral Nutrition and Physical Activity, 4*, 51.

Rhodes, R. E., Courneya, K. S., & Hayduk, L. A. (2002). Does personality moderate the theory of planned behavior in the exercise domain? *Journal of Sport and Exercise Psychology, 24*, 120–132.

Rhodes, R. E., Courneya, K. S., & Jones, L. W. (2002). Personality, the theory of planned behavior, and exercise: The unique role of extroversion's activity facet. *Journal of Applied Social Psychology, 32*, 1721–1736.

Rhodes, R. E., Courneya, K. S., & Jones, L. W. (2003). Translating exercise intentions into behavior: Personality and social cognitive correlates. *Journal of Health Psychology, 8*, 447–458.

Rhodes, R. E., Courneya, K. S., & Jones, L. W. (2004). Personality and social cognitive influences on exercise behavior: Adding the activity trait to the theory of planned behavior. *Psychology of Sport and Exercise, 5*, 243–254.

Rhodes, R. E., Courneya, K. S., & Jones, L. W. (2005). The theory of planned behavior and lower-order personality traits: Interaction effects in the exercise domain. *Personality and Individual Differences, 38*, 251–265.

Rhodes, R. E., & Pfaeffli, L. A. (2009). Mediators of physical activity behaviour change among adult non-clinical populations: A review update. *Annals of Behavioral Medicine, 37*, s85.

Rhodes, R. E., & Plotnikoff, R. C. (2006). Understanding action control: Predicting physical activity intention–behavior profiles across six months in a Canadian sample. *Health Psychology, 25*, 292–299.

Rhodes, R. E., Plotnikoff, R. C., & Courneya, K. S. (2008). Predicting the physical activity intention–behaviour profiles of adopters and maintainers using three social cognition models. *Annals of Behavioral Medicine, 36*, 244–252.

Rhodes, R. E., & Smith, N. E. I. (2006). Personality correlates of physical activity: A review and meta-analysis. *British Journal of Sports Medicine, 40*, 958–965.

Rimmele, U., Seiler, R., Marti, B., Wirtz, P. H., Ehlert, U., & Heinrichs, M. (2009). The level of physical activity affects adrenal and cardiovascular reactivity to psychosocial stress. *Psychoneuroendocrinology, 34*, 190–198.

Roberts, B. W., Bogg, T., Walton, K. E., Chernyshenko, O. S., & Stark, S. E. (2004). A lexical investigation of the lower-order structure of conscientiousness. *Journal of Research in Personality, 38*, 164–178.

Rutledge, T., & Linden, W. (2000). Defensiveness status predicts 3-year incidence of hypertension. *Journal of Hypertension, 18*, 153–159.

Saklofske, D. H., Austin, E. J., Rohr, B. A., & Andrews, J. J. W. (2007). Personality, emotional intelligence and exercise. *Journal of Health Psychology, 12*, 937–948.

Sale, C., Guppy, A., & El-Sayed, M. (2000). Individual differences, exercise and leisure activity in predicting affective well-being in young adults. *Ergonomics, 43*, 1689–1697.

Spano, L. (2001). The relationship between exercise and anxiety, obsessive compulsiveness, and narcissism. *Personality and Individual Differences, 30*, 87–93.

Stokols, D. (1996). Translating social ecological theory into guidelines for community health promotion. *American Journal of Health Promotion, 10*, 282–298.

Symons Downs, D., & Hausenblas, H. A. (2005). Exercise behavior and the theories of reasoned action and planned behavior: A meta-analytic update. *Journal of Physical Activity and Health, 2*, 76–97.

Szabo, A. (1992). Habitual participation in exercise and personality. *Perceptual and Motor Skills, 74*, 978.

Trost, S. G., Owen, N., Bauman, A., Sallis, J. F., & Brown, W. (2002). Correlates of adults' participation in physical activity: Review and update. *Medicine & Science in Sports & Exercise, 34*, 1996–2001.

U.S. Department of Health and Human Services. (1996). *Physical activity and health: A report of the Surgeon General.* Atlanta, GA: National Center for Chronic Disease Prevention and Health Promotion, Centers for Disease Control and Prevention.

van Loon, A. J. M., Tijhuis, M., Surtees, P., & Ormel, J. (2001). Personality and coping: Their relationship with lifestyle risk factors for cancer. *Personality and Individual Differences, 31*, 541–553.

Warburton, D. E. R., Katzmarzyk, P., Rhodes, R. E., & Shephard, R. J. (2007). Evidence-informed physical activity guidelines for Canadian adults. *Applied Physiology, Nutrition and Metabolism, 32*, S16–S68.

Warburton, D. E. R., Nicol, C. W., & Bredin, S. S. (2006). Health benefits of physical activity: The evidence. *Canadian Medical Association Journal, 174*, 801–809.

Welsh, M. C., Labbe, E. E., & Delaney, D. (1991). Cognitive strategies and personality variables in adherence to exercise. *Psychological Reports, 68*, 1327–1335.

Wiebe, D. J., & Smith, T. W. (1997). Personality and health: Progress and problems in psychosomatics. In R. Hogan, J. Johnson, & S. Briggs (Eds.), *Handbook of personality psychology* (pp. 891–918). San Diego, CA: Academic Press.

Psychosocial Influence

Martin S. Hagger

Abstract

Theories of psychosocial influence identify important psychological factors that influence exercise behavior and outline the mechanisms and processes by which these factors exert their influence. This chapter summarizes the psychosocial influences on exercise behavior using two popular theoretical approaches from social psychology: social cognitive theory and the theories of reasoned action and planned behavior. Synthesizing research from these theories has identified self-efficacy, attitudes, and perceived behavioral control as key factors influencing exercise intentions and behavior and has labeled them as targets for interventions to promote exercise behavior. The effects of other factors, such as personality and implicit variables, and features of the constructs, such as intention stability, are also reviewed. Implementation intentions are identified as important means to address the intention–behavior gap. The implications of the research for the development of interventions to most effectively promote exercise participation are considered.

Key Words: social cognition, self-efficacy, planned behavior, intention, attitude, implementation intentions, implicit processes, theoretical integration, intervention.

Introduction

Psychologists attempting to understand people's participation in exercise have focused on two global aims: (1) identifying the psychological factors that influence physical activity participation and (2) identifying the mechanisms and processes by which these factors influence participation. As exercise is primarily a *social* behavior, the dominant approach to understanding this set of behaviors has been through the adoption and application of social psychological theories and models. This chapter reviews the dominant social psychological approaches to understanding exercise behavior and review both the pioneering and contemporary research that has aimed to provide explanations of the influences and accompanying mechanisms. After briefly outlining the assumptions associated with the social cognitive approach, this chapter

identifies two of the dominant models that have contributed to identifying the key constructs that influence exercise behavior and have been most effective in explaining variance in physical activity behavior. The two approaches are Bandura's (1977b, 1986, 1997) social cognitive theory and Ajzen and Fishbein's (Ajzen, 1985; Ajzen & Fishbein, 1980) theories of reasoned action and planned behavior and their derivatives. A review the research adopting these approaches and an evaluation of their importance and level of contribution to the exercise psychology literature will be presented. In addition, this chapter outlines their shortcomings and limitations and identifies how innovative new approaches, such as incorporating the role of implicit factors, planning and implemental strategies, and integrated motivational models, are advancing and broadening knowledge in this area. Finally, conclusions and highlights of how the field is likely to develop in the future are presented.

Assumptions

The dominant approach to understanding the psychosocial influences on exercise behavior and their associated mechanisms is the adoption of social cognitive models derived from the field of social psychology. The theories reviewed in this chapter all originate from this approach, and it is important to identify and highlight the assumptions associated with such models (Hagger & Chatzisarantis, 2009a). This will delineate the boundary conditions of the factors and processes identified in the current review.

First, exercise is considered an intentional set of activities under the volitional control of the individual. This means that intentions are primarily responsible for the uptake, often referred to as *adoption*, and maintenance, often referred to as *adherence* or *compliance*, of exercise behavior. Second, the social psychological approaches assume that individuals process social information and form intentions to engage in exercise behavior in the same way. This *information processing* approach is common to many models and theories in social psychology. Central to this approach is that given the same set of circumstances in terms of internal social psychological states and environmental conditions, all individuals will respond in an identical manner. As a consequence, knowledge of the social factors and conditions that lead to exercise behavior is derived from group-level or interindividual data focusing on the factors common to all individuals of a particular group or population. Third, the approach assumes that people can reliably report their internal states through carefully developed and presented psychometric instruments and measures. These serve as the primary source of information on the social psychological factors that influence exercise behavior. Such self-reported data is central to social cognitive models of exercise behavior. Finally, the approach does not eschew the influence of individual differences or implicit, nonintentional factors, but considers such factors as distal influences on behavior or factors that moderate the effect of the immediate psychosocial factors.

Social Cognitive Theory

Social cognitive theory is one of the most influential theories in social psychology and has inspired an entire literature on *social cognition*. The theory is synonymous with three important tenets: reciprocal determinism, vicarious experience or observational learning, and self-efficacy. The architect of social cognitive theory, Bandura (1977b, 1986, 1997), proposed that experience and behavior, beliefs and knowledge, and environmental factors all act as mutual causes of each other. This premise is known as *reciprocal determinism* and acknowledges that people's internal and external factors influence their behavior just as their behavior also influences their environment in a dynamic, interactive process. This illustrates the importance of context as well as experience as important factors influencing behaviors like exercise. Two processes have been shown to be important environmental and intrapersonal influences on behavior. First, people tend to learn behavioral responses from experience, whether firsthand or by watching others, known in the latter case as *vicarious experience*. Second, such experiences, if successful, promote confidence, known as *self-efficacy*, in the ability to produce the appropriate action to achieve a particular goal or outcome. Bandura (1986) defines self-efficacy as "people's judgements of their capabilities to organise and execute courses of action required to attain designated types of performances. It is concerned not with the [actual] skills one has but with judgements of what one can do with whatever skills one possesses" (p. 391). Self-efficacy has also been defined by some authors as "situation-specific self-confidence" (Feltz & Chase, 1998, p. 60). In addition, a distinction is frequently made between self-efficacy beliefs and outcome expectations, where beliefs reflect perceptions regarding the capacity to produce outcomes by performing a specific behavior or action, and outcome expectations reflect perceptions of the expected costs and benefits of performing the behavior or outcome. Research in the exercise field has largely focused on the role of self-efficacy as a predictor of exercise behavior, although there is also research that has looked at the role of outcome expectations (Dzewaltowski, 1989; Dzewaltowski, Noble, & Shaw, 1990). This chapter will focus on the roles that self-efficacy and outcome expectations have in exercise behavior as well as the factors that lead to the development of self-efficacy and outcome expectations.

With regard to exercise participation, both self-efficacy and outcome expectations are considered to be likely important antecedent factors (Rodgers & Brawley, 1991). Unsurprisingly, both constructs have been the subject of enquiry in exercise psychology (McAuley & Blissmer, 2000, 2002; Teixeira, Going, Sardinha, & Lohman, 2005). Perceptions of self-efficacy are likely to be influential in the adoption of exercise, yet it is also likely that outcome expectations will affect exercise compliance and provide the internal "reinforcement" necessary for exercise maintenance (Anderson, Wojcik, Winett, & Williams, 2006). In addition to their predictive effects, Bandura (1986, 1997) suggested that self-efficacy and outcome expectations are influenced by four factors: prior success and performance attainment, imitation and modeling, verbal and social persuasion, and judgments of physiological states.

Examining each of these influences in turn, *prior experience and performance accomplishment* represent previous personal success with a target behavior and act as a source of information for the formation of self-efficacy. Importantly, it is *successful* previous experience with the behavior that is influential in developing self-efficacy. Such experiences are viewed as the most important predictor of self-efficacy in social cognitive theory (Bandura, 1977a). *Imitation or modeling* of others' behavior (vicarious experiences) has also been found to affect self-efficacy. Observing the successful execution of an action or behavior is proposed to reinforce the action in the individual and contribute to self-efficacy for future performance. For example, observing others perceived to be competent or skilled demonstrating exercise participation is likely to increase self-efficacy in novices or less competent exercisers. The effects of the vicarious experiences are likely to be more pervasive if the model has similar characteristics to the observer. The provision of *verbal and social persuasive* messages, whether external information like positive feedback or technical commentary from a credible source or person-centered information such as imagery or self-talk, is likely to foster increased self-efficacy. Finally, judgments of *physiological states* such as arousal and affect are likely to affect self-efficacy. Therefore feedback from the autonomic system regarding physiological states is likely to influence self-efficacy. These sources of information contribute synergistically to self-efficacy beliefs.

The effects of these sources of self-efficacy in an exercise context were summarized by Ewart (1989): "The most effective way to encourage patients to adopt exercise activities for which they lack self-efficacy is to expose them to the recommended activity in gradually increasing doses, arrange for them to see others similar to themselves performing the activity; have respected health care providers offer encouragement by providing reassurance and emphasizing the patient's accomplishments, and arrange the setting of the activity so as to induce a relaxed but 'upbeat' mood" (p. 684). This statement accurately and comprehensively captures the different sources of self-efficacy in terms of prior successful experience (emphasizing accomplishments), vicarious experience (arranging to see others performing the activity), verbal persuasion (offering encouragement), and physiological states (inducing "upbeat" mood).

Self-Efficacy in Exercise

Research on self-efficacy in the context of exercise has focused on it as an antecedent of exercise behavior and also examined it as an important mediator of interventions to change exercise behavior in clinical and nonclinical populations. For example, in clinical populations self-efficacy has been examined as a predictor of exercise adherence among patients undergoing recovery from cardiovascular disease (myocardial infarction) (Mildestvedt, Meland, & Eide, 2008; Woodgate & Brawley, 2008) and other chronic illnesses (Motl, McAuley, Doerksen, Hu, & Morris, 2009; Park & Gaffey, 2007; Shaughnessy & Resnick, 2009; Sweet et al., 2009). Such research has demonstrated that self-efficacy predicts changes in exercise behavior and has also shown that self-efficacy changes as a result of exercise experience, demonstrating the importance of past experience as an influential factor on the development of self-efficacy perceptions. In nonclinical populations, self-efficacy has been shown to predict exercise in adult and older adult samples (McAuley, 1992; McAuley & Blissmer, 2002; McAuley & Courneya, 1993), has discriminated adherers from dropouts in exercise-based weight loss programs (Rodgers & Brawley, 1993), and has predicted positive affect after exercise (Bozoian, Rejeski, & McAuley, 1994). Research has also consistently found that self-efficacy for exercise was increased through competence-based exercise interventions (Luszczynska & Haynes, 2009) and is a significant mediator of the effects of interventions on exercise participation (Costanzo & Walker, 2008; Hortz & Petosa, 2008; Toft et al., 2007; Umstattd, Wilcox, Saunders, Watkins, & Dowda, 2008). In summary, studies investigating the effects of self-efficacy on exercise behavior have demonstrated a consistent relationship between self-efficacy beliefs and exercise participation.

The Legacy of Social Cognitive Theory

Social cognitive theory in general and the construct of self-efficacy specifically have had an indelible influence on theoretical research in social psychology applied to exercise contexts. The consistent relationship between self-efficacy and exercise behavior and its role as a mediator of the effects of intervention on exercise participation and adherence demonstrate its effectiveness as a psychological driving force behind behavior. A vast literature has demonstrated its importance as a construct and mechanism in a multitude of other behaviors. Therefore the construct serves an important role in exercise psychology and is still a frequent basis for interventions in exercise. Interventions to change self-efficacy and behavior in an exercise context frequently focus on strategies that provide experiences and perceptions that target the antecedent factors of self-efficacy listed earlier. However, research has demonstrated that self-efficacy is but one factor that influences exercise behavior, and there are numerous others such as attitudes and social support (Petter, Blanchard, Kemp, Mazoff, & Ferrier, 2009). This has led people to develop hybrid, integrated theoretical approaches that incorporate self-efficacy alongside other factors to predict and change behavior (Hagger, 2010). Examples of such theoretical approaches include protection motivation theory (Rogers, 1975), the transtheoretical model (Prochaska & DiClemente, 1982; Prochaska & Markus, 1994), and the theory of planned behavior (Ajzen, 1985, 1991). All of these theories include variants of the self-efficacy construct, demonstrating the importance of Bandura's (1977b, 1986, 1997) theory and thinking in social psychology applied to exercise behavior. In the next section, I review the research on a leading approach to exercise behavior, comprising the theory of reasoned action and the theory of planned behavior. The latter theory incorporates self-efficacy as part of a perceived behavioral control component.

A limitation of self-efficacy, and indeed many other psychosocial influences on exercise behavior, is that it may not account for more implicit or "habitual" factors that influence behavior. For example, self-efficacy seems to be most effective on behaviors that require considerable effort, overcoming barriers, and self-regulation (Lee, Arthur, & Avis, 2008; Poag & McAuley, 1992). Habitual behaviors that are under the control of nonconscious or habitual factors, such as toothbrushing, are less likely to be predicted by self-efficacy. In contrast, behaviors that require considerable effort, deliberation, and planning and involve overcoming obstacles and barriers are more susceptible to self-efficacy influences. This is probably why self-efficacy has been shown to be a consistent influence on exercise behaviors. However, it may be less influential among people

who have made decisions to exercise in the past and already have high self-efficacy. In such contexts, implicit processes and situational conditions that help people enact their intentions or motivations may be more effective. This topic is covered in a subsequent section of this chapter.

The Theories of Reasoned Action and Planned Behavior

The *theory of reasoned action* (Ajzen & Fishbein, 1980; Fishbein & Ajzen, 2009) is a widely adopted social cognitive theory aimed at explaining intentional behavior. It has been applied to many health-related behaviors, including exercise. The model has largely been superseded in the contemporary social psychology literature by an updated version; the theory of planned behavior (Ajzen, 1985). In the theory of reasoned action, intention is considered a motivational construct and represents the degree of planning and effort people are willing to invest in performing any future planned action or behavior. Intention is conceptualized within the theory as the most proximal psychosocial influence on behavior and is a function of a set of personal and normative belief-based social cognitive constructs regarding the performance of the future behavior, termed *attitudes* and *subjective norms*, respectively. Attitudes refer to an individual's overall evaluation of the behavior and are frequently measured *directly* using psychometric scales (Ajzen, 2003). However, the direct attitude measure is hypothesized to be underpinned by the individual's sets of personal beliefs that the target behavior will result in outcomes (behavioral beliefs) and by whether such outcomes are salient to the individual (outcome expectations). These beliefs can also be measured individually for each belief and outcome and are considered *indirect* measures of attitude. Similarly, subjective norms are typically measured directly as a person's overall evaluation that significant others would want them to engage in exercise behavior. As with attitudes, subjective norms are derived indirectly from sets of beliefs that reflect expectations that significant others will exert pressure or cajole the individual to engage in the target behavior (normative beliefs) and the individual's propensity to comply with those significant others (motivation to comply). In the theory, the more favorable an individual's attitudes and subjective norms are, the stronger his or her intentions to perform the behavior will be. In terms of process and the operationalization of the model, intentions are hypothesized to lead directly to behavior and to mediate the effects of attitudes and subjective norms on behavior. This means that intentions *explain* the attitude–behavior and subjective norm–behavior relationships. Intentions are therefore necessary to convert attitudes and subjective norms into behavior.

The major hypotheses of the theory of reasoned action have been supported in numerous studies across a number of different behaviors (Armitage & Conner, 2001; Godin & Kok, 1996; Sheppard, Hartwick, & Warshaw, 1988), including exercise (Hagger, Chatzisarantis, & Biddle, 2002b). Specifically, tests of the model have provided evidence for the overall predictive value of intentions and that attitudes have a pervasive effect on intentions, with the influence of subjective norms being considerably weaker and more variable (Hagger et al., 2002b). In addition, studies adopting cross-lagged panel designs in which the theory constructs are measured at two points in time have indicated that the effects of attitudes on intentions remain relatively strong and stable over time (Chatzisarantis, Hagger, Biddle, & Smith, 2005; Hagger, Chatzisarantis, Biddle, & Orbell, 2001). The latter designs indicate that it is the most proximal or recently formed perceptions that seem to have the most pervasive influence on exercise behavior. From an intervention or behavior change perspective this is very relevant, because it implies that immediacy of messages is important and also indicates that previous decision making has an influence, but only through change in the relevant constructs rather than direct effects independent of current perceptions. For a full account of the importance and relevance of such designs, readers are directed to the primary source adopting this approach for the theory in an exercise context (Hagger, Chatzisarantis, Biddle, & Orbell, 2001).

In addition, the most frequently cited or "modal" beliefs that underpin the attitude and subjective norms constructs in exercise contexts have been identified. Such beliefs are typically elicited from pilot research using open-ended measures that are content-analyzed to provide sufficient information to develop the salient outcomes for the behavioral belief and outcome evaluation measures and the salient referents for the normative belief and motivation-to-comply measures (Ajzen & Fishbein, 1980). Research in exercise has typically identified the following salient outcomes: "good companionship," "weight control," "benefit health," "take too much time," "have fun," "get fit," "stay in shape," "improve skills," "get an injury," and "getting hot and sweaty" (Hagger, Chatzisarantis, & Biddle,

2001). Similarly, important referents identified include friends, colleagues, and family members like parents, grandparents, and siblings (Hagger, Chatzisarantis, & Biddle, 2001). The comparatively limited research examining relations between the indirect belief-based measures and the direct measures suggests that multiplicative composites of the belief and value systems do not account for a high degree of variance in the direct measures of attitudes and subjective norms (Hagger, Chatzisarantis, & Biddle, 2001). Few definitive solutions have been put forward for this problem, and the role of beliefs and expectancy-value models within the theory of planned behavior is an area of surprisingly sparse attention in the literature (Ajzen & Fishbein, 2008; Bagozzi, 1984; French & Hankins, 2003).

The theory of reasoned action has received some criticism in the literature. For example, critics have suggested that the constructs in the theory merely represent a "snapshot" of a decision-making process that is state-like and therefore dynamic and changing (Hagger & Chatzisarantis, 2005b). The model, they argue, therefore does not capture the true fluctuations and variations in the beliefs and perceptions that influence exercise behavior over time. In addition, there are numerous boundary conditions of the theory in terms of which measures of constructs need to correspond in terms of the specific target behavior, the time frame in which it will be conducted, and the context in which it will be conducted (Ajzen, 1991; Chatzisarantis & Biddle, 1998). These conditions constrain the flexibility of the model to account for spontaneous behavioral engagement and possible changes in the context and time frame of the behavior. It also means that the model is not very effective in adapting to changing contexts and environments. Criticism has also been leveled at the adoption of the belief-based measures and the expectancy-value model that underpins these beliefs (French & Hankins, 2003). In addition, insufficient attention has been paid to the measurement of behavior within the theory of reasoned action. Without an accurate measure of behavior, the principle of correspondence cannot be applied (Ogden, 2003). This criticism casts doubt on several studies, such as those where assessment has relied on nonvalidated self-reports or used inappropriate "objective" measures, such as pedometers for people who are physically active predominantly through cycling or swimming. The theory allows the investigation of the interrelationships among attitudes, subjective norms, intentions, and a single behavior. It does not account for behavioral alternatives or competing activities. However, people are often confronted with many behavioral alternatives that may compete for time and motivational resources, and it may be that such alternatives lead to intentions for exercise being suppressed in favor of alternative actions.

The Theory of Planned Behavior

A further limitation of the theory of reasoned action, noted by Ajzen (1985), is that not all behaviors are under volitional control. In response to this, Ajzen developed an alternative, the *theory of planned behavior* which extended the theory of reasoned action to include an additional, control-related psychosocial determinant of intention (Ajzen, 1985). As with the theory of reasoned action, the central premise of the theory of planned behavior is that intention is the proximal predictor of behavior. However, an additional factor, termed *perceived behavioral control*, was introduced as an antecedent of intentions alongside attitudes and subjective norms. The construct of perceived behavioral control encompasses control-related perceptions with respect to the target behavior, including actual barriers and personal evaluations of limitation or capacity with respect to the behavior. Ajzen noted that the construct contains elements of Bandura's (1977b) self-efficacy constructs, in that it captures judgments of how well one can execute required actions to produce important outcomes. This has led some commentators to claim that the theory is really a partial integration of the theory of reasoned action with social cognitive theory (Hagger, 2009). As with attitudes and subjective norms, the construct of perceived behavioral control is underpinned by a set of beliefs (Ajzen, 1985). *Control beliefs* refer to the perceived presence of factors that may facilitate or impede performance of behavior, and *perceived power* refers to the perceived impact that facilitative or inhibiting factors may have on such performance (Ajzen & Driver, 1991). In the same way that an expectancy-value model is used to form indirect antecedents of attitudes and subjective norms, an indirect measure of perceived behavioral control is formed from the composite of the control beliefs multiplied by the perceived power associated with the beliefs (Ajzen & Driver, 1991).

Perceived behavioral control is an important factor in the model because it reflects the salient personal and environmental factors that influence behavior (Ajzen, 1985). Ajzen predicted that the effects of perceived behavioral control that are mediated by intention reflect the level of volitional control an individual has over the performance of the behavior in the future, similar to self-efficacy. However, if perceived behavioral control had a direct effect on behavior unmediated by intention, it would serve as a proxy for actual control and reflect the degree to which participation in the behavior is impaired by real environmental barriers or impedances. There is therefore the potential within the theory for direct and indirect effects of perceived behavioral control on exercise behavior.

Comparison studies have shown the theory of planned behavior to be more effective in explaining variance in exercise behavior than the theory of reasoned action (e.g., Dzewaltowski et al., 1990; Hagger et al., 2002b). Specifically, such research has demonstrated that attitude and perceived behavioral control predict intentions and explain approximately equal proportions of the variance in exercise behavior (Hagger & Chatzisarantis, 2005a; Hagger et al., 2002b). The research has also identified a lesser role for subjective norms, as in the theory of reasoned action. Studies have also identified the modal control beliefs, including barriers and facilitators, that underpin the direct measure of perceived behavioral control: "bad weather," "age," "heart pain," "costs," "fatigue," and "having no time" (Godin, Valois, Jobin, & Ross, 1991; Hagger, Chatzisarantis, & Biddle, 2001). As with behavioral and normative beliefs, research shows that control beliefs demonstrate considerable variance across populations and behaviors. For example, studies in the physical activity domain have identified "age" and "fear of having a heart attack" among the control beliefs for older and clinical populations (Godin et al., 1991), but these beliefs do not feature among the control beliefs of younger populations, who focus more on inclement weather and lack of time (Hagger, Chatzisarantis, & Biddle, 2001).

In addition to individual empirical studies, a meta-analysis of 72 studies applying the theory of planned behavior in exercise contexts has been conducted (Hagger et al., 2002b). Findings supported the major premises of the theory. A meta-analytic path analysis demonstrated that intention was the sole proximal predictor of exercise and that the effects of attitudes and perceived behavioral control on intentions were moderate and stronger than the effects of subjective norms. Included in the analysis were studies that separated measures of self-efficacy (reflecting personal capacity and confidence estimates) and perceived controllability (reflecting perceived barriers). Self-efficacy explained additional variance in the prediction of both intentions and behavior. In addition, past behavior predicted all of the theory constructs and attenuated their effects on intention and behavior. However, the influences of the social cognitive constructs remained significant. This result indicated that the variables in the model accounted for previous decision-making processes, but the most recent decision-making variables were nevertheless salient in explaining exercise intentions and behavior. In conclusion the authors stated: "While past behavior had a significant and direct influence on intention, attitude, perceived behavioral control, and self-efficacy, these cognitions are also necessary for translating past decisions about behavioral involvement into action. This is consistent with the notion that involvement in volitional behaviors such as regular physical activity involves both conscious and automatic influences" (Hagger et al., 2002b, p. 23).

The theory of planned behavior has received considerable attention in the social psychology literature, and this has been reflected in the exercise psychology literature. This attention is attributable to the theory's effectiveness in accounting for variance in exercise intention and behavior as well as its relative parsimony and role as a flexible framework for the study of psychosocial influences and processes that underpin exercise behavior. For example, its role as a flexible framework is supported by research that has shown the attitude, subjective norm, and perceived behavioral control constructs mediate the effects on intentions and behavior of distal constructs such as personality (Bozionelos & Bennett, 1999; Chatzisarantis & Hagger, 2008; Conner & Abraham, 2001; Conner, Rodgers, & Murray, 2007; Hoyt, Rhodes, Hausenblas, & Giacobbi, 2009; Rhodes & Courneya, 2003; Rhodes, Courneya, & Jones, 2002, 2003) and other individual-differences variables (Chatzisarantis & Hagger, 2007; Fitch & Ravlin, 2005; Hagger, Anderson, Kyriakaki, & Darkings, 2007). However, researchers have also indicated that the theory does not account for all of the variance in intention and behavior, nor does it mediate the effects of certain "external variables" on intentions and behavior (e.g., Bagozzi & Kimmel, 1995; Conner & Abraham, 2001; Conner & Armitage, 1998; Rhodes & Courneya, 2003; Rhodes et al., 2002). Paradoxically, this "weakness" has become the theory's greatest strength. Ajzen (1991) states that the theory should be viewed as a flexible framework into which other variables can be incorporated provided that they make meaningful and unique contributions to the prediction of intentions and that there is theoretical precedence for their inclusion.

As a consequence of its considerable flexibility, the theory has been adopted by researchers as a general framework with which to investigate the effects of a number of additional social cognitive constructs on intention and behavior (Conner & Armitage, 1998). To the extent that such a construct has a unique effect on intention or behavior and is not mediated by the core theory variables of attitude, subjective norms, and perceived behavioral control, the researcher has evidence to support its inclusion within the theory. A number of constructs have been found to have a unique effect on intentions, behavior, or both, including anticipated affect and attitude ambivalence (Armitage & Conner, 2000), anticipated regret (Sheeran & Orbell, 1999a), cultural norms and ethnicity (Blanchard et al., 2003, 2008, 2009; Van Hooft & De Jong, 2009; Walker, Courneya, & Deng, 2006), descriptive norms (Sheeran & Orbell, 1999a), group norms and membership (Terry, Hogg, & White, 2000; White, Hogg, & Terry, 2002), health locus of control (Armitage, 2003; Hagger & Armitage, 2004), moral norms (Godin, Conner, & Sheeran, 2005; Lam, 1999), past behavior (Aarts, Verplanken, & van Knippenberg, 1998; Albarracín & Wyer, 2000; Conner, Warren, Close, & Sparks, 1999; Hagger, Chatzisarantis, & Biddle, 2001), prototypes (Norman, Armitage, & Quigley, 2007), self-identity (Hagger & Chatzisarantis, 2006), and self-schemas (Sheeran & Orbell, 2000a).

In addition to the effects of other constructs, the influence of variations in the characteristics and nature of the core constructs of the theory of planned behavior on intentions, and of intention itself, on behavior have been investigated (Sheeran, 2002). Examples include the stability of intentions (Sheeran, Orbell, & Trafimow, 1999), the accessibility of attitudes (Doll & Ajzen, 1992; Verplanken, Hofstee, & Janssen, 1998), and hypothetical bias (Ajzen, Brown, & Carvahal, 2004). In addition, researchers have sought to differentiate between the independent and fundamental concepts within each of the psychosocial components that predict intentions. For example, attitudes have been differentiated into cognitive or instrumental attitudes and affective attitudes (Lowe, Eves, & Carroll, 2002; Trafimow & Sheeran, 1998), subjective norms have been differentiated into injunctive norms and descriptive norms (Rivis & Sheeran, 2003), and as mentioned previously, perceived behavioral control has been differentiated into self-efficacy and perceived controllability (Armitage & Conner, 1999a,

1999b; Hagger, Chatzisarantis, & Biddle, 2001; Povey, Conner, Sparks, James, & Shepherd, 2000; Sniehotta, Scholz, & Schwarzer, 2005; Terry & O'Leary, 1995). Even intentions have been distinguished from desires, the latter being "emotional" forms of intention (Perugini & Bagozzi, 2001, 2004). In the same vein, researchers have also investigated the extent to which individuals are oriented toward or base their intentions on each of the core theory constructs (Sheeran, Trafimow, Finlay, & Norman, 2002; Trafimow & Finlay, 1996).

These modifications suggest that the antecedents of volitional behaviors like physical activity may be more complex than originally conceived by the theory (Conner & Armitage, 1998). However, many of these modifications make relatively modest increases in the strength of the predictions within the model, and the separation of the theory components into more specific, differentiated constructs does not appear to affect the prediction of intentions and behavior at the global level (Hagger & Chatzisarantis, 2005a). Notwithstanding these modifications, the theory still performs relatively well in explaining exercise behavior and in its most parsimonious form can inform successful interventions to promote exercise (e.g., Chatzisarantis & Hagger, 2005; Darker, French, Eves, & Sniehotta, 2010).

Limitations

Although the theory of planned behavior has demonstrated considerable success in predicting exercise behavior in numerous contexts and groups, the theory and the research that has adopted it does have considerable documented limitations. First, the relationship between intentions and behavior is far from perfect. In fact, it falls considerably short of a large effect size; meta-analytic studies have typically indicated that the relationship between intentions and behavior is relatively modest (Hagger et al., 2002b), perhaps medium in size according to Cohen's (1987) taxonomy of effect sizes. Numerous reasons have been cited for this problem, such as a lack of correspondence between the measures of intention and behavior, the relative instability of intentions, and the moderating effect of numerous individual-difference factors such as self-schema. These issues have been frequently investigated, and research has shown that the intention–behavior "gap" is diminished under conditions of high intention stability and among self-schematics (Sheeran & Orbell, 2000a). However, the relationship remains relatively modest in effect size, which means that

people frequently do not convert their good intentions to engage in exercise into actual behavior.

A further limitation is that researchers have become fixated on a particular method of measuring and testing the theory, namely, using direct measures of the components in prospective studies. While these measures are useful, they do not provide a complete picture, particularly of the belief components that underpin and serve as the origin of the direct, global measures of attitudes, subjective norms, and perceived behavioral control. As a consequence, few studies truly demonstrate the origin of the antecedents of exercise behavior using the theory of planned behavior. This is problematic, particularly for people using the theory of planned behavior as a framework for the development of exercise interventions. Such interventions need to target the beliefs that underpin attitudes, subjective norms, and perceived behavioral control/self-efficacy to change the global construct and effect a concomitant change in intentions and behavior. As a result, interventions based on the theory have frequently not met with success (Hardeman et al., 2002), and research has also shown that interventions to change intentions often do not effect large changes in behavior (Webb & Sheeran, 2006). In addition, few studies have systematically targeted beliefs from each of the theory components and used them in controlled experimental or intervention designs to evaluate their effectiveness (Sniehotta, 2009). This presents a problem for the theory, and research needs to identify and map the specific beliefs that underpin the direct measures within the theory far more comprehensively and consistently to provide people wishing to use the theory as a template to develop interventions.

Implicit Theories

Research in social psychology over the past 10 years has begun to shift away from models that focus solely on deliberative, intentional, and explicit influences on behavior and has sought to develop theories that account for the nonconscious, impulsive, and implicit influences on human behavior (Bargh & Chartrand, 1999; Greenwald et al., 2002; Kehr, 2004; Nosek, Greenwald, & Banaji, 2007; Strack & Deutsch, 2004). Such approaches have given rise to so-called *dual route* models of motivation in recognition that behavior is a function of deliberative, volitional, and planned influences as well as those that are automatic, nonconscious, and unplanned (Hofmann, Friese, & Wiers, 2008; Strack & Deutsch, 2004). Interest in automatic and implicit processes has been mirrored by concomitant advances in methods to measure them. Research adopting measures of implicit processes alongside more traditional self-report measures of cognition has illustrated that behavior is influenced by both explicit and implicit social cognitive variables and that these effects are relatively independent (Perugini, 2005; Spence & Townsend, 2007). For example, research has demonstrated that implicit attitudes toward health-related behaviors predict behavior independent of explicit attitudes measured using traditional psychometric scales (Perugini, 2005).

These results suggest that exercise behavior may be a function of both explicit influences, similar to those captured by social cognitive theory and the theory of planned behavior, and implicit influences. Some individuals may be more implicitly biased toward engaging in exercise than others. This was shown by Calitri, Lowe, Eves, and Bennett (2009), who found significant relationships between previous exercise experience and responses to implicitly presented cues regarding exercise. This research also demonstrated that explicit attitudes moderated this effect, indicating that the effect of explicit and implicit attitudes on behavioral decisions is interactive. These findings indicate that people involved with promoting exercise should consider the effects of implicitly presented messages regarding exercise as well as the presentation of information and messages about exercise using traditional means of delivery such as persuasive communication, which target explicit perceptions.

Planning and Implemental Approaches

One approach that has shown efficacy in resolving the intention–behavior "gap" has been the adoption of action planning and implemental strategies as interventions. Heckhausen and Gollwitzer (1987) conceptualized intentional behavior such as exercise as having two stages leading to enactment: an intentional (motivational) phase and an implemental (volitional) phase. The intentional phase delineates the formation of intentions to engage in exercise behavior captured by the components of the theory of planned behavior. However, according to Heckhausen and Gollwitzer's model, intentions are necessary but not sufficient conditions for engaging in exercise behavior. The implemental phase, therefore, outlines how critical cues in the environment assist individuals in enacting their intentions by promoting links between an environmental event (cue) and the action (exercise behavior). Inducing

the individual to identify the key cues that highlight the important environmental contexts and activity associated with the initiation of a behavior is effective in promoting behavioral engagement. This identification of cues, known as an *implementation intention,* is done by having individuals write down when and where they will carry out the behavior (e.g., "*if* I am at work and 12 p.m. rolls around, *then* I will collect my kit bag and make my way to the gym"). Such strategies lead to increased accessibility of the cue in the environment and, from there, the recall of the associated action (Aarts, Dijksterhuis, & Midden, 1999; Brandstätter, Lengfelder, & Gollwitzer, 2001).

Providing opportunities for individuals to form implementation intentions results in increased engagement in health-related behaviors (Chapman, Armitage, & Norman, 2009; Orbell, Hodgkins, & Sheeran, 1997; Prestwich, Ayres, & Lawton, 2008; Prestwich et al., 2005; Prestwich, Perugini, & Hurling, 2009; Scholz, Schuz, Ziegelmann, Lippke, & Schwarzer, 2008; Sheeran & Orbell, 2000b; van Osch et al., 2009; Verplanken & Faes, 1999), including exercise (Arbour & Martin Ginis, 2009; Chatzisarantis, Hagger, & Thøgersen-Ntoumani, 2008; De Vet, Oenema, Sheeran, & Brug, 2009; Luszczynska, 2006; Milne, Orbell, & Sheeran, 2002; Prestwich, Lawton, & Conner, 2003; Sniehotta, Scholz, Schwarzer et al., 2005). A meta-analysis of implementation intention research demonstrated that the effect of such strategies on behavior is strong and consistent (Gollwitzer & Sheeran, 2006). In terms of mechanisms, research has revealed that implementation intentions do not result in changes in intentions or in variables of the theory of planned behavior but rather are mediated by planning and memory recall (Orbell et al., 1997; Scholz et al., 2008; Sheeran & Orbell, 1999b). The identification of such psychosocial mediators is salient, because it provides information on the processes responsible for the effect (Michie, 2008).

Integrated Approaches

Recently, researchers have sought to integrate psychosocial models such as the theory of planned behavior with other motivational theories, such as self-determination theory (Deci & Ryan, 1985, 2000), that are deemed to provide complementary explanations of the processes that underlie motivated behavior (Hagger, 2009). With regard to the theory of planned behavior, such integration can provide information regarding the origins of the attitudes, subjective norms, and perceived behavioral control constructs. Several researchers have used integrated approaches in mediational models to illustrate the processes that lead to decisions to engage in social behavior. For example, self-determined or autonomous motives from self-determination theory have been shown to directly predict behavioral intentions (Chatzisarantis, Hagger, Biddle, & Karageorghis, 2002; Hagger, Chatzisarantis, & Biddle, 2002a; Standage, Duda, & Ntoumanis, 2003; Wilson & Rodgers, 2004). However, some researchers have tested a more complete model in which different styles of self-determined and non-self-determined motivations from self-determination theory predict intentions via the mediation of attitudes and perceived behavioral control. This motivational sequence has been supported in a number of studies (Chatzisarantis et al., 2002; Hagger, Chatzisarantis, Barkoukis, Wang, & Baranowski, 2005; Hagger et al., 2002a; Hagger, Chatzisarantis, Culverhouse, & Biddle, 2003; Hagger, Chatzisarantis, & Harris, 2006). (For a detailed explanation of self-determination theory, readers are directed to Hagger and Chatzisarantis, 2008.)

The proposition that self-determination theory (Deci & Ryan, 1985, 2000) can augment social cognitive theories such as the theory of planned behavior has been suggested by previous researchers and theorists but has only recently received empirical support. Numerous authors have proposed that motivational, organismic theories such as self-determination theory could offer explanations for the origins of constructs in social cognitive theories. As Andersen, Chen, and Carter (2000) state, "most information processing [social cognitive] models are silent on matters central to self-determination theory" (p. 272). Deci and Ryan (1985) suggested that social cognitive theories identify the immediate antecedents of behavior but neglect the origins of the antecedents: "Cognitive theories begin their analysis with what Kagan (1972) called a motive, which is a cognitive representation of some future desired state. What is missing, of course, is the consideration of the conditions of the organism that makes these future states desired" (p. 228). Constructs such as attitudes, perceived behavioral control, and intentions from social cognitive theories like the theory of planned behavior are measured as explicitly stated expectancies regarding future behavioral engagement. Therefore the integration of social cognitive theories with other motivational theories may offer more information in regard to the mechanisms that underlie intentional social and health behavior.

The integration of the theory of planned behavior and self-determination theory is based on two key premises. The first premise is the hypothesis that the relationship between autonomous motives from self-determination theory and the constructs from the theory of planned behavior is a *formative* one. Central to self-determination theory is the distinction between self-determined, or *autonomous,* forms of motivation and non-self-determined, or *controlling,* forms of motivation. Self-determined motives are closely associated with increased persistence, enjoyment, and engagement in tasks and behaviors in the absence of external contingencies, while non-self-determined motives are associated with decreased motivation and persistence when external contingencies are lacking. People who have high levels of autonomous motivation in a given domain are likely to experience their behavior in that domain as personally relevant and valued, in that it is concordant with their psychological need for self-determination (Sheldon, 2002). As a consequence, autonomously motivated people will have a greater tendency to critically examine the importance and value of the outcomes of engaging in any future target behavior. In the case of exercise, autonomously motivated people will be likely to find information that points to the importance of these health behaviors and thus form a positive attitude toward future participation in them. In contrast, people who report high levels of controlled forms of motivation will tend to focus on external contingencies of future engagement in a target behavior, which are likely to have little to do with the valued consequences of the behavior. Individuals with high levels of autonomous motivation are likely to feel more confident of reaching their goals and to engage in behavior to satisfy those goals because such behavior quenches their need for competence. Links have been found between autonomous motivation and perceived competence (e.g., Williams, Gagne, Ryan, & Deci, 2002; Williams, McGregor, Zeldman, & Freedman, 2004).

The second premise relates to the relative degree of generality reflected by the constructs from the two theories. The autonomous motives from self-determination theory reflect dispositional motivational orientations in a particular context and are therefore expected to predict behavioral engagement across all forms of behavior in that context. Vallerand (2000) labels this form of motivation *contextual-level motivation.* However, the constructs from the theory of planned behavior are *expectations* about engaging in the behavior in the future, and measures of these constructs therefore specify explicitly the behavior and the time frame of the bout of that behavior. Vallerand suggested that contextual-level motivation affects motivational orientations at the situational level in a top-down fashion (see also Guay, Mageau, & Vallerand, 2003). Intentions in the theory of planned behavior are hypothesized to be located at this level because they reflect expectations about engaging in a specific target behavior at a specific future time. They are therefore conceptualized as orientations to engage in a behavior at the situational level. Vallerand also hypothesized that contextual-level motivation would also influence cognitions at the situational level. It is therefore expected that motivation at the contextual level would influence the beliefs that underlie engagement in specific bouts of a behavior in the future, which according to the theory of planned behavior are constructs like attitudes and perceived behavioral control. In accordance with this theory, it would be expected that contextual-level motives would predict the performance of behavior at the situational level and its antecedents.

Empirical Support for the Theoretical Integration

A growing body of research has supported the integration of the theory of planned behavior and self-determination theory. The development of research in this area began with Chatzisarantis, Biddle, and Meek (1997), who found that intentions based on self-determination theory (autonomous intentions) were a better predictor of behavior than "traditional" forms of intentions. Similarly, Sheeran, Norman, and Orbell (1999) found that intentions based on attitudes were more likely to predict behavior than intentions based on subjective norms. They suggested that intentions based on attitudes reflected pursuing behaviors for personally valued outcomes (akin to an identified regulation) and therefore for more autonomous reasons than intentions based on subjective norms, which reflected more controlling aspects of motivation (such as external or introjected regulations). Together these results paved the way for more comprehensive studies in which the effects of self-determined forms of motivation influenced behavior.

Since these pioneering studies, researchers have been committed to comprehensive tests that adopt hypotheses from both component theories to address hypotheses relating to social behavior in numerous contexts. Prominent among these studies are those that outline a clear motivational sequence in which

the generalized motivational orientations from self-determination theory influence constructs from the theory of planned behavior (e.g., Chatzisarantis et al., 2002; Hagger et al., 2002a). In such studies, the theory of planned behavior acts as a conduit for the effects of autonomous forms of motivation on motivated behavior. The decision-making constructs from the theory of planned behavior reflect the formation of plans to engage in a behavior in the future and represent situational motivational orientations toward that target behavior. The self-determination theory motives serve to indicate a source of information that influences the decision-making process. For example, autonomous forms of motivation from self-determination theory are hypothesized to influence attitudes from the theory of planned behavior as autonomous motivational dispositions in a particular domain and are likely to be impetuses to the formation of attitudes oriented toward serving personally valued goals and to mediate the effects of autonomous motivation on intention.

Hagger, Chatzisarantis, and Biddle (2002a) found that self-determined forms of motivation affected intentions to engage in physical activity behavior, but only via the mediation of attitudes and perceived behavioral control. This result provided support for the hypothesis that autonomous forms of motivation bias individuals' decision making in favor of forming attitudes congruent with their personal goals (attitudes) and perceptions that the behavior will lead to competence-related outcomes (perceived behavioral control). This hypothesis was corroborated in a subsequent study that extended these findings to actual behavior. Autonomous motives affected behavior via a motivational sequence beginning with autonomous forms of motivation and ending with behavioral engagement mediated by attitudes, perceived behavioral control, intentions, and effort (Chatzisarantis et al., 2002). Since this initial research, several studies have corroborated the indirect effect of autonomous motives from self-determination theory on intentions and behavior as stipulated by the proposed motivational sequence. A recent meta-analysis of all studies adopting these theories and testing some of the components of the integrated motivational sequence has provided further support for the sequence (Hagger & Chatzisarantis, 2009b). The meta-analysis demonstrated that across 36 studies, the majority of which were in an exercise context, the effects of self-determined motivation on behavior were mediated by the variables from the theory of planned behavior. This finding provides useful information about the process by which social contexts influence behavior and suggests recommendations for intervention. For example, it has been shown that interventions can be designed in such a way as to change perceptions at any stage of the motivational sequence, targeting either autonomous motives as a distal influence on intentions or attitudes and perceived control as a proximal influence. This may lead to hybrid interventions that adopt techniques from both self-determination theory (Chatzisarantis & Hagger, 2009) and the theory of planned behavior (Chatzisarantis & Hagger, 2005) to promote increased exercise participation.

Conclusion

This chapter outlined the importance of psychosocial factors in exercise behavior. Central to this review is the notion of identifying not only the factors that influence exercise but the mechanisms and processes by which those factors exert their influence. These processes were identified and reviewed with respect to two key psychosocial theories that have been applied to the understanding of exercise behavior: social cognitive theory and the theory of planned behavior. It was illustrated that self-efficacy is a pervasive influence on exercise behavior and has been incorporated into the reasoned action approach (Ajzen & Fishbein, 1980; Fishbein & Ajzen, 2009) to provide a comprehensive model of exercise behavior, the theory of planned behavior (Ajzen, 1985, 1991). The theory has demonstrated efficacy in explaining exercise behavior and as the basis of interventions, but it has limitations that include the relatively modest intention–behavior relationship and its omission of other variables, including implicit factors. Also presented was new and innovative research in the field that has attempted to address the intention–behavior gap and augment these theories, including work involving implementation intentions, implicit constructs, and the incorporation of hypotheses from other theories.

The present review provides a brief summary of the large body of research examining the psychosocial influences on physical activity behavior. The literature is continually being augmented and updated with innovative new studies that aim to understand the various influences on exercise and the processes associated with these influences. This research should form the basis of new and innovative interventions and public health messages to promote increased physical activity among clinical and sedentary adult and child populations. Developing interventions on the basis of this cutting-edge research will lead to programs with the greatest probability of success.

Future Directions

Research examining the psychosocial influences on exercise behavior should focus on addressing the following key questions:

• What are the key behavioral beliefs, outcome evaluations, normative beliefs, motivations to comply, control beliefs, and power-of-control beliefs for exercise behavior for different populations? Can these be mapped onto interventions to change each of the direct measures of the constructs from the theory of planned behavior?

• Can we develop further full-factorial experimental tests of the theory of planned behavior in leisure-time exercise contexts, similar to those conducted by Sniehotta and colleagues (Sniehotta, 2009)?

• To what extent are the beliefs that underpin attitudes, intentions, and perceived behavioral control self-determined (or autonomous) or non-self-determined (or controlling) in accordance with self-determination theory?

• What is the contribution of implicit social cognitive variables like self-efficacy and motivation to exercise behavior relative to explicit influences?

References
Entries marked with an asterisk are recommended for further reading.

Aarts, H., Dijksterhuis, A., & Midden, C. (1999). To plan or not to plan? Goal achievement or interrupting the performance of mundane behaviors. *European Journal of Social Psychology, 29*, 971–979.

Aarts, H., Verplanken, B., & van Knippenberg, A. (1998). Predicting behavior from actions in the past: Repeated decision-making or a matter of habit? *Journal of Applied Social Psychology, 28*, 1355–1374.

*Ajzen, I. (1985). From intentions to actions: A theory of planned behavior. In J. Kuhl & J. Beckmann (Eds.), *Action-control: From cognition to behavior* (pp. 11–39). Heidelberg: Springer-Verlag.

Ajzen, I. (1991). The theory of planned behavior. *Organizational Behavior and Human Decision Processes, 50*, 179–211.

Ajzen, I. (2003, April 14). *Constructing a TPB questionnaire: Conceptual and methodological considerations*. Retrieved September 1, 2009, from http://www-unix.oit.umass.edu/~aizen

Ajzen, I., Brown, T. C., & Carvahal, F. (2004). Explaining the discrepancy between intentions and actions: The case of hypothetical bias in contingent valuation. *Personality and Social Psychology Bulletin, 30*, 1108–1121.

Ajzen, I., & Driver, B. E. (1991). Prediction of leisure participation from behavioral, normative, and control beliefs: An application of the theory of planned behavior. *Leisure Sciences, 13*, 185–204.

Ajzen, I., & Fishbein, M. (1980). *Understanding attitudes and predicting social behavior*. Upper Saddle River, NJ: Prentice Hall.

Ajzen, I., & Fishbein, M. (2008). Scaling and testing multiplicative combinations in the expectancy-value model of attitudes. *Journal of Applied Social Psychology, 38*, 2222–2247.

Albarracín, D., & Wyer, R. S. (2000). The cognitive impact of past behavior: Influences on beliefs, intentions, and future behavioral decisions. *Journal of Personality and Social Psychology, 79*, 5–22.

Andersen, S. M., Chen, S., & Carter, C. (2000). Fundamental human needs: Making social cognition relevant. *Psychological Inquiry, 4*, 269–275.

Anderson, E. S., Wojcik, J. R., Winett, R. A., & Williams, D. M. (2006). Social-cognitive determinants of physical activity: The influence of social support, self-efficacy, outcome expectations, and self-regulation among participants in a church-based health promotion study. *Health Psychology, 25*, 510–520.

Arbour, K. P., & Martin Ginis, K. A. (2009). A randomised controlled trial of the effects of implementation intentions on women's walking behaviour. *Psychology and Health, 24*, 49–65.

Armitage, C. J. (2003). The relationship between multidimensional health locus of control and perceived behavioural control: How are distal perceptions of control related to proximal perceptions of control? *Psychology and Health, 18*, 723–738.

Armitage, C. J., & Conner, M. (1999a). Distinguishing perceptions of control from self-efficacy: Predicting consumption of a low fat diet using the theory of planned behavior. *Journal of Applied Social Psychology, 29*, 72–90.

Armitage, C. J., & Conner, M. (1999b). The theory of planned behavior: Assessment of predictive validity and 'perceived control.' *British Journal of Social Psychology, 38*, 35–54.

Armitage, C. J., & Conner, M. (2000). Attitudinal ambivalence: A test of three key hypotheses. *Personality and Social Psychology Bulletin, 26*, 1421–1432.

Armitage, C. J., & Conner, M. (2001). Efficacy of the theory of planned behaviour: A meta-analytic review. *British Journal of Social Psychology, 40*, 471–499.

Bagozzi, R. P. (1984). Expectancy-value attitude models: An analysis of critical measurement issues. *International Journal of Research in Marketing, 1*, 295–310.

Bagozzi, R. P., & Kimmel, S. K. (1995). A comparison of leading theories for the prediction of goal directed behaviours. *British Journal of Social Psychology, 34*, 437–461.

Bandura, A. (1977a). Self-efficacy: Toward a unifying theory of behavioral change. *Psychological Review, 84*, 191–215.

Bandura, A. (1977b). *Social learning theory*. Englewood Cliffs, NJ: Prentice Hall.

Bandura, A. (1986). *The foundations of thought and action*. Englewood Cliffs, NJ: Prentice Hall.

*Bandura, A. (1997). *Self-efficacy: The exercise of control*. New York: Freeman.

Bargh, J. A., & Chartrand, T. L. (1999). The unbearable automaticity of being. *American Psychologist, 54*, 462–479.

Blanchard, C. M., Kupperman, J., Sparling, P. B., Nehl, E., Rhodes, R. E., Courneya, K. S., & Baker, F. (2009). Do ethnicity and gender matter when using the theory of planned behavior to understand fruit and vegetable consumption? *Appetite, 52*, 15–20.

Blanchard, C. M., Kupperman, J., Sparling, P., Nehl, E., Rhodes, R. E., Courneya, K. S., Baker, F., & Rupp, J. C. (2008). Ethnicity and the theory of planned behavior in an exercise context: A mediation and moderation perspective. *Psychology of Sport and Exercise, 9*, 527–545.

Blanchard, C. M., Rhodes, R. E., Nehl, E., Fisher, J., Sparling, P., & Courneya, K. S. (2003). Ethnicity and the theory of planned behavior in the exercise domain. *American Journal of Health Behavior, 27*, 579–591.

Bozionelos, G., & Bennett, P. (1999). The theory of planned behaviour as predictor of exercise: The moderating influence of beliefs and personality variables. *Journal of Health Psychology, 4*, 517–529.

Bozoian, S., Rejeski, W. J., & McAuley, E. (1994). Self-efficacy influences feeling states associated with acute exercise. *Journal of Sport and Exercise Psychology, 16*, 326–333.

Brandstätter, V., Lengfelder, A., & Gollwitzer, P. M. (2001). Implementation intentions and efficient action initiation. *Personality and Social Psychology Bulletin, 81*, 946–960.

Calitri, R., Lowe, R., Eves, F. F., & Bennett, P. (2009). Associations between visual attention, implicit and explicit attitude and behaviour for physical activity. *Psychology and Health, 24*, 1105–1123.

Chapman, J., Armitage, C. J., & Norman, P. (2009). Comparing implementation intention interventions in relation to young adults' intake of fruit and vegetables. *Psychology and Health, 24*(3), 317–332. doi:10.1080/08870440701864538

Chatzisarantis, N. L. D., & Biddle, S. J. H. (1998). Functional significance of psychological variables that are included in the theory of planned behaviour: A self-determination theory approach to the study of attitudes, subjective norms, perceptions of control and intentions. *European Journal of Social Psychology, 28*, 303–322.

Chatzisarantis, N. L. D., Biddle, S. J. H., & Meek, G. A. (1997). A self-determination theory approach to the study of intentions and the intention–behaviour relationship in children's physical activity. *British Journal of Health Psychology, 2*, 343–360.

Chatzisarantis, N. L. D., & Hagger, M. S. (2005). Effects of a brief intervention based on the theory of planned behavior on leisure time physical activity participation. *Journal of Sport and Exercise Psychology, 27*, 470–487.

Chatzisarantis, N. L. D., & Hagger, M. S. (2007). Mindfulness and the intention–behavior relationship within the theory of planned behavior. *Personality and Social Psychology Bulletin, 33*, 663–676.

Chatzisarantis, N. L. D., & Hagger, M. S. (2008). Influences of personality traits and continuation intentions on physical activity participation within the theory of planned behaviour. *Psychology and Health, 23*, 347–367.

Chatzisarantis, N. L. D., & Hagger, M. S. (2009). Effects of an intervention based on self-determination theory on self-reported leisure-time physical activity participation. *Psychology and Health, 24*, 29–48.

Chatzisarantis, N. L. D., Hagger, M. S., Biddle, S. J. H., & Karageorghis, C. (2002). The cognitive processes by which perceived locus of causality predicts participation in physical activity. *Journal of Health Psychology, 7*, 685–699.

Chatzisarantis, N. L. D., Hagger, M. S., Biddle, S. J. H., & Smith, B. (2005). The stability of the attitude–intention relationship in the context of physical activity. *Journal of Sport Sciences, 23*, 49–61.

Chatzisarantis, N. L. D., Hagger, M. S., & Thøgersen-Ntoumani, C. (2008). Effects of implementation intentions and self concordance on health behavior. *Journal of Applied Biobehavioral Research, 13*, 198–214.

Cohen, J. (1987). *Statistical power analysis for the behavioral sciences* (2nd ed.). Hillsdale, NJ: Erlbaum.

Conner, M., & Abraham, C. (2001). Conscientiousness and the theory of planned behavior: Toward a more complete model of the antecedents of intentions and behavior. *Personality and Social Psychology Bulletin, 27*, 1547–1561.

Conner, M., & Armitage, C. J. (1998). Extending the theory of planned behavior: A review and avenues for further research. *Journal of Applied Social Psychology, 28*, 1429–1464.

Conner, M., Rodgers, W., & Murray, T. (2007). Conscientiousness and the intention–behavior relationship: Predicting exercise behavior. *Journal of Sport and Exercise Psychology, 29*, 518–533.

Conner, M., Warren, R., Close, S., & Sparks, P. (1999). Alcohol consumption and the theory of planned behavior: An examination of the cognitive mediation of past behavior. *Journal of Applied Social Psychology, 29*, 1676–1704.

Costanzo, C., & Walker, S. N. (2008). Incorporating self-efficacy and interpersonal support in an intervention to increase physical activity in older women. *Women & Health, 47*, 91–108.

Darker, C. D., French, D. P., Eves, F. F., & Sniehotta, F. F. (2010). An intervention to promote walking amongst the general population based on an 'extended' theory of planned behaviour: A waiting list randomised controlled trial. *Psychology and Health, 25*, 71–88.

Deci, E. L., & Ryan, R. M. (1985). *Intrinsic motivation and self-determination in human behavior*. New York: Plenum Press.

Deci, E. L., & Ryan, R. M. (2000). The "what" and "why" of goal pursuits: Human needs and the self-determination of behavior. *Psychological Inquiry, 11*, 227–268.

De Vet, E., Oenema, A., Sheeran, P., & Brug, J. (2009). Should implementation intentions interventions be implemented in obesity prevention: The impact of if–then plans on daily physical activity in Dutch adults. *International Journal of Behavioral Nutrition and Physical Activity, 6*, 11.

Doll, J., & Ajzen, I. (1992). Accessibility and stability of predictors in the theory of planned behavior. *Journal of Personality and Social Psychology, 63*, 754–765.

Dzewaltowski, D. A. (1989). Toward a model of exercise motivation. *Journal of Sport and Exercise Psychology, 11*, 252–269.

Dzewaltowski, D. A., Noble, J. M., & Shaw, J. M. (1990). Physical activity participation: Social cognitive theory vs. the theories of reasoned action and planned behavior. *Journal of Sport and Exercise Psychology, 12*, 388–405.

Ewart, C. K. (1989). Psychological effects of resistive weight training—implications for cardiac patients. *Medicine & Science in Sports & Exercise, 21*, 683–688.

Feltz, D. L., & Chase, M. A. (1998). The measurement of self-efficacy and confidence in sport. In J. L. Duda (Ed.), *Advances in sport and exercise psychology measurement* (pp. 65–80). Morgantown, WV: Fitness Information Technology.

Fishbein, M., & Ajzen, I. (2009). *Predicting and changing behavior*. New York: Psychology Press.

Fitch, J. L., & Ravlin, E. C. (2005). Willpower and perceived behavioral control: Influences on the intention–behavior relationship and postbehavior attributions. *Social Behavior and Personality, 33*, 105–123.

French, D. P., & Hankins, M. (2003). The expectancy-value muddle in the theory of planned behaviour—and some proposed solutions. *British Journal of Health Psychology, 8*, 37–55.

Godin, G., Conner, M., & Sheeran, P. (2005). Bridging the intention–behaviour 'gap': The role of moral norm. *British Journal of Social Psychology, 44*, 497–512.

Godin, G., & Kok, G. (1996). The theory of planned behavior: A review of its applications to health related behaviors. *American Journal of Health Promotion, 11*, 87–98.

Godin, G., Valois, R., Jobin, J., & Ross, A. (1991). Prediction of intention to exercise of individuals who have suffered from coronary heart disease. *Journal of Clinical Psychology, 47*, 762–772.

*Gollwitzer, P. M., & Sheeran, P. (2006). Implementation intentions and goal achievement: A meta-analysis of effects and processes. *Advances in Experimental Social Psychology, 38*, 69–119.

Greenwald, A. G., Banaji, M. R., Rudman, L. A., Farnham, S. D., Nosek, B. A., & Mellott, D. S. (2002). A unified theory of implicit attitudes, stereotypes, self-esteem, and self-concept. *Psychological Review, 109*, 3–25.

Guay, F., Mageau, G. A., & Vallerand, R. J. (2003). On the hierarchical structure of self-determined motivation: A test of top-down, bottom-up, reciprocal, and horizontal effects. *Personality and Social Psychology Bulletin, 29*, 992–1004.

*Hagger, M. S. (2009). Theoretical integration in health psychology: Unifying ideas and complementary explanations. *British Journal of Health Psychology, 14*, 189–194.

Hagger, M. S. (2010). Current issues and new directions in psychology and health: Physical activity research showcasing theory into practice. *Psychology and Health, 25*, 1–5.

Hagger, M. S., Anderson, M., Kyriakaki, M., & Darkings, S. (2007). Aspects of identity and their influence on intentional behaviour: Comparing effects for three health behaviours. *Personality and Individual Differences, 42*, 355–367.

Hagger, M. S., & Armitage, C. (2004). The influence of perceived loci of control and causality in the theory of planned behavior in a leisure-time exercise context. *Journal of Applied Biobehavioral Research, 9*, 45–64.

Hagger, M. S., & Chatzisarantis, N. L. D. (2005a). First- and higher-order models of attitudes, normative influence, and perceived behavioural control in the theory of planned behaviour. *British Journal of Social Psychology, 44*, 513–535.

*Hagger, M. S., & Chatzisarantis, N. L. D. (2005b). *The social psychology of exercise and sport*. Buckingham, UK: Open University Press.

Hagger, M. S., & Chatzisarantis, N. L. D. (2006). Self-identity and the theory of planned behaviour: Between- and within-participants analyses. *British Journal of Social Psychology, 45*, 731–757.

Hagger, M. S., & Chatzisarantis, N. L. D. (2008). Self-determination theory and the psychology of exercise. *International Review of Sport and Exercise Psychology, 1*, 79–103.

Hagger, M. S., & Chatzisarantis, N. L. D. (2009a). Assumptions in research in sport and exercise psychology. *Psychology of Sport and Exercise, 10*, 511–519.

Hagger, M. S., & Chatzisarantis, N. L. D. (2009b). Integrating the theory of planned behaviour and self-determination theory in health behaviour: A meta-analysis. *British Journal of Health Psychology, 14*, 275–302.

Hagger, M. S., Chatzisarantis, N. L. D., Barkoukis, V., Wang, C. K. J., & Baranowski, J. (2005). Perceived autonomy support in physical education and leisure-time physical activity: A cross-cultural evaluation of the trans-contextual model. *Journal of Educational Psychology, 97*, 376–390.

Hagger, M. S., Chatzisarantis, N., & Biddle, S. J. H. (2001). The influence of self-efficacy and past behaviour on the physical activity intentions of young people. *Journal of Sports Sciences, 19*, 711–725.

Hagger, M. S., Chatzisarantis, N. L. D., & Biddle, S. J. H. (2002a). The influence of autonomous and controlling motives on physical activity intentions within the theory of planned behaviour. *British Journal of Health Psychology, 7*, 283–297.

*Hagger, M. S., Chatzisarantis, N. L. D., & Biddle, S. J. H. (2002b). A meta-analytic review of the theories of reasoned action and planned behavior in physical activity: Predictive validity and the contribution of additional variables. *Journal of Sport and Exercise Psychology, 24*, 3–32.

Hagger, M. S., Chatzisarantis, N., Biddle, S. J. H., & Orbell, S. (2001). Antecedents of children's physical activity intentions and behaviour: Predictive validity and longitudinal effects. *Psychology and Health, 16*, 391–407.

Hagger, M. S., Chatzisarantis, N. L. D., Culverhouse, T., & Biddle, S. J. H. (2003). The processes by which perceived autonomy support in physical education promotes leisure-time physical activity intentions and behavior: A trans-contextual model. *Journal of Educational Psychology, 95*, 784–795.

Hagger, M. S., Chatzisarantis, N. L. D., & Harris, J. (2006). From psychological need satisfaction to intentional behavior: Testing a motivational sequence in two behavioral contexts. *Personality and Social Psychology Bulletin, 32*, 131–138.

Hardeman, W., Johnston, M., Johnston, D. W., Bonetti, D., Wareham, N. J., & Kinmonth, A. L. (2002). Application of the theory of planned behaviour in behaviour change interventions: A systematic review. *Psychology and Health, 17*, 123–158.

Heckhausen, H., & Gollwitzer, P. M. (1987). Thought contents and cognitive functioning in motivational and volitional states of mind. *Motivation and Emotion, 11*, 101–120.

Hofmann, W., Friese, M., & Wiers, R. W. (2008). Impulsive versus reflective influences on health behavior: A theoretical framework and empirical review. *Health Psychology Review, 2*, 111–137.

Hortz, B., & Petosa, R. L. (2008). Social cognitive theory variables mediation of moderate exercise. *American Journal of Health Behavior, 32*, 305–314.

Hoyt, A. L., Rhodes, R. E., Hausenblas, H. A., & Giacobbi, P. R., Jr. (2009). Integrating five-factor model facet-level traits with the theory of planned behavior and exercise. *Psychology of Sport and Exercise, 10*, 565–572.

Kehr, H. M. (2004). Implicit/explicit motive discrepancies and volitional depletion among managers. *Personality and Social Psychology Bulletin, 30*, 315–327.

Lam, S. (1999). Predicting intentions to conserve water from the theory of planned behavior, perceived moral obligation, and perceived water right. *Journal of Applied Social Psychology, 29*, 1058–1071.

Lee, L. L., Arthur, A., & Avis, M. (2008). Using self-efficacy theory to develop interventions that help older people overcome psychological barriers to physical activity: A discussion paper. *International Journal of Nursing Studies, 45*, 1690–1699.

Lowe, R., Eves, F., & Carroll, D. (2002). The influence of affective and instrumental beliefs on exercise intentions and behavior: A longitudinal analysis. *Journal of Applied Social Psychology, 32*, 1241–1252.

Luszczynska, A. (2006). An implementation intentions intervention, the use of a planning strategy, and physical activity after myocardial infarction. *Social Science & Medicine, 62*, 900–908.

Luszczynska, A., & Haynes, C. (2009). Changing nutrition, physical activity and body weight among student nurses and midwives: Effects of a planning intervention and self-efficacy beliefs. *Journal of Health Psychology, 14*, 1075–1084.

McAuley, E. (1992). The role of efficacy cognitions in the prediction of exercise behavior in middle-aged adults. *Journal of Behavioral Medicine, 15*, 65–88.

McAuley, E., & Blissmer, B. (2000). Self-efficacy determinants and consequences of physical activity. *Exercise and Sport Science Reviews, 28*, 85–88.

McAuley, E., & Blissmer, B. (2002). Self-efficacy and attributional processes in physical activity. In T. S. Horn (Ed.), *Advances in Sport Psychology* (pp. 185–206). Champaign, IL: Human Kinetics.

McAuley, E., & Courneya, K. S. (1993). Adherence to exercise and physical activity as health-promoting behaviors. *Applied and Preventive Psychology, 2*, 65–77.

Michie, S. (2008). What works and how? Designing more effective interventions needs answers to both questions. *Addiction, 103*, 886–887.

Mildestvedt, T., Meland, E., & Eide, G. E. (2008). How important are individual counselling, expectancy beliefs and autonomy for the maintenance of exercise after cardiac rehabilitation? *Scandinavian Journal of Public Health, 36*, 832–840.

Milne, S. E., Orbell, S., & Sheeran, P. (2002). Combining motivational and volitional interventions to promote exercise participation: Protection motivation theory and implementation intentions. *British Journal of Health Psychology, 7*, 163–184.

Motl, R. W., McAuley, E., Doerksen, S., Hu, L., & Morris, K. S. (2009). Preliminary evidence that self-efficacy predicts physical activity in multiple sclerosis. *International Journal of Rehabilitation Research, 32*, 260–263.

Norman, P., Armitage, C. J., & Quigley, C. (2007). The theory of planned behavior and binge drinking: Assessing the impact of binge drinker prototypes. *Addictive Behaviors, 32*, 1753–1768.

Nosek, B. A., Greenwald, A. G., & Banaji, M. R. (2007). The Implicit Association Test at age 7: A methodological and conceptual review. In J. A. Bargh (Ed.), *Automatic processes in social thinking and behavior* (pp. 265–292). New York: Psychology Press.

Ogden, J. (2003). Some problems with social cognition models: A pragmatic and conceptual basis. *Health Psychology, 22*, 424–428.

Orbell, S., Hodgkins, S., & Sheeran, P. (1997). Implementation intentions and the theory of planned behavior. *Personality and Social Psychology Bulletin, 23*, 945–954.

Park, C. L., & Gaffey, A. E. (2007). Relationships between psychosocial factors and health behavior change in cancer survivors: An integrative review. *Annals of Behavioral Medicine, 34*, 115–134.

*Perugini, M. (2005). Predictive models of implicit and explicit attitudes. *British Journal of Social Psychology, 44*, 29–45.

Perugini, M., & Bagozzi, R. P. (2001). The role of desires and anticipated emotions in goal-directed behaviours: Broadening and deepening the theory of planned behavior. *British Journal of Social Psychology, 40*, 79–98.

Perugini, M., & Bagozzi, R. P. (2004). The distinction between desires and intentions. *European Journal of Social Psychology, 34*, 69–84.

Petter, M., Blanchard, C., Kemp, K. A. R., Mazoff, A. S., & Ferrier, S. N. (2009). Correlates of exercise among coronary heart disease patients: review, implications and future directions. *European Journal of Cardiovascular Prevention & Rehabilitation, 16*, 515–526.

Poag, K., & McAuley, E. (1992). Goal setting, self-efficacy and exercise behavior. *Journal of Sports and Exercise Psychology, 14*, 352–360.

Povey, R., Conner, M., Sparks, P., James, R., & Shepherd, R. (2000). Application of the theory of planned behaviour to two dietary behaviours: Roles of perceived control and self-efficacy. *British Journal of Health Psychology, 5*, 121–139.

Prestwich, A., Ayres, K., & Lawton, R. (2008). Crossing two types of implementation intentions with a protection motivation intervention for the reduction of saturated fat intake: A randomized trial. *Social Science & Medicine, 67*, 1550–1558.

Prestwich, A., Conner, M., Lawton, R., Bailey, W., Litman, J., & Molyneaux, V. (2005). Individual and collaborative implementation intentions and the promotion of breast self-examination. *Psychology and Health, 20*, 743–760.

Prestwich, A., Lawton, R., & Conner, M. (2003). The use of implementation intentions and the decision balance sheet in promoting exercise behaviour. *Psychology and Health, 10*, 707–721.

Prestwich, A., Perugini, M., & Hurling, R. (2009). Can the effects of implementation intentions on exercise be enhanced using text messages? *Psychology and Health, 24*, 677–687.

Prochaska, J. O., & DiClemente, C. C. (1982). Trans-theoretical theory: Towards a more integrated model of change. *Journal of Consultative Clinical Psychology, 19*, 276–288.

Prochaska, J. O., & Markus, B. H. (1994). The transtheoretical model: Applications to exercise. In R. K. Dishman (Ed.), *Advances in exercise adherence* (pp. 161–180). Champaign, IL: Human Kinetics.

Rhodes, R. E., & Courneya, K. S. (2003). Relationships between personality, an extended theory of planned behaviour model and exercise behaviour. *British Journal of Health Psychology, 8*, 19–36.

Rhodes, R. E., Courneya, K. S., & Jones, L. W. (2002). Personality, the theory of planned behavior, and exercise: A unique role for extroversion's activity facet. *Journal of Applied Social Psychology, 32*, 1721–1736.

Rhodes, R. E., Courneya, K. S., & Jones, L. W. (2003). Translating exercise intentions into behavior: Personality and social cognitive correlates. *Journal of Health Psychology, 8*, 449–460.

Rivis, A., & Sheeran, P. (2003). Descriptive norms as an additional predictor in the theory of planned behaviour: A meta-analysis. *Current Psychology, 22*, 218–233.

Rodgers, W. M., & Brawley, L. R. (1991). The role of outcome expectations in participation motivation. *Journal of Sport and Exercise Psychology, 13*, 411–427.

Rodgers, W. M., & Brawley, L. R. (1993). Using both self-efficacy theory and the theory of planned behavior to discriminate adherers and dropouts from structured programs. *Journal of Applied Sport Psychology, 5*, 195–206.

Rogers, R. W. (1975). A protection motivation theory of fear appeals and attitude change. *Journal of Psychology, 91*, 93–114.

Scholz, U., Schuz, B., Ziegelmann, J. R., Lippke, S., & Schwarzer, R. (2008). Beyond behavioural intentions: Planning mediates between intentions and physical activity. *British Journal of Health Psychology, 13*, 479–494.

Shaughnessy, M., & Resnick, B. M. (2009). Using theory to develop an exercise intervention for patients post stroke. *Topics in Stroke Rehabilitation, 16*, 140–146.

Sheeran, P. (2002). Intention–behavior relations: A conceptual and empirical review. In W. Stroebe & M. Hewstone (Eds.), *European Review of Social Psychology* (Vol. 12, pp. 1–36). London: Wiley.

Sheeran, P., Norman, P., & Orbell, S. (1999). Evidence that intentions based on attitudes better predict behaviour than intentions based on subjective norms. *European Journal of Social Psychology, 29*, 403–406.

Sheeran, P., & Orbell, S. (1999a). Augmenting the theory of planned behavior: Roles for anticipated regret and descriptive norms. *Journal of Applied Social Psychology, 29*, 2107–2142.

Sheeran, P., & Orbell, S. (1999b). Implementation intentions and repeated behaviour: Augmenting the predictive validity of the theory of planned behaviour. *European Journal of Social Psychology, 29*, 349–369.

Sheeran, P., & Orbell, S. (2000a). Self schemas and the theory of planned behaviour. *European Journal of Social Psychology, 30*, 533–550.

Sheeran, P., & Orbell, S. (2000b). Using implementation intentions to increase attendance for cervical cancer screening. *Health Psychology, 19*, 283–289.

Sheeran, P., Orbell, S., & Trafimow, D. (1999). Does the temporal stability of behavioral intentions moderate intention–behavior and past behavior–future behavior relations? *Personality and Social Psychology Bulletin, 25*, 721–730.

Sheeran, P., Trafimow, D., Finlay, K. A., & Norman, P. (2002). Evidence that the type of person affects the strength of the perceived behavioural control–intention relationship. *British Journal of Social Psychology, 41*, 253–270.

Sheldon, K. M. (2002). The self-concordance model of health goal striving: When personal goals correctly represent the person. In E. L. Deci & R. M. Ryan (Eds.), *Handbook of self-determination research* (pp. 65–86). Rochester, NY: University of Rochester Press.

Sheppard, B. H., Hartwick, J., & Warshaw, P. R. (1988). The theory of reasoned action: A meta-analysis of past research with recommendation and future research. *Journal of Consumer Research, 15*, 325–343.

Sniehotta, F. F. (2009). An experimental test of the theory of planned behavior. *Applied Psychology: Health and Well-being, 1*, 257–270.

Sniehotta, F. F., Scholz, U., & Schwarzer, R. (2005). Bridging the intention–behaviour gap: Planning, self-efficacy, and action control in the adoption and maintenance of physical exercise. *Psychology and Health, 20*, 143–160.

Sniehotta, F. F., Scholz, U., Schwarzer, R., Fuhrmann, B., Kiwus, U., & Voller, H. (2005). Long-term effects of two psychological interventions on physical exercise and self-regulation following coronary rehabilitation. *International Journal of Behavioral Medicine, 12*, 244–255.

Spence, A., & Townsend, E. (2007). Predicting behaviour towards genetically modified (GM) food using implicit and explicit attitudes. *British Journal of Social Psychology, 46*, 437–457.

Standage, M., Duda, J. L., & Ntoumanis, N. (2003). A model of contextual motivation in physical education: Using constructs from self-determination and achievement goal theories to predict physical activity intentions. *Journal of Educational Psychology, 95*, 97–110.

Strack, F., & Deutsch, R. (2004). Reflective and impulsive determinants of social behavior. *Personality and Social Psychology Review, 8*, 220–247.

Sweet, S. N., Fortier, M. S., Guerin, E., Tulloch, H., Sigal, R. J., Kenny, G. P., & Reid, R. D. (2009). Understanding physical activity in adults with type 2 diabetes after completing an exercise intervention trial: A mediation model of self-efficacy and autonomous motivation. *Psychology, Health & Medicine, 14*, 419–429.

Teixeira, P. J., Going, S. B., Sardinha, L. B., & Lohman, T. G. (2005). A review of psychosocial pre-treatment predictors of weight control. *Obesity Reviews, 6*, 43–65.

Terry, D. J., Hogg, M. A., & White, K. M. (2000). Attitude–behavior relations: Social identity and group membership. In D. J. Terry & M. A. Hogg (Eds.), *Attitudes, behavior, and social context: The role of norms and group membership* (pp. 67–93). Mahwah, NJ: Erlbaum.

Terry, D. J., & O'Leary, J. E. (1995). The theory of planned behaviour: The effects of perceived behavioural control and self-efficacy. *British Journal of Social Psychology, 34*, 199–220.

Toft, U. N., Kristoffersen, L. H., Aadahl, M., Smith, L. V. H., Pisinger, C., & Jorgensen, T. (2007). Diet and exercise intervention in a general population mediators of participation and adherence: The Inter99 study. *European Journal of Public Health, 17*, 455–463.

Trafimow, D., & Finlay, K. A. (1996). The importance of subjective norms for a minority of people: Between-subjects and within-subjects effects. *Personality and Social Psychology Bulletin, 22*, 820–828.

Trafimow, D., & Sheeran, P. (1998). Some tests of the distinction between cognitive and affective beliefs. *Journal of Experimental Social Psychology, 34*, 378–397.

Umstattd, M. R., Wilcox, S., Saunders, R., Watkins, K., & Dowda, M. (2008). Self-regulation and physical activity: The relationship in older adults. *American Journal of Health Behavior, 32*, 115–124.

Vallerand, R. J. (2000). Deci and Ryan's self-determination theory: A view from the hierarchical model of intrinsic and extrinsic motivation. *Psychological Inquiry, 11*, 312–318.

Van Hooft, E. A. J., & De Jong, M. (2009). Predicting job seeking for temporary employment using the theory of planned behaviour: The moderating role of individualism and collectivism. *Journal of Occupational and Organizational Psychology, 82*, 295–316.

van Osch, L., Beenackers, M., Reubsaet, A., Lechner, L., Candel, M., & de Vries, H. (2009). Action planning as predictor of health protective and health risk behavior: An investigation of fruit and snack consumption. *International Journal of Behavioral Nutrition and Physical Activity, 6*, 69.

Verplanken, B., & Faes, S. (1999). Good intentions, bad habits, and effects of forming implementation intentions on healthy eating. *European Journal of Social Psychology, 29*, 591–604.

Verplanken, B., Hofstee, G., & Janssen, H. (1998). Accessibility of affective versus cognitive components of attitudes. *European Journal of Social Psychology, 28*, 23–35.

Walker, G. J., Courneya, K. S., & Deng, J. (2006). Ethnicity, gender, and the theory of planned behavior: The case of playing the lottery. *Journal of Leisure Research, 38*, 224–248.

Webb, T. L., & Sheeran, P. (2006). Does changing behavioral intentions engender behavior change? A meta-analysis of the experimental evidence. *Psychological Bulletin, 132*, 249–268.

White, K. M., Hogg, M. A., & Terry, D. J. (2002). Improving attitude–behavior correspondence through exposure to normative support from a salient ingroup. *Basic and Applied Social Psychology, 24*, 91–103.

Williams, G. C., Gagne, M., Ryan, R. M., & Deci, E. L. (2002). Facilitating autonomous motivation for smoking cessation. *Health Psychology, 21*, 40–50.

Williams, G. C., McGregor, H. A., Zeldman, A., & Freedman, Z. R. (2004). Testing a self-determination theory process model for promoting glycemic control through diabetes self-management. *Health Psychology, 23*, 58–66.

Wilson, P. M., & Rodgers, W. M. (2004). The relationship between perceived autonomy support, exercise regulations and behavioral intentions in women. *Psychology of Sport and Exercise, 5*, 229–242.

Woodgate, J., & Brawley, L. R. (2008). Self-efficacy for exercise in cardiac rehabilitation—review and recommendations. *Journal of Health Psychology, 13*, 366–387.

Theoretical Approaches to Exercise Promotion

David M. Williams *and* Bess H. Marcus

Abstract

In the field of exercise promotion, theory provides a bridge between basic behavioral science and applied intervention research. This chapter reviews theories of exercise promotion. The theories most often used in exercise promotion emphasize cognitive factors and are grounded in expectancy-value formulations. Some newer theoretical approaches also emphasize environmental or affective processes. To advance the science of behavior change, further expansion of theory is needed, as well as continued testing and refinement of existing theory. Such advances can only be accomplished through the interplay between basic and applied research. More funding is needed to support the continuation of quality basic research. Applied research must emphasize theoretical fidelity and the translation of core scientific principles into corresponding behavior change tactics in diverse contexts and populations.

Key Words: theory-related terminology, basic and applied research, affective processes, ecological framework, theoretical fidelity.

Introduction

The field of exercise psychology deals with the interplay between exercise and psychological phenomena (e.g., perception of internal and external stimuli, cognition, affect, interpersonal interactions, and behavior). Theory is important to exercise psychology, because it represents a bridge between scientific knowledge (what determines [exercise] behavior) and applied problems (how can we help people engage in exercise behavior?). Specifically, theory (a) helps us to predict whether or not exercise behavior will occur, (b) helps us to explain how or why exercise behavior occurs (or does not occur), (c) provides guidelines for designing interventions to promote exercise behavior, (d) represents an accumulation of shared knowledge that saves us from having to rediscover that knowledge each time we seek answers to new scientific and practical questions, and (e) provides a common language for communication among researchers and practitioners.

Research in exercise psychology can be categorized into research in which the dependent variable is exercise behavior (e.g., the effects of attitudes about exercise on exercise behavior) or research in which the dependent variable is psychological phenomena (e.g., the effects of exercise on depression or cognitive symptoms of dementia). Because this chapter is on theoretical approaches to exercise promotion, we focus on exercise psychology research in which exercise behavior is the outcome of interest. We begin with a discussion of theory-related terminology. This is followed by brief summaries of the theories used most often in exercise promotion research and new trends in theories of exercise promotion. We end with recommendations regarding further application, testing, and refinement of theory in the context of exercise promotion research.

Terminology
Theories, Models, and Frameworks

The terms *theory*, *model*, and *framework* are often used interchangeably. Moreover, such terms are often combined in phrases such as *theoretical model*, *theoretical framework*, *conceptual model*, or *conceptual framework*. We attempt herein to distinguish among these terms based mostly on the definitions set forth by Glanz, Rimer, and Viswanath (2008). To begin with, "a theory is a set of interrelated concepts, definitions, and propositions that present a *systematic* view of events or situations by specifying relations among variables, in order to *explain* and *predict* the events or situations" (Glanz, Rimer, & Viswanath, 2008, p. 26; italics in original). Theories are sufficiently broad in scope that they are capable of explaining (often multiple) outcomes of interest (e.g., health behaviors) in *multiple and diverse contexts*. Good theories are internally consistent, parsimonious, falsifiable, and explanatory as well as predictive.

Whereas theories explain (often multiple) outcomes of interest (e.g., multiple health behaviors) in a wide range of contexts, models are specific to a particular outcome (e.g., exercise behavior) in a particular context. Thus models do not necessarily differ from theories in content or structure but do differ in relevance to the specific outcome and context to be studied (Glanz et al., 2008). Models can be complete replications of individual theories, or models can include some aspects of individual theories (representing some but not all of their constructs and their interrelationships), combinations of aspects from multiple theories, concepts that are not inherent to any existing theories, or any combination of the above. Researchers (or practitioners) create models for what they expect will happen in their research (or practice); such models may or may not be derived from (or completely replicate) one or more theories. Specific hypotheses should be derivable from both theories and models.

When a model is formally specified in one or more publications, is proposed to be relevant to a broad range of outcomes, and is tested repeatedly in multiple research studies, the distinction between model and theory becomes blurred. For example, the health belief model and the transtheoretical model were originally based on constructs from multiple theories and designed to explain specific outcomes (vaccinations [Rosenstock, 1966] and smoking cessation [Prochaska & DiClemente,

1983], respectively) but have since been used to explain a broader range of outcomes, including exercise promotion, and thus are categorized herein as theories.

A *framework* is a set of concepts that are proposed to influence each other in some way (Glanz et al., 2008). Frameworks provide broad ways of viewing one or more related outcomes (e.g., multiple health behaviors) and thus provide guidelines for the development or refinement of theories and models. Unlike theories, however, frameworks do not specifically delineate how concepts are interrelated and thus cannot provide testable hypotheses. According to this definition of framework, the ecological model, the biopsychosocial model, and the biomedical model are frameworks and are referred to as such hereafter.

Theories, models, and frameworks can be mutually influential. For example, a researcher, informed by the ecological *framework*, may test a *model* in which environmental variables (e.g., residential neighborhood type) add to the prediction of exercise behavior beyond the variables from the *theory* of planned behavior. If the proposed *model* is supported, it may lead to the refinement of the *theory*.

Concepts, Constructs, and Variables

Psychological concepts, constructs, and variables are the building blocks of theories, models, and frameworks (Glanz et al., 2008) and thus require their own definitions. To again borrow from Glanz and colleagues (2008), *concepts* are ideas that exist outside the context of a theory. For example, a familiar psychological concept is that people have expectations about future events. When concepts are labeled and described in the context of a theory they are referred to as *constructs* (Glanz et al., 2008). Thus, in the context of social learning theory the concept of expected future events is represented by the theoretical construct *expectancy* (Rotter, 1954). Concepts and constructs typically refer to psychological phenomena that are socially *constructed* and thus not amenable to direct observation (e.g., expectancy) rather than objectively observed (e.g., body weight), although this distinction is often fuzzy (e.g., race or ethnicity).

Finally, *variables* are observable operationalizations of concepts or constructs (Glanz et al., 2008). An example of an expectancy variable is the mean numerical response to a ten-item questionnaire assessing expected likelihood of ten potential outcomes of beginning a program of regular exercise in the next three months. Researchers may examine the relationships among *variables* that represent specific *constructs* according to a particular theory. Such examinations can tell us something about the underlying theory, but only to the extent that variables are operationalized in a way that is consistent with the definition of the construct (i.e., valid) and reliably measured.

In the next section, we provide a historically driven review of the theories most often used in exercise promotion research.

Review of Exercise Psychology Theories

A recent systematic review (Painter, Borba, Hynes, Mays, & Glanz, 2008) showed that four of the most commonly used theories in health behavior research are the transtheoretical model (Prochaska & DiClemente, 1984), social cognitive theory (Bandura, 1986), the health belief model (Rosenstock, 1966), and the theory of planned behavior/reasoned action (Ajzen, 1991; Fishbein & Ajzen, 1975). These theories are also often used in the narrower domain of exercise promotion research. Each of these theories is rooted in (a) behavioral learning theories emphasizing classical and operant conditioning, (b) expectancy-value theories such as social learning theory, and (c) the social cognitive framework. What follows is a roughly chronological account of the foundations of these four theories, along with summaries of these and associated theories often used in exercise psychology research.

Theoretical Foundations
BEHAVIORAL LEARNING THEORY

Learning theory is broad and encompasses various perspectives, including behavioral, cognitive, and constructivist. However, within exercise psychology research, learning theory usually refers to behavioral approaches chiefly characterized by operant conditioning (Bolles, 1979). Behavioral learning theory is not often explicitly tested in exercise psychology research or explicitly named as the foundation for exercise promotion interventions. However, the implicit impact of learning theory is pervasive, particularly to the extent that it serves as the foundation for social learning theory. For example, the implicit idea that people will be more likely to exercise when reinforced (i.e., rewarded) for doing so underlies the outcome expectancy construct prominent in many exercise psychology theories (Maddux, 1993). Likewise, the notion that

expected outcomes of exercise are more likely to influence behavior as they become more temporally proximal (Williams, 2008) is based on theoretical tenets of behavioral learning theory.

SOCIAL LEARNING THEORY

Rotter's (1954) social learning theory (SLT) was one of several expectancy-value theories first proposed in the 1950s in which theorists began to consider cognitive mechanisms underlying the stimulus–response relationships that dominated behaviorism (for a review see Kirsch, Lynn, Vigorito, & Miller, 2004). Specifically, in SLT, Rotter proposed that the likelihood of a behavior is a function of the aggregation of the product of expected outcomes of the behavior and their subjective value. This relationship underlies many of the theories used in exercise psychology research (Maddux, 1993). Rotter (1966) later added to SLT the construct of locus of control, which is the extent to which one believes one's actions are determined by one's behavior (internal locus) or by other, chance factors (external locus).

Belief-based Theories Rooted in SLT
HEALTH BELIEF MODEL

The health belief model (HBM) was originally conceived to understand variability in illness detection behaviors and was published by Rosenstock in 1966. The HBM includes five constructs fully grounded in behavioral learning theory and SLT. Specifically, perceived susceptibility and perceived severity represent the expected likelihood and severity of disease, respectively, given continuation of the current course of action (i.e., an unhealthy behavior is continued or a healthy behavior is not adopted). Second, perceived benefits and costs represent expected positive and negative outcomes of engaging in the recommended health behavior (or cessation of unhealthy behavior). Finally, cues to action represent environmental stimuli that might trigger the healthy behavior. Thus cues to action are consistent with the concept of stimulus control in operant conditioning, in which behavior is rewarded when certain stimuli are present. Given the broad applicability of the HBM and its considerable empirical support, it is best considered a theory rather than a model.

PROTECTION MOTIVATION THEORY

Protection motivation theory (PMT) was conceived by Rogers in 1975 to explain the process through which fear-arousing communications affect behavior. As with the HBM, PMT includes expected negative outcomes of the unhealthy behavior and corresponding outcome values (perceived susceptibility to and severity of disease), as well as expected positive and negative outcomes of the recommended health behavior (benefits and costs). In PMT perceived benefits of healthy behavior are focused on disease avoidance and are labeled response efficacy, which is the expectation that the recommended health behavior will decrease the risk of disease. Additionally, PMT includes the perceived extrinsic and intrinsic rewards of engaging in the unhealthy behavior, that is, the factors that are presumed to be motivating the current level of unhealthy behavior. Thus as with the HBM, early versions of PMT were firmly rooted in the expectancy-value formulation proposed in SLT.

THEORY OF REASONED ACTION

Also proposed in 1975, the theory of reasoned action (TRA) was conceived by Fishbein and Ajzen to formally conceptualize how attitudes about behavior and social norms influence behavior. Unlike the HBM and PMT, TRA was not specific to health behavior. However, as with the HBM and PMT, TRA was grounded in SLT. Specifically, in TRA expected outcomes of the target behavior and their corresponding values underlie attitudes toward the behavior, whereas expectations of how other people would view one's behavior and one's motivation to comply with those views underlie social norms. Attitudes and social norms are theorized to influence intentions to perform the behavior, which is considered the proximal determinant of behavior.

The Social Cognitive Framework, Social Cognitive Theory, and Self-Efficacy Theory

In 1977 Bandura (1977b) extended SLT and laid the foundations for what he would later label social cognitive theory (Bandura, 1986). The label *social cognitive theory* (SCT) is sometimes used to refer to a framework (referred to hereafter as the *social cognitive framework*) grounded in five core assumptions: (a) People are capable of symbolic and abstract reasoning; (b) human behavior is goal directed and guided by forethought; (c) people are capable of internal regulation of their behavior (self-regulation); (d) people can learn by observing the behavior of others and its consequences (vicarious learning); and (e) environmental (e.g., built and social environment), personal (e.g., cognitive and demographic), and behavioral (e.g., previous and current behavior)

factors are mutually influential (Bandura, 1986; for early foundations of these principles see Bandura, 1977b). The social cognitive framework underlies the family of "social cognitive theories" (HBM, PMT, and TRA), which all share these common principles (Maddux, 1993).

Also in 1977, Bandura (1977a) introduced the concept of self-efficacy, which is one's perceived capability to perform a behavior and is likely the single most researched theoretical construct in exercise psychology. Bandura (1986) posits that self-efficacy is influenced by four factors: exposure to modeling of the target behavior, verbal persuasion to perform the behavior, previous success in performing the behavior, and physiological and affective states at the time the behavior is to be performed. Likely due to its substantial predictive power (for a meta-analysis see Moritz, Feltz, Fahrbach, & Mack, 2000), the self-efficacy construct was added to each of the previously discussed belief-based theories—HBM, PMT, and TRA—that are based on expectancy-value formulations (Ajzen, 1991; Rogers, 1983; Strecher, DeVellis, Becker, & Rosenstock, 1986). (With this change, the TRA was relabeled the theory of planned behavior [TPB].)

The label *social cognitive theory* (as opposed to *social cognitive framework*) is perhaps more appropriately reserved for Bandura's (2004) causal theory of behavior, in which self-efficacy is posited to influence behavior directly and through its influence on outcome expectancies, perceived barriers to the target behavior, and frequency and type of proximal goals that one sets for performing the behavior. Finally, *self-efficacy theory* (SET) is a component of social cognitive theory focusing on the relationship between self-efficacy, outcome expectancy, and behavior (Bandura, 1997).

Theories That Posit a Larger Role for Affective Processes

THE PARALLEL PROCESS MODEL

The HBM, PMT, TRA/TPB, and SCT/SET all subscribe to the social cognitive framework and focus on the role of cognition in understanding health behavior. The parallel process model (PPM), however, posits that health behaviors are a function of simultaneous cognitive and affective processing of health-related information. The PPM was originally formulated as a way to better understand the impact of fear appeals on health behavior (Leventhal, 1970). In the PPM, fear-eliciting stimuli (e.g., pictures of diseased lungs or teeth) influence health-related behavior through parallel but interacting affective (e.g., fear or worry) and cognitive (e.g., expectancies, plans, or goals) processes. For example, worry about the outcomes of a cancer screening can directly influence whether one undergoes the screening, especially if one does not expect clear benefits from the screening. A number of theories have grown out of the PPM that share its emphasis on both affective and cognitive processing of health-related stimuli (Diefenbach et al., 2008). These theoretical derivatives are more detailed than the PPM, have subtle differences regarding the interrelationships between affect and cognition (Leventhal, Diefenbach, & Leventhal, 1992; Witte, 1992), and place greater emphasis on cancer-related outcomes (Miller, Shoda, & Hurley, 1996). While these theories are not often applied to exercise behavior, they potentially could be, and their emphasis on affective processes serves as a foundation for some newer theoretical approaches to exercise promotion (see below).

SELF-DETERMINATION THEORY

Self-determination theory (SDT), originally formulated in 1985 (Deci & Ryan, 1985), has received considerable recent attention in exercise psychology (Hagger & Chatzisarantis, 2007; Ryan, Williams, Partrick, & Deci, 2009; Wilson, Mack, & Grattan, 2009). In contrast to the family of social cognitive theories, which focus mostly on cognitive determinants of behavior, SDT focuses on the distinction between intrinsic and extrinsic motivation, their social and cognitive antecedents, and their relative effects on behavior (Ryan & Deci, 2000). Intrinsically motivated behavior is performed for the inherent enjoyment and satisfaction associated with the behavior and, in turn, is more likely to lead to continuation of the behavior (e.g., adherence to exercise programs). Extrinsically motivated behavior is performed for the purposes of obtaining external rewards or avoiding punishment, consistent with behavioral learning theory. However, extrinsic motivation can also lead to continued behavior to the extent that it is more internally than externally regulated. Ranging from most internally to most externally regulated, extrinsic motivation is further subdivided into integrated regulation (where expected behavioral outcomes are incorporated with personal goals), identified regulation (where expected behavioral outcomes have personal importance), introjected regulation (where the individual is self-regulated via guilt, pride, etc.), and external regulation (where the individual complies solely for external rewards).

According to SDT, the quality of human motivation is based on psychological needs for competence, autonomy, and relatedness, which are akin to the concepts of self-efficacy, locus of control, and social support or norms, respectively, from SLT, SCT, and TRA. Generally speaking, perceptions of greater competence, autonomy, and relatedness are likely to lead to intrinsic motivation or more internally regulated extrinsic motivation. Finally, motivation subtypes (i.e., intrinsic, integrated, identified, introjected, and external) are dependent on expected outcomes of behavior (Ryan & Deci, 2000).

Stage Theories

THE TRANSTHEORETICAL MODEL

The transtheoretical model (TTM), which was introduced in 1983 (Prochaska & DiClemente, 1983), has two features that distinguish it from the theories discussed above. First, whereas each of the above theories posits the same determinants of behavior at all points in the behavior change process, the TTM is based on the premise that different factors are important at different points in the behavior change process. According to the TTM, individuals progress through stages of change: precontemplation, contemplation, preparation, action, and maintenance. As the TTM is applied to exercise behavior, precontemplators do not currently exercise and do not intend to start in the next six months; contemplators do not exercise but intend to start in the next six months; those in preparation exercise, but not regularly; those in the action stage exercise regularly but have done so for less than six months; and finally, those in the maintenance stage exercise regularly and have done so for six months or longer (Marcus, Rossi, Selby, Niaura, & Abrams, 1992).

The second distinguishing feature of the TTM is the incorporation of multiple processes of change, from diverse theories of human behavior, as determinants of progression across the stages of change. Processes of change are divided into two categories: cognitive and behavioral. The cognitive processes for exercise are consciousness raising, dramatic relief, environmental reevaluation, self-reevaluation, and social liberation. The behavioral processes for exercise are counterconditioning, helping relationships, reinforcement management, self-liberation, and stimulus control. (For application of these concepts to exercise behavior see Marcus & Forsyth, 2008; Marcus et al., 1992.) Use of the specific processes of change depends on the individual's stage of change. Use of the cognitive processes tends to peak in the preparation stage, and use of the behavioral processes tends to peak in the action stage (Prochaska, DiClemente, & Norcross, 1992). Also included in the TTM are decisional balance, which is weighing of the pros and cons of the behavior as in decision theory (Janis & Mann, 1977), and self-efficacy.

THE HEALTH ACTION PROCESS APPROACH

The health action process approach (HAPA) is another stage theory that has seen increasing use in exercise promotion research (e.g., Schwarzer, Luszczynska, Ziegelmann, Scholz, & Lippke, 2008). Unlike the TTM, the HAPA is explicitly derived from the family of social cognitive theories. Indeed, it was originally proposed, in 1992, as a stage-based derivation of existing social cognitive theories, including the HBM, SET, TRA/TPB, and PMT (Schwarzer, 1992). However, the HAPA distinguishes between the processes that determine intention to perform a behavior (motivation phase) and the processes that determine performance of the behavior (action or volition phase). Specifically, in the motivation phase intentions are determined by perceived threat (a function of perceived vulnerability and severity of disease as in the HBM and PMT), expected outcomes (i.e., SLT, SCT, and TPB), and self-efficacy (i.e., SCT), whereas in the volition phase adoption and maintenance of behavior is determined by plans for initiating the behavior (action plans) and perceived capability to follow through with such plans (self-efficacy), as well as perceived and actual physical and social environmental barriers (Schwarzer, 1992; Schwarzer et al., 2008).

ROTHMAN'S MAINTENANCE STAGE THEORY

Rothman and colleagues (Rothman, 2000; Rothman, Baldwin, & Hertel, 2004) have also posited a stage theory grounded in the social cognitive framework. In general, the theory states that traditional social cognitive constructs such as self-efficacy and outcome expectancies are important for behavior initiation, but that once the behavior has been initiated it is one's satisfaction with the outcomes of the behavior that determines whether the behavior will be maintained. That is, the outcomes that one *expects* as a result of the behavior drive initial behavior, but the outcomes that one *experiences* after performing the behavior determine continuation of the behavior.

New Trends in Theories of Exercise Promotion

The theories reviewed above are some of the most often used theories in exercise psychology. Despite the great strides that have been made in theory development in the past three to four decades, there is always room for improvement. For example, our theories are not as highly predictive or explanatory as they might be (Baranowski, Anderson, & Carmack, 1998). And although theory-based exercise promotion interventions tend to be successful in the short term, they tend not to be effective in promoting sustained regular exercise behavior (Marcus et al., 2006).

One oft-cited weakness of the theories most prominently featured in exercise psychology research (SCT, TPB/TRA, the HBM, and the TTM) is their considerable conceptual overlap (Baranowski et al., 1998; Maddux, 1993). Indeed, multiple theories include cognitive constructs of personal control over behavior (e.g., self-efficacy and perceived behavioral control), intention or goals for performing a behavior (e.g., behavioral intention and proximal goals), expected outcomes of behavior (e.g., outcome expectancy, behavioral beliefs, and perceived susceptibility), perceived value of potential outcomes (e.g., outcome value, outcome evaluations, and perceived severity), or constructs that reflect both expectancy and value (e.g., attitudes and perceived benefits and costs). While the focus has mainly been on these cognitive constructs, SCT, TRA/TPB, and the TTM also include constructs related to social processes (social support, social norms, and helping relationships, respectively).

Some theorists have argued that the overlap among the theoretical constructs that make up these theories is an indication that there is consensus regarding the determinants of health behavior and that further theorizing on the determinants of health behavior is not necessary (Fishbein, 2008). However, others have argued that further theoretical refinement and development is necessary (Michie, Rothman, & Sheeran, 2007), as evidenced by our inability to explain a meaningful amount of variance in behavior change and our inability to consistently produce sustained health behavior change (Baranowski et al., 1998; Mielewczyk & Willig, 2007). This section discusses two new trends in exercise promotion research that involve a greater focus on environmental and affective concepts in addition to the more traditional focus on cognitive and social factors.

The Ecological Framework

Several independent groups of researchers have proposed an ecological framework for health behavior in which behavior is best understood by considering constructs on multiple levels including biological, intrapersonal, interpersonal, community, policy, and physical environmental (for a review see Sallis, Owen, & Fisher, 2008). The ecological framework builds on the dominant social cognitive framework, which includes a prominent role for the environment in its broadest formulation (Bandura, 1986) but has spurred causal theories and corresponding research that focus mostly on the intrapersonal (e.g., self-efficacy and outcome expectancy) and interpersonal (e.g., social support and social norms) levels (e.g., Bandura, 2004).

The ecological framework has encouraged new streams of research, particularly with respect to community, policy, and physical environmental influences on exercise behavior (Sallis et al., 2006). As noted by King and colleagues (King, Stokols, Talen, Brassington, & Killingsworth, 2002), there is a need for more integration between research on the role of policy and environmental factors and theories that focus on intrapersonal factors. Such integration may lead to development of more specified causal theories of how these variables interact.

The Role of Affective Processes in Exercise Promotion

Following in the tradition of the PPM, a number of researchers have posited a greater role for affect in determining exercise behavior. *Affect* is used herein as an umbrella term for an evaluative neurobiological response to an external or internal stimulus that is manifested in (a) coordinated patterns of physiological (e.g., release of hormones, increased heart rate) and involuntary behavioral (e.g., facial expression, vocalization) changes, *and/or* (b) subjective experiential feelings (e.g., pleasure/displeasure) (Berridge, 2003). Affect includes isolated experiences of *core affect* (e.g., pleasure or displeasure) as well as more differentiated and complex moods and emotions characterized by combinations of core affect, cognitive appraisals of the internal and external environment, and physiological and behavioral responses (e.g., anger, sadness, and pride; Russell & Barrett, 1999). Research on affective determinants of exercise has involved affective experiences about or in response to exercise behavior as well as cognitive expectations about such affective responses. Such research should be distinguished from research in which the affective response to exercise is the outcome of interest (dependent variable), such as studies of exercise as a tool for treating clinical depression (Dunn, Trivedi, Kampert, Clark, & Chambliss, 2005).

Much of the research on affective determinants of exercise behavior has been conducted in the context of the TPB. Specifically, both *anticipated affect* in response to exercise (e.g., anticipated regret for not exercising; van der Pligt & de Vries, 1998) and *affective attitudes* about exercise (e.g., exercise is miserable versus enjoyable; Rhodes & Courneya, 2003) have been examined in the context of the TPB as examples of behavioral beliefs and attitudes, respectively, and have been shown to be predictive of exercise behavior (Rhodes, Fiala, & Conner, 2009). Additionally, Kiviniemi, Voss-Humke, & Seifert (2007) have shown that *affective associations*—how someone feels when considering (i.e., thinking about) exercise—are cross-sectionally associated with level of exercise behavior and mediate the influence of traditional TPB variables (i.e., attitudes and social norms) on exercise behavior. Affective associations are actual affective responses to the thought of exercise and should be distinguished from cognitive expectations (e.g., anticipated affect) or affective attitudes about exercise.

Yet another affective variable that has recently been theorized to influence exercise behavior is acute affective response to exercise (as distinguished from anticipated affect, affective attitudes, and affective associations). This growing line of research has been heavily influenced by the insight that the traditional notion that exercise makes people feel good is inconsistent with data on the prevalence of regular exercise and rates of attrition from exercise programs (Backhouse, Ekkekakis, Bidle, Foskett, & Williams, 2007). Specifically, while people tend to feel good when they finish a bout of exercise, affective valence *during* exercise depends on the intensity of the exercise and, at moderate intensities, depends on the characteristics of the person (e.g., fitness level or thoughts about exercise) and the exercise environment (Ekkekakis & Acevedo, 2006). This important insight has led to theory and research suggesting that the variability in acute affective response during exercise may be predictive of future exercise behavior (Bryan, Hutchison, Seals, & Allen, 2007; Ekkekakis & Lind, 2006; Williams, 2008). For example, Williams (2008) has argued that acute affective response to past exercise affects future exercise behavior via anticipation of affective response.

Bryan and colleagues (2007) have posited that acute affective response to exercise interacts with genetic, physiological, environmental, and traditional cognitive factors to influence exercise behavior. Such integrative theorizing is consistent with the ecological framework discussed above and represents an important step toward a more comprehensive understanding of the factors that influence exercise behavior.

Concluding Remarks
Need for Further Expansion and Refinement of Existing Theory

Many of the most often used theories in exercise psychology (i.e., the HBM, SET, TRA/TPB) are grounded in the social cognitive framework and reflect the emphasis on cognitive processes that has dominated the more general field of psychology in the last few decades. Recent strides have been made in expanding the scope of theoretical inquiry to environmental and affective issues (see above); however, better understanding of the determinants of exercise behavior requires further expansion into new domains. For example, there is need for greater focus on temporal issues related to exercise behavior. Temporal issues have been partially addressed in the context of stage theories, which differentiate among the factors that influence intention formation, exercise initiation, and exercise maintenance; however, further theorizing on the influence of immediate versus distal outcomes of exercise is needed. The negative outcomes of exercise, such as displeasure, inconvenience, and response cost (things that one could have otherwise done) are temporally proximal, whereas positive outcomes of exercise, such as potential weight loss, health outcomes, and social approval are temporally distal. Hall and Fong (2007) have proposed a new temporal self-regulation theory, which addresses these issues and has considerable promise for application to exercise promotion.

In addition to expanding theory, we must continue to test traditional theories and refine them when they do not stand up to conceptual and empirical scrutiny (Ogden, 2003). For example, recent research has shown that exercise self-efficacy, which is causally prior to outcome expectancies in SCT/SET, may instead be largely determined by expected outcomes of exercise (Council, Ahern, Follick, & Kline, 1988; Rhodes & Blanchard, 2007; for a full discussion see Williams, 2010b). Such refinement of existing theories has significant implications for

theoretical expansion as well as the design of exercise promotion programs.

Need for More Basic Behavioral Research

Theoretical expansion and refinement can best be accomplished through the interplay between basic and applied behavioral research (Rothman & Salovey, 2007). However, the different primary goals of basic and applied research often conflict. For example, basic research often requires homogeneous conditions and study samples and highly structured and rigid experimental manipulations. Applied research, on the other hand, often requires demonstrating that interventions can be effectively delivered by a range of practitioners to diverse participants in diverse conditions. Additionally, basic research requires careful isolation of independent variables, whereas to be funded and published, applied research often must include multifaceted interventions that are likely to have a statistically significant effect on exercise behavior relative to the comparison condition (Williams, 2010a). Research funding is often heavily weighted toward applied research that pursues advances in behavioral (and biological) outcomes rather than the theoretical processes behind those outcomes. As a result, most basic research in exercise psychology is either unfunded or involves secondary analysis of theoretical variables from research primarily intended to address practical questions.

Use of mediation analysis in the context of applied health behavior intervention research represents a hybrid of basic and applied research (Rothman, 2004). Specifically, mediation research informs researchers as to whether or not they successfully manipulated psychological phenomena and whether those psychological phenomena in turn affected behavior as theorized. One strength of mediation research is that theoretical variables are experimentally manipulated by the presence or absence of an exercise promotion intervention intended to affect such variables. Moreover, mediation analysis often has relatively high external validity, because the data are obtained in a field-based intervention setting rather than in a laboratory setting.

Nonetheless, mediation analysis is not a substitute for tightly controlled basic experimental research, for at least two reasons. First, when mediation analysis is applied to behavioral intervention research, it is often the case that many variables are manipulated at once through the implementation of a multifaceted intervention; thus it is difficult to isolate the effects of a particular theoretical variable or to know which variable changed first (Weinstein, 2007; Williams & Dunsiger, 2007). Second, mediation analysis can answer basic theoretical questions only to the extent that the critical theoretical variables were successfully manipulated. Mediation analysis in which the target theoretical variables are not successfully manipulated is akin to experimental research in which the manipulation check fails. Researchers should be careful not to conclude that a theory lacks utility based on null mediation analysis when the targeted theoretical constructs were not effectively changed.

Thus while mediation research is undoubtedly critical to advancing health behavior theory, basic behavioral research, in which the primary goal is to understand rather than change human behavior, is needed for continued development of the theories on which applied research and practice are based. The recent creation of the Basic Behavioral and Social Science Opportunity Network (OppNet) is an important step toward recognizing and funding such basic research. The National Institutes of Health web site states: "OppNet advances basic behavioral and social science research through activities and initiatives that build a body of knowledge about the nature of behavior and social systems. OppNet prioritizes activities and initiatives that focus on basic mechanisms of behavior and social processes; that are relevant to the missions and public health challenges of multiple NIH Institutes, Centers and Offices (ICOs); and that build upon existing NIH investments without replicating them" (http://opp-net.nih.gov/about-mission.asp). Although OppNet is a significant step in the right direction, additional and sustained funding for basic behavioral research is needed.

Need for Theoretical Fidelity in Applied Exercise Promotion Research

Behavioral interventions that are tested in applied research contexts are often unlikely to be fully replicated in the real world because of funding constraints, lack of trained staff, and inability to replicate what are often complex, multifaceted intervention programs. When applied behavioral research interventions are atheoretical or lack theoretical fidelity, they resemble practice (focusing on helping those enrolled in the study) more than scientific research (adding to the scientific body of knowledge). To advance behavioral science, it is critical that applied behavioral (e.g., exercise) research test theoretical principles in applied contexts. In this way, theoretical principles—derived from basic research and tested

in applied research—can ultimately be applied in diverse real-world settings.

For this to work, we must advance the science of implementing behavioral principles. For example, it is one thing to know that affective attitudes are important determinants of exercise behavior, but it is another thing to understand how best to change affective attitudes (Fishbein, 2008; Slater, 2006). Michie and colleagues' program of research (Abraham & Michie, 2008; Michie, Abraham, Whittington, McAteer, & Gupta, 2009; Michie et al., 2005; Michie & Prestwich, 2010) is dedicated to growing the systematic science of the implementation of health behavior theory. Continued research testing theoretical principles is needed to reinforce the bridge between the science of human behavior and its application to public health.

References

Abraham, C., & Michie, S. (2008). A taxonomy of behavior change techniques used in interventions. *Health Psychology, 27*, 379–387.

Ajzen, I. (1991). The theory of planned behavior. *Organizational Behavior and Human Decision Processes, 50*, 179–211.

Backhouse, S. H., Ekkekakis, P., Bidle, S. J., Foskett, A., & Williams, C. (2007). Exercise makes people feel better but people are inactive: Paradox or artifact? *Journal of Sport and Exercise Psychology, 29*, 498–517.

Bandura, A. (1977a). Self-efficacy: Toward a unifying theory of behavioral change. *Psychological Review, 84*, 191–215.

Bandura, A. (1977b). *Social learning theory*. Upper Saddle River, NJ: Prentice Hall.

Bandura, A. (1986). *Social foundations of thought and action: A social cognitive theory*. Englewood Cliffs, NJ: Prentice Hall.

Bandura, A. (1997). *Self-efficacy: The exercise of control*. New York: W. H. Freeman.

Bandura, A. (2004). Health promotion by social cognitive means. *Health Education and Behavior, 31*, 143–164.

Baranowski, T., Anderson, C., & Carmack, C. (1998). Mediating variable framework in physical activity interventions: How are we doing? How might we do better? *American Journal of Preventive Medicine, 15*, 266–297.

Berridge, K.C. (2003). Pleasures of the brain. *Brain and Cognition, 52*,106-128.

Bolles, R. C. (1979). *Learning theory* (2nd ed.). New York: Holt, Rinehart & Winston.

Bryan, A., Hutchison, K. E., Seals, D. R., & Allen, D. L. (2007). A transdisciplinary model integrating genetic, physiological, and psychological correlates of voluntary exercise. *Health Psychology, 26*, 30–39.

Council, J. R., Ahern, D. K., Follick, M. J., & Kline, C. L. (1988). Expectancies and functional impairment in chronic low back pain. *Pain, 33*, 323–331.

Deci, E. L., & Ryan, R. M. (1985). *Intrinsic motivation and self-determination in human behavior*. New York: Plenum.

Diefenbach, M. A., Miller, S. M., Porter, M., Peters, E., Stefanek, M., & Leventhal, H. (2008). Emotions and health behavior: A self-regulation perspective. In M. Lewis, J. M. Haviland-

Jones, & L. F. Barrett (Eds.), *Handbook of emotions* (3rd ed., pp. 645–660). New York: Guilford Press.

Dunn, A. L., Trivedi, M. H., Kampert, J. B., Clark, C. G., & Chambliss, H. O. (2005). Exercise treatment for depression: Efficacy and dose response. *American Journal of Preventive Medicine, 28*, 1–8.

Ekkekakis, P., & Acevedo, E. O. (2006). Affective responses to acute exercise: Toward a psychobiological dose–response model. In E. O. Acevedo & P. Ekkekakis (Eds.), *Psychobiology of physical activity* (pp. 91–109). Champaign, IL: Human Kinetics.

Ekkekakis, P., & Lind, E. (2006). Exercise does not feel the same when you are overweight: The impact of self-selected and imposed intensity on affect and exertion. *International Journal of Obesity, 30*, 652–660.

Fishbein, M. (2008). A reasoned action approach to health promotion. *Medical Decision Making, 28*(6), 834–844.

Fishbein, M,, & Aizen, I. (1975). *Belief, attitude, intention, and behavior: An introduction to theory and research.* Reading, MA: Addison-Wesley.

Glanz, K., Rimer, B. K., & Viswanath, K. (2008). Theory, research and practice in health behavior and health education. In K. Glanz, B. K. Rimer, & K. Viswanath (Eds.), *Health behavior and health education: Theory, research and practice* (pp. 23–40). San Francisco, CA: Jossey-Bass.

Hagger, M. S., & Chatzisarantis, N. L. D. (2007). Advance in self-determination theory research in sport and exercise. *Psychology of Sport & Exercise, 8*, 597–599.

Hall, P. A., & Fong, G. T. (2007). Temporal self-regulation theory: A model for individual health behavior. *Health Psychology Review, 1*, 6–52.

Janis, I., & Mann, L. (1977). *Decision making: A psychological analysis of conflict, choice, and commitment.* New York: Free Press.

King, A. C., Stokols, D., Talen, E., Brassington, G. S., & Killingsworth, R. (2002). Theoretical approaches to the promotion of physical activity: Forging a transdisciplinary paradigm. *American Journal of Preventive Medicine, 23*, S15–S25.

Kirsch, I., Lynn, S. J., Vigorito, M., & Miller, R. R. (2004). The role of cognition in classical and operant conditioning. *Journal of Clinical Psychology, 60*, 369–392.

Kiviniemi, M. T., Voss-Humke, A. M., & Seifert, A. L. (2007). How do I feel about the behavior? The interplay of affective associations with behaviors and cognitive beliefs as influences on physical activity behavior. *Health Psychology, 26*, 152–158.

Leventhal, H. (1970). Findings and theory in the study of fear communications. In L. Berkowitz (Ed.), *Advances in experimental social psychology* (pp. 119–186). New York: Academic Press.

Leventhal, H., Diefenbach, M. A., & Leventhal, E. A. (1992). Illness cognition: Using common sense to understand treatment adherence and affect–cognition interactions. *Cognitive Therapy and Research, 16*, 143–163.

Maddux, J. E. (1993). Social cognitive models of health and exercise behavior: An introduction and review of conceptual issues. *Journal of Applied Sport Psychology, 5*, 116–140.

Marcus, B. H., & Forsyth, L. A. (2008). *Motivating people to be physically active* (2nd ed.). Champaign, IL: Human Kinetics.

Marcus, B. H., Rossi, J. S., Selby, V. C., Niaura, R. S., & Abrams, D. B. (1992). The stages and processes of exercise adoption and maintenance in a worksite sample. *Health Psychology, 11*, 386–395.

Marcus, B. H., Williams, D. M., Dubbert, P. M., Sallis, J. F., King, A. C., Yancey, A. K.,...Claytor, R. P. (2006). Physical activity intervention studies: What we know and what we need to know. A scientific statement from the American Heart Association Council on Nutrition, Physical Activity, and Metabolism (Subcommittee on Physical Activity); Council on Cardiovascular Disease in the Young; and the Interdisciplinary Working Group on Quality of Care and Outcomes Research. *Circulation, 114*, 2739–2752.

Michie, S., Abraham, C., Whittington, C., McAteer, J., & Gupta, S. (2009). Effective techniques in healthy eating and physical activity interventions: A meta-regression. *Health Psychology, 28*, 690–701.

Michie, S., Johnston, M., Abraham, C., Lawton, R., Parker, D., & Walker, A. (2005). Making psychological theory useful for implementing evidence based practice: A consensus approach. *Quality Safe Health Care, 14*, 26–33.

Michie, S., & Prestwich, A. (2010). Are interventions theory-based? Development of a theory coding scheme. *Health Psychology, 29*, 1–8.

Michie, S., Rothman, A. J., & Sheeran, P. (2007). Current issues and new directions in psychology and health: Advancing the science of behavior change. *Psychology and Health, 22*, 249–253.

Mielewczyk, F., & Willig, C. (2007). Old clothes and an older look: The case for a radical makeover in health behaviour research. *Theory and Psychology, 17*, 811–837.

Miller, S. M., Shoda, Y., & Hurley, K. (1996). Applying cognitive-social theory to health-protective behavior: Breast self-examination in cancer screening. *Psychological Bulletin, 119*, 70–94.

Moritz, S. E., Feltz, D. L., Fahrbach, K. R., & Mack, D. E. (2000). The relation of self-efficacy measures to sport performance: A meta-analytic review. *Research Quarterly for Exercise and Sport, 71*, 280–294.

Ogden, J. (2003). Some problems with social cognition models: A pragmatic and conceptual analysis. *Health Psychology, 22*, 424–428.

Painter, J. E., Borba, C. P., Hynes, M., Mays, D., & Glanz, K. (2008). The use of theory in health behavior research from 2000 to 2005: A systematic review. *Annals of Behavioral Medicine, 35*, 358–362.

Prochaska, J. O., & DiClemente, C. C. (1983). Stages and processes of self-change of smoking: Toward an integrative model of change. *Journal of Consulting and Clinical Psychology, 51*, 390–395.

Prochaska, J. O., & DiClemente, C. C. (1984). *The transtheoretical approach: Crossing the traditional boundaries of therapy.* Homewood, IL: Dow Jones, Irwin.

Prochaska, J. O., DiClemente, C. C., & Norcross, J. C. (1992). In search of how people change: Applications to addictive behaviors. *American Psychologist, 47*(9), 1102–1114.

Rhodes, R. E., & Blanchard, C. M. (2007). What do confidence items measure in the physical activity domain? *Journal of Applied Social Psychology, 37*, 759–774.

Rhodes, R. E., & Courneya, K. S. (2003). Investigating multiple components of attitude, subjective norm, and perceived control: An examination of the theory of planned behaviour in the exercise domain. *British Journal of Social Psychology, 42*, 129–146.

Rhodes, R. E., Fiala, B., & Conner, M. (2009). A review and meta-analysis of affective judgments and physical activity in adult populations. *Annals of Behavioral Medicine, 38*, 180–204.

Rogers, R. W. (1975). A protection motivation theory of fear appeals and attitude change. *Journal of Psychology, 91*, 93–114.

Rogers, R. W. (1983). Cognitive and physiological processes in fear appeals and attitude change: A revised theory of protection motivation. In J. T. Cacioppo & R. E. Petty (Eds.), *Social psychophysiology: A sourcebook* (pp. 153–176). New York: Guilford.

Rosenstock, I. M. (1966). Why people use health services. *Milbank Memorial Fund Quarterly, 44*, S94–S127.

Rothman, A. J. (2000). Toward a theory-based analysis of behavioral maintenance. *Health Psychology, 19*, S64–S69.

Rothman, A. J. (2004). "Is there nothing more practical than a good theory?": Why innovations and advances in health behavior change will arise if interventions are used to test and refine theory. *International Journal of Behavioral Nutrition and Physical Activity, 1*, 11.

Rothman, A. J., Baldwin, A., & Hertel, A. (2004). Self-regulation and behavior change: Disentangling behavioral initiation and behavioral maintenance. In K. Vohs & R. Baumeister (Eds.), *Handbook of self-regulation* (pp. 130–148). New York: Guilford Press.

Rothman, A. J., & Salovey, P. (2007). The reciprocal relation between principles and practice: Social psychology and health behavior. In A. Kruglanski & E. T. Higgins (Eds.), *Social psychology: Handbook of basic principles* (2nd ed., pp. 826–849). New York: Guilford Press.

Rotter, J. B. (1954). *Social learning and clinical psychology.* Englewood Cliffs, NJ: Prentice-Hall.

Rotter, J. B. (1966). Generalized expectancies for internal versus external control of reinforcement. *Psychological Monographs, 80*, 1–28.

Russell, J. A., & Barrett, L. F. (1999). Core affect, prototypical emotional episodes, and other things called emotion: Dissecting the elephant. *Journal of Personality and Social Psychology, 76*, 805–819.

Ryan, R. M., & Deci, E. L. (2000). Self-determination theory and the facilitation of intrinsic motivation, social development, and well-being. *American Psychologist, 55*, 68–78.

Ryan, R. M., Williams, G. C., Partrick, H., & Deci, E. L. (2009). Self-determination theory and physical activity: The dynamics of motivation in development and wellness. *Hellenic Journal of Psychology, 6*, 107–124.

Sallis, J. F., Cervero, R. B., Ascher, W., Henderson, K. A., Kraft, M. K., & Kerr, J. (2006). An ecological approach to creating active living communities. *Annual Review of Public Health, 27*, 297–322.

Sallis, J. F., Owen, N., & Fisher, E. B. (2008). Ecological models of health behavior. In K. Glanz, B. K. Rimer, & K. Viswanath (Eds.), *Health behavior and health education: Theory, research and practice* (pp. 465–485). San Francisco, CA: Jossey-Bass.

Schwarzer, R. (1992). Self-efficacy in the adoption and maintenance of health behaviors: Theoretical approaches and a new model. In R. Schwarzer (Ed.), *Self-efficacy: Thought control of action* (pp. 217–243). New York: Taylor and Francis.

Schwarzer, R., Luszczynska, A., Ziegelmann, J. P., Scholz, U., & Lippke, S. (2008). Social-cognitive predictors of physical exercise adherence: Three longitudinal studies in rehabilitation. *Health Psychology, 27*, S54–S63.

Slater, M. D. (2006). Specification and misspecification of theoretical foundations and logic models for health communication campaigns. *Health Communications, 20*, 149–157.

Strecher, V. J., DeVellis, B. M., Becker, M. H., & Rosenstock, I. M. (1986). The role of self-efficacy in achieving health behavior change. *Health Education Quarterly, 13*, 73–92.

van der Pligt, J. & de Vries, N. K. (1998). Expectancy-value models of health behavior: The role of salience and anticipated affect. *Psychology and Health, 13*, 289–305.

Weinstein, N. D. (2007). Misleading tests of health behavior theories. *Annals of Behavioral Medicine, 33*, 1–10.

Williams, D. M. (2008). Exercise, affect, and adherence: An integrated model and a case for self-paced exercise. *Journal of Sport and Exercise Psychology, 30*, 471–496.

Williams, D. M. (2010a). Importance of the nature of comparison conditions for testing theory-based interventions: Comment on Michie and Prestwich (2010). *Health Psychology, 29*, 467.

Williams, D. M. (2010b). Outcome expectancy and self-efficacy: Theoretical implications of an unresolved contradiction. *Personality and Social Psychology Review, 14*, 417–425.

Williams, D. M., & Dunsiger, S. (2007). Suggestions for testing health behavior theories: Implications for mediator analysis. *Annals of Behavioral Medicine, 34*(2), 223.

Wilson, P. M., Mack, D. E., & Grattan, K. P. (2009). Understanding motivation for exercise: A self-determination theory perspective. *Canadian Psychology, 49*, 250–256.

Witte, K. (1992). Putting the fear back into fear appeals: The extended parallel process model. *Communication Monographs, 59*, 329–349.

Theoretical Approaches to Physical Activity Intervention

Claudio R. Nigg *and* Karly S. Geller

Abstract

There is nothing as practical as a good theory. A good theory explains a phenomenon, predicts relationships and outcomes, is testable (falsifiable), is parsimonious, is generalizable (transferable), and encourages productivity. Physical activity is a complex behavior. Applying theory properly to physical activity will lead to a greater understanding of the important variables and mechanisms involved, guide interventions, and ultimately lead to better public health practices. This chapter presents several theories being used in physical activity in the context of a research article structure. This allows us to describe several theories and to illustrate how theory is part of all aspects of the research process.

Key Words: theory, model, framework, physical activity, exercise, intervention.

Introduction

Before we formally begin this chapter, we would like you to meet a 12-year-old boy named Sam. Sam, an only child, lives with his parents in a safe, middle-class neighborhood. Sam's father is the local high school football coach, and his mother a successful pediatrician. Sam plays on the middle school football team, practicing with his team five times a week during the football season and playing with his dad in the backyard during the off-season. For his 12th birthday, his mom brought home a shiny red bike, and Sam can't get enough of it. After he walks home from school, he meets his best friend on the corner and they bike around their neighborhood and to the park, where they play football until around the time their parents return from work. Luckily the fast-forward button on our remote control is working, and we can also see Sam as a healthy adult, engaging regularly in physical activity.

Sounds lovely—however, let's see what happens after some adjustments to Sam's environment and surrounding influences. The same 12-year-old boy now lives with only his mother in a small, one-

bedroom apartment. As a single parent, his mother works two minimum-wage jobs, returning home late from work each night. Because the neighborhood is unsafe, Sam rides the school bus home each day and is not allowed to play outside unsupervised. Instead, Sam spends his after-school time inside the apartment of a trusted neighbor, where he finishes his homework and watches television until his mother gets home. With transportation and financial constraints, there is no football or shiny red bike for Sam. Do we dare push the fast-forward button? If we did, what do you think we would see about Sam's health and physical activity habits?

This chapter presents several behavioral and social science theories that each provide a unique platform for understanding why individuals may or may not engage in regular physical activity behavior. These theories would attempt to explain, predict, or change Sam's physical activity levels by taking into account the individual, familial, social, and cultural factors that influence his choice or opportunities to be active (or both). For instance, what changed in the second scenario that affected Sam's physical activity? How influential was the shiny red bike on Sam's future physical activity behavior? Does living in a safe environment or having a physically active role model predict children's activity levels?

Imagine now that Sam is a girl or that his best friend has an Xbox video game system instead of a bike. We can see how physical activity behavior is multifaceted, including direct influences from single factors as well as indirect impact from a combination of influences. Clearly, some sort of guidance is required if we are to conceptualize and examine the complexity of these relationships as they affect physical activity behavior, with the aim of advancing the success of future interventions. Traditionally, guidance such as this is rooted in theory development and application. In short, theory provides an applicable template for systematically collecting facts, formulating hypotheses, and extending the knowledge base (King, 1978). As we proceed through this chapter, whose structure resembles that of a research article, you will notice the emergence of theory at each stage of the research process, assisting in the description, prediction, or change of physical activity behavior. However, in an effort to present a basis from which to examine physical activity participation, we will first discuss the state of physical activity behavior in the United States, asking: So what? What's the problem?

Physical Activity Promotion: So What? What's the Problem?

To effectively launch any scientific examination, one must first describe the main focus or problem being addressed and provide evidence to validate the significance and expected contribution of the study. For instance, the forerunner of most research on physical activity promotion is evidence supporting associations between physical activity behavior and health improvements—the "So what?" Immediately this calls for presentation of the current *problem*, which establishes the appropriateness of the study's purpose and rationale.

Regular physical activity is associated with both physiological and psychological health benefits. Physiologically, regular physical activity is related to decreased risk of coronary heart disease (J. Lee, Sparrow, Vokonas, Landsberg, & Weiss, 1995; Manson et al., 1999; Morris, Clayton, Everitt, Semmence, & Burgess, 1990; Paffenbarger & Hyde, 1984; Paffenbarger, Hyde, Hsieh, & Wing, 1986; Powell, Thompson, Caspersen, & Kendrick, 1987), hypertension, type 2 diabetes mellitus (Albright et al., 2000; Grundy et al., 1999; Hu et al., 1999;

Paffenbarger, Wing, Hyde, & Jung, 1983), various cancers (I. M. Lee, 2003), and overall mortality (I. M. Lee & Skerrett, 2001). Specific to youth, regular physical activity has a demonstrated association with increased bone mass, aerobic fitness, and levels of high-density lipoproteins as well as reduced risk for hypertension, obesity, and diabetes (Myers, Strikmiller, Webber, & Berenson, 1996). Further, increased physical activity is related to increased concentration, academic achievement (Sallis et al., 1999), higher confidence, stronger self-image, reduced disruptive behavior, and lower levels of depression (Dowling, 2000).

In addition, the United States has experienced a dramatic rise in the prevalence of obesity, to the point where it has become an epidemic and public health concern. Specifically, from 1980 to 2008 obesity increased from 7% to 20% among children aged 6–11 years and from 5% to 18% among adolescents aged 12–19 years (Ogden, Carroll, Curtin, Lamb, & Flegal, 2010). Obese children have a greatly increased risk of becoming obese adults, and more than 34% of United States adults are already obese, while another 34% are overweight (Flegal, Carroll, Ogden, & Curtin, 2010). These high rates are a serious concern considering obesity's association with the premature development of chronic diseases including heart disease, stroke, osteoarthritis, and some forms of cancer (U.S. Surgeon General, 2001). The International Agency for Research on Cancer estimates that 25% of cancer cases worldwide are due to overweight, obesity, or a sedentary lifestyle (Vaninio & Bianchini, 2002). Among the culprits blamed for the obesity epidemic are decreasing levels of physical activity and increasingly sedentary lifestyles (Kohl & Hobbs, 1998; Prentice & Jebb, 1995). Conversely, scientific evidence has given hope by demonstrating the critical role of regular physical activity in obesity prevention and recovery (Katzymaryk, Gledhill, & Shephard, 2000; Strong et al., 2005).

Given the compelling evidence for the protective role of physical activity against obesity and other chronic diseases, the United States Department of Health and Human Services (USDHHS) (2009) has developed guidelines for youth and adults. These recommend that youth engage in 60 or more minutes of moderate-to-vigorous physical activity each day and adults in at least 150 minutes of moderate-intensity or 75 minutes of vigorous-intensity activity each week. Despite these recommendations, only 42% of children aged 6–11 years and 8% of adolescents meet this standard (Troiano et al., 2008).

Adults are similarly deficient, with 39% being completely sedentary and 61% never engaging in vigorous-intensity physical activity (Pleis & Lucas, 2009). Moreover, the amount of time spent engaging in physical activity decreases continuously from childhood to older adulthood (Barnes, 2007; Pratt, Macera, & Blanton, 1999; Sallis, 1993; Trost et al., 2002). In view of the numerous health benefits of physical activity, inactivity in America has become a public health concern and needs to be addressed in both research and practice.

We hope the above description of the association between physical activity and disease constitutes an appropriate discussion of "So what?" and "What's the problem?" The remainder of this chapter outlines several theoretical approaches to physical activity promotion, intending to advance the reader's understanding of the role of theory in both research investigations and intervention implementation and evaluation. We begin with a broad definition of *theory* as it relates to physical activity and proceed with a thorough discussion of its role throughout the research process. The subsequent sections are designed to mimic a manuscript appropriate for submission to a scientific journal, with the purpose of summarizing several theoretical approaches to physical activity promotion while providing an informative template for the dissemination of scientific research.

Theory Application in Physical Activity Research

With its numerous health benefits but opposing low prevalence, physical activity has become a high research priority in the United States. In fact, its adoption of physical activity has been emphasized in reports from the United States Surgeon General (USDHHS, 2001) and specifically targeted in the Healthy People 2010 Objectives (USDHHS, 2000). In turn, physical activity promotion research that implements various intervention components and evaluates their impact on specific behavioral and health outcomes has become prominent. Intervention studies are asking *how*: How can we (i.e., collaborative research efforts) most efficiently promote physical activity? However, research application in the form of program implementation often occurs in the final stages of the research process. Before developing and testing physical activity programs, research must first illuminate the mechanisms underlying physical activity behavior, asking what factors influence people's decisions to engage in physical activity. These factors can be personal to the individual (gender, ethnicity, age, etc.), psychological (attitudes, self-efficacy, etc.), social (family, peer role modeling, etc.), or environmental (accessible bike paths, gymnasium, etc.). It is these factors or mechanisms that research should initially examine and eventually target in physical activity interventions.

Theory development is a systematic way of organizing and testing the numerous factors influencing people's physical activity behavior. Theory has been defined as a proposed description or model to explain a phenomenon, allowing the formation of testable predictions of future occurrences or observations (Kerlinger, 1973). Theories of physical activity or inactivity conceptualize what factors influence physical activity and how they interact to encourage or discourage it. By proposing and organizing these relationships, a theory generates predictions and facilitates empirical examinations that can support or falsify them. Repeated theoretical investigation highlights the most significant influences on physical activity, enabling later advances in the effectiveness of exercise promotions, interventions, or programs.

Theory application contributes to two general approaches to research: exploratory research and intervention evaluation. As mentioned earlier, empirical examinations of the potential determinants of physical activity are a necessity for the development of effective promotional programs. These types of studies can range from qualitative focus groups to quantitative longitudinal investigations, in addition to measurement validation studies and various group comparisons. Regardless of intent or design, each theory-based examination contributes a brick to the foundation of knowledge specific to physical activity behavior. This continually growing foundation is the origin of descriptive and empirical evidence for future examinations or intervention studies.

Overall, exploratory research in the physical activity context intends to describe or predict various factors related to this multifaceted behavior, asking the "W" questions: where, what, when and why. Behavioral theory provides the platform that fosters these types of examinations, initiating the basic idea for a study and contributing to the development of hypotheses, study design, study procedures, statistical application, and interpretation of results. The outcome(s) of theory-based examinations then provides the evidence that supports or refutes theoretical expectations to further develop the evidenced-based knowledge foundation. For example, research may intend to describe *who* is meeting the physical activity guidelines, leading to exploring the possibility that age, gender, ethnicity, and socioeconomic status play a role in predicting physical activity levels. Results of a study may indicate that socioeconomic status does not predict physical activity levels, refuting expectations stemming from previous research based on the ecological model (explained later in this chapter). Although repetition of this examination would be needed before any final conclusions are drawn, such studies provide the bricks from which effective physical activity interventions are built.

As with exploratory research, theory application is extremely helpful during intervention evaluation studies, guiding the processes of study design, program implementation, data interpretation, and program evaluation. Physical activity intervention research extends previous examinations of the various "W" questions to intervention or program evaluations. Thus previous descriptive or predictive research informs intervention development about the factors contributing to physical activity behavior, which are applied in actual promotional programs and later evaluated. Intervention research asks *how*: How can these theoretical constructs be implemented to effectively promote physical activity? For instance, from examination research of the social cognitive model we may expect self-efficacy (i.e., *what*) to predict physical activity behavior. This is useful knowledge; however, to increase levels of regular physical activity and improve public health, intervention research needs to determine *how* to intervene to most effectively improve program participants' self-efficacy so as to increase their level of physical activity.

The second half of this chapter describes the application of several distinct theories to research on physical activity, highlighting the large range of theoretical approaches to describing the nature of this behavior. The complexity of behavioral science has encouraged a multidisciplinary approach incorporating ideas from various sciences. For example, a human developmental scientist may expect early childhood experiences to predict adult physical activity behaviors, while an ecological scientist hypothesizes that environment change predicts physical activity. A genetic scientist could be interested in the idea of a "physical activity gene," and a social scientist might believe that higher income levels provide the physical activity opportunities that predict this behavior. Theory development unifies these diverse approaches into a set of theoretical propositions, formulating a parsimonious system by which to explain, predict, or change physical activity behavior (Crosby, Kegler, & DiClemente, 2002).

Theory-based research on physical activity has become widespread, evolving from traditional approaches to behavioral science and progressing to a newer generation of conceptualizations. In addition to their own distinct explanations for human behavior, traditional theories provide evidenced-based templates for novel developments. As our society advances from one generation to the next, the mechanisms determining human behavior also evolve, illuminating the need for theoretical updates. Novel theoretical approaches that respond to ongoing societal changes and encompass factors relevant to current events are critical. For example, a newer theoretical model may borrow the traditional idea that behavior is a consequence of one's environment but update it to include developments in a new generation (e.g., Xbox video games.). On the other hand, it is important to distinguish between durable societal changes and short-lived fads. Thus there is a partnership between traditional and novel theoretical approaches, with one grounded in empirical evidence and the other responding to social evolution.

In this chapter we describe examples of both traditional and novel theoretical approaches to physical activity behavior, demonstrating their unique service to behavioral science as they advance research from accurate descriptions of *what*, *where*, *when*, and *why* to effective implementations of the *how*. The remaining sections of this chapter are designed like an actual research manuscript. Our dual intention is to present the constructs from both traditional and novel theoretical approaches to physical activity behavior and to give examples of their direct application to the process.

Introduction

All research articles begin with an introduction section that outlines the relevant background information, the research aim(s) or purpose(s), the study's expected contribution, and the hypothesized outcomes. The introduction section should begin with an evidence-based presentation that explains the rationale for the study. The discussion should begin by presenting the research within a broad context and then become more specialized, ending with a presentation of the specific research question and hypotheses. It is critical to include a theoretical basis for the investigation and hypotheses. Good theory is both generalizable and testable: generalizable in that the same ideas are applicable across diverse populations and settings, and testable in that hypotheses can be empirically examined. Thus the introduction of a research manuscript must provide a platform based on theory and supported or refuted with relevant evidence. This facilitates the presentation of a testable hypothesis that can be compared or contrasted with what other researchers have reported, potentially advancing knowledge in the field of physical activity promotion.

Let's return to the story of Sam. A good literature review for a study would begin broadly, describing the association between physical activity and the health of youth along with reporting the inadequate physical activity levels among youth, thus presenting the problem the research study addresses—the "So what?" The role modeling construct and its relationship to youth physical activity level has been tested in previous research using the theoretical framework of social cognitive theory; thus application of this model to the study facilitates development of a testable hypothesis that can advance current knowledge. Following an introduction of social cognitive theory and the role modeling construct, one would then present what is already known regarding the influence of parent role modeling on youth physical activity levels. Finally, one would narrow the discussion to reflect the uniqueness of the study. What brick does it add to the current knowledge structure? How will the results advance the field? It might be that most investigations of the influence of role modeling are limited to Caucasians, and this research has been done among a more diverse population. Further, maybe the study uses an objective measure of physical activity (e.g., accelerometry), and the previous research has been limited to youth or parent self-report measures.

Incorporating novelty into studies that mimic portions of previous studies plays an important role in advancing research. Repetition in research provides supportive evidence, furthering our confidence in previous conclusions, while novel elements may illuminate variables that affect the relationship under study that were overlooked or not considered in previous examinations. For example, a strong positive relationship between role modeling and physical activity may already be established. However, in addition to supporting this finding, new results may suggest that age moderates this relationship, demonstrating a decreased role modeling effect as children develop into adolescence.

Overall, theory organizes the introduction of a research article's topic within a generalizable and testable framework that operates as a communication tool between previous and future research. In the following sections, we introduce a number of physical activity theories, both traditional and novel, and provide examples of their application to physical activity intervention research. For this youthful area of investigation (Nigg & Jordan, 2005), we define traditional theories as those introduced to the physical activity area more than a decade ago and novel theories as having been introduced within the last decade.

The Traditional Theories

SELF-EFFICACY THEORY

Self-efficacy theory (SET) was originally developed as a general approach to understanding human behavior (Bandura, 1997) and has since been adapted specifically to physical activity research, where it is has been applied in over 100 publications (McAuley & Mihalko, 1998). SET explains behavior as a consequence of one's perceived self-efficacy and outcome expectancies. *Perceived self-efficacy* is defined as one's belief that one has the capability to perform a behavior that will result in an expected outcome, whereas *outcome expectancies* are the outcome(s) expected to result from performing that behavior (Bandura, 1997). Outcome expectancies can be either positive or negative, and each can increase or decrease in response to physical activity participation. According to SET, self-efficacy and outcome expectancy directly affect physical activity behavior, with physical activity expected to increase as self-efficacy and positive outcome expectancies increase and negative outcome expectancies decrease.

The distinction between self-efficacy and outcome expectancies is important in developing physical activity interventions. Self-efficacy is one's belief that one is skilled enough to achieve a specific outcome, while an expectancy is a likely consequence of that behavior. Thus 12-year-old Sam may have strong self-efficacy in that he believes he has the basketball-playing ability to make the middle school team; however, his outcome expectancy may be low because there are limited available spots on the team. Given this, Sam's high self-efficacy may interact with his outcome expectancy to discourage him from trying out for the team. According to SET, physical activity occurs when both self-efficacy and positive outcome expectancies are high, which is hypothesized to result from four underlying factors: mastery experiences, vicarious experiences,

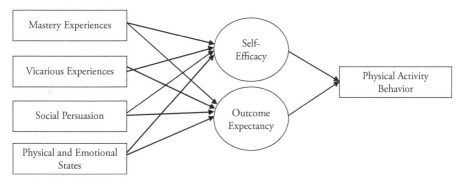

Figure 14.1 Theoretical relationship between constructs of self-efficacy theory.

verbal persuasion, and interpretation of emotional or physiological arousal (see Figure 14.1).

To improve self-efficacy and outcome expectancy, SET-based interventions would target these four underlying mechanisms. *Mastery experiences,* referring to past performances that are successful or unsuccessful, are theorized to have the greatest impact on self-efficacy. Thus an exercise program for patients recovering from heart surgery might start out with short-term goals that gradually progress from simple to more challenging, which will likely ensure initial successes. As these successful mastery experiences accumulate, self-efficacy and positive expectations are expected to improve and ultimately encourage habitual physical activity.

The second underlying influence according to SET is *vicarious experiences,* or social modeling. When individuals witness a successful performance by another person who is of equal competence to themselves, their efficacy and positive expectancies are expected to increase. For example, including older adult participants in a preexisting aerobic exercise program where adults of similar age and ability are successfully completing each workout should improve the former participants' efficacy and expectancies, leading to a higher prevalence of habitual physical activity. Introducing older adults into an aerobic class made up mostly of college students is likely to not have the same positive outcome.

Social persuasion, the next construct that can influence self-efficacy, includes encouragement and feedback from credible sources. Thus, if 12-year-old Sam values the opinion of his father, who tells him that he has the ability to be on the middle school football team, Sam's efficacy should improve and increase the likelihood of him trying out for the team. The level of influence would not be as strong if Sam received this persuasion from someone he had just met or someone he does not respect.

The final construct underlying self-efficacy and expectancies is the interpretation of *physical and emotional states,* with stronger emotional states having a greater influence on physical activity behavior. For example, a physical activity intervention targeting older adults would need to be sensitive to their potential fears of falling or heart attack (since physical activity increases heart rate) by providing initial educational experiences and hands-on guidance during introduction to the exercise program.

SOCIAL COGNITIVE THEORY

Social cognitive theory (SCT) defines human behavior as a reciprocal interaction among personal, behavioral, and environmental factors (Bandura, 1986, 1989; Bandura, Adams, & Beyer, 1977) (see Figure 14.2). Personal factors reside within an individual and include psychological factors (e.g., self-efficacy and self-regulation) and biological features (e.g., hormones and height). Behavioral factors are behaviors performed by the individual, and environmental factors are characteristics of situations that reside outside of an individual (e.g., peers and weather conditions). According to SCT it is not the individual influence of personal, behavioral, and environmental factors that affects physical activity behavior, but rather their interaction, or *reciprocal determinism.* For example, Carol's decision to walk to work in the morning rather than take her car is likely influenced by personal, environmental, and behavioral factors combined. She may be confident in her ability (personal factor) to walk that far, but not if the streets are covered with ice (environmental factor). If Carol attempts the walk and falls numerous times (behavioral factor), her confidence regarding her ability to walk to work may be altered.

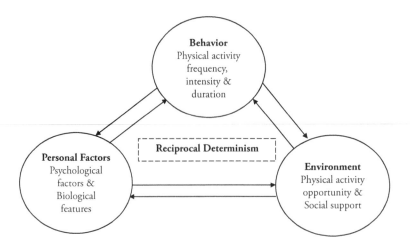

Figure 14.2 Theoretical relationships between constructs of social cognitive theory.

According to SCT, promotion interventions can increase levels of habitual physical activity by targeting underlying mechanisms that uniquely influence personal, environmental, or behavioral factors. The most frequently studied personal construct of social cognitive theory is perceived self-efficacy, which influences the type of activities chosen, the level of exerted effort, and perseverance in the face of obstacles. (See the previous section on SET for a description of the underlying mechanisms determining one's self-efficacy.) Individuals who are more efficacious are more likely than their counterparts to attempt novel activities, to exert more effort, and to sustain their activities (Bandura, 1986; Bandura et al., 1977).

Additional personal factors outlined by SCT include behavioral capability, self-control, expectations and expectancies, and emotional coping responses. *Behavioral capability,* or the knowledge and skill to perform physical activity, is expected to increase when promotional programs include skills training that offers participants numerous opportunities for mastery experiences. The *self-control* construct of SCT refers to individuals' personal regulation of goal-directed behaviors, which is expected to improve as individuals are provided opportunities to learn and practice specific skills including self-monitoring, goal setting, problem solving, and self-reward. *Expectations and expectancies* refer to the anticipated outcomes of a behavior and the values that an individual places on those outcomes, respectively. To improve expectations and expectancies, physical activity interventions may include exposure to individuals who model positive outcomes of physical activity (positive expectations) that have functional meaning to the

participant (expectancies). Finally, *emotional coping responses,* or the coping strategies used to deal with emotional stimuli, could be improved with training in problem solving and stress management.

Along with personal factors, SCT outlines specific characteristics of the environment, both social and physical, that are expected to influence physical activity levels. Social environmental factors may include family members, friends, and work colleagues, while physical environmental factors include conditions such as how walkable one's neighborhood is, the weather, and accessibility of physical activity opportunities (e.g., a gymnasium or recreational facility). Physical activity promotion programs may improve the social environment by targeting social support, observational learning, reinforcement, or any combination thereof. These types of interventions require compliance from the individuals who are the source of social influence. For example, sustained improvement in children's habitual physical activity is unlikely without consideration of the social entities that shape their environment. Intervention efforts to increase children's knowledge of the health benefits of physical activity are in vain if their parents continually model sedentary behavior or if the physical education programs at their schools are continually reduced or even eliminated.

Efforts to promote physical activity through environmental factors may target increases in participants' awareness of physical activity opportunities or in the actual provision of opportunities. For example, program components may target participants' perception of physical activity opportunities by providing information on local recreation facilities or gymnasiums. Additionally, a promotional program may intervene by including opportunities or training for participants to overcome opportunity barriers (e.g., walking programs or opportunities for physical activity at home). More concrete promotion interventions may aim to build or rebuild environments to directly increase opportunities for physical activity. For example, exploratory research may one day illuminate optimal neighborhood and playground designs to facilitate the highest levels of physical activity; intervention research would then aim to disseminate these designs within future neighborhood and playground developments.

TRANSTHEORETICAL MODEL

The transtheoretical model (TTM) was developed as a comprehensive model of behavior change, incorporating cognitive, behavioral, and temporal aspects into a unified approach (Prochaska & DiClemente, 1983; Prochaska, Redding, & Evers, 1996). The constructs outlined in the TTM consist of the stages of change, the processes of change, decisional balance, self-efficacy, and temptation. *Stage of change* classifies individuals according to their progression toward habitual physical activity and is hypothesized to relate to the other TTM constructs. Thus individuals' processes of change, decisional balance, self-efficacy, and temptation are expected to change as they move through the stages of change.

The stage-of-change construct breaks the time or readiness dimension into five progressive stages along which behavior change occurs. The first stage is precontemplation, which includes those individuals with no intention to engage in regular physical activity. The second stage is contemplation, or the intent to engage in regular physical activity within the next six months. This is followed the preparation stage, in which individuals have immediate intentions and commitments to engage in regular physical activity (i.e., within the next 30 days). Individuals who have initiated regular physical activity behavior have advanced to the action stage. Finally, once an individual has persisted in habitual physical activity behavior for more than six months, he or she has entered the maintenance stage.

The *processes of change* are the strategies theorized to aid in stage progression and are labeled as either experiential or behavioral. Experiential processes occur through personal experiences and include consciousness raising, dramatic relief, environmental reevaluation, self-reevaluation, and social liberation. In complement with the experiential processes, the behavioral processes arise from the environment and through action and include counterconditioning, helping relationships, reinforcement management, self-liberation, and stimulus control. Table 14.1

Table 14.1. Processes of Change Defined for Physical Activity according to the Transtheoretical Model

Experimental processes	Definition
Consciousness raising	Seek new information about physical activity
Dramatic relief	Experience and express intense feelings/emotions about not engaging in physical activity
Environmental reevaluation	Assess how physical activity affects the physical and social environment
Self-reevaluation	Cognitive and emotional reappraisal of values regarding inactivity
Social liberation	Develop awareness and acceptance of lifestyles that include physical activity
Behavioral processes	**Definition**
Counterconditioning	Substitute alternatives for sedentary behavior
Helping relationships	Seek support from others to adopt and continue exercising
Reinforcement management	Change contingencies; reward physical activity
Self-liberation	Choose and commit to physical activity; belief that one can change
Stimulus control	Control situations and cues that deter physical activity

Note. Adapted with permission from "Theories of Exercise Behavior," by S. J. H. Biddle and C. R. Nigg, 2000, *International Journal of Sport Psychology, 31*, pp. 290–304.

presents definitions of each process of change as they relate to physical activity. According to the theory, a person's stage of change directly relates to certain processes of change, such that experiential processes benefit progression through the earlier stages of change while behavioral processes emerge during later stages. This interplay between the stages and processes of change is of considerable use in constructing interventions for physical activity promotion, providing information with which to more efficiently tailor intervention strategies to the individual.

Decisional balance is an individual's evaluation of the costs (cons) and benefits (pros) of engaging in a behavior, and stage progression is suggested to occur as pros increase and cons decrease (Marshall & Biddle, 2001; Prochaska et al., 1996). Much as in SET, self-efficacy is defined as an individual's confidence, while *temptations* are the negative urges that distract or deter the individual from engaging in physical activity. Figure 14.3 depicts how the TTM constructs are theoretically related. The processes of change are listed according to their application to the theorized stages, with more behavioral processes in advanced stages. Decisional balance is expected to have the strongest relationship with the earlier stages of change. Thus, as individuals progress toward preparation, they evolve from perceiving greater cons related to physical activity (precontemplation) to rating the pros and cons more equally (contemplation and preparation). Also depicted in Figure 14.3 are the increase in self-efficacy and decrease in temptations that are expected to occur as one progresses through the stages.

A major strength of the TTM is the potential to tailor its constructs to fit an individual's readiness to begin physical activity behavior. Different people are going to be at different levels of readiness to begin physical activity. For example, some people are only thinking about beginning an exercise program, and others may be searching for ways to make maintenance of their morning walks easier. Both these types of individuals share the goal of physical activity; however, they are clearly at different stages of change and require different intervention approaches. The tailoring capability of the TTM is helpful not only for targeting different people at different stages of readiness for physical activity but also for adapting strategies to the same individual over time. For example, a promotion program targeting sedentary adults would first apply intervention strategies tailored to the precontemplation stage; however, these strategies would adjust gradually over time to become tailored to the action or maintenance stages as the same adults work toward habitual physical activity.

In addition to the potential it offers for a population-based intervention approach, the TTM is clear enough to be used by virtually any type of practitioner or researcher. The TTM has the capacity to combine clinical and public health interventions to maximize success in health behavior change (Prochaska et al., 1996). In that sense, it may be feasible in the future for doctors, nurses, social workers, psychologists, and other health care professionals to have access to materials that bring the TTM model into their offices. For example, a health practitioner could quickly assess a client's stage-of-change status for physical activity and efficiently counsel him or her on specific techniques most beneficial to progress toward higher stages.

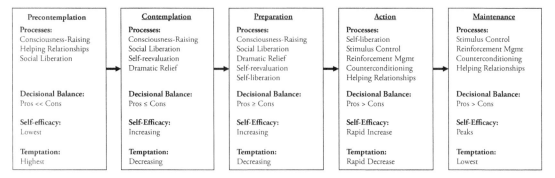

Precontemplation	Contemplation	Preparation	Action	Maintenance
Processes: Consciousness-Raising Helping Relationships Social Liberation	**Processes:** Consciousness-Raising Social Liberation Self-reevaluation Dramatic Relief	**Processes:** Consciousness-Raising Social Liberation Dramatic Relief Self-reevaluation Self-liberation	**Processes:** Self-liberation Stimulus Control Reinforcement Mgmt Counterconditioning Helping Relationships	**Processes:** Stimulus Control Reinforcement Mgmt Counterconditioning Helping Relationships
Decisional Balance: Pros << Cons	**Decisional Balance:** Pros ≤ Cons	**Decisional Balance:** Pros ≥ Cons	**Decisional Balance:** Pros > Cons	**Decisional Balance:** Pros > Cons
Self-efficacy: Lowest	**Self-Efficacy:** Increasing	**Self-Efficacy:** Increasing	**Self-Efficacy:** Rapid Increase	**Self-Efficacy:** Peaks
Temptation: Highest	**Temptation:** Decreasing	**Temptation:** Decreasing	**Temptation:** Rapid Decrease	**Temptation:** Lowest

Figure 14.3 Theoretical relationship between stages of change, processes of change, decisional balance, self-efficacy, and temptation in the transtheoretical model. Adapted with permission from "Overview of the Transtheoretical Model," by G. J. Burkholder and C. R. Nigg, 2002, in P. Burbank and D. Riebe (Eds.), *Promoting exercise and behavior change in older adults: Interventions with the transtheoretical model* (pp. 57–84). New York: Springer.

THEORY OF REASONED ACTION AND PLANNED BEHAVIOR

The theory of reasoned action (TRA) is based on the general assumption that *intention* directly determines behavior and is influenced by attitude and subjective (social) normative factors (Ajzen, 1985). The theory of planned behavior (TPB) augments TRA to include the influence of *perceived behavioral control* (Ajzen, 1988). Perceived behavioral control was added to account for behaviors with lower decisional control; for example, 12-year-old Sam may have strong intentions to attend football practice every afternoon, but he knows his parents can take him only twice a week. Taken together, TRA and TPB theorize that attitudes, subjective norms, and perceived behavioral control influence behavioral intention, which in turn determines behavior (Ajzen, 1991) (see Figure 14.4).

The *attitude* construct of TRA/TPB is determined in part by one's beliefs about physical activity as well as the expected likely outcomes of engaging in physical activity. These behavioral beliefs are combined with judgments regarding the value of each expected outcome of the behavior to form the attitude construct (Ajzen, 1988). Thus, to improve participants' attitudes toward physical activity, intervention strategies would emphasize the healthy consequences of physical activity as well as the importance and value of being healthy. According to the theory, the resulting improved attitude toward physical activity would be followed by increased intention and ultimately increases in physical activity behavior.

Subjective norms are determined by normative beliefs and the motivation to comply. Normative beliefs concern one's perception that individuals or groups approve or disapprove of engaging in physical activity. These normative beliefs are coupled with one's motivation to comply with those people or their beliefs to form the subjective norm construct. Application of subjective norms in physical activity promotion may expose participants to credible sources expressing healthy normative beliefs. For example, a program targeting increased physical activity among obese families may intervene through having family pediatricians illuminate the health risks of obesity and promoting the health benefits of physical activity.

HEALTH BELIEF MODEL

The health belief ,model (HBM) was originally developed as an integrative approach to explain why individuals do or do not undertake various preventative health behaviors (Barker et al., 1977). The behaviors targeted in the HBM include clinic visits, self-screening, vaccinations, specific dietary behaviors, and regular physicals. According to the theory, for individuals to seek out preventative health behaviors, they must have health knowledge and motivation, perceive themselves as vulnerable to the health problem, view the health condition as threatening, believe in the intervention program's effectiveness, and perceive few difficulties with engaging in the specific health behavior(s). Individuals' willingness to increase their time spent engaging in physical activity is primarily influenced by their perceived threat of disease, perceived benefits and barriers, and self-efficacy. Figure 14.5 depicts the relationship among the constructs within the HBM.

Perceived susceptibility refers an individual's perceived risk of contracting a health condition, and *perceived severity* is determined by their level of concern regarding the seriousness of the health condition and the risk of leaving it untreated. The theoretical expectation is that people will begin to change their health behaviors when they become aware or begin to perceive that their own health is at risk. To target perceptions of susceptibility and severity, HBM-based physical activity interventions may work to build awareness of the health risks associated with inactivity by providing information that is directly relevant to the participant.

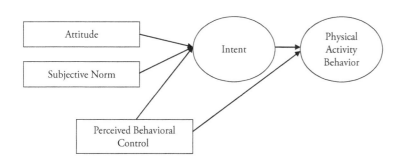

Figure 14.4 Theoretical relationships between constructs of the theories of planned behavior and reasoned action. Adapted with permission from "Theories of Exercise Behavior," by S. J. H. Biddle and C. R. Nigg, 2000, *International Journal of Sport Psychology, 31,* pp. 290–304.

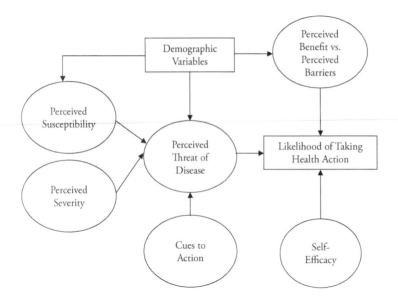

Figure 14.5 Theoretical relationships between constructs of the health belief model. Adapted with permission from "Theories of Exercise Behavior," by S. J. H. Biddle and C. R. Nigg, 2000, *International Journal of Sport Psychology, 31*, pp. 290–304.

Perceived benefits are defined as an individual's beliefs in the effectiveness of strategies to reduce risk of disease or illness, while *perceived barriers* are potential negative consequences of adopting a specific health action and include both physical and social factors. The likelihood of an individual's engaging in physical activity behavior is enhanced when the perceived benefits outweigh the perceived barriers. To target these perceptions, intervention strategies may include educational experiences presenting the positive health outcomes associated with regular physical activity as well as strategies to overcome common barriers to regular physical activity (e.g., money and time).

In addition to cognitive desires to change one's behavior, the HBM recognizes the critical role of additional factors necessary to progress individuals from wanting to take action to actually taking action. In this light, the HBM incorporates two additional elements into predicting the likelihood that behavior change will occur: *cues to action* and *self-efficacy*. Cues to action are situations external to an individual that prompt their desire to make the associated behavior change. Physical activity promotion programs may facilitate cues to action by sending e-mails or letters to participants reminding them of reasons to begin regular physical activity that are personalized to their own health concerns or goals. The HBM concept of self-efficacy is similar to that in previous models, being defined as an individual's belief in his or her ability to make a health-related change.

ECOLOGICAL MODEL

The ecological model systematically classifies health-related factors into five levels of influence (McLeroy, Bibeau, Steckler, & Glanz, 1988). As Figure 14.6 depicts, the model organizes its constructs similarly to the layers of an onion, surrounding each individual with both proximal and distal influences. Closest to the individual are *intrapersonal* factors or characteristics of that individual, including demographic classifications and personal beliefs and attitudes. Ecologically based interventions at this level are concerned with behavioral differences based on variables such as gender or ethnicity as well as individuals' beliefs such as perceived benefits versus perceived costs. Just outside of these individual characteristics are *interpersonal* processes, which include both formal and informal social networks of

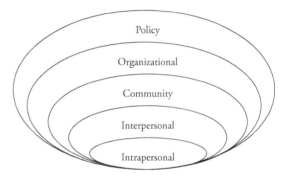

Figure 14.6 Levels of influence on individuals' health behavior in the ecological model.

support. Promotion programs concerned with this layer of influence may intervene within the family, peer system, coworkers, or a combination.

The third layer of influence in the ecological model is represented by the *community,* or institutional factors surrounding an individual. Influencing characteristics within this layer include community characteristics and rules that either encourage and support or deter specific behaviors. For example, the type of training and information provided to physical education teachers has the potential to affect the physical activity opportunities provided to their students, indirectly influencing the students' physical activity levels. The fourth, *organizational* layer contains extended community factors, including the relationships among organizations and social networks. An example of this layer is the United States federal government's giving priority to health promotion and dispensing larger funding to agencies supporting related research (e.g., the Centers for Disease Control and the Department of Health and Human Services).

At the outermost layer of the ecological model are public *policies* and laws at the local, regional, and national levels. Theoretical strategies at this level could target influences ranging from punitive reactions to proactive legislation. For example, health insurance policy responding to the current obesity epidemic might increase monthly rates for adults whose body mass index exceeds their healthy range. More proactive approaches might include removing machines vending sugary sodas and calorically dense snacks from schools or mandating increased time for students in physical education classes.

Novel Theoretical Approaches
THE PRECAUTION ADOPTION PROCESS MODEL

The precaution adoption process model (PAPM) is another stage-based model. Figure 14.7 illustrates the seven stages of the PAPM. Rather than classifying the majority of physical activity behaviors as either taking place or not, the PAPM conceptualizes changes as occurring more dynamically over time (Blalock et al., 1996). The PAPM hypothesizes that individuals who are at different points along the precaution adoption process will likely behave in qualitatively different ways. In light of this expectation, PAPM-based interventions are adapted to an individual's classification into one of the seven stages, specifically tailoring intervention strategies to facilitate advancement toward the action stage (Weinstein, 1988).

In contrast with the TTM, the PAPM does not theorize that different variables enter at different stages or foster progression through the stages; rather, changes in an individual's cognitions (i.e., health beliefs and perceptions) are expected to determine their advancement toward the acting stage. The PAPM is also more absolute than the TTM, assuming that individuals do not skip any stage. An additional contrast to the TTM is the absence of time specifications and broader expectations of relapse between stages (Weinstein, 1988).

Stage 1 of the PAPM includes individuals who are unfamiliar with physical activity and unaware of its relatedness to their personal health. Once individuals learn about the negative health consequences of sedentary behavior, the protective nature of regular physical activity, or both, they advance to stage 2 of the model. It is important to distinguish stage 2's condition of awareness without action from the unawareness in stage 1. The theoretical supposition is that knowledge will likely develop from thinking about engaging in physical activity, which has the potential to improve the likelihood of eventual action. Second, perceived outcomes and attitudes relative to physical activity will likely change as a consequence of one's new cognitions. Therefore, these new cognitions become potential indirect predictors of future physical activity behavior.

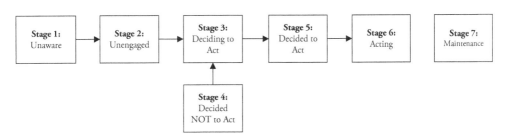

Figure 14.7 Theoretical relationships between constructs of the precaution adoption process model.

The next two stages include individuals who are deciding to begin physical activity (stage 3) or have decided not to (stage 4). Because individuals in stage 4 have reached a definite decision, they are theorized to respond differently to promotional techniques, demonstrating greater resistance to persuasion strategies (Brockner & Rubin, 1985; Cialdini, 1988). Stages 5 and 6 of the PAPM represent having decided to be physical active and actually beginning physical activity, respectively. The distinction between these two stages is similar to that in the TPB, hypothesizing a clear difference between intentions to act and actually engaging in physical activity. Finally, initial engagement in physical activity (stage 6) is hypothesized as a separate stage from maintenance (stage 7), or the long-term sustainment of physical activity.

THE ELABORATION LIKELIHOOD MODEL OF PERSUASION

The central focus of the elaboration likelihood model (ELM) is an individual's attitude toward engaging in a behavior. According to the theory, attitude encompasses individuals' general evaluations about themselves, others, objects, or issues that relate to various behavioral, cognitive, and affective experiences and that ultimately persuade them to engage (or not) in behaviors. The ELM was initially developed to resolve previous inconsistencies in studies researching attitudes and behavior. Rather than focusing on a single process, the ELM outlines the process of promotion as involving two distinct routes by which one's attitude is influenced: the central route and the peripheral route (Petty, Barden, & Wheeler, 2002).

The central route is relevant in situations where an individual expresses cognitive thoughts or concerns about the targeted behavior. In contrast, the peripheral route requires minimal thought but instead involves altering attitudes through simple associations or mental shortcuts. According to the ELM, persuasion occurs along an elaboration continuum, stretching from the extreme central route to the extreme peripheral route—from processes requiring careful consideration to those requiring no cognition; along most of this continuum, both routes can influence attitudes simultaneously (Petty, 1994). It is how an individual interprets information rather than the information per se that is hypothesized to influence behavior (Petty, Wheeler, & Bizer, 1999). Figure 14.8 illustrates the central and peripheral processes along the continuum,

showing certain variables hypothesized to influence one's motivation to think or one's ability to think, which include but are not limited to the quality of the delivered message, previous attitudes, thought rehearsal, identification with the message delivery source, and counterpersuasions.

Physical activity interventions developed to target the central or effortful processes require the presence of two conditions to effectively change attitude to promote action. First, the recipient of the message must be motivated to interpret the message, which can be dependent on the recipient's perception of the message's personal relevance (Petty & Cacioppo, 1999). For instance, a physical activity message presented to older adults at an assisted-living community would be more effective when related to quality-of-life health benefits then when linked to athletic performance benefits. The second condition relates to the recipient's ability to think, which can be influenced by variables such as the level of distraction (Petty, Wells, & Brock, 1976) and how often the message is repeated (Cacioppo & Petty, 1979). Thus a physical activity promotion message for older adults would need to consider potentially distracting factors such as small, unreadable print in advertisements or inappropriate presentation timing that results in sensory overload.

Methods

The methods section describes specifically how the research or intervention study was performed. The general goal is to present this information concisely but clearly enough that future research can replicate the study. It is important to find an appropriate middle ground between too little detail and an overload of information. For both exploratory and intervention research, this section is typically divided into subsections that cover the participants and setting, measures, design, and procedure. The order of these subsections is usually arbitrary; however, it is important that the presentation be organized and readable. Theory offers helpful guidance for the specifics of one's study plan, which we describe in the following subsections. In general, application of a relevant theory helps to ensure that a study's approach matches the intentions of the research, so as to optimally address the specific research questions. The optimal research design will allow accurate assessment of the targeted population in a way that produces interpretable outcomes with high internal and external validity.

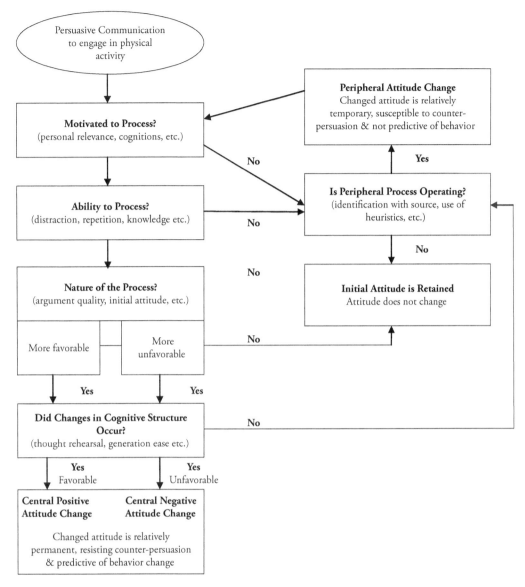

Figure 14.8 Theoretical relationships between constructs of the elaboration likelihood model.

Participants and Setting

This section provides details about the sample of participants included in the research study and the setting in which the study takes place. Details such as selection criteria, study dropout statistics, and location (e.g., rural or urban) are directly relevant to data interpretation and for comparison with previous and future research reports.

The theoretical approach guiding the explanation or promotion of physical activity behavior is directly relevant to characteristics of the people and environment being studied. Given the uniqueness of individuals' characteristics and beliefs, along with demographic diversity, the mechanisms driving the decision to engage in physical activity behavior are likely to vary. Correspondingly, differences in the environment may also determine variability in individuals' physical activity behavior. As mentioned in our introduction to the various theories, many documented conceptualizations of behavior consider both the person and the environment. These factors thus bear on both research design and data interpretation. For example, in SCT individual characteristics and the surrounding environment are theorized to interact in the determination of behavior. Thus in developing a SCT-based research design to examine the prevalence of weight lifting, one should consider assessing the socioeconomic status of participants, as some may not have the necessary finances or transportation to the facility.

In addition to guiding exploratory research, theory is critical to the processes involved in intervention development and dissemination. Exploratory research may indicate that certain theoretical components are more influential among certain subgroups to be considered during intervention development. For example, physical activity behaviors among youth under the age of 18 years may be more sensitive to vicarious experiences or role modeling than are behaviors of older adults. Thus interventions based on SET would need to consider this distinction when targeting the self-efficacy of individuals in these age groups.

From a broader perspective, different theories may indicate distinct research intentions relative to population characteristics and specific interventions. For example, for interventions guided by the HBM or the TPB, initial assessments of the targeted subgroup(s) are needed to tailor intervention components for optimal effectiveness for their specific needs; thus these approaches are more appropriate for smaller-scale programs in a specific area or clinical setting. Larger-scale interventions aimed at affecting health behavior at the population level require tailoring strategies that are more generalizable and can be determined more efficiently, such as components from the TTM or the PAPM.

Applying theory during intervention development also aids the institution or staff participating in program implementation. For instance, an exercise promotion program in a clinical setting may work through pediatricians providing information to parents regarding the health consequences of inactivity and the benefits of regular exercise. Compare this with an exercise intervention implemented during after-school programs by part-time college-age student employees. Intervention components implemented in a clinical setting would need to consider the time limitations of the medical doctors, who would have to provide quick assessments and predetermined promotional strategies. Here a helpful theoretical guide may be the TTM, which can provide a quick assessment of each patient's readiness to change and tailored strategies that the doctor can administer efficiently. On the other hand, if youth spend two or more hours daily in an after-school program, an intervention program can exploit the prolonged contact time to target several mechanisms to increase physical activity. For example, a

SCT-based intervention may implement strategies to improve youth self-efficacy as well as target the after-school environment by increasing opportunities for youth to be active (e.g., activity demanding equipment and better playgrounds). Also in the after-school case, an ecologically based program might implement strategies targeting each individual child (e.g., improving self-efficacy), the after-school program leaders (e.g., offering social support and positive role modeling), the surrounding community (e.g., providing a walkable path to and from school), and school policy (e.g., requiring programs to provide at least one hour of recreational time to participating students).

Measures

The measurement section specifies how the data were obtained and should include as many details as possible or a citation for the measurement scales used. This not only ensures appropriate replication and comparability of the study in future research but also validates the conclusions drawn from the data. By proposing and outlining the specific phenomena that influence behavior, theory facilitates the operationalization of theorized constructs into measurement scales. The process of establishing the specific elements that define or make up a theoretical factor (operationally defined as questionnaire items) is an integral part of high-quality research and is sometimes taken too casually. Without valid and reliable measures, one cannot determine what is being compared.

For example, one might conclude that the intervention being studied improved older adults' attitude toward physical activity, increasing their intention to exercise and their actual exercise behavior. However, such a conclusion depends on measuring attitude and intention accurately, with measurement scales generalizable to diverse adults from potentially unique backgrounds. Further, if one were examining change in attitude and intention across time (e.g., from baseline to 6 months after intervention implementation), it is important to be certain that any differences are due to actual change in participants' attitudes and intentions rather than shifts in measurement validity due to time. Accurate and consistent measures based on concepts originated from theory provide the foundation for effective research.

Given that many of the theoretical mechanisms expected to influence physical activity behavior are products of personal perceptions, data derived from the operationalizations of these concepts (i.e., measurement scales) are likely based on self-report. Self-report has the potential to result in numerous biases that need to be considered in behavioral research. These may include recall bias, response bias, reporting bias, selection bias, sampling bias, measurement bias, and bias due to participant withdrawal. One type of recall bias is forgetfulness, which becomes a prominent accuracy problem when one asks children to remember and report the type and amount of their daily physical activity. Reporting bias may occur when participants report inaccurate information because of social desirability. For instance, parents may exaggerate the level of social support given toward their children's physical activity because they believe this will impress others. Bias due to subject attrition may degrade generalizations made at the population level. For instance, differences in self-efficacy for physical activity between those who remained in the study and those who dropped out may bias the interpretation of data from only the participants who remained. The possibility of bias should be controlled as much as possible and considered throughout study development and data reporting.

The rigorous statistical techniques needed to critically examine the accuracy and consistency of a measurement scale are out of this chapter's scope, and we direct the reader to the studies referenced in each theory description for details of the corresponding scales. While there have been extensive examinations of measurement instruments related to physical activity behavior; there is never a perfect measurement scale and preliminary tests of reliability and validity are essential for every research application and report.

Procedures or Intervention Components

The procedures or intervention section of a research manuscript should describe the purpose and use of any materials, tests or measurements, or equipment (e.g., accelerometers or physical activity logs). Furthermore, each step in the execution of the study should be carefully summarized, indicating the details of each intervention session. This would include specifically describing any instructions, training, or treatment(s) received by the participants. When conducting a comparison between a control group and an intervention group, it is necessary to also provide details regarding the control group.

It is this section of the manuscript that considers the "nuts and bolts" of an intervention. These must be shown to clearly relate to the theorized mechanisms that motivate or sustain behavior (i.e., theoretical constructs). Theory provides concepts and ideas, but it is left to the researcher to develop the real-life strategies that will be promoted or implemented within an intervention in hopes of actually improving levels of physical activity. For example, the TPB emphasizes intention as the mechanism directly underlying an individual's physical activity behavior. Therefore, to encourage habitual exercise, TPB followers would design promotion interventions that target individual intentions.

The real-life strategies implemented in a promotional program will differ based on the choice of theory and the intended outcome. For example, a TTM-based intervention might target a large number of participants initially determined to be in stage 2 of readiness (contemplation) and implement tailored strategies with the intent of advancing participants to stage 3 (preparation). The most efficient intervention strategies to facilitate this change among a large group could involve providing promotional materials via e-mail or in pamphlet form. Counter to this approach would be a HBM-based group intervention targeting obese adults who proactively pursued a physical activity program. Intervention strategies for this situation would be more reactive, helping individuals recover from already existing health conditions. Intervention strategies using concepts from the HBM may be more intense than those of the TTM-based intervention. For example, with the intent of increasing levels of physical activity, participants might receive individualized counseling about strategies to increase their perceived threat of disease (so as to increase their perceived benefits of exercise), in addition to knowledge about physical activity and available opportunities to increase their self-efficacy.

Intervention Dissemination

In theory-based intervention evaluations it is important to consider the intervention's potential to be disseminated. In addition to generating empirical evidence, dissemination of effective interventions to impact public health must be a primary research goal. Given the current economic crisis, rise in chronic disease, and obesity epidemic, intervention studies have an ethical responsibility to aspire toward dissemination of successful programs to populations similar to those studied. It is never too early in the research process to consider the dissemination of a successful program. Evaluating a program's promise for successful dissemination also relates to the efficacy of certain theoretical applications. For example, evaluating a theory-based intervention in this way provides evidence regarding optimal dissemination for specific populations or settings. For example, a PAPM approach may be disseminated best within clinical settings, whereas the optimal dissemination of a SCT approach for youth would be in the school or after-school setting.

Depending on population characteristics, some interventions may be easier to disseminate. The Reach, Effectiveness, Adoption, Implementation, and Maintenance (RE-AIM) framework offers techniques for evaluating the efficiency and efficacy of a physical activity promotion program with respect to public health (Glasgow, Lichtenstein, & Marcus, 2003; Glasgow, Vogt, & Boles, 1999). The framework includes five dimensions. The *reach* of a program is determined by dividing the number of participants by the number recruited, and *effectiveness* is the size of the effect the program components had on participants' physical activity behavior (Glasgow, Klesges, Dzewaltowski, Estabrooks, & Vogt, 2006). For example, a program may have large effectiveness but poor reach or vice versa. *Adoption* represents the number of settings and clinicians who participate and should be analyzed with consideration for participant characteristics that may moderate program success (e.g., past experience and motivation). The *implementation* score indicates the extent of equivalence between the actual delivery of program components and the predetermined program protocol (Glasgow et al., 2006). An implementation calculation provides insight as to how easily the program is adapted to various contexts or among different practitioners. Finally, a *maintenance* score represents the long-term physical activity of the participants as well as the long-term sustainability of the program. Each of the RE-AIM dimensions can be examined individually; however, combinations of two or more dimensions provide better public health information for future policy decisions (see Glasgow et al., 2006).

Design and Data Analysis

The design and data analysis section outlines how the data collected in the study were summarized, compared, and analyzed. This portion of a research manuscript translates the previously described intervention concepts into measurable data that will be analyzed to reach a conclusion about the research question or evaluate the outcomes of the intervention. A good description of the data clarifies the independent and dependent variables, indicating the levels of the independent variables—whether the measured concept(s) were repeated, matched, or autonomous. Further, the section describes how the participants were assigned to groups and any control procedures used. For example, the gold standard in research is a randomized controlled study, involving completely random assignment of participants, groups, schools, neighborhoods, and so forth to either the intervention group(s) or the control group. Finally, the section describes all statistical analyses performed, which can range from qualitative analyses for a focus group interview to multivariate longitudinal growth curve modeling. It is also necessary to provide details regarding the statistical package(s) used for the analysis (i.e., name, company, and location of the company). This is an important detail, because packages may offer distinct approaches to data analysis, providing somewhat different outcome data.

The data design and statistical procedures should be consistent with the initial conceptualization of the study's intent. In other words, the theoretical basis for the research question(s) or study intention is very relevant to the planned data analyses. For example, suppose the original intent was to compare the frequency of meeting physical activity guidelines between participants categorized as intending to engage in regular physical activity and those who do not have that intention (as might be the case in research using the TRA/TPB). One could then summarize the data as percentages and test whether or not the observed frequency distribution differs from what is theoretically expected (a higher frequency of meeting guidelines among individuals intending habitual physical activity). Compare this with evaluating the impact on youth body mass index (BMI) of an ecologically based physical activity promotion program that included components that intervened at the community level, the school level, and the individual level. The data design and analysis of this study would be considerably more complicated. For example, analyses would need to consider the BMI associations within youth at the same school site and within the same community (the interclass correlations) and adjust for this type of clustered data structure using a three-level mixed model design (community, school, and individual).

Results

The presentation of research results requires careful consideration of the optimum description and analysis. Tables, figures, or both are helpful to illustrate the main findings. The following are some general guidelines. When presenting means also present a measure of variability (e.g., standard deviation or standard error). When summarizing nominal or ordinal data, proportions or percentages are more useful than frequencies, as they are independent of sample size. For inferential outcomes, provide the statistical value, degrees of freedom (df), probability value (p value), and an estimate of effect size.

It is important to emphasize only the meaning of the statistics rather than their implications. Result interpretations are reserved for the following, discussion section. In light of this, the results section need not reflect on theory or theoretical constructs. On the other hand, it is beneficial to keep theory in mind while writing this section, as it has guided the research process up to now. The writer must take a long look at the data, bearing in mind the characteristics of the participants, the theoretical constructs addressed and their meaning, the research question(s) or intervention components, and the data design and statistical analysis—all of which arose from applying a particular theory.

Discussion

The purpose of the discussion section is to evaluate and interpret the results, with special consideration for the initial study purpose and research question(s). This section should begin with a brief restatement of the purpose and a nontechnical summary of the results, presenting the main findings or outcomes without use of statistical terminology. This is followed with more specific discussion of what each result implies, relating what was found to the literature presented in the introduction section. It is now appropriate to emphasize the theoretical implications of the results. Depending on the specific application of the theory, it may be necessary to discuss whether the results support or contradict the theory. This type of discussion will move the current knowledge structure forward, by advancing understanding of physical activity behavior mechanisms, improving predictability of physical activity behavior, or advancing research efforts to determine the causation of physical activity behavior.

For instance, the discussion section of a randomized controlled trial study that evaluated a TTM-based physical activity intervention could potentially provide three general types of conclusions. The first is a description, which might summarize the sample's or sample subgroups' levels of physical activity or proportions of readiness to change as well as levels of each process of change, decisional balance, self-efficacy, and temptation. Second, the discussion could address the predictability of each TTM construct for physical activity, supporting or refuting implications of the theory. For instance, do the results support the theoretical expectation that higher levels of self-efficacy and lower levels of temptation are both predictive of increased levels of physical activity? The third potential contribution of this study is insight into the *how* question. With a randomized controlled trial intervention study one can draw inferences about causation. In other words, conclusions can be made as to whether or not the theory-based intervention components increased the intervention participants' physical activity compared with the control group participants. Overall, the application of theory in this hypothetical study would contribute to the knowledge structure by addressing numerous "W" questions as well as providing insight into *how*.

The discussion section should also address any noteworthy limitations of the study in addition to any suggestions for future research. Although the study results may make a large contribution to physical activity research, it is essential to mention any and all possible study characteristics that may limit the accuracy or generalizability of the results. For instance, the data may well have relied on participants' self-reports, which introduces the likelihood of several biases that would need to be mentioned. Or the study might have been carried out among a sample of college students, who were 85% Caucasian. Thus caution should be raised about the external validity or generalizability of the results to individuals of other ages and ethnicities. Finally, it is important to always take the advancement of current knowledge into account by providing suggestions as to how future theory-based physical activity examination or intervention studies can build on the study's findings.

Conclusions

The final section of any good manuscript ends with approximately one to three paragraphs that include a final summary of the conclusions. It may also be relevant to comment on the significance of the findings, discussing how the conclusions relate to the "big picture." Further, it is a researcher's responsibility to consider the application of results: What is the take-home message for researchers, practitioners, or policy makers? This type of discussion builds a bridge between research and real-world settings (e.g., clinics, schools, and community centers) to better the health of our population.

The application of theory to increase physical activity and reduce inactivity requires much further exploration and evaluation. As the low prevalence of physical activity and the obesity epidemic in the United States suggest, the current knowledge structure is clearly anemic. Additional exploratory studies, addressing all appropriate "W" questions, are needed to describe and predict reasons people adopt physical activity. A second future agenda is the evaluation of theory-based physical activity interventions applying experimental designs that can empirically provide understanding of the components that enter into increasing activity and decreasing inactivity. Such work may reveal one of three conclusions: (1) Existing theories and models are applicable; (2) revisions to existing theories and models are required; or (3) existing theories and models are simply not appropriate.

For physical activity research to progress, researchers must keep in mind the "big picture" of theory application as it relates to physical activity and sedentary behaviors. In the social and behavioral sciences there is an overabundance of theories, and deciding which theory works and in what population is a significant challenge. Therefore, good researchers begin by asking themselves several questions: (1) Are the current behavioral theories adequate approaches to behavior change? (2) How complicated is each approach, and is the effort worth the outcome? (3) Are revisions to the theory needed before application to physical activity behavior? (4) How can my research aid in the appropriate modification, extension, integration, or potential abandonment of a specific theory? (5) Are more complicated statistical designs and analyses needed to adequately test physical activity behavior theories and associated measurement scales? (6) Are there simple, naturally occurring examples that we can learn from and expand upon?

Within the view of the history of science advanced by Kuhn (1970), we are in the early stages of scientific development or the preparadigm stage as we directly apply theoretical approaches from different fields to describe or interpret phenomena in the physical activity context. Scientific knowledge develops slowly during these stages, because there is often little agreement among scientists owing to the development of theory and research and power struggles among factions within the discipline (Hardy, 1978). On the other hand, even with physical activity research being at the earliest stages of scientific development, it has taken great strides toward identifying the determinants of physical activity behavior. Considerably more high-quality research is needed to better our understanding of the mechanisms underlying physical activity. With the boost of a solid theoretical basis, we can begin to focus our efforts to highlight and disseminate the most appropriate applications of theory to increase physical activity and aid in improving the health of our population.

A Note on Evaluating the Use of Theory

The following questions should be considered to determine if a theory has been used properly:

- Is a theory identified and described?
- Is it fully translated into the intervention components?
- Are all components implemented and assessed?
- Do the theory variables match the outcomes?
- Did the intervention change the theory variables and the outcomes?

Readers are referred to a "litmus test" by Nigg and Paxton (2008) that details these concepts.

References

Ajzen, I. (1985). From intentions to actions: A theory of planned behavior. In J. Kuhl & J. Beckmann (Eds.), *Action control: From cognition to behavior* (pp. 11–39). New York: Springer-Verlag.

Ajzen, I. (1988). *Attitudes, personality, and behavior*. Chicago, IL: Dorsey Press.

Ajzen, I. (1991). The theory of planned behavior. *Organizational Behavior and Human Decision Processes, 50*(2), 179–211.

Albright, A., Franz, M., Hornsby, G., Kriska, A., Marrero, D., Ullrich, I., & Verity, L. S. (2000). American College of Sports Medicine position stand. Exercise and type 2 diabetes. *Medicine & Science in Sport & Exercise, 32*(7), 1345–1360.

Bandura, A. (1986). *Social foundations of thought and action: A social cognitive theory*. Englewood Cliffs, NJ: Prentice Hall.

Bandura, A. (1989). Human agency in social cognitive theory. *American Psychologist, 44*(9), 1175–1184.

Bandura, A. (1997). *Self-efficacy: The exercise of control*. New York: Freeman.

Bandura, A., Adams, N. E., & Beyer, J. (1977). Cognitive processes mediating behavioral change. *Journal of Personality and Social Psychology, 35*(3), 125–139.

Barker, M. H., Haefner, D. P., Kasl, S. V., Kirscht, J. P., Maiman, L. A., & Rosenstock, I. M. (1977). Selected psychosocial models and correlates of individual health-related behaviors. *Medical Care, 15*(5), 27–46.

Barnes, P. (2007). *Physical activity among adults: United States, 2000 and 2005*. Hyattsville, MD: National Center for Health Statistics, U.S. Department of Health and Human Services, Centers for Disease Control.

Biddle, S. J. H., & Nigg, C. R. (2000). Theories of exercise behavior. *International Journal of Sport Psychology, 31*, 290–304.

Blalock, S. J., DeVellis, R. F., Giorgino, K. B., DeVellis, B. M., Gold, D., Dooley, M. A.,…Smith, S. L. (1996). Osteoporosis prevention in premenopausal women: Using a stage model approach to examine the predictors of behavior. *Health Psychology, 15*, 84–93.

Brockner, J., & Rubin, J. Z. (1985). *Entrapment in escalating conflicts: A social psychological analysis.* New York: Springer-Verlag.

Burkholder, G. J., & Nigg, C. R. (2002). Overview of the transtheoretical model. In P. Burbank & D. Riebe (Eds.), *Promoting exercise and behavior change in older adults: Interventions with the transtheoretical model* (pp. 57–84). New York: Springer.

Cacioppo, J. T., & Petty, R. E. (1979). Effects of message repetition and position on cognitive response, recall, and persuasion. *Journal of Personality and Social Psychology, 37,* 97–109.

Cialdini, R. B. (1988). *Influence: Theory and practice.* Glenview, IL: Scott, Foresman.

Crosby, R. A., Kegler, M. C., & DiClemente, R. J. (2002). Understanding and applying theory in health promotion practice and research. In R. J. DiClemente, R. A. Crosby, & M. C. Kegler (Eds.), *Emerging theories in health promotion practice and research* (pp. 1–15). San Francisco, CA: Jossey-Bass.

Dowling, C. (2000). Getting them out of the doll corner *The frailty myth: Redefining the physical potential of women and girls* (pp. 84–112). New York: Random House.

Flegal, K. M., Carroll, M. D., Ogden, C. L., & Curtin, L. R. (2010). Prevalence and trends in obesity among U.S. adults, 1999–2008. *JAMA, 303*(3), 235–241.

Glasgow, R. E., Klesges, L. M., Dzewaltowski, D. A., Estabrooks, P. A., & Vogt, T. M. (2006). Evaluating the impact of health promotion programs: Using the RE-AIM framework to form summary measures for decision making involving complex issues. *Health Education Research, 21*(5), 688–694.

Glasgow, R. E., Lichtenstein, E., & Marcus, A. C. (2003). Why don't we see more translation of health promotion research to practice? Rethinking the efficacy-to-effectiveness transition. *American Journal of Public Health, 93*(8), 1261–1267.

Glasgow, R. E., Vogt, T. M., & Boles, S. M. (1999). Evaluating the public health impact of health promotion interventions: The RE-AIM framework. *American Journal of Public Health, 89*(9), 1322–1327.

Grundy, S. M., Blackburn, G., Higgins, M., Lauer, R., Perri, M. G., & Ryan, D. (1999). Physical activity in the prevention and treatment of obesity and its comorbidities: Evidence report of independent panel to assess the role of physical activity in the treatment of obesity and its comorbidities. *Medicine & Science in Sport & Exercise, 31*(11), 1493–1500.

Hardy, M. (1978). Evaluating nursing theory. In J. G. Paterson (Ed), *Theory development: What, why, how?* (pp. 75–86). New York: National League for Nursing.

Hu, F. B., Sigal, R. J., Rich-Edwards, J. W., Colditz, G. A., Solomon, C. G., Willett, W. C.,…Manson, J. E. (1999). Walking compared with vigorous physical activity and risk of type 2 diabetes in women: A prospective study. *JAMA, 282*(15), 1433–1439.

Katzmaryk, P. T., Gledhill, N., & Shephard, J. (2000). The economic burden of physical inactivity in Canada. *Canadian Medical Association Journal, 163,* 1435–1440.

Kerlinger, F. N. (1973). *Foundations of behavioral research.* New York: Holt, Rinehart, & Winston.

King, I. (1978). The "why" of theory development. In J. G. Paterson (Ed.), *Theory development: What, why, how?* (pp. 11–16). New York: National League for Nursing.

Kohl, H. W., 3rd, & Hobbs, K. E. (1998). Development of physical activity behaviors among children and adolescents. *Pediatrics, 101*(3 Pt. 2), 549–554.

Kuhn, T. S. (1970). *The structure of scientific revolutions.* Chicago: University of Chicago Press.

Lee, I. M. (2003). Physical activity and cancer prevention—data from epidemiologic studies. *Medicine & Science in Sport & Exercise, 35*(11), 1823–1827.

Lee, I. M., & Skerrett, P. J. (2001). Physical activity and all-cause mortality: What is the dose–response relation? *Medicine & Science in Sport & Exercise, 33*(6 Suppl.), S459–S471; discussion S493–S454.

Lee, J., Sparrow, D., Vokonas, P. S., Landsberg, L., & Weiss, S. T. (1995). Uric acid and coronary heart disease risk: Evidence for a role of uric acid in the obesity–insulin resistance syndrome. The Normative Aging Study. *American Journal of Epidemiology, 142*(3), 288–294.

Manson, J. E., Hu, F. B., Rich-Edwards, J. W., Colditz, G. A., Stampfer, M. J., Willett, W. C.,…Hennekens, C. H. (1999). A prospective study of walking as compared with vigorous exercise in the prevention of coronary heart disease in women. *New England Journal of Medicine, 341*(9), 650–658.

Marshall, S. J., & Biddle, S. J. (2001). The transtheoretical model of behavior change: A meta-analysis of applications to physical activity and exercise. *Annals of Behavioral Medicine, 23*(4), 229–246.

McAuley, E., & Mihalko, S. L. (1998). Measuring exercise-related self-efficacy. In J. L. Duda (Ed.), *Advances in sport and exercise psychology measurement* (pp. 371–390). Morgantown, WV: Fitness Information Technology.

McLeroy, K. R., Bibeau, D., Steckler, A., & Glanz, K. (1988). An ecological perspective on health promotion programs. *Health Education Quarterly, 15*(4), 351–377.

Morris, J. N., Clayton, D. G., Everitt, M. G., Semmence, A. M., & Burgess, E. H. (1990). Exercise in leisure time: Coronary attack and death rates. *British Heart Journal, 63*(6), 325–334.

Myers, L., Strikmiller, P. K., Webber, L. S., & Berenson, G. S. (1996). Physical and sedentary activity in school children grades 5–8: The Bogalusa Heart Study. *Medicine & Science in Sport & Exercise, 28*(7), 852–859.

Nigg, C. R., & Jordan, P. J. (2005). It's a difference of opinion that makes a horserace…. *Health Education Research, 20,* 291–293.

Nigg, C. R., & Paxton, R. (2008). Conceptual perspectives used to understand youth physical activity and inactivity. In A. L. Smith & S. J. H. Biddle (Eds.), *Youth physical activity and inactivity: Challenges and solutions* (pp. 79–113). Champaign, IL: Human Kinetics.

Ogden, C. L., Carroll, M. D., Curtin, L. R., Lamb, M. M., & Flegal, K. M. (2010). Prevalence of high body mass index in US children and adolescents, 2007–2008. *JAMA, 303*(3), 242–249.

Paffenbarger, R. S., Jr., & Hyde, R. T. (1984). Exercise in the prevention of coronary heart disease. *Preventive Medicine, 13*(1), 3–22.

Paffenbarger, R. S., Jr., Hyde, R. T., Hsieh, C. C., & Wing, A. L. (1986). Physical activity, other life-style patterns, cardiovascular disease and longevity. *Acta Medica Scandinavica Supplementum, 711,* 85–91.

Paffenbarger, R. S., Jr., Wing, A. L., Hyde, R. T., & Jung, D. L. (1983). Physical activity and incidence of hypertension in college alumni. *American Journal of Epidemiology, 117*(3), 245–257.

Petty, R. E. (1994). Two routes to persuasion: State of the art. In G. d'Ydewalle & P. Eelen (Eds.), *International perspectives on psychological science* (Vol. 2, pp. 229–247). Hillsdale, NJ: Erlbaum.

Petty, R. E., Barden, J., & Wheeler, C. (2002). The elaboration likelihood model of persuasion: Health promotions that yield sustained behavior change. In R. J. DiClemente, R. A. Crosby, & M. C. Kegler (Eds.), *Emerging theories in health promotion practice and research* (pp. 185–214). San Francisco, CA: Jossey-Bass.

Petty, R. E., & Cacioppo, J. T. (1999). Issue involvement can increase or decrease persuasion by enhancing message-relevant cognitive responses. *Journal of Personality and Social Psychology, 37*, 1915–1926.

Petty, R. E., Wells, G. L., & Brock, T. C. (1976). Distraction can enhance or reduce yielding to propaganda: Thought disruption versus effort justification. *Journal of Personality and Social Psychology, 34*, 874–884.

Petty, R. E., Wheeler, S. C., & Bizer, G. Y. (1999). Is there one persuasion process of more? Lumping versus splitting in attitude theories. *Psychological Inquiry, 10*, 156–163.

Pleis, J. R., & Lucas, J. W. (2009). Summary health statistics for U.S. adults: National Health Interview Survey, 2007. *Vital and Health Statistics Series, 10, 240*, 1–159.

Powell, K. E., Thompson, P. D., Caspersen, C. J., & Kendrick, J. S. (1987). Physical activity and the incidence of coronary heart disease. *Annual Review of Public Health, 8*, 253–287.

Pratt, M., Macera, C. A., & Blanton, C. (1999). Levels of physical activity and inactivity in children and adults in the United States: Current evidence and research issues. *Medicine & Science in Sport & Exercise, 31*(11 Suppl.), S526–S533.

Prentice, A. M., & Jebb, S. A. (1995). Obesity in Britain: Gluttony or sloth? *British Medical Journal, 311*(7002), 437–439.

Prochaska, J. O., & DiClemente, C. C. (1983). Stages and processes of self-change of smoking: Toward an integrative model of change. *Journal of Consulting and Clinical Psychology, 51*(3), 390–395.

Prochaska, J. O., Redding, C. A., & Evers, K. E. (1996). The transtheoretical model and stages of change. In F. Glanz, Marcus Lewis, F., & Rimer, B.K. (Eds.), *Health behavior and health education: Theory, research, and practice* (pp. 60–84). San Francisco, CA: Jossey-Bass.

Sallis, J. F. (1993). Epidemiology of physical activity and fitness in children and adolescents. *Critical Reviews of Food Science and Nutrition, 33*(4–5), 403–408.

Sallis, J. F., McKenzie, T. L., Kolody, B., Lewis, M., Marshall, S., & Rosengard, P. (1999). Effects of health-related physical education on academic achievement: Project SPARK. *Research Quarterly of Exercise and Sport, 70*(2), 127–134.

Strong, W. B., Malina, R. M., Blimkie, C. J., Daniels, S. R., Dishman, R. K., Gutin, B.,...Trudeau, F. (2005). Evidence based physical activity for school-age youth. *Journal of Pediatrics, 146*(6), 732–737.

Troiano, R. P., Berrigan, D., Dodd, K. W., Masse, L. C., Tilert, T., & McDowell, M. (2008). Physical activity in the United States measured by accelerometer. *Medicine & Science in Sport & Exercise, 40*(1), 181–188.

Trost, S. G., Pate, R. R., Sallis, J. F., Freedson, P. S., Taylor, W. C., Dowda, M., & Sirard, J. (2002). Age and gender differences in objectively measured physical activity in youth. *Medicine & Science in Sport & Exercise, 34*(2), 350–355.

U.S. Department of Health and Human Services. (2000, November). *Healthy people 2010* (2nd ed.). With *Understanding and improving health and objectives for improving health.* 2 vols. Washington, DC: U.S. Government Printing Office.

U.S. Department of Health and Human Services. (2001). The Surgeon General's call to action to prevent and decrease overweight and obesity. Rockville, MD: U.S. Department of Health and Human Services, Public Health Service, Office of the Surgeon General. Available from U.S. Government Printing Office, Washington, DC.

U.S. Department of Health and Human Services (2008). *2008 physical activity guidelines for Americans.* Washington, DC: U.S. Department of Health and Human Services. Retrieved May 13, 2009, from http://www.health.gov/paguidelines/pdf/paguide.pdf

U.S. Surgeon General. (2001). *Overweight and obesity: Health consequences.* Rockville, MD: U.S. Department of Health and Human Services.

Vaninio, H., & Bianchini, F. (2002). *Weight control and physical activity.* Lyon, France: IARC Press.

Weinstein, N. D. (1988). The precaution adoption process. *Health Psychology, 7*(4), 355–386.

Social Cognitive Models

Ryan E. Rhodes *and* Rachel Mark

Abstract

This chapter provides an overview of the five most prominent social cognitive theories applied to understand exercise and physical activity: the theory of planned behavior, social cognitive theory, the transtheoretical model of behavior change, self-determination theory, and the health belief model/protection motivation theory. Each theory is reviewed in terms of its history, concepts, and application to physical activity. Relevant advances and future directions conclude each section. All theories have shown some utility in explaining physical activity, but intervention studies employing these models in a mediation capacity remain elusive. Still, it is apparent that the health belief model/protection motivation theory may have the least utility for continued application in the physical activity domain.

Key Words: social cognition, theory, physical activity, exercise, future directions.

Introduction

The health benefits of regular physical activity are well established and linked to over 25 chronic conditions (Bouchard & Shephard, 1994). Moreover, the list of documented health benefits seems to grow on an almost daily basis (Warburton, Nicol, & Bredin, 2006). Physical activity is important in the prevention and rehabilitation of many serious physical health conditions, such as cardiovascular disease, diabetes, some cancers, osteoporosis, and obesity (Warburton et al., 2006). It is also linked to psychological benefits through its ability to reduce depression, anxiety, and stress as well as enhance self-confidence, self-esteem, and cognitive functioning (Colcombe & Kramer, 2003; Warburton, Katzmarzyk, Rhodes, & Shephard, 2007). Indeed, it is irrefutable that regular physical activity is a foundational behavior for human health and well-being.

Despite this evidence, the majority of individuals in developed countries remain insufficiently active in terms of intensity, frequency, and duration to accrue positive health benefits (Canadian Fitness and Lifestyle Research Institute, 2004; Centers for Disease Control, 2005). There is also ample evidence that most people struggle to maintain their regular exercise programs regardless of the demographic profile of the group or the purpose of the exercise (Dishman & Buckworth, 1996; Foster, Hillsdon, & Thorogood, 2005). Motivating individuals to adopt and maintain regular physical activity therefore is a major challenge for health professionals.

The low prevalence of physical activity, compounded by the difficulties in behavioral adherence, suggests that well-founded interventions to promote physical activity are of paramount importance. The development of interventions is likely facilitated by a sound understanding of the determinants of physical activity (Baranowski, Anderson, & Carmack, 1998). That is, unless we know the factors that influence behavioral adoption and maintenance, we will not be able to intervene in any effective way.

A common first step in understanding any behavior is to determine what variables are correlated with it. Correlates do not necessarily denote any causal relationship with the behavior but they may create a basic platform for understanding factors associated with it. In early exercise psychology research it was common to assess a large collection of eclectic variables and examine each in turn for its correlation with exercise behavior, but make no attempt to understand how the various correlates might be interrelated (Dishman, 1990; Trost, Owen, Bauman, Sallis, & Brown, 2002). For example, correlates of exercise behavior include age, sex, education, income, ethnicity, body weight, climate, smoking status, health status, attitudes, perceived control, self-efficacy, intentions, motivation, commitment, perceived barriers, knowledge, skills, distance from a fitness facility, aesthetics, having home exercise equipment, amount of park space, time spent outdoors, spousal support, number of children at home, extraversion, neuroticism, exercise intensity, exercise type, cohesion, group norms, class size, muscle fiber type, and genetic predispositions. This approach may classify groups of correlates (demographic, personal, social, environmental, etc.), but it attempts no other model reduction or model depth.

Theoretical models, on the other hand, specify depth and breadth among correlates in a schematic manner that attempts to be comprehensive yet parsimonious. The importance of theory in guiding the development of interventions is generally well recognized by researchers (Baranowski et al., 1998; Lewis, Marcus, Pate, & Dunn, 2002; Rhodes & Pfaeffli, 2010). Accordingly, most recent research into the antecedents of exercise behavior has adopted a theoretical model to guide the inquiry. To date, the two categories of exercise correlates that have received the most theoretical attention are the intrapersonal/ psychological, or cognitive, category and the interpersonal, or social, category. Models that combine these two categories have been labeled social cognitive models.

Many of the currently popular theoretical models applied to exercise behavior are social cognitive theories or contain social cognitive elements (Hagger & Chatzisarantis, 2007; Stokols, 1996). That is, the models theorize primarily about the relationships among variables at the inter- and intrapersonal levels of correlates. The purpose of the present chapter is to provide an overview of the major social cognitive models that have been applied in the physical activity domain. While a host of social cognitive models

have been applied to physical activity, the literature is most robust for five models: the theory of planned behavior (Ajzen, 1985, 1991), social cognitive theory (Bandura, 1977), the transtheoretical model (Prochaska & DiClemente, 1982), self-determination theory (Deci & Ryan, 1985), and protection motivation theory (Rogers, 1983). In the following sections, we review these models, appraise the evidence for their explaining and changing physical activity, and outline their specific adaptations and future in this domain.

Theory of Planned Behavior
Background

The theory of planned behavior (TPB) was developed as an extension of the theory of reasoned action (TRA) (Ajzen & Fishbein, 1980), which is grounded in the attitude–behavior literature (Fishbein, 1967). The TRA suggests that two constructs, attitude and subjective norm, predict behavioral intention, which is the proximal predictor of behavior. Attitude can be defined as the overall appraisal or evaluation that an individual has concerning a behavior (Ajzen, 2006). It can include the benefits and costs of the behavior and the value the individual places on these positive or negative appraisals. The second construct thought to predict intention, subjective norm, refers to the perceived social influence or pressure that other people (family, friends, doctor, etc.) place on an individual to perform a given behavior (Ajzen, 2006).

Adding Perceived Behavioral Control

The TRA was developed to predict volitional behaviors, those behaviors a person can enact without constraint. It became evident, both conceptually and through the validation of other models that, included Bandura's (1977) self-efficacy construct, that many behaviors of interest are not under pure volitional control. Because of this limitation, the TPB was developed to incorporate the prediction of behaviors that are not completely volitional (Ajzen, 1991). The TPB maintains the structure of the TRA in that attitude and subjective norm are predictors of intention and in that intention remains the proximal predictor of behavior. However, a third construct, perceived behavioral control (PBC), is also used to predict intention within the model (see Figure 15.1). PBC refers to an individual's perception of the ability that they have to perform a behavior. This can involve, among other things, barriers or facilitators to behavior, such as resources, skills, and

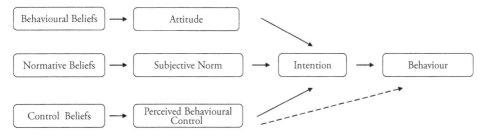

Figure 15.1. The theory of planned behavior. This model suggests that intention is the proximal predictor of behavior and that attitude, subjective norm, and perceived behavior control contribute to the formation of intention. These three predictors of intention are each formed by the summation of salient beliefs about a given behavior.

opportunities (e.g., time, fatigue, weather, access to facilities, and money). Ajzen (1991) comments that of the different elements of behavioral control used throughout behavioral theories, PBC is most similar to Bandura's (1977) definition of self-efficacy in highlighting the judgments that an individual holds about how well they can execute a given action to deal with different situations.

While PBC is thought to influence intention in conjunction with attitude and subjective norm (thereby indirectly predicting behavior), it is also thought to predict behavior directly. Ajzen (1991) outlines two reasons why PBC can directly inform behavior. First, even when a person has a strong intention to perform a behavior, if there are perceived barriers or low levels of confidence, this intention is less likely to be translated into an actual behavior. The second reason is that PBC acts as a proxy measure of actual behavioral control.

Symons Downs and Hausenblas (2005b) summarize the assumptions of the TPB as follows: A person will strongly intend to engage in a behavior if they evaluate it in a positive manner (attitude), believe that individuals important to them want them to engage in the behavior (subjective norm), and perceive themselves to have control over performing the behavior (PBC). As a consequence, they state, individuals with high levels of intention and PBC will have a greater likelihood of engaging in the behavior.

Ajzen (1991, 2006) points out that the relative weights of attitude, subjective norm, and PBC in the formation of intention, and the influence that intention and PBC have on behavior, can vary by behavior and by individual. For example, one behavior may be almost completely motivational (i.e., intentional), with the motivation stemming from one's attitudes, while another behavior may be almost entirely based on PBC.

Antecedents of Theory Constructs

The appraisal that an individual makes of the costs and benefits of performing a specific behavior forms the attitude construct. This overall appraisal comprises salient beliefs that an individual holds, which for the attitude construct are known as behavioral beliefs. These behavioral beliefs differ depending on the behavior being performed. For example, the beliefs that an individual holds in relation to the act of voting in a municipal election (e.g., "it is my civic duty") are different from the beliefs an individual holds about participating in daily physical activity (e.g., it is fun and helps with stress relief).

Based on an expectancy-value model, the strength of each belief and the outcome expectation of each belief can be used to compute a belief composite that equates to the attitude toward the behavior (Ajzen, 2006). The mathematical notation for this is

$$A_B \alpha \sum b_i \, e_i$$

where A_B is the attitude towards the behavior, b_i is the behavioral belief strength, and e_i is the outcome expectation. That is, belief strength and outcome expectation are multiplied and then summed across each behavioral belief.

Subjective norm refers to the social pressures to perform a given behavior that an individual perceives. As with the attitude construct, subjective norm is made up of a number of salient beliefs, known as normative beliefs. The individual roles that different people play in creating the total social pressure perceived differ according to the behavior. For example, a physician may play a greater role from an individual's partner in the pressure that individual feels to appropriately manage a chronic disease such as diabetes. However when looking at safe sex behavior, an individual may feel greater pressure from the partner.

The measurement of normative beliefs according to an expectancy-value model follows a similar design to that for behavioral beliefs. Here, the normative belief strength for each referent (spouse, doctor, etc.) is multiplied by the motivation of the individual to comply with the desires of each referent (Ajzen, 2006). The equation for the summation of normative beliefs is

$$ SN \; \alpha \; \sum n_i \; m_i $$

where SN is subjective norm, n_i is the normative belief strength, and m_i is the motivation to comply.

The perceived ease or difficulty of performing a behavior makes up the PBC construct. The salient beliefs contributing to this construct are known as control beliefs. These can be seen as facilitators or barriers to performing a behavior. The strength that individual barriers or facilitators have on behavior varies depending on the behavior. These barriers can also be quite specific. For example, if an individual wants to go for a run outside, weather may be a barrier, as the individual may be less likely to run outside if the weather is poor. However, still looking at exercise behavior, if an individual is going to take an aerobics class, the poor weather is less likely to act as a barrier if the class is indoors; however, the proximity of the facility hosting the exercise class to the individual's home may play a limiting role if it is too far.

The composite level of PBC is calculated in a fashion similar to those for attitude and subjective norm. In the expectancy-value model, the PBC composite is developed by multiplying c_i, the strength of each control belief, by p_i, the control belief power (the effect that holding this belief would have on behavior) (Ajzen, 2006):

$$ PBC \; \alpha \; \sum c_i \; p_i $$

Ajzen (2002a) suggests that for interventions using the TPB to be successful, they must change the salient beliefs an individual holds that make up the attitude, subjective norm, and PBC constructs, which ultimately determine intention and behavior. A few steps must be performed before the development of an intervention. Pilot work should be performed to identify the salient beliefs for a given population and behavior. The pilot study can be a series of open-ended questions obtained by written response or orally through interview or focus group settings. From this work, questionnaires may be developed

that include the salient beliefs identified in the pilot. This helps to determine the weight of each construct in the prediction of behavior. From the questionnaire and after determining which salient beliefs will be targeted, an intervention may be developed.

The TPB and Exercise Behavior
META-ANALYTIC FINDINGS

Over 200 studies have applied the TPB within the exercise domain to predict and explain physical activity (Biddle & Nigg, 2000). A number of meta-analytic reviews have also been conducted of studies using the TPB within the exercise domain (Hagger, Chatzisarantis, & Biddle, 2002; Hausenblas, Carron, & Mack, 1997; Symons Downs & Hausenblas, 2005b). The most recent such meta-analysis was conducted by Symons Downs and Hausenblas (2005b). This meta-analysis examined 83 studies using the TPB and 28 studies using the TRA. Among these studies, significant effect sizes were found for the relationships between all of the constructs of the TPB, including that between intention and behavior. Large mean effect sizes were found between intention and exercise (d = 1.01), intention and PBC (d = 0.90), and intention and attitude (d = 1.07) (Symons Downs & Hausenblas, 2005b). Moderate mean effect sizes were found between PBC and behavior (d = 0.51) as well as between intention and subjective norm (d = 0.59). The sizes of the effects of attitude and PBC on intention indicate that these are the key antecedents of intention. Furthermore, these moderate-to-large effect sizes for all constructs suggest that the TPB can provide a successful framework for predicting physical activity.

ELICITED BELIEFS

As mentioned previously, individuals hold a number of salient behavioral, normative, and control beliefs that contribute to the aggregate constructs of attitude, subjective norm, and PBC, respectively. These beliefs are specific to each type of behavior. Symons Downs and Hausenblas (2005a) conducted a review to assess the behavioral, normative, and control beliefs most commonly elicited in 47 TPB elicitation studies in the exercise domain. Table 15.1 lists the top five beliefs from each construct.

TPB and Other External Variables

The initial TPB conceptualization was very open to augmentation if sound empirical evidence for additional predictors not listed in TPB could be

Table 15.1. Commonly Elicited Theory of Planned Behavior Beliefs

Belief type	Top beliefs
Behavioral beliefs (advantages)	1. Improves physical and psychological health 2. Weight control 3. Improves daily functioning 4. Increases energy 5. Relieves stress and promotes relaxation
Behavioral beliefs (disadvantages)	1. Health issues 2. Tired 3. Time 4. Inconvenience 5. Expensive
Normative beliefs	1. Family members 2. Friends 3. Health care professionals 4. School and work site personnel 5. Community
Control beliefs (barriers)	1. Health issues 2. Inconvenience 3. Lacking motivation and energy 4. Time 5. Lacking social support
Control beliefs (facilitators)	1. Convenience 2. Pleasure 3. Social support 4. Exercise experience 5. Health

Adapted with permission from "Elicitation Studies and the Theory of Planned Behavior: A Systematic Review of Exercise Beliefs," by D. Symons Downs and H. A. Hausenblas, 2005, *Psychology of Sport and Exercise, 6*, pp. 1–31.

demonstrated (Ajzen, 1991). Further, Ajzen (1991) provided a distinct structure in which to test the model. External variables—those variables not covered in the measurement domains of the TPB proper—are hypothesized to be mediated through the structure of the TPB. For example, education is thought to affect behavior through attitudes, subjective norm, and PBC. Ajzen (1991) was less specific about a second route. This would be where external variables could conceivably affect behavior through moderation of TPB structure (Blanchard et al., 2008). Many tests have been conducted to examine the mediating and moderating capacity of the TPB in health behaviors (Ajzen & Fishbein, 2005; Conner & Armitage, 1998). Overall, the model has stood up well to these challenges, providing support for its conceptual structure. There are, however, some specific advances to the TPB in the physical activity domain that warrant mention as the model moves forward in the 21st century.

Moving Forward and Adapting the TPB to Exercise and Physical Activity

There is considerable support for the predictive validity of the TPB for exercise and physical activity (Hagger et al., 2002), but its use in this domain is marked by changing model depth and breadth and challenges for its applicability in behavior change.

MODEL BREADTH

In terms of model breadth, several studies have examined whether the TPB proper mediates other constructs. These studies test whether TPB is sufficient as the proximal predictor of behavior. While various factors predict physical activity independent of the TPB, such as habit (Gardner, 2009), personality (Rhodes & Smith, 2006), and the perceived environment (Rhodes, Courneya, Blanchard, & Plotnikoff, 2007), these often explain minor variance in behavior when compared with intention.

Instead, the largest impact on the breadth of TPB structure has come from within the measurement domains of the TPB constructs themselves.

Ajzen (2006) openly acknowledged that attitude, subjective norm, and PBC may have multicomponent structures rather than simple unidimensional structures. In particular, attitude was conceived as having affective (pleasure or enjoyment) and instrumental (utility or benefit) qualities; subjective norm was considered to have injunctive (perceptions of what others want) and descriptive (perceptions of what others do) components; and PBC was considered to have self-efficacy and controllability components, although these have not been clearly defined or delineated (Ajzen, 2002a, 2002b; Rhodes & Courneya, 2003c).

Tests of this multicomponent model with physical activity have shown clear distinctions between all of these concepts (Hagger & Chatzisarantis, 2005; Rhodes & Courneya, 2003a). In terms of predictive validity, however, affective and instrumental attitudes have shown the greatest and most reliable differences (Rhodes, Fiala, & Conner, 2009). Affective attitude is generally the largest predictor of intention. The two normative constructs often fail to predict intention independent of attitude and PBC (Hagger & Chatzisarantis, 2005; Rhodes, Blanchard, & Matheson, 2006; Rhodes & Courneya, 2003a), and thus their separate structures appear less consequential. The multicomponent structure of the PBC construct is more problematic. Use of the two-component model results in multicollinearity (Rhodes & Blanchard, 2006; Rhodes & Courneya, 2003a), and phrases that discount motivation such as "if I wanted to" reduce the PBC items to a single construct (Courneya, Conner, & Rhodes, 2006; Rhodes & Courneya, 2004).

In summary, TPB breadth has advanced most in the physical activity domain via partitions of the theory's own constructs and not through augmentation with other constructs. While continued testing is needed, the current conceptualization of affective and instrumental attitude, subjective norm, and PBC appears sound.

MODEL DEPTH

While model breadth tests the TPBs mediation capacity and sufficiency, adding depth to the model complements this approach by examining the antecedents and consequences of TPB structure. Two prominent examples are present in the physical activity literature. The first involves the antecedents of TPB belief formation, and the second involves the translation of intentions into behavior.

Unlike Bandura (1977), Ajzen (1991) has been obscure about how underlying behavioral, normative, and control beliefs are formed. The formation of beliefs is considered the consequence of exposure to variables outside the TPB structure, and no process for their formation or specific external factors have been outlined clearly. Thus some researchers have examined potential antecedents via mediation models with the TPB. Rhodes and colleagues, for example, have demonstrated that extraversion (Rhodes & Courneya, 2003b) and the built environment (Rhodes et al., 2007) may form or shape physical activity attitudes and perceptions of control. Chatzisarantis and Hagger (2005) have shown that beliefs may be changed through persuasive appeals, and Rhodes, Warburton, and Bredin (2009) have shown that new exercise experiences may affect beliefs. These studies demonstrate that belief formation may involve a mixture of disposition, environment, education/information, and experience. Perhaps most interesting in this area of adding depth to the antecedents of TPB beliefs is the integration of self-determined needs as the foundation of belief structure (Hagger & Chatzisarantis, 2007). In a series of studies by Hagger and colleagues (Hagger & Chatzisarantis, 2007), the TPB mediated the need for autonomy support and competence when predicting physical activity. Thus people's beliefs about physical activity are the result of how the behavior meets their basic needs for self-determination. This research is in its early phases, but the collection of belief antecedents points to the complexity of how physical activity belief systems, as per the TPB, may be formed.

At the other end of the TPB, some researchers have been examining model depth at the level of the intention–behavior connection. While the relationship between intention and physical activity is reliable and of large magnitude (Hagger et al., 2002; Symons Downs & Hausenblas, 2005b), there is considerable intention–behavior discordance. The point estimate correlation is approximately $r = .50$, and this is reduced to $r = .20$ in intervention studies (Webb & Sheeran, 2006). This suggests that considerable variance remains unexplained in physical activity after application of the TPB. Indeed, a recent Canadian survey found that although 87% of adults intend to be active, only 43% were achieving this sought-after goal (Canadian Fitness and

Lifestyle Research Institute, 2004). Thus closing this intention–behavior "gap" is a timely pursuit for health promoters (Rhodes, Plotnikoff, & Courneya, 2008; Sniehotta, 2009).

At the forefront of this research is the concept of regulatory strategies and planning (Sniehotta, 2009). Ajzen (2006) openly admits that the TPB lacks a planning construct. The TPB structure suggests that motivation, in the form of intent, is the primary cause of behavior. Recent theorizing, led initially by Gollwitzer and Brandstatter (1997), suggests that behavioral enactment may have both motivational and volitional phases. TPB may explain behavioral motivation, but behavioral self-regulation may be needed to translate this motivation into behavior. This premise has been supported by meta-analysis (Gollwitzer & Sheeran, 2006). Planning itself (for how, when, and where an individual will perform what behavior) may have a minor impact on physical activity independent of motivation (Rhodes & Dickau, in press), but the self-regulation around barriers may be critical to behavioral attainment despite positive intentions (Lewis et al., 2002; Rhodes & Pfaeffli, 2010; Rhodes & Plotnikoff, 2006; Sniehotta, 2009; Sniehotta, Scholz, & Schwarzer, 2005, 2006). Further research is needed to create a construct to measure self-regulation distinct from motivation (Rhodes, Blanchard, Matheson, & Coble, 2006). Such a construct would be a useful addition to the TPB structure.

TPB AND INTERVENTION

The TPB and TRA emerged from a desire to understand and predict behavior but not necessarily to change behavior. Thus the theories' adoption in interventions in any behavioral domain has been slow despite hundreds of correlational prediction studies. In physical activity research, the foundation for using theory is its pragmatic application to promotion and behavior change (Baranowski et al., 1998; Rhodes & Pfaeffli, 2010). However, almost no physical activity interventions using TPB have been conducted. Initial attempts to intervene with children (Chatzisarantis & Hagger, 2005) and special populations (Vallance, Courneya, Plotnikoff, & Mackey, 2008) have had modest success. Three studies have employed the TPB with sedentary adults (Jones, Sinclair, Rhodes, & Courneya, 2004; Parrott, Tennant, Olejnik, & Poudevigne, 2008; Reger, Cooper, Booth-Butterfield, Smith, & Bauman, 2002), and two of these studies showed null results (Jones et al., 2004; Reger et al., 2002).

Overall, the paucity of research and lack of behavior change in the interventions provides too limited evidence on which to make a judgment of the effectiveness of TPB in physical activity interventions. Clearly, the new challenge for TPB is to demonstrate its utility in such interventions.

Social Cognitive Theory
Background

A shift in behavioral theorizing from a behavioral focus to a cognitive focus sparked the development of the social cognitive theory (SCT) by Bandura in the 1970s. The basis of the SCT is a system of reciprocal causation such that behavior is a complex interaction among the individual, the environment, and behavior (Bandura, 1977; see Figure 15.2). Bandura (2004) highlights that knowledge is the precursor to the possibility of behavior change. Without awareness of how their current behavior is influencing health, individuals have no basis for behavior change. After acquiring knowledge, individuals must believe that they have the capability to change their behavior. This situation-specific self-confidence is known as self-efficacy. Bandura defines self-efficacy as "beliefs in one's capabilities to organize and execute the courses of action required to produce given levels of attainment." (Bandura, 1977, p. 193) If individuals do not feel that they possess the ability to change their behavior, they have little motivation to attempt to change it. Self-efficacy is described in greater detail below.

Outcome expectations are also central to the SCT. These refer to the expectations an individual has about the outcomes of a behavior. These are in part influenced by an individual's level of self-efficacy. Sociostructural factors (i.e., facilitators and barriers) also play a role in behavior change. The individual must hold a strong enough level of self-efficacy to overcome these barriers. Personal goals related to behavior can be formed through the combination of self-efficacy, outcome expectations, and sociostructural factors. Bandura (2004) suggests that short-term goals are the most manageable than long-term goals and are more linked to success than long-term goals. Outcome expectations are outlined in greater detail below.

Self-Efficacy

Self-efficacy is situation specific: The ability that an individual perceives him- or herself to have for one behavior will be different from the ability perceived for a different behavior. In contrast to

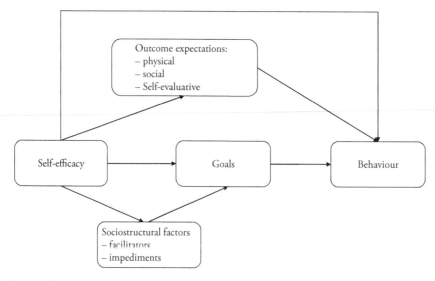

Figure 15.2. The social cognitive theory. This theory suggests that self-efficacy and outcome expectations are the key constructs influencing behavior. Self-efficacy can influence behavior through the self-regulatory processes that create goals. These goals can also be influenced by factors the individual perceives as facilitators of and barriers to performing the behavior.

self-confidence, self-efficacy relates more to the perceptions that an individual has that he or she can perform a specific behavior successfully (Bandura, 1998). Therefore, the degree of self-efficacy individuals perceive themselves to have relates to the skills that they believe themselves to have. These skills include the ability to employ coping mechanisms, the confidence to overcome barriers, and the confidence to draw upon available resources.

Bandura (1977) outlined four key constructs contributing to the degree of self-efficacy that an individual has for a given behavior: past performance accomplishments, vicarious experience, social persuasion, and physiological and affective states (see Figure 15.3). Bandura states that these factors have different amounts of influence on self-efficacy, with past performance accomplishments contributing the most and physiological and affective experiences contributing the least.

Past performance accomplishments or *mastery* refers to the success that an individual has had in the past in performing either the specific behavior or one similar to it. Repeated success will increase self-efficacy levels, whereas unsuccessful attempts or failures will lower efficacy levels (Bandura, 1977). For example, if an adult had high levels of accomplishment playing basketball as a teenager, then she may have a higher level of self-efficacy for joining an adult basketball team. With this construct, the more similar that the past behavior is to the present behavior, the greater effect the past accomplishment

will have on the current level of self-efficacy. This factor is thought to play the greatest role in an individual's perceived self-efficacy because it is based on the individual's own accomplishments.

Vicarious experience or *modeling* refers to the individual's viewing the same behavior being performed by another individual. The more similar the model is to the individual, the more successful the modeling mechanism will be. The individual does not necessarily need to know the model; however, he or she should perceive some degree of similarity. If the model is similar to the individual and is successful in completing the behavior, the individual will likely have a greater level of self-efficacy with respect to the behavior. This contribution to overall self-efficacy is weaker than that of personal accomplishment because the experience of success is indirect.

Social persuasion refers to verbal or nonverbal persuasion received in relation to performing a given behavior. This can come through many sources, including advertising, health care practitioners, friends, and spouses. The persuasion is more effective when the individual doing the persuading is seen as being knowledgeable (e.g., a doctor, fitness instructor, or dietitian). For the same reasons as vicarious experience, social persuasion contributes less to self-efficacy levels than personal experience (Bandura, 1977).

Physiological and affective states are the last factor contributing to self-efficacy. Physiological states

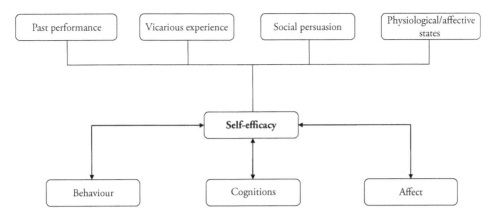

Figure 15.3. Self-efficacy component of the social cognitive theory. Self-efficacy is influenced by four factors: past performance, vicarious experience, social persuasion, and physiological and affective states. Self-efficacy also interacts reciprocally with behavior, cognitions, and affect.

are feeling states within the body. For example, with vigorous exercise, these can include sweating, rapid heartbeat, muscle stiffness and fatigue. Individuals who are not familiar with exercising at a vigorous intensity may find these physiological responses scary and may doubt their ability to perform vigorous exercise correctly. Affective states are emotional feelings and responses. When the affective response to the behavior is positive (e.g., happiness or a decrease in stress), the level of perceived self-efficacy increases. However, when the affective response is negative, the level of self-efficacy may decrease.

Outcome Expectations

Another construct key to SCT is that of outcome expectations, the perceived outcomes or consequences of performing a given behavior (Bandura, 1977). Bandura (1998) outlines three types of outcome expectations: physical outcome expectations, social outcome expectations, and self-evaluative outcome expectations. Physical outcome expectations are the anticipated short- or long-term physical consequences of performing a behavior. For example, in relation to exercise, a short-term physical outcome expectation could be fatigue and muscle soreness, but a long-term expectation could be decreased risk of heart disease if the exercise behavior is maintained regularly. Social outcome expectations are the anticipated social consequences of performing a behavior. An overweight woman may anticipate support and encouragement from her spouse if she begins to eat more fruits and vegetables and decreases her consumption of high-fat foods. The last type of outcome expectation, self-evaluative, refers to the individual's anticipated feelings about

having performed a behavior. These could include guilt, esteem, embarrassment, or shame.

The SCT and Exercise

Rather than the entire SCT, the theory's central concept of self-efficacy has been its main contribution to the literature in the physical activity and exercise domain. Because of the reciprocal nature of the SCT, self-efficacy is viewed as both a determinant and consequence of physical activity participation (McAuley & Blissmer, 2000). As a determinant, self-efficacy showed an overall correlation of $r = .35$ with physical activity behavior in a recent meta-analysis (Spence et al., 2006); this represents a medium effect size (Cohen, 1992) and one of the largest overall correlations with physical activity (Trost et al., 2002).

In a review paper on self-efficacy and exercise, this significant positive relationship has been illustrated among a variety of populations (clinical and nonclinical) and ages (ranging from adolescents to older adults) (McAuley & Blissmer, 2000). The strength of the relationship between self-efficacy and physical activity, however, has been shown to vary depending on the stage of uptake of the behavior (Oman & King, 1998; Sallis et al., 1986). Specifically, self-efficacy may play a greater role in exercise behavior adoption and uptake than in behavior maintenance. Oman and King (1998) conducted a two-year randomized trial in which 63 participants were randomly assigned to one of three conditions of participation in an aerobic exercise program (higher-intensity home-based exercise, higher-intensity class-based exercise, or lower-intensity home-based exercise). Independent of treatment group, baseline self-efficacy was a significant predictor of exercise behavior during the adoption stage but not during the maintenance phase.

Self-efficacy as a consequence of physical activity has been shown in numerous studies to significantly influence physical activity participation (McAuley & Blissmer, 2000). For example, a study of 174 older adults participating in an exercise program (randomized to an aerobic exercise group or a stretching-and-toning group) measured both exercise self-efficacy and physical efficacy levels across a 12-month trial (McAuley et al., 1999). Results showed a curvilinear growth of self-efficacy across the trial, with declines at the follow-up stage. Participants therefore had increases in both exercise and physical self-efficacy throughout the program, but declines occurred following the program. As a result of the interplay between physical activity participation and self-efficacy, it is essential for practitioners to develop physical activity opportunities that help to build personal self-efficacy levels.

The literature on physical activity interventions using the SCT (and not solely the self-efficacy construct) is limited and offers mixed support for its use (Rhodes & Pfaeffli, 2010). For example, Cramp and Brawley (2006) performed a randomized controlled trial with 57 new mothers. Participants were randomized to either a standard exercise program (control) or the same program with the addition of group-mediated cognitive behavioral counseling that provided information and support on self-regulatory processes to overcome barriers, self-monitor, and set goals (intervention). The results indicated that there were significant treatment effects in favor of the intervention group for proximal outcome expectations, barrier efficacy, and self-reported moderate-intensity physical activity. Another study, by Hallam and Petosa (2004), included an intervention in a work site setting where participants attended four education sessions aimed at increasing self-regulatory tools, teaching about safely engaging in exercise, and describing the outcomes associated with regular physical activity. The comparison group received standard information from a fitness facility (fitness center orientation and education on how to use the equipment). Measures were obtained for outcome expectations, self-efficacy, and use of self-regulatory strategies. Self-regulation was found to be significantly higher for the intervention group at baseline, six-week follow-up, six-month follow-up and 12-month follow-up. Significant differences between groups were found for outcome expectations at baseline and were found to increase at six

weeks for the intervention group but then decrease at other follow-ups. For self-efficacy, there were no significant differences between the groups; however, there were significant increases for the intervention group across the follow-ups. Exercise frequency was not significantly different between groups until the 12-month follow-up, where the intervention group had a significantly higher number of weekly exercise sessions; however, there were significant increases in exercise frequency for the intervention group across the follow-ups. The study showed support for self-regulation's acting as a mediator for exercise behavior at the 12-month follow-up; other measured SCT variables did not emerge as mediators.

Thus while studies offer some support for the use of SCT in exercise interventions, more research is needed.

Moving Forward and Adapting the SCT to Exercise and Physical Activity

The SCT is a difficult model to test because of its principle of reciprocal determinism. As demonstrated with self-efficacy, the construct poses itself as both an antecedent and a consequence of behavior, the individual, and the environment. Longitudinal panel models and intervention studies such as the ones reviewed above appear necessary to gaining a better understanding of the theory. Unfortunately, these are relatively scant. Related to this, few studies have intervened on self-efficacy using the very clear processes and antecedents proposed by Bandura (1977, 1997). Doing so is essential to testing the veracity of the model.

Perhaps most important in future research is to test the full model of the SCT proposed by Bandura (1998). Numerous studies claim to have examined the SCT but merely applied self-efficacy, and few studies have applied the full SCT model. This obvious shortcoming provides an important impetus for future work.

MULTIPLE EFFICACIES AND PHYSICAL ACTIVITY

An early debate among self-efficacy theorists centered around the role of self-efficacy in repeated and complex behaviors (Bandura, 1995; Kirsch, 1995; Maddux, 1995). The focus was on whether self-efficacy is about the confidence to perform an act itself (e.g., walking involves putting one foot in front of the other) or the confidence to regulate the action. In physical activity, this distinction has given rise to the idea that there are two types of self-efficacy, commonly called barrier or coping efficacy and task efficacy (Blanchard et al., 2007). Barrier efficacy is the confidence to overcome and navigate the possible barriers that interfere with performing repeated bouts of physical activity, while task efficacy is the confidence to perform the physical activity act itself. In general, it appears that barrier efficacy is the principal predictor of physical activity participation, except among clinical or physically compromised populations (Blanchard et al., 2007; Blanchard, Rodgers, Courneya, Daub, & Knapik, 2002), where task self-efficacy appears to be the best predictor. This exception makes theoretical sense, as confidence in performing the task itself would seem necessary before one can concern oneself with regulating the daily barriers to action. Several other self-efficacy measures have emerged in the physical activity literature with respect to specific barriers or behaviors that contribute to regular physical activity participation (e.g., scheduling and planning). Because self-efficacy is situation and behavior specific, multiple efficacies are theoretically valid. Continued research is needed, however, to decide upon the most important efficacies that predict physical activity.

SELF-EFFICACY AND MOTIVATION

Related to the issue multiple self-efficacies, it has been debated whether the construct of self-efficacy has a meaning independent of outcome expectations and motivation (Cahill, Gallo, Lisman, & Weinstein, 2006; Kirsch, 1982; Rhodes & Blanchard, 2007b). Cahill et al. (2006) reflected on Bandura's (1977) assertions that behavioral actions were regulated and influenced by the anticipation of negative emotional consequences of those actions (e.g., anxiety and fear). Such consequences, Cahill et al. argued, amount to an outcome expectancy, the influence of which can be assuaged given stronger self-efficacy to perform the desired behavior (Bandura, 1977). Similarly, Rhodes and colleagues have argued and demonstrated that including "confidence" items in a self-efficacy measure without a motivational qualifier (e.g., "if I wanted to") effectively measures motivation more than ability (Rhodes & Blanchard, 2007b; Rhodes & Courneya, 2003c, 2004). These researchers argued that it was essential to discriminate between a person's being willing and being able to perform a task (Cahill et al., 2006). If a person had the requisite skills for a specific behavior (able) and chose not to perform the behavior (not willing), this could imply that outcome expectancies (negative ones) were driving that person's actions.

Outcome expectancies have been shown to influence self-efficacy statements. When confidence items were used to measure self-efficacy for performing physical activity, Rhodes and Blanchard (2007b) demonstrated that positive outcome expectancies and motivation did, in part, influence personal judgments of confidence. The challenge for physical activity scientists remains to separate motivation and outcome expectancies from self-efficacy expectations.

The Transtheoretical Model
Background

The transtheoretical model (TTM) was developed by Prochaska and DiClemente (1982) specifically to study behavior change in individuals who were quitting smoking via clinical observations. However, this theory has now been widely applied to a number of other health behaviors, including safe sex practices, cancer screening behavior, dietary and nutrition habits, and physical activity and exercise behavior (Spencer, Adams, Malone, Roy, & Yost, 2006). The TTM is a stage-based behavior change model that incorporates factors from different theoretical frameworks. The premise of the framework is that people progress slowly through six stages (precontemplation, contemplation, preparation, action, maintenance, and termination) and that instead of the movement between stages being linear (i.e., only forward), it is dynamic and can be cyclical (i.e., forward or backward). In addition to the six stages of behavioral change, the model is made up of ten processes of change, a decisional balance of change (i.e., the pros and cons of change), and an element of self-efficacy including confidence and the ability to overcome temptation (see Figure 15.4).

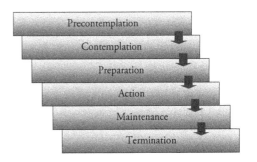

Figure 15.4. The transtheoretical model. This model is a stage-based approach to behavior change, beginning with precontemplation, where the individual is not considering behavior change, and ending with termination, where the new behavior is habitual and does not even need to be thought about.

The Six Stages of Change

PRECONTEMPLATION

The first stage of the model is precontemplation. At this stage, the individual is not considering any sort of behavior change over the next six months. The decisional balance is weighted more toward cons of behavior change than pros, possibly because of a lack of knowledge of the importance of changing behavior.

CONTEMPLATION

In the contemplation stage, the individual has developed an intention to change his or her behavior over the next six months but is not currently pursuing any action to start this change. The pros and cons of the behavior are equally weighted; the individual is aware of the benefits of behavior change but is also still considering the cons. It is often recommended that intervention take place at this stage, because without an additional push toward behavior change, the individual may stay ambivalent toward the change and remain in this stage for a long period.

PREPARATION

At the third stage, preparation, individuals have created an intention to change their behavior within the next month. The pros of behavior change outweigh the cons, and the individual is beginning to make preparations for carrying out the change. These can include actions such as buying running shoes, looking at gym memberships, finding recipes for healthy cooking, or finding the appropriate tools to assist in quitting smoking. In the preparation stage, the individual may also begin to take small steps toward the behavior change (e.g., eating more green vegetables or walking to the grocery store instead of driving).

ACTION

This fourth stage, action, is where the major behavioral change takes place. Here, the individual has changed behavior and is working optimally to maintain behavior. The pros of the behavior change clearly outweigh the cons. However, this stage is the most unstable of the six stages, as the individual is working hard to avoid relapsing into past behavior.

MAINTENANCE

In the maintenance stage, the individual has sustained the change in behavior for at least six months. The pros of behavior change still far outweigh the cons. The individual still needs to work to maintain the behavior change; however, the chance of relapse is less than in the action stage.

TERMINATION

In termination, the final stage of the model, there is no chance that the individual will return to the previous unhealthy behavior. The new behavior has become so habitual and ingrained in the individual's life that the thought of going back does not even exist. Prior to entering this final stage, the maintenance stage should have lasted approximately five years.

The Processes of Change

The progression through the six stages of the TTM is based on ten processes of change. Of these, five are experiential processes that focus on increasing awareness of behavior change (consciousness raising, self-reevaluation, environmental reevaluation, dramatic relief, and social liberation). The other five are behavioral processes that are based on actions carried out to augment the environment to support behavior change (self-liberation, counterconditioning, stimulus control, reinforcement management, and helping relationships). Table 15.2 describes these processes in greater depth.

Self-Efficacy

The self-efficacy component in the TTM is similar to the self-efficacy construct from the SCT (Bandura, 1977). Self-efficacy is a task-specific form of confidence in being able to accomplish the task at hand. This situation-specific confidence aids individuals in progressing through the six stages. The relationship is considered linear: As an individual progresses through the stages, self-efficacy for behavior change increases as well.

The TTM and Physical Activity

A number of literature reviews on the TTM and exercise behavior have been published (Adams & White, 2002; Marshall & Biddle, 2001; Spencer et al., 2006). The most recent review paper, by Spencer and colleagues (2006), examined 150 studies: 38 intervention studies, 70 population studies, and 42 validation studies. Of the 38 intervention studies, the majority (32) were stage-matched. These interventions were delivered in a number of ways, including print, in person, over the phone, and with a computer. The most successful studies were those that were stage-matched and offered short- or long-term support rather than single contacts. Cross-sectional

Table 15.2. Processes of Change in the Transtheoretical Model

Process	Description and example
Experiential	
Consciousness raising	Increasing awareness and knowledge about the behavior change; e.g., reading informational materials and speaking with health care practitioners
Self-reevaluation	Consideration of how much the behavior and behavior change is a part of one's identity; e.g., consideration of one's values and what role the behavior plays in them
Environmental reevaluation	Evaluation of the physical and social environment in relation to the unhealthy behavior; e.g., evaluating the effects of secondhand smoke on others or the health care cost of obesity.
Dramatic relief	Experiencing of negative emotions or feelings associated with an unhealthy behavior; e.g., being embarrassed about being overweight or feeling guilty for smoking
Social liberation	Finding information about social and environmental support for the behavior change; e.g., finding a friend to exercise with or joining a support group of individuals attempting to quit smoking
Behavioral	
Self-liberation	Making a firm commitment to chang; e.g., telling others about the change or making a pact with someone else trying to change behavior
Counterconditioning	Substituting a healthy behavior for an unhealthy behavior; e.g., eating a piece of fruit for a snack rather than a chocolate bar, taking the stairs instead of the elevator, or going for a bike ride instead of watching television
Stimulus control	Controlling cues in the environment to prevent falling back into the unhealthy behavior; e.g., placing gym clothes by the front door the night before to remember to take them to work so that one can exercise afterward, or making a set exercise schedule with days, times, and locations
Reinforcement management	Providing oneself with rewards for complying with the healthy behavior change (which should themselves rewards support the change); e.g., **buying yourself a present** if one eats healthily for one week (not being able to eat a chocolate bar if one eats healthily for one week)
Helping relationships	Seeking out social support for assistance in the behavior change; e.g., finding a running group or having a coworker remind one to take the stairs instead of the elevator at work.

American community-based samples suggested that stage membership was predictive of exercise level (Armstrong & Sallis, 1993). In clinical adult populations, forward progression through the stages was associated with cardiac therapy (Jue & Cunningham, 1998) and adherence to exercise (Hellman, 1997).

A number of studies included in the Spencer et al. (2006) review addressed construct validity. Marcus and Simkin (1993) created an algorithm called the Stage of Exercise Behavior Change that was based on the standard measure created by Prochaska and DiClemente (1982) and included the first five stages of the TTM. Cardinal (1995) developed a ladder format to represent the five stages of change (called the Stages of Exercise Scale). The concurrent validity of this scale was illustrated using self-reported and biometric exercise measures. A strength of Cardinal's study was the clear definition of exercise. Another study, by Reed, Velicer, Prochaska, Rossi, and Marcus (1997), compared eight exercise stage algorithms and found that the most successful one defined exercise traditionally and used a five-item questionnaire where participants chose the statements that best suited them.

Despite support for the application of the TTM to exercise behavior, there have been a number of criticisms. Reviews of the TTM in physical activity interventions (Adams & White, 2002; Bridle et al., 2005) have looked at how effective the TTM may be in actual physical activity behavior change. These reviews concluded that while the TTM may be somewhat effective in changing physical activity behavior, there is little support for the model in terms of adherence to physical activity behavior. Adams and White (2003) suggested that physical activity behavior is more complex than behaviors such as smoking cessation, for which the model was developed. As a result, interventions using the TTM and treating physical activity behavior as a simpler, single behavior may not be targeting the many facets of the behavior that need to be changed. Another limitation to this model has to do with the ability to place individuals in the correct stage of change. There is inconsistency in the construct validity of the algorithms used to place individuals in the stages (Bunton, Baldwin, Flynn, & Whitelaw, 2000). Another limitation noted by Adams and White (2005) is that there are a number of factors, such as demographics and environmental factors, that the model does not take into account. Spencer et al. (2006) also point out that the TTM-based physical activity research has been done primarily with Caucasian, female, middle-class samples.

Moving Forward and Adapting the TTM to Physical Activity

Despite over 100 studies having used the TTM to understand physical activity, very few advances that are physical activity specific have been made to the model since its original adaptation from smoking behavior (Marcus, Selby, Niaura, & Rossi, 1992). There has not been strong evidence that the termination stage applies to physical activity (Courneya & Bobick, 2000b), and other constructs, such as those in the TPB, have been applied using the stage algorithm with better success than the original constructs (Armitage, 2009; Courneya & Bobick, 2000a). The theory itself has undergone extensive criticism based on the argument that the concept of a stage may not be appropriate for repeated, life-long health behaviors like physical activity (Adams & White, 2002; Bandura, 1998). The thesis of this criticism is that true stages of change need to be discrete with discrete antecedents, whereas the TTM stages may be linear intention/behavior constructions rather than discrete stages.

Independent of the stages-of-change controversy, TTM's processes of change represent the novel contribution of the model. While theories like the TPB, protection motivation theory, and self-determination theory (both discussed below) focus primarily on why people perform behaviors, TTM focuses on how people change. The processes may be one of the most important contributions of the model (Armitage, 2009), but they have been given little scrutiny. Ten processes are unlikely to transfer directly from smoking to physical activity; indeed, confirmatory analyses of the processes of change have shown that only some have utility in the latter context (Rhodes, Berry, Naylor, & Wharf Higgins, 2004). Future research focused on how many of the processes of change are viable for physical activity is warranted. Some evidence suggests that only a few, such as self-monitoring, may be needed (Michie, Abraham, Whittington, McAteer, & Gupta, 2009).

Self-Determination Theory

Background

The self-determination theory (SDT) was developed in 1985 by Deci and Ryan to help explain achievement-oriented behaviors. The overall premise of the model is that humans have three innate psychological needs that influence behavior: competence, autonomy, and relatedness. The degree to which these needs are met influences the type of motivation that an individual has to perform a behavior. The model proposes that there are three types of motivation: intrinsic motivation, extrinsic motivation, and amotivation. Depending on which type of motivation the individual has, the motives for performing the behavior will vary. The highest level of self-determined motivation is intrinsic motivation: An intrinsically motivated individual performs the behavior for his or her own pleasure and satisfaction. Figure 15.5 depicts the structure of the SDT.

Three Psychological Needs

The three psychological needs that must be met for self-determined behavior to be performed are competence, autonomy, and relatedness. Competence is similar to self-efficacy and refers to the individual's task-specific level of confidence that he or she can complete the behavior successfully. Autonomy refers to the the individual's feeling of being able to choose to perform the behaviors that he or she wants to perform. Lastly, the need for relatedness refers to the individual's need to feel a

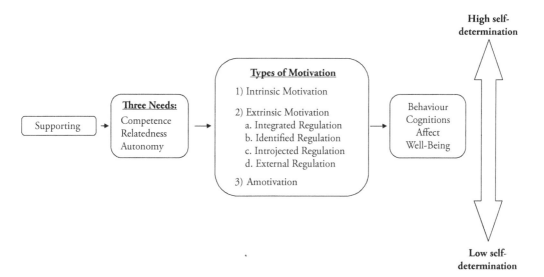

Figure 15.5. The self-determination theory. This theory states that individuals are more likely to perform a behavior if there is a high level of self-determined motivation. The continuum of self-determined motivation ranges from intrinsic motivation (the highest) to amotivation (the lowest). The type of motivation an individual has is based on whether the three innate psychological needs of competence, relatedness, and autonomy are being met.

sense of security and involvement with social groups and to feel that he or she has the self-confidence and ability to perform the behavior with others.

Three Types of Motivation

INTRINSIC MOTIVATION

Having the three needs met leads to the highest level of self-determined behavior, that which is intrinsically motivated (Deci & Ryan, 1985). Being intrinsically motivated means that the individual is performing the behavior for pure pleasure and personal satisfaction and not for any external factor such as rewards, obligation, or avoiding punishment. Intrinsic motivation will be maximized if the behavior provides an optimal level of challenge and the opportunity to feel successful (Deci & Ryan, 2000).

EXTRINSIC MOTIVATION

When an individual is motivated to perform a behavior for an external reason, the action is considered to be extrinsically motivated. There are four levels of extrinsic motivation, which lie on a continuum based on the degree to which the behavior is self-determined. The type of extrinsic motivation with the greatest level of self-determination is integrated regulation. This type of regulation coincides with the individual's sense of self and value system (Hagger & Chatzisarantis, 2007). The second type of extrinsic motivation on the continuum is

identified regulation, when the behavior is performed to achieve one's personal goals. Ryan and Deci (2000) state that with identified regulation, the individual identifies with the values and purpose of the behavior. The third type is introjected regulation. An individual controlled by introjected regulation engages in the behavior out of internal contingencies. For example, the individual might reward him- or herself for performing the behavior successfully or engage in the behavior out of a sense of obligation. The last type of extrinsic motivation. and the lowest on the continuum for self-determination, is external regulation. Externally regulated behavior is performed to gain some sort of external reward or to avoid a punishment.

AMOTIVATION

The third type of motivation, amotivation, is said to occur when the individual has no sort of motivation at all for the given behavior. Individuals may be amotivated to engage in a behavior when the three needs are not met, when the behavior does not provide optimal challenge, or when the individual does not see any utility to the behavior.

The SDT and Exercise Behavior

Self-determination theory one of the newer theories in its application to exercise psychology, and as such, a greater amount of research is needed to understand its full potential in this domain.

Research in both exercise and physical education has supported the use of SDT when the three psychological needs are met (Hagger & Chatzisarantis, 2007). In correlational studies within the exercise domain, meeting the need for autonomy has been associated with exercise uptake and maintenance over time (Chatzisarantis, Hagger, Biddle, Smith, & Wang, 2003). In a study by Wilson, Rodgers, Blanchard, and Gessell (2003), perceived competence had a large correlation with intrinsic motivation, whereas perceived autonomy had only a moderate correlation with identified regulation. The third need, relatedness, was not significantly correlated with any type of behavioral regulation. This study also showed that intrinsic regulation of exercise was a significant predictor of attitudes toward exercise behavior. In another correlational study, Wilson, Rodgers, Fraser, and Murray (2004) found that higher levels of self-determined motivation were associated with increased exercise frequency, increased effort in exercise, and greater intentions to exercise.

In a physical education context, intrinsic motivation has been associated with increased physical activity, increased learning, and improved attitude toward physical activity (Standage, Gillison, & Treasure, 2007). In a study of adolescents in a physical education context, Lim and Wang (2009) found that perceived autonomy was positively associated with intrinsic motivation and negatively correlated with amotivation. This study also highlighted that intrinsic motivation was positively correlated with the adolescents' intention to be physically active outside of the school setting.

Very few studies have employed the SDT model as a framework for interventions (Rhodes & Pfaeffli, 2010). Fortier, Sweet, O'Sullivan, and Williams (2007) conducted a randomized controlled trial using constructs of the SDT. Results indicated that autonomous support and perceived competence significantly predicted physical activity behavior for the experimental group at 13 weeks. The study also showed that the experimental group had higher levels of physical activity than a control group at 13 weeks, as well as higher levels of autonomous motivation at six weeks. On the other hand, a study by Levy and Cardinal (2004) used a mail intervention where an intervention group was given print materials with information on the three SDT needs as they relate to physical activity. The study showed no significant differences between the intervention and control groups, offering no support for the SDT intervention. From these mixed results, it is clear that further research employing SDT interventions is needed in the exercise domain.

Moving Forward and Adapting the SDT to Exercise and Physical Activity

Given the relative newcomer status of the SDT in the physical activity domain, most research has focused on direct application of the model to predict or change behavior. There have been some demonstrations of model integration providing evidence that the psychological needs in SDT are mediated by the more proximal social cognitions of TPB (Hagger & Chatzisarantis, 2007). Wilson et al. (2004) have similarly augmented the theory to include attitudes, motives, and intentions. Adapting SDT to physical activity may require additional considerations in measurement. The regulation constructs, particularly intrinsic and identified regulation, have high collinearity, suggesting that some adaptation is necessary (Rhodes et al., 2009).

Health Belief Model and Protection Motivation Theory
The Health Belief Model

The health belief model (HBM) is an expectancy-value model developed by American public health researchers to enhance the effectiveness of their health education programs (Hochbaum, 1958). This development was driven by the understanding that individuals' demographic variables could not be effectively modified to increase the effect of health education, and therefore other psychological variables would need to be investigated. These psychological variables tapped into individuals' beliefs about whether a behavior was desirable to perform or not, a concept referred to as valence (Lewin, 1951).

The two main components of the HBM are threat perception and behavioral evaluation, which each also comprise two types of beliefs (see Figure 15.6). Threat perception is made up of beliefs concerning perceived susceptibility to illness and beliefs concerning the anticipated severity of the consequences of illness. Behavioral evaluation comprises beliefs about the efficacy of performing a recommended health behavior and the barriers to performing the behavior. Also included in the HBM are cues to action, which are triggers capable of bringing about a behavior shift if the individual holds appropriate beliefs (e.g., health campaigns and social influence). The final construct of the HBM, health motivation, is defined as an individual's general concern with health matters (Becker, Haefner, & Maiman, 1977).

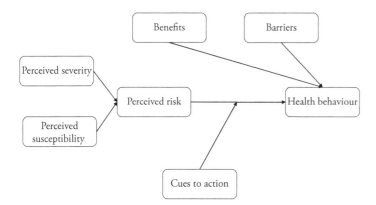

Figure 15.6. The health belief model. The premise of this model is that the uptake of a new health behavior is influenced by the perceived risk of an unhealthy behavior. Perceived risk is influenced by perceived severity and perceived susceptibility. Uptake of the health behavior is also influenced by barriers to and benefits of this behavior. Cues to action can also act as triggers to influence behavior change.

Harrison, Mullen, and Green (1992) conducted a meta-analysis of studies using the HBM with adults. They concluded that the six constructs of the HBM lack standardized definitions and as a result the strength of the theory as a psychological framework is limited. The review found small and varied effect sizes for the HBM constructs. It found that retrospective studies had significantly larger effect sizes than prospective studies.

Protection Motivation Theory

The protection motivation theory (PMT) was developed to gain a better understanding of the impact of fear appeals (Rogers, 1975). Rogers (1983) later revised the model to include the cognitive processes of behavior change as they relate to fear appeals. The basis of the theory is the belief that fear appeals may in fact alter or mediate attitudes and behavior. Rogers (1975) based the PMT on three variables that Hovland, Janis, and Kelley (1953) proposed as the components of a fear appeal: the magnitude of the severity of an event, the probability that the event will occur if no protective behavior is employed or the current behavior is not modified, and the perceived efficacy of a coping response to reduce or eliminate the event. Rogers (1975) adapted these variables to correspond to mediating cognitive processes of perceived severity, perceived vulnerability, and response efficacy.

The main constructs within the model have been divided into threat appraisal and coping appraisal. Threat appraisal consists of perceived severity and perceived vulnerability. Coping appraisal is also made up of two components: response efficacy and the individual's perceived level of self-efficacy. As well, the proximal predictor of protection behavior is protection motivation, which is measured similarly to behavioral intention. In the full model,

protection motivation is calculated from the four cognitive constructs by subtracting threat appraisal from intrinsic or extrinsic rewards and subtracting response costs from coping appraisal (Plotnikoff & Trinh, 2010). While the main model employs this subtractive method, the majority of PMT research concerns itself with the effects of the four components of the model on protective behavior (see Figure 15.7).

PMT and Exercise Intentions and Behavior

The PMT has been used in the physical activity domain across a number of populations (e.g., adults, youth, diabetes patients, and cardiac patients) (Plotnikoff & Trinh, 2010). Examples of both cross-sectional and experimental studies are highlighted below.

Among 800 randomly sampled adults considered to be at high risk for heart disease, Plotnikoff and Higginbotham (1998) found that coping appraisal constructs were strongly correlated with both exercise intention and behavior, while the threat appraisal constructs had only a small association with behavioral intention. As well, the results from this study indicated that perceived vulnerability was negatively associated with intentions and behavior, which could be explained by the defensive mechanisms (e.g., avoidance) that individuals may employ if they feel vulnerable to a disease.

In a prospective design, Blanchard et al. (2009) studied 76 cardiac patients engaged in a home-based cardiac rehabilitation program. The study showed that both three- and six-month exercise behavior were significantly predicted by self-efficacy and that response efficacy was the primary predictor of three- and six-month exercise intentions.

In experimental studies, the results have been mixed. Three construct manipulation studies have

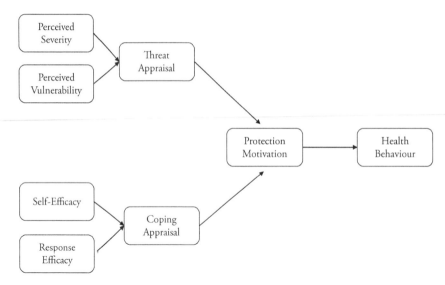

Figure 15.7. The protection motivation theory. This model states that the uptake of a health behavior is based on protection motivation, which is similar to behavioral intention. Protection motivation comprises threat appraisal (made up of perceived severity and perceived vulnerability) and coping appraisal (made up of self-efficacy and response efficacy).

been conducted among college students where exercise behavior was promoted as the primary means of prevention for health-related conditions (Plotnikoff & Trinh, 2010). There is also mixed evidence for the utility of PMT in behavioral interventions (Milne, Orbell, & Sheeran, 2002; Plotnikoff, McCargar, Wilson, & Loucaides, 2005). For example, Milne, Orbell, and Sheeran (2000) found significant increases in intention among an undergraduate experimental group in comparison with a control group as a consequence of a PMT-based health education intervention; however, changes in behavior were not significantly different between the groups.

Conclusions

Theories of exercise and physical activity have received enormous attention in the last two decades. Much of this work has focused on social cognition models applied from other disciplines. The models reviewed in this chapter—the TPB, SCT, TTM, SDT, and HBM/PMT—represent the bulk of this applied work. All have shown some utility in explaining physical activity, but there have been few intervention studies employing these models in a mediation capacity (Rhodes & Pfaeffli, 2010). Further, the redundancy among the model constructs is well noted (Bandura, 1998, 2004; Fishbein et al., 2001); many of them represent the same wine with different labels. Integrated models of these constructs need to pay careful attention to potential construct redundancies (Bandura, 1998, 2004;

Fishbein et al., 2001). With this point in mind, it is apparent that the HBM/PMT may have the least utility for continued application in the physical activity domain. The model assumes that disease threat is a primary motivator for behavioral action, yet many other physical activity motives are evident from the literature (social factors, fun, achievement, aesthetics, etc.). The TPB has shown strong predictive capacity, but the model needs to cross the hurdle from basic prediction to applied behavior modification if it is to show true worth in physical activity. The SCT, on the other hand, appears to need more conceptual studies that examine relevant subcomponent self-efficacy structures (task versus coping, etc.) as well as a full test of the model. The TTM has undergone the most critical scrutiny (Adams & White, 2002), but it has also been applied the most to physical activity and has shown utility (Spencer et al., 2006). Continued work examining marked stages of physical activity and processes of change appears warranted. Finally, the SDT has emerged recently as a viable model in the physical activity domain, yet more validation of its several regulation constructs and efficacy in interventions is required.

Other research avenues may have utility for advancing social cognitive theories in physical activity. First, targeting interventions to various populations and contexts seems important but has received limited support (Rhodes & Blanchard, 2007a; Rhodes, Blanchard, & Blacklock, 2008; Wankel & Mummery, 1993; Wankel, Mummery, Stephens, &

Craig, 1994). Evidence for differences across these theories by population and context is required. Second, better measures of all theoretical constructs, including exercise as an outcome itself, is an ongoing challenge that deserves continual attention. Finally, even though developing and implementing intervention strategies (e.g., cognitive behavioral, social, and environmental) that map onto theoretical models is the ultimate goal of exercise behavior research, it receives far less attention than it should. Indeed, short of validating measures and the initial relative contributions of a model, experimental designs should be the norm for theory testing (Weinstein, 2007).

References

Adams, J., & White, M. (2002). Are activity promotion interventions based on the transtheoretical model effective? A critical review. *British Journal of Sports Medicine, 37*, 106–114.

Ajzen, I. (1985). From intentions to actions: A theory of planned behavior. In J. Kuhl & J. Beckman (Eds.), *Action control: From cognition to behavior* (pp. 11–39). Heidelberg: Springer-Verlag.

Ajzen, I. (1991). The theory of planned behavior. *Organizational Behavior and Human Decision Processes, 50*, 179–211.

Ajzen, I. (2002a). *Construction of a theory of planned behavior intervention.* Retrieved April 4, 2007, from http://www-unix.oit.umass.edu/~aizen/pdf/tpb.intervention.pdf

Ajzen, I. (2002b). Perceived behavioral control, self-efficacy, locus of control, and the theory of planned behavior. *Journal of Applied Social Psychology, 32*, 665–683.

Ajzen, I. (2006). *Constructing a TPB questionnaire: Conceptual and methodological considerations.* Retrieved April 7, 2007, from http://www-unix.oit.umass.edu/~aizen/pdf/tpb.measurement.pdf

Ajzen, I., & Fishbein, M. (1980). *Understanding attitudes and predicting social behavior.* Englewood Cliffs, NJ: Prentice Hall.

Ajzen, I., & Fishbein, M. (2005). The influence of attitudes on behavior. In D. Albarracín, B. T. Johnson, & M. P. Zanna (Eds.), *Handbook of attitudes* (pp. 173–221). Mahwah, NJ: Erlbaum.

Armitage, C. J. (2009). Is there utility in the transtheoretical model? *British Journal of Health Psychology, 14*, 195–210.

Armstrong, C. A., & Sallis, J. F. (1993). Stages of change, self-efficacy, and the adoption of vigorous exercise: A prospective analysis. *Journal of Sport and Exercise Psychology, 15*, 390–403.

Bandura, A. (1977). Self-efficacy: Toward a unifying theory of behavioral change. *Psychological Review, 84*, 191–215.

Bandura, A. (1995). On rectifying conceptual ecumenism. In J. E. Maddux (Ed.), *Self-efficacy, adaptation, and adjustment: Theory, research, and application* (pp. 347–376). New York: Plenum.

Bandura, A. (1997). *Self-efficacy: The exercise of control.* New York: Freeman.

Bandura, A. (1998). Health promotion from the perspective of social cognitive theory. *Psychology and Health, 13*, 623–649.

Bandura, A. (2004). Health promotion by social cognitive means. *Health Education and Behavior, 31*, 143–164.

Baranowski, T., Anderson, C., & Carmack, C. (1998). Mediating variable framework in physical activity interventions: How are we doing? How might we do better? *American Journal of Preventive Medicine, 15*, 266–297.

Becker, M. H., Haefner, D. P., & Maiman, L. A. (1977). The health belief model in the prediction of dietary compliance: A field experiment. *Journal of Health and Social Behaviour, 18*, 348–366.

Biddle, S. J. H., & Nigg, C. R. (2000). Theories of exercise behavior. *International Journal of Sport Psychology, 31*, 290–304.

Blanchard, C. M., Fisher, J., Sparling, P., Nehl, E., Rhodes, R. E., Courneya, K. S., . . . Rupp, J. C.(2008). Ethnicity and the theory of planned behavior in an exercise context: A mediation and moderation perspective in college students. *Psychology of Sport and Exercise, 9*, 527–545.

Blanchard, C. M., Fortier, M. S., Sweet, S. N., O'Sullivan, T. L., Hogg, W., Reid, R. D., . . . Sigal, R. J. (2007). Explaining physical activity levels from a self-efficacy perspective: The Physical Activity Counseling Trial. *Annals of Behavioral Medicine, 34*, 323–328.

Blanchard, C. M., Reid, R. D., Morrin, L. I., McDonnell, L., McGannon, K., Rhodes, R. E., . . . Edwards, N. (2009). Does protection motivation theory explain exercise intentions and behavior during home-based cardiac rehabilitation? *Journal of Cardiopulmonary Rehabilitation and Prevention, 29*, 188–192.

Blanchard, C. M., Rodgers, W., Courneya, K. S., Daub, B., & Knapik, G. (2002). Does barrier efficacy mediate the gender/exercise adherence relationship during phase II cardiac rehabilitation? *Rehabilitation Psychology, 47*, 106–120.

Bouchard, C., & Shephard, R. J. (1994). Physical activity fitness and health: the model and key concepts. In: C. Bouchard, & R. J. Shephard, T. Stephens (Eds). *Physical activity fitness and health: International proceedings and consensus statement* (pp. 77–88). Champaign, IL: Human Kinetics.

Bridle, C., Riemsma, R. P., Pattenden, J., Sowden, A. J., Mather, L., & Watt, I. S. (2005). Systematic review of the effectiveness of health behavior interventions based on the transtheoretical model. *Psychology and Health, 20*, 283–301.

Bunton, R., Baldwin, S., Flynn, D., & Whitelaw, S. (2000). The "stages of change" model in health promotion: Science and ideology. *Critical Public Health, 10*, 55–69.

Cahill, S. P., Gallo, L. A., Lisman, S. A., & Weinstein, A. (2006). Willing or able? The meanings of self-efficacy. *Journal of Social and Clinical Psychology, 25*, 196–209.

Canadian Fitness and Lifestyle Research Institute. (2004). *Increasing physical activity: Trends for planning effective communication.* Retrieved February 24, 2006, from http://www.cflri.ca/eng/statistics/surveys/capacity2004.php

Cardinal, B. J. (1995). The Stages of Exercise Scale and stages of exercise behavior in female adults. *Journal of Sports Medicine and Physical Fitness, 35*, 87–92.

Centers for Disease Control. (2005). Trends in leisure-time physical activity by age, sex, and race/ethnicity—United States, 1994–2004. *Morbidity & Mortality Weekly Report, 54*, 991–994.

Chatzisarantis, N. L. D., & Hagger, M. S. (2005). Effects of a brief intervention based on the theory of planned behavior on leisure-time physical activity participation. *Journal of Sport and Exercise Psychology, 27*, 470–487.

Chatzisarantis, N. L. D., Hagger, M. S., Biddle, S. J. H., Smith, B., & Wang, J. C. K. (2003). A meta-analysis of perceived locus of causality in exercise, sport, and physical education contexts. *Journal of Sport and Exercise Psychology, 25*, 284–306.

Cohen, J. (1992). A power primer. *Psychological Bulletin, 112,* 155–159.

Colcombe, S. J., & Kramer, A. F. (2003). Fitness effects on the cognitive function of older adults: A meta-analytic study. *Psychological Science, 14,* 125–130.

Conner, M., & Armitage, C. J. (1998). Extending the theory of planned behavior: A review and avenues for further research. *Journal of Applied Social Psychology, 28,* 1429–1464.

Courneya, K. S., & Bobick, T. M. (2000a). Integrating the theory of planned behavior with the processes and stages of change in the exercise domain. *Psychology of Sport and Exercise, 1,* 41–56.

Courneya, K. S., & Bobick, T. M. (2000b). No evidence for a termination stage in exercise behaviour change. *Avante, 6,* 75–85.

Courneya, K. S., Conner, M., & Rhodes, R. E. (2006). Effects of different measurement scales on the variability and predictive validity of the "two-component" model of the theory of planned behavior in the exercise domain. *Psychology and Health, 21,* 557–570.

Cramp, A. G., & Brawley, L. R. (2006). Moms in motion: A group-mediated cognitive-behavioral physical activity intervention. *International Journal of Behavioral Nutrition and Physical Activity, 3,* 1479.

Deci, E. L., & Ryan, R. M. (1985). *Intrinsic motivation and self-determination in human behavior.* New York: Plenum.

Deci, E. L., & Ryan, R. M. (2000). The "what" and "why" of goal pursuits: Human needs and the self-determination of behaviour. *Psychological Inquiry, 11,* 227–268.

Dishman, R. K. (1990). Determinants of participation in physical activity. In C. Bouchard (Ed.), *Exercise, fitness and health: A consensus of current knowledge* (pp. 214–238). Champaign, IL: Human Kinetics.

Dishman, R. K., & Buckworth, J. (1996). Increasing physical activity: A quantitative synthesis. *Medicine & Science in Sports & Exercise, 28,* 706–719.

Fishbein, M. (1967). Attitude and the prediction of behavior. In M. Fishbein (Ed.), *Readings in attitude theory and measurement* (pp. 477–492). New York: Wiley.

Fishbein, M., Triandis, H. C., Kanfer, F. H., Becker, M., Middlestadt, S. E., & Eichler, A. (2001). Factors influencing behavior and behavior change. In A. Baum & T. A. Revenson (Eds.), *Handbook of health psychology* (pp. 3–17). Mahwah, NJ: Erlbaum.

Fortier, M. S., Sweet, S. N., O'Sullivan, T. L., & Williams, G. C. (2007). A self-determination process model of physical activity adoption in the context of a randomized controlled trial. *Psychology of Sport and Exercise, 8,* 741–757.

Foster, C., Hillsdon, M., & Thorogood, M. (2005). Interventions for promoting physical activity: *Cochrane Database of Systematic Reviews,* (1), CD003180.pub2. doi: 10.1002/14651858

Gardner, B. (2009). Modelling motivation and habit in stable travel mode contexts. *Transportation Research, 12,* 68–76.

Gollwitzer, P. M., & Brandstatter, V. (1997). Implementation intentions and effective goal pursuit. *Journal of Personality and Social Psychology, 73,* 186–199.

Gollwitzer, P. M., & Sheeran, P. (2006). Implementation intentions and goal achievement: A meta-analysis of effects and processes. *Advances in Experimental Social Psychology, 38,* 69–119.

Hagger, M., & Chatzisarantis, N. L. D. (2005). First- and higher-order models of attitudes, normative influence, and perceived behavioural control in the theory of planned behaviour. *British Journal of Social Psychology, 44,* 513–535.

Hagger, M., & Chatzisarantis, N. L. D. (Eds.). (2007). *Intrinsic motivation and self-determination in exercise and sport.* Champaign, IL: Human Kinetics.

Hagger, M., Chatzisarantis, N. L. D., & Biddle, S. J. H. (2002). A meta-analytic review of the theories of reasoned action and planned behavior in physical activity: Predictive validity and the contribution of additional variables. *Journal of Sport and Exercise Psychology, 24,* 1–12.

Hallam, J. S., & Petosa, R. (2004). The long-term impact of a four-session work-site intervention on selected social cognitive theory variables linked to adult exercise adherence. *Health Education and Behavior, 31,* 88–100.

Harrison, J. A., Mullen, P. D., & Green, L. W. (1992). A meta-analysis of studies of the health belief model with adults. *Health Education Research, 7,* 107–116.

Hausenblas, H. A., Carron, A. V., & Mack, D. E. (1997). Application of the theories of reasoned action and planned behavior to exercise behavior: A meta-analysis. *Journal of Sport and Exercise Psychology, 19,* 36–51.

Hellman, E. A. (1997). Use of the stages of change in exercise adherence model among older adults with a cardiac diagnosis. *Journal of Cardiopulmonary Rehabilitation, 17,* 145–155.

Hochbaum, G. M. (1958). *Public participation in medical screening programs: A socio-psychological study.* Washington, DC: United States Government Printing Office.

Hovland, C., Janis, I. L., & Kelley, H. (1953). *Communication and persuasion.* New Haven, CT: Yale University Press.

Jones, L. W., Sinclair, R. C., Rhodes, R. E., & Courneya, K. S. (2004). Promoting exercise behaviour: An integration of persuasion theories and the theory of planned behaviour. *British Journal of Health Psychology, 9,* 505–521.

Jue, N. H., & Cunningham, S. L. (1998). Stages of exercise behaviour change at two time periods following coronary artery bypass graft surgery. *Progress in Cardiovascular Nursing, 13,* 23–33.

Kirsch, I. (1982). Efficacy expectations or response predictions: The meaning of efficacy ratings as a function of task characteristics. *Journal of Personality and Social Psychology, 42,* 132–136.

Kirsch, I. (1995). Self-efficacy and outcome expectancy: A concluding commentary. In J. E. Maddux (Ed.), *Self-efficacy, adaptation, and adjustment: Theory, research, and application* (pp. 331–346). New York: Plenum.

Levy, S. S., & Cardinal, B. J. (2004). Effects of a self-determination theory-based mail-mediated intervention on adults' exercise behavior. *American Journal of Health Promotion, 18,* 345–349.

Lewin, R. W. (1951). *Field theory in social science.* New York: Harper.

Lewis, B. A., Marcus, B., Pate, R. R., & Dunn, A. L. (2002). Psychosocial mediators of physical activity behavior among adults and children. *American Journal of Preventive Medicine, 23*(2 Suppl.), 26–35.

Lim, B. S. C., & Wang, C. K. J. (2009). Perceived autonomy support, behavioural regulations in physical education, and physical activity intention. *Psychology of Sport and Exercise, 10,* 52–60.

Maddux, J. E. (1995). Looking for common ground: A comment on Kirsch and Bandura. In J. E. Maddux (Ed.), *Self-efficacy, adaptation, and adjustment: Theory, research, and application* (pp. 377–386). New York: Plenum.

Marcus, B. H., Selby, V. C., Niaura, R. S., & Rossi, J. S. (1992). Self-efficacy and the stages of exercise behavior change. *Research Quarterly for Exercise and Sport, 63,* 60–66.

Marcus, B. H., & Simkin, L. R. (1993). The stages of exercise behavior. *Journal of Sports Medicine and Physical Fitness, 33*, 83–88.

Marshall, S. J., & Biddle, S. J. H. (2001). The transtheoretical model of behavior change: A meta-analysis of applications to physical activity and exercise. *Annals of Behavioral Medicine, 23*, 229–246.

McAuley, E., & Blissmer, B. (2000). Self-efficacy determinants and consequences of physical activity. *Exercise and Sport Sciences Reviews, 28*, 85–88.

McAuley, E., Katula, J. A., Mihalko, S. L., Blissmer, B., Duncan, T. E., Pena, M., Dunn, E. (1999). Mode of physical activity and self-efficacy in older adults: A latent growth curve analysis. *Journals of Gerontology, Series B: Psychological Sciences and Social Sciences, 54B*, 283–292.

Michie, S., Abraham, C., Whittington, C., McAteer, J., & Gupta, S. (2009). Effective techniques in healthy eating and physical activity interventions: A meta-regression. *Health Psychology, 28*, 690–701.

Milne, S., Orbell, S., & Sheeran, P. (2000). Prediction and intervention in health-related behavior: A meta-analytic review of protection motivation theory. *Journal of Applied Social Psychology, 30*, 106–143.

Milne, S., Orbell, S., & Sheeran, P. (2002). Combining motivational and volitional interventions to promote exercise participation: Protection motivation theory and implementation intentions. *British Journal of Health Psychology, 7*, 163–184.

Oman, R. F., & King, A. C. (1998). Predicting the adoption and maintenance of exercise prediction using self-efficacy and previous exercise participation rates. *American Journal of Health Promotion, 12*, 154–161.

Parrott, M. W., Tennant, L. K., Olejnik, S., & Poudevigne, M. S. (2008). Theory of planned behavior: Implications for an email-based physical activity intervention. *Psychology of Sport and Exercise, 9*, 511–526.

Plotnikoff, R. C., & Higginbotham, N. (1998). Protection motivation theory and the prediction of exercise and low-fat diet behaviors among Australian cardiac patients. *Psychology and Health, 13*, 411–429.

Plotnikoff, R. C., McCargar, L. J., Wilson, P. M., & Loucaides, C. A. (2005). Efficacy of an email intervention for the promotion of physical activity and nutrition behavior in the workplace context. *American Journal of Health Promotion, 19*, 422–429.

Plotnikoff, R. C., & Trinh, L. (2010). Protection motivation theory: Is this a worthwhile theory for physical activity promotion? *Exercise and Sport Sciences Reviews, 38*, 91–98.

Prochaska, J. O., & DiClemente, C. C. (1982). Transtheoretical therapy: Toward a more integrative model of change. *Psychotherapy: Theory, Research & Practice, 19*, 276–288.

Reed, G. R., Velicer, W. F., Prochaska, J. O., Rossi, J. S., & Marcus, B. H. (1997). What makes a good staging algorithm: Examples from regular exercise. *American Journal of Health Promotion, 12*, 57–66.

Reger, B., Cooper, L., Booth-Butterfield, S., Smith, H., & Bauman, A. (2002). Wheeling walks: A community campaign using paid media to encourage walking among sedentary older adults. *Preventive Medicine, 35*, 285–292.

Rhodes, R. E., Berry, T., Naylor, P. J., & Wharf Higgins, S. J. (2004). Three-step validation of exercise processes of change in an adolescent sample. *Measurement in Physical Education and Exercise Science, 8*, 1–20.

Rhodes, R. E., & Blanchard, C. M. (2006). Conceptual categories or operational constructs? Evaluating higher order theory of planned behavior structures in the exercise domain. *Behavioral Medicine, 31*, 141–150.

Rhodes, R. E., & Blanchard, C. M. (2007a). Just how special are the physical activity cognitions in diseased populations? Preliminary evidence for integrated content in chronic disease prevention and rehabilitation. *Annals of Behavioral Medicine, 33*, 302–312.

Rhodes, R. E., & Blanchard, C. M. (2007b). What do confidence items measure in the physical activity domain? *Journal of Applied Social Psychology, 37*, 753–768.

Rhodes, R. E., Blanchard, C. M., & Blacklock, R. E. (2008). Do physical activity beliefs differ by age and gender? *Journal of Sport and Exercise Psychology, 30*, 412–423.

Rhodes, R. E., Blanchard, C. M., & Matheson, D. H. (2006). A multi-component model of the theory of planned behavior. *British Journal of Health Psychology, 11*, 119–137.

Rhodes, R. E., Blanchard, C. M., Matheson, D. H., & Coble, J. (2006). Disentangling motivation, intention, and planning in the physical activity domain. *Psychology of Sport and Exercise, 7*, 15–27.

Rhodes, R. E., & Courneya, K. S. (2003a). Investigating multiple components of attitude, subjective norm, and perceived behavioral control: An examination of the theory of planned behavior in the exercise domain. *British Journal of Social Psychology, 42*, 129–146.

Rhodes, R. E., & Courneya, K. S. (2003b). Relationships between personality, an extended theory of planned behaviour model, and exercise behaviour. *British Journal of Health Psychology, 8*, 19–36.

Rhodes, R. E., & Courneya, K. S. (2003c). Self-efficacy, controllability, and intention in the theory of planned behavior: Measurement redundancy or causal independence? *Psychology and Health, 18*, 79–91.

Rhodes, R. E., & Courneya, K. S. (2004). Differentiating motivation and control in the theory of planned behavior. *Psychology, Health and Medicine, 9*, 205–215.

Rhodes, R. E., Courneya, K. S., Blanchard, C. M., & Plotnikoff, R. C. (2007). Prediction of leisure-time walking: An integration of social cognitive, perceived environmental, and personality factors. *International Journal of Behavioral Nutrition and Physical Activity, 4*, 51.

Rhodes, R. E., & Dickau, L. (in press). Moderators of the intention–behaviour relationship in the physical activity domain: A review. *British Journal of Sports Medicine*.

Rhodes, R. E., Fiala, B., & Conner, M. (2009). Affective judgments and physical activity: A review and meta-analysis. *Annals of Behavioral Medicine, 38*, 180–204.

Rhodes, R. E. & Pfaeffli, L. A. (2010). Mediators of behaviour change among adult non-clinical populations: A review update. *International Journal of Behavioral Nutrition and Physical Activity, 7*(37), 1–11.

Rhodes, R. E., & Plotnikoff, R. C. (2006). Understanding action control: Predicting physical activity intention–behavior profiles across six months in a Canadian sample. *Health Psychology, 25*, 292–299.

Rhodes, R. E., Plotnikoff, R. C., & Courneya, K. S. (2008). Predicting the physical activity intention–behaviour profiles of adopters and maintainers using three social cognition models. *Annals of Behavioral Medicine, 36*, 244–252.

Rhodes, R. E., & Smith, N. E. I. (2006). Personality correlates of physical activity: A review and meta-analysis. *British Journal of Sports Medicine, 40,* 958–965.

Rhodes, R. E., Warburton, D. E. R., & Bredin, S. S. (2009). Predicting the effect of interactive video bikes on exercise adherence: An efficacy trial. *Psychology, Health and Medicine, 14*(6), 631–641.

Rogers, R. W. (1975). A protection motivation theory of fear appeals and attitude change. *Journal of Psychology, 91,* 93–114.

Rogers, R. W. (1983). Cognitive and physiological processes in fear appeals and attitude change: A revised theory of protection motivation. In J. T. Cacioppo & R. E. Petty (Eds.), *Social psychophysiology* (pp. 153–176). New York: Guilford Press.

Sallis, J. F., Haskell, W. L., Fortman, S. P., Vranizan, K. M., Taylor, C. B., & Solomon, D. S. (1986). Predictors of adoption and maintenance of physical activity in a community sample. *Preventive Medicine, 15,* 331–341.

Sniehotta, F. F. (2009). Towards a theory of intentional behaviour change: Plans, planning, and self-regulation. *British Journal of Health Psychology, 14,* 261–273.

Sniehotta, F. F., Scholz, U., & Schwarzer, R. (2005). Bridging the intention–behaviour gap: Planning, self-efficacy, and action control in the adoption and maintenance of physical exercise. *Psychology and Health, 20,* 143–160.

Sniehotta, F. F., Scholz, U., & Schwarzer, R. (2006). Action plans and coping plans for physical exercise: A longitudinal intervention study in cardiac rehabilitation. *British Journal of Health Psychology, 11,* 23–37.

Spence, J. C., Burgess, J. A., Cutumisu, N., Lee, J. G., Moylan, B., Taylor, L.,...Witcher, C. S.(2006). Self-efficacy and physical activity: A quantitative review. *Journal of Sport and Exercise Psychology, 28,* S172.

Spencer, L., Adams, T. B., Malone, S., Roy, L., & Yost, E. (2006). Applying the transtheoretical model to exercise: A systematic and comprehensive review of the literature. *Health Promotion Practice, 7,* 428–443.

Standage, M., Gillison, F., & Treasure, D. C. (2007). Self-determination and motivation in physical education. In M. Hagger & N. L. Chatzisarantis (Eds.), *Intrinsic motivation and self-determination in exercise and sport* (pp. 71–83). Champaign, IL: Human Kinetics.

Stokols, D. (1996). Translating social ecological theory into guidelines for community health promotion. *American Journal of Health Promotion, 10,* 282–298.

Symons Downs, D., & Hausenblas, H. A. (2005a). Elicitation studies and the theory of planned behavior: A systematic review of exercise beliefs. *Psychology of Sport and Exercise, 6,* 1–31.

Symons Downs, D., & Hausenblas, H. A. (2005b). Exercise behavior and the theories of reasoned action and planned behavior: A meta-analytic update. *Journal of Physical Activity and Health, 2,* 76–97.

Trost, S. G., Owen, N., Bauman, A., Sallis, J. F., & Brown, W. (2002). Correlates of adults' participation in physical activity: Review and update. *Medicine & Science in Sports & Exercise, 34,* 1996–2001.

Vallance, J. K., Courneya, K. S., Plotnikoff, R. C., & Mackey, J. R. (2008). Analyzing theoretical mechanisms of physical activity behavior change in breast cancer survivors: Results from the Activity Promotion (ACTION) Trial. *Annals Of Behavioral Medicine, 35*(2), 150–158.

Wankel, L. M., & Mummery, K. (1993). Using national survey data incorporating the theory of planned behavior: Implications for social marketing strategies in physical activity. *Journal of Applied Sport Psychology, 5,* 158–177.

Wankel, L. M., Mummery, W. K., Stephens, T., & Craig, C. L. (1994). Prediction of physical activity intention from social psychological variables: Results from the Campbell's Survey of Well-Being. *Journal of Sport and Exercise Psychology, 16,* 56–69.

Warburton, D. E. R., Katzmarzyk, P., Rhodes, R. E., & Shephard, R. J. (2007). Evidence-informed physical activity guidelines for Canadian adults. *Applied Physiology, Nutrition and Metabolism, 32,* S16–S68.

Warburton, D. E. R., Nicol, C. W., & Bredin, S. S. (2006). Health benefits of physical activity: The evidence. *Canadian Medical Association Journal, 174,* 801–809.

Webb, T. L., & Sheeran, P. (2006). Does changing behavioral intentions engender behavior change? A meta-analysis of the experimental evidence. *Psychological Bulletin, 132,* 249–268.

Weinstein, N. D. (2007). Misleading tests of health behavior theories. *Annals of Behavioral Medicine, 33,* 1–10.

Wilson, P. M., Rodgers, W. M., Blanchard, C. M., & Gessell, J. (2003). The relationship between psychological needs, self-determined motivation, exercise attitudes, and physical fitness. *Journal of Applied Social Psychology, 33,* 2373–2392.

Wilson, P. M., Rodgers, W. M., Fraser, S. N., & Murray, T. C. (2004). Relationships between exercise regulations and motivational consequences in university students. *Research Quarterly for Exercise & Sport, 75*(1), 81–91.

Exercise Is a Many-Splendored Thing, but for Some It Does Not Feel So Splendid: Staging a Resurgence of Hedonistic Ideas in the Quest to Understand Exercise Behavior

Panteleimon Ekkekakis *and* Manolis Dafermos

Abstract

Contemporary theories of exercise behavior have been the products of the so-called cognitive revolution, which has shaped the dominant paradigm in psychology over the past several decades. Cognitive theories rely on the assumption that, in making behavioral decisions, humans collect relevant information and make their selections on the basis of a more-or-less rational analysis of this information. Although the dominance of cognitive theories in the field of exercise psychology is unquestionable, evidence suggests that they leave most of the variance in exercise behavior unaccounted and interventions based on them are of limited effectiveness in changing exercise behavior. This chapter reviews the history and evaluates the potential of an alternative approach, namely the hedonic theory of motivation. This idea, long neglected due the fascination of psychologists with information-processing models of the mind, attributes a substantial portion of the variance in decision-making to affective processes. Modern iterations of the idea emerging from the fields of neurology and behavioral economics reaffirm the ancient thesis that, in the long run, humans tend to repeat what makes them feel better and tend to avoid what makes them feel worse. Evidence from studies in the context of exercise suggests that affective responses to exercise vary greatly between individuals. Furthermore, despite a still-evolving methodological platform, preliminary studies show that affective responses to exercise predict subsequent exercise behavior. This line of research and theorizing offers a novel and intriguing perspective on the mechanisms underlying behavioral decision-making in the context of exercise. The literature reviewed in this chapter highlights the need for further research on the motivational implications of affective processes and lays the foundation for the development of a hedonic theory of exercise behavior.

Key Words: hedonic theory, affect heuristic, information processing, rationality assumption, epistemology

Ah, the truth about exercise? . . . The real value of it is not in terms of abstract health benefits like longevity—an extra few hours or maybe months—but because it feels good when you do it or when it's over. To hell with Hygeia, the truth lies in the pleasure.
—Excerpt from a letter by Drs. Richard A, Friedman and Fred Charatan to the *British Medical Journal* (Vol. 328, p. 1315, 2004)

For my sixty-fifth birthday this year, my wife purchased a week of personal training at the local health club for me. Although I am still in great shape since playing on my college tennis team 45 years ago, I decided it would be a good idea to go ahead and give it a try. ... [After two workouts] The only way I can brush my teeth is by laying on the toothbrush on the counter and moving my mouth back and forth over it. ... My chest hurt when I got on the treadmill, so Belinda put me on the stair monster. ... Belinda told me it would help me get in shape and enjoy life. She said some other [expletive deleted] too. [After four workouts] I hate that witch Belinda more than any human being has ever hated any other human being in the history of the world. ... If there was a part of my body I could move without unbearable pain, I would beat her with it. [At the end of the first week] I'm having the church van pick me up for services today so I can go and thank God that this week is over. I will also pray that next year my wife will choose a gift for me that is fun—like a root canal or a vasectomy.

—Excerpt from a widely circulated e-mail message, forwarded to one of the authors (P.E.) by a former student

Exercise psychology is a scientific field in the midst of a Kuhnian crisis. An old paradigm, according to which behavioral decisions (such as the decision to engage in, adhere to, or disengage from physical activity) are guided by the rational cognitive analysis of available information, has started to show its weaknesses. Over the past 20 years, a period during which more information about the health benefits of physical activity has become available than ever before, the percentage of people engaging in regular physical activity has remained stagnant. Cognitive models typically account for less than 25% of the variation in physical activity behavior. It would be hard to deny that there must be additional sources of variance and that these should be explored. This chapter is about the untapped potential represented by one such variable—namely, affect.

On the Brink of a Kuhnian Revolution?

To place the current situation in exercise psychology in historical context and to better understand the underlying intellectual conflict between the old and new paradigm, it is useful to revisit some of Thomas Kuhn's timeless insights about the emergence of scientific revolutions. According to Kuhn (1962/1996), "normal science" is a label that describes "research firmly based upon one or more past scientific achievements, achievements that some particular scientific community acknowledges for a time as supplying the foundation for its further practice" (p. 10). Normal science operates on the basis of "paradigms." A paradigm is a combination of theory, practice, and instrumentation that acts as an accepted example of scientific practice. Paradigms serve a crucial function in the scientific enterprise because they "provide models from which spring particular coherent traditions of scientific research" (p. 10).

Once a paradigm is established, the main function of "normal-scientific" research is "the articulation of those phenomena and theories that the paradigm already supplies" (Kuhn, 1962/1996, p. 24). What normal science does not do is to observe and consider new phenomena ("indeed those that will not fit the box are often not seen at all," p. 24) and to develop new theories (scientists are even "often intolerant of those invented by others," p. 24). According to Kuhn, "normal science does not aim at novelties of fact or theory and, when successful, finds none" (p. 52). In the process of articulating the components of the paradigm, scientists develop increasingly elaborate instruments, an increasingly esoteric vocabulary, an increasingly complex skill set, and increasingly refined concepts. The unintended consequences of these developments are the "immense restriction of the scientist's vision" and a "considerable resistance to paradigm change." In essence, science becomes "increasingly rigid" (p. 64).

How, then, does progress occur? According to Kuhn, a mature paradigm, despite its rigidity and resistance to change, is a prerequisite for change. The reason is that a paradigm precisely specifies what is anticipated. For example, it leads to the development of instruments specifically engineered to find the "anticipated" result and trains researchers to detect even the most intricate matches between paradigm-based predictions and observations. This situation creates the conditions for the observation of "anomalies," the engine of scientific progress. Kuhn (1962) defined an "anomaly" as "nature's failure to conform entirely to expectation" (p. 762). Anomalies appear "only against the background provided by the paradigm," and in fact, "the more precise and far-reaching that paradigm is, the more sensitive an indicator it provides of anomaly and hence of an occasion for paradigm change" (Kuhn, 1962/1996, p. 65).

Clearly, not all anomalies result in progress. The vast majority are ignored. When an anomaly persists over an extended period of time, the most common effect is that scientists will attempt to alter their instrumentation in a way that makes the anomaly disappear or they will try to make the anomaly fit within the paradigm (i.e., modify the expectation and thus make the former anomaly seem expected). According to Kuhn (1962/1996), "they will devise numerous articulations and ad hoc modifications of their theory in order to eliminate any apparent conflict" (p. 78). In general, "when confronted by even severe and prolonged anomalies" that make them "begin to lose faith [and] consider alternatives," scientists "do not renounce the paradigm that has led them into crisis" (p. 77). The main reason is that "as in manufacture so in science—retooling is an extravagance to be reserved for the occasion that demands it. The significance of crises is the indication they provide that an occasion for retooling has arrived" (p. 76).

In rare cases, an anomaly results in a "crisis." The forces that can convert an anomaly to a crisis are many, and usually several of them must co-occur. For example, a persistent anomaly may call into question some of the most fundamental tenets of the paradigm. In other cases, the paradigm predicts that an application should be ineffective when long practice has clearly established its utility (or conversely, the paradigm predicts that an application should be effective when practice reliably demonstrates its failure). As a result of such discrepancies, the anomaly becomes more widely recognized (e.g., replicated and confirmed by a broader circle of scientists) and even catches the attention of prominent figures in the field. The anomaly then becomes "the new fixation point of scientific scrutiny" (Kuhn, 1962/1996, p. 83) and its resolution becomes a shared goal. One of the defining features of a field in crisis is the emergence of multiple and divergent attempts to resolve the anomaly. As these attempts multiply, they also become more diversified. Although early attempts may follow the rules of the paradigm closely, the persistence of the anomaly begs "ad hoc adjustments" (p. 83) of the paradigm that are increasingly bold and unruly. Thus "the rules of normal science become increasingly blurred. Though there still is a paradigm, few practitioners prove to be entirely agreed about what it is. Even formerly standard solutions of solved problems are called in question" (p. 83).

A crisis is a powerful transformative force, because it brings forth critical thinking and creativity. According to Kuhn (1962/1996), "the transition from a paradigm in crisis to a new one from which a new tradition of normal science can emerge is far from a cumulative process, one achieved by an articulation or extension of the old paradigm" (pp. 84–85). Instead, a crisis forces "a reconstruction of the field from new fundamentals, a reconstruction that changes some of the field's most elementary theoretical generalizations as well as many of its paradigm methods and applications" (p. 85). Such "reconstructions" progress slowly and usually against considerable resistance. Formerly dominant paradigms do not just collapse or disappear overnight:

> Once it has achieved the status of paradigm, a scientific theory is declared invalid only if an alternate candidate is available to take its place. ... The act of judgment that leads scientists to reject a previously accepted theory is always based upon more than a comparison of that theory with the world. The decision to reject one paradigm is always simultaneously the decision to accept another, and the judgment leading to that decision involves the comparison of both paradigms with nature and with each other.
> (Kuhn, 1962/1996, p. 77)

Much like political revolutions, scientific revolutions "are inaugurated by a growing sense, ... often restricted to a narrow subdivision of the scientific community, that an existing paradigm has ceased to function adequately in the exploration of an aspect of nature to which that paradigm itself had previously led the way" (p. 92). Scientific revolutions, therefore, are "those non-cumulative developmental episodes in which an older paradigm is replaced in whole or in part by an incompatible new one" (p. 92).

What Is the Dominant Paradigm in Exercise Psychology?

All currently prominent models of physical activity or exercise behavior are exemplars of the same paradigm. The health belief model (Rosenstock, Strecher, & Becker, 1988), the theory of planned behavior (Ajzen, 1991), the social cognitive theory (Bandura, 1986), and (to a large extent) the transtheoretical model (Prochaska & DiClemente, 1982) are all products of the so-called cognitive revolution. As such, they all rely on the fundamental assumption that in making behavioral decisions, people collect and analyze the relevant information that is available to them, rationally weigh pros and cons, and make complicated probabilistic predictions about the future consequences of their actions.

For example, according to the theories of reasoned action and planned behavior, "people think and act in more or less logical ways" (Ajzen, 2005, p. 29). Human behavior "can be described as reasoned" (Ajzen & Fishbein, 2005, p. 203) in the sense that the decision to act "rests ultimately on the information people have relevant to the behavior" (Ajzen & Fishbein, 2005, p. 195). In social cognitive theory, cognitive processing also plays the central role in decision making. People are described as data processors, constantly engaged in collecting and analyzing information:

> Many activities involve inferential judgments about conditional relations between events in probabilistic environments. Discernment of predictive rules requires cognitive processing of multidimensional information that contains many ambiguities and uncertainties. In ferreting out predictive rules, people must draw on their state of knowledge to generate hypotheses about predictive factors, to weight and integrate them into composite rules, to test their judgments against outcome information, and to

remember which notions they had tested and how well they had worked.
> (*Bandura*, 1989, p. 1176)

Similarly, according to the transtheoretical model, in approaching the decision to change their behavior, people are constantly engaged in analyzing and comparing pros and cons and make decisions on that basis: "for most problem behaviors people will decide that the pros of changing the behavior outweigh the cons before they take action to modify their behavior" (Prochaska et al., 1994, p. 44).

It is also striking that within the framework of these popular theories, all of which have been adopted from social and health psychology to account for exercise behavior, exercise is considered just another variant of health behavior (similar to practicing safe sex, brushing one's teeth, or eating fruits and vegetables). Yet exercise appears to have near-zero correlations with other health behaviors, suggesting that its underlying regulatory mechanisms are, at least in part, distinct (Newsom, McFarland, Kaplan, Huguet, & Zani, 2005). Nevertheless, popular broad-scope theories do not take this uniqueness of exercise into consideration. Acknowledging this point, Rhodes and Nigg (2011) write that "there is adequate, if not overwhelming, evidence to suggest that unique theories of [physical activity] should be pursued" (p. 114).

Anomalies in the Paradigm

The "physical activity paradox" is one of the most frustrating phenomena in public health. On the one hand, physical activity is arguably, as the late Jeremy Morris (1994) famously put it, "today's best buy in public health." This characterization is convincingly supported by compelling epidemiologic and experimental evidence across a broad range of conditions (Miles, 2007; Pedersen & Saltin, 2006; Warburton, Katzmarzyk, Rhodes, & Shephard, 2007). On the other hand, promoting physical activity to the public has proven a very "tough sell" (Dishman, 2001). This situation challenges the notion that human beings make decisions on the basis of rational information processing. However, that idea is a core assumption of most contemporary theories of health (and physical activity) behavior. Such theories are built on the belief that when presented with a behavioral option that can credibly lower the risk of an important negative outcome (e.g., death), most people, thinking and acting rationally, will select that option.

For example, according to the theory of planned behavior, "attitude toward a behavior is determined by accessible beliefs about the consequences of the behavior, termed *behavioral beliefs*. Each behavioral belief links the behavior to a certain outcome. The attitude toward the behavior is determined by the person's evaluation of the outcomes associated with the behavior and by the strength of these associations" (Ajzen, 2005, p. 123). Thus recognizing that physical activity can be beneficial in lowering the risk of cardiovascular disease is expected to improve the attitude toward physical activity. In turn, this should lead to the formation of an intention to be physically active. Similarly, in social cognitive theory, realizing that physical activity can bring about the important outcome of maintaining cardiovascular health should increase the chance of someone's becoming physically active. According to Bandura (2001), "people ... anticipate the likely consequences of prospective actions, and select and create courses of action likely to produce desired outcomes and avoid detrimental ones. Through the exercise of forethought, people motivate themselves and guide their actions in anticipation of future events" (p. 7). In the transtheoretical model, increasing the perceived pros (such as recognizing that exercise can lower the risk of death from cardiovascular disease) is a prerequisite for moving from "precontemplation" to later stages of change. Furthermore, "to move to action, pros should be higher than cons" (Prochaska, Redding, & Evers, 2008, p. 104). From a rational standpoint, it would be hard to imagine a "con" that could outweigh the "pro" of staying alive.

If these assumptions are correct, it follows that in societies inundated with messages about the health benefits of physical activity, the population should be, for the most part, physically active. In the United States, a country in which the population is routinely exposed to media messages about the health benefits of physical activity. Morrow, Jackson, Bazzarre, Milne, and Blair (1999) surveyed 2,002 adults representing the 48 contiguous states and the District of Columbia. Of them, 84% knew that physical inactivity was related to the development of heart disease. In another analysis of the same data set, Martin, Morrow, Jackson, and Dunn (2000) reported that of the 2,002 respondents, 97% identified physical inactivity as a health risk factor (52% as "very important," 37% as "important," and 8% as "somewhat important"). Nevertheless, 68.1% did not meet the minimum physical activity guidelines (Pate et al., 1995). Even of those who rated physical inactivity as a "very important" health risk factor, about two-thirds (64.2%) did not engage in the minimum recommended levels of activity.

In other words, despite the fact that "message penetration" about the health benefits of physical activity in U.S. society seems excellent (at rates of 85–95%), participation in physical activity remains low. Just how low became evident with the publication of results from the first nationwide study of accelerometry-based activity monitoring. Troiano et al. (2008) reported that among adults between the ages of 20 and 59 years, only 3.5% (3.8% of men, 3.2% of women) participated in bouts of at least moderate-intensity physical activity totaling at least 30 minutes per day on at least 5 days per week. For those over the age of 60 years, the percentage was even lower, at 2.4% (2.5% of men, 2.3% of women). A latent class analysis of the same data set showed that when every minute of activity was considered, 78.7% of the population was included in the two least active classes (33.6% averaging 5.3 minutes and 45.1% averaging 21.0 minutes of moderate-to-vigorous physical activity per day). When only activity performed in bouts of at least 10 minutes was considered (during which at least 70% of the accelerometer counts were above the threshold for moderate-to-vigorous activity), 93.5% of the population was included in the two least active classes (56.1% averaging nearly zero and 37.4% averaging 10.3 minutes of moderate-to-vigorous physical activity per day). The data for vigorous activity are even more disconcerting. On 91.1% of all days, participants accumulated less than 1 minute of vigorous physical activity on average. Of 3,462 participants who provided valid data for at least three days, only 23 (0.66%) registered 20 minutes of vigorous physical activity on at least three days per week (Metzger et al., 2008).

In Australia, another country with social marketing campaigns promoting the health benefits of physical activity, the results have been similar. According to data from the National Physical Activity Survey, nearly all adults (92%) said that they knew they would get health benefits if they did at least 30 minutes of moderate physical activity per day (Armstrong, Bauman, & Davies, 2000). Nevertheless, over 50% did not reach this criterion (15% reported no leisure-time physical activity during the previous week, and another 40% accumulated fewer than 150 minutes of activity). From 1997 to 1999, knowledge about the health benefits of physical activity increased nationwide, but the percentage of people satisfying the guidelines decreased (Bauman et al., 2003). Specifically, the percentage of people who knew that being more active is good for health increased from 85.0% to 88.1%, and those who knew that brisk walking for half an hour daily is good for health increased from 90.3% to 92.1%. At the same time, the percentage who reported at least 150 minutes of physical activity on at least five days per week decreased from 50.9% to 45.2%.

Within specific studies, the results have been similarly discordant with rationality assumptions. For example, patients in cardiac rehabilitation (N = 353) were asked questions related to their perceived risk (e.g., "If I keep my lifestyle the way it was prior to the acute treatment, I will suffer from coronary health problems") (Schwarzer, Luszczynska, Ziegelmann, Scholz, & Lippke, 2008). Their answers indicated that they were well aware of their elevated level of risk (M = 3.10 out of 4.00). However, the correlation of risk perception to the intention to be physically active (e.g., "I intend to become physically active on a regular basis") was only r = .09. Outcome expectancy (e.g., "If I would exercise on a regular basis, then I would feel balanced in my daily life"; M = 3.60 out of 4.00) was also weakly related to intention (r = .29). Similarly, patients in orthopedic rehabilitation (N = 368) reported high risk perception (e.g., "likelihood that you will ever suffer from chronic pain"; M = 2.96 out of 5.00) and outcome expectancy (e.g., "If I would engage in physical exercise on 2 or more days per week, for at least 20 minutes each time, then I would be doing something good for my health"; M = 3.19 out of 4.00). However, neither variable correlated with intention (r = .03 and .11, respectively).

These and numerous other studies with similar results suggest that it might be erroneous to assume that the decision to engage in or adhere to an exercise program depends solely on the rational analysis and evaluation of information. The corollary is that appealing to the public's knowledge and rational reasoning as the cornerstone of intervention efforts, as is commonly the case (e.g., enumerating the health benefits of activity and the risks of inactivity), is unlikely to be very effective (e.g., Dishman & Buckworth, 1996).

In fact, a growing number of theorists have questioned the ability of human beings to collect, process, and apply information in the manner described by cognitive models of health behavior. Herbert Simon, the 1978 Nobel laureate in economics ("for his pioneering research into the decision-making process within economic organizations"), argued that "human beings have neither the facts nor the consistent structure of values nor the reasoning power at their disposal that would be required" to perform the kinds of computations that cognitive models entail (Simon, 1983, p. 17). Instead, Simon suggested that "human rationality is very limited, very much bounded by the situation and by human computational powers" (p. 34), a notion now referred to as "bounded rationality." Other researchers have also criticized the assumptions of cognitive theories, focusing on the substantial deviations that human judgments and behavioral choices often exhibit compared with standard models of rationality (e.g., Stanovich & West, 2000). These researchers have proposed that rather than being determined by a thorough and truly reasoned analysis, human decisions are aided by a set of "heuristics" (shortcuts or simplified rules) that, although frequently flawed and biased, bring the complexity of problems down to the scale of human reasoning abilities and ultimately help people navigate their world.

The Hedonic Perspective as an Emerging Alternative

Many authors who question the exclusive reliance of decision making on cognitive analysis tend to assign an important role to affective influences, reminding us that people generally tend to do what makes them feel better and tend to avoid what makes them feel worse. For example, following his strong argument for bounded rationality, Simon (1983) suggested that "in order to have anything like a complete theory of human rationality, we have to understand what role emotion plays in it" (p. 29). Before him, Young (1959) had argued that "any theory of behavior which ignores the concept of affectivity will be found inadequate as an explanation of the total facts" (p. 106). Along the same lines, in a thought-provoking and highly influential article that ignited a famous debate with Richard Lazarus, Robert Zajonc (1980) wrote: "We sometimes delude ourselves that we proceed in a rational manner and weigh all the pros and cons of the various alternatives. But this is probably seldom the actual case. Quite often 'I decided in favor of X' is no more than 'I liked X'" (p. 155). Similarly, in the introduction of his landmark book *Descartes'*

Error: Emotion, Reason, and the Human Brain, Damasio (1994) wrote:

> I began writing this book to propose that reason may not be as pure as most of us think it is or wish it were, that emotions and feelings may not be intruders in the bastion of reason at all: they may be enmeshed in its networks, for worse *and* for better. The strategies of human reason probably did not develop, in either evolution or any single individual, without the guiding force of the mechanisms of biological regulation, of which emotion and feeling are notable expressions. Moreover, even after reasoning strategies become established in the formative years, their effective deployment probably depends, to a considerable extent, on a continued ability to experience feelings.
>
> (p. xii)

In the view of these prominent theorists, models of decision making based exclusively on information processing are bound to be deficient. To quote Bettman (1993), such models "are overbearingly cognitive; like the tin man in the Wizard of Oz, these models have no heart" (p. 8).

Heeding such calls, authors have proposed that one of the heuristics that people use to facilitate decision making is the "affect heuristic" (e.g., Kahneman, 1999; Slovic, Finucane, Peters, & MacGregor, 2002; 2007). The basic tenet of the affect heuristic, heralded as "probably the most important development in the study of judgment heuristics in the past few decades" (Kahneman, 2003, p. 710), is that "positive and negative affective feelings ... guide and direct judgments and decisions" (Finucane, Peters, & Slovic, 2003, pp.340–341). Specifically, affect "facilitates information integration in judgments and decisions, guides reason, ... gives priorities among multiple goals," and is "a powerful motivator of behavior" (p. 341). As explained in the next section, this idea is certainly not new, since its historic origins can be traced to Epicurean philosophy, and well-known revivals can be found in Bentham's "hedonic calculus" and Freud's "pleasure principle." Recently, the idea has reappeared in diverse scientific fields, including social psychology (Baumeister, Vohs, DeWall, & Zhang, 2007; Emmons & Diener, 1986), behavioral economics (Kahneman, 1999; Loewenstein & Lerner, 2003; Mellers, 2004), affective neuroscience (Bechara, Damasio, & Damasio, 2000; Damasio, 1996; Naqvi, Shiv, & Bechara, 2006), and experimental physiology (Cabanac, 1992).

It is noteworthy that the idea that affect can be "a powerful motivator of behavior" seems to be much more influential in fundamentally interdisciplinary research fields than those that adhere closely to paradigms dictated by "mainstream" psychology. In effect, interdisciplinary fields have operated unrestrained by the influence of the cognitive tradition, which within psychology proper seems to have imposed an "immense restriction of the scientist's vision," to use Kuhn's (1962/1996, p. 64) words. For example, that eating behavior and food choices are driven at least in part by the rewarding effects of food (Lutter & Nestler, 2009; Moore & O'Donohue, 2008; Stroebe, Papies, & Aarts, 2008) has come to be regarded as almost self-evident. By extension, we readily accept that the pleasure associated with eating has contributed to the problem of obesity (Kishi & Elmquist, 2005; Rolls, 2007). Similarly, few would question that the addictive effects of drugs of abuse are mediated by pleasurable feelings (Bechara, 2005; Koob, 2008; Robinson & Berridge, 2008).

In decision research, although most researchers still subscribe to information processing models, the role of affect has been gaining considerable ground. In a major review, Weber and Johnson (2009) noted the following: "Though successful in many ways, the cognitive revolution may have been too focused on analytic and computational processes. The emotions revolution of the past decade or so has tried to correct this overemphasis by documenting the prevalence of affective processes, depicting them as automatic and essentially effort-free inputs that orient and motivate adaptive behavior" (p. 65). Nevertheless, within the core of psychology, as acknowledged by Ajzen and Fishbein (2005), "much of the research [stemming from cognitive theories of motivation and behavior] has devoted little attention to the role of emotion in the prediction of intentions and actions" (p. 203).

Overview of the Long History of Psychological Hedonism

The present generation of researchers in exercise psychology has been educated in an academic culture that is almost entirely devoid of information about the role of affect as a motivating force in human behavior. Tracing the historical origins and subsequent evolution and refinement of the idea of "psychological hedonism" by relying solely on the contemporary literature. However, the value of having this type of historical perspective cannot be overemphasized. First, it is crucial for researchers to appreciate that this is an idea that, despite ups and downs, has remained alive amid radical and tumultuous changes in philosophical and metatheoretical currents over the past 25 centuries. Second, it is important, as the phoenix of affect in psychological thought rises from the ashes once again, to avoid the pitfall of rediscovering the wheel by reigniting debates that have already taken place. Third, a solid understanding of the historical journey of the idea of psychological hedonism will inevitably reveal both its limitations and its strengths and will thus help contemporary researchers formulate modern iterations of the essential themes that are more robust and more relevant to today's psychology. For these reasons, in this section, we trace the time line of this idea over the course of the past 25 centuries by concentrating on select works of figures whose views have proven to be of landmark significance from a historical perspective.

"Hedonism" is generally defined as the pursuit of pleasure. However, an important distinction must be drawn between hedonism as a doctrine in ethical philosophy and so-called psychological or motivational hedonism. Hedonism as an ethical philosophy advances the view that pleasure is the only ultimate good and that only pleasant states are desirable in themselves. This position can be taken as tantamount to the controversial claim that any pursuit of pleasure, from physical to spiritual and from individual to societal, must be condoned, regardless of the cost to others. Psychological or motivational hedonism, on the other hand, refers to the doctrine that behavior is motivated by the desire for pleasure and the avoidance of displeasure (Mees & Schmitt, 2008). Pleasure and displeasure may result immediately or in the long run (and may thus serve as either *proximal* or *distal* motives). Furthermore, as emphasized by Sober and Wilson (1998), pleasure and displeasure may range from purely corporeal sensations (e.g., the pleasure of quenching one's thirst or the pain of an injury) to feelings embedded within cognitively enriched states such as attitudes or emotions (e.g., the pleasure of pride or the displeasure of embarrassment). In its extreme version, this type of hedonism implies that *all* human behavior is carried out with the intent to either seek pleasure or avoid displeasure. In other words, according to this perspective, the pursuit of pleasure and the avoidance of displeasure are the *only* ultimate human motives.

Aristippus (435–366 BCE), the founder of the Cyrenaic school, proposed a body-centered, radical version of hedonism. He taught that the goal of all human actions is to seek pleasure. According to Diogenes Laertius (trans. 1972), "he derived pleasure from what was present, and did not toil to procure the enjoyment of something not present" (*Lives of Eminent Philosophers*, Book II, Chapter 8, line 66). Aristippus and the other Cyrenaics held that there are two emotional states of the mind, pleasure and pain. Pleasure comes from bodily stimuli that are agreeable or attractive, whereas pain is associated with bodily symptoms that are aversive or repellent. Diogenes Laertius described the belief of the Cyrenaics in psychological hedonism in these words: "That pleasure is the end is proved by the fact that from our youth up we are instinctively attracted to it, and, when we obtain it, seek for nothing more, and shun nothing so much as its opposite, pain" (Book II, Chapter 8, line 88). Cyrenaics also believed that "bodily pleasures are far better than mental pleasures, and bodily pains far worse than mental pains" (Diogenes Laertius, *Lives of Eminent Philosophers*, Book II, Chapter 8, line 90). So a crucial characteristic of the Cyrenaic school is that it elevated rather than suppressed the pleasures of the body over those of the mind.

Plato's (428–348 BCE) view of pleasure is complex. In *Protagoras*, Plato defended a prohedonistic position. On the other hand, in *Gorgias*, *Phaedo*, and *The Republic*, he introduced a contrast between reason and bodily pleasure. The antihedonistic ideas of the Pythagoreans may have influenced Plato's soul–body dualism and his treatment of desires as irrational, dark forces of the soul (Gosling & Taylor, 1982). According to Plato (trans. 1997), "there is a dangerous, wild and lawless form of desire in everyone, even in those of us who seem to be entirely moderate or measured" (*Republic*, IX, 572b). In *Philebus*, Plato presented a discussion between Rotarchus and Socrates about the nature of the supreme good. The conclusion was that the life that combines wisdom and pleasure is better than the life that excludes one or the other. A life of pleasure would not be desirable without wisdom, nor could a life of wisdom exist without pleasure. Plato divided pleasures into various types, such as the intellectual pleasure of learning, the pleasure of honor and dignity, and the bodily pleasures, such as food, drink, and sex (*Republic*, XI, 580e–581a). There is a correspondence between these types of pleasure and parts of the soul (i.e., the rational, emotional, and appetitive). Although Plato is often thought of as a dualist, he believed that it was necessary to keep harmony and integration between the parts of the human soul. However, Plato also held that there could be internal conflict between different sorts of desires and pleasures: "Some of our unnecessary pleasures and desires seem to me to be lawless. They are probably present in everyone, but they are held in check by the laws and by the better desires in alliance with reason. In a few people, they have been eliminated entirely or only a few weak ones remain, while in others they are stronger and more numerous" (*Republic*, IX, 571b). Plato's views on the tensions between different kinds of pleasures is important in the history of hedonistic ideas because it foreshadows the notion of internal conflicts in later psychodynamic theories in psychology.

Aristotle (384–322 BCE) accepted that "people who fall short with regard to pleasures and delight in them less than they should are hardly found; for such insensibility is not human" (*Nicomachean Ethics*, III, 1119a, 5, trans. 1984). Endorsing an essential hedonistic position, he believed that the pleasure associated with an activity is a crucial determinant of how this activity will be prioritized, since "the more pleasant activity drives out the other activity" whereas "when an activity causes pain, this pain destroys it" (*Nicomachean Ethics*, X, 1175b, 4–23). However, Aristotle also maintained that the ultimate goal of human life is not pleasure per se but *eudaimonia*, defined as the state of personal well-being in a holistic sense. Thus Aristotle rejected the idea that pleasure in general is the aim of all human actions and the purpose of human life. Instead, he elevated the significance of pleasure that is specifically connected with the intellectual life: "For, while there is pleasure in respect of any sense, and in respect of thought and contemplation no less, the most complete is pleasantest, and that of a well-conditioned organ in relation to the worthiest of its objects is the most complete; and the pleasure completes the activity" (*Nicomachean Ethics*, X, 1174b, 20–23). Thus in Aristotle's view, not all pleasures have the same value; the value of pleasure depends on the value of the activity from which the pleasure arises.

Epicurus (341–270 BCE) held that the goal of human life is pleasure. He called pleasure both the starting point and the culmination of a blessed life. Epicurus believed that a pleasant life is not defined by festivities and entertainment, sexual love, or enjoyment of a plentiful table. He held that human beings cannot lead a life of pleasure if it is not also a life of prudence, honor, and justice. According to Diogenes Laertius (trans. 1925),

Epicurus believed that the "misfortune of the wise is better than the prosperity of the fool" (*Lives of Eminent Philosophers*, X, 134). For the Cyrenaics, pleasure referred to cyclical and transient states, such as satiety after a meal. While Epicurus did not deny this type of pleasure, he argued that this is only one type and that a more important type is the pleasure that is enduring. Examples of this latter type include serenity and peace of mind, friendship, and being fearless in the face of death. All these, according to Epicurus, contribute to the highly desirable state of "rest." This concept refers to serenity of the soul, the absence of trouble and unrest of the psyche, and should not be confused with inactivity or indolence of the body. The antitheses to this concept of rest are the ideas of "motion" and "activity," but again these do not refer to the movement of the body but rather to a state of debauchery and consumerism. According to Epicurus, "peace of mind and freedom from pain are pleasures which imply a state of rest; joy and delight are seen to consist in motion and activity" (Diogenes Laertius, *Lives of Eminent Philosophers*, X, 136). Thus pleasure does not mean sensual enjoyment but freedom from pain in the body and from trouble in the mind (*Lives of Eminent Philosophers*, X, 131–132). Epicurus also disagreed with the Cyrenaics in that he believed the "pains of the mind" to be worse than the "pains of the body" because "the flesh endures the storms of the present alone, the mind those of the past and future as well as the present" (*Lives of Eminent Philosophers*, X, 137).

During the Middle Ages, hedonism was rejected as incompatible with Christian values. The humanistic scholars were those who revisited the idea of hedonism. Erasmus (1466–1536) and Thomas More (1478–1535) proposed their own versions of hedonism. In Thomas More's *Utopia*, for example, people called Utopians believed that pleasure was the ultimate goal of all their activities and that health was the foundation of all pleasures.

René Descartes (1596–1650), as a rationalist, did not accept the version of hedonism according to which pleasure is the most important element in human life. Descartes was, of course, a dualist who believed not only that mind and body are distinct entities but also that one (the mind) must have commanding control over the other (the body). He held that pleasure and pain, as well as what he characterized as "passions" (what would be referred to as "emotions" today), are caused by the flow of animal spirits in the body. They can intrude into and disrupt the function of the ethereal mind, in what

Descartes acknowledged as perhaps the main threat to his concept of substance dualism. Nevertheless, despite these intrusions and disruptions, Descartes adopted the position of the Stoics that the mind must exert control over passions and desires. In his words, "what we call 'titillation' or 'pleasurable sensation' occurs when the objects of the senses produce some movement in the nerves which would be capable of harming them if they did not have enough strength to resist it or if the body was not in a healthy condition" (*The Passions of the Soul*, 94/399, trans. 1985).

Thomas Hobbes (1588–1679) adopted a hedonistic approach to human motivation. In his view, human behavior is directed by self-interest and self-protection. Hobbes held that humans are thus stimulated by appetites, which bring forth a movement toward an object, and aversions, which induce a movement away from an object: "And in animal motion this is the very first endeavor, and found even in the embryo; which while it is in the womb, moveth its limbs with voluntary motion, for the avoiding of whatsoever troubleth it, or for the pursuing of what pleaseth it. And this first endeavor, when it tends towards such things as are known by experience to be pleasant, is called *appetite*, that is, an approaching; and when it shuns what is troublesome, *aversion*, or flying from it" (Hobbes, 1655/1839, p. 407). The Latin-origin words *appetitive* and *aversive* signify approach and withdrawal, and for Hobbes all the passions of the mind consist of appetite and aversion. Hobbes distinguished between different types of pleasures: "Of pleasures or delights, some arise from the sense of an object present; and those may be called pleasure of sense ... Others arise from the expectation that proceeds from foresight of the end or consequence of things; whether those things in the sense please or displease. And these are pleasures of the mind of him that draweth consequences, and are generally called 'joy.'" (Hobbes, 1651/1839, pp. 42–43).

David Hume (1711–1776) also adopted the basic hedonistic doctrine: "Tis obvious, that when we have the prospect of pain or pleasure from any object, we feel a consequent emotion of aversion or propensity, and are carry'd to avoid or embrace what will give us this uneasiness or satisfaction" (Hume, 1740/1978, p. 414). Hume proposed a division of passions into "direct" (e.g., desire, aversion, grief, joy, hope, fear, despair, and security) and "indirect" (e.g., pride, humility, ambition, vanity, love, hatred, envy, pity, malice, generosity, and their variants). The direct passions "arise immediately from good or evil, from pain or pleasure," whereas the indirect passions "proceed from the same principles, but by the conjuction of other qualities" (Hume, 1740/1978, p. 276). Although the criteria upon which this division is based are not entirely clear (McIntyre, 2000), a central consideration appears to be the degree of cognitive involvement or elaboration. Hume recognized that "bodily pains and pleasures are the source of many passions ... but arise originally ... in the body ... without any preceding thought or perception" (p. 276). On the other hand, other passions arise from ideas and reflections and are therefore enriched by cognition. Hume did not accept the view that reason should control the passions: "reason is, and ought only to be slave of the passions, and can never pretend to any other office than to serve and obey them" (Hume, 1740/1978, p. 415). He also did not agree with the view that reason alone can be a motive to volition and action. The impulse of actions, he held, arises not from reason but from passion (Watson, 1895).

Julien Offray de La Mettrie (1709–1751) was a physician by training who opposed the dualistic view of emotions and passions (including pleasure) as detached from the body. Introducing an innovative mechanistic view based on classical Newtonian physics, he famously likened humans to complicated machines. Associated with La Mettrie's materialism were his prohedonism views. He maintained that pleasures (such as those associated with sex or taking opium) and pains (such as hunger) are very powerful motives for human actions. Furthermore, in his book *Man as Machine*, La Mettrie wrote that "We were not originally made to be wise and we have perhaps become so by a sort of misuse of our organic faculties ... Nature created us all solely to be happy – yes, all, from the worm crawling on the ground to the eagle soaring on high" (La Mettrie, 1748/1996, p. 22) Later, in his work *Anti-Seneca* (also known as *Discourse on Happiness*), Le Mettrie was even more explicit in his views about the role of pleasure and pain: "We shall be Anti-Stoics! Those philosophers ... appear impervious to pleasure or pain; we shall glory in feeling both ... We shall not try to control what rules us; we shall not give orders to our sensations. We shall recognize their dominion and our slavery and try to make it pleasant for us, convinced as we are that happiness in life lies there" (La Mettrie, 1750/1996, p. 119).

For **Claude Adrien Helvétius (1715–1771),** pleasure and pain are the ruling motives of human behavior: "pleasure and pain are, and always will be, the only principles of action in man" (M. Helvétius, 1777/1810, p. 146). Following La Mettrie, Helvétius assigned a central role to the pleasures and pains of the body but also acknowledged that pleasure and pain may derive from thought: "I know but two sorts of pain, that we feel and that we foresee. I die of hunger; I feel a present pain. I foresee that I shall soon die of hunger. ... There are two sorts of pleasures, as there are two sorts of pains: the one is the present bodily pleasure, the other is that of foresight" (M. Helvétius, 1777/1810, pp. 126–129).

Jeremy Bentham (1748–1832) is perhaps the best known representative of the school of English utilitarianism. He accepted psychological hedonism, stating that "nature has placed mankind under the governance of two sovereign masters, pain and pleasure. It is for them alone to point out what we ought to do, as well as to determine what we shall do" (Bentham, 1789/1948, p. 1). He also believed that individual interest supersedes all others. In Bentham's utilitarianism, everything is judged by its utility, which in turn translates to pleasure. Bentham proposed that pleasures and pains can be quantified and developed a "hedonic calculus" according to which actions are evaluated by the net amount of pleasure (minus pain) that they generate.

John Stuart Mill (1806–1873) was also a proponent of utilitarianism who equated the concept of utility with that of pleasure: "Those who know anything about the matter are aware that every writer, from Epicurus to Bentham, who maintained the theory of utility, meant by it, not something to be contradistinguished from pleasure, but pleasure itself, together with exemption from pain" (*Utilitarianism*, Chapter II). Mill accepted fundamental tenets of hedonism, writing, for example, that "pleasure, and freedom from pain, are the only things desirable as ends; and that all desirable things ... are desirable either for the pleasure inherent in themselves, or as means to the promotion of pleasure and the prevention of pain" (*Utilitarianism*, Chapter II). He countered the opinions of those who had taken hedonism to be a "doctrine worthy only of swine" by emphasizing that there are qualitative differences between pleasures, with those pleasures that involve distinctively human faculties, such as the intellect, the feelings, the imagination, and the moral sentiments, being superior to others (West, 2004).

Herbert Spencer's (1820–1903) work holds a special place in the history of hedonistic ideas because he was the first to articulate the function of pleasure and pain within an evolutionary framework, and did so even before Darwin's *On the Origin of Species*. He maintained that "there exists a primordial connection between pleasure-giving acts and continuance or increase of life, and, by implication, between pain-giving acts and decrease or loss of life" (Spencer, 1879, p. 82). In his two-volume opus *The Principles of Psychology*, Spencer wrote that "pains are the correlatives of actions injurious to the organism, while pleasures are the correlatives of actions conducive to its welfare. ... It is an inevitable deduction from the hypothesis of Evolution, that races of sentient creatures could have come into existence under no other conditions" (Spencer, 1905, p. 279). Evolution linked pleasure to approach and pain to avoidance, and consequently "it is undeniable that every animal habitually persists in each act which gives pleasure, so long as it is does so, and desists from each act which gives pain" (p. 280). These links must be reliable and powerful. Any creature that departs from this cardinal rule becomes extinct: "if the states of consciousness which a creature endeavors to maintain are the correlatives of injurious actions, and if the states of consciousness which it endeavors to expel are the correlatives of beneficial actions, it must quickly disappear" (p. 280). Thus "conduct conducive to life" can only be the conduct "that is conducive to a surplus of pleasures over pains" (Spencer, 1879, p. 45).

Alexander Bain (1818–1903) endorsed Spencer's views on the function of pleasure and pain in evolution: "states of pleasure are connected with an increase, states of pain with an abatement, of some, or all, of the vital functions" (Bain, 1879, p. 283). Interestingly, throughout his work, Bain used "the pleasure of healthy exercise" and "the pain of fatigue" to illustrate his points. Thus immediately after the aforementioned excerpt, he wrote: "it is known that exercise is pleasurable only when we are expending surplus energy, and thereby making the blood to course through the system more rapidly. ... Let the stage of fatigue, however, be reached, and let the spur to exertion be still continued, we then witness the concurring circumstances of the sense of pain, and the lowering of vital energy" (p. 283). In turn, the "increase in vital power," according to Bain, must be one of the reasons for the "love of exercise for its own sake, or apart from the ends of productive industry, and the preservation of health" (p. 81). Bain also echoed the basic premise of psychological hedonism, linking pleasure to the pursuit and displeasure to the avoidance of action: "when movement concurs with pain, the pain arrests the movement through its general depressing agency; as, on the other hand, a movement bringing pleasure is sustained and promoted through the connection between pleasure and exalted energy" (p. 302). Bain incorporated these ideas into a theory of voluntary action. He proposed that behavior results from two innate sources, namely spontaneous acts and pleasure. Specifically, beings have an initial propensity for spontaneous behavior, and of the resulting random or accidental actions, some yield pleasure. Once a pleasant experience has occurred, the pleasure transforms that formerly spontaneous behavior to voluntary behavior.

William James's (1842–1910) appraisal of hedonistic ideas is measured and nuanced. In agreement with Spencer, James believed that pleasure signals benefit and pain signals harm, thus facilitating adaptation within an evolutionary framework: "It is a well-known fact that pleasures are generally associated with beneficial, pains with detrimental, experiences. All the fundamental vital processes illustrate this law. Starvation, suffocation, privation of food, drink and sleep, work when exhausted, burns, wounds, inflammation, the effects of poison, are as disagreeable as filling the hungry stomach, enjoying rest and sleep after fatigue, exercise after rest, and a sound skin and unbroken bones at all times, are pleasant" (James, 1890a, p. 143). Moreover, James accepted that pleasure and displeasure can have powerful motivational effects: "As present pleasures are tremendous reinforcers, and present pains tremendous inhibitors of whatever action leads to them, so the thoughts of pleasures and pains take rank amongst the thoughts which have most impulsive and inhibitive power. ... If a movement feels agreeable, we repeat and repeat it as long as the pleasure lasts. If it hurts us, our muscular contractions at the instant stop" (James, 1890b, p. 550). However, James distanced himself from Bain's "premature philosophy," according to which pleasure and pain "are our only spurs to action." In James's view, although the thought of pleasure or pain can provide the stimulus for many human actions and ongoing pleasure and pain can modulate behavior, "they are far from being our only stimuli. ... If the thought of pleasure can impel to action, surely other thoughts may. Experience only can decide which thoughts do" (James, 1890b, pp. 550–552).

In the early 1900s, probably influenced by the writings of Bentham and other proponents of utilitarianism, **Sigmund Freud (1856–1939)** postulated the existence of psychic processes aimed at reducing or eliminating sources of tension that result in displeasure and selecting memories of pleasurable experiences. In 1911, these ideas found direct expression in what became known as the "pleasure principle," promoted by Freud as one of the fundamental mechanisms of human behavior: "The sovereign tendency obeyed by the [unconscious mental processes] is easy of recognition; it is called the pleasure-pain principle (*lust-unlust* in German, or pleasure-displeasure, but translated as pleasure-pain, to highlight Freud's influence from Bentham), or more shortly the pleasure principle. These processes strive toward gaining pleasure; from any operation which might arouse unpleasantness ('pain'), mental activity draws back (repression)" (Freud, 1911/1946, p 14) The counterpart of the pleasure principle in psychoanalytic theory is the reality principle, according to which maturing human beings learn to control their ids, defer gratification, and endure pain. However, the salience of the pleasure principle is such that it never really succumbs to the reality principle; essentially, the role of the reality principle is to ensure the achievement of pleasure (even if delayed or somewhat reduced) by taking account of the constraints imposed by reality.

The advent of behaviorism created an adverse intellectual environment for hedonistic ideas and essentially set into motion the gradual disappearance of emotions from mainstream psychological research and theorizing. Behaviorists rejected the notion that "inner states," such as pleasant and unpleasant emotions, can be meaningful objects of study for a science of human behavior. According to **B. F. (Burrhus Frederic) Skinner (1904–1990),** for example, the proper subject matter of the study of emotion consists of (a) the emotional behavior and (b) the conditions that precipitated the behavior. It is indeed a testament to the robustness of hedonistic principles that they survived (of course, described in different terms) even in this environment. Specifically, among several laws theorized to govern the process of learning, **Edward Lee Thorndike (1874–1949)** proposed the so-called law of effect. Consistent with hedonistic ideas, this law suggests that when a behavior is paired with pleasure it becomes more likely to be repeated, whereas if it is paired with displeasure it becomes more likely to be avoided: "of several responses made to the same situation, those which are accompanied or closely followed by satisfaction to the animal will, other things being equal, be more firmly connected with the situation, so that, when it recurs, they will be more likely to recur; those which are accompanied or closely followed by discomfort to the animal will, other things being equal, have their connections with that situation weakened, so that, when it recurs, they will be less likely to occur. The greater the satisfaction or discomfort, the greater the strengthening or weakening of the bond" (Thorndike, 1911, p. 244). The law of effect was supported by some behaviorists, including **Clark L. Hull (1884–1952)** and Skinner, who incorporated reinforcement in operant conditioning, but not others, including **Edward C. Tolman (1886–1959),** who showed that learning can also occur without reinforcement.

During the 20th century, references to hedonistic ideas can be found in the works of a relatively few motivation researchers, including **Leonard T. Troland (1889–1932)**, **Paul T. Young (1892–1978)**, and **David C. McClelland (1917–1998)**. For example, Troland identified the senses of "beneception" and "nociception" as powerful motivators. Young wrote that one cannot fully understand learning and motivation without taking affective processes into account. McClelland theorized that positive and negative affect are primary states, which become associated with internal or environmental cues and later activate affective states similar to the primary affect but anticipatory in nature.

Hedonistic ideas received more attention and recognition in the writings of emotion theorists in the later part of the 20th century. **Silvan S. Tomkins (1911–1991)**, mentor to scholars who revived the study of emotion such as Paul Ekman and Carroll Izard, reintroduced the idea of affect as the primary motivational system. Acknowledgments of the role of affect in behavior can also be found in the work of cognitivists. However, the importance of affect is portrayed as minor compared with the commanding role of cognition. As one example, in **Albert Bandura's (1925–)** theory of self-efficacy, emotional arousal is postulated to influence behavior, albeit not directly but rather through the cognitive interpretation of its significance for one's efficacy. The recent renewal of scientific interest in the role of affect in human behavior should be attributed primarily to the work of researchers who are active outside the narrow confines of psychology proper. Such high-profile proponents of hedonistic ideas include **Michel Cabanac (1934–)** in physiology, **Daniel Kahneman (1934–)** in behavioral economics, and **Antonio Damasio (1944–)** in neurology.

Having concluded this historical overview, it is instructive to consider the criticisms that have been leveled against hedonism over the years. For example, James (1890b) referred to some of Bain's positions as the "silliness of the old-fashioned pleasure-philosophy" (p. 551). William McDougall (1916) called them "absurdities" (p. 43). However, it is important to decipher which specific hedonistic ideas the critics opposed. A major source of contention was the entanglement of hedonism with moral philosophy, principally in the writings of the utilitarians, who equated all good with pleasure and argued that the pursuit of pleasure should be life's ultimate objective. McDougall (1916), for example, charged that such a view "in reducing all morality to hedonism ... grossly libels human nature" (p. 190). He went on to say that "surely it is obvious that men do often carry through a line of action which is to them painful in every phase, in the contemplation of it, in deciding upon it, and in its execution and achievement!" (p. 374). Another problem was the claim in the writings of some ardent proponents of hedonism, such as Bain, that the pursuit of (proximal or distal) pleasure and the avoidance of (proximal or distal) displeasure was the motive behind *all* human action. Considering how absolute this claim was, it is not surprising that it was targeted by skeptics. James (1890b), for example, wrote: "Who smiles for the pleasure of the smiling, or frowns for the pleasure of the frown? Who blushes to escape the discomfort of not blushing? Or who in anger, grief, or fear is actuated to the movements which he makes by the pleasures which they yield?" (p. 550).

Nevertheless, the fundamental tenets of motivational hedonism have remained unscathed. There have not been serious attacks against the core idea that pleasure is generally associated with beneficial courses of action, whereas displeasure is typically associated with harm. Furthermore, there is little resistance to the notion that human beings, in most cases, tend to repeat behaviors associated with pleasure and tend to avoid behaviors linked to displeasure. James Mark Baldwin (1891), for example, argued that "this fact, that our most abstract acts of volition are strongly influenced by subconscious affective conditions, is only beginning to have the recognition it deserves" (p. 320) and acknowledged that "it is probable that we make no deliberate decisions whatever in which our own happiness has not been a factor of influence" (p. 327). McDougall (1916), one of the most vocal opponents of psychological hedonism, accepted that "pleasure [tends] to sustain and prolong any mode of action, pain to cut it short" (p. 43). As for the tendency to "seek pleasure and ... try to avoid pain," McDougall characterized this as an "undeniable fact" (p. 364). Thus, it is crucial for contemporary readers to understand that although the idea that pleasure and displeasure represent powerful motivational forces in human behavior may have lost some of its prominence over the past few decades, it remains essentially unchallenged. Except for some of its most extreme or controversial variants, there have not been devastating conceptual attacks against it. There have not been empirical findings showing that pleasure and displeasure do not account for meaningful portions of behavioral variance; quite the contrary. The idea has remained standing in the very competitive arena of psychological ideas for over 25 centuries. To understand why hedonism is not included in the tables of contents of contemporary psychological textbooks, one must first understand Kuhn.

Hedonistic Ideas and Exercise Behavior

The idea that exercise must be pleasant or else it is unlikely to be continued was promoted by Robert Roberts, a director of a Young Men's Christian Association (YMCA) gymnasium in Boston in the late 1800s and one of the pioneers of the physical training movement. According to what became known as Roberts's "platform," all exercises should be "safe, short, easy, beneficial, and pleasing" to keep the exercisers coming back (Leonard, 1915, p. 124). The idea reappeared in the writings of the some of the pioneers of contemporary exercise science. According to William Morgan (1977),

> It seems reasonable to assume that [individuals] must experience some form of positive reinforcement from the outset. In other words, if the experience is not pleasurable, one should expect the volunteer to drop out. The exercise must not be perceived as primarily noxious, and it also must be sufficiently pleasurable to compete successfully with other pleasurable options available to the exerciser.
> (p. 244)

Similarly, Pollock, Wilmore, and Fox (1978) wrote that exercise programs should "meet the criteria for improving and maintaining a sufficient level of physical fitness" but must also be "enjoyable," "rewarding to the participant," and "preferably … fun" (pp. 121–122). The reason is that "people participate in programs they enjoy" (Pollock, 1978, p. 59). Dishman, Sallis, and Orenstein (1985) noted that "feelings of enjoyment and well-being seem to be stronger motives for continued participation" than "knowledge of and belief in the health benefits of physical activity" (p. 162), as well as "more

important to maintaining activity than concerns about health" (p. 166). Later, Dishman (1990) suggested that affective variables are probably more important determinants of physical activity participation in the long run than cognitive variables: "Knowledge and belief in the health benefits of physical activity may motivate initial involvement and return to activity following relapse, but feelings of enjoyment and well-being seem to be stronger motives for continued participation" (p. 83). Along similar lines, Biddle (2000) argued that "how people feel during and after activity may be critical in determining whether they continue. Hence, emotion and mood may be motivational" (p. 269).

Despite such calls, the idea that the pleasure or displeasure that exercisers derive from their participation might influence their subsequent behavior (to continue exercising or drop out) has yet to be fully accepted by a broad circle of researchers within exercise psychology. According to Dishman (2003),

> Though physical activity arguably offers more opportunities for pleasure than do most other health-related behaviors (compared to brushing, flossing, buckling up, and seeing the doctor, for example), we, ironically, have learned very little about intrinsic reinforcements (e.g., enjoyment of physical activity) for continued participation.
> (p. 46)

It is again interesting to note that authors in interdisciplinary fields outside exercise psychology, especially those with close ties between research and practice, have been more active in promoting the idea of an affect–behavior connection than authors within exercise psychology. For example, in cardiac rehabilitation, exercise leaders are urged to pay close attention to such factors as "anxieties from the fear of overexertion causing an event, and attaining enjoyment from the exercise." Otherwise, "the required longer-term changes of behavior for maintaining physical activity at appropriate levels are less likely" (Buckley, 2006, p. 48). Similarly, in physical therapy, researchers and practitioners have noted that patients with chronic pain and fatigue tend to develop a fear of physical movement out of concerns that their symptoms might be exacerbated or their injury might reoccur. This fear, termed "kinesiophobia," has been found to be negatively associated with physical activity and positively associated with self-rated disability (Elfving, Andersson, & Grooten, 2007; Nijs, De Meirleir, & Duquet, 2004).

Missed Clues

The inattention to the motivational implications of affective constructs within exercise psychology contrasts rather sharply with the results of numerous interview-based studies inquiring about the reasons why people adhere to or disengage from exercise. In these studies, themes such as "fun," "pleasure," "energy," and "enjoyment" typically emerge as some of the top reasons people present for adhering to exercise, and conversely themes such as "fear," "pain," "boredom," or "discomfort" emerge as some of the key reasons leading to nonadherence and dropout. Studies yielding such themes have been conducted with children (Kientzler, 1999), adolescents (Daley, Copland, Wright, & Wales, 2008; Flintoff & Scraton, 2001; Loman, 2008), middle-aged adults (Currie, Amos, & Hunt, 1991; Gauvin, 1990; Huberty et al., 2008; Laverie, 1998; Nies & Motyka, 2006; Vanden Auweele, Rzewnicki, & van Mele, 1997), older adults (Fox, Stathi, McKenna, & Davis, 2007; Henderson & Ainsworth, 2003; Lee, Avis, & Arthur, 2007; Lees, Clark, Nigg, & Newman, 2005; O'Brien Cousins, 2000; Wilcox, Oberrecht, Bopp, Kammermann, & McElmurray, 2005), and adults suffering from heart failure (Tierney et al., 2011), arthritis (Hendry, Williams, Markland, Wilkinson, & Maddison, 2006), diabetes (Ferrand, Perrin, & Nasarre, 2008), low back pain (Slade, Molloy, & Keating, 2009), and other conditions (Graham, Kremer, & Wheeler, 2008). According to a review of this literature, affective constructs such as fun and enjoyment "were reported more often as predictors of participation and non-participation than perceived health benefits" (Allender, Cowburn, & Foster, 2006, p. 832).

Moreover, it is fairly well established that affective traits are significantly related to physical activity participation. Depression, trait anxiety, neuroticism, perceived stress, and negative affectivity have been found to predict less activity (e.g., Delahanty, Conroy, & Nathan, 2006; Dergance, Mouton, Lichtenstein, & Hazuda, 2005; Hamid, 1990; Herman et al., 2002; Roshanaei-Moghaddam, Katon, & Russo, 2009; Stetson, Rahn, Dubbert, Wilner, & Mercury, 1997; Yeung & Hemsley, 1997a, 1997b), whereas positive affect has been found to predict more activity (Carels, Coit, Young, & Berger, 2007; Kelsey et al., 2006).

Furthermore, several studies have shown that the pairing of exercise with pleasant or unpleasant affect in one's memory is a significant correlate and predictor of exercise behavior. For example, affective associations (whether respondents associated physical activity with descriptors like "happy," "joy," or "delighted" as opposed to "sad," "sorrow," or "annoyed") not only directly accounted for significant portions of the variance in self-reported physical activity but also mediated the links between cognitive variables (e.g., anticipated benefits and barriers, cognitive attitudes, perceived behavioral control) and physical activity (Kiviniemi, Voss-Humke, & Seifert, 2007). In a study using a priming paradigm to assess automatic evaluations of exercise stimuli (e.g., "athletic" versus "exhausted"), physically active participants responded significantly faster to positive words after exercise primes, whereas inactive participants responded more rapidly to negative words (Bluemke, Brand, Schweizer, & Kahlert, 2010). In another study, the affective component of attitude (rating physical activity and exercise as "enjoyable" versus "not enjoyable") showed much stronger relations (in fact, in most cases, at least twice as strong) with the self-reported frequency of physical activity and exercise a month later than the cognitive component of attitude (rating physical activity and exercise as "beneficial" versus "harmful") (Lawton, Conner, & McEachan, 2009). Another recent study showed that the anticipation of positive (but not negative) affective responses stemming from "successfully engaging in regular physical activity" for 90 days (i.e., "delighted," "happy," "fulfilled," "calm," "relaxed," or "at ease") was associated with a greater likelihood of initiating physical activity for those participants who were inactive and a greater likelihood of continuing participation for those who were already active (Fridlund Dunton & Vaughan, 2008). In a sample of 389 women between the ages of 18 and 68 years, self-reported physical activity was significantly related to the self-conscious emotions of body-related pride ($r = .27$) and shame ($r = -.23$), as well as shame-free guilt ($r = .32$) and guilt-free shame ($r = -.39$) (Sabiston et al., 2010). In children between the ages of 8 and 12 years, the combination of ratings of "liking" (on a visual analog scale ranging from "don't like at all" to "like very much") and evidence of the relative rewarding value of physical activity (i.e., willingness to press a button to obtain access to one's favorite physical activity as opposed to watching a cartoon) was a significant predictor of minutes spent in moderate-to-vigorous physical activity (assessed by accelerometry) during a week (Roemmich et al., 2008). In a sample of psychiatric patients, those who endorsed the statement "exercise gives me pleasure" were 21 times more likely to exercise than those who answered negatively (Sorensen, 2006).

Overall, the inattention to affect as a motivational force in exercise behavior cannot be attributed to a lack of relevant clues in the literature. If one cares to look, the clues are present. If they have not been more widely noticed, this is probably due to the fact that exercise psychology, under the cognitivist paradigm, seems to have become "increasingly rigid" (Kuhn, 1962/1996, p. 64). In other words, the clues have been missed because findings attributing a powerful role to affective influences on behavior simply fall outside the scope of the dominant paradigm of the past decades.

Stumbling Blocks

When a paradigm ascends to the status of "normal science," it starts to dictate an "orthodox" way of thinking that transcends a broad range of domains of academic life, from what is publishable or fundable to what is worth teaching in undergraduate and postgraduate curricula. As more and more generations of students are indoctrinated within an academic culture that endorses the assumption of rationality and models of human behavior based entirely on information processing, alternative or complementary perspectives become marginalized, rejected, or eventually eradicated from the "mainstream" literature. A reflection of this process, as noted earlier, is that most contemporary textbooks in exercise psychology contain nothing on the role of affect in exercise behavior.

Consequently, graduates of exercise science programs have no knowledge about the importance of affect in shaping decisions about exercise and, more importantly, have not been taught how to optimize the affective experiences derived from exercise participation, with the goal of improving long-term adherence to improve the chances of long-term adherence. Instead, they are instructed only to provide information about the benefits associated with exercise participation (e.g., weight loss outcomes) and to boost self-perceptions that are considered relevant (e.g., self-efficacy), along with a few behavioral techniques (e.g., placement of behavioral prompts at points of decision). References to the role of affect in exercise behavior are absent from almost all major recent reviews on mediators of exercise initiation and maintenance, such as the reports of the Task Force on Community Preventive Services (Kahn et al., 2002) and the American Heart Association Council on Nutrition, Physical Activity, and Metabolism (Marcus et al., 2006), as well as from recently proposed theoretical models that focus specifically on exercise behavior

(e.g., Nigg, Borrelli, Maddock, & Dishman, 2008; Schwarzer, 2008).

The marginalization of a potential mechanism in the literature, along with the promotion of theoretical models from which this mechanism is absent or with which this mechanism is seen as incompatible, gradually bring about the elimination of the mechanism from current thinking. Associated concepts and terms are removed from the professional vernacular and forgotten. As the mechanism is given insufficient attention or is altogether ignored, new generations of researchers assume that it either does not exist or does not matter. A weak evidence base weakens the interest of scientists, and in turn weakened interest results in even fewer studies designed to investigate the mechanism, thus perpetuating a vicious cycle. Ultimately, a potentially useful idea may be condemned to obscurity or oblivion.

While reviews have consistently identified enjoyment as a significant correlate of physical activity behavior (Bauman, Sallis, Dzewaltowski, & Owen, 2002; Dishman, 1988, 1990; Dishman et al., 1985; Sallis & Hovell, 1990; Sallis & Owen 1999; Trost, Owen, Bauman, Sallis, & Brown, 2002), at least until recently, if one were to scrutinize the evidence base, one would uncover only weak sources of evidence, such as anecdotal accounts, retrospective surveys, and expert opinions (e.g., Shephard, 1988; Stones, Kozma, & Stones, 1987; Wankel, 1985, 1993). Thus according to a review of factors that mediate physical activity behavior change, "past research provides no support that enjoyment is a mediator of physical activity" (Lewis, Marcus, Pate, & Dunn, 2002, p. 32). The basis for this conclusion was that intervention studies in which enjoyment was examined as a possible mediator of physical activity behavior change showed that enjoyment did not improve as a result of the intervention, regardless of whether physical activity increased or not (Calfas et al., 2000; Neumark-Sztainer, Story, Hannan, Tharp, & Rex, 2003; Nichols et al., 2000; Schneider Jamner, Spruit-Metz, Bassin, & Cooper, 2004). In fact, in some studies the intervention *reduced* enjoyment (Castro, Sallis, Hickman, Lee, & Chen, 1999; Stevens, Lammink, van Heuvelen, de Jong, & Rispens, 2003). Other interventions were observed to reduce perceived autonomy, a theorized powerful mediator of intrinsic motivation (Wilson, Rodgers, Blanchard, & Gessell, 2003). Thus perhaps more than anything else, what the current evidence indicates is that exercise science knows little or nothing about how to enhance the affective experience of physical activity or exercise. Consequently, to date, no intervention studies have been designed to test whether enhancing the affective responses to physical activity or exercise can improve adherence and retention.

Although the literature examining the effects of physical activity or exercise on affective variables (e.g., mood and anxiety) is extensive and continues to grow, the role of these effects in subsequent physical activity or exercise behavior remains largely unexplored. This could be due to a variety of reasons. First, the main objective of most of this research has been to examine the potential of exercise as a safe, inexpensive, and effective method of improving mental health. Until the last decade or so, the relevance of the "feel better" effects of exercise for enhancing intrinsic motivation and adherence had not been given more than cursory consideration.

A second possible reason is that within exercise psychology there is a strong belief that the "feel better" effect is nearly universal. If that were true, there would be no reason to even contemplate a link between exercise-associated affect and subsequent exercise behavior, simply because there would not be enough variability in the postulated predictor to account for the variability in the criterion. Commenting on this issue, Morgan and O'Connor (1988) wrote:

> To argue that people who feel good following exercise would be more likely to adhere than those who do not may be intuitively defensible, but such a view is simplistic because it is quite probable that many or most individuals who discontinue may do so even though they too enjoy an improved mood state following exercise. This hypothesis could be tested empirically but it is probably not necessary because roughly 80% to 90% of individuals in exercise programs report within 8–10 weeks that exercise makes them feel better, but 50% drop out within a few months.
>
> (p. 116)

The "80% to 90%" estimate was based on anecdotal accounts collected after a six-week exercise intervention from a sample of healthy male professors (Morgan, Roberts, Brand, & Feinerman, 1970). This intervention failed to lower self-reported depression, but approximately 85% of the participants "spontaneously volunteered to participate in subsequent exercise studies" because they perceived that they "felt better" (p. 216). However, the validity of this figure can be questioned given the susceptibility of retrospective accounts to bias (Henry, Moffitt, Caspi, Langley, & Silva, 1994).

Rethinking the Exercise–Affect Link

Researchers in recent years have started to place the exercise–affect connection under a new, more critical light. Reexamining this issue has necessitated an overhaul of the conceptual and methodological approach on which previous studies were based. The fundamental assumption behind the new approach was that the exercise–affect relationship is more intricate and multifaceted than just the "feel better" effect. This includes the possibility that some individuals may not feel better when they exercise and that some may even feel worse. As de Geus and de Moor (2008) put it, "we need to reach out to these people through other means than just repeating over and over that 'exercise will make you feel better'" (p. 58).

The first step was to rebuild the methodological platform to ensure that any nonpositive affective changes would not escape detection (Backhouse, Ekkekakis, Biddle, Foskett, & Williams, 2007; Ekkekakis, Parfitt, & Petruzzello, 2011; Ekkekakis & Petruzzello, 1999). This required (a) implementing a measurement approach that encompasses negative in addition to positive affective states, (b) tracking affective changes throughout the entire exercise episode, including the duration of the exercise bout itself, as well as the recovery period, (c) increasing statistical power by reducing error variance due to incomplete standardization of exercise intensity across participants, and (d) examining changes at the level of individuals and subgroups rather than exclusively at the level of group means.

The second step was to develop a new, broad theoretical framework that goes beyond the "feel better" effect and acknowledges the possibility of negative effects and individual variability, makes testable predictions about dose–response patterns, and postulates a specific mechanistic basis. This new framework has been named the dual-mode theory (Ekkekakis, 2003, 2005, 2009a; Ekkekakis & Acevedo, 2006; Ekkekakis, Hall, & Petruzzello, 2005b). From the perspective of this theory, affective responses to exercise are considered evolutionary adaptations, shaped through natural selection to promote Darwinian fitness within the specific context of exercise. The theory postulates that affective responses to exercise are determined by the continuous interplay between two factors, namely "top-down" cognitive parameters (e.g., appraisals of physical self-efficacy and self-presentational concerns) and "bottom-up" interoceptive cues (e.g., signals from chemoreceptors, baroreceptors, thermoreceptors, mechanoreceptors, and various visceroceptors in the heart, lungs, and internal organs). The relative importance of these two factors is theorized to change systematically as a function of exercise intensity. Specifically, cognitive factors are expected to be the dominant determinants of affect at intensities below and (mainly) near the ventilatory or lactate threshold (VT/LT), where the intensity begins to pose a challenge. On the other hand, interoceptive cues will gain greater salience at intensities that significantly exceed the VT/LT and a physiological steady state becomes difficult or impossible to maintain.

Within the framework of the dual-mode theory, affective responses to different levels of exercise intensity must be meaningfully linked to the adaptational outcomes associated with these intensities. Specifically, exercise performed at a level of intensity below the VT/LT can be sustained for a long time without causing major homeostatic perturbations and without threatening general health and well-being (assuming a healthy organism). Moreover, given the ability to carry out such activity for prolonged periods, it is reasonable to conclude that this is probably the level of physical exertion that was most common in ancestral environments characterized by hunting and gathering activities occupying large parts of daily life. Since these subsistence activities directly affected survival and the ability to find mates and raise viable children (i.e., the two components of Darwinian fitness), it is reasonable to suggest that a mechanism might have evolved to promote or reward such activities. The most likely candidate for providing such a reward is pleasure (Cabanac, 1992, 2002, 2006, 2010; Panksepp, 1998). This is not an implausible argument, since it is readily accepted in regard to the pleasure that accompanies other human activities of significant adaptational value, such as eating appetizing food when hungry, drinking fresh water when thirsty, or engaging in sexual relationships (e.g., Berridge & Kringelbach, 2008; Denton, McKinley, Farrell, & Eagan, 2009). Thus the dual-mode theory predicts that exercise intensities below the VT/LT should be associated with increases in pleasure among the majority of participants.

Consistent with this prediction, exercise bouts performed below the VT/LT have been shown to improve affect at the level of entire groups (e.g., Bixby, Spalding, & Hatfield, 2001) or at least within subgroups (e.g., Ekkekakis, Hall, & Petruzzello, 2008; Parfitt, Rose, & Burgess, 2006; Rose & Parfitt, 2007). Especially when walking at a self-selected

pace, most individuals tend to report increases in pleasure and energy (Ekkekakis, 2009c; Ekkekakis, Backhouse, Gray, & Lind, 2008; Ekkekakis, Hall, Van Landuyt, & Petruzzello, 2000). A meta-analysis (Reed & Ones, 2006) showed that the average effect size for the improvement in states that combine pleasure with high perceived activation (e.g., energy or vigor) was nearly twice as high ($d = 0.57$) in studies that employed low intensity (15–39% VO_2 reserve) than studies that employed moderate ($d = 0.35$, 40–59% VO_2 reserve) or high intensity ($d = 0.31$, 60–85% VO_2 reserve).

An exception to this general trend is seen when the individuals involved in exercise are chronically inactive, obese, or both (e.g., Ekkekakis, Lind, & Vazou, 2010; Sheppard & Parfitt, 2008; Welch, Hulley, Ferguson, & Beauchamp, 2007). These physical and lifestyle characteristics render such individuals evolutionary rarities, but unfortunately they now represent the majority of the population in industrialized countries. Among such samples, a decline in pleasure is found even when the intensity is below the VT/LT. Both physical and cognitive mechanisms may account for this finding. Physically, the performance of a body long subjected to sedentary living and further burdened by excess adiposity may be limited by factors besides the cardiorespiratory system. These may include joint stiffness, muscle atrophy, knee and backaches, or ineffective thermoregulation. Likewise, these individuals may cognitively appraise the exercise stimulus in conjunction with the exercise context as posing an evaluative threat. Individuals who are out of shape, overweight, or both are usually aware of their physical condition and appearance, especially in comparison with idealized normative standards. Thus they may feel apprehensive when placed in a situation in which their poor state is likely to be noticed and criticized by others (e.g., in a crowded gymnasium or during an exercise test in a laboratory). These physical and cognitive mechanisms may influence affective responses throughout the entire range of exercise intensity, including below the VT/LT.

When the intensity of physical activity reaches the VT/LT, it starts to pose a substantial physiological challenge to most individuals, regardless of their physical condition. Displeasure is the vehicle by which significant physiological perturbations enter conscious awareness (Cabanac, 2006). Data about the physiological state of the organism are no longer handled only by automatic regulatory loops that operate largely outside conscious awareness but also begin to generate increasingly salient negative affective experiences. These data, which include acidosis (a drop of pH), hyperventilation, secretion of stress hormones (i.e., epinephrine and cortisol), and numerous other changes, once they exceed critical thresholds, act as "danger signals," and physiological challenges thus become affective challenges. Information about the physiological condition of the body is continuously collected by primary afferent neurons throughout the body and forwarded to the brain via spinal pathways and the vagus nerve (Craig, 2002, 2006).

What probably differentiates intensities near the VT/LT from intensities that exceed the VT/LT is that the intensification of these signals causes additional neural gates to open, allowing this information to reach levels beyond the homeostatic areas of the brain stem, medulla, and hypothalamus. Areas known to be involved in the processing of aversive bodily cues and the generation of affective responses include the amygdala, the insula, and the periaqueductal gray (Cameron, 2009; Carretié, Albert, López-Martín, & Tapia, 2009; Ekkekakis & Acevedo, 2006). As with all varieties of negative affect, the generation of negative affective reactions to exercise calls forth cognitive mechanisms, most likely situated in parts of the anterior cingulate and prefrontal cortices, aimed at controlling this negative response (Feldman Barrett, Mesquita, Ochsner, & Gross, 2007; Ochsner & Gross, 2005, 2008).

The effectiveness of these cortical regulatory mechanisms in controlling negative affective responses depends on an individual's developmental history (i.e., the learning of such coping skills as reappraisal, suppression, or attentional distraction) and on genetically determined individual differences in neural parameters that provide the biological substrate of cognitive control (such as differences in the anatomical size of cortical areas, receptor density, or level of oxygenation; see Hariri & Forbes, 2007). As a result of these differences, some individuals will be more effective in regulating negative affect than others. In turn, these differences may influence the level of exercise intensity than an individual prefers or can tolerate (de Geus & de Moor, 2008; Ekkekakis, 2008; Ekkekakis, Hall, & Petruzzello, 2005a). Thus the dual-mode theory predicts that at intensities proximal to the VT/LT, affective responses will vary, with some individuals reporting increases and others decreases in pleasure.

From an evolutionary standpoint, variable affective responses signal the absence of a direct or unambiguous role in adaptation, including the possibility that the response entails a trade-off between benefits and risks. In the case of exercise, the ability to control negative affect in the presence of a homeostatic perturbation probably entails such a trade-off. On the one hand, being able to do more work (e.g., cover more ground in pursuit of prey) or being able to continue working under environmentally adverse conditions yields an evolutionary advantage; one is more likely to be a reliable provider of nourishment for oneself, one's mate, and one's progeny. On the other hand, consistently "pushing the envelope" by bringing the organism close to its biological limits is tantamount to challenging one's fate. Given the low tolerance of many physiological systems to deviations from normalcy (e.g., hyper- or hypothermia, metabolic acidosis, or myocardial or cerebrovascular ischemia), operating near the limit raises the risk of sudden death or an incapacitating injury. Therefore, on balance, the ability to regulate the negative affective response to exercise at intensities proximal to the VT/LT is probably neither consistently advantageous nor consistently harmful.

Consistent with theoretical predictions, affective changes at intensities proximal to the VT/LT have been shown to be highly variable (Ekkekakis et al., 2005b; Ekkekakis, Hall, & Petruzzello, 2008; Parfitt et al., 2006; Rose & Parfitt, 2007; Welch et al., 2007). Self-reported individual differences in preference for and tolerance of exercise intensity have been found to account for approximately 20–25% of the variance in ratings of pleasure vs. displeasure during exercise performed at the VT (Ekkekakis et al., 2005a). Similarly, individual differences in situational appraisals of exercise self-efficacy have been found to account for approximately 20–30% of the variance in affective valence at this intensity (Ekkekakis, 2003).

When exercise intensity substantially exceeds the VT/LT and a physiological steady state can no longer be maintained, the adaptational implications are unambiguous: This level of exercise intensity is not only unsustainable but also risky. Exercise must soon stop or the intensity must be reduced to avoid collapse, a system-wide bioenergetic crisis, and possibly irreparable harm. For this to happen, the affective directive to consciousness must be intense, immediate, unequivocal, and irrepressible. Much like intense pain, a strong negative affective response to strenuous exercise has evolved to act as a lifesaver, a fail-safe mechanism that protects the health and long-term well-being of the individual by causing an immediate behavioral withdrawal from the precipitating stimulus. Thus the dual-mode theory predicts a universal decline in pleasure when exercise intensity exceeds the VT/LT and precludes the maintenance of a physiological steady state.

Consistent with this prediction, there is compelling evidence of declines in pleasure above the VT/LT (Bixby et al., 2001; Bixby & Lochbaum, 2006; Ekkekakis, Hall, & Petruzzello, 2008; Kilpatrick Kraemer, Bartholomew, Acevedo, & Jarreau, 2007; Rose & Parfitt, 2007; Sheppard & Parfitt, 2008). Such declines are reported by all or nearly all individuals. Moreover, at such intensities reports of affective valence develop strong negative correlations with markers of physiological strain such as oxygen uptake, level of lactate accumulation, and the respiratory exchange ratio (e.g., Acevedo, Kraemer, Haltom, & Tryniecki, 2003; Acevedo, Rinehardt, & Kraemer, 1994; Ekkekakis, 2003; Hardy & Rejeski, 1989). These findings suggest a transition to a mode of affect generation in which affective responses become a direct reflection of the perturbed internal environment. As the dual-mode theory predicts, the interoceptive cues evidently become the dominant determinants of the affective state.

Initially it was believed that this might happen as a result of the intensification of these interoceptive cues at supra-VT/LT intensities (Ekkekakis & Acevedo, 2006). For example, as ventilation becomes deeper and more frequent, core temperature rises, and the muscles become more acidic, the corresponding afferent cues might simply overpower the top-down prefrontal control over the affective centers of the brain. More recently, however, an additional possibility emerged. In neuroimaging studies, it was observed that "when humans have strong affective experiences, higher cortical regions tend to shut down" (Panksepp & Panksepp, 2000, p. 115). In both acute (e.g., induction of transient emotions by various experimental manipulations) and chronic paradigms (e.g., depressed patients or individuals suffering from posttraumatic stress), various subdivisions of the prefrontal cortex (often bilaterally) show reduced metabolic activity, usually in conjunction with increased activity in the amygdala (Quirk & Beer, 2006). Although neuroimaging during vigorous exercise with a method that provides good temporal and spatial resolution, such as functional magnetic resonance, remains technically unfeasible, approximately 30 studies using near-infrared spectroscopy of the prefrontal cortex have shown an increase in oxygenation with low-to-moderate levels of exercise intensity but a decrease with high exercise intensity, particularly beyond the respiratory compensation point (see Ekkekakis, 2009b, for a review). These findings suggest that the intensification of the bodily signals at intensities above the VT/LT might not be the only mechanism that precipitates the "switch" to a mode of affect induction in which interoceptive cues become the dominant determinants. A complementary mechanism might consist of a transient hypometabolism in the prefrontal cortex, the main neural substrate for the regulation of negative affect. The existence of such a mechanism would make adaptational sense, inasmuch as the mediation or control of affect by cognition could introduce distortions in the relationship between the homeostatic perturbation and the negative affective response. The vital importance of this mechanism can be appreciated if one considers what would happen if it did not exist: The "effective" use of a cognitive coping technique, if taken to extremes, would result in death.

If this mechanism is confirmed, it could have important practical implications. It would mean that an exerciser's capacity to cognitively modify his or her affective response during exercise above the VT/LT would be diminished, regardless of the level of experience in using cognitive techniques. For example, an exerciser might be taught to cognitively reframe (reappraise) the unpleasant affective responses as signs of a body that is getting stronger, to counter the negative affect with a bolstered appraisal of efficacy, or to divert his or her attention away from the unpleasant bodily sensations and toward a distracting external stimulus (e.g., a music or television program). These interventions, all cognitive in nature (i.e., manipulating the input and interpretation of information relevant to the affective state), might maintain their effectiveness in influencing the affective response only up to the level of exercise intensity that precipitates a decline in prefrontal oxygenation. The few studies that have examined the role of exercise intensity in the effectiveness of cognitive techniques in influencing subjective responses to exercise support this notion (see Lind, Welch, & Ekkekakis, 2009, for a review).

In closing this section, it is important to underscore that exercise intensity is certainly not the only variable that can influence affective responses. Research has uncovered a multitude of additional variables that play a role, including the sense of efficacy (e.g., Jerome et al., 2002), the satisfaction of basic psychological needs (e.g., Wilson, Mack, Blanchard, & Gray, 2009), self-presentational concerns (e.g., Focht & Hausenblas, 2006; Martin Ginis, Burke, & Gauvin, 2007), and exercise leader behavior (e.g., Loughhead, Patterson, & Carron, 2008).

Some Realistic Examples to Bring Things into Perspective

When discussing vigorous or strenuous exercise, one might tend to visualize Olympic-caliber athletes and herculean-scale athletic endeavors, such as running a marathon. However, it is crucial to remember how relative the concept of intensity is. To bring things into perspective, consider an example of a 45-year-old woman who decides to reinitiate physical activity after a couple of decades of mostly sedentary living due to work or family obligations. Let us assume that she presents with a body mass index of 30 kg/m^2 (on the cusp between being categorized as overweight or obese), a maximal oxygen uptake of 18 ml·kg^{-1}·min^{-1}, and a VT at 55% of maximal aerobic capacity (i.e., at approximately 10 ml·kg^{-1}·min^{-1}). These are typical values for middle-aged sedentary women (e.g., see Ekkekakis & Lind, 2006; Ekkekakis et al., 2010). These numbers suggest that the woman in this example would reach her VT at less than three metabolic equivalents (METs) and her maximal capacity at approximately five METs.

A juxtaposition of these values with the Compendium of Physical Activities (Ainsworth et al., 2011) suffices to illustrate the enormous challenge of exercise prescription with this typical individual. Activities corresponding to 2.8 METs (sufficient to reach VT) include standing, light play with children, or a slow walk (2.5 mph), but only on a downhill slope. An intensity of 4.0 METs (close to 80% of maximal capacity and probably close to the respiratory compensation point or the maximal lactate steady state) corresponds to such activities as bicycling slowly (<10 mph), doing water calisthenics, sweeping the garage or the sidewalk, walking or running intermittently at a moderate pace while playing with children, or raking the lawn and sacking leaves. As these examples illustrate, for many (perhaps most) sedentary middle-aged or older individuals, a level of exercise intensity that exceeds the VT/LT corresponds to nothing more than common everyday tasks and is certainly far from anything involving herculean effort.

According to the results of recent studies on the exercise–affect link, the woman in the example would not only feel worse while performing an activity as seemingly innocuous as raking and sacking leaves (Ekkekakis et al., 2010) but might also be unable to cognitively control this negative affective response. While it seems reasonable to publicly proclaim that physical activity should be "enjoyable" to be maintained, exercise scientists are only now beginning to come to terms with the magnitude of the challenge inherent in making this proclamation a reality for the majority of sedentary adults.

Most exercise guidelines still appear strangely oblivious to this challenge. For example, according to the data from the 2000 Behavioral Risk Factor Surveillance System, no more than 3.0% of obese women and 6.4% of obese men trying to lose weight report engaging in physical activity of at least 60 minutes daily (which is what current guidelines recommend) in addition to restricting their caloric intake (Bish et al., 2005). One might start to wonder about the true public health relevance of a recommendation that almost no one seems willing (or able) to follow.

Perhaps the following data might provide an indication of the magnitude of the challenge faced by exercise practinioners. The American College of Sports Medicine (2010) recommends that the initial intensity of activity for obese adults be no more than 40–60% of maximal oxygen uptake reserve. Over time, obese adults are encouraged to exercise for 60–90 minutes. While designing a study to investigate the affective responses of sedentary obese women, Ekkekakis and colleagues (2010) needed to identify a level of treadmill speed that would be appropriate as a warm-up. According to previous studies by Browning and Kram (2005) and Browning, Baker, Herron, and Kram (2006), obese middle-aged women self-select treadmill speeds of approximately 1.40 m/s. Therefore, Ekkekakis et al. set the warm-up speed below this level, at 1.11 m/s (2.50 mph), with the grade at 0%. The obese women in the sample (with an average age of 44.7 years and average body mass index of 35 kg/m^2) had already reached 61% of their maximal aerobic capacity after walking at this speed for only 2 minutes. These results are not unique. The 55 obese women tested by Mattsson, Larsson, and Rössner (1997), who were more physically active and fit than the women in the study by Ekkekakis et al. (2010), approached the upper limit of the recommended intensity range (56% VO$_2$max) after walking at a self-selected "comfortable" speed (1.18 m/s, or 2.65 mph) for only 4 minutes. Therefore, at least while performing weight-bearing activities such as walking, obese women seem unable to maintain a physiological steady state within the recommended range of 40–60% of maximal oxygen uptake reserve. Even within 2–4 minutes, the intensity will probably exceed 60% and, in all likelihood, the VT. Thus it is perhaps unsurprising that obese women report no increase in pleasure in response to exercise

(Ekkekakis et al., 2010) or that they are highly unlikely to satisfy the current recommendation of 60 minutes of daily moderate-intensity physical activity (Bish et al., 2005).

Are Affective Responses Related to Subsequent Physical Activity Behavior?

In previous sections, it was shown that (a) exercise, depending on its intensity, can reduce pleasure and (b) different individuals exhibit different affective changes in response to exercise. It is important to reiterate that these are recent findings. Before the last decade or so, neither the variability of affective responses nor the fact that people can feel worse during (intense) exercise had been demonstrated reliably (Van Landuyt, Ekkekakis, Hall, & Petruzzello, 2000). Both of these elements are crucial, because if the only effect of exercise were to increase pleasure and if this effect were shared by all, or nearly all, people, then there would be no reason to examine whether affective responses could account for behavioral variance. So these recent findings have laid the foundation for the examination of the role of affective responses in subsequent physical activity and exercise behavior.

The implications of the "feel worse" effect documented by several of the studies reviewed above should be considered in the context of the observation that what seems to determine whether an activity registers in memory as pleasant or unpleasant is not necessarily the absolute level of pleasure but rather "the change (for better or worse) that it represents, and how it compares with alternative outcomes" (Varey & Kahneman, 1992, p. 179), such as those associated with sedentary behaviors. In other words, if an exercise bout makes people feel worse (less pleasure) than they did before the bout (even if they do not rate the affect during exercise as "bad") or if exercise makes people feel less pleasure than alternative options (e.g., watching television or playing video games), this suffices to reduce the likelihood of exercise being their preferred behavioral option.

With evidence of variability in affective responses to exercise, including a "feel worse" effect, investigating whether affective responses to exercise are related to exercise participation seems fully warranted. As shown in Table 16.1, this question has so far been addressed in 11 known studies. While studies conducted in recent years have tended to be more conceptually and methodologically sophisticated than those conducted in the 1990s, it is clear that this line of research is still developing and is still exploring the best avenues for accomplishing its goal. For example, in some studies affect was assessed in terms of a few distinct states, whereas in others it was assessed in terms of broad dimensions. In some studies the intensity of exercise was determined by perceptions of exertion, in others as a percentage of maximal capacity, and in others in relation to the VT. In some studies physical activity was defined by the number of gymnasium visits (i.e., session attendance), whereas in others it was defined as total free-living activity. Of the studies in the latter category, in some cases activity was assessed by a standardized questionnaire or interview, in others by nonvalidated rating scales, and in others by accelerometry. So clearly the standards of "best practice" are still evolving.

It is also important to point out that all the studies in this area have been correlational (although, to their credit, most have been prospective rather than cross-sectional). Given how little is known about possible methods of improving affective responses to exercise, especially among high-risk groups such as individuals who are sedentary, obese, or in less than perfect health, it is perhaps not surprising that no studies so far have attempted any experimental manipulations of the affective responses with the purpose of assessing their mediational effects on physical activity participation, exercise adherence, or dropout. Perhaps the most obvious candidate for such a manipulation would be the intensity of exercise, since more information is available about this independent variable than any other (Ekkekakis et al., 2011).

The 11 studies summarized in Table 16.1 provide preliminary support for a link between affective responses and exercise behavior. Most notably, the most recent studies, which incorporated several conceptual and methodological innovations, all found evidence of statistically significant associations between affective responses and measures of exercise behavior (Kwan & Bryan, 2010; Schneider, Dunn, & Cooper, 2009; Williams et al., 2008). The common characteristic of these recent studies is that they all included assessments of affect during the exercise bouts. Although the treatment of these data differed among studies (i.e., as absolute scores, as changes from baseline, or as individual linear slopes over time), as did the measures of affect that were used (i.e., a single-item rating scale of pleasure–displeasure or a multi-item questionnaire), these studies support the idea that affective responses during exercise are more variable and perhaps more closely linked to decisions regarding

Table 16.1 Studies Examining the Relation between Affective Responses to Bouts of Exercise and Exercise Participation, Adherence, or Attendance

Study	Sample	Design	Measure	Findings
Annesi, 2002a	69 (20 men, 49 women), mean age 37.9 years (range 20–61 years)	Prospective, 14-week intervention	EFI	Attendance ranged from 17% to 100%. Changes in EFI scores from before to after sessions during weeks 1, 3, 5, 8, 11, and 14 were averaged for each participant. For a subsample ($n = 24$) with low self-motivation, there were significant correlations between attendance and changes in Positive Engagement (.48), Revitalization (.47), Tranquility (.41), and Physical Exhaustion (-.62). However, for participants with medium self-motivation, the correlations were nonsignificant, and for those with high self-motivation, the correlations were in the opposite direction. Change scores in EFI subscales accounted for less than 1% of the variance in attendance but the interactions with self-motivation were significant ($R^2 = .23$ for Positive Engagement; .22 for Revitalization; .20 for Tranquility; .27 for Physical Exhaustion).
Annesi, 2002b	72 (32 men, 40 women), mean age 37.6 years (range 21–54 years)	Prospective, 15-week intervention	EFI	Attendance ranged from 17% to 100%. Changes in EFI scores from before to after nine sessions (one every 3 weeks) were averaged for each participant. Participants were then classified as showing a positive ($n = 36$) or a nonpositive ($n = 36$) pattern of change on the EFI overall (where positive meant increases in Positive Engagement, Revitalization, and Tranquility, and a decrease in Physical Exhaustion) or only on the Physical Exhaustion subscale (42 positive and 30 nonpositive). The positive or nonpositive pattern of change in the EFI overall or in the Physical Exhaustion subscale explained less than 1% of the variance in attendance. However, controlling for differences in self-motivation raised these percentages to 10% (significant) and 7% (nonsignificant), respectively.
Annesi, 2005	66 (20 men, 46 women), mean age 38.2 years (range 22–60 years)	Prospective, 14-week intervention	EFI	Both attendance (%) and the numbers of days until cessation of exercise (for 4 consecutive weeks) were monitored. A six-item scale was constructed based on the EFI by summing the Revitalization and reversed Physical Exhaustion item scores. This scale was administered before and after 6 exercise sessions (weeks 2, 4, 6, 8, 10, and 12). Attendance ranged from 24% to 100%. One-third of the participants dropped out, and length of adherence ranged from 21 to 98 days. On average, participants reported positive changes on the six-item scale in 73.2% of their exercise sessions (range from 0% to 100%). The percentage of sessions with positive changes correlated significantly with session attendance (.36) and with length of adherence (.37).

(Continued)

Table 16.1 (Continued)

Study	Sample	Design	Measure	Findings
Annesi, 2006	50 women, mean age 38.8 years (range 22–60 years)	Prospective, 12-week intervention	EFI	Only the Revitalization and Physical Exhaustion subscales of the EFI were included. Changes from before to after 6 exercise sessions (weeks 1, 3, 5, 7, 9, and 11) were averaged for each participant. An aggregate score was also derived by summing the Revitalization and reversed Physical Exhaustion scores. Increases in Revitalization were reported by 38 women (76%), and decreases in Physical Exhaustion were reported by 34 women (68%). Attendance ranged from 29% to 100%. Changes in both Revitalization (.31) and Physical Exhaustion (−.28) were significantly related to attendance. Attendance was also significantly predicted by the combination of changes in Revitalization (but not Physical Exhaustion) with both self-motivation (R^2 = .12) and with perceived physical condition (R^2 = .13). Using changes in the aggregate Revitalization–Exhaustion score increased the percentages of predicted variance (R^2 = .19 and .17, respectively).
Berger, Darby, Owen, & Carels, 2010	32 obese, sedentary women (25 completed the program, 7 dropped out)	Prospective, 6-month behavioral weight loss intervention	POMS	Among women who completed the program, the intervention did not alter the changes in the POMS factor scores from before to after a graded exercise test. These mood changes were also unrelated to the duration of the exercise tests or the changes in body mass, body mass index, percentage body fat, or exercise enjoyment. The 7 dropouts showed mood changes in opposite directions from those of the 25 completers (increases in tension, depression, anger, fatigue, and confusion and a decrease in vigor; also, a larger increase in fatigue).
Berger & Owen, 1992	87 college students (59 intervention, 28 control)	Prospective, 14-week intervention	POMS, STAI	Students completed the POMS and STAI before and after workouts (swimming and yoga classes) on weeks 1, 6, and 12. A mean change score was computed by subtracting postexercise from pre-exercise scores on the 6 POMS scales and STAI and adding the difference scores from the three assessments. Students attended 91% of the classes. The scores of the six POMS subscales and STAI were used as predictors and the number of absences from class was used as the criterion in a multiple regression. More positive changes significantly predicted fewer absences (R = .49).

Author	Sample	Design	Measure	Results
Carels, Berger, & Darby, 2006	25 obese, sedentary, postmenopausal women, mean age 53.9 years	6-month behavioral weight loss intervention	POMS	The women completed the POMS before and after a graded submaximal exercise test (up to about 75% of age-predicted heart rate reserve) performed at the beginning and end of a weight loss intervention. Change scores in POMS subscales were computed by subtracting postexercise scores from pre-exercise scores. After controlling for income, education, change in body mass index during the intervention, and physical activity or VO_2max at baseline, changes in mood were not significantly related to physical activity (assessed by accelerometry, diaries, or questionnaire) or VO_2max at the end of the intervention. However, women who reported more time in planned exercise (assessed by diary) during the middle and final 8 weeks of the intervention reported more pretest (.54, .57) and posttest vigor (.51, .68) and less posttest confusion (-.58, -.67). Similarly, women who reported more postexercise fatigue (-.60) reported less time in planned exercise during the final 8 weeks. No mood states were significantly correlated with calories expended in leisure-time physical activity (assessed by questionnaire or accelerometry). Contrary to hypotheses, women who reported more posttest depression and anger had higher postintervention VO_2max after controlling for baseline VO_2max.
Klonoff, Annechild & Landrine, 1994	23 women	Prospective, 10-week intervention	9-point scales of happiness, euphoria	Before and after an initial aerobics class, the women were asked, "How happy are you?" and "How euphoric are you?" on 9-point rating scales ranging from "Not at all" to "Extremely." Increases were reported on both scales (from 6.18 to 7.45 and from 4.38 to 6.31). Three classes were offered each weekday for 10 weeks (total of 123 possible sessions). Of these, the women attended on average 10.3 sessions (approximately 1 per week) but with great interindividual differences. Paradoxically, attending more sessions was associated with higher anxiety (.42), more reported physical symptoms (.56), and higher body weight (.52). Changes in happiness, euphoria, and the average of the two scales were unrelated to the number of exercise sessions attended. Similarly, blood levels of beta-endorphin and changes in these levels from before to after the initial exercise session were unrelated to attendance.
Kwan & Bryan, 2010	129 nonsedentary, nonathletic adults (62 men, 67 women), mean age 22.4 years	Baseline assessment and 3-month follow-up	PAAS	A measure of the frequency of physical activity was derived by standardizing and averaging the participants' reports of (a) how often they engaged in aerobic exercise in the past 3 months, (b) the average number of days per week they engaged in aerobic exercise in the past 3 months, and (c) how many days they engaged in aerobic exercise in the past week. The PAAS was administered at minutes 5, 10, 20, and 30 of a 30-min treadmill bout at 65% VO_2max and minutes 15 and 30 of recovery. On average, the participants reported increases in positive affect and decreases in negative affect, tranquility, and exhaustion during exercise. Post exercise, positive affect and tranquility increased, whereas negative affect and fatigue decreased. The participants reported 3.83 days of aerobic exercise per week at baseline and 3.60 days at 3-month follow-up. Larger increases in positive affect and larger decreases in exhaustion during exercise were associated with more frequent aerobic exercise at follow-up (3% and 6% of the variance, respectively) after controlling for pre-exercise affect and baseline level of vigorous physical activity. Similarly, more tranquility and less fatigue at minute 15 of recovery were related to more frequent aerobic exercise at follow-up (5% and 4% of the variance, respectively).

(Continued)

Table 16.1 (Continued)

Study	Sample	Design	Measure	Findings
Schneider et al., 2009	124 adolescents (67 boys, 57 girls), mean age 14.78 years (range 14–16 years)	Cross-sectional, correlational	FS	The participants completed one 30-min cycle-ergometer ride at 80% of the ventilatory threshold (VT) and another at 50% of the distance between VT and VO_2max. Physical activity was assessed by accelerometry over one week. For the participants who wore the accelerometers for at least 8 hours per day on at least 4 days, the proportion of days on which the participant did at least 60 min of moderate-to-vigorous physical activity (MVPA) was calculated. Boys met this criterion on 32% of the days and girls on 17%. Changes in FS from baseline to the average of minutes 10 and 20 during exercise and to the average of minutes 0 and 10 of postexercise recovery were also calculated. The 22% of participants with improved FS scores during sub-VT exercise averaged 54.25 min of daily MVPA, the 22% with no change averaged 46.94 min, and the 56% with declines averaged 39.83 min. Moreover, participants with improved FS scores met the 60-min/day guideline on 36% of days, compared with 22% of those with declines or no change. After controlling for aerobic fitness and sex, a 1-unit increase in FS during exercise was associated with 4.18 min of additional daily MVPA ($R^2 = .03$), 3.23 min of additional moderate activity ($R^2 = .03$), and a 5% increase in the number of days meeting the 60-min/day guideline ($R^2 = .06$). Changes in FS during supra-VT exercise and changes from before to after exercise were not significantly related to physical activity.
Williams et al., 2008	37 sedentary adults (8 men, 29 women), mean age 43.92 years	Prospective, with 6-month and 12-month follow-ups	FS	The FS was administered every 2 min during a submaximal treadmill protocol (up to 85% of age-predicted maximal heart rate). The first FS scores after the participants reached 64% of age-predicted maximal heart rate were recorded; 27.0% reported an increase, 29.7% a decline, and 43.2% no change. Only 31 participants completed assessments of physical activity (physical activity recall interview) at the 6- and 12-month follow-ups. FS scores during moderate intensity were significantly correlated with physical activity at the 6-month (.50) and 12 month (.47) follow-ups. The relationships remained significant after controlling for baseline levels of physical activity and baseline FS. A 1-unit increase in FS was associated with 38 additional minutes of at least moderate physical activity per week at the 6-month follow-up and 41 additional minutes per week at the 12-month follow-up.

Note. EFI = Exercise-induced Feeling Scale (Gauvin & Rejeski, 1993); FS = Feeling Scale (Hardy & Rejeski, 1989); PAAS = Physical Activity Affect Scale (Lox, Jackson, Tuholski, Wasley, & Treasure, 2000); POMS = Profile of Mood States (McNair, Lorr, & Droppleman, 1970); STAI = State–Trait Anxiety Inventory (Spielberger, Gorsuch, & Lushene, 1970).

subsequent exercise behavior than postexercise responses.

For example, Schneider et al. (2009) reported that during a 30-minute bout of exercise at 80% of the VT, 22% of their adolescent participants reported increases in pleasure, 22% reported no change, and 56% reported decreases. These variable changes were significantly related to moderate-to-vigorous free-living physical activity, moderate-intensity physical activity, and the proportion of days that the adolescents satisfied the current recommendation of 60 minutes of physical activity daily (with betas of .18, .17, and .24, respectively). In contrast, changes from before to after the exercise bout were considerably less variable, with 90% reporting increases in pleasure, 4% reporting no change, and 6% reporting decreases. Not surprisingly, these relatively more homogeneous changes were unrelated to physical activity. Similarly, when the intensity was set so high (50% of the distance between VT and VO_2max) that 85% of the participants felt worse during exercise, the affective changes were again unrelated to physical activity.

These data complement the results of a meta-analysis on the relation between enjoyment-related constructs and physical activity. Specifically, Rhodes, Fiala, and Conner (2009) analyzed studies in which the correlate of physical activity was enjoyment, intrinsic motivation, or the affective component of attitude measured separately from the cognitive or instrumental component. Despite the different labels given to these constructs, they are all assessed by questions referring to whether respondents find physical activity enjoyable, likable, or fun to do. Rhodes et al. collectively called these constructs "affective judgments," a new term with clear cognitive connotations that the authors defined as referring to "*judgments* about the overall pleasure/displeasure, enjoyment, and feeling states expected from enacting physical activity" (p. 181, italics added). According to Rhodes et al., "core affect or generalized feeling states" (i.e., the immediate and short-term affective responses examined in this section) do not belong in this category (p. 182). Nevertheless, these "affective judgments" had an average correlation of $r = .38$ with physical activity participation. Rhodes et al. concluded that this renders these enjoyment-related constructs among the strongest known correlates of physical activity behavior (at least on par with self-efficacy and stronger than the built-environment, social, sociodemographic, and personality variables). Although enjoyment is a broad and multifarious construct, it

is important to note that it shows significant overlap with affective responses to exercise (Focht, 2009; Motl, Berger, & Leuschen, 2000; Raedeke, 2007; Robbins, Pis, Pender, & Kazanis, 2004).

Setting the Stage for a Hedonic Theory of Exercise Behavior

The central theme of this chapter is that the "affect heuristic" might be a powerful, albeit currently underappreciated and underexploited, mechanism that shapes the decision to remain physically active or to drop out. As more information accumulates on the influence of exercise on pleasure and displeasure, the basic idea of an affect–behavior link will have to be elaborated upon and developed into a formal, testable theory of exercise behavior. The main objective of this chapter was to set the stage for this advance. In conjunction with other recent works (Backhouse et al., 2007; Ekkekakis, Hall, & Petruzzello, 2008; Parfitt & Hughes, 2009; Williams, 2008), the evidence discussed in the previous sections supports the development of a model of behavioral decision making that explicitly acknowledges and incorporates affective influences.

As suggested previously, perhaps the main reason for the inattention to the role of affect in theoretical efforts to predict and explain exercise behavior has been the dominating influence of the cognitivist zeitgeist. In a classic article, Loewenstein (1996) made a similar point. He argued that decision-making approaches based on the assumption of rationality fall short in the treatment of motivation and effort because they fail to take into account the impact of affective or visceral factors. In his words, such approaches make "no qualitative distinction between choosing, say one car over another, or 'deciding' to pick up one's pace in the last mile of a marathon; both are simply decisions" (p. 287). As an example, he noted that because of the tendency to underestimate the power of affective influences, one might find it difficult to understand why Olympic speed skaters "fail to maintain their pace in the face of such overwhelming incentives" (p. 287). According to Loewenstein, "physical effort ... often produces an aversive sensation referred to as fatigue or, at higher levels, exhaustion. Like other visceral factors, fatigue and exhaustion are directly aversive and alter the desirability of different activities; most prominently, they decrease the desirability of further increments of effort" (p. 287). His conclusion was that "with all its cleverness ... decision theory is somewhat crippled emotionally, and thus detached from the emotional and visceral richness of life" (p. 289).

Although these might seem like compelling arguments, it is clear that considerable conceptual groundwork remains to be completed before a formal hedonic theory of exercise behavior can be proposed. Some of the key ideas are highlighted below.

Core Affect or Emotions?

When a participant reports that he or she "feels good" or "feels bad" when exercising, this "good" or "bad" feeling could reflect a response emanating from various levels along the hierarchically organized domain of affect. At the most basic level, which has been called "core affect" (Russell, 2003), this could describe a primitive, automatic, and cognitively unmediated feeling of pleasure or displeasure. Examples of such pleasure include the pure sense of energy and bodily exhilaration that accompanies a brisk walk, a bicycle ride, or a swim on a beautiful day. Examples of such displeasure include the feeling of struggle and distress when one is pushed to the limit of one's endurance capacity or the sense of complete energy drain after a tiring run in hot and humid conditions. These feelings have a distinctly affective character (are unmistakably pleasant or unpleasant, respectively), but they probably do not require an antecedent cognitive appraisal, nor can they be significantly altered by cognition. For example, a 1500-m runner can do very little to change the sense of tension and fatigue during the final lap, despite a genetic predisposition for high tolerance to fatigue. Likewise, a severely deconditioned obese exerciser cannot freely dissociate his or her attention away from (or cognitively reframe) his or her feeling of exhaustion halfway through an aerobics class.

At the other end of the affective spectrum, there are pleasant and unpleasant emotional states that are highly complex, intrinsically culture bound, cognitively induced, and cognitively modifiable. Examples of positive emotions include the contentment and personal satisfaction associated with reaching one's weight loss goal or the sense of pride and empowerment experienced by a formerly sedentary older person after being able to walk briskly for 30 minutes for the first time in many years. Examples of negative emotions include the worry and embarrassment felt by someone with high social physique anxiety when exercising in a gymnasium, surrounded by mirrors and fit people in tight clothing, or the deep fear felt by a patient in cardiac rehabilitation when starting to exercise after a heart attack. In these cases, the positive or negative

emotions follow directly from cognitive appraisals, such as the realization that one has reached a personally important and challenging goal or that one's self-image or physical being is threatened. With appropriate interventions, these cognitive appraisals can be modified and, consequently, the ensuant emotional reactions can be altered.

A hedonic theory of exercise behavior should acknowledge and incorporate the important distinctions between core or basic affect on the one hand and emotions on the other (also see Baumeister et al., 2007; Kahneman, 2003; Shiv, Fedorikhin, & Nowlis, 2005). For some authors, what is most important for determining the motivational implications of a stimulus (such as exercise) is its position along the fundamental dimension of pleasure–displeasure (e.g., Kahneman, 1999; Kahneman, Wakker, & Sarin, 1997; Slovic, Peters, Finucane, & MacGregor, 2005). For example, according to Kahneman et al. (1997),

> Pleasure is evidently a "go" signal, which guides the organism to continue important activities such as foreplay or consuming sweet, energy-rich food. Pain is a "stop" signal, which interrupts activities that are causing harm, such as placing weight on a wounded foot. The common characteristic of the basic forms of pleasure and distress is that they regulate the response to the current situation.
> (p. 379)

Similarly, episodes of pleasure and displeasure upon exposure to affect-inducing stimuli shape positive or negative memories of these events. In turn, these memories influence the decision on whether to approach or avoid future encounters with these stimuli. According to Kahneman et al. (1997),

> Remembered utilities also have an adaptive function: they determine whether a situation experienced in the past should now be approached or avoided. Unlike pain and pleasure, which control behavior in the current situation, learned attractions and aversions adjust current behavior to the remembered evaluations of events in the past.
> (p. 380)

Other authors have argued that the affective impact of various activities should be assessed not in terms of a single dimension (such as pleasure–displeasure) but rather in terms of specific emotions (Fredrickson, 2000; Lerner & Keltner, 2000). The main argument for this position is that not all pleasures and displeasures have the same personal significance. Instead, if pleasure (or displeasure) is experienced as part of a highly personally meaningful emotion, it may have a larger impact on future behavior than the pleasure (or displeasure) that is not a component of such an emotion (such as the purely somatic pleasures or displeasures). According to Fredrickson (2000), "affective states most closely linked with future-oriented social relations and/or personal growth carry relatively high meaning (e.g. love and shame), whereas those most closely linked with immediate individual survival carry relatively low meaning (e.g. pleasure and pain)" (p. 595). Consequently, she predicts the following:

> Normal individuals strive harder—and suffer more costs—to repeat experiences that include high meaning positive affects (e.g. love, interest/flow) than to repeat those that include only low meaning positive affect (e.g. pleasure, comfort). Likewise, they most actively avoid experiences that include high meaning negative affects (e.g. shame, remorse), but may routinely endure those that include only low meaning negative affect (e.g. anxiety, disgust).
> (p. 595)

This position has also been espoused in reference to exercise behavior. According to Rose and Parfitt (2007), "the cognitive appraisal that generates the affective response at various exercise intensities is likely to be more critical to the affect-adherence relationship than the quantitative measure of [Feeling Scale] that results" (p. 306). In other words, "knowing why someone feels the way he or she does during exercise ... could be just as important as knowing how he or she feels" (p. 306). Thus one challenge as this line of research moves forward is to investigate the salient types of cognitive appraisals and ensuant emotions that occur in the context of exercise and then to explore their relative impact on subsequent exercise behavior.

Peak Rule, End Rule, and Duration Neglect

In a remarkably insightful series of studies, Kahneman and coworkers used momentary ratings to track the dynamics of pleasure–displeasure, pain, or discomfort during various pleasant or unpleasant procedures (Fredrickson & Kahneman, 1993; Kahneman, Fredrickson, Schreiber, & Redelmeier, 1993; Redelmeier & Kahneman, 1996; Redelmeier, Katz, & Kahneman, 2003; Varey & Kahneman, 1992). These studies have revealed three important principles that influence how the affective responses experienced during an activity relate to the positive or negative memories formed of that activity and the likelihood of repeating the activity in the

future. According to these principles, what has the largest impact on how an event registers in memory and influences future behavioral choices is the peak (positive or negative) affect experienced during the event (the so-called peak rule) and the affect experienced at the end (the so-called end rule). On the other hand, the duration of the experience seems inconsequential (a phenomenon called "duration neglect").

In an application of these ideas to exercise, Brewer, Manos, McDevitt, Cornelius, and Van Raalte (2000) found that respondents rated as less aversive a hypothetical bout of exercise that was described as 33% longer (20 minutes vs. 15 minutes) if it ended with a reduction in intensity (ratings of perceived exertion of 8, 13, 17, and 11 on the 6–20 scale at the 5th, 10th, 15th, and 20th minutes, respectively, vs. 8, 13, and 17 at the 5th, 10th, and 15th minutes). In a second study, the authors reported that an actual bout of exercise that was 20 minutes long but ended with reduced intensity (heart rate of 120, 140, 160, and 130 beats/min at the 5th, 10th, 15th, and 20th minutes, respectively) was selected for repetition nearly twice as frequently (65% to 35%) as a 15-minute bout that ended with high intensity (heart rate of 120, 140, and 160 beats/min at the 5th, 10th, and 15th minutes).

The Conflict between Affect and Reason

Assuming that the role of affective constructs in shaping behavioral decisions is acknowledged, a larger and arguably even more challenging issue will be to delineate the relative contributions of affect and reason. Both seem important, but how do they interact? Theorists have proposed that the system responsible for judgment and reasoning is characterized by a dual-layer architecture (S. Epstein, 1994; Evans, 2003, 2008; Kahneman, 2003; Sloman, 1996; Stanovich & West, 2000). The evolutionarily more primitive "System 1" is rapid, effortless, inflexible, and automatic. The outcomes of this system include instinctive responses that are innately programmed. For the most part, System 1 processes are theorized to be impervious to volitional control. System 1 relies heavily on affect, opting for choices that are positively laden and avoiding choices that are negatively laden. On the other hand, "System 2" is slower, more effortful, and flexible. Its major advantage compared with System 1 is that it allows abstract reasoning, future projections, hypothesis testing, and other executive processes. Its operations are typically under volitional control and therefore modifiable.

Authors have speculated that in some situations behavioral decisions are made following a conflict between System 1 and System 2 processes (Finucane et al., 2003; Stanovich & West, 2000; Svenson, 2003). Such conflicts have been explored for smoking (Slovic, 2001) and food choice (Shiv & Fedorikhin, 1999, 2002) but not for exercise. However, in anecdotal accounts, many people describe their effort to maintain an exercise program as a "struggle" or an internal conflict, saying, for example, "I know I should be exercising, but ..." or "I wish I was taking better care of myself." What statements such as these seem to imply is that although most people are aware of the benefits associated with exercise and, within the bounds of human rationality, can probably infer the long-term negative consequences of sedentary behavior, their behavior is also subject to certain inhibitory or counteracting forces. Affect-based System 1 processes are a likely candidate for this role.

S. Epstein (1994) considered the affect-based experiential system to be the "default option" (p. 716), because it is less effortful and more efficient than the rational system. Moreover, he argued that the affective nature of the experiential system itself makes it "more compelling than is dispassionate logical thinking" (p. 716). Finally, because the workings of the experiential system remain largely outside of conscious awareness, it is very difficult for the rational system to exert control over them. Similar views have been expressed by authors investigating the causes of obesity, addictions, and other problems assumed to have an affective, experiential, or "visceral" component (Loewenstein, 1996, 2001; Slovic, 2001; Slovic et al., 2007). According to Slovic et al. (2007),

> The affect heuristic enables us to be rational actors in many important situations. But not in all situations. It works beautifully when our experience enables us to anticipate accurately how we will like the consequences of our decisions. It fails miserably when the consequences turn out to be much different in character than we anticipated.
>
> (p. 1350)

Somatic Markers

Besides the data on exercise-induced affective responses that were reviewed in previous sections, several other pieces of evidence from the literature seem to indicate that exercise may not register as a particularly pleasant stimulus in the memory of many people. The fact that displeasure, discomfort,

and pain are frequently raised as perceived barriers to exercise participation in interview studies is a strong indicator. Furthermore, adult nonobese women consistently chose sedentary options (watching a comedy show, reading a magazine, doing a crossword puzzle, or playing a computer game) over exercise even though they had rated the sedentary and exercise options as equally "liked" and they were allowed to select their own exercise intensity (Vara & Epstein, 1993). This preference for sedentary options over active ones has also been observed among children (L. H. Epstein, Smith, Vara, & Rodefer, 1991; Roemmich et al., 2008). For people who are chronically inactive or obese, the preference for sedentary options may be accentuated (L. H. Epstein, 1998; L. H. Epstein & Saelens, 2000). Very obese children, for example, do not opt for exercise even when gaining access to the sedentary option is made difficult whereas access to exercise is without any cost (L. H. Epstein et al., 1991). This finding is consistent with data showing lowered pleasure ratings during exercise among obese individuals (Ekkekakis & Lind, 2006; Ekkekakis et al., 2010).

Especially considering that the majority of adults are inadequately active and overweight, we hypothesize that even a few attempts to exercise, if they led to experiences of diminished pleasure, might suffice to build a negatively laden memory trace for exercise. This proposition is similar to Damasio's (1994, 1996) idea of a somatic marker. According to Damasio (1994), somatic markers are "a special instance of feelings [which] have been connected by learning to predicted future outcomes of certain scenarios" (p. 174). When a positive somatic marker is juxtaposed to a certain future outcome, "it becomes a beacon of incentive" (p. 174). Conversely,

> When the choice of option X, which leads to bad outcome Y, is followed by punishment and thus painful body states, the somatic-marker system acquires the hidden, dispositional representation of this experience-driven, noninherited arbitrary connection. Re-exposure of the organism to option X, or thoughts about outcome Y, will now have the power to reenact the painful body state and thus serve as an automated reminder of bad consequences to come.
>
> (p. 180)

Damasio (1994) also examined the possibility that certain actions may have an immediate consequence that is unpleasant but a future outcome that is positive. Interestingly, he offered jogging (along with surgery, graduate school, and medical school) as one such example. In such cases, the only way to override the tendency to avoid the immediately unpleasant option is if, somehow, the positivity of the future outcome prevails. If it does not, inaction will ensue. Evidence suggests that often the prospect of immediate displeasure is a powerful deterrent. For example, inactivity in patients suffering from chronic fatigue (Nijs et al., 2004) or back pain (Elfving et al., 2007), who are probably well informed about the benefits of regular physical activity, is associated with an acquired fear of movement ("kinesiophobia") that presumably developed as a result of unpleasant or painful prior experiences. The fascinating experimental studies of Shiv and Fedorikhin (1999, 2002; see Shiv et al., 2005, for a review) on the choice between a chocolate cake (rated more favorably from an affective standpoint but less favorably from a cognitive standpoint) and a fruit salad (with the converse ratings) have shown that the likelihood of choosing the option that offers the promise of a future positive outcome is lessened when information processing capacity is compromised (e.g., by limited knowledge, stress, competing considerations, or time pressure).

Conclusion

The evidence discussed in this chapter suggests that the foundation has now been laid for the development of a hedonic theory of exercise behavior. Findings show that affective responses to exercise vary between individuals and include decreases in pleasure (in addition to increases). These changes could reflect processes at any level of the hierarchy that extends from core affect to emotions. "Peak" and "end" affective experiences (positive or negative) are particularly likely to play a key role in how exercise episodes register in memory and thus in shaping a theorized "somatic marker" associated with the concept of exercise. If a positively laden (System 1) somatic marker co-occurs with a positive (System 2) cognitive evaluation of exercise and its meaning (e.g., its long-term health benefits), the chances of exercise participation should be increased. Conversely, the co-occurrence of a negatively laden somatic marker with a negative (or even a neutral or indifferent) cognitive evaluation should suffice to lower the chances of exercise participation.

There is also the possibility of a conflict between the two processes underlying decision making. Presumably such conflicts occur often. It is possible that in most cases, such conflicts involve a positive cognitive evaluation ("I know exercise would be good for me") but a negative somatic marker derived from prior experiences (e.g., exercise is something that on a previous attempt felt unpleasant, uncomfortable, painful, boring, or embarrassing). In such cases, the behavioral choice would probably depend on which of the two counteracting forces is stronger (with the weighing possibly taking place outside conscious awareness). On the one hand, there are the questions of (a) how convinced one is that exercise would yield the desired outcomes and (b) how personally meaningful those outcomes are. On the other hand, there is the issue of the consistency of unpleasant affective experiences during prior exercise attempts.

In the short run, small imbalances would probably allow at least a few additional exercise attempts (which may or may not modify the somatic marker for exercise). If, however, the negativity of prior experiences is strong enough to tilt the scale heavily, the likelihood of exercise participation would be diminished. Theorists predict that in the long run, affective, "visceral," or "experiential" factors are more likely to prevail over "cognitive" or "rational" ones (S. Epstein, 1994; Loewenstein, 1996; Slovic, 2001; Slovic et al., 2007). In other words, as long as prior exercise experiences have formed a somatic marker charged with negative affect (and additional attempts have failed to alter it to any significant extent), no cognitive evaluation or rational thinking, no matter how positive, might be strong enough to keep a person on the path to long-term exercise adherence. This is especially likely if the efficacy or efficiency of System 2 is compromised (beyond its already limited capacity) by factors that occur commonly in modern life, such as incomplete information, stress, or time pressure (Shiv et al., 2005).

References

Acevedo, E. O., Kraemer, R. R., Haltom, R. W., & Tryniecki, J. L. (2003). Perceptual responses proximal to the onset of blood lactate accumulation. *Journal of Sports Medicine and Physical Fitness, 43,* 267–273.

Acevedo, E. O., Rinehardt, K. F., & Kraemer, R. R. (1994). Perceived exertion and affect at varying intensities of running. *Research Quarterly for Exercise and Sport, 65,* 372–376.

Ainsworth, B. E., Haskell, W. L., Herrmann, S. D., Meckes, N., Bassett, D. R., Jr., Tudor-Locke, C., … Leon A. S. (2011). 2011 Compendium of Physical Activities: A second update of codes and MET values. *Medicine & Science in Sports & Exercise, 43,* 1575–1581.

Ajzen, I. (1991). The theory of planned behavior. *Organizational Behavior and Human Decision Processes, 50,* 179–211.

Ajzen, I. (2005). *Attitudes, personality and behaviour* (2nd ed.). Berkshire, England: Open University Press.

Ajzen, I., & Fishbein, M. (2005). The influence of attitudes on behavior. In D. Albarracín, B. T. Johnson, & M. P. Zanna (Eds.), *The handbook of attitudes* (pp. 173–221). Mahwah, NJ: Lawrence Erlbaum.

Allender, S., Cowburn, G., & Foster, C. (2006). Understanding participation in sport and physical activity among children and adults: A review of qualitative studies. *Health Education Research: Theory and Practice, 21*, 826–835.

American College of Sports Medicine (2010). *ACSM's guidelines for exercise testing and prescription* (8th ed.). Philadelphia, PA: Lippincott Williams & Wilkins.

Annesi, J. J. (2002a). Relationship between changes in acute exercise-induced feeling states, self-motivation, and adults' adherence to moderate aerobic exercise. *Perceptual and Motor Skills, 94*, 425–439.

Annesi, J. J. (2002b). Self-motivation moderates effect of exercise-induced feelings on adherence. *Perceptual and Motor Skills, 94*, 467–475.

Annesi, J. J. (2005). Relationship between before-to-after-exercise feeling state changes and exercise session attendance over 14 weeks: Testing principles of operant conditioning. *European Journal of Sport Science, 5*, 159–163.

Annesi, J. J. (2006). Relations of self-motivation, perceived physical condition, and exercise-induced changes in revitalization and exhaustion with attendance in women initiating a moderate cardiovascular exercise regimen. *Women and Health, 42*, 77–93.

Aristotle (trans. 1984). Nicomachean ethics (W. D. Ross & J. O. Urmson, Trans.). In J. Barnes (Ed.), *The complete works of Aristotle: The revised Oxford translation* (Vol. 2, pp. 1729–1867). Princeton, NJ: Princeton University Press.

Armstrong, T., Bauman, A., & Davies, J. (2000). *Physical activity patterns of Australian adults: Results of the 1999 National Physical Activity Survey*. Canberra: Australian Institute of Health and Welfare.

Backhouse, S. H., Ekkekakis, P., Biddle, S. J. H., Foskett, A., & Williams, C. (2007). Exercise makes people feel better but people are inactive: Paradox or artifact? *Journal of Sport and Exercise Psychology, 29*, 498–517.

Bain, A. (1879). *The senses and the intellect* (3rd ed.). New York: Appleton.

Baldwin, J. M. (1891). *Handbook of psychology: Feeling and will*. New York: Henry Holt.

Bandura, A. (1986). *Social foundations of thought and action: A social cognitive theory*. Englewood Cliffs, NJ: Prentice Hall.

Bandura, A. (1989). Human agency in social cognitive theory. *American Psychologist, 44*, 1175–1184.

Bandura, A. (2001). Social cognitive theory: An agentic perspective. *Annual Review of Psychology, 52*, 1–26.

Bauman, A., Armstrong, T., Davies, J., Owen, N., Brown, W., Bellew, B., & Vita, P. (2003). Trends in physical activity participation and the impact of integrated campaigns among Australian adults, 1997–99. *Australia and New Zealand Journal of Public Health, 27*, 76–79.

Bauman, A. E., Sallis, J. F., Dzewaltowski, D. A., & Owen, N. (2002). Toward a better understanding of the influences on physical activity: The role of determinants, correlates, causal variables, mediators, moderators, and confounders. *American Journal of Preventive Medicine, 23*(Suppl. 2), 5–14.

Baumeister, R. F., Vohs, K. D., DeWall, C. N., & Zhang, L. (2007). How emotion shapes behavior: Feedback, anticipation, and reflection, rather than direct causation. *Personality and Social Psychology Review, 11*, 167–203.

Bechara, A. (2005). Decision making, impulse control and loss of willpower to resist drugs: A neurocognitive perspective. *Nature Neuroscience, 8*, 1458–1463.

Bechara, A., Damasio, H., & Damasio, A. R. (2000). Emotion, decision making and the orbitofrontal cortex. *Cerebral Cortex, 10*, 295–307.

Bentham, J. (1948). *An introduction to the principles of morals and legislation*. New York: Hafner. (Original work published 1789.)

Berger, B. G., Darby, L. A., Owen, D. R., & Carels, R. A. (2010). Implications of a behavioral weight loss program for obese, sedentary women: A focus on mood enhancement and exercise enjoyment. *International Journal of Sport and Exercise Psychology, 8*, 10–23.

Berger, B. G., & Owen, D. R. (1992). Mood alteration with yoga and swimming: Aerobic exercise may not be necessary. *Perceptual and Motor Skills, 75*, 1331–1343.

Berridge, K. C., & Kringelbach, M. L. (2008). Affective neuroscience of pleasure: Reward in humans and animals. *Psychopharmacology, 199*, 457–480.

Bettman, J. R. (1993). The decision maker who came in from the cold. *Advances in Consumer Research, 20*, 7–11.

Biddle, S. J. H. (2000). Exercise, emotions, and mental health. In Y. L. Hanin (Ed.), *Emotions in sport* (pp. 267–291). Champaign, IL: Human Kinetics.

Bish, C. L., Michels Blanck, H., Serdula, M. K., Marcus, M., Kohl, H. W. III., & Kettel Khan, L. (2005). Diet and physical activity behaviors among Americans trying to lose weight: 2000 Behavioral Risk Factor Surveillance System. *Obesity Research, 13*, 596–607.

Bixby, W. R., & Lochbaum, M. R. (2006). Affect responses to acute bouts of aerobic exercise in fit and unfit participants: An examination of opponent-process theory. *Journal of Sport Behavior, 29*, 111–125.

Bixby, W. R., Spalding, T. W., & Hatfield, B. D. (2001). Temporal dynamics and dimensional specificity of the affective response to exercise of varying intensity: Differing pathways to a common outcome. *Journal of Sport and Exercise Psychology, 23*, 171–190.

Bluemke, M., Brand, R., Schweizer, G., & Kahlert, D. (2010). Exercise might be good for me, but I don't feel good about it: Do automatic associations predict exercise behavior? *Journal of Sport and Exercise Psychology, 32*, 137–153.

Brewer, B. W., Manos, T. M., McDevitt, A. V., Cornelius, A. E., & Van Raalte, J. L. (2000). The effect of adding lower intensity work on perceived aversiveness of exercise. *Journal of Sport and Exercise Psychology, 22*, 119–130.

Browning, R. C., Baker, E. A., Herron, J. A., & Kram, R. (2006). Effects of obesity and sex on the energetic cost of preferred speed of walking. *Journal of Applied Physiology, 100*, 390–398.

Browning, R. C., & Kram, R. (2005). Energetic cost and preferred speed of walking in obese vs. normal weight women. *Obesity Research, 13*, 891–899.

Buckley, J. (2006). Exercise physiology and monitoring of exercise in cardiac rehabilitation. In M. K. Thow (Ed.), *Exercise leadership in cardiac rehabilitation: An evidence-based approach* (pp. 47–95). Chichester, UK: John Wiley & Sons.

Cabanac, M. (1992). Pleasure: The common currency. *Journal of Theoretical Biology, 155*, 173–200.

Cabanac, M. (2002). What is emotion? *Behavioural Processes, 60*, 69–83.

Cabanac, M. (2006). Exertion and pleasure from an evolutionary perspective. In E. O. Acevedo & P. Ekkekakis (Eds.), *Psychobiology of physical activity* (pp. 79–89). Champaign, IL: Human Kinetics.

Cabanac, M. (2010). The dialectics of pleasure. In M. L. Kringelbach & K. C. Berridge (Eds.), *Pleasures of the brain* (pp. 113–124). New York: Oxford University Press.

Calfas, K. J., Sallis, J. F., Nichols, J. F., Sarkin, J. A., Johnson, M. F., Caparosa, S., ... Alcaraz, J. E. (2000). Project GRAD: Two-year outcomes of a randomized controlled physical activity intervention among young adults. *American Journal of Preventive Medicine, 18*, 28–37.

Cameron, O. G. (2009). Visceral brain–body information transfer. *NeuroImage, 47*, 787–794.

Carels, R. A., Berger, B., & Darby, L. (2006). The association between mood states and physical activity in postmenopausal, obese, sedentary women. *Journal of Aging and Physical Activity, 14*, 12–28.

Carels, R. A., Coit, C., Young, K., & Berger, B. (2007). Exercise makes you feel good, but does feeling good make you exercise? An examination of obese dieters. *Journal of Sport and Exercise Psychology, 29*, 706–722.

Carretié, L., Albert, J., López-Martín, S., & Tapia, M. (2009). Negative brain: An integrative review on the neural processes activated by unpleasant stimuli. *International Journal of Psychophysiology, 71*, 57–63.

Castro, C. M., Sallis, J. F., Hickman, S. A., Lee, R. E., & Chen, A. H. (1999). A prospective study of psychosocial correlates of physical activity for ethnic minority women. *Psychology and Health, 14*, 277–293.

Craig, A. D. (2002). How do you feel? Interoception: The sense of the physiological condition of the body. *Nature Reviews Neuroscience, 3*, 655–666.

Craig, A. D. (2006). Physical activity and the neurobiology of interoception. In E. O. Acevedo & P. Ekkekakis (Eds.), *Psychobiology of physical activity* (pp. 15–28). Champaign, IL: Human Kinetics.

Currie, C. E., Amos, A, & Hunt, S. M. (1991). The dynamics and processes of behavioural change in five classes of health-related behaviour: Findings from qualitative research. *Health Education Research: Theory and Practice, 6*, 443–453.

Daley, A. J., Copland, R. J., Wright, N. P., & Wales, J. K. H. (2008). "I can actually exercise if I want to; it isn't as hard as I thought": A qualitative study of the experiences and views of obese adolescents participating in an exercise therapy intervention. *Journal of Health Psychology, 13*, 810–819.

Damasio, A. R. (1994). *Descartes' error: Emotion, reason, and the human brain*. New York: Putnam.

Damasio, A. R. (1996). The somatic marker hypothesis and the possible functions of the prefrontal cortex. *Philosophical Transactions of the Royal Society of London, Series B, 351*, 1413–1420.

de Geus, E. J. C., & de Moor, M. H. M. (2008). A genetic perspective on the association between exercise and mental health. *Mental Health and Physical Activity, 1*, 53–61.

Delahanty, L. M., Conroy, M. B., & Nathan, D. M. (2006). Psychological predictors of physical activity in the Diabetes Prevention Program. *Journal of the American Dietetic Association, 106*, 698–705.

Denton, D. A., McKinley, M. J., Farrell, M., & Eagan, G. F. (2009). The role of primordial emotions in the evolutionary origin of consciousness. *Consciousness and Cognition, 18*, 500–514.

Dergance, J. M., Mouton, C. P., Lichtenstein, M. J., & Hazuda, H. P. (2005). Potential mediators of ethnic differences in physical activity in older Mexican Americans and European Americans: Results from the San Antonio Longitudinal Study of Aging. *Journal of the American Geriatrics Society, 53*, 1240–1247.

Descartes, R. (trans. 1985). The passions of the soul (R. Stoothoff, Tans.). In *The philosophical writings of Descartes* (Vol. 1, pp. 325–404). Cambridge, UK: Cambridge University Press.

Diogenes Laertius (trans. 1925). *Lives of eminent philosophers* (Vol. 2, R. D. Hicks, Trans.). Cambridge, MA: Harvard University Press.

Diogenes Laertius (trans. 1972). *Lives of eminent philosophers* (Vol. 1, R.D. Hicks, Trans.). Cambridge, MA: Harvard University Press.

Dishman, R. K. (1988). Exercise adherence research: Future directions. *American Journal of Health Promotion, 3*, 52–56.

Dishman, R. K. (1990). Determinants of participation in physical activity. In C. Bouchard, R. J. Shephard, T. Stephens, J. R. Sutton, & B. D. McPherson (Eds.), *Exercise, fitness, and health: A consensus of current knowledge* (pp. 75–101). Champaign, IL: Human Kinetics.

Dishman, R. K. (2001). The problem of exercise adherence: Fighting sloth in nations with market economies. *Quest, 53*, 279–294.

Dishman, R. K. (2003). The impact of behavior on quality of life. *Quality of Life Research, 12*(Suppl. 1), 43–49.

Dishman, R. K., & Buckworth, J. (1996). Increasing physical activity: A quantitative synthesis. *Medicine & Science in Sports & Exercise, 28*, 706–719.

Dishman, R. K., Sallis, J. F., & Orenstein, D. R. (1985). The determinants of physical activity and exercise. *Public Health Reports, 100*, 158–171.

Ekkekakis, P. (2003). Pleasure and displeasure from the body: Perspectives from exercise. *Cognition and Emotion, 17*, 213–239.

Ekkekakis, P. (2005). The study of affective responses to acute exercise: The dual-mode model. In R. Stelter & K. K. Roessler (Eds.), *New approaches to sport and exercise psychology* (pp. 119–146). Oxford, UK: Meyer & Meyer Sport.

Ekkekakis, P. (2008). The genetic tidal wave finally reached our shores: Will it be the catalyst for a critical overhaul of the way we think and do science? *Mental Health and Physical Activity, 1*, 47–52.

Ekkekakis, P. (2009a). The Dual-Mode Theory of affective responses to exercise in metatheoretical context: I. Initial impetus, basic postulates, and philosophical framework. *International Review of Sport and Exercise Psychology, 2*, 73–94.

Ekkekakis, P. (2009b). Illuminating the black box: Investigating prefrontal cortical hemodynamics during exercise with near-infrared spectroscopy. *Journal of Sport and Exercise Psychology, 31*, 505–553.

Ekkekakis, P. (2009c). Let them roam free? Physiological and psychological evidence for the potential of self-selected exercise intensity in public health. *Sports Medicine, 39*, 857–888.

Ekkekakis, P., & Acevedo, E. O. (2006). Affective responses to acute exercise: Toward a psychobiological dose–response model. In E. O. Acevedo & P. Ekkekakis (Eds.), *Psychobiology of physical activity* (pp. 91–109). Champaign, IL: Human Kinetics.

Ekkekakis, P., Backhouse, S. H., Gray, C., & Lind, E. (2008). Walking is popular among adults but is it pleasant? A framework for clarifying the link between walking and affect as illustrated in two studies. *Psychology of Sport and Exercise, 9*, 246–264.

Ekkekakis, P., Hall, E. E., & Petruzzello, S. J. (2005a). Some like it vigorous: Individual differences in the preference for and tolerance of exercise intensity. *Journal of Sport and Exercise Psychology, 27*, 350–374.

Ekkekakis, P., Hall, E. E., & Petruzzello, S. J. (2005b). Variation and homogeneity in affective responses to physical activity of varying intensities: An alternative perspective on dose-response based on evolutionary considerations. *Journal of Sports Sciences, 23*, 477–500.

Ekkekakis, P., Hall, E. E., & Petruzzello, S. J. (2008). The relationship between exercise intensity and affective responses demystified: To crack the forty-year-old nut, replace the forty-year-old nutcracker! *Annals of Behavioral Medicine, 35*, 136–149.

Ekkekakis, P., Hall, E. E., Van Landuyt, L. M., & Petruzzello, S. J. (2000). Walking in (affective) circles: Can short walks enhance affect? *Journal of Behavioral Medicine, 23*, 245–275.

Ekkekakis, P., & Lind, E. (2006). Exercise does not feel the same when you are overweight: The impact of self-selected and imposed intensity on affect and exertion. *International Journal of Obesity, 30*, 652–660.

Ekkekakis, P., Lind, E., & Vazou, S. (2010). Affective responses to increasing levels of exercise intensity in normal-weight, overweight, and obese middle-aged women. *Obesity, 18*, 79–85.

Ekkekakis, P., Parfitt, G., & Petruzzello, S. J. (2011). The pleasure and displeasure people feel when they exercise at different intensities: Decennial update and progress towards a tripartite rationale for exercise intensity prescription. *Sports Medicine, 41*, 641–671.

Ekkekakis, P., & Petruzzello, S. J. (1999). Acute aerobic exercise and affect: Current status, problems, and prospects regarding dose-response. *Sports Medicine, 28*, 337–374.

Elfving, B., Andersson, T., & Grooten, W. J. (2007). Low levels of physical activity in back pain patients are associated with high levels of fear-avoidance beliefs and pain catastrophizing. *Physiotherapy Research International, 12*, 14–24.

Emmons, R. A., & Diener, E. (1986). A goal-affect analysis of everyday situational choices. *Journal of Research in Personality, 20*, 309–326.

Epstein, L. H. (1998). Integrating theoretical approaches to promote physical activity. *American Journal of Preventive Medicine, 15*, 257–265.

Epstein, L. H., & Saelens, B. E. (2000). Behavioral economics of obesity: Food intake and energy expenditure. In W. K. Bickel & R. E. Vuchinich (Eds.), *Reframing health behavior change with behavioral economics* (pp. 293–311). Mahwah, NJ: Lawrence Erlbaum.

Epstein, L. H., Smith, J. A., Vara, L. S., & Rodefer, J. S. (1991). Behavioral economic analysis of activity choice in obese children. *Health Psychology, 10*, 311–316.

Epstein, S. (1994). Integration of the cognitive and the psychodynamic unconscious. *American Psychologist, 49*, 709–724.

Evans, J. St. B. T. (2003). In two minds: Dual-process accounts of reasoning. *Trends in Cognitive Sciences, 7*, 454–459.

Evans, J. St. B. T. (2008). Dual-processing accounts of reasoning, judgment, and social cognition. *Annual Review of Psychology, 59*, 255–278.

Feldman Barrett, L., Mesquita, B., Ochsner, K. N., & Gross, J. J. (2007). The experience of emotion. *Annual Review of Psychology, 58*, 373–403.

Ferrand, C., Perrin, C., & Nasarre, S. (2008). Motives for regular physical activity in women and men: A qualitative study in French adults with type 2 diabetes, belonging to a patients' association. *Health and Social Care in the Community, 16*, 511–520.

Finucane, M. L., Peters, E., & Slovic, P. (2003). Judgment and decision making: The dance of affect and reason. In S. L. Schneider & J. Shanteau (Eds.), *Emerging perspectives on judgment and decision research* (pp. 327–364). New York: Cambridge University Press.

Flintoff, A., & Scraton, S. (2001). Stepping into active leisure? Young women's perceptions of active lifestyles and their experiences of school physical education. *Sport, Education and Society, 6*, 5–21.

Focht, B. C. (2009). Brief walks in outdoor and laboratory environments: Effects on affective responses, enjoyment, and intentions to walk for exercise. *Research Quarterly for Exercise and Sport, 80*, 611–620.

Focht, B. C., & Hausenblas, H. A. (2006). Exercising in public and private environments: Effects on feeling states in women with social physique anxiety. *Journal of Applied Biobehavioral Research, 11*, 147–165.

Fox, K. R., Stathi, A., McKenna, J., & Davis, M. G. (2007). Physical activity and mental well-being in older people participating in the Better Ageing Project. *European Journal of Applied Physiology, 100*, 591–602.

Fredrickson, B. L. (2000). Extracting meaning from past affective experiences: The importance of peaks, ends, and specific emotions. *Cognition and Emotion, 14*, 577–606.

Fredrickson, B. L., & Kahneman, D. (1993). Duration neglect in retrospective evaluations of affective episodes. *Journal of Personality and Social Psychology, 65*, 45–55.

Freud, S. (1946). Formulations regarding the two principles in mental functioning (J. Riviere, Trans.). In *Collected papers* (Vol. IV, pp. 13–21). London: Hogarth. (Original work published 1911)

Fridlund Dunton, G., & Vaughan, E. (2008). Anticipated affective consequences of physical activity adoption and maintenance. *Health Psychology, 27*, 703–710.

Gauvin, L. (1990). An experiential perspective on the motivational features of exercise and lifestyle. *Canadian Journal of Sport Sciences, 15*, 51–58.

Gauvin, L., & Rejeski, W. J. (1993). The Exercise-induced Feeling Inventory: Development and initial validation. *Journal of Sport and Exercise Psychology, 15*, 403–423.

Gosling, J. C., & Taylor, C. C. (1982). *The Greek pleasure.* Oxford: Oxford University Press.

Graham, R., Kremer, J., & Wheeler, G. (2008). Physical exercise and psychological well-being among people with chronic illness and disability: A grounded approach. *Journal of Health Psychology, 13*, 447–458.

Hamid, P. N. (1990). Positive and negative affectivity and maintenance of exercise programs. *Perceptual and Motor Skills, 70*, 478.

Hardy, C. J., & Rejeski, W. J. (1989). Not what, but how one feels: The measurement of affect during exercise. *Journal of Sport and Exercise Psychology, 11*, 304–317.

Hariri, A. R., & Forbes, E. E. (2007). Genetics of emotion regulation. In J. J. Gross (Ed.), *Handbook of emotion regulation* (pp. 110–132). New York: Guilford.

Helvétius, M. (1810). *A treatise on man; his intellectual faculties and his education* (Vol. 1, W. Hooper, Trans.). London: Albion Press. (Original work published 1777.)

Henderson, K. A., & Ainsworth, B. E. (2003). A synthesis of perceptions about physical activity among older African American and American Indian women. *American Journal of Public Health, 93*, 313–317.

Hendry, M., Williams, N. H., Markland, D., Wilkinson, C., & Maddison, P. (2006). Why should we exercise when our knees hurt? A qualitative study of primary care patients with osteoarthritis of the knee. *Family Practice, 23*, 558–567.

Henry, B., Moffitt, T. E., Caspi, A., Langley, J., & Silva, P. A. (1994). On the "remembrance of things past": A longitudinal evaluation of the retrospective method. *Psychological Assessment, 6*, 92–101.

Herman, S., Blumenthal, J. A., Babyak, M., Khatri, P., Craighead, W. E., Krishnan, K. R., & Doraiswamy, P. M. (2002). Exercise therapy for depression in middle-aged and older adults: Predictors of early dropout and treatment failure. *Health Psychology, 21*, 553–563.

Hobbes, T. (1839). Elements of philosophy: The first section. In W. Molesworth (Ed. and Trans.), *The English works of Thomas Hobbes of Malesbury* (Vol. 1, Ch. 25, pp. 387–410). London: John Bohn. (Original work published 1655.)

Hobbes, T. (1839). Leviathan or the matter, form, and power of a commonwealth ecclesiastical and civil. In W. Molesworth (Ed.), *The English works of Thomas Hobbes of Malesbury* (Vol. 3, Ch. 6, pp. 38–51). London: John Bohn. (Original work published 1651.)

Huberty, J. L., Ransdell, L. B., Sidman, C., Flohr, J. A., Shultz, B., Grosshans, O., & Durrant, L. (2008). Explaining long-term exercise adherence in women who complete a structured exercise program. *Research Quarterly for Exercise and Sport, 79*, 374–384.

Hume, D. (1978). Of the passions. In P. H. Nidditch (Ed.), *A treatise of human nature: Being an attempt to introduce the experimental method of reasoning into moral subjects* (2nd Ed., p. 275–454). Oxford, UK: Oxford University Press. (Original work published 1740.)

James, W. (1890a). *The principles of psychology* (Vol. 1). London: Macmillan.

James, W. (1890b). *The principles of psychology* (Vol. 2). London: Macmillan.

Jerome, G. J., Marquez, D. X., McAuley, E., Canaklisova, S., Snook, E., & Vickers, M. (2002). Self-efficacy effects on feeling states in women. *International Journal of Behavioral Medicine, 9*, 139–154.

Kahn, E. B., Ramsey, L. T., Brownson, R. C., Heath, G. W., Howze, E. H., Powell, K. E., … Corso, P. (2002). The effectiveness of interventions to increase physical activity: A systematic review. *American Journal of Preventive Medicine, 22*(Suppl. 4), 73–107.

Kahneman, D. (1999). Objective happiness. In D. Kahneman, E. Diener, & N. Schwarz (Eds.), *Well-being: The foundation of hedonic psychology* (pp. 3–25). New York: Sage.

Kahneman, D. (2003). A perspective on judgment and choice: Mapping bounded rationality. *American Psychologist, 58*, 697–720.

Kahneman, D., Fredrickson, B. L., Schreiber, C. A., & Redelmeier, D. A. (1993). When more pain is preferred to less: Adding a better end. *Psychological Science, 4*, 401–405.

Kahneman, D., Wakker, P. P., & Sarin, R. (1997). Back to Bentham? Explorations of experienced utility. *Quarterly Journal of Economics, 112*, 375–405.

Kelsey, K. S., McEvoy DeVellis, B., Begum, M., Belton, L., Gerken Hooten, E., & Kramish Campbell, M. (2006). Positive affect, exercise and self-reported health in blue-collar women. *American Journal of Health Behavior, 30*, 199–207.

Kientzler, A. L. (1999). Fifth- and seventh-grade girls' decisions about participation in physical activity. *Elementary School Journal, 99*, 391–414.

Kilpatrick, M. W., Kraemer, R. R., Bartholomew, J. B., Acevedo, E. O., & Jarreau, D. (2007). Affective responses to exercise are dependent on intensity rather than total work. *Medicine & Science in Sports & Exercise, 39*, 1417–1422.

Kishi, T., & Elmquist, J. K. (2005). Body weight is regulated by the brain: A link between feeding and emotion. *Molecular Psychiatry, 10*, 132–146.

Kiviniemi, M. T., Voss-Humke, A. M., & Seifert, A. L. (2007). How do I feel about the behavior? The interplay of affective associations with behaviors and cognitive beliefs as influences on physical activity behavior. *Health Psychology, 26*, 152–158.

Klonoff, E. A., Annechild, A., & Landrine, H. (1994). Predicting exercise adherence in women: The role of psychological and physiological factors. *Preventive Medicine, 23*, 257–262.

Koob, G. F. (2008). Hedonic homeostatic dysregulation as a driver for drug-seeking behavior. *Drug Discovery Today: Disease Models, 5*, 207–215.

Kuhn, T. S. (1962) Historical structure of scientific discovery. *Science, 136*, 760–764.

Kuhn, T. S. (1996). *The structure of scientific revolutions* (3rd ed.). Chicago: University of Chicago Press. (Original work published 1962)

Kwan, B. M., & Bryan, A. (2010). In-task and post-task affective response to exercise: Translating exercise intentions into behaviour. *British Journal of Health Psychology, 15*, 115–131.

La Mettrie, J. O. (1996). Machine man. In A. Thomson (Ed. and Trans.), *Machine man and other writings* (pp. 1–39). Cambridge, UK: Cambridge University Press. (Original work published 1748.)

La Mettrie, J. O. (1996). Anti-Seneca or the sovereign good. In A. Thomson (Ed. and Trans.), *Machine man and other writings* (pp. 117–143). Cambridge, UK: Cambridge University Press. (Original work published 1750.)

Laverie, D. A. (1998). Motivations for ongoing participation in a fitness activity. *Leisure Sciences, 20*, 277–302.

Lawton, R., Conner, M., & McEachan, R. (2009). Desire or reason: Predicting health behaviors from affective and cognitive attitudes. *Health Psychology, 28*, 56–65.

Lee, L. L., Avis, M., & Arthur, A. (2007). The role of self-efficacy in older people's decisions to initiate and maintain regular walking as exercise: Findings from a qualitative study. *Preventive Medicine, 45*, 62–65.

Lees, F. D., Clark, P. G., Nigg, C. R., & Newman, P. (2005). Barriers to exercise behavior among older adults: A focus group study. *Journal of Aging and Physical Activity, 13*, 23–33.

Leonard, F. E. (1915). *Pioneers of modern physical training* (2nd ed.). New York: Association Press.

Lerner, J. S., & Keltner, D. (2000). Beyond valence: Toward a model of emotion-specific influences on judgement and choice. *Cognition and Emotion, 14*, 473–493.

Lewis, B. A., Marcus, B. H., Pate, R. R., & Dunn, A. L. (2002). Psychosocial mediators of physical activity behavior among adults and children. *American Journal of Preventive Medicine, 23*(Suppl. 2), 26–35.

Lind, E., Welch, A. S., & Ekkekakis, P. (2009). Do "mind over muscle" strategies work? Examining the effects of attentional association and dissociation on exertional, affective, and physiological responses to exercise. *Sports Medicine, 39,* 743–764.

Loewenstein, G. (1996). Out of control: Visceral influences on behavior. *Organizational Behavior and Human Decision Processes, 65,* 272–292.

Loewenstein, G. (2001). A visceral account of addiction. In P. Slovic (Ed.), *Smoking: Risk, perception, and policy* (pp. 188–215). Thousand Oaks, CA: Sage.

Loewenstein, G., & Lerner, J. S. (2003). The role of affect in decision making. In R. J. Davidson, K. R. Scherer, & H. H. Goldsmith (Eds.), *Handbook of affective sciences* (pp. 619–642). New York: Oxford University Press.

Loman, D. G. (2008). Promoting physical activity in teen girls: Insight from focus groups. *MCN: The American Journal of Maternal/Child Nursing, 33,* 294–299.

Loughhead, T. M., Patterson, M. M., & Carron, A. V. (2008). The impact of fitness leader behavior and cohesion on an exerciser's affective state. *International Journal of Sport and Exercise Psychology, 6,* 53–28.

Lox, C. L., Jackson, S., Tuholski, S. W., Wasley, D., & Treasure, D. C. (2000). Revisiting the measurement of exercise-induced feeling states: The Physical Activity Affect Scale (PAAS). *Measurement in Physical Education and Exercise Science, 4,* 79–95.

Lutter, M., & Nestler, E. J. (2009). Homeostatic and hedonic signals interact in the regulation of food intake. *Journal of Nutrition, 139,* 629–632.

Marcus, B. H., Williams, D. M., Dubbert, P. M., Sallis, J. F., King, A. C., Yancey, A. K., ... Claytor, R. P. (2006). Physical activity intervention studies: What we know and what we need to know. *Circulation, 114,* 2739–2752.

Martin, S. B., Morrow, J. R., Jackson, A. W., & Dunn, A. L. (2000). Variables related to meeting the ACSM/CDC physical activity guidelines. *Medicine & Science in Sports & Exercise, 32,* 2087–2092.

Martin Ginis, K. A., Burke, S. M., & Gauvin, L. (2007). Exercising with others exacerbates the negative effects of mirrored environments on sedentary women's feeling states. *Psychology and Health, 22,* 945–962.

Mattsson, E., Larsson, U. E., & Rössner, S. (1997). Is walking for exercise too exhausting for obese women? *International Journal of Obesity, 21,* 380–386.

McDougall, W. (1916). *An introduction to social psychology* (10th ed.). London: Methuen.

McIntyre, J. L. (2000). Hume's passions: Direct and indirect. *Hume Studies, 26,* 77–86.

McNair, D. M., Lorr, M., & Droppleman, L. F. (1971). *Manual for the Profile of Mood States.* San Diego, CA: Educational and Industrial Testing Service.

Mees, U., & Schmitt, A. (2008). Goals of action and emotional reasons for action: A modern version of the theory of ultimate psychological hedonism. *Journal for the Theory of Social Behavior, 38,* 157–178.

Mellers, B. A. (2004). Pleasure, utility, and choice. In A. S. R. Manstead, N. Frijda, & A. Fischer (Eds.), *Feelings and emotions: The Amsterdam symposium* (pp. 282–300). New York: Cambridge University Press.

Metzger, J. S., Catellier, D. J., Evenson, K. R., Treuth, M. S., Rosamond, W. D., & Siega-Riz, A. M. (2008). Patterns of objectively measured physical activity in the United States. *Medicine & Science in Sports & Exercise, 40,* 630–638.

Miles, L. (2007). Physical activity and health. *Nutrition Bulletin, 32,* 314–363.

Moore, B. A., & O'Donohue, W. T. (2008). Hedonic approach to pediatric and adolescent weight management. In W. T. O'Donohue, B. A. Moore, & B. J. Scott (Eds.), *Handbook of pediatric and adolescent obesity treatment* (pp. 143–151). New York: Routledge.

Morgan, W. P. (1977). Involvement in vigorous physical activity with special reference to adherence. In L. I. Gedvilas & M. E. Kneer (Eds.), *Proceedings of the National College Physical Education Association for Men/National Association for Physical Education of College Women national conference* (pp. 233–246). Chicago, IL: National College Physical Education Association for Men.

Morgan, W. P., & O'Connor, P. J. (1988). Exercise and mental health. In R. K. Dishman (Ed.), *Exercise adherence: Its impact on public health* (pp. 91–121). Champaign, IL: Human Kinetics.

Morgan, W. P., Roberts, J. A., Brand, F. R., & Feinerman, A. D. (1970). Psychological effect of chronic physical activity. *Medicine and Science in Sports, 2,* 213–217.

Morris, J. N. (1994). Exercise in the prevention of coronary heart disease: Today's best buy in public health. *Medicine & Science in Sports & Exercise, 26,* 807–814.

Morrow, J. R., Jackson, A. W., Bazzarre, T. L., Milne, D., & Blair, S. N. (1999). A one-year follow-up to *Physical activity and health: A report of the Surgeon General. American Journal of Preventive Medicine, 17,* 24–30.

Motl, R. W., Berger, B. G., & Leuschen, P. S. (2000). The role of enjoyment in the exercise–mood relationship. *International Journal of Sport Psychology, 31,* 347–363.

Naqvi, N., Shiv, B., & Bechara, A. (2006). The role of emotion in decision making: A cognitive neuroscience perspective. *Current Directions in Psychological Science, 15,* 260–264.

Neumark-Sztainer, D., Story, M., Hannan, P. J., Tharp, T., & Rex, J. (2003). Factors associated with changes in physical activity. *Archives of Pediatric and Adolescent Medicine, 157,* 803–810.

Newsom, J. T., McFarland, B. H., Kaplan, M. S., Huguet, N., & Zani, B. (2005). The health consciousness myth: Implications of the near independence of major health behaviors in the North American population. *Social Science and Medicine, 60,* 433–437.

Nichols, J. F., Wellman, E., Caparosa, S., Sallis, J. F., Calfas, K. J., & Rowe, R. (2000). Impact of a worksite behavioral skills intervention. *American Journal of Health Promotion, 14,* 218–221.

Nies, M. A., & Motyka, C. L. (2006). Factors contributing to women's ability to maintain a walking program. *Journal of Holistic Nursing, 24,* 7–14.

Nigg, C. R., Borrelli, B., Maddock, J., & Dishman, R. K. (2008). A theory of physical activity maintenance. *Applied Psychology, 57,* 544–560.

Nijs, J., De Meirleir, K., & Duquet, W. (2004). Kinesiophobia in chronic fatigue syndrome: Assessment and associations with disability. *Archives of Physical Medicine and Rehabilitation, 85,* 1586–1592.

O'Brien Cousins, S. (2000). "My heart couldn't take it": Older women's beliefs about exercise benefits and risks. *Journal of Gerontology, 55B*, P283–P294.

Ochsner, K. N. & Gross, J. J. (2005). The cognitive control of emotion. *Trends in Cognitive Sciences, 9*, 242–249.

Ochsner, K. N. & Gross, J. J. (2008). Cognitive emotion regulation: Insights from social cognitive and affective neuroscience. *Current Directions in Psychological Science, 17*, 153–158.

Panksepp, J. (1998). *Affective neuroscience: The foundations of human and animal emotions*. New York: Oxford University Press.

Panksepp, J., & Panksepp, J. B. (2000). The seven sins of evolutionary psychology. *Evolution and Cognition, 6*, 108–131.

Parfitt, G., & Hughes, S. (2009). The exercise intensity–affect relationship: Evidence and implications for exercise behavior. *Journal of Exercise Science & Fitness, 7*, S34–S41.

Parfitt, G., Rose, E. A., & Burgess, W. M. (2006). The psychological and physiological responses of sedentary individuals to prescribed and preferred intensity exercise. *British Journal of Health Psychology, 11*, 39–53.

Pate, R. R., Pratt, M., Blair, S. N., Haskell, W. L., Macera, C. A., Bouchard, C., ... Wilmore, J. A. (1995). Physical activity and public health: A recommendation from the Centers for Disease Control and Prevention and the American College of Sports Medicine. *Journal of the American Medical Association, 273*, 402–407.

Pedersen, B. K., & Saltin, B. (2006). Evidence for prescribing exercise as therapy in chronic disease. *Scandinavian Journal of Medicine and Science in Sports, 16*(Suppl. 1), 3–63.

Plato (trans. 1997). Republic (G. M. A. Grube & C. D. C. Reeve, Trans.). In J. M. Cooper (Ed.), *Plato: Complete works* (pp. 971–1223). Indianapolis, IN: Hackett.

Pollock, M. L. (1978). How much exercise is enough? *Physician and Sportsmedicine, 6*, 50–64.

Pollock, M. L., Wilmore, J. H., & Fox, S. M. (1978). *Health and fitness through physical activity*. New York: John Wiley & Sons.

Prochaska, J. O., & DiClemente, C. C. (1982). Transtheoretical therapy: Toward a more integrative model of change. *Psychotherapy: Theory, Research & Practice, 19*, 276–288.

Prochaska, J. O., Redding, C. A., & Evers, K. E. (2008). The transtheoretical model and stages of change. In K. Glanz, B. K. Rimer, & K. Viswanath (Eds.), *Health behavior and health education: Theory, research, and practice* (4th ed., pp. 97–121). San Francisco: Jossey-Bass.

Prochaska, J. O., Velicer, W. F., Rossi, J. S., Goldstein, M. G., Marcus, B. H., Rakowski, W., ... Rossi, S. R. (1994). Stages of change and decisional balance for 12 problem behaviors. *Health Psychology, 13*, 39–46.

Quirk, G. J., & Beer, J. S. (2006). Prefrontal involvement in the regulation of emotion: Convergence of rat and human studies. *Current Opinion in Neurobiology, 16*, 723–727.

Raedeke, T. D. (2007). The relationship between enjoyment and affective responses to exercise. *Journal of Applied Sport Psychology, 19*, 105–115.

Redelmeier, D. A., & Kahneman, D. (1996). Patients' memories of painful medical treatments: Real-time and retrospective evaluations of two minimally invasive procedures. *Pain, 66*, 3–8.

Redelmeier, D. A., Katz, J., & Kahneman, D. (2003). Memories of colonoscopy: A randomized trial. *Pain, 104*, 187–194.

Reed, J., & Ones, D. S. (2006). The effect of acute aerobic exercise on positive activated affect: A meta-analysis. *Psychology of Sport and Exercise, 7*, 477–514.

Rhodes, R. E., Fiala, B., & Conner, M. (2009). A review and meta-analysis of affective judgments and physical activity in adult populations. *Annals of Behavioral Medicine, 38*, 180–204.

Rhodes, R. E., & Nigg, C. R. (2011). Advancing physical activity theory: A review and future directions. *Exercise and Sport Sciences Reviews, 39*, 113–119.

Robbins, L. B., Pis, M. B., Pender, N. J., & Kazanis, A. S. (2004). Exercise self-efficacy, enjoyment, and feeling states among adolescents. *Western Journal of Nursing Research, 26*, 699–715.

Robinson, T. E., & Berridge, K. C. (2008). The incentive sensitization theory of addiction: Some current issues. *Philosophical Transactions of the Royal Society of London, Series B, 363*, 3137–3146.

Roemmich, J. N., Barkley, J. E., Lobarinas, C. L., Foster, J. H., White, T. M., & Epstein, L. H. (2008). Association of liking and reinforcing value with children's physical activity. *Physiology and Behavior, 93*, 1011–1018.

Rolls, E. T. (2007). Understanding the mechanisms of food intake and obesity. *Obesity Reviews, 8*(Suppl. 1), 67–72.

Rose, E. A., & Parfitt, G. (2007). A quantitative analysis and qualitative explanation of the individual differences in affective responses to prescribed and self-selected exercise intensities. *Journal of Sport and Exercise Psychology, 29*, 281–309.

Rosenstock, I. M., Strecher, V. J., & Becker, M. H. (1988). Social learning theory and the health belief model. *Health Education Quarterly, 15*, 175–183.

Roshanaei-Moghaddam, B., Katon, W. J., & Russo, J. (2009). The longitudinal effects of depression on physical activity. *General Hospital Psychiatry, 31*, 306–315.

Russell, J. A. (2003). Core affect and the psychological construction of emotion. *Psychological Review, 110*, 145–172.

Sabiston, C. M., Brunet, J., Kowalski, K. C., Wilson, P. M., Mack, D. E., & Crocker, P. R. E. (2010). The role of body-related self-conscious emotions in motivating women's physical activity. *Journal of Sport and Exercise Psychology, 32*, 417–437.

Sallis, J. F., & Hovell, M. F. (1990). Determinants of exercise behavior. *Exercise and Sport Sciences Reviews, 18*, 307–330.

Sallis, J. F., & Owen, N. (1999). *Physical activity and behavioral medicine*. Thousand Oaks, CA: Sage.

Schneider, M., Dunn, A., & Cooper, D. (2009). Affect, exercise, and physical activity among healthy adolescents. *Journal of Sport and Exercise Psychology, 31*, 706–723.

Schneider Jamner, M., Spruit-Metz, D., Bassin, S., & Cooper, D. M. (2004). A controlled evaluation of a school-based intervention to promote physical activity among sedentary adolescent females: Project FAB. *Journal of Adolescent Health, 34*, 279–289.

Schwarzer, R. (2008). Modeling health behavior change: How to predict and modify the adoption and maintenance of health behaviors. *Applied Psychology, 57*, 1–29.

Schwarzer, R., Luszczynska, A., Ziegelmann, J. P., Scholz, U., & Lippke, S. (2008). Social-cognitive predictors of physical exercise adherence: Three longitudinal studies in rehabilitation. *Health Psychology, 27*, S54–S63.

Shephard, R. J. (1988). Exercise adherence in corporate settings: Personal traits and program barriers. In R. K. Dishman (Ed.),

Exercise adherence: Its impact on public health (pp. 305–319). Champaign, IL: Human Kinetics.

Sheppard, K. E., & Parfitt, G. (2008). Patterning of physiological and affective responses during a graded exercise test in sedentary men and boys. *Journal of Exercise Science & Fitness, 6*, 121–129.

Shiv, B., & Fedorikhin, A. (1999). Heart and mind in conflict: The interplay of affect and cognition in consumer decision making. *Journal of Consumer Research, 26*, 278–292.

Shiv, B., & Fedorikhin, A. (2002). Spontaneous versus controlled influences of stimulus-based affect on choice behavior. *Organizational Behavior and Human Decision Processes, 87*, 342–370.

Shiv, B., Fedorikhin, A., & Nowlis, S. M. (2005). Interplay of the heart and the mind in decision-making. In S. Ratneshwar & D. G. Mick (Eds.), *Inside consumption: Consumer motives, goals, and desires* (pp. 166–184). London: Routledge.

Simon, H. A. (1983). *Reason in human affairs*. Stanford, CA: Stanford University Press.

Slade, S. C., Molloy, E., & Keating, J. L. (2009). People with chronic low back pain who have participated in exercise programs have preferences about exercise: A qualitative study. *Australian Journal of Physiotherapy, 55*, 115–121.

Sloman, S. A. (1996). The empirical case for two systems of reasoning. *Psychological Bulletin, 119*, 3–22.

Slovic, P. (2001). Cigarette smokers: Rational actors or rational fools? In P. Slovic (Ed.), *Smoking: Risk, perception, and policy* (pp. 97–124). Thousand Oaks, CA: Sage.

Slovic, P., Finucane, M. L., Peters, E., & MacGregor, D. G. (2002). The affect heuristic. In T. Gilovich, D. Griffin, & D. Kahneman (Eds.), *Heuristics and biases: The psychology of intuitive judgment* (pp. 397–420). New York: Cambridge University Press.

Slovic, P., Peters, E., Finucane, M. L., & MacGregor, D. G. (2005). Affect, risk, and decision-making. *Health Psychology, 24*, S35–S40.

Slovic, P., Finucane, M. L., Peters, E., & MacGregor, D. G. (2007). The affect heuristic. *European Journal of Operational Research, 177*, 1333–1352.

Sober, E., & Wilson, D. S. (1998). *Unto others: The evolution and psychology of unselfish behavior*. Cambridge, MA: Harvard University Press.

Sorensen, M. (2006). Motivation for physical activity of psychiatric patients when physical activity was offered as part of treatment. *Scandinavian Journal of Medicine and Science in Sports, 16*, 391–398.

Spencer, H. (1879). *The data of ethics*. New York: Appleton.

Spencer, H. (1905). *The principles of psychology* (3rd ed., Vol. 1). New York: Appleton.

Spielberger, C. D., Gorsuch, R. L., & Lushene, R. E. (1970). *Manual for the State–Trait Anxiety Inventory*. Palo Alto, CA: Consulting Psychologists Press.

Stanovich, K. E., & West, R. F. (2000). Individual differences in reasoning: Implications for the rationality debate? *Behavioral and Brain Sciences, 23*, 645–726.

Stetson, B. A., Rahn, J. M., Dubbert, P. M., Wilner, B. I., & Mercury, M. G. (1997). Prospective evaluation of the effects of stress on exercise adherence in community-residing women. *Health Psychology, 16*, 515–520.

Stevens, M., Lammink, K. A. P. M., van Heuvelen, M. J. G., de Jong, J., & Rispens, P. (2003). Gronningen Active Living Model (GALM): Stimulating physical activity in sedentary older adults: Validation of the behavioral change model. *Preventive Medicine, 37*, 561–570.

Stones, M. J., Kozma, A., & Stones, L. (1987). Fitness and health evaluations by older exercisers. *Canadian Journal of Public Health, 78*, 18–20.

Stroebe, W., Papies, E. K., & Aarts, K. (2008). From homeostatic to hedonic theories of eating: Self-regulatory failure in food-rich environments. *Applied Psychology, 57*, 172–193.

Svenson, O. (2003). Values, affect, and processes in human decision making: A differentiation and consolidation theory perspective. In S. L. Schneider & J. Shanteau (Eds.), *Emerging perspectives on judgment and decision research* (pp. 287–326). New York: Cambridge University Press.

Thorndike, E. L. (1911). *Animal intelligence: Experimental studies*. New York: Macmillan.

Tierney, S., Mamas, M., Skelton, D., Woods, S., Rutter, M. K., Gibson, M., … Deaton, C. (2011). What can we learn from patients with heart failure about exercise adherence? A systematic review of qualitative papers. *Health Psychology, 30*, 401–410.

Troiano, R. P., Berrigan, D., Dodd, K. W., Mâsse, L. C., Tilert, T., & McDowell, M. (2008). Physical activity in the United States measured by accelerometers. *Medicine & Science in Sports & Exercise, 40*, 181–188.

Trost, S. G., Owen, N., Bauman, A. E., Sallis, J. F., & Brown, W. (2002). Correlates of adults' participation in physical activity: Review and update. *Medicine & Science in Sports & Exercise, 34*, 1996–2001.

Vanden Auweele, Y., Rzewnicki, R., & van Mele, V. (1997). Reasons for not exercising and exercise intentions: A study of middle-aged sedentary adults. *Journal of Sports Sciences, 15*, 151–165.

Van Landuyt, L. M., Ekkekakis, P., Hall, E. E., & Petruzzello, S. J. (2000). Throwing the mountains into the lakes: On the perils of nomothetic conceptions of the exercise–affect relationship. *Journal of Sport and Exercise Psychology, 22*, 208–234.

Vara, L. S., & Epstein, L. H. (1993). Laboratory assessment of choice between exercise or sedentary behaviors. *Research Quarterly for Exercise and Sport, 64*, 356–360.

Varey, C., & Kahneman, D. (1992). Experiences extended across time: Evaluation of moments and episodes. *Journal of Behavioral Decision Making, 5*, 169–185.

Wankel, L. M. (1985). Personal and situational factors affecting exercise involvement: The importance of enjoyment. *Research Quarterly for Exercise and Sport, 56*, 275–282.

Wankel, L. M. (1993). The importance of enjoyment to adherence and psychological benefits from physical activity. *International Journal of Sport Psychology, 24*, 151–169.

Warburton, D. E. R., Katzmarzyk, P. T., Rhodes, R. E., & Shephard, R. J. (2007). Evidence-informed physical activity guidelines for Canadian adults. *Applied Physiology, Nutrition, and Metabolism, 32*, S16–S68.

Watson, J. (1895). *Hedonistic theories from Aristippus to Spencer*. New York: Macmillan.

Weber, E. U., & Johnson, E. J. (2009). Mindful judgment and decision making. *Annual Review of Psychology, 60*, 53–85.

Welch, A. S., Hulley, A., Ferguson, C., & Beauchamp, M. R. (2007). Affective responses of inactive women to a maximal incremental exercise test: A test of the dual-mode model. *Psychology of Sport and Exercise, 8*, 401–423.

West, H. R. (2004). *An introduction to Mill's utilitarian ethics*. New York: Cambridge University Press.

Wilcox, S., Oberrecht, L., Bopp, M., Kammermann, S. K., & McElmurray, C. T. (2005). A qualitative study of exercise in older African American and white women in rural South Carolina: Perceptions, barriers, and motivations. *Journal of Women and Aging, 17,* 37–53.

Williams, D. M. (2008). Exercise, affect, and adherence: An integrated model and a case for self-paced exercise. *Journal of Sport and Exercise Psychology, 30,* 471–496.

Williams, D. M., Dunsiger, S., Ciccolo, J. T., Lewis, B. A., Albrecht, A. E., & Marcus, B. H. (2008). Acute affective response to a moderate-intensity exercise stimulus predicts physical activity participation 6 and 12 months later. *Psychology of Sport and Exercise, 9,* 231–245.

Wilson, P. M., Mack, D. E., Blanchard, C. M., & Gray, C. E. (2009). The role of perceived psychological need satisfaction in exercise-related affect. *Hellenic Journal of Psychology, 6,* 183–206.

Wilson, P. M., Rodgers, W. M., Blanchard, C. M., & Gessell, J. (2003). The relationship between psychological needs, self-determined motivation, exercise attitudes, and physical fitness. *Journal of Applied Social Psychology, 33,* 2373–2392.

Yeung, R. R., & Hemsley, D. R. (1997a). Exercise behaviour in an aerobics class: The impact of personality traits and efficacy cognitions. *Personality and Individual Differences, 23,* 425–431.

Yeung, R. R., & Hemsley, D. R. (1997b). Personality, exercise and psychological well-being: Static relationships in the community. *Personality and Individual Differences, 22,* 47–53.

Young, P. T. (1959). The role of affective processes in learning and motivation. *Psychological Review, 66,* 104–125.

Zajonc, R. B. (1980). Feeling and thinking: Preferences need no inferences. *American Psychologist, 35,* 151–175.

PART 5

Exercise Psychology in Special Populations

Exercise Psychology and Physical Disability

Jeffrey J. Martin

Abstract

Enhanced fitness can prevent or attenuate disability and associated secondary conditions. This chapter reviews the psychosocial research on physical activity (PA) engagement by people with physical disabilities. Included are sections addressing the psychosocial benefits of PA, levels of PA engagement, barriers to PA (e.g., medical, environmental, and social), and predictors of PA participation. The chapter incorporates subsections for children/adolescents and for adults. In addition, research findings are categorized as individual, social, or environmental. It is clear that barriers to PA can be grounded in individual-level considerations ranging from the nature of a person's disability and attendant factors (e.g., pain) to the individual's social networks, such as parents in the case of children and health personnel in the case of adults living in health care facilities. The built environment can also constrain PA.

Key Words: Disability, physical activity, exercise, sport, health, adapted, social psychology.

The purpose of this chapter is to review the psychosocial research on physical activity (PA) engagement by people with physical disabilities. The chapter is organized into five sections; for purposes of discussion, the research findings are subdivided into two populations: children/adolescents and adults. The first section of the chapter presents the various benefits of PA participation for individuals with disabilities. Second is a section that includes a brief presentation of PA participation rates of individuals with disabilities. The third section examines the barriers that individuals with disabilities face when attempting to be physically active. The fourth section discusses predictors of PA. The concluding section presents directions for future research.

Benefits of Physical Activity

A major argument for the value of PA is the multiple benefits associated with it across diverse domains (i.e., physiological, social, cognitive, and emotional). Like nondisabled individuals, people with disabilities can improve their fitness in programs that are home based (Keyser, Rasch, Finley, & Rodgers, 2003), community centered (Allen, Dodd, Taylor, McBurney, & Larkin, 2004), or parts of randomized controlled trials (Hicks et al., 2003). In particular, an often cited benefit of enhanced fitness is its role in preventing or attenuating disability and associated secondary conditions. For instance, in a three-year longitudinal study of over 1,300 older (>65 years) Taiwanese individuals (S. C. Wu, Leu, & Li, 1999), those who exercised were less likely to become chronically disabled (i.e., disabled for more than three months). Although delaying impaired function and enjoying physiological benefits are important, this chapter focuses on the psychosocial benefits of PA.

Children and Adolescents

INDIVIDUAL

Competence

Taub and Greer (2000) interviewed 22 school-children/adolescents with disabilities enrolled in grades 4–12 to determine how they felt about their PA involvement. A clear theme in their answers was that PA enhanced their perceptions of competence, with three mechanisms noted. First, children's increased strength and fitness as a result of PA led to increased competence. Second, children's opportunities to portray their abilities helped counter negative stereotypes held by their peers. Third, PA engagement expanded children's vision of their potential future competencies. Some children experienced anxiety as a result of not feeling skilled in some sports (e.g., volleyball). Participants also reported growth in their overall self-esteem. Taub and Greer (2000) viewed children's increased competence and self-esteem as legitimizing their social identities and contributing to reduced stigmatization and a sense of being "normal."

Perceived competence was also the focus of a study examining the impact of a one-week summer sport camp for children with visual impairments (Shapiro, Moffett, Lieberman, & Dummer, 2005). Shapiro and colleagues (2005) found a gender–time interaction effect, with girls increasing their competence over time. A consistent pattern of increases in social acceptance, athletic competence, and physical appearance was evident in the girl's mean scores. The authors speculated that girls' relationships with the camp counselors were stronger than boys', and that the girls may have been more open to competence-enhancing feedback. Both mechanisms may have then resulted in girls' improving where boys did not. Clearly, both social dynamics and mastering sporting activities may have jointly affected the girls' perceptions of competence (Shapiro et al., 2005). Groff and Kleiber (2001) interviewed 11 youth with cerebral palsy (CP) or spina bifida (SB) who participated in an after-school adapted-sport program. Respondents also indicated that their sport experiences led to confidence in other areas of their lives.

Independence and Normality

Anderson, Bedini, and Moreland (2005) interviewed fourteen 10- to 16-year-old girls to determine their perceptions of the benefits associated with PA. Respondents indicated that PA aided in minimizing the influence of their disability on their mental and physical health. For instance, a girl named Jan indicated that she felt most "normal" when she was "playing sports" (Anderson et al., 2005, p. 91). Jan also noted that she felt "free when I'm doing them [sports]" (Anderson et al., 2005, p. 91). Another theme by Anderson et al. (2005) was that children attributed increased feelings of independence to their sport involvement. Given that independence is a critical psychological need (Deci & Ryan, 1985), giving individuals choices can help them feel independent. Mandigo and Natho (2005) examined the value of choice and quality of experience when they assessed the quality of summer camps (offering sailing, ropes courses, etc.). Participants reported higher levels of competence, enjoyment, optimal challenge, and skills for programs that they chose to do than for programs that were required.

SOCIAL

Peers

Martin and Smith (2002) and Martin (2005) reported that youth athletes with disabilities derived a variety of social benefits from having a best friend on their sport team, and females tended to report greater benefits than did males. In Groff and Kleiber's (2001) study, virtually every participant in the after-school adapted-sport program commented on the value of being able to connect with other youth who had disabilities. In turn, this sense of connectedness helped them "be themselves" (Groff & Kleiber, 2001, p. 326). Groff and Kleiber surmised that it was specifically the adapted nature of the sport program that was critical in providing an atmosphere that allowed the youth to be "personally expressive" (p. 328). Taub and Greer (2000) also noted increased social integration among youth athletes with disabilities. Participating in PA increased their opportunities to interact with classmates who were both able bodied and who had a disability. Their increased interaction strengthened their social bonding and broadened their friendship networks. Although Taub and Greer (2000) painted an encouraging picture of how PA can be a "salient normalizing experience" (p. 410), they were careful to point out that some children had negative experiences, such as being excluded from physical education (PE) classes, not being selected for teams, and being teased. Thus while PA and PE can be positive psychosocial vehicles, there is also the potential for negative consequences.

In Anderson et al.'s (2005) study, participants cited a benefit not frequently mentioned: PA as an opportunity to be with friends while simultaneously being away from home. Individuals with disabilities face more barriers to travel and have fewer opportunities to see the world than youngsters without disabilities. Thus it seems very understandable that children with disabilities might cherish PA as an opportunity to see the world with friends (i.e., teammates).

Peers and Reciprocity

Schleien, Green, and Stone (2003) suggested that friendships developed in inclusive recreation settings may not always be true friendships. Green and Schleien (1991) likewise reported that the major relationships of individuals with disabilities are with family, caregivers, and others with disabilities, and that these individuals may mistake those relationships, which are often partly founded on a sense of obligation, for true friendships. Place and Hodge (2001) also posited that interactions among adolescents in PE may reflect a sense of moral obligation rather than expressions of friendship. They further maintained that individuals with disabilities may have trouble providing reciprocity and accepting friendship responsibilities, which are critical to authentic friendships. Additionally, Place and Hodge suggested that people with disabilities may not have well-developed skills for promoting and maintaining friendships in inclusive settings. Schleien et al. (2003) reasoned that if their portrayal of individuals with disabilities was accurate, those individuals' misperceptions of what constitutes a friendship and their lack of friendship-generating skills might present barriers to their ability to form authentic friendships in inclusive PA settings.

Some limited convergent evidence for this viewpoint is offered by George and Duquette's (2006) single-case study of Eric, an 11-year-old boy with low vision. He was well liked by his peers except during PE class. During sports, classmates picked him last for their teams, often became impatient with him, and frequently excluded him. His low vision limited his ability to engage in spontaneous games such as hide-and-seek and chasing. In his mother's words,

> He thinks that he needs to be friends with a certain group of kids and I wonder if he's missing out on the ones who really do enjoy his company because to Eric, they're not the ones he wants to be friends with. To me, he wants to be friends with the ones who are athletic. I know who he thinks are his friends, but I don't know if they are his friends. Because to be a best friend has to be something that is reciprocated, and I don't know if that's necessarily the case.
> (*George & Duquette*, 2006, p. 156)

Eric's teachers confirmed that he was less popular during PE class than in other settings. Fortunately, although his PE and sport setting friendships were conditional, in other contexts George and Duquette asserted that he was fully accepted by his peers. They concluded that Eric was considered an "acquaintance" by the able-bodied athletic boys and that his real friendships were rooted in the classroom, with "academic" children.

Adults

INDIVIDUAL

Self-Efficacy and Competence

The strong theme of involvement in sports resulting in competence is not new. For instance, Farias-Tomaszewski, Jenkins, and Keller (2001) evaluated the benefits derived from therapeutic horseback riding. They obtained measures of physical and global self-efficacy and behavioral confidence before and after a 12-week riding program provided to 22 adults with physical disabilities. The efficacy measures were self-report scales, whereas behavioral confidence reflected assessments by a research assistant (blind to the study purposes) and the riding instructor of observable behaviors (e.g., reluctance to mount the horse or need for assistance by the riding instructor). Although global self-efficacy did not change, both physical self-efficacy and behavioral confidence increased over the course of the intervention. While the study did not use a control group, the converging results from three different assessments (by the participant, riding instructor, and research assistant) supporting gains in efficacy and confidence give the findings greater validity than those of research that relies, as is common, on a single source of self-report data.

Enjoyment

Other researchers have investigated the relationship between exercise and mood. For instance, individuals with disabilities (mostly spinal cord injury [SCI]) reported increased positive affect and decreased negative affect after exercising (Giacobbi et al., 2006). Furthermore, the relationships between exercise and positive and negative affect were consistent regardless of whether respondents reported negative or positive life events. Thus exercise was helpful in mood management not only when participants had a good day but also when they had a bad day. There was also some suggestion that individuals predisposed to experiencing negative affect (i.e., neurotic individuals) may derive greater mood-enhancing benefits from PA (Giacobbi et al., 2006).

Kosma, Ellis, Cardinal, Bauer, and McCubbin (2007) examined 143 adults with disabilities and found that participants reported a number of advantages to engaging in PA that reflected their beliefs about the beneficial outcomes of PA. The biggest benefit, noted by almost half the respondents (48.0%) was enhanced emotional functioning. In a study by Allen et al. (2004), adults with CP also reported enjoying PA and more specifically their experiences with strength training For instance, according to nine of the 10 participants, the major reason that they viewed strength training as positive was because it was enjoyable. Their enjoyment was largely grounded in their social interactions with both the other participants and the staff managing the program.

Quality of Life

Martin Ginis, Latimer, and colleagues have conducted a number of quality-of-life studies examining the impact of PA on mood, stress, depression, pain, life satisfaction, and subjective well-being in mostly male adults with SCI (Ditor et al., 2003; Hicks et al., 2003, 2005; Latimer, Martin Ginis, & Craven, 2004; Latimer, Martin Ginis, & Hicks, 2005; Latimer, Martin Ginis, Hicks, & McCartney, 2004; Martin Ginis & Hicks, 2005; Martin Ginis & Latimer, 2006; Martin Ginis et al., 2002, 2003). Their research agenda targets the benefits of PA ranging from acute to chronic programs. Because virtually all of their research studies are prospective, randomized controlled trials, their findings command greater confidence than those of cross-sectional correlational designs.

In a study examining the impact of acute (i.e., single episodes of) treadmill exercise they found that individuals who experienced the greatest reductions in pain while exercising also had the strongest improvement in feeling states (Martin Ginis & Latimer, 2006). However, some participants experienced increased pain during exercise.

Martin Ginis et al. (2003) examined the role of chronic (three months) exercise. More specifically, they examined if reduced perceptions of pain and stress and increased feelings of control and efficacy mediated improvements in subjective well-being and quality of life. Thirty-four individuals with SCI participated in a randomized controlled trial that consisted of stretching, aerobic arm ergometry, and resistance training (e.g., weight lifting). Participants in the exercise group experienced increased subjective well-being and physical self-concept and reduced pain, stress, and depression compared with the controls. Additionally, partial support was found for a meditational model, as stress and pain (but not control and efficacy) mediated the influence of exercise on quality of life. This latter result suggests that exercise improved quality of life because it reduced stress and pain.

Latimer, Martin Ginis, et al. (2004) examined the benefits of a nine-month, twice weekly program of resistance and aerobic exercise. They found that exercise reduced stress through a reduction in pain. Stated differently, a decrease in pain as a result of exercise led to decreased stress. The authors speculated that improved muscle function in injury-prone muscle groups may have alleviated pain, which in turn reduced stress. Similar to the exercise-pain stress link, a reduction in stress due to exercise resulted in lower depression. Latimer, Martin Ginis, et al. suggested that perceptions of increased physical capability for activities of daily living led to a decrease in stress about managing difficult activities of this sort. In turn, reduced stress caused participants to experience fewer symptoms of depression. Martin Ginis et al. (2002) conducted focus group interviews with 15 individuals, 10 of whom were in their nine-month study to understand the benefits of PA. The most to least cited benefits were that wheeling and activities of daily living became easier (n = 4), reduced feelings of being disabled (n = 2), the experience of a challenge (n = 2), that wheelchair transfers became easier (n = 2), that muscles and joints loosened (n = 2), and that PA was a vehicle for social interaction (n = 2). A clear theme is that PA made daily life easier. Hicks et al. (2003) also examined the psychological and physiological effects of a nine-month, twice weekly exercise program. They found that participants (N = 21), relative to the control group (N = 13), had increases in upper body strength; reported less pain, stress, and depression; and showed greater satisfaction with quality of life and physical function.

The Hicks et al. (2003) study had a dropout rate of nearly half (48%). Therefore Ditor et al. (2003) decided to conduct a three-month follow-up study of seven individuals who completed the nine-month Hicks et al. (2003) investigation. A critical finding from this follow-up study was that the nine-month exercise-related benefits were not maintained. Another valuable finding was the participant's report of pain after the initial nine-month study was negatively related to their adherence over the course of the three-month study and predicted 83% of the variance in adherence. In other words, less pain was related to greater adherence.

Latimer et al. (2005) conducted a secondary analysis of the Hicks et al. (2003) data to determine if exercise mediated the effects of stress on well-being in individuals with SCI. The participants represented all the individuals from the Hicks et al. study ($N = 34$) who completed all the measures for the first six months of that nine-month study. Participants in this randomized controlled trial were assessed at zero, three, and six months and were in an exercise ($n = 13$) or control ($n = 10$) group. Baseline results indicated that participants reporting more stress also reported more depression. Similarly, at baseline, stress and quality of life were negatively related: Participants who reported a high quality of life also reported low stress. In general, at subsequent measurements, the stress–depression relationship and the stress–quality of life relationship disappeared for the exercise condition but remained for the control group. Given this differential pattern of associations over time for the two groups, Latimer et al. (2005) concluded that their findings provided preliminary support for the value of PA in buffering stress and enhancing quality of life.

Hicks et al. (2005) examined SCI adults ($N = 13$) who participated in a 12-month-long program of body weight–supported treadmill training. They also collected data at eight months' post training. Participants walked three times a week and in each session walked 5–15 minutes three times. As expected, participant's ability to walk improved (more on the treadmill than over the ground), as did their life and physical function satisfaction. Gains in satisfaction were correlated with treadmill walking ability: As participants became better at walking, they became more satisfied with life.

In brief, Martin Ginis, Latimer, and colleagues (Ditor et al., 2003; Hicks et al., 2003, 2005; Latimer, Martin Ginis, & Craven, 2004; Latimer et al., 2005; Latimer, Martin Ginis, et al., 2004; Martin Ginis & Latimer, 2006; Martin Ginis et al., 2002, 2003) have assembled an impressive body of research providing strong support for quality-of-life benefits of PA for SCI individuals.

Tasiemski, Kennedy, Gardner, and Taylor (2005) were interested in determining if PA was positively related to multidimensional life satisfaction for wheelchair users with SCI living in the U.K. About half of their participants ($N = 985$) participated in sport, and they were compared on life satisfaction scales with those participants who did not participate in sport or PA. A clear pattern was found that physically active individuals had higher levels of general life satisfaction, ability to care for themselves, and satisfaction with leisure, sex, financial issues, vocational issues, and family and friends. Regression analyses indicated that sport participation, along with mood, marital status and extent of loss of independence, predicted general life satisfaction.

Warms, Belza, Whitney, Mitchell, and Stiens (2004) examined 16 individuals with SCI in a six-week intervention that lacked a control group. They found that participants increased their upper body strength and reported enhanced exercise self-efficacy, a reduction in motivational barriers, and increases in self-rated health status. While the intervention seemed to reduce internal barriers (i.e., lack of motivation), it predictably did not lead to any discernible reduction in participants' perceptions of external barriers.

Muraki, Tsunawake, Hiramatsu, and Yamasaki (2000) divided 169 SCI athletes into four groups based on their PA. They found that the most active group (more than three days a week of PA) reported the lowest levels of depression and trait anxiety and conversely scored the highest on a measure of vigor. There was a clear linear trend across all four groups (high active, middle active, low active, and inactive) in the mean scores for these three measures, in the expected direction. This finding not only further supports the value of PA but demonstrates a dose–response relationship.

SOCIAL

Relationship Complexity

PA does not automatically confer social benefits on participants, whether they are able-bodied or have a disability (Taub & Greer, 2000). For instance, Devine (2004) examined 14 adults, many with a disability (e.g., CP and spina bifida), who participated in an inclusive recreation program. The three themes she gleaned from her data quite succinctly portrayed the range, from positive to neutral to negative, of their social experiences. For instance, on the positive side participants viewed their leisure activity as helping to bridge barriers between themselves and fellow participants without disabilities. A participant named Judy, for example, indicated that the adaptive equipment she used was accepted and that her peers were "really cool about it and all. They even named the stuff ya know and all" (Devine, 2004, p. 148).

Comments by Aaron, a 33-year-old with a SCI, illustrate the dynamic and positive influence that being proactive can have on recreation personnel and, in turn, how they can influence able-bodied participants:

> I think they really picked up on how he [recreation staff member] treated me. They all seemed willing to play [sport] with me and joke with me. I think he really set the tone, if ya know what I mean. I mean when I first started [in the recreation program] I gave [staff] a heads-up to not be soft on me or anything and I'm here to tell ya he wasn't and I think it really made a difference on the others.
>
> (*Devine*, 2004, p. 149)

For a small number of participants the leisure context was neutral. Participants perceived able-bodied individuals as feeling ambivalent or uninterested in them. Andrew indicated that at a fitness club people appeared afraid to talk to him, yet he still perceived them as nice. Perhaps his own words, in response to whether he felt accepted, do the best job of portraying this category of neutrality: "Sometimes, but I really don't know. I don't know if they like me or want me here or not. I can't tell" (Devine, 2004, p. 153). A parallel framework for understanding this category may be found in the friendship literature, where Asher and Dodge (1986) distinguish between children who clearly feel rejected and children who are ignored or neglected.

Devine (2004) labeled her last type of participants "distancers." Participants with more severe disabilities tended to exemplify this type more than those with milder disabilities. Jan, for instance, reported feeling invisible, whereas Elvis, who had CP, told a story of being mocked for his speech. Similar to numerous reports in the literature, Jordan indicated that recreation staff were overprotective when he came to bat during a baseball game. Jordan reported that "I felt like everyone treated me like a baby then, like they had to take care of me and I was already 21 years old" (Devine, 2004, p. 152).

Socially Grounded Competence

Page, O'Conner, and Peterson (2001) interviewed six high-level athletes with disabilities (e.g., Paralympians). A consistent theme emerging from their data was the importance of the presence of other people. Similar to many findings in this area, the opportunity to construct relationships by being on a team was an major benefit of PA. However, contrary to many findings related to the social benefits of disability sport, participants did not cite the value of social interaction per se as the only socially grounded benefit. Instead, the opportunity to demonstrate competence to others, even if they did not know who the others were, was of value. Page et al. report that "virtually any individual, just by being in the presence of a participant, was a significant other in the eyes of the participant" (p. 45). Furthermore, part of the participants' drive to demonstrate competence was the perception that because of their disability, they were often viewed as incompetent.

Converging evidence for the value of competence and the importance of the perceptions of others can be found in the work of Arbour, Latimer, Martin Ginis, and Jung (2007). Arbour and colleagues found that nondisabled individuals (*N* = 446) viewed physically active individuals with disabilities more favorably than they did nonactive individuals. For instance, exercisers were viewed more favorably on a variety of personality dimensions (e.g., friendly, self-reliant, persistent, independent, self-confident, and happy) and physical dimensions (e.g., healthy, muscular, fit, and physically strong) than were non-exercising and control groups.

Family

As Lyons, Sullivan, Ritvo, and Coyne (1995) note, disability is an interpersonal issue and family relationships are critical. A small but growing body of research exists on how PA experiences affect the family as a unit and children, siblings, and parents separately. This research has documented the relational benefits grounded in PA that families experience. As noted by Mactavish, Schleien, and Tabourne (1997), researchers examining family recreation and PA experiences (e.g., Mactavish & Schleien, 2000; Orthner & Mancini, 1990) have shown that such involvement enhances family quality of life.

Zabriskie, Lundberg, and Groff (2005) asked 129 participants, most of whom (70%) were under the age of 18, to report how their adaptive skiing or horseback riding experiences affected their family quality of their life. Nearly 70% agreed or strongly agreed that their experiences in these sports enhanced their family life. Additionally, almost 80% of the participants agreed or strongly agreed that skiing or riding with family members added or contributed to the meaning of the activity. This finding is supported by Mactavish and Schleien (2004), who found that parents (particularly mothers) in families that have children with disabilities often engaged in PA (e.g., swimming or bike riding) with their children to enhance family relationships. Mactavish et al. (1997) interviewed 65 families with children who had a variety of disabilities (e.g., CP).

Most families engaged in recreation at home or in the community (e.g., through church).

Most families ($n = 61$) indicated that one of three patterns of involvement typified their PA engagement: all family members, a subgroup such as one parent and all children, or an alternating pattern involving the first two groups. The most prevalent scenario was one parent (typically the mother) and one child with a disability or all children engaging in some form of recreational activity. In most cases mothers consciously planned activities as a way to overcome various barriers (e.g., busy schedules or competing demands) that would have otherwise prevented PA experiences. Engaging in recreation and PA activities was also more manageable with small groups, especially if the child had a significant developmental disability that required much attention. To summarize, the PA and recreation experiences of families that included a child with a disability tended to be child centered and typically organized by mothers.

Siblings without disabilities also contributed to generating play opportunities for their brothers or sisters with a disability by adapting how they played, particularly if they enjoyed the activity too (Pit-Ten Cate & Loots, 2000). In contrast, siblings of children with disabilities have also noted that outdoor games (e.g., football) were unpleasant experiences because of the difficulty of playing together (Pit-Ten Cate & Loots, 2000). As children with and without disabilities grow older, disparities in abilities become more evident. As a result there is potential for the equitable horizontal friendship relationship to be replaced by the inequitable vertical supervisory relationship common in siblings of differing capabilities and ages (Harry, Day, & Quist, 1998).

However, even this characterization is incomplete and lacks the complexity found in the day-to-day interactions among siblings in play settings. For instance, Harry et al. (1998) observed Raul, a 12-year-old boy with Down syndrome, and his three brothers over a four-year period. Many of their observations revolved around informal play in neighborhood parks and during basketball as well as in physical education class. In brief, they found that Raul's siblings engaged in four types of play: "big brothering" play, facilitating play that helped Raul, parallel play, and reciprocal play. Furthermore, the relative amounts of the above play patterns differed among siblings. Older brothers engaged in more big-brothering than a brother who was close in age to Raul.

Scholl, McAvoy, Rynders, and Smith (2003) examined the ramifications of an inclusive four-day outdoor skill training program, followed by a three- to five-day outdoor adventure trip, on families that included a child with a disability. Parents reported that their involvement in the project helped them overcome or eliminate constraints they typically experienced in finding ways for their children to be physically active. Both qualitative and quantitative results indicated that parents believed the experience enhanced family interactions and promoted greater family cohesion. Kristén, Patriksson, and Fridlund (2003) studied 20 Swedish families' involvement in their children's PA (orienteering, golf, or archery). One of the themes that emerged was that children's involvement in sport allowed the family to "experience a feeling of togetherness" (Kristén et al., 2003, p. 30). In brief, PA-oriented experiences are vehicles that enhance the psychosocial functioning of families.

Parent Benefits

The benefits of PA extend beyond the participants to the parents in what might be viewed as unintended beneficial consequences. For instance, Castañeda and Sherrill (1999) examined family participation in Challenger baseball, which is an adapted form of baseball so children with disabilities can play. They followed 15 families over a two-year period and summarized the five major benefits of Challenger baseball as noted by the parents. The third most prominent theme was how bringing their children to games and practices also provided parents with a ready-made support group. For instance, one mother noted:

> You get to be around other families that also share some of the stressful situations that go along with managing children with special needs. It makes that family feel very welcome in the sense that they can live a normal life; they can participate in normal activities.
>
> (*Castañeda & Sherrill*, 1999, p. 383)

Summary: Benefits of Physical Activity

In summary, the body of research reviewed highlights that PA does not inherently confer benefits on participants with disabilities. Rather, the participation and support of other individuals (e.g., parents, peers, and health care personnel) contributes greatly to the quality of the experience. Furthermore, the benefits of PA may be enhanced when participants are able to be active with similar others (e.g., in disability-specific programs), valued peers (e.g., a best friend), and significant adults (e.g., parents). The benefits of PA involvement can also extend to individuals without disabilities (e.g., parents) when they can derive social support from individuals in similar life circumstances. In some cases PA experiences can be detrimental, as when exercising too much causes pain or when peers in PE settings engage in hurtful teasing. Finally, work by Martin Ginis and colleagues suggests that quality-of-life benefits (e.g., reduced depression) may be a function of reduced stress and pain resulting from exercise.

Physical Activity Participation

Appropriate PA engagement is important for everyone given the numerous psychological, social, and physiological benefits associated with it. It is particularly critical for individuals with disabilities (Rimmer, 2005). For example, children, adolescents, and adults with disabilities are all at greater risk for overweight and obesity than nondisabled individuals (Rimmer, Rowland, & Yamaki, 2007).

Existing research clearly indicates that most individuals with physical disabilities engage in minimal PA. This pattern cuts across virtually all major demographic categories. Low levels of PA have been documented in the U.S. (Schenker, Coster, & Parush, 2005), Canada (Longmuir & Bar-Or, 1994), Israel (Margalit, 1981), the Netherlands (van den Berg-Emons et al., 1995), Japan (Suzuki et al., 1991), and Rwanda (Amosun, Mutimura, & Frantz, 2005). Children and adolescents (Brown & Gordon, 1987) as well as adults (Martin, 2007) engage in less PA than able-bodied individuals.

The pattern of low PA also exists across settings and types of PA. Children with disabilities obtain less PA in school (Schenker et al., 2005) irrespective of whether the location is the gym, recess, PE, or the playground (Simeonsson, Carlson, Huntington, McMillen, & Brent, 2002). Lifestyle PA is also limited for children (Margalit, 1981) and for adults (Shumway-Cook et al., 2002). The finding of low PA holds true for nearly all disability types: It has been observed in SCI (Suzuki et al., 1991), CP (Margalit, 1981), spina bifida (Brown & Gordon, 1987), Duchenne muscular dystrophy (McDonald, Widman, Walsh, Walsh, & Abresch, 2005), amputees (Amosun et al., 2005), visual impairments (Kozub, 2006), developmental disabilities (Levinson & Reid, 1991), and mixed-disability groups (Martin, 2007). One exception is hearing-impaired children (Suzuki et al., 1991). Findings of low PA are also consistent regardless of the measure used: self-report (Longmuir & Bar-Or, 1994), pedometers (Lieberman, Stuart, Hand, & Robinson, 2006), total daily energy expenditure (Buchholz, McGillivray, & Pencharz (2003), accelerometers (Kozub & Oh, 2004), or doubly labeled water (van den Berg-Emons et al., 1995)

In summary, most people with disabilities obtain less PA than individuals without disabilities. There are, however, differences within disability. People who have more severe disabilities, are older, or are of lower socioeconomic status (SES) obtain less PA than individuals who have less severe disabilities, are younger, or are from upper SES brackets (Rimmer, Riley, Wang, Rauworth, & Jurkowski, 2004). Finally, deaf individuals often do not obtain less PA than able-bodied individuals. (Deaf individuals often do not see themselves as having a disability but rather consider themselves to have a different mode of communication.)

Barriers to Physical Activity

The life-changing nature of acquiring a disability has led researchers to become interested in barriers to PA. It is critical to understand what prevents people with disabilities from obtaining PA in order to obviate the sense of hopelessness exemplified by the finding that 95% of Canadians with a disability who are sedentary believed that "nothing" would increase their PA (Canadian Fitness Survey, 1983).

Children and Adolescents

INDIVIDUAL

Disability

It should be obvious that disability influences PA choices. For instance, children without the use of their legs (e.g., amputee or quadriplegic children) are unable to run. Thirty-three percent of the parents of 54 deaf-blind children believed that their child's disability was the most common barrier to engagement in activities such as swimming or bicycling (Lieberman & MacVicar, 2003). In regard to disability severity, parents of children who were blind noted far more barriers than parents of children with low vision (Nixon, 1988). Clearly, it is difficult for children with severe disabilities to engage in PA.

Pain and Fatigue

Children report "pain or discomfort" as a major barrier to PA (Kang, Zhu, Ragan, & Frogley, 2007). As many as two-thirds of children with CP experience pain, especially children with moderate and severe CP (Hadden & von Baeyer, 2002; Tervo, Symons, Stout, & Novacheck, 2006). Tervo et al. (2006) indicated that pain was correlated with walking ability: Parents who reported more pain in their children also reported that their children were worse at walking than did parents of children experiencing less pain. With respect to specific activities that pain interfered with, over a third of the parents indicated that pain interfered with running short distances, riding a bike, climbing stairs, walking, and participating in recreation and in PE. Out of 31 specific activities examined, pain interfered the most with recreation participation (cited by 45.5% of parents). The physical discomfort of PA has also been noted as a barrier for adolescents with hearing loss (Tsai & Fung, 2005).

SOCIAL

Parents

Many children are reliant on their parents to encourage, transport them to, pay for, and facilitate their PA involvement. This dependence on adults is heightened for children with disabilities, as they often cannot take advantage of informal opportunities for PA. For instance, a child in a wheelchair cannot easily go outside and spontaneously play in the snow. Scholl et al. (2003) examined the PA barriers faced by 24 families. Five general categories of barriers emerged. First, parents faced emotional, economic, and physical challenges related specifically to their children's disabilities. One mother often found it difficult to come up with creative activities for her nonverbal and passive son. Another family spent $100,000 on making their home accessible. Second, parents had to juggle caregiving responsibilities so that they did not neglect their children without disabilities. Third, parents experienced stress when monitoring their children's play engagement. For example, parents were sensitive to how others might react negatively to their children's disabilities.

Fourth, parents were concerned for their children's safety when playing. Ironically, in the Kang et al. (2007) study, children indicated that three of the top five "nonbarriers" to PA were fears about injury during PA, about getting hurt during transportation, and about being safe in general. A participant in the Anderson et al. study (2005) stated her parents were "scared [she] might break" (p. 92). In brief, although parents are concerned about their children's safety during PA, their children often do not share that worry. The fifth and last theme in the Scholl et al. (2003) study was the parents' perception that many community recreation personnel lacked disability awareness.

Community Personnel

The criticism of community recreation personnel by parents in the Scholl et al. (2003) is not uncommon. In a study of children with hearing impairments, parents perceived that a major barrier to PA was community facility staff who were unfamiliar with their children's disability (Lieberman & MacVicar, 2003). Parents noted that other barriers included lack of knowledge about appropriate adaptations, programming ideas, how to communicate, and accessibility issues.

Physical Education Personnel

Stuart, Lieberman, and Hand (2006) reported that parents also believed that PE teachers lacked training in dealing with children with disabilities. PE teachers themselves reported their own lack of professional preparation as the top barrier to teaching PE to children with disabilities (Lieberman, Houston-Wilson, & Kozub, 2002). A lack of equipment (e.g., auditory balls) and inadequate programming were two more barriers. Fitzgerald (2005) reported that some boys with disabilities felt ignored in PE.

Oh, Ozturk, and Kozub (2004) examined 19 visually impaired students in PE and found most of them to be insufficiently active. Most notable was a lack of any sustained large-limb movement. Exacerbating this troublesome picture was an obvious absence of any significant social engagement. For instance, over half (11/19) of the participants were engaged with adults, peers, or materials less than 20% of the time.

Lieberman and Houston-Wilson (1999) classified PE barriers in three areas: teachers, students, and administrative. Many teachers expressed that they lacked professional preparation. Activities (e.g., football) were often not suitable unless modified. In addition, the pace of the lessons was often too fast, and teachers viewed children with visual impairments as safety threats. The second category of barriers lay in the students themselves. Many students were viewed by their teachers as being overprotected by their parents and lacking in confidence as a result of limited experiences. As a result they often came to class fearful, short on skills, and lacking confidence. The last category reflects administrative barriers. PE is frequently replaced by therapy, mobility training, or Braille class even though to do so is against American law (i.e., the Individuals with Disabilities

Education Act (IDEA) Amendment, 1997). Costly adapted equipment (e.g., auditory balls) is often needed to accommodate students with disabilities. PE participation is also restricted by unnecessary blanket medical excuses from doctors.

In conclusion, the most serious problem in PE is that many students are excluded by PE teachers because of their impairment (Lieberman, Robinson, & Rollheiser, 2006).

Peers

Levinson and Reid (1991) reported that a lack of friends was a barrier to PA. Kang et al. (2007) reported that "a lack of a place to exercise with peers" was in the top five (out of 45) obstacles to PA. Stuart et al. (2006) also found that parents of children with low vision, and the children themselves, viewed a lack of peers to play with as a major barrier. Adolescents with severe or profound hearing loss also reported that a lack of friends to engage in leisure-time PA with was a barrier (Tsai & Fung, 2005). Finally, children's treatment by peers can be a barrier. Taub and Greer (2000) pointed out that some children in their study were not allowed to participate in PE classes, were teased, and were not picked for teams. Boys in PE in Fitzgerald's study (2005) similarly reported being called names by other children.

ENVIRONMENT

Institutional

Young girls with disabilities have reported that there are limited places to engage in PA (Anderson et al., 2005). Parents of blind children viewed a lack of opportunity as one of the top three barriers to PA for their children (Stuart et al., 2006). Children have also noted having "no activities" to do as a barrier (Stuart et al., 2006). Scholl et al. (2003) reported that as children got older the limited PA opportunities dwindled further and were often restricted to competitive sport. Even when opportunities exist, they can be illusionary. Wheelchair basketball leagues sometimes prevent children who use motorized chairs from playing (Anderson et al., 2005). Finally, Tsai and Fung (2005) reported that even when PA facilities are available, they can be inconveniently located.

Physical

Built-environment barriers are physical constraints such as a lack of a curb cut, which can prevent wheelchair users from crossing the street. Built-environment barriers can also be subtle. For instance, in a U.K. study, although many sport centers offered swimming for individuals with disabilities, the water was often too cold to swim in (French & Hainsworth, 2001).

Adults

INDIVIDUAL

Disability

In adults, much as in children and adolescents, the nature of a person's disability is itself a barrier to PA (e.g., Finch, Owen, & Price, 2001). Ellis, Kosma, Cardinal, Bauer, and McCubbin (2007) found that adults reported disability and related symptoms as the foremost barrier (cited by 20.6% of participants).

Another way to examine the impact of disability is to examine PA levels before and after injury. Tasiemski, Kennedy, and Gardner (2006) found that among their 985 participants, only 43% of those who played sports prior to their SCI continued playing after injury. Also, as might be expected, the number of hours engaged in sport dropped after participants experienced a SCI.

In a somewhat paradoxical finding, Chaves and colleagues (2005) found that the number-one PA barrier among 70 SCI individuals was their wheelchair—even more than their physical impairment. Thus although the wheelchair is considered a significant aid to SCI individual's ability to move about, it is ironically also viewed as a major limitation. A major difficulty noted was an uncomfortable fit, which is not surprising given that most suppliers and clinicians have limited training in prescribing wheelchairs. In a related finding, the wheelchair was the biggest factor subjects reported as "limiting their access" to leaving home and using transportation, with the physical environment a close second (Chaves, Boninger, Cooper, Fitzgerald, Gray, & Cooper, 2004). According to Chaves et al., many SCI individuals find manual wheelchairs heavy, hard to manipulate, and often too wide for home use.

In regard to disability severity, individuals with paraplegia were more likely to be physically active than those with quadriplegia (Manns & Chad, 1999). Over half of the 2,298 Australians surveyed by Finch et al. (2001) reported that their injury or disability was the major barrier preventing them from increasing their PA. In support of this finding, Manns and Chad (1999) examined 38 men and women with SCI and found that leisure-time PA was correlated with their level of disability. Individuals with lower levels of disability were more active than those with more severe disabilities.

Furthermore, the relationship between disability level and PA was stronger for quadriplegics than paraplegics. Finally, participants' "impairment" was also the most common "external" barrier to exercise cited by 113 American adults (Kinne, Patrick, & Maher, 1999).

Pain and Fatigue

Another common barrier to PA is pain. Henderson and Bedini (1995) reported that, according to their participants, the most important factor limiting their PA was pain, lack of energy, or both. Often women would describe the need to "pace themselves" to avoid excessive tiredness. Feelings of limited energy have also been reported elsewhere (Rimmer, Rubin, Braddock, & Hedman, 2000). In fact, many women would make daily assessments of their energy level and feelings of fatigue or pain before deciding on their activity level (Hendersen & Bedini, 1995). Goodwin and Compton (2004) found pain to be a dominant theme in their study of six active women with disabilities. In fact pain was at times more limiting to their PA than their disability. Ironically, pain could result from both too much and too little PA. In brief, the women had to consistently manage their disability, pain, and their PA on a regular basis.

Rollins and Nichols (1994) reported that 28% of the participants in their study indicated that PA was "at least somewhat" painful. Wilber and colleagues (2002) reported that chronic pain and fatigue are two of the most common secondary conditions associated with disability. Gardner et al. (2007) found that fatigue and pain were the third and fourth most common barriers to PA (reported by 16.6% and 13.9% of participants, respectively). Lack of energy was also reported by Rimmer, Rubin, and Braddock (2000) and Scelza, Kalpakjian, Zemper, and Tate (2005). Pain may be a particularly relevant barrier for individuals with a SCI compared with, for instance, visually impaired individuals. Ninety-four percent of people with SCI indicate that they have pain (Martin Ginis et al., 2003).

Illness and Injury

As adults age, they are more likely to cite disease and injury as a barrier to PA. For instance, older (75–81 years) Finnish adults with mobility limitations reported "poor health" as the biggest barrier to exercise, especially if they had a severe mobility limitation (Rasinaho, Hirvensalo, Leinonen, Lintunen, & Rantanen, 2006). In a study of over 6,000 British residents, Chinn, White, Harland,

Drinkwater, and Raybould (1999) found that while illness and disability were barriers for only 4% of 16- to 24-year-olds, that figure increased to 20% and 52% for adults 45–54 and 65–75 years old, respectively. Gardner et al. (2007) found that injury or illness was one of the top 10 reasons (cited by 11.2%) that their respondents did not engage in PA. K. O. O'Neill and Reid (1991) reported that 40% of their older (55–90 years) Canadian participants were prevented from exercising by illness or disability. As Rimmer (2005) cogently points out, older people with disabilities have to simultaneously manage their primary disability, associated secondary conditions (e.g., obesity), and health-related aspects of aging (e.g., more illness).

Knowledge

Heller, Ying, Rimmer, and Marks (2002) examined barriers to exercise for adults with CP living in nursing or group home environments. One of the most significant barriers was a lack of knowledge about exercise locations (cited by 34.5% of participants). Rimmer, Rubin, and Braddock (2000) noted that 58% of older (35–64 years) low-income urban African American women with severe disabilities did not know where to exercise. Similar findings have been reported for individuals with SCI (Scelza et al., 2005). Amosun et al. (2005) reported on the barriers faced by SCI adults living in Rwanda. The top two were a lack of knowledge about where to exercise (32%) and a lack of motivation (22%).

Fear

Fear was noted as a "very important" barrier to PA by 12% of the participants in a study by Rollins and Nichols (1994). Fear is a particularly prominent barrier for those who are most limited in mobility (Rasinaho et al., 2006). Fear of developing tight muscles or joints has been noted by individuals with SCI (Martin Ginis et al., 2003). Finally, Rimmer, Rubin, et al. (2000) found that 40% of their respondents were afraid to leave their homes for fear of crime and fear of falling, which may reflect the urban setting in which they lived.

Time

A common barrier to PA among nondisabled people is a lack of time (Schifflet, Cator, & Megginson, 1994), and a shortage of time also limits PA for adults with disabilities. Rollins and Nichols (1994) reported a lack of time due to work (cited by 27.6% of respondents), family (16.6%), and other interests (8.0%) as being "very important" barriers. Zhu

(2001) found that a lack of time was the second most severe barrier to PA; another highly ranked barrier was "lack of a block of time." The latter finding suggests that respondents viewed a set amount of time as a prerequisite, or at least important, for PA. This perception runs counter to the U.S. national recommendation for daily PA, which conveys the appropriateness of obtaining PA in small chunks of time (e.g., 10 minutes) over the course of a day (U.S. Department of Health and Human Services, 1996). In contrast to the above findings, Rimmer, Rubin, et al. (2000) found that most of their respondents (92%) did not view a lack of time as a barrier, a result that might reasonably be viewed as indicative of their unemployed status.

Economics

Rimmer, Rubin, et al. (2000) found that two of the top four barriers to PA were the cost of an exercise program (cited by 84% of respondents) and a lack of transportation (61%). Rimmer, Riley, Wang, and Rauworth (2004) likewise noted that people with disabilities cited the costs of transportation and memberships to exercise clubs as barriers to PA. Other researchers have also noted a lack of transportation and prohibitive cost as barriers to PA engagement (Martin Ginis et al., 2002; Scelza et al., 2005). Levin, Redenbach, and Dyck (2004) write that a lack of finances for adaptive equipment is also an obstacle to sport participation.

SOCIAL
Health Care Personnel

Heller et al. (2002) examined barriers to PA for adults with CP. They found that half the caregivers did not believe an exercise program would help their residents, and about a third of those residents themselves believed exercise would not help their CP. Some caregivers (16.1%) thought that exercise would make their clients' CP worse. These results suggest that the significant others (e.g., caregivers) who should be helping their clients becoming more active and healthier do not believe exercise is beneficial and may, in fact, be harmful.

A recent report would seem to partly substantiate the Heller et al. (2002) results. In a survey of physical medicine and rehabilitation resident physicians, Staley and Worsowicz (2005) found that fewer than half had attended a class or lecture on disability sport and PA, and only a little over half had received information on those topics from an attending doctor. Fortunately, 88% indicated they were interested in learning more.

Levins et al. (2004) interviewed eight adults with SCI in order to understand influences on their PA. Most participants suggested that their experiences in rehabilitation did not prepare them for PA. For instance, they reported not having access to information about or resources (e.g., facilities) for PA. A common theme emerging from the study by Scelza et al. (2005) was a sense among individuals with disabilities that their physical abilities were underestimated, even by their physical therapists.

Fitness Facility Personnel

Rimmer, Riley, Wang, and Rauworth (2005) reported that individuals with disabilities perceived that owners and employees of fitness centers viewed accessibility as a "necessary evil" (p. 423) or as unimportant. Similarly, Rimmer et al. found that focus group members in the fitness profession cited fitness professional's negative attitudes, lack of work ethic, and liability concerns as barriers. These same focus group members also noted that fitness and recreation facilities often lacked policies related to disabilities. For instance, open swim periods were not long enough to take into account the extra transportation, changing, and access time that individuals with disabilities need to be ready to swim. Members of all focus group, that included individuals with disabilities, city planners, architects, and fitness professionals cited a lack of PA programming as a barrier for individuals with disabilities.

ENVIRONMENT
Institutional

Rimmer and colleagues (2005) evaluated the accessibility of 35 U.S. health clubs in urban and suburban settings across six areas: built environment, swimming pool, equipment, information, policies, and professional behavior. Most facilities had helpful assistive devices such as grab bars in the showers or automatic entrance doors. In contrast, most facilities did not have curb cuts for easy access or paths to lockers that were not blocked. Most facilities also did not allow adequate room for transfers from wheelchairs to exercise equipment, but they did have adequate access to the exercise area in general.

It would be costly to fix many of the exercise facility shortcomings, such as a lack of adaptive exercise equipment. In other areas, such as some staff members appearing to be uncomfortable with dealing directly with individuals with disabilities, improvement would be cost free. However, Rimmer et al. found that most staff (more than 85%) provided helpful assistance and made direct eye contact with clients with disabilities. Rimmer et al. concluded that people with mobility disabilities and visual impairments would "have difficulty accessing various areas of fitness facilities and health clubs" (p. 2022). Martin Ginis and colleagues (2003) affirmed that sentiment by noting that 10 of 15 SCI participants cited inaccessible facilities or equipment as a barrier to PA. Schifflet et al. (1994) also found that individuals with disabilities viewed a lack of access to PA facilities to be an impediment to maintaining an active lifestyle.

Barriers found in the built environment extend beyond barriers found in exercise facilities. Older people often use malls to obtain PA through walking. Unfortunately the same opportunity for PA is restricted for individuals with disabilities. McClain (2000) studied three large shopping malls in the southwestern U.S. to determine their compliance with the Americans with Disabilities Act of 1990. She examined the parking lots, elevators, ramps, restrooms, food courts, telephones, dressing rooms, store aisles, and store shelf heights. She obtained mixed results, with compliance ranging from 0% to 100% depending on the feature. For example, although the malls all had ramps for wheelchairs, ramps at two of the three malls had too steep slopes. No food court tables had adequate knee space for wheelchair users.

French and Hainsworth (2001) noted that members of disabled sport groups cited difficulties accessing and using toilet and changing facilities in sport facilities as their number-one complaint. A lack of ramps and insufficient room to accommodate a wheelchair were also common barriers. Rimmer, Riley, Wang, and Rauworth (2004) surveyed architects, recreation and fitness professionals, park managers, and city managers and thus were able to obtain unique information from individuals who were directly or indirectly responsible for building facilities or developing programs. Similar to what prior research had reported, they were told of barriers in the built environment (e.g., no elevators in fitness facilities). In their study of SCI adults living in the U.K., Tasiemski and colleagues (2005) reported that the second most significant barrier to participating in sports was a lack of accessible facilities.

Clearly the built environment (and perceptions of the built environment) should be construed as barriers to PA for persons with disabilities.

Neighborhood

Even outdoor areas designed for PA can inadvertently present barriers to individuals with disabilities. For example, poorly lit walking paths or wooded walking trails with rocks or fallen branches can be barriers to individuals with vision loss (Rimmer, 2006). A lack of audible signals at traffic lights and curb cuts that do not have high-contrast color markings that make them distinctly visible are also barriers for individuals with vision loss (Rimmer, 2006).

Other researchers have substantiated the shortcomings noted by Rimmer (2006). For instance, Spivock, Gauvin, and Brodeur (2007) surveyed 112 neighborhoods in Montreal, Canada, to determine if the environment made it easy or difficult for people with disabilities to integrate PA into their everyday lives. They assessed walking surfaces (e.g., whether paths were wide enough for a wheelchair), signage (e.g., whether crosswalks had auditory signals) and surroundings (e.g., whether access ramps and parking for people with disabilities were present). Mean scores for the various features were low in absolute terms (under the midpoint of the scale). In relative terms, they were significantly lower than reference question scores for the active-living friendliness of neighborhoods for nondisabled individuals.

Opportunity

French and Hainsworth (2001) interviewed individuals representing various sport and PA organizations (e.g., national disability sport organizations) as well as individuals with disabilities in the U.K. Many comments reflected a belief that the demand for disability sport opportunities was minimal. At the local government level a common approach to providing PA and sport opportunities was to schedule a "taster day or session" to introduce sport to people with disabilities. Representatives of local governments sponsoring these activities often commented that although the events were heavily publicized, attendance was typically low, which likely contributed to a belief that demand is not high. A lack of opportunity has also been noted in the U.S. For instance, Gardner et al.'s (2007) participants reported that a lack of access to programs, equipment, and fitness sites was one of the top 10 barriers to PA (cited by 17% of the respondents).

Summary: Barriers to Physical Activity

It is clear that barriers to PA can be grounded in issues ranging from individual-level considerations such as the nature of a person's disability and attendant factors (e.g., pain) to members of individuals' social networks, such as parents in the case of children and health personnel in the case of adults living in health care facilities. The built environment can also constrain PA.

The complexity of pinpointing a set of specific factors that might be considered the most important barriers is illuminated by four examples. First, in the French and Hainsworth (2001) study, sport center representatives recognized that access to their facilities was woefully inadequate and presumably realized how such a barrier would limit participation. However, the representatives also assumed that low participation reflected a lack of interest as opposed to an inability to participate (due to, e.g., a lack of transportation). This highlights two opposing views that could both be correct for different groups of people in different settings.

Second, the influence of a barrier (or barriers) is not uniform and can interact with other important factors. For instance, as Cardinal, Kosma, and McCubbin (2004) point out, the impact of a barrier depends on a person's readiness to engage in PA. Barriers may be irrelevant for individuals who have no intention to engage in PA, whereas for those individuals in the maintenance stage of exercise (i.e., who are engaged in regular PA), barriers have presumably been successfully managed. In contrast to these two examples, barriers may be quite salient and important for people who are contemplating or preparing to engage in PA or are newly engaged in regular PA.

Third, participants in Kinne et al.'s (1999) study noted a variety of common barriers such as their impairment, a shortage of accessible facilities, a lack of money, and a lack of information. However, external barriers such as a lack of access to facilities did not differentiate between participants who maintained exercise and those who did not. This finding indicates that some individuals are able to overcome their barriers to regularly engage in PA.

Fourth, Scelza et al. (2005) used the same barrier scale as Rimmer, Rubin, and Braddock (2000) but with a much different sample. Their results for the top barriers were identical: the cost of an exercise program, lack of energy, lack of transportation, and not knowing where to exercise. However, the percentages of participants reporting those factors as barriers were higher in the Rimmer et al. study. The participants in the Rimmer et al. study were older, lower-SES African American women from the inner city with chronic illnesses (e.g., stroke). In contrast, Scelza et al. (2005) studied younger, higher-SES,

mostly male SCI adults living in a much smaller university community setting. Despite two vastly different samples and settings the barriers were quite similar in type—but they were dissimilar in degree.

In summary, there is no shortage of barriers to PA for individuals with disabilities, and different barriers exist for different people. Barriers range from common impediments experienced by all people (e.g., a lack of time) to barriers related specifically to a person's disability (e.g., pain and wheelchairs). As such, no common set of barriers can be identified with any certainty at this time.

Predictors of Physical Activity

While understanding the roadblocks to PA for people with disabilities is important, it is also valuable to know what factors enable or facilitate PA. A clear understanding of such factors can refine theory, aid researchers in designing PA intervention studies, and inform health care professionals.

Children and Adolescents

INDIVIDUAL

Self-Efficacy and Competence

In a study of PA in children with developmental coordination disorder (DCD), Cairney, Hay, Faught, Mandigo, and Flouris (2005) found that children with DCD had lower PA self-efficacy than children without DCD. In a similar study Cairney and colleagues found that preference, confidence, and enjoyment accounted for 28% of the variance in PA (Cairney, Hay, Faught, Wade, et al., 2005). It should be noted that in both studies, the self-efficacy measure was confounded with task value and enjoyment items, making attributing results solely to self-efficacy problematic.

In a related study Cairney and colleagues (2007) also examined the role of perceived competence in PA for children with DCD in PE. They found that children with DCD were heavier, less fit, and expressed less competence about their physical abilities than children without DCD.

Enjoyment and Value

Children in the Cairney et al. (2007) study reported less enjoyment of PE than children without DCD but still had relatively high absolute enjoyment scores. The key finding from the Cairney et al. (2007) study was that DCD children's lesser enjoyment of PE was mostly the result of having lower competence for PA, rather than of being heavier or less fit.

Martin (2005) reported that enjoyment was the major predictor of sport commitment in a sample of international youth athletes. Sport commitment was defined as a desire to continue sport involvement in the future. Stuart et al. (2006) found that parent's expectations for their children to successfully engage in PA were significantly related to children's expectations of PA success and how much they valued PA. Value and expectations are primary predictors of behavior and have been supported as such in PA research with children without disabilities. Thus it is plausible that parent's expectations contributed to PA engagement in children with disabilities through the development of children's positive value and expectancy judgments.

ENVIRONMENT: INSTITUTIONAL

School participation often involves high levels of activity as students move throughout the day among school locations (e.g., library, cafeteria, classroom, playground, gym, hallways, and parking lot). Recess time, the playground, and PE class are all locations where PA is also often the norm but can be avoided.

Initial research regarding levels of PA by children with disabilities is not encouraging. For instance, Eriksson, Welander, and Granlund (2007) observed 33 children with and without disabilities and found that children with disabilities had lower PA participation rates than children without disabilities. Eriksson et al. noted that children with disabilities would, for example, stay in a classroom while the other children played outside. Furthermore, when children with disabilities played outdoors they often engaged in different activities from their peers. Eriksson et al. noted that lower PA engagement of children with disabilities typically occurred when peers excluded them during unstructured activities (e.g., recess).

Almqvist and Granlund (2005) sought to determine the qualities of the person and the environment that predicted high levels of school PA participation. For environmental variables, they assessed the availability of school activities such as athletics, school dances, and outdoor play. They also measured the physical and social school environment, assessing, for example, whether the school was perceived as safe and whether the outdoor environment was adapted to facilitate PA. For the personal variables they measured social interaction and perceptions of autonomy. Almqvist and Granlund concluded from their results that high levels of positive interactions between students with disabilities and their teachers and peers, coupled with a strong sense of autonomy, contributed to active living while at school.

Disability type and severity were unrelated to participation. However, because of the complexity of their analyses (i.e., different variables in different clusters predicted participation), Almqvist and Granlund noted that "participation can be built from different patterns or combinations of variables" (p. 312). Their reluctance to dismiss the value of any variable is understandable, as variables may differ in their importance for different children.

Adults
INDIVIDUAL
Prior Experience

Ponchillia, Strause, and Ponchillia (2002) found results supporting the value of PE and PA in young adults. For instance, participating in PE in high school was positively related to college sports participation. In turn, 75% of their participants who participated in college sport teams participated in sporting events after college, compared with 40% for those who did not take part in college sports. In brief, school sporting activities tracked PA engagement later in life.

In a study of 33 SCI individuals, those who exercised prior to their injury were more likely to be physically active than those who had not been active (S. B. O'Neill & Maguire, 2004). S. B. O'Neill and Maguire (2004) also reported that 12 of their 14 active subjects were male, suggesting that gender differences in PA among people with disabilities may mimic the gender differences in PA found among individuals without disabilities.

Hedrick and Broadbent (1996) also found support for the value of prior PA experience in PA engagement after disability. They examined 229 university alumni with disabilities and found that college-level PA was the best predictor of current PA, accounting for 18% of the variance. An additional 6% of the variance was due to perceived disability severity. Interestingly, subjective disability severity accounted for variance whereas objective functional disability type did not. This result suggests that perceived limitations play at least as important a role in PA behavior as objective limitations due to a disability.

Finally, S. K. Wu and Williams (2001) examined 143 SCI wheelchair athletes from the U.K. Individuals who had been active prior to their injury engaged in regular sport participation an average of almost three years sooner ($M = 4.5$ years) after the injury than participants who had been inactive ($M = 7.3$ years). As the means illustrate the different of almost 3 years is not trivial.

Collectively, these findings illustrate the value of sport as a vehicle for PA.

Self-Efficacy and Self-Concept

In a study of 224 middle-aged adults with disabilities, Kosma, Gardner, Cardinal, Bauer, and McCubbin (2006) were able to predict 18% of the variance in self-reported PA. Individuals employing both behavioral and cognitive processes of change and who were high in self-efficacy reported more PA than individuals lower in efficacy and using fewer cognitive and behavioral strategies. For instance, participants who reported scheduling time for PA (a behavioral process) or reading to learn about PA (a cognitive process) engaged in more PA than people who did not use such change strategies.

Bean, Bailey, Kiely, and Leveille (2007) assessed exercise self-efficacy, readiness to exercise, and physical performance in a sample of low-income seniors who varied in their disability status as defined by activities of daily living (e.g., dressing) and instrumental activities of daily living (e.g., shopping). Participants with the highest scores for physical performance and both types of activities for daily living also reported the strongest exercise self-efficacy. That is, participants who were least disabled (e.g., had no difficulty in performing activities of daily living) also were most ready to exercise.

In a study examining the relationship between physical self-concept and PA, Martin (2007) found that sport competence, endurance, coordination, strength, and flexibility self-concepts and general self-concept were all positively related to exercise. In a multiple regression analysis the six variables together accounted for 56% of the variance in PA, with general physical self-concept and strength making the greatest contributions to the regression equation. Participants with better physical self-concepts and perceptions of strength reported more exercise than respondents with weaker perceptions in these areas. Given that physical self-concept and self-efficacy are similar (i.e., both are physical self-perceptions), both the Martin (2007) and Kosma et al. (2006) results support the potentially important function of physical self-perceptions in promoting PA.

Kerstin, Gabriele, and Richard (2006) interviewed 16 physically active people with SCI to ascertain their perceptions of the factors that helped them become physically active. Participants identified cognitive strategies reflecting self-efficacy, such as watching other SCI people be active (i.e., role models) and recalling their own PA mastery experiences and the positive affect associated with them.

Intentions and Control

Continuing their research, Kosma and colleagues (Kosma, Gardner, Cardinal, Bauer, & McCubbin, 2007) examined the ability of the theory of planned behavior (TPB) and the TPB along with the stages-of-change construct from the transtheoretical model to predict PA in individuals with disabilities. Participants (N = 143) were white and of middle SES. When using the TPB model alone Kosma et al. were able to predict 16% of the variance in PA. Findings from the second model revealed that stage of change was a stronger predictor of PA than intention. This finding supports the importance of understanding individuals' readiness to be active in order to stage-match intervention programs.

In a second study using the TPB to examine PA, Gardner et al. (2007) sought to examine the PA beliefs underlying participants' perceived behavioral control (PBC) that facilitated their PA involvement. The top three responses to the question "What factors or circumstances would enable you to participate in PA?" were access to programs, fitness sites, and equipment (22.3%); help (15.6%); and inexpensive activities or more money (12.1%).

Latimer, Martin Ginis, and Craven (2004) used the TPB to investigate PA engagement among SCI individuals. They found that the TPB varied in its ability to predict PA depending on whether participants were quadriplegics or paraplegics. In general, more and stronger relationships were found between TPB variables and PA for quadriplegic than paraplegic SCI participants. Multiple regression results revealed that TPB variables did not predict intentions or PA for paraplegic participants. For quadriplegic individuals PBC predicted intentions and moderate-intensity PA. Latimer and colleagues concluded that lesion level moderated the role of PBC. They reasoned that quadriplegics face more barriers to exercise than paraplegics. Thus PBC, which partially reflects feelings of confidence, becomes an important cognition promoting intentions.

In a follow-up study using the TPB, Latimer and Martin Ginis (2005) reported that intentions accounted for 16% of the variance in leisure-time PA of SCI individuals. To explain this low number, Latimer and Martin Ginis noted that their measure of PBC might not have fully captured the beliefs about the numerous factors that promote and hinder PA engagement. This suggestion seems plausible when one compares the content of their measure of PBC with the plethora of beliefs facilitating and preventing PA reported by respondents in the Gardner et al. (2007) study. Latimer and Martin Ginis (2005) also insightfully noted that barriers are not static and can change over time (e.g., bladder infection).

The weak relationship found between intentions and PA by Latimer, Martin Ginis, and Craven (2004) motivated Latimer, Martin Ginis, and Arbour (2006) to examine whether an intervention designed to help participants implement their intentions would help. When scheduling 30 minutes of PA three days a week, participants in the experimental group also had to specify where and when they would be active. Additional details were also required, such as the specific type of PA and how hard and long they would work out. The intervention was effective: The experimental group engaged in more PA than the control group, and their intentions were stronger predictors of PA. The intervention was also successful in helping participants enhance their efficacy to overcome scheduling barriers.

Using the theory of reasoned action, a forerunner of the TPB, Godin, Colantonio, Davis, Shephard, and Simard (1986) examined leisure-time PA among lower-limb-disabled adults. Intention was the strongest predictor of PA, accounting for 35% of the variance. Habit accounted for 7% of the variance, suggesting that leisure-time PA had not become a "lifestyle" for these individuals.

In a second study, using the TPB, Godin, Shephard, Davis, and Simard (1989) examined whether acquired versus congenital disability might differentially influence leisure-time PA among young male adults with lower-limb disabilities (e.g., paraplegia). For individuals with a congenital disability, intention was the only significant predictor of PA, accounting for 55% of the variance. In contrast, a combination of having established a habit of exercising, less education, and a lower-level lesion predicted 40% of the variance in PA for individuals with an acquired disability. It is plausible that individuals born with a disability have developed coping strategies to overcome barriers to PA that allow them to implement their intentions. In contrast, individuals experiencing an injury later in life may rely on a previously established PA lifestyle and a commensurate PA identity to aid them in their efforts to be active. The finding that participants with less education were more active is contrary to much research indicating that more educated people tend to be more active. Godin and colleagues speculated that less educated individuals might have more free time for PA and that strong-armed "blue collar" workers might find wheelchair ambulation easier and thus engage in it more.

SOCIAL: HEALTH CARE PERSONNEL

As described earlier, Heller et al. (2002) examined predictors of PA in adults with CP living mostly in nursing or group homes. A key predictor of exercise participation, accounting for 8% of the variance, was caregivers' perceptions that exercise was helpful. This result suggests that the knowledge and attitudes of significant others (e.g., caregivers) influence a person's PA participation.

Summary: Predictors of Physical Activity

Most researchers examining predictors of PA have focused on individual-level constructs using social cognitive theories such as self-efficacy theory and the TPB. Most of the researchers using these theories have also tended to emphasize the cognitive part of "social cognitive." As a result, research is lacking on the social and environmental predictors of PA. It should also be recognized that often barriers and predictors are simply opposite sides of the same coin. For instance, a supportive PE teacher can facilitate PA (i.e., be a predictor), whereas an untrained PE teacher can hinder PA (i.e., be a barrier). Sometimes the same construct can be both a barrier and a predictor. For example, a wheelchair that is too wide may prevent someone from entering an exercise facility (i.e., be a barrier). At the same time, that same wheelchair may allow the person to wheel him- or herself to the grocery store (i.e., be a predictor) when a caregiver might have had to do the shopping if the person did not own a wheelchair. Finally, a single incident of lifestyle PA might reasonably be attributed to different causes. For instance, if someone cannot wheel him- or herself up a ramp to an exercise facility, the cause could be located in the wheelchair (too heavy), the person (not strong enough), a lack of aid (no social support), or the environment (a poorly designed ramp). This example illustrates the complexities involved in understanding the factors that influence PA.

Future Research Directions

Potential research directions in this field are numerous; I will briefly note four. First, a few sport and exercise psychology researchers have investigated the important role that efficacy and competence play in sport and PA. However, only limited theory-based lines of research have been developed. Self-concept theory (Marsh & Redmayne,

1994) and self-determination theory (Hagger & Chatzisarantis, 2008) are just two examples of theories that have been employed extensively in attempts to understand sport behavior among able-bodied youth, but they have rarely been used to understand sport among youth with disabilities. Hence, using self-concept theory and self-determination theory to study individuals with disabilities and PA is recommended.

Second, it seems particularly critical to understand the ways in which PA can help mitigate the high rates of unemployment, depression, and loneliness and the reduced social networks of people with disabilities. The social benefits of sport for able-bodied youth have been pretty well substantiated by researchers, but few researchers have examined how disability youth sport can enhance friendships and reduce loneliness in children. Similarly, few researchers have documented how group PA experiences can do the same for adults with disabilities.

Third, although Martin Ginis and colleagues have conducted an excellent line of research using randomized controlled trials on PA in individuals with SCI (Ditor et al., 2003; Hicks et al., 2003, 2005; Latimer, Martin Ginis, & Craven, 2004; Latimer, Martin Ginis, & Hicks, 2005; Latimer, Martin Ginis, et al., 2004; Martin Ginis & Hicks, 2005; Martin Ginis & Latimer, 2006; Martin Ginis et al., 2002, 2003), similar lines of research with individuals with different disabilities (e.g., amputees and the visually impaired) are rare. Women, older individuals, groups with rarer disabilities (e.g., dwarfism), and individuals with severe disabilities are underresearched, and we know little about their PA experiences. Research is needed in all these areas.

Fourth, according to Rimmer et al. (2007) the recent explosion of research examining the alarming increase of overweight and obesity in children has targeted able-bodied children. We know very little about the relative influences of individual, social, and environmental factors on youth with disabilities, who have even higher rates of obesity and overweight than those without disabilities. Clearly, research is needed examining the antecedents of PA and its link to overweight and obesity among children with disabilities. Similar research is needed with adults with disabilities, as they also have higher rates of overweight and obesity as well as more complicating secondary conditions (e.g., diabetes) than nondisabled individuals.

References

Allen, J., Dodd, K. J., Taylor, N. F., McBurney, H., & Larkin, H. (2004). Strength training can be enjoyable and beneficial for adults with cerebral palsy. *Disability and Rehabilitation, 26*(19), 1121–1127.

Almqvist, L., & Granlund, M. (2005). Participation in school environment of children and youth with disabilities: A person-oriented approach. *Scandinavian Journal of Psychology, 46*, 305–314.

Amosun, S. L., Mutimura, E., & Frantz, J. M. (2005). Health promotion needs of physically disabled individuals with lower limb amputation in Rwanda. *Disability and Rehabilitation, 27*(14), 837–847.

Anderson, D. M., Bedini, L. A., & Moreland, L. (2005). Getting all girls into the game: Physically active recreation for girls with disabilities. *Journal of Park and Recreation Administration, 23*(4), 78–103.

Arbour, K. P., Latimer, A. E., Martin Ginis, K. A., & Jung, M. E. (2007). Moving beyond the stigma: The impression formation benefits of exercise for individuals with a physical disability. *Adapted Physical Activity Quarterly, 24*, 144–159.

Asher, S. R., & Dodge, K. A. (1986). Identifying children who are rejected by their peers. *Developmental Psychology, 22*, 444–449.

Bean, J. F., Bailey, A., Kiely, D. K., & Leveille, S. G. (2007). Do attitudes toward exercise vary with differences in mobility and disability status? A study among low-income seniors. *Disability and Rehabilitation, 29*(15), 1215–1220.

Brown, M., & Gordon, W. A. (1987). Impact of impairment on activity patterns of children. *Archives of Physical Medicine and Rehabilitation, 68*, 828–832.

Buchholz, A. C., McGillivray, C. F., & Pencharz, P. B. (2003). Physical activity levels are low in free-living adults with chronic paraplegia. *Obesity Research, 11*(4), 563–570.

Cairney, J., Hay, J., Faught, B., Mandigo, J., & Flouris, A. (2005). Developmental coordination disorder, self-efficacy toward physical activity and play: Does gender matter? *Adapted Physical Activity Quarterly, 22*, 67–82.

Cairney, J., Hay, J., Faught, B., Wade, T. J., Corna, L., & Flouris, A. (2005b). Developmental coordination disorder, generalized self-efficacy toward physical activity and participation in organized and free play activities. *Journal of Pediatrics, 147*, 515–520.

Cairney, J., Hay, J., Mandigo, J., Wade, T., Faught, B. E., & Flouris, A. (2007). Developmental coordination disorder and reported enjoyment of physical education in children. *European Physical Education Review, 13*, 81–98.

Canada Fitness Survey. (1983). *Fitness and lifestyle in Canada.* Ottawa: Canada Fitness Survey.

Cardinal, B. J., Kosma, M., & McCubbin, J. A. (2004). Factors influencing the exercise behavior of adults with physical disabilities. *Medicine & Science in Sports & Exercise, 36*(5), 868–875.

Castañeda, L., & Sherrill, C. (1999). Family participation in Challenger baseball: Critical theory perspectives. *Adapted Physical Activity Quarterly, 16*, 372–388.

Chaves, E. S., Boninger, M. L., Cooper, R., Fitzgerald, S. G., Gray, D. B., & Cooper, R. A. (2005). Assessing the influence of wheelchair technology on perception of participation in spinal cord injury. *Archives of Physical Medicine and Rehabilitation, 85*, 1854–1858.

Chinn, D., White, M., Harland, J., Drinkwater, C., & Raybould, S. (1999). Barriers to physical activity and socioeconomic position: Implications for health promotion. *Journal of Epidemiology and Community Health, 53,* 191–192.

Deci, E. L., & Ryan, R. M. (1985). *Intrinsic motivation and self-determination in human behavior.* New York: Plenum.

Devine, M. A. (2004). Being a "doer" instead of a "viewer": The role of inclusive leisure contexts in determining social acceptance for people with disabilities. *Journal of Leisure Research, 36*(2), 137–159.

Ditor, D. S., Latimer, A. E., Martin Ginis, K. A., Arbour, K. P., McCartney, N., & Hicks, L. (2003). Maintenance of exercise participation in individuals with spinal cord injury: Effects on quality of life, stress and pain. *Spinal Cord, 41*(8), 446–450.

Ellis, R. E., Kosma, M., Cardinal, B. J., Bauer, J. J., & McCubbin, J. A. (2007). Physical activity beliefs and behaviors of adults with physical disabilities. *Disability and Rehabilitation, 29,* 1221–1227.

Eriksson, L., Welander, J., & Granlund, M. (2007). Participation in everyday school activities for children with and without disabilities. *Journal of Developmental and Physical Disabilities, 19,* 485–502.

Farias-Tomaszewski, S., Jenkins, S. R., & Keller, J. (2001). An evaluation of therapeutic horseback riding programs for adults with physical impairments. *Therapeutic Recreation Journal, 35*(3), 250–257.

Finch, C., Owen, N., & Price., R. (2001). Current injury or disability as a barrier to being more physically active. *Medicine & Science in Sports & Exercise, 33*(5), 778–782.

Fitzgerald, H. (2005). Still feeling like a spare piece of luggage? Embodied experiences of (dis)ability in physical education and school sport. *Physical Education and Sport Pedagogy, 10*(1), 41–59.

French, D., & Hainsworth, J. (2001). "There aren't any buses and the swimming pool is always cold!": Obstacles and opportunities in the provision of sport for disabled people. *Managing Leisure, 6,* 35–49.

George, A. L., & Duquette, C. (2006). The psychosocial experiences of a student with low vision. *Journal of Visual Impairment & Blindness, 100*(3), 152–163.

Giacobbi, P. R., Hardin, B., Frye, N., Hausenblas, H. A., Sears, S., & Stegelin, A. (2006). A multi-level examination of personality, exercise, and daily life events for individuals with physical disabilities. *Adapted Physical Activity Quarterly, 23,* 129–147.

Godin, G., Colantonio, A., Davis, G. M., Shephard, R. J., & Simard, C. (1986). Prediction of leisure time exercise behavior among a group of lower-limb disabled adults. *Journal of Clinical Psychology, 42,* 272–279.

Godin, G., Shephard, R. J., Davis, G. M., & Simard, C. (1989). Prediction of exercise in lower-limb disabled adults: The influence of cause of disability (traumatic or atraumatic). *Journal of Social Behavior and Personality, 4*(5), 615–623.

Goodwin, D. L., & Compton, S. G. (2004). Physical activity experiences of women aging with disabilities. *Adapted Physical Activity Quarterly, 21,* 122–138.

Green, F. P., & Schleien, S. J. (1991). Understanding friendship and recreation: A theoretical sampling. *Therapeutic Recreation Journal, 25,* 29–40

Groff, D. G., & Kleiber, D. A. (2001). Exploring the identity formation of youth involved in an adapted sports program. *Therapeutic Recreation Journal, 35*(4), 318–332.

Hadden, K. L., & von Baeyer, C. L. (2002). Pain in children with cerebral palsy: Common triggers and expressive behaviors. *Pain, 99,* 281–288.

Hagger, M., & Chatzisarantis, N. (2008). Self-determination theory and the psychology of exercise. *International Review of Sport and Exercise Psychology, 1,* 79–103.

Harry, B., Day, M., & Quist, F. (1998). "He can't really play": An ethnographic study of sibling acceptance and interaction. *Journal of the Association for Persons with Severe Handicaps, 23*(4), 289–299.

Hedrick, B. N., & Broadbent, E. (1996). Predictors of physical activity among university graduates with physical disabilities. *Therapeutic Recreation Journal, 30*(2), 137–148.

Heller, T., Ying, G., Rimmer, J. H., & Marks, B. A. (2002). Determinants of exercise in adults with cerebral palsy. *Public Health Nursing, 19*(3), 223–231.

Henderson, K. A., & Bedini, L. A. (1995). "I have a soul that dances like Tina Turner but my body can't": Physical activity and women with mobility impairments. *Research Quarterly for Exercise and Sport, 66*(2), 151–161.

Hicks, A. L., Adams, M. M., Martin Ginis, K., Giangregorio, L., Latimer, A., Phillips, S. M., & McCartney, N. (2005). Long-term body-weight supported treadmill training and subsequent follow-up in persons with chronic SCI: Effects on functional walking ability and measures of subjective well-being. *Spinal Cord, 43,* 291–298.

Hicks, A. L., Martin Ginis, K., Ditor, D. S., Latimer, A., Craven, C., Bugarest, J., & McCartney, N. (2003). Long-term exercise training in persons with spinal cord injury: Effects on strength, arm ergometry performance and psychological well-being. *Spinal Cord, 41,* 34–43.

Kang, M., Zhu, W., Ragan, B. G., & Frogley, M. (2007). Exercise barrier severity and perseverance of active youth with physical disabilities, *Rehabilitation Psychology, 52*(2), 170–176.

Kerstin, W., Gabriele, B., & Richard, L. (2006). What promotes physical activity after spinal cord injury? An interview study from a patient perspective. *Disability and Rehabilitation, 28*(8), 481–488.

Keyser, R. E., Rasch, E. K., Finley, M., & Rodgers, M. M. (2003). Improved upper-body endurance following a 12-week home exercise program for manual wheelchair users. *Journal of Rehabilitation Research and Development, 40*(6), 501–510.

Kinne, S., Patrick, D. L., & Maher, E. J. (1999). Correlates of exercise maintenance among people with mobility impairments. *Disability and Rehabilitation, 21*(1), 15–22.

Kosma, M., Gardner, R. E., Cardinal, B. J., Bauer, J. J., & McCubbin, J. A. (2006). Psychosocial determinants of stages of change and physical activity among adults with disabilities. *Adapted Physical Activity Quarterly, 23,* 49–64.

Kosma, M., Gardner, R. E., Cardinal, B. J., Bauer, J. J., & McCubbin, J. A. (2007). The mediating role of intention and stages of change in physical activity among adults with physical disabilities: An integrative framework. *Journal of Sport and Exercise Psychology, 29,* 21–38.

Kozub, F. M. (2006). Motivation and physical activity in adolescents with visual impairments. *RE:view, 37*(4), 149–160.

Kozub, F. M., & Oh, H. K. (2004). An exploratory study of physical activity levels in children and adolescents with visual impairments. *Clinical Kinesiology, 58*(3), 1–7.

Kristén, L., Patriksson, G., & Fridlund, B. (2003). Parents' conceptions of the influences of participation in a sports programme on their children and adolescents with physical disabilities. *European Physical Education Review, 9*(1), 23–41.

Latimer, A. E., & Martin Ginis, K. A. (2005). The theory of planned behavior in prediction of leisure time physical activity among individuals with spinal cord injury. *Rehabilitation Psychology, 50,* 389–396.

Latimer, A. E., Martin Ginis, K. A., & Arbour, K. P. (2006). The efficacy of an implementation intention intervention for promoting physical activity among individuals with spinal cord injury: A randomized controlled trial. *Rehabilitation Psychology, 51*(4), 273–280.

Latimer, A. E., Martin Ginis, K. A., & Craven, B. C. (2004). Psychosocial predictors and exercise intentions and behavior among individuals with spinal cord injury. *Adapted Physical Activity Quarterly, 21,* 71–85.

Latimer, A. E., Martin Ginis, K. A., & Hicks, A. L. (2005). Buffering the effects of stress on well-being among individuals with spinal cord injury: A potential role for exercise. *Therapeutic Recreation Journal, 39*(2), 131 138.

Latimer, A. E., Martin Ginis, K. A., Hicks, A. L., & McCartney, N. (2004). An examination of the mechanisms of exercise induced change in psychological well-being among people with spinal cord injury. *Journal of Rehabilitation Research and Development, 41*(5), 643–652.

Levins, S. M., Redenbach, D. M., & Dyck, I. (2004). Individual and societal influences on participation in physical activity following spinal cord injury: A qualitative study. *Physical Therapy, 84*(6), 496–509.

Levinson, L. J., & Reid, G. R. (1991, Summer). Patterns of physical activity among youngsters with developmental disabilities. *Canadian Association of Health, Physical Education and Recreation Journal, 3,* 24–28.

Lieberman, L. J., & Houston-Wilson, C. (1999). Overcoming the barriers to including students with visual impairments and deaf-blindness in physical education. *RE:view, 31*(3), 129–138.

Lieberman, L. J., Houston-Wilson, C., & Kozub, F. M. (2002). Perceived barriers to including students with visual impairments in general physical education. *Adapted Physical Activity Quarterly, 19,* 364–377.

Lieberman, L. J., & MacVicar, J. M. (2003). Play and recreational habits of youth who are deaf-blind. *Journal of Visual Impairment & Blindness, 97*(12), 755–768.

Lieberman, L. J., Robinson, B. L., & Rollheiser, H. (2006). Youth with visual impairments: Experiences in general physical education. *RE:view, 38*(1), 35–48.

Lieberman, L. J., Stuart, M. E., Hand, K., & Robinson, B. (2006). An investigation of the motivational effects of talking pedometers among children with visual impairments and deaf-blindness. *Journal of Visual Impairment & Blindness, 100*(12), 726–736.

Longmuir, P. E., & Bar-Or, O. (1994). Physical activity of children and adolescents with a disability: Methodology and effects of age and gender. *Pediatric and Exercise Science, 6,* 168–177.

Lyons, R. F., Sullivan, M. J. L., Ritvo, P. G., & Coyne, J. C. (1995). *Relationships in chronic illness and disability.* Thousand Oaks, CA: Sage.

Mactavish, J. B., & Schleien, S. J. (2000). Exploring family recreation activity in families that include children with developmental disabilities. *Therapeutic Recreation Journal, 34*(2), 133–153.

Mactavish, J. B., & Schleien, S. J. (2004). Re-injecting spontaneity and balance in family life: Parents' perspectives on recreation in families that include children with developmental disability. *Journal of Intellectual Disability Research, 48*(2), 123–141.

Mactavish, J. B., Schleien, S. J., & Tabourne, C. (1997). Patterns of family recreation in families that include children with a developmental disability. *Journal of Leisure Research, 29*(1), 21–46.

Mandigo, J. L., & Natho, K. (2005). Examining summer campers' quality of experience. *Palaestra, 21*(2), 26–31.

Manns, P. J., & Chad, K. E. (1999). Determining the relation between quality of life, handicap, fitness, and physical activity for persons with spinal cord injury. *Archives of Physical Medicine and Rehabilitation, 80,* 1566–1571.

Margalit, M. (1981). Leisure activities of cerebral palsied children. *Israeli Journal of Psychiatry and Related Sciences, 18*(3), 209–214.

Marsh, H. W., & Redmayne, R. (1994). A multidimensional physical self-concept and its relations to multiple components of fitness. *Journal of Sport and Exercise Psychology, 16,* 270–305.

Martin, J. J. (2005). Psychosocial aspects of youth disability sport. *Adapted Physical Activity Quarterly, 23,* 65–77.

Martin, J. J. (2007). Physical activity and physical self-concept of individuals with disabilities: An exploratory study. *Journal of Human Movement Studies, 52,* 37–48.

Martin, J. J., & Smith, K. (2002). Friendship quality in youth disability sport: Perceptions of a best friend. *Adapted Physical Activity Quarterly, 19,* 472–482.

Martin Ginis, K. A., & Hicks, A. L. (2005). Exercise research issues in the spinal cord injured population. *Exercise and Sport Science Reviews, 33,* 49–53.

Martin Ginis, K. A., & Latimer, A. E. (2006). The effects of single bouts of body-weight supported treadmill training on the feeling states of people with spinal cord injury. *Spinal Cord, 45,* 112–115.

Martin Ginis, K. A., Latimer, A. E., Francoeur, C., Hanley, H., Watson, K., Hicks, A. L., & McCartney, N. (2002). Sustaining exercise motivation and participation among people with spinal cord injuries: Lessons learned from a 9 month intervention. *Palaestra, 18*(1), 38–40, 51.

Martin Ginis, K. A., Latimer, A. E., McKenzie, K., Ditor, D. S., McCartney, N., Hicks, A. L., Bugaresti, J., & Craven, B. C. (2003). Using exercise to enhance subjective well-being among people with spinal cord injury: The mediating influences of stress and pain. *Rehabilitation Psychology, 48,* 157–164.

McClain, L. (2000). Shopping center wheelchair accessibility: Ongoing advocacy to implement the Americans with Disabilities Act of 1990. *Public Health Nursing, 17*(3), 178–186.

McDonald, C. M., Widman, L. M., Walsh, D. D., Walsh, S. A., & Abresch, R. T. (2005). Use of step activity monitoring for continuous physical activity assessment in boys with Duchenne muscular dystrophy. *Archives of Physical Medicine and Rehabilitation, 86,* 802–808.

Muraki, S., Tsunawake, N., Hiramatsu, S., & Yamasaki, M. (2000). The effect of frequency and mode of sports activity on the psychological status of tetraplegics and paraplegics. *Spinal Cord, 38,* 309–314.

Nixon, H. (1988). Getting over the worry hurdle: Parental encouragement and the sports involvement of visually impaired children and youth. *Adapted Physical Activity Quarterly*, 5, 29–43.

Oh, H., Ozturk, M. A., & Kozub, F. M. (2004). Physical activity and social engagement patterns during physical education of youth with visual impairments. *RE:view, 36*(1), 39–48.

O'Neill, K. O., & Reid, G. (1991). Barriers to physical activity by older adults. *Canadian Journal of Public Health, 82,* 392–396.

O'Neill, S. B., & Maguire, S. (2004). Patient perception of the impact of sporting activity on rehabilitation in a spinal cord injuries unit. *Spinal Cord, 42,* 627–630.

Orthner, D. K., & Mancini, J. A. (1990). Leisure impacts on family interaction and cohesion. *Journal of Leisure Research, 22*(2), 125–137.

Page, S. J., O'Conner, E., & Peterson, K. (2001). Leaving the disability ghetto. *Journal of Sport and Social Issues, 25*(1), 40–55.

Pit-Ten Cate, I. M., & Loots, G. M. P. (2000). Experiences of siblings of children with physical disabilities. *Disability and Rehabilitation, 22*(9), 399–408.

Place, K., & Hodge, S. R. (2001). Social inclusion of students with physical disabilities in general physical education. *Adapted Physical Activity Quarterly, 18,* 389–404.

Ponchillia, P. E., Strause, B., & Ponchillia, S. V. (2002). Athletes with visual impairments: Attributes and sports participation. *Journal of Visual Impairment & Blindness, 96*(4), 267–272.

Rasinaho, M., Hirvensalo, M., Leinonen, R., Lintunen, T., & Rantanen, T. (2006). Motives for and barriers to physical activity among older adults with mobility limitations. *Journal of Aging and Physical Activity, 15,* 90–102.

Rimmer, J. H. (2005). Exercise and physical activity in persons aging with a disability. *Physical Medicine and Rehabilitation Clinics of North America, 16,* 41–56.

Rimmer, J. H. (2006). Building inclusive physical activity communities for people with vision loss. *Journal of Visual Impairment & Blindness, 100,* 863–865.

Rimmer, J. H., Riley, B., Wang, E., & Rauworth, A. (2004). Development and validation of AIMFREE: Accessibility Instruments Measuring Fitness and Recreation Environments. *Disability and Rehabilitation, 26*(18), 1087–1095.

Rimmer, J. H., Riley, B., Wang, E., & Rauworth, A. (2005). Accessibility of health clubs for people with mobility disabilities and visual impairments. *American Journal of Public Health, 95*(11), 2022–2028.

Rimmer, J. H., Rowland, J. L., & Yamaki, K. (2007). Obesity and secondary conditions in adolescents with disabilities: Addressing the needs of an underserved population. *Journal of Adolescent Health, 41,* 224–229.

Rimmer, J. H., Rubin, S. S., & Braddock, D. (2000). Barriers to exercise in African American women with physical disabilities. *Archives of Physical Medicine and Rehabilitation, 81,* 182–188.

Rimmer, J. H., Rubin, S. S., Braddock, D., & Hedman, G. (2000). Physical activity patterns of African-American women with physical disabilities. *Medicine & Science in Sports & Exercise, 31,* 613–618.

Rollins, R., & Nichols, D. (1994). Leisure constraints, attitudes and behavior of people with activity restricting physical disabilities. In I. Henry (Ed.), *Leisure: Modernity, postmodernity and lifestyles* (pp. 277–290). Colchester, UK: Leisure Studies Association.

Scelza, W. M., Kalpakjian, C. Z., Zemper, E. D., & Tate, D. G. (2005). Perceived barriers to exercise in people with spinal cord injury. *American Journal of Physical Medicine and Rehabilitation, 84,* 576–583.

Schenker, R., Coster, W., & Parush, S. (2005). Participation and activity performance of students with cerebral palsy within the school environment. *Disability and Rehabilitation, 27*(10), 539–552.

Schifflet, B., Cator, C., & Megginson, N. (1994). Active lifestyle adherence among individuals with and without disabilities. *Adapted Physical Activity Quarterly, 11,* 359–367.

Schleien, S. J., Green, F. P., & Stone, C. F. (2003). Making friends within inclusive community recreation programs. *American Journal of Recreation Therapy, 2*(1),7–16.

Scholl, K., McAvoy, L., Rynders, J., & Smith, J. (2003). The influence of an inclusive outdoor recreation experience on families that have a child with a disability. *Therapeutic Recreation Journal, 37*(1), 38–57.

Shapiro, D. R., Moffett, A., Lieberman, L. J., & Dummer, G. M. (2005). Perceived competence of children with visual impairments. *Journal of Visual Impairment & Blindness, 99*(1), 15–25.

Shumway-Cook, A., Patla, A. E., Stewart, A., Ferrucci, L., Ciol, M. A., & Guralnik, J., M. (2002). Environmental demands associated with community mobility in older adults with and without mobility disabilities. *Physical Therapy, 82*(7), 670–681.

Simeonsson, R. J., Carlson, D., Huntington, G. S., McMillen, J. S., & Brent, J. L. (2001). Students with disabilities: A national survey of participation in school activities. *Disability and Rehabilitation, 23*(2), 49–63.

Spivock, M., Gauvin, L., & Brodeur, J. J. (2007). Neighborhood-level active living buoys for individuals with physical disabilities. *American Journal of Preventive Medicine, 32*(3), 224–230.

Staley, J. T., & Worsowicz, G. (2005). Survey of physical medicine and rehabilitation resident physicians awareness of sport and leisure activities for the disabled. *Archives of Physical Medicine and Rehabilitation, 86,* E28.

Stuart, M. E., Lieberman, L., & Hand, K. (2006). Beliefs about physical activity among children who are visually impaired and their parents. *Journal of Visual Impairment & Blindness, 100*(4), 223–234.

Suzuki, M., Saitoh, S., Tasaki, Y., Shimomura, Y., Makishima, R., & Hosoya, N. (1991). Nutritional status and daily physical activity of handicapped students in Tokyo metropolitan schools for deaf, blind, mentally retarded, and physically handicapped individuals. *American Journal of Clinical Nutrition, 54,* 1101–1111.

Tasiemski, T., Kennedy, P., & Gardner, B. P. (2006). Examining the continuity of recreation engagement in individuals with spinal cord injuries. *Therapeutic Recreation Journal, 40*(2), 77–93.

Tasiemski, T., Kennedy, P., Gardner, B. P., & Taylor, N. (2005). The association of sports and physical recreation with life satisfaction in a community sample of people with spinal cord injuries. *Neurorehabilitation, 20,* 253–265.

Taub, D. E., & Greer, K. R. (2000). Physical activity as a normalizing experience for school-age children with physical disabilities. *Journal of Sport and Social Issues, 24*(4), 395–414.

Tervo, R. C., Symons, F., Stout, J., & Novacheck, T. (2006). Parental report of pain and associated limitations in ambulatory children with cerebral palsy. *Archives of Physical Medicine and Rehabilitation, 87,* 928–934.

Tsai, E., & Fung, L. (2005). Perceived constraints to leisure time physical activity participation of students with hearing impairment. *Therapeutic Recreation Journal, 39*(3), 192–206.

van den Berg-Emons, H. J. G., Saris, W. H. M., de Barbanson, D. C., Westerterp, K. R., Huson, A., & van Baak, M. A. (1995). Daily physical activity of schoolchildren with spastic diplegia and of healthy control subjects. *Journal of Pediatrics, 127*(4), 578–584.

U.S. Department of Health and Human Services. (1996). *Physical activity and health: A report of the Surgeon General.* Atlanta, GA: U.S. Department of Health and Human Services, Centers for Disease Control and Prevention, National Center for Chronic Disease Prevention and Health Promotion.

Warms, C. A., Belza, B. L., Whitney, J. D., Mitchell, P. H., & Stiens, S. A. (2004). Lifestyle physical activity for individuals with spinal cord injury: A pilot study. *American Journal of Health Promotion, 18*(4), 288–291.

Wilber, N., Mitra, M., Walker, D. K., Allen, D. A., Meyers, A. R., & Tupper, P. (2002). Disability as a public health issue: Findings and reflections from the Massachusetts Survey Of Secondary Conditions. *Milbank Quarterly, 80,* 393–421.

Wu, S. C., Leu, S. Y., & Li, C. Y. (1999). Incidence of and predictors for chronic disability in activities of daily living among older people in Taiwan. *Journal of the American Geriatrics Society, 47*(9), 1082–1086.

Wu, S. K., & Williams, T. (2001). Factors influencing sport participation among athletes with spinal cord injury. *Medicine & Science in Sports & Exercise, 33*(2), 177–182.

Zabriskie, R. B., Lundberg, N. R., & Groff, D. G. (2005). Quality of life and identity: The benefits of a community-based therapeutic recreation and adaptive sports program. *Therapeutic Recreation Journal, 39*(3), 176–191.

Zhu, W. (2001). Calibration of the barrier instrument using the Rasch rating scale model. *Research Quarterly for Exercise and Sport, 72*(1), A-98.

Physical Activity and Exercise in Older Adults

Louis Bherer

Abstract

In today's societies, the proportions of older and very old individuals have grown considerably. However, this positive evolution brings with it certain drawbacks. For example, aging is accompanied by physiological changes that may affect health, cognitive functioning, and psychological well-being. In recent decades, an increasing number of studies have suggested that people should adopt physical activity and exercise as part of their lifestyle to alleviate the negative impact of aging on the body and mind. This chapter presents evidence that physical activity and exercise can play a positive role in improving psychological health and cognitive functioning by enhancing brain integrity in healthy older adults and in geriatric patients suffering from chronic diseases, geriatric syndromes, mild cognitive impairment, and dementia.

Key Words: physical activity, exercise, aging, chronic diseases, psychological well-being, cognition, dementia.

Introduction

Over the last century, improvements in living conditions, health, and medical care have led to a substantial increase in life expectancy. Moreover, this trend appears to have accelerated, with a gain of almost six years of life in the last 20 years. Average life expectancy at birth was 68 years worldwide in 2008, ranging from 57 to 80 across countries (Hutton, 2008). The World Health Organization predicts that the number of people aged 60 years and older, currently estimated at 600 million, will double by 2025 and will reach two billion by 2050. In the United States, 13% of the population is aged 65 and over, compared with 4% at the beginning of the 20th century. This proportion is expected to reach approximately 20% by 2030. In Canada, the aging population is estimated to increase from 4.2 to 9.8 million by 2036, when one out of four Canadians will be over 65 years old (Statistics Canada, 2008).

Aging involves many physical changes at both the molecular and cellular level in organs and in overall body composition (Harman, 2003; Manini, 2010; Zafon, 2007). These changes can dramatically alter the quality of life (Yazdanyar & Newman, 2009). Demographic aging is therefore a major economic and health concern. Biological changes associated with chronological aging, or senescence, are associated with an increased risk of chronic conditions and diseases such as cognitive impairment, cardiovascular disease, and metabolic syndrome (a cluster of the following reversible metabolic risk factors: glucose intolerance, abdominal obesity, dyslipidemia, and hypertension). Age-related diseases have increased by alarming proportions in recent decades (Wang et al., 2010). This concern is exacerbated by the fact that medical conditions can sometimes interact. For instance, as will be further discussed in this chapter, coronary heart disease has been associated with increased risk of developing mild cognitive impairment and dementia.

In the last decade, many studies have suggested that lifestyle factors have a significant impact on how people age. A key finding that is highly relevant to this chapter and the topic of this text is that age-related cognitive decline can be slowed by certain lifestyle factors. In a recent literature review, Fratiglioni, Paillard-Borg, and Winblad (2004) reported that three lifestyle factors can play a significant role in slowing the rate of cognitive decline and preventing dementia: a socially integrated network, cognitive leisure activity, and regular physical activity. More importantly, in this review and others (Hertzog, Kramer, Wilson, & Lindenberger, 2008; Kramer, Bherer, Colcombe, Dong, & Greenough, 2004), physical activity shows the most promise for protecting against the deleterious effects of age on health and cognition.

For many years, an increasing number of studies have suggested that regular physical activity maintained throughout life is associated with lower incidence and prevalence of chronic diseases such as cancer, diabetes, and cardiovascular and coronary heart diseases (Booth, Gordon, Carlson, & Hamilton, 2000; Myers et al., 2002) and may help protect against dementia (Larson et al., 2006). However, we still do not understand exactly how physical activity performed throughout life, or even for a relatively short period (i.e., a few months to a year), affects the rate of cognitive decline. Important issues are still under investigation, such as the dose–response relationship, the level of change or protection provided by physical activity, and whether physical activity can be beneficial despite chronic medical conditions, neurological syndromes such as dementia, and the physical limitations of frail patients. Although recent advances in brain imaging techniques and genetics have opened new research avenues, more studies are required to find definitive answers to these important questions.

This chapter reviews the literature on physical activity as an effective way to alleviate the burden of aging. It does not claim to be an exhaustive review of the effects of physical activity and exercise on older adults. Rather, it aims to provide an overview of the advances in knowledge, based on studies that have attempted to assess whether and how physical activity and exercise positively affects older adults at any age and with various physical and psychological conditions. This chapter discusses the impact of physical activity on cognition, physical resources, and psychological well-being in older

adults who are healthy, who have chronic diseases or geriatric syndromes, or who suffer from cognitive impairment. In each case, this chapter distinguishes between evidence from cross-sectional comparative studies based on age or health status, evidence from longitudinal studies (following the same individuals over many years), and evidence from intervention studies (comparing exercise programs to no-intervention conditions or other types of training).

Physical Activity and Aging Demographics

Broadly defined, physical activity encompasses a wide range of activities by which to achieve an active lifestyle. Studies showing the benefits of physical activities refer to "physical activity," "exercise," and "physical fitness." The strong similarity between these terms makes it difficult to tell them apart. *Physical activity* refers to any activity that involves bodily movements, and more precisely, the use of skeletal muscles. It usually is classified as requiring either high or low energy expenditure. *Physical exercise* refers to a subcategory of physical activity that is planned, structured, repetitive, and purposive. The aim is to improve or maintain one or more components of physical fitness (Caspersen, Powell, & Christenson, 1985). *Physical fitness* has been defined as "the ability to carry out daily tasks with vigor and alertness, without undue fatigue and with ample energy to enjoy leisure-time pursuits and to meet unforeseen emergencies" (Caspersen et al., 1985, p. 128).

For many people, growing older seems to involve an inevitable loss of health (fitness, strength, or energy). However, even with declining physical capacities, no one is too old to enjoy the benefits of regular physical activity. Unfortunately, despite the growing evidence for the health benefits of physical activity, elderly persons tend to be physically inactive and do not get enough leisure-time physical activity. Indeed, few older adults achieve the minimum recommended 30 or more minutes of moderate physical activity five or more days per week (Nelson et al., 2007). According to the Centers for Disease Control and Prevention (CDC), 28–34% of adults aged 65–74 and 35–44% of adults aged 75 years or older are inactive, which means that they engage in virtually no leisure-time physical activity (CDC, 1996). Inactivity is more common in older than middle-aged people. Moreover, women are more likely than men to report no leisure-time activity. In the United States, only 31% of individuals aged 65–74 report participating in 20 minutes of moderate physical activity three or more days per week, and even fewer (16%) report 30 minutes of moderate activity five or more days per week (U.S. Department of Health and Human Services, 2000). For those aged 75 and older, activity levels are even lower; 23% engage in moderate activity for 20 minutes three or more days per week, and only 12% participate in moderate activity for 30 minutes five or more days per week.

Vigorous physical activity that causes heavy sweating or significantly raises the heart rate has long been recommended to maintain and enhance cardiorespiratory fitness. Nevertheless, relatively few older persons engage in regular vigorous activity (i.e., three times per week or more), and the numbers decline steadily with age. The U.S. Department of Health and Human Services (2000) estimated that only 13% of individuals between ages 65 and 74—and only 6% of those over 75 years old—engaged in vigorous physical activity for 20 minutes three or more days per week. More recently, the CDC (2006) reported that in the United States, estimates of rates of leisure-time physical activity ranged from 10% to 43%. It therefore appears that there has been no appreciable improvement in levels of physical activity among older adults in the past decade. However, the prevalence of regular physical activity is expected to increase in the near future, from 43% to 45% for men and from 32% to 36% for women (CDC, 2007).

The level of physical activity varies according to sociocultural factors, including ethnicity. For example, when longitudinal changes in physical activity were measured in Mexican American and European American adult women based on recall interviews administered at baseline and seven years later, European American women reported more vigorous leisure activity than Mexican Americans (Sallis et al., 2001). Several factors can be associated with the choice of an active or inactive lifestyle. King et al. (2000) explored personal and environmental factors associated with physical inactivity across ethnic groups in the United States. In a sample of 2,900 middle-aged and older women, they noted that American Indian status, older age, little education, lack of energy, and lack of hills, enjoyable scenes, and other persons exercising in the neighborhood are associated with inactivity. Caregiving duties and lack of energy were the most frequent barriers to an active lifestyle. Crespo, Smit, Andersen, Carter-Pokras, and Ainsworth (2000) observed that physical inactivity is more prevalent in ethnic minorities than Caucasians, independently of social class. Crespo et al. concluded that more research was needed to examine the effect of other constructs than social class, such as acculturation, safety, social support, and environmental barriers, on promoting successful interventions to increase physical activity in these populations. These observations are in line with a recent recommendation by Wang et al. (2010) that it is critical to consider lifestyle differences across American ethnic subgroups (Asian American, Mexican-Hispanic American, African American, and Caucasian-European-White American) to develop effective health policies and educational campaigns.

In the United States, there appears to be enormous variability across regions and states in rates of participation in physical activity. In a study by Hawkins, Cockburn, Hamilton, and Mack (2004), only 11% of responders in California reported no moderate physical activity and only 27% reported no vigorous physical activity—a substantially lower prevalence of sedentary behavior than nationwide numbers. Hawkins et al. attributed this difference to differences in age and education. It follows that such variations should be considered when planning guidelines to improve physical activity in older adults.

Although most studies and surveys have examined physical activity in the broad sense, sometimes with a more specific interest in vigorous aerobic exercise, strength training has recently received increasing attention. Strength training is intended to increase muscle strength and mass. Adults who engage in strength training are less likely to experience loss of muscle mass, functional decline, and fall-related injuries than adults who do not train. The health benefits of strength training have led authorities and scientific boards to promote nationwide strength training exercise in both the United States (American College of Sports Medicine, 1998) and Canada (Canadian Society for Exercise Physiology, 2011). Data from the National Health Interview Survey suggest that the prevalence of strength training in U.S. adults increased slightly from 1998 to 2004 (CDC, 2006). However, in 2004 only 22% of men and 18% of women reported doing strength training two or more times per week, substantially lower than the national 2010 objective of 30% (CDC, 2006). This finding underscores the need for additional programs to increase strength training by adults.

Measuring Physical Activity And Cardiorespiratory Fitness In Older Adults

A major challenge in the study of exercise in older adults is how to measure physical activity in a heterogeneous population that often presents physical limitations. Moreover, because of the large variety of activities practiced by community-dwelling older persons, it is difficult to assess physical activity with standard methods. Nevertheless, the importance of physical activity and exercise and the implications for public health call for the identification of valid assessment methods at both the individual and population levels. As argued by Dishman (2006), determining the causes and health outcomes of physical activity in older adults requires the use of valid assessment methods that are reliable and practical to administer.

A wide range of methods and approaches have been used to assess physical activity in older adults (Dishman, 2006), from direct observation and self-report questionnaires on leisure-time activity, to direct biological markers to assess energy expenditure (oxygen consumption, direct and indirect calorimetry, dietary measures, doubly labeled water, and heart rate monitoring), to physical performance and cardiorespiratory fitness tests. Motion sensors and movement counters are other objective approaches to assessing physical activity in a free-living environment. They can be used in combination with self-reports and biological markers of physical activity. These devices vary widely in methodology and accuracy, from electronic pedometers that count steps to accelerometers that record the frequency and intensity of movements. Newly designed accelerometers that store and collect data over long periods are also available but are expensive to use in large-scale studies.

Many studies, especially those involving large numbers of participants, estimate physical activity level using self-report questionnaires. Several self-report measures have been designed and validated for use with older adult populations. The benefits, drawbacks, and limitations of this approach have been the focus of scientific investigations for many years. *Medicine & Science in Sports & Exercise* (Kriska, 1997) published a special edition on this issue. Recent comprehensive reviews on measurement issues in aging and physical activity are also available (Dishman, 2006; Zhu & Chodzko-Zajko, 2006). A questionnaire that is frequently cited in the literature on aging is the Yale Physical Activity Survey (Dipietro, Caspersen, Ostfeld, & Nadel, 1993). It was specifically designed for older adults and allows assessing physical activity in the broad sense, including domestic tasks and activities, leisure activities, and sports. It also estimates activity intensity (light, moderate, or vigorous). Dipietro et al.

(1993) reported that the summary index obtained with the Yale survey is significantly related to direct maximum oxygen consumption (VO_2max) tests. However, self-report questionnaires tend to overestimate activity level and in some cases cannot replace direct measures of physical fitness. Nevertheless, physical activity questionnaires provide a useful alternative when physical condition or functional limitations preclude direct physical testing.

In an increasing number of studies, physical fitness is measured directly by graded physical exercise tests or submaximal walking tests. These tests are often used in combination with self-report physical activity questionnaires to assess the level of daily activity and associated cardiorespiratory function. Submaximal walking tests and graded physical exercise tests have become increasingly popular because they can accurately measure cardiorespiratory fitness by estimating VO_2max, or the ability to transport and use oxygen during intense effort (Betik & Hepple, 2008). Accurate VO_2max measurement requires a physical effort that is sufficient in duration and intensity to fully tax the aerobic energy system. In general clinical and athletic testing, this usually involves a graded exercise test (on either a treadmill or a cycle ergometer) during which exercise intensity is progressively increased while ventilation and oxygen and carbon dioxide concentrations of the inhaled and exhaled air are measured (Betik & Hepple, 2008). VO_2max is reached when oxygen consumption remains at steady state despite an increased workload. This measure of aerobic capacity reflects physical fitness and therefore functional capacity. Low VO_2max is associated with increased risk of chronic diseases such as cardiovascular diseases and increased risk of death (Betik & Hepple, 2008).

Reduction in the body's maximal rate of oxygen utilization has become an important issue in aging research. Whereas in most healthy young individuals this measure is not a practical concern, except for endurance athletes participating in specific training programs, it is of primary importance for older adults, for whom performing everyday tasks is dependent on VO_2max (Betik & Hepple, 2008). Following more than 300 Canadians aged between 55 and 86 years over eight years, Paterson et al. (2004) showed that lower cardiorespiratory fitness was a significant predictor of becoming dependent on an assisting living. Many studies have tried to assess changes in VO_2max with age. Cross-sectional and longitudinal studies suggest that VO_2max decreases by approximately 10% per decade in sedentary individuals but only 5% in highly active individuals, even after controlling for changes in physical activity (Stathokostas, Jacob-Johnson, Petrella, & Paterson, 2004). Moreover, the decline does not appear to be linear. According to a recent study in 810 healthy men and women followed over eight years, decline in VO$_2$max was approximately 3–6% per decade from ages 20 to 30 years, but reached 20% per decade after 70 years of age (Fleg et al., 2005).

When the appropriate apparatus or medical supervision is unavailable or when participants suffer from a medical condition that renders the maximal graded exercise test inappropriate, submaximal field tests offer a useful alternative. The Rockport one-mile test is a submaximal test that is widely used to assess cardiorespiratory fitness in older adults (Kline et al., 1987). Participants are instructed to walk one mile without stopping, as fast as possible. The time required to complete the distance is recorded on a stopwatch, and heart rate is recorded at the end of the test. VO$_2$max is estimated using equations that take into account participants' weight, age, sex, cardiac frequency post exercise, and time taken to cover the one-mile distance. Kline et al. (1987) reported a strong correlation ($r = 0.88$) between the estimated Rockport VO$_2$max and a direct measure of VO$_2$max during an increment test on a treadmill.

Measuring cardiorespiratory fitness with the gold standard graded exercise test can be challenging in older adults because of time constraints and health risks as well as lack of resources and trained staff. In older adults, VO$_2$max testing involves risks including injury, heart attack, stroke, and even death. Even submaximal field walking tests like the Rockport one-mile test are not without risk for elderly adults, as these tests might push them to near maximal effort. The significant relationship between cardiorespiratory fitness and several health indicators in older adults (e.g., chronic conditions, mortality rate, and cognitive decline) thus calls for valid alternative methods for testing cardiorespiratory fitness. In a recent study, Mailey et al. (2010) tested the construct validity of a nonexercise test to estimate cardiorespiratory fitness in a sample of community-dwelling older adults. Based on a previous study by Jurca and colleagues (2005) in middle-aged, relatively fit adults, the authors used a regression equation that included participants' demographic and health characteristics, for example, age, sex, body mass index, resting heart rate, and physical activity assessed by self-report questionnaires. The equation-predicted cardiorespiratory fitness in

metabolic equivalent units (METs) was significantly correlated with the graded exercise test results (.67) and the Rockport one-mile submaximal test results (.66). Mailey et al. concluded that nonexercise estimates of cardiorespiratory fitness are valid for use in older populations. Moreover, they reported that the estimated METs were at least as effective as METs obtained with the graded and submaximal tests in predicting cardiovascular conditions.

A significant relationship between equation-based and direct exercise tests is compelling evidence that cardiorespiratory fitness can be validly estimated with low-risk equation-based tests. However, it remains debatable whether this approach is sensitive enough to detect changes or differences in cognitive functions or psychological variables that have been associated with direct measures of cardiorespiratory functions. This question was addressed by McAuley et al. (2011) in a recent study in 86 older adults aged about 65. The participants completed an equation-based nonexercise assessment of cardiorespiratory fitness, as validated in Mailey et al.'s (2010) study; underwent neurocognitive tests of processing speed and spatial working memory; filled out a self-report on memory complaints; and received a structural brain scan. McAuley et al. reported that the equation-based estimate was significantly correlated with measures of processing speed and spatial working memory, memory complaints, and structural volume of the hippocampus. In general, the same relationship was observed between neurocognitive measures and the direct maximal and submaximal walking tests. However, the correlation between the submaximal Rockport test and spatial working memory was not significant. Further research is needed to provide a definitive explanation for this result. Nonetheless, the results of McAuley et al. (2011) suggest that the equation-based test could provide a valid alternative means to assess cardiorespiratory fitness when costly or time-consuming direct assessments cannot be performed.

Physical Activity and Psychological Health in Seniors

A complete description of the psychological aspects of aging is beyond the scope of this chapter. Therefore this chapter presents a brief overview of the psychological challenges that frequently accompany aging to provide a general understanding of the benefits of physical activity and exercise for psychological aging. The most common chronic psychological conditions whose prevalence increases with age are depression, anxiety, and reduced quality of life and well-being. Of these, depression is one of the most prevalent mental disorders in older adult populations, and depressive symptoms can be predictors of cognitive decline and preclinical dementia (Djernes, 2006). Depression is defined as a state of great sadness and apprehension. It is marked by symptoms of depressed mood and a loss of interest in, or of the ability to experience pleasure in response to, normally stimulating, positive events.

It is estimated that in any given year, 6.5–10.1% of the adult U.S. population suffers from depression. For older individuals, the U.S. prevalence rates are 5% or less (Gurland, Cross, & Katz, 1996). In fact, it has been commonly shown that older adults are less likely to be diagnosed with depression than their younger counterparts but that they are more likely to report depressive symptoms, particularly physical symptoms (U.S. Department of Health and Human Services, 1999). In other words, geriatric depression tends to be more somatic (body related) and less ideational (perceived).

Epidemiological studies worldwide report prevalence rates of major depression ranging from 1.1% to 28.0% (Angst et al., 2002; Gureje, Kola, & Afolabi, 2007; Gureje, Uwakwe, Oladeji, Makanjuola, & Esan, 2010; McDougall et al., 2007; Preville et al., 2008; Steffens et al., 2000; Streiner, Cairney, & Veldhuizen, 2006; Tintle, Bacon, Kostyuchenko, Gutkovich, & Bromet, 2011). Prevalence rates of major depression are higher in clinical settings (6–48%) than in community-based cohorts (Ansseau, Fischler, Dierick, Mignon, & Leyman, 2005; Jongenelis et al., 2004; Kramer, Allgaier, Fejtkova, Mergl, & Hegerl, 2009; Levin et al., 2007; Martin-Merino, Ruigomez, Johansson, Wallander, & Garcia-Rodriguez, 2010; Teresi, Abrams, Holmes, Ramirez, & Eimicke, 2001). Studies also suggest that depressive symptoms that do not meet the criteria of the American Psychiatric Association's *Diagnostic and Statistical Manual of Mental Disorders* (DSM) for major depression are common among older adults across living arrangements (e.g., personal residence, nursing home, or long-term care), with prevalence rates of 50% or higher (Heun, Papassotiropoulos, & Ptok, 2000; Jongenelis et al., 2004; Meeks, Vahia, Lavretsky, Kulkarni, & Jeste, 2011; Teresi et al., 2001; Yunming et al., 2011).

Depression can severely alter cognition, and its effects have been observed on selective attention and working memory (Landro, Stiles, & Sletvold, 2001), verbal memory (Fossati, Amar, Raoux, Ergis, & Allilaire, 1999), immediate memory (Lauer et al.,

1994), performance on the Stroop color-word test (Degl'Innocenti, Agren, & Backman, 1998), vigilance tasks (Christensen, Griffiths, Mackinnon, & Jacomb, 1997), academic performance (Haines, Norris, & Kashy, 1996), and spatial processing and learning (Benedict, Dobraski, & Goldstein, 1999). In fact, the range of deficits is overwhelming and has been compared to that seen in moderately severe traumatic brain injury (Veiel, 1997).

Anxiety disorders are another common psychological condition in community-dwelling older adults, with prevalence estimates of 0.1% to 15% (Beekman et al., 1998; Bryant, Jackson, & Ames, 2008; Grenier et al., 2011; Gum, King-Kallimanis, & Kohn, 2009; Kessler et al., 2005; Mackenzie, Reynolds, Chou, Pagura, & Sareen, 2011; Riedel-Heller, Busse, & Angermeyer, 2006; Ritchie et al., 2004). In clinical settings (e.g., nursing homes and primary care), the prevalence of late-life anxiety disorders is even higher, with rates varying between 1.0% and 28% (Bryant et al., 2008; Parmelee, Lawton, & Katz, 1998; Smalbrugge, Jongenelis, Pot, Beekman, & Eefsting, 2005; Tolin, Robison, Gaztambide, & Blank, 2005). Studies also suggest that subclinical anxiety (i.e., symptoms not meeting the threshold for a formal DSM diagnosis) should not be neglected in older adult populations, where prevalence is estimated at up to 56% (Bryant et al., 2008; Grenier et al., 2011; Heun et al., 2000; Rivas-Vazquez, Saffa-Biller, Ruiz, Blais, & Rivas-Vazquez, 2004).

Furthermore, both depression and anxiety (at the clinical or subclinical level) are associated with impaired quality of life (Beard, Weisberg, & Keller, 2010; Lima & Fleck, 2011; Meeks et al., 2011; Michalak et al., 2004; Spitzer et al., 1995; Stein & Barrett-Connor, 2002). In fact, both disorders (at a clinical or subclinical level) have been associated with several chronic physical health problems that characterize aging, such as type 2 diabetes (Huang, Chiu, Lee, & Wang, 2011; Khuwaja et al., 2010; Sulaiman, Hamdan, Tamim, Mahmood, & Young, 2010), multiple sclerosis (M. N. Burns, Siddique, Fokuo, & Mohr, 2010; Dahl, Stordal, Lydersen, & Midgard, 2009; Julian & Arnett, 2009), heart diseases (Huffman, Celano, & Januzzi, 2010; Phillips et al., 2009; Rutledge et al., 2009; Vogelzangs et al., 2010), Parkinson's disease (Dissanayaka et al., 2010; Nuti et al., 2004; Reiff et al., 2011), and mild cognitive impairment (Apostolova & Cummings, 2008; Gallagher et al., 2011; Geda et al., 2008; Muangpaisan, Intalapaporn, & Assantachai, 2008; Rozzini et al., 2009). The presence of neuropsychiatric symptoms (i.e., anxiety and depression) may increase the risk of conversion of mild cognitive impairment to Alzheimer's disease (Devier et al., 2009; Modrego & Ferrandez, 2004; Palmer et al., 2007), although results are inconsistent. Epidemiological studies indicate that depression and anxiety often co-occur and that their coexistence may lead to more severe health complications (Beekman et al., 2000; Brown, Campbell, Lehman, Grisham, & Mancill, 2001; King-Kallimanis, Gum, & Kohn, 2009; Lenze et al., 2000; Mehta et al., 2003; Preisig, Merikangas, & Angst, 2001; Prina, Ferri, Guerra, Brayne, & Prince, 2011).

Several studies suggest that physical activity is associated with better general physical and mental health, particularly in older populations (Bertheussen et al., 2010). Some studies suggest that physical activity is an effective treatment for depression and anxiety (Conn, 2010b; Fox, 1999; Paluska & Schwenk, 2000; Pasco et al., 2011; Penedo & Dahn, 2005). The use of exercise therapy as an alternative to antidepressants in older populations has long been recommended (Babyak et al., 2000; Blumenthal et al., 1999), and it has been successful in reducing relapses of depressive episodes in older adults (Babyak et al., 2000; Singh, Clements, & Singh, 2001). Most studies to date have focused on aerobic exercise, with results suggesting that moderate- to high-intensity exercise training can reduce symptoms of depression in older adults. Further research is needed to investigate the potential benefits of resistance training in depression.

In a meta-analysis of randomized trials on the antidepressive effects of exercise, Rethorst, Wipfli & Landers (2009) reviewed 58 trials (n = 2982) and found an overall effect size of −0.80. The authors also assessed clinical significance in trials with clinically depressed patients and found that nine of 16 exercise treatment groups were classified as "recovered" at posttreatment, with another three groups classified as "improved." The effect sizes were larger in clinical than nonclinical populations with depressive symptoms. Moreover, dropout rates for the exercise treatment were about the same as those found in usual-care treatments (i.e., psychotherapeutic and drug interventions). Greater benefits were observed when the exercise program involved a combination of aerobic and resistance exercises lasting 10–16 minutes. Some studies have shown inconclusive findings. Indeed, a recent Cochrane Review (Mean, Morley et al., 2009) found that the effect sizes are moderate and statistically nonsignificant when considering methodologically robust trials only. Nevertheless, the review's authors concluded that exercise appears to improve symptoms of depression in people with a diagnosis of depression, although the evidence suggests that long-term exercise is required for benefits on mood.

Physical activity also appears to be an effective prevention tool and treatment alternative for anxiety symptoms and disorders. In a meta-analytic study using data synthesized across 3,289 participants from 19 eligible studies, Conn (2010a) found that physical activity can effectively reduce anxiety in healthy seniors. However, the magnitude of the effect is slightly smaller than the values reported in meta-analyses including participants with clinical anxiety disorders, and the anxiolytic effects may be more pronounced in clinical and subclinical populations (Salmon, 2001; Wipfli, Rethorst, & Landers, 2008). Nevertheless, these findings suggest that even healthy adults could reduce their anxiety through diverse unsupervised and supervised physical activity interventions. However, Conn concluded that supervised moderate-intensity and high-intensity physical activity at a fitness center may be more effective, by providing participants with explicit guidelines for exercise intensity, duration, and frequency. It would also encourage social interaction, which could improve program adherence. Moreover, although the exercise dose was not associated with change in anxiety (for a similar dose–response analysis, see the meta-analysis by Wipfli et al., 2008), Conn (2010a) concluded that low-intensity physical activity may not provide enough stimulus to improve anxiety.

In a recent prospective study, Pasco et al. (2011) examined habitual physical activity and the risk of de novo depression and anxiety disorders in adults aged 60 and older. Physical activity was measured using a validated questionnaire, and psychiatric interviews were conducted four years later (excluding participants with depressive or anxiety disorders at baseline). Pasco et al. found that physical activity protected against the likelihood of depressive and anxiety disorders and that each standard-deviation increase in the transformed physical activity score reduced the risk of depressive or anxiety disorders by half.

Quality of life and well-being are two distinct but closely related psychological constructs that are of primary importance for older adults. A recent systematic review of the literature concluded that higher levels of physical activity were consistently associated with better scores on a variety of health-related quality-of-life dimensions (Klavestrand &

Vingard, 2009). The effect of physical activity on mental well-being has been widely studied in cardiac patients. In particular, structured exercise training (i.e., aerobic and isometric exercises) involving 36 sessions over a three-month period appears to be an effective method to treat depressive symptoms and to improve quality of life in patients with heart failure (Milani, Lavie, Mehra, & Ventura, 2011). Furthermore, it appears that both aerobic interval training and continuous moderate exercise can improve health-related quality of life after coronary artery bypass grafting (Moholdt et al., 2009). In another study, a six-week cardiac rehabilitation program involving 12 individually tailored aerobic exercise sessions significantly improved quality of life, physical activity status, anxiety, and depression in patients with cardiac disease. Gains were maintained at 12 months (Yohannes, Doherty, Bundy, & Yalfani, 2010). In sum, physical activity targets not only cardiac improvement but also comorbid conditions (i.e., depression and anxiety) that may adversely affect the prognosis of heart disease. A recent study has observed improvements in several aspects of quality of life after only three months of structured physical exercise training in frail older adults (Langlois et al., 2010). This suggests that even in the presence of functional limitations and reduced physical capacities, physical exercise can lead to a significantly improved quality of life in older adults. Physical activity is related to psychological well-being independently of age, gender, length of program, or study design (Rejeski & Mihalko, 2001).

A recent meta-analysis evaluated the impacts of physical activity interventions on psychological well-being in people aged 65 years and older living in the community or in residential care homes (Windle, Hughes, Linck, Russell, & Woods, 2010). Different types of intervention were included in the analysis (aerobics, yoga, tai chi, and combinations of various types of exercise). Results showed an overall significant beneficial effect of physical training on well-being (effect size = 0.27), as determined by the SF-36 mental health score and a self-esteem questionnaire (Brazier et al., 1992). However, according to the authors, there was no clear pattern with respect to the number of sessions per week or physical exercise dose required to improve well-being, nor with respect to the long-term effects of the intervention.

The mechanisms by which exercise and physical activity improve psychological well-being are not fully understood. Direct effects on brain structure and functions likely come into play, as discussed below. However, indirect psychological benefits such as improved self-efficacy and stress management are probably involved as well (Berchtold, 2008). Regular physical activity leads to higher self-efficacy, positive well-being, less perceived fatigue, less anxiety, and less psychological distress. The social context of the physical activity also plays an important role. A socially enriched and positive leadership style for group physical activity enhances feelings of revitalization and positive engagement. Social relationships play an important role in quality of life and well-being.

McAuley, Elavsky, Jerome, Konopack, and Marquez (2005) investigated social influences on the effects of physical activity on well-being in older adults. They hypothesized that physical activity would enhance positive feelings and reduce negative feeling states across multiple assessments during a six-month exercise trial. They observed that individuals who exercised more frequently during the program, who were more efficacious, and who received more exercise-related social support at baseline also showed higher well-being at the end of the first trial month. Both exercise frequency and change in well-being played significant roles in predicting self-efficacy at program end. This result suggests that physical activity enhances self-efficacy. However, McAuley & Elavsky (2008) recently suggested that self-efficacy can influence the initiation of and continuous participation in physical activities, and that the relationship between physical activity and self-efficacy is therefore bidirectional.

Physical Activity and Cognition in Healthy Seniors

It is generally assumed that age brings with it declines in performance in a multitude of cognitive tasks that require a variety of perceptual and cognitive processes (for extensive literature reviews, see Craik & Salthouse, 2008; Hertzog et al., 2008; Reuter-Lorenz & Park, 2010). However, it has also generally been observed that knowledge-based or crystallized abilities (i.e., those largely based on culture and experience), such as verbal knowledge and comprehension, are maintained or improved over the life span. This is in contrast to process-based abilities (i.e., reasoning, speed, and other basic abilities not dependent on experience), which display age-related declines. More specifically, it has been frequently reported that processing speed declines early in aging, and this decrease has recently been associated with loss of white matter integrity.

Working memory, or the ability to maintain and consciously manipulate information, is also highly age sensitive. The age-related difference in working memory tends to be greater in tasks that require executive control processes such as inhibition, updating, and manipulation, and even greater if the memory load (i.e., the number of items to be maintained) is high. In brain imaging studies, age-related working memory deficits have been associated with reduced task-related activation in frontal regions of the cerebral cortex in older compared with younger adults. Older adults also tend to show lower inhibition than younger adults. As a result, they are more distracted by irrelevant information and more affected by proactive interference (i.e., interference induced by current learning on further encoding of new information). Furthermore, decline in episodic memory is a well-known effect of aging. Compared with younger adults, older adults tend to show reduced recall on all memory tasks (e.g., verbal or visual). This decrease has been associated with poor encoding strategies, less use of environmental support, and deficits in binding new information with existing knowledge during encoding.

Many theoretical accounts have been put forward to explain the cognitive changes that occur with age. Recent advances in structural and functional brain imaging techniques have provided insight into potential brain mechanisms of aging. For instance, significant changes in the central nervous system that accompany aging can potentially account for age-related cognitive declines. Changes in brain volume occur faster in adults after 50 years of age, with an annual decline of 0.35% as compared with 0.12% in young adults (for reviews see Dennis & Cabeza, 2008; Raz, 2005). The rate of ventricle dilatation can approximate 4.25% per year at 70 years of age, compared with 0.43% in young adults. The volume of the hippocampus, a cerebral structure that plays a major role in memory, is very sensitive to age, with a mean annual decline of 0.86% per year from 26 to 82 years of age. Moreover, the rate of hippocampal volume loss increases with age, going from 1.18% per year after 50 years to 1.85% per year after 70 years.

The rate of brain structural change is sometimes difficult to document across studies because few have followed participants longitudinally. In a recent study, Raz, Ghisletta, Rodrigue, Kennedy, and Lindenberger (2010) followed participants of 49 years and older over 30 months and observed that some structures showed changes after only 15 months, such as the hippocampus, the entorhinal cortex, the orbital–frontal cortex, and the cerebellum. Other structures showed shrinking after 30 months, including the caudate nucleus, the prefrontal subcortical white matter, and the corpus callosum. However, some brain structures showed almost no change (the primary visual cortices, the putamen, and the pons).

In addition, aging brings overall changes in white matter integrity (e.g., leukoaraiosis), with greater changes occurring after the seventh decade and localized preferentially in the anterior (frontal and prefrontal) regions (Dennis & Cabeza, 2008). These changes are more pronounced in patients with vascular diseases such as hypertension and type 2 diabetes. Not only does aging alter cerebral structures at the macro- and microanatomic levels; it also causes changes in cerebral metabolism, such as reduced regional cerebral metabolic rates for glucose and oxygen and decreases in cerebral blood flow. Although it is frequently assumed that structural changes are associated with declines in brain metabolism, recent evidence suggests otherwise. For example, Chen, Rosas, and Salat (2010) observed that in some brain regions, age-associated reductions in cerebral blood flow can be independent of regional atrophy.

A major contemporary finding was that age-related cognitive decline is heterogeneous across older individuals and that lifestyle factors such as physical exercise can modulate the impact of aging on cognition (Hertzog et al., 2008; Kramer et al., 2004). The evidence that physical exercise might help prevent age-related cognitive decline comes from cross-sectional, longitudinal, and intervention studies.

For many years, studies have suggested that physical activity is a significant moderator of age-related cognitive decline. In cross-sectional designs that compare older to younger adults, the age-related difference in cognitive performance tends to be less when the study involves high-fit rather than low-fit or sedentary older adults. Reaction time (RT) tasks are often used to assess the relationship between physical fitness and cognitive performance. Spirduso (1975) compared the performance of younger and older adults who were either regular racket and handball players or nonactive. They found that nonactive older adults had slower responses than younger active, younger nonactive, and older active individuals on both simple and choice RT tasks. Clarkson-Smith and Hartley (1989) also compared the performance of physically active and sedentary elderly participants (aged 55–91 years) and observed faster responses by active participants on both simple and choice RT tasks. Moreover, increasing response choices induced larger increases in RT in sedentary than in active individuals. Abourezk and Toole (1995) also observed better performance by active than nonactive women aged 60 years and older, but only on a choice RT task.

More recent studies have deepened our understanding of the cognitive processes by which physical fitness maintains performance in RT tasks with aging. In a cross-sectional study, Hillman, Weiss, Hagberg, and Hatfield (2002) observed reduced amplitude of the contingent negative variation, an electrophysiological marker of response preparation, in young and older physically fit participants compared with sedentary participants. They argued that older adults who were more aerobically fit used fewer cognitive resources than sedentary individuals to prepare a speeded response. This finding suggests that in aging populations physical fitness exercise could maintain preparatory processes, which are a voluntary or attention-demanding set of strategic behaviors that support an optimal processing state prior to the execution of movement (Stuss, Shallice, Alexander, & Picton, 1995). In a more recent study, Renaud, Bherer, and Maquestiaux (2010) observed better response preparation in high-fit than low-fit older adults, particularly when response preparation had to be maintained over several seconds. Renaud et al. assessed the relationship between cardiovascular fitness and temporal preparation in 110 elderly persons from two age groups (60–69 and 70–79 years). The results suggested that high-fit individuals can better maintain preparation over time (up to 9 s). Moreover, an age-by-fitness interaction was reported for motor speed, which suggests that maintaining high physical fitness has a protective effect on motor slowing with aging. As a whole, these cross-sectional studies suggest that cardiorespiratory fitness is associated with more efficient response preparation processes. However, the conclusions that can be drawn from the results of cross-sectional studies are limited, and these studies cannot be taken to support a causal link between physical fitness training and cognitive improvement.

Longitudinal and intervention studies provide more compelling evidence. In longitudinal studies, older adults who participate in physical activity show less cognitive decline over two- to 10-year follow-up periods than nonactive older adults. For instance, Barnes, Yaffe, Satariano, and Tager (2003) assessed cardiorespiratory fitness in participants aged 55 and older and observed that baseline fitness level predicts cognitive performance six years later in a variety of cognitive domains (working memory, processing speed, attention, and general mental functioning). More recently, Aichberger et al. (2010) investigated the effects of physical inactivity on cognitive performance in nationally representative samples of non-institutionalized persons aged 50 years and older across 11 European countries (Austria, Germany, Sweden, Denmark, Switzerland, the Netherlands, Belgium, France, Spain, Italy, and Greece), controlling for the most commonly reported predictors of cognitive decline. They found that individuals who participated in any type of regular physical activity showed less cognitive decline than nonactive individuals after 2.5 years of follow-up, especially when they engaged in vigorous activities more than once a week.

Further evidence for the moderating effect of physical activity on age-related cognitive decline stems from intervention studies, which generally show enhanced cognitive performance in older adults who have completed a physical activity program that produces significant increases in cardiorespiratory fitness (indexed by direct measures or estimation of VO_2max). Dustman et al. (1984) compared middle-aged and older individuals who completed a four-month aerobic training program with age-matched controls who participated in strength and flexibility exercises and controls who did not exercise. Only the training group showed improved cardiorespiratory function, along with improvements on a simple RT task. Similar results were obtained in women aged 57–85 years old following a three-year physical training program (Rikli & Edwards, 1991). Hawkins, Kramer, and Capaldi (1992) reported that in older adults, a 10-week aquatic fitness program led to greater improvement in task conditions that tap dual-task and task-switching abilities than in conditions that do not require executive or attentional control processes. In a study by Kramer et al. (1999), older adults who completed a six-month aerobic training program (walking) showed a significant improvement in cognitive performance, unlike those who completed a stretching program. Cognitive improvement was greater in tasks that tapped attentional control or executive control functions, as required to inhibit a prepotent response or to divide attention between concurrent tasks. Cognitive improvement was correlated with observed improvement in VO_2max. Several meta-analyses have confirmed that aerobic training induces greater improvement in executive control than in other cognitive domains (Colcombe & Kramer, 2003; but see Etnier, Nowell, Landers, & Sibley, 2006, for different conclusions).

The selective benefit of aerobic exercise for tasks that tap executive control was also observed in another more recent study (Smiley-Oyen, Lowry, Francois, Kohut, & Ekkekakis, 2008), where 57 older adults completed a 10-month training program of either aerobic or strength-and-flexibility exercise. A positive effect on executive control (as indexed by a Stroop color-word test) was observed after aerobic training only. However, changes in cognitive performance were not related to changes in aerobic fitness. In a more recent meta-analytic review of randomized controlled trials of aerobic exercise on neurocognitive functions, Smith et al. (2010) examined 29 studies conducted between 1966 and 2009 (including more than 2,000 participants and 234 effect sizes). They found that individuals who were randomly assigned to receive aerobic exercise training showed modest improvements in attention, processing speed, executive function, and memory, with less convincing effects on working memory. These results, along with those from Colcombe and Kramer (2003), suggest a selective effect of aerobic exercise on neurocognitive functions.

In a recent study of the effects of aerobic exercise on attentional control and executive functions, Renaud, Maquestiaux, Joncas, Kergoat, and Bherer (2010) assessed the effect of three months of aerobic training on response preparation in older adults. Participants were assigned to either a three-month aerobic training group or a control group. The training group participated in an aerobic training program consisting of three 60-minute sessions per week. Results indicated that 12 weeks of aerobic training induced a significant improvement in cardiorespiratory capacity (estimated VO_2max) along with enhanced preparation, such that participants maintained preparation over time more efficiently after the training program. These results provide additional support for the notion that improving aerobic fitness may enhance attentional control mechanisms in older adults.

Physical Activity and Brain Structures and Functions in Older Adults

The biological mechanisms by which physical exercise training enhances cognition remain to be completely elucidated, although the number of studies that have tried to better identify these mechanisms has exploded in the last 10 years. Studies that support the notion that physical exercise has an impact on brain functions can be divided into two main groups (Spirduso, Francis, & MacRae, 2005): those that investigated the direct biological effects of exercise using animal or human models, and those showing indirect effects on cognition through the benefits of exercise for health conditions (stress and sleep) and chronic diseases (coronary heart diseases) that affect neurocognitive functions.

The first evidence for the direct effects of exercise on the brain came from animal studies showing that the basic neurobiological mechanisms associated with exercise can occur at two levels, supramolecular and molecular (see Lista & Sorrentino, 2010, for a review). At the supramolecular level, physical activity has been found to induce angiogenesis, or the physiological process by which new blood vessels grow from preexisting vessels (Black, Isaacs, Anderson, Alcantara, & Greenough, 1990; Isaacs, Anderson, Alcantara, Black, & Greenough, 1992). Physical activity has also been associated with neurogenesis, or neural cell proliferation, in the hippocampus in elderly rats (van Praag, Shubert, Zhao, & Gage, 2005). Although the functional significance of this effect remains unclear, there is evidence that newly formed neurons can integrate into a neural network and become functional (Lledo, Alonso, & Grubb, 2006). Exercise-induced synaptogenesis has also been reported (Eadie, Redila, & Christie, 2005; Hu, Ying, Gomez-Pinilla, & Frautschy, 2009).

The molecular mechanisms by which exercise induces angiogenesis, neurogenesis, and synaptogenesis have received growing attention in the last few years. Again, the evidence comes mainly from animal studies, which have shown exercise-associated changes in molecular growth factors such as brain-derived neurotrophic factor (BDNF), which plays a crucial role in neuroplasticity and neuroprotection, and increased production of insulin-like growth factor 1, which is involved in both neurogenesis and angiogenesis. Moreover, neurotransmitter systems also seem to be modulated through exercise (see Lista & Sorrentino, 2010 for a review). Until very recently, evidence for the molecular and supramolecular effects of exercise came exclusively from animal studies. However, a very innovative study (Erickson et al., 2011) recently showed increased BDNF plasma levels in older adults after aerobic exercise (compared with stretching), which were associated with increased hippocampal volume. If reproduced, these results would confirm that physical exercise induces genuine neurotrophic effects on brain structures and functions at the molecular, supramolecular, and structural levels.

In humans, several studies using structural and functional brain imaging or electrophysiological measures of brain activity suggest that physical exercise induces transient and permanent changes at the structural and functional levels in the aging brain (Erickson & Kramer, 2009; Hillman, Erickson, & Kramer, 2008; Kramer, Erickson, & Colcombe, 2006; Voelcker-Rehage, Godde, & Staudinger, 2010). Recent findings using voxel-based morphometry (a type of detailed image segmentation of high-resolution brain scans) indicated that a higher cardiorespiratory fitness level (VO_2 max) was associated with a reduced loss of gray and white matter in the frontal, prefrontal, and temporal regions in older adults (Colcombe et al., 2003). In another study, Erickson et al. (2009) performed a region-of-interest analysis on magnetic resonance images in 165 nondemented older adults and found that higher fitness levels were associated with larger left and right hippocampi and were correlated with better spatial memory performance. These findings suggest that aerobic fitness is associated with changes in brain structures that translate into better cognitive function in older adults (see also Erickson et al., 2011).

Even more striking evidence of the benefits of fitness for brain functions comes from functional brain imaging (fMRI) studies. It has been shown that enhanced cardiovascular functions after aerobic training are associated with greater task-relevant activity in brain areas recruited in an attentional control task (Colcombe et al., 2004). More recently, Voss et al. (2010) found changes in functional connectivity after aerobic exercise training in older adults: Twelve months of training led to increased connectivity among regions that support the default-mode network and the frontal executive network. Changes in these large-scale brain networks have received increasing attention in aging neuroscience, as they indicate massive changes in brain systems. For instance, Voss et al.'s (2010) study suggests that physical exercise has a restorative effect on large-scale brain circuitry.

A complete understanding of the potential for physical activity to protect the brain from the effects of age would require investigating the indirect influences of exercise on cognition. There is growing evidence that exercise has indirect beneficial effects on cognition through its impact on factors that are known to alter neurocognitive integrity (Spirduso, Poon, & Chodzko-Zajko, 2008). Spirduso et al. (2008) suggest three groups of potential mediators in the relationship between exercise and cognition:

physical resources, chronic diseases or states, and mental resources. The effect of physical exercise on mental resources has been addressed in discussions of the benefits of exercise for managing depression (Bartholomew & Ciccolo, 2008), anxiety, and chronic stress, and for enhancing self-efficacy (McAuley & Elavsky, 2008). Physical activity has been suggested to have an impact on physical resources through its effects on diet (Joseph, 2008) and sleep (Lopez, 2008; Vitiello, 2008).

The next section details how many studies suggest that physical activity and exercise can heighten cognitive functions through indirect biological mechanisms, by reducing the risk of chronic diseases and conditions such as hypertension (Tanaka & Cortez-Cooper, 2008), type 2 diabetes (Royall, 2008), and chronic obstructive pulmonary disease (Emery, 2008). Against this background, metabolic syndrome and coronary heart diseases have recently received increasing attention because of their high prevalence in aging populations.

Physical Activity and Chronic Medical Conditions

Most of the studies that have been published on fitness and cognition in older adults involved generally healthy community dwellers. In many such cases, participants present few medical conditions or risk factors, virtually no limiting factors for exercise, and no signs of cognitive impairment. Although these seminal studies have allowed us to conclude that physical exercise at any age can provide substantial and appreciable benefits for psychological health and neurocognitive functions, it has not been definitively determined whether physical exercise can prevent or treat chronic diseases and complex geriatric syndromes. Metabolic syndrome and coronary heart diseases are two chronic medical conditions that occur frequently in aging populations. According to the Heart and Stroke Foundation of Canada (2006), 90% of older adults have at least one cardiovascular disease risk factor, and 1 out of 10 adults has three or more factors. In 2006, cardiovascular diseases accounted for 30% of all deaths in Canada. More importantly, 54% of these deaths were due to coronary heart disease (Heart and Stroke Foundation of Canada, 2006). The prevalence of obesity continues to rise at epidemic proportions in both North America and Europe, with estimates that over 50% of adults above the age of 50 in the United States have metabolic syndrome, a very common consequence of obesity (Ford, Giles, & Mokdad, 2004). The impacts of metabolic syndrome and coronary heart disease on psychological health and cognition have been well documented. It has also been observed that both syndromes can be improved through physical exercise. The following section focuses on the impacts of these diseases on psychological health and cognition, and the potential of physical activity to alleviate those symptoms.

Metabolic syndrome is a clustering of reversible metabolic risk factors (glucose intolerance, abdominal obesity, dyslipidemia, and hypertension). There is growing interest in the relationship between metabolic syndrome and late-life cognitive impairment. Individuals with metabolic syndrome are at increased risk of developing cardiovascular disease (Eckel, Grundy, & Zimmet, 2005) and at higher risk of Alzheimer's disease (Stampfer, 2006). Komulainen and colleagues (2007) tested the hypothesis that metabolic syndrome predicts cognitive impairment in a 12-year follow-up study of a sample of 101 women aged 60–70 years. They found that women with metabolic syndrome at baseline had a higher risk of poor memory at follow-up than those without initial metabolic syndrome after adjustments for age, education, and depression. Yaffe et al. (2007) investigated the effect of metabolic syndrome on cognitive functions in 718 Latino adults aged 60 and older using the Modified Mini-Mental State Examination and a verbal memory test. They found that people with metabolic syndrome showed greater decline on both tests and concluded that metabolic syndrome may accelerate cognitive decline through mechanisms related to micro- and macrovascular damage, insulin resistance, adiposity, and inflammation.

More recently, Solfrizzi et al. (2009) investigated the relationship between metabolic syndrome and its individual components and the incidence of mild cognitive impairment (MCI) and its progression to dementia in a longitudinal study. MCI patients with metabolic syndrome had a higher risk of progression to dementia than individuals without metabolic syndrome over 3.5 years of follow-up. Segura et al. (2009) used a more extensive neuropsychological battery of tests to assess cognitive impairment in metabolic syndrome and reported specific deficits in processing speed and executive functions after controlling for education and gender. These authors suggested that metabolic syndrome may be a prodromal state of vascular cognitive impairment.

Individuals with coronary heart disease also show cognitive deficits. Coronary heart disease has been associated with loss of gray matter in various brain regions, including some that play significant roles in cognitive function and behavior (Almeida et al., 2008). Coronary heart disease has also been associated with increased amounts of cerebral amyloid deposits, which might increase the risk of dementia and Alzheimer's disease (Soneira & Scott, 1996; Sparks et al., 1990). It was recently suggested that coronary heart disease could be a marker of subclinical cerebrovascular disease and mild cognitive impairment (Roberts et al., 2010). Although the underlying neural mechanisms remain to be understood, many studies have associated coronary heart disease with cognitive impairment in normal cognitive aging (Breteler, Claus, Grobbee, & Hofman, 1994; Singh-Manoux, Britton, & Marmot, 2003) and with nonamnesic mild cognitive impairment (Roberts et al., 2010). (Nonamnesic cognitive decline refers to decline in attention and executive control functions rather than loss of memory functions as in more typical amnesic cognitive decline.)

Physical activity is widely promoted to improve vascular risk factors, including those associated with metabolic syndrome and coronary heart diseases. Many epidemiological studies have reported that physical activity in older adults is significantly associated with cardiorespiratory fitness measures and insulin resistance as well as most other components of the metabolic syndrome. Exercise training has been shown to improve the metabolic profile of insulin-resistant individuals and to restrain disease progression in type 2 diabetic patients (Ostergard et al., 2006). In the HERITAGE Family Study (Katzmarzyk et al., 2003), 20 weeks of aerobic training decreased the percentage of participants with high triglyceride levels, high blood pressure, high glucose, and high waist circumference. Progressive resistance training for five months has been shown to improve insulin sensitivity (–46.3%), total cholesterol (–12%), LDL-cholesterol (–14%), and triglyceride levels (–20%) and to decrease abdominal fat in older adults. In addition, the DARE study (Sigal et al., 2007) showed that aerobic training and resistance training independently improved glycemic control and that the combination of the two improved glycemic control further. It can therefore be hypothesized that exercise training decreases the risk of metabolic disorders by improving insulin sensitivity, fat distribution, muscle strength, and maximal oxygen consumption (VO_2max).

Several meta-analyses have revealed a positive influence of exercise on individuals with coronary heart disease. Hagberg, Eshani, and Holloszy

(1983) demonstrated that a 12-month exercise program increased VO$_2$max by 39% and stroke volume by 18%. They thereby confirmed that when coronary heart disease patients followed an exercise program, the resultant increase in VO$_2$max was caused by cardiac rather than peripheral adaptations. These results also demonstrated that for the same workload, the heart consumes less oxygen after a training program. These cardiac improvements allow for much greater workloads to be performed before the occurrence of the ischemic threshold, ECG anomalies (arrhythmia), and angina (Casillas, Gremeaux, Damak, Feki, & Pérennou, 2007). Other studies have suggested an improvement in the ratio between myocardial oxygen contribution and demand after an aerobic exercise program, notably due to an increase in coronary blood flow. Regular physical activity in coronary heart disease patients can also positively influence heart rate variability by increasing parasympathetic and decreasing sympathetic tone at rest. This improved autonomic nervous control proves to be an effective and nonpharmacological way to enhance cardiac electrical stability, thereby protecting against sudden cardiac death (Billman, 2002).

Although exercise has been proven beneficial for patients, the type and intensity of the exercise must be optimized. Current guidelines recommend moderate-to-vigorous aerobic exercise at 10 beats beneath the ischemic threshold to ensure optimal safety during training. However, studies have shown that aerobic exercise above this threshold does not cause ischemic myocardial damage (Juneau, Roy, Nigam, Tardif, & Larivee, 2009; Noël et al., 2007). In light of these results, new studies have focused on different types of exercise to optimize training in individuals with coronary heart disease. A recent meta-analysis of prospective cohort studies evaluated the relationship between physical activity and the risk of developing coronary heart disease (Sofi, Capalbo, Cesari, Abbate, & Gensini, 2008). In all, 26 studies were analyzed (n = 513,472 individuals), with follow-up periods ranging from 4 to 25 years. Results showed that individuals who reported performing moderate or high level of physical activity had a significantly lower risk of coronary heart disease than those who reported little or no physical activity.

A recent randomized controlled study evaluated the effects of physical activity and diet on blood pressure in overweight, unmedicated outpatients aged 35 years and older with high blood pressure (Blumenthal et al., 2010). The participants were randomly assigned to three groups: (1) their usual diet with no change in lifestyle (n = 49), (2) a diet plan to lower hypertension (DASH) (n = 46), and (3) DASH combined with physical aerobic exercise (n = 49). Physical training consisted of aerobic exercises three times a week over four months at 70–85% maximal heart rate reserve. Results showed that the DASH diet can significantly improve blood pressure in overweight adults. Moreover, adding aerobic exercise can lead to greater improvements in blood pressure as well as cardiorespiratory fitness (VO$_2$ peak). These clearly documented cardiovascular benefits associated with physical activity suggest that vascular adaptations may also be occurring in the brain, directly or indirectly benefiting brain function.

Physical Activity and Geriatric Syndromes

With increasing age, and specifically with advanced age (over 75 years), many individuals eventually develop one or more of a group of related medical problems referred to as geriatric syndromes. Perceptual limitations (vision and hearing problems), urinary incontinence, falls, delirium, and dementia are example of geriatric syndromes. They are characterized by having more than one cause and involving several body systems. Moreover, one geriatric syndrome often contributes to another. For instance, urinary incontinence may lead to falls, which in turn may lead to cognitive complications, and so forth.

Frailty is an emerging, complex geriatric syndrome that appears particularly relevant to our purpose here, as it apparently limits physical activity and exercise. Moreover, frailty has gained increased attention among health professionals because it offers an important frame of reference for risk quantification and prognosis in elderly populations (Lekan, 2009). Frailty is defined as a complex health state of increased vulnerability to stressors due to impairments in multiple systems. It has been associated with adverse outcomes such as disability, falls, hospitalization, and death (Fried et al., 2001). With aging, the prevalence of frailty increases from 7% in older adults aged between 65 and 74 years to 18% between 75 and 84 years to 37% at age 85 years and older (Rockwood et al., 2004). Frailty is a heterogeneous clinical syndrome that can include several medical conditions, including cardiovascular diseases, musculoskeletal disorders (arthritis, osteoporosis, or fractures), gastrointestinal diseases (intestinal difficulties, pyrosis, or reflux), and cognitive impairment (Rockwood et al., 2005). Physical inactivity is a major risk factor for frailty (Fried et al., 2001).

In a cross-sectional study, Cesari and colleagues (2006) investigated the associations between frailty, muscle density, and fat mass in 923 older adults aged 65 years and older. Participants were defined as frail if they presented three or more of the following criteria: weight loss, exhaustion, low walking speed, low handgrip strength, and physical inactivity. According to these criteria, 81 participants (8.8%) were frail. Results showed that compared with non-frail participants, frail participants had lower muscle density and muscle mass and higher fat mass. Of the frailty criteria, physical inactivity showed the strongest correlation with body composition (percentage of fat, muscle, and bone). The cognitive profile associated with frailty remains poorly documented. Some studies report reduced cognitive performance in frail older adults (Avila-Funes et al., 2009; Fried et al., 2001; Rochat et al., 2010) and that individual frailty status can be a strong predictor of cognitive decline (Samper-Ternent, Al Snih, Raji, Markides, & Ottenbacher, 2008).

Results from longitudinal studies show that physical activity and exercise can prevent frailty in older adults. In a recent study, 2,964 older adults were followed for five years to determine the relationship between physical activity and the risk of becoming frail (Peterson et al., 2009). Results showed that individuals who regularly exercised at baseline were less likely to develop frailty within the five-year period than sedentary individuals, even after adjustment for baseline health conditions and demographic characteristics.

It is important to note that frailty is not a contraindication for physical activity. On the contrary, it may be one of the most compelling reasons to prescribe physical exercise (Landi et al., 2010). Intervention studies suggest that physical activity can improve several frailty syndrome components, especially sarcopenia (reduction in skeletal muscle mass) and functional impairment (Landi et al., 2010). As previously mentioned, regular exercise and greater aerobic fitness are associated with a decrease in all-cause mortality and morbidity and have been proven to reduce disease and disability and improve quality of life in older persons (U.S. Department of Health and Human Services, 2008).

A recent randomized controlled trial assessed the effects of a three-month physical training intervention on quality of life in 77 physically frail persons aged 75 years and older (Helbostad, Sletvold, & Moe-Nilssen, 2004). Participants were randomized between two experimental groups: one that did functional exercises twice a day to improve balance and lower-extremity muscle strength, and another that did the same exercises plus strength training twice a week. Results showed improved psychological well-being in the second group, particularly in physical functioning, emotion, and mental health.

Another recent study has demonstrated that physical exercise training can have positive effects on frail individuals (Langlois et al., 2010). Only three months of training resulted in significant improvement in frail older adults not only in physical capacity but also in cognitive performance (executive functions, processing speed, and working memory). Quality of life was also significantly improved, in terms of leisure activities and satisfaction with physical capacity.

Physical Activity in Older Adults with Cognitive Impairment

In 2011, an estimated 5.4 million Americans of all ages had Alzheimer's disease, the most common form of dementia (Alzheimer's Association, 2011). Of these, 5.2 million were aged 65 and older. However, 200,000 suffered from the younger-onset form of the disease, which occurs before 65 years. According to the American Alzheimer's Association (2011), one in eight people aged 65 and older (13%) and 43% of people 85 and older have Alzheimer's disease. A dramatic increase in prevalence occurs after the age of 75. Of those with Alzheimer's disease, 4% are under age 65, 6% are between 65 and 74, 45% are between 75 and 84, and 45% are over 85 years old. Currently, there is no cure for Alzheimer's disease. However, research has suggested that lifestyle factors can significantly reduce the risk of developing dementia. These factors include continuous cognitive stimulation, balanced nutrition, social interaction, and regular physical activity.

In a recent cross-sectional study, Geda et al. (2010) explored whether physical activity was associated with decreased risk of MCI, considered by many as the prodromal phase of dementia. Participants completed a self-report questionnaire concerning the physical exercise they had performed within one year of cognitive assessment (late-life physical exercise) and between the ages of 50 and 65 years (midlife physical exercise). A total of 198 subjects with MCI were compared with 1,126 with normal cognition. Results showed that moderate activity during midlife was associated with a 39%

lower risk of having mild cognitive impairment in later life. Similarly, late-life moderate exercise was associated with a 32% lower risk for MCI.

Burns et al. (2008) explored the effect of exercise on cognitively impaired individuals and found an association between direct measures of cardiorespiratory fitness (VO_2 peak) and cognition (neuropsychological test battery) in normal older participants and patients in the early stage of Alzheimer's dementia (AD). Results showed that cardiorespiratory fitness was modestly reduced in patients with AD compared with participants without dementia. Although no significant association was found between cardiorespiratory fitness and brain volume in participants without dementia, higher fitness levels in early AD participants were associated with larger brain volume (less brain atrophy), even when age, sex, dementia severity, and physical frailty were controlled for.

A recent cross-sectional study compared cognitive functions and activities of daily living between adults without dementia and sedentary or active older adults with Alzheimer's dementia (Arcoverde et al., 2008). Results showed that in the sedentary group, the best predictor of cognitive performance (as measured using the Mini-Mental State Examination) was disease duration. However, in the active group, scores on activities of daily living were the best predictor of cognitive performance. According to the authors, this results means that autonomy, provided by maintaining an active exercise lifestyle, might have positively influenced cognitive maintenance. However, the strength of the conclusions that one can draw from this study is limited by the small number of participants in each group.

A recent longitudinal study examined the association between midlife physical activity and late-life cognitive function and dementia (Chang et al., 2010). Results showed that being active (around 5 hours per week) was associated with higher scores in processing speed, memory, and executive functions, even after demographic and cardiovascular factors were controlled for. Moreover, participants who reported being active were significantly less likely to have dementia in later life. In a recent prospective study, 1,740 persons older than 65 years without cognitive impairment were followed for 6.2 years (Larson et al., 2006). Results showed a 32% reduction in risk for dementia in individuals who exercised three or more times a week: Those participants had a dementia incidence of 13 per 1,000 person-years, as compared with 19.7 per 1,000 person-years in those who exercised fewer than three times a week.

Muscle strength has also been reported to be correlated with risk of Alzheimer's disease and rate of cognitive decline. Boyle, Buchman, Wilson, Leurgans, and Bennett (2010) followed 900 community-based older persons without dementia at baseline and found a lower rate of global cognitive decline, mild cognitive impairment, and Alzheimer's dementia in older adults with higher muscle strength. The protective effects remained after adjustment for several covariates, including body mass index, physical activity, pulmonary function, vascular risk factors, vascular diseases, and apolipoprotein E4 status. Furthermore, in a recent meta-analysis that covered 15 prospective studies (12 cohorts) and 33,816 nondemented individuals, 3,210 of whom showed cognitive decline during the 1- to 12-year follow-ups, Sofi et al. (2010) observed that physical activity significantly and consistently reduced cognitive decline. Individuals who were highly physically active showed 38% less risk of cognitive decline than the whole sample, and those who did low- to moderate-level exercise also showed significantly less risk (35%). A meta-analysis of randomized controlled trials (2,020 participants; 30 trials) by Heyn, Abreu, & Ottenbacher (2004) reported beneficial effects of physical activity on physical fitness (effect size = 0.69) and cognitive function (effect size = 0.57) in adults with cognitive impairment (MCI and dementia). However, other studies have reported modest benefits (Lautenschlager et al., 2008) or no appreciable effect (Eggermont, Swaab, Hol, & Scherder, 2009) of physical activity on cognition in patients with cognitive impairment.

A recent randomized clinical study evaluated the impact of a six-month aerobic exercise intervention in individuals with MCI (Baker et al., 2010). Thirty-three older adults (17 women) with amnestic MCI ranging in age from 55 to 85 years were randomized to either a high-intensity aerobic exercise (75–85% of heart rate capacity) or a control stretching group. Results showed beneficial effects of aerobic exercise, especially on executive functioning. Effects were more pronounced for women than men, despite comparable gains in cardiorespiratory fitness. In another randomized controlled study, Kemoun et al. (2010) examined the benefits of a 15-week physical activity program in 31 subjects with a mean age of 82 years. They reported that the physical activity program slowed cognitive decline and improved quality of walking in elderly persons with dementia. A more recent study compared cognitive effects in a Tai Chi intervention group (n = 171) and a stretching-and-toning group (n = 218) of older adults with cognitive impairment (Lam et al., 2011). Results showed that both groups improved in global cognitive function, delayed recall, and subjective cognitive complaints. However, improvements in balance, visual span, and clinical dementia rating scores were observed in the intervention group only.

Physical exercise can enhance not only cognition but also mood and well-being in geriatric patients. A recent randomized controlled trial evaluated the effects of physical training on depressive symptoms and psychological well-being in older people who were dependent in activities of daily living and were living in residential care facilities (Conradsson, Littbrand, Lindelof, Gustafson, & Rosendahl, 2010). Participants were 191 people aged between 65 and 100 years. Fifty-two percent of the participants had been diagnosed with a dementia disorder. Participants were randomly assigned to two groups: a physical training intervention group and a group who did control activities (e.g., watching films, singing, reading, and conversation). The exercise program consisted of high-intensity functional weight-bearing exercises designed to improve lower-limb strength, balance, and gait ability. Results showed that high-intensity exercise produced positive effects on physical capacity. However, no significant between-group effects were found on depressive symptoms or well-being either in all participants or in people with dementia alone.

Conclusion

As the first decade of the 21st century came to a close, the populations of most countries were aging rapidly. Although this is by far the most positive result of advances in modern science and improvements in health care policies, demographic aging imposes significant economic burdens on societies. Moreover, people who enjoy a long life expectancy also have to face increasing risks of suffering from chronic diseases, psychological distress, and cognitive declines. All these drawbacks of living a longer life have been associated with physical inactivity. In other words, being physically active lowers the chances of facing the negative consequences of aging. In 2001, a "National Blueprint" was released in the United States to recognize the substantial body of scientific evidence that physical activity leads to health benefits at any age (Chodzko-Zajko, 2006). In seniors, immediate and long-term benefits can be seen at the physiological level, such as improved

sleep and cardiovascular functions. Regular exercise can also positively alter psychological aspects of aging. Physical activity reduces depression and anxiety symptoms, enhances well-being, and improves quality of life. Furthermore, physical exercise can improve sociocultural aspects of aging by increasing social contact, preventing loneliness, and maintaining long-term social networks.

For the most part, the literature supports the notion that regular exercise, more specifically aerobic exercise that helps maintain cardiorespiratory fitness, plays a positive role in adapting to the changes that occur with age. Further research is needed to better document the effects of other forms of exercise as well as the dose–response relationships that govern the positive effects of exercise in all the domains in which benefits have been reported. Nevertheless, a plethora of evidence supports the promotion of health policies that target inactivity in individuals of all ages and with any medical condition who are able to safely participate in physical activity.

Physical activity guidelines were recently proposed by an advisory committee to the U.S. Department of Health and Human Services (U.S. Department of Health and Human Services, 2008). The committee, composed of 13 leading experts in exercise science and public health, rated the scientific evidence of the health benefits of physical activity as strong, moderate, or weak. To do so, the committee considered the type, number, and quality of studies available as well as the consistency of findings across studies that addressed each outcome. According to the committee, there is strong evidence that physical activity can significantly lower the risks of early death, coronary heart disease, stroke, high blood pressure, adverse blood lipid profile, type 2 diabetes, metabolic syndrome, colon cancer, and breast cancer. It can also help prevent weight gain and falls, facilitate weight loss, reduce depression, and improve cardiorespiratory and muscular fitness. The committee determined that there is moderate-to-strong evidence that physical activity is associated with better functional health in older adults and reduced abdominal obesity. In addition, there is moderate evidence that physical activity can lower the risk of hip fracture, lung cancer, and endometrial cancer and that it can facilitate weight maintenance after weight loss, increase bone density, and improve sleep quality. The committee set forth a series of recommendations that are particularly relevant for health care workers who deal with seniors and frail individuals. These recommendations suggest that if they are able to, all adults with disabilities should do at least 150 minutes a week of moderate-intensity aerobic exercise or 75 minutes a week of vigorous-intensity aerobic exercise. The aerobic exercise should be performed in sessions of at least 10 minutes, preferably spread over the week. Exercise programs should also include moderate- or high-intensity muscle-strengthening activities that involve all the major muscle groups on two or more days a week. All individuals unable to meet these guidelines should engage in regular physical activity according to their abilities and should avoid inactivity.

Hopefully, these guidelines will encourage people of all ages to participate in safe physical activity, regardless of medical conditions, chronic diseases, or limited physical capacities. Future studies could determine whether physical activity can further reduce the prevalence of age-associated diseases and increase the quality of life for the seniors of tomorrow, who will be living even longer than those of today.

Acknowledgment

The authors wish to thank Francis Langlois, Sébastien Grenier and Florian Bobeuf for their help in the preparation of this manuscript. The author is supported by the Canadian research chair program.

References

Abourezk, T., & Toole, T. (1995). Effect of task complexity on the relationship between physical fitness and reaction time in older women. *Journal of Aging and Physical Activity, 3*, 251–260.

Aichberger, M. C., Busch, M. A., Reischies, F. M., Ströhle, A., Heinz, A., & Rapp, M. A. (2010). Effect of physical inactivity on cognitive performance after 2.5 years of follow-up: Longitudinal results from the Survey of Health, Ageing, and Retirement (SHARE). *GeroPsych: The Journal of Gerontopsychology and Geriatric Psychiatry, 23*(1), 7–15.

Almeida, O. P., Garrido, G. J., Beer, C., Lautenschlager, N. T., Arnolda, L., Lenzo, N. P.,…Flicker, L. (2008). Coronary heart disease is associated with regional grey matter volume loss: Implications for cognitive function and behaviour. *Internal Medicine Journal, 38*(7), 599–606.

Alzheimer's Association. (2011). Alzheimer's disease facts and figures. *Alzheimer's & Dementia, 7*(2), 1–68.

American College of Sports Medicine. (1998). American College of Sports Medicine position stand: Exercise and physical activity for older adults. *Medicine & Science in Sports & Exercise, 30*(6), 992–1008.

Angst, J., Gamma, A., Gastpar, M., Lepine, J. P., Mendlewicz, J., & Tylee, A. (2002). Gender differences in depression: Epidemiological findings from the European DEPRES I and II studies. *European Archives of Psychiatry and Clinical Neuroscience, 252*(5), 201–209.

Ansseau, M., Fischler, B., Dierick, M., Mignon, A., & Leyman, S. (2005). Prevalence and impact of generalized anxiety disorder and major depression in primary care in Belgium and Luxemburg: The GADIS study. *European Psychiatry, 20*(3), 229–235.

Apostolova, L. G., & Cummings, J. L. (2008). Neuropsychiatric manifestations in mild cognitive impairment: A systematic review of the literature. *Dementia and Geriatric Cognitive Disorders, 25*(2), 115–126.

Arcoverde, C., Deslandes, A., Rangel, A., Pavao, R., Nigri, F., Engelhardt, E., & Laks, J. (2008). Role of physical activity on the maintenance of cognition and activities of daily living in elderly with Alzheimer's disease. *Arquivos de Neuro-Psiquiatria, 66*(2B), 323–327.

Avila-Funes, J. A., Amieva, H., Barberger-Gateau, P., Le Goff, M., Raoux, N., Ritchie, K.,…Dartigues, J. F. (2009). Cognitive impairment improves the predictive validity of the phenotype of frailty for adverse health outcomes: The three-city study. *Journal of the American Geriatrics Society, 57*(3), 453–461.

Babyak, M., Blumenthal, J. A., Herman, S., Khatri, P., Doraiswamy, M., Moore, K.,…Krishnan, K. R. (2000). Exercise treatment for major depression: Maintenance of therapeutic benefit at 10 months. *Psychosomatic Medicine, 62*(5), 633–638.

Baker, L. D., Frank, L. L., Foster-Schubert, K., Green, P. S., Wilkinson, C. W., McTiernan, A.,…Craft, S. (2010). Effects of aerobic exercise on mild cognitive impairment: A controlled trial. *Archives of Neurology, 67*(1), 71–79.

Barnes, D. E., Yaffe, K., Satariano, W. A., & Tager, I. B. (2003). A longitudinal study of cardiorespiratory fitness and cognitive function in healthy older adults. *Journal of the American Geriatrics Society, 51*(4), 459–465.

Bartholomew, J., & Ciccolo, J. (2008). Exercise, depression, and cognition. In W. Spirduso, L. Poon, & W. Chodzko-Zajko (Eds.), *Exercise and its mediating effects on cognition* (pp. 33–46). Champaign, IL: Human Kinetics.

Beard, C., Weisberg, R. B., & Keller, M. B. (2010). Health-related quality of life across the anxiety disorders: Findings from a sample of primary care patients. *Journal of Anxiety Disorders, 24*(6), 559–564.

Beekman, A. T., Bremmer, M. A., Deeg, D. J., van Balkom, A. J., Smit, J. H., de Beurs, E.,…van Tilburg, W. (1998). Anxiety disorders in later life: A report from the Longitudinal Aging Study Amsterdam. *International Journal of Geriatric Psychiatry, 13*(10), 717–726.

Beekman, A. T., de Beurs, E., van Balkom, A. J., Deeg, D. J., van Dyck, R., & van Tilburg, W. (2000). Anxiety and depression in later life: Co-occurrence and communality of risk factors. *American Journal of Psychiatry, 157*(1), 89–95.

Benedict, R. H., Dobraski, M., & Goldstein, M. Z. (1999). A preliminary study of the association between changes in mood and cognition in a mixed geriatric psychiatry sample. *The Journals of Gerontology Series B Psychological Sciences and Social Sciences, 54*(2), P94–P99.

Berchtold, N. (2008). Exercise, stress mechanisms, and cognition. In W. Spirduso, L. Poon, & W. Chodzko-Zajko (Eds.), *Exercise and its mediating effects on cognition* (pp. 47–67). Champaign, IL: Human Kinetics.

Bertheussen, G. F., Romundstad, P. R., Landmark, T., Kaasa, S., Dale, O., & Helbostad, J. L. (2010). Associations between physical activity and physical and mental health—a HUNT 3 study. *Medicine & Science in Sports & Exercise, 43*(7), 1220–1228.

Betik, A. C., & Hepple, R. T. (2008). Determinants of VO2 max decline with aging: An integrated perspective. *Applied Physiology, Nutrition, and Metabolism, 33*(1), 130–140.

Billman, G. E. (2002). Aerobic exercise conditioning: A non-pharmacological antiarrhythmic intervention. *Journal of Applied Physiology, 92*(2), 446–454.

Black, J. E., Isaacs, K. R., Anderson, B. J., Alcantara, A. A., & Greenough, W. T. (1990). Learning causes synaptogenesis, whereas motor activity causes angiogenesis, in cerebellar cortex of adult rats. *Proceedings of the National Academy of Sciences of the United States of America, 87*(14), 5568–5572.

Blumenthal, J. A., Babyak, M. A., Hinderliter, A., Watkins, L. L., Craighead, L., Lin, P. H.,...Sherwood, A. (2010). Effects of the DASH diet alone and in combination with exercise and weight loss on blood pressure and cardiovascular biomarkers in men and women with high blood pressure: The ENCORE study. *Archives of Internal Medicine, 170*(2), 126–135.

Blumenthal, J. A., Babyak, M. A., Moore, K. A., Craighead, W. E., Herman, S., Khatri, P.,...Krishnan, K. R. (1999). Effects of exercise training on older patients with major depression. *Archives of Internal Medicine, 159*(19), 2349–2356.

Booth, F. W., Gordon, S. E., Carlson, C. J., & Hamilton, M. T. (2000). Waging war on modern chronic diseases: Primary prevention through exercise biology. *Journal of Applied Physiology, 88*(2), 774–787.

Boyle, P. A., Buchman, A. S., Wilson, R. S., Leurgans, S. E., & Bennett, D. A. (2010). Physical frailty is associated with incident mild cognitive impairment in community-based older persons. *Journal of the American Geriatrics Society, 58*(2), 248–255.

Brazier, J. E., Harper, R., Jones, N. M., O'Cathain, A., Thomas, K. J., Usherwood, T., & Westlake, L. (1992). Validating the SF-36 health survey questionnaire: New outcome measure for primary care. *British Medical Journal, 305*(6846), 160–164.

Breteler, M. M., Claus, J. J., Grobbee, D. E., & Hofman, A. (1994). Cardiovascular disease and distribution of cognitive function in elderly people: The Rotterdam Study. *British Medical Journal, 308*(6944), 1604–1608.

Brown, T. A., Campbell, L. A., Lehman, C. L., Grisham, J. R., & Mancill, R. B. (2001). Current and lifetime comorbidity of the DSM-IV anxiety and mood disorders in a large clinical sample. *Journal of Abnormal Psychology, 110*(4), 585–599.

Bryant, C., Jackson, H., & Ames, D. (2008). The prevalence of anxiety in older adults: Methodological issues and a review of the literature. *Journal of Affective Disorders, 109*(3), 233–250.

Burns, J. M., Cronk, B. B., Anderson, H. S., Donnelly, J. E., Thomas, G. P., Harsha, A.,...Swerdlow, R. H. (2008). Cardiorespiratory fitness and brain atrophy in early Alzheimer disease. *Neurology, 71*(3), 210–216.

Burns, M. N., Siddique, J., Fokuo, J. K., & Mohr, D. C. (2010). Comorbid anxiety disorders and treatment of depression in people with multiple sclerosis. *Rehabilitation Psychology, 55*(3), 255–262.

Canadian Society for Exercise Physiology. (2011). *Canadian physical activity guidelines: Clinical practice guideline development report*. Retrieved on December 2, 2011 from http://www.csep.ca/english/view.asp?x=898

Casillas, J. M., Gremaux, V., Damak, S., Feki, A., & Pérennou, D. (2007). Exercise training for patients with cardiovascular disease. *Annales de Readaptation et de Médecine Physique, 50*(6), 403–418.

Caspersen, C. J., Powell, K. E., & Christensen, G. M. (1985). Physical activity, exercise, and physical fitness: Definitions and distinctions for health-related research. *Public Health Reports, 100*(2), 126–131.

Centers for Disease Control and Prevention. (1996). *Physical activity and health: A report of the Surgeon General*. Atlanta, GA: U.S. Department of Health and Human Services, National Center for Chronic Disease Prevention and Health Promotion.

Centers for Disease Control and Prevention. (2006). Trends in strength training—United States, 1998–2004. *Morbidity and Mortality Weekly Report, 55*(28), 769–772.

Centers for Disease Control and Prevention. (2007). Prevalence of regular physical activity among adults—United States, 2001 and 2005. *Morbidity and Mortality Weekly Reportp, 56*(46), 1209–1212.

Cesari, M., Leeuwenburgh, C., Lauretani, F., Onder, G., Bandinelli, S., Maraldi, C.,...Ferrucci, L. (2006). Frailty syndrome and skeletal muscle: Results from the Invecchiare in Chianti study. *American Journal of Clinical Nutrition, 83*(5), 1142–1148.

Chang, M., Jonsson, P. V., Snaedal, J., Bjornsson, S., Saczynski, J. S., Aspelund, T.,...Launer, L. J. (2010). The effect of midlife physical activity on cognitive function among older adults: AGES—Reykjavik Study. *The Journals of Gerontology Series A: Biological Sciences and Medical Sciences, 65*(12), 1369–1374.

Chen, J. J., Rosas, H. D., & Salat, D. H. (2011). Age-associated reductions in cerebral blood flow are independent from regional atrophy. *Neuroimage, 55*(2), 468–478.

Chodzko-Zajko, W. (2006). National Blueprint: Increasing physical activity among adults 50 and older. Implications for future physical activity and cognitive functioning research. In W. Poon, W. Chodzko-Zajko, & P. Tomporowski (Eds.), *Active living, cognitive functioning, and aging* (pp. 1–14). Champaign, IL: Human Kinetics.

Christensen, H., Griffiths, K., Mackinnon, A., & Jacomb, P. (1997). A quantitative review of cognitive deficits in depression and Alzheimer-type dementia. *Journal of the International Neuropsychical Society, 3*(6), 631–651.

Clarkson-Smith, L., & Hartley, A. A. (1989). Relationships between physical exercise and cognitive abilities in older adults. *Psychology and Aging, 4*(2), 183–189.

Colcombe, S. J., Erickson, K. I., Raz, N., Webb, A. G., Cohen, N. J., McAuley, E., & Kramer, A. F. (2003). Aerobic fitness reduces brain tissue loss in aging humans. *The Journals of Gerontology Series A: Biological Sciences and Medical Science, 58*(2), 176–180.

Colcombe, S., & Kramer, A. F. (2003). Fitness effects on the cognitive function of older adults: A meta-analytic study. *Psychological Science, 14*(2), 125–130.

Colcombe, S. J., Kramer, A. F., Erickson, K. I., Scalf, P., McAuley, E., Cohen, N. J.,...Elavsky, S. (2004). Cardiovascular fitness, cortical plasticity, and aging. *Proceedings of the National Academy of Sciences of the United States of America, 101*(9), 3316–3321.

Conn, V. S. (2010a). Anxiety outcomes after physical activity interventions: Meta-analysis findings. *Nursing Research, 59*(3), 224–231.

Conn, V. S. (2010b). Depressive symptom outcomes of physical activity interventions: Meta-analysis findings. *Annals of Behavioral Medicine, 39*(2), 128–138.

Conradsson, M., Littbrand, H., Lindelof, N., Gustafson, Y., & Rosendahl, E. (2010). Effects of a high-intensity functional exercise programme on depressive symptoms and psychological well-being among older people living in residential care facilities: A cluster-randomized controlled trial. *Aging & Mental Health, 14*(5), 565–576.

Craik, F. I. M., & Salthouse, T. A. (2008). *Handbook of aging and cognition* (3rd ed.). New York: Psychology Press.

Crespo, C. J., Smit, E., Andersen, R. E., Carter-Pokras, O., & Ainsworth, B. E. (2000). Race/ethnicity, social class and their relation to physical inactivity during leisure time: Results from the Third National Health and Nutrition Examination Survey, 1988–1994. *American Journal of Preventive Medicine, 18*(1), 46–53.

Dahl, O. P., Stordal, E., Lydersen, S., & Midgard, R. (2009). Anxiety and depression in multiple sclerosis: A comparative population-based study in Nord-Trondelag County, Norway. *Multiple Sclerosis, 15*(12), 1495–1501.

Degl'Innocenti, A., Agren, H., & Backman, L. (1998). Executive deficits in major depression. *Acta Psychiatrica Scandinavica, 97*(3), 182–188.

Dennis, N. A., & Cabeza, R. (2008). Neuroimaging of healthy cognitive aging. In F. I. M. Craik & T. A. Salthouse (Eds.), *Handbook of aging and cognition* (3rd ed., pp. 1–54). New York: Psychology Press.

Devier, D. J., Pelton, G. H., Tabert, M. H., Liu, X., Cuasay, K., Eisenstadt, R.,...Devanand, D. P. (2009). The impact of anxiety on conversion from mild cognitive impairment to Alzheimer's disease. *International Journal of Geriatric Psychiatry, 24*(12), 1335–1342.

Dipietro, L., Caspersen, C. J., Ostfeld, A. M., & Nadel, E. R. (1993). A survey for assessing physical activity among older adults. *Medicine & Science in Sports & Exercise, 25*(5), 628–642.

Dishman, R. (2006). Measurement of physical activity. In W. Poon, W. Chodzko-Zajko, & P. Tomporowski (Eds.), *Active living, cognitive functioning, and aging* (pp. 91–111). Champaign, IL: Human Kinetics.

Dissanayaka, N. N. W., Sellbach, A., Matheson, S., O'Sullivan, J. D., Silburn, P. A., Byrne, G. J.,...Mellick, G. D. (2010). Anxiety disorders in Parkinson's disease: Prevalence and risk factors. *Movement Disorders, 25*(7), 838–845.

Djernes, J. K. (2006). Prevalence and predictors of depression in populations of elderly: A review. *Acta Psychiatrica Scandinavica, 113*(5), 372–387.

Dustman, R. E., Ruhling, R. O., Russell, E. M., Shearer, D. E., Bonekat, H. W., Shigeoka, J. W.,...Bradford, D. C. (1984). Aerobic exercise training and improved neuropsychological function of older individuals. *Neurobiology of Aging, 5*(1), 35–42.

Eadie, B. D., Redila, V. A., & Christie, B. R. (2005). Voluntary exercise alters the cytoarchitecture of the adult dentate gyrus by increasing cellular proliferation, dendritic complexity, and spine density. *Journal of Comparative Neurology, 486*(1), 39–47.

Eckel, R. H., Grundy, S. M., & Zimmet, P. Z. (2005). The metabolic syndrome. *Lancet, 365*(9468), 1415–1428.

Eggermont, L. H., Swaab, D. F., Hol, E. M., & Scherder, E. J. (2009). Walking the line: A randomised trial on the effects of a short term walking programme on cognition in dementia. *Journal of Neurology, Neurosurgery & Psychiatry, 80*(7), 802–804.

Emery, C. (2008). Exercise, chronic obstructive pulmonary disease, and cognition. In W. Spirduso, L. Poon, & W. Chodzko-Zajko (Eds.), *Exercise and its mediating effects on cognition* (pp. 197–210). Champaign, IL: Human Kinetics.

Erickson, K. I., & Kramer, A. F. (2009). Aerobic exercise effects on cognitive and neural plasticity in older adults. *British Journal of Sports Medicine, 43*(1), 22–24.

Erickson, K. I., Prakash, R. S., Voss, M. W., Chaddock, L., Hu, L., Morris, K. S.,...Kramer, A. F. (2009). Aerobic fitness is associated with hippocampal volume in elderly humans. *Hippocampus, 19*(10), 1030–1039.

Erickson, K. I., Voss, M. W., Prakash, R. S., Basak, C., Szabo, A., Chaddock, L.,...Kramer, A. F. (2011). Exercise training increases size of hippocampus and improves memory. *Proceedings of the National Academy of Sciences of the United States of America, 108*(7), 3017–3022.

Etnier, J. L., Nowell, P. M., Landers, D. M., & Sibley, B. A. (2006). A meta-regression to examine the relationship between aerobic fitness and cognitive performance. *Brain Research Reviews, 52*(1), 119–130.

Fleg, J. L., Morrell, C. H., Bos, A. G., Brant, L. J., Talbot, L. A., Wright, J. G., & Lakatta, E. G. (2005). Accelerated longitudinal decline of aerobic capacity in healthy older adults. *Circulation, 112*(5), 674–682.

Ford, E. S., Giles, W. H., & Mokdad, A. H. (2004). Increasing prevalence of the metabolic syndrome among U.S. adults. *Diabetes Care, 27*(10), 2444–2449.

Fossati, P., Amar, G., Raoux, N., Ergis, A. M., & Allilaire, J. F. (1999). Executive functioning and verbal memory in young patients with unipolar depression and schizophrenia. *Psychiatry Research, 89*(3), 171–187.

Fox, K. R. (1999). The influence of physical activity on mental well-being. *Public Health Nutrition, 2*(3A), 411–418.

Fratiglioni, L., Paillard-Borg, S., & Winblad, B. (2004). An active and socially integrated lifestyle in late life might protect against dementia. *Lancet Neurology, 3*(6), 343–353.

Fried, L. P., Tangen, C. M., Walston, J., Newman, A. B., Hirsch, C., Gottdiener, J.,...McBurnie, M. A. (2001). Frailty in older adults: Evidence for a phenotype. *The Journals of Gerontology Series A: Biological Sciences and Medical Sciences, 56*(3), M146–M156.

Gallagher, D., Coen, R., Kilroy, D., Belinski, K., Bruce, I., Coakley, D.,...Lawlor, B. A. (2011). Anxiety and behavioural disturbance as markers of prodromal Alzheimer's disease in patients with mild cognitive impairment. *International Journal of Geriatric Psychiatry, 26*(2), 166–172.

Geda, Y. E., Roberts, R. O., Knopman, D. S., Christianson, T. J., Pankratz, V. S., Ivnik, R. J.,...Rocca, W. A. (2010). Physical exercise, aging, and mild cognitive impairment: A population-based study. *Archives of Neurology, 67*(1), 80–86.

Geda, Y. E., Roberts, R. O., Knopman, D. S., Petersen, R. C., Christianson, T. J. H., Pankratz, V. S.,...Rocca, W. A. (2008). Prevalence of neuropsychiatric symptoms in mild cognitive impairment and normal cognitive aging: Population-based study. *Archives of General Psychiatry, 65*(10), 1193–1198.

Grenier, S., Préville, M., Boyer, R., O'Connor, K., Béland, S.-G., Potvin, O.,...Brassard, J. (2011). The impact of DSM-IV symptom and clinical significance criteria on the prevalence estimates of subthreshold and threshold anxiety in the older adult population. *American Journal of Geriatric Psychiatry, 19*(4), 316–326.

Gum, A. M., King-Kallimanis, B., & Kohn, R. (2009). Prevalence of mood, anxiety, and substance-abuse disorders for older Americans in the National Comorbidity Survey-Replication. *American Journal of Geriatric Psychiatry, 17*(9), 769–781.

Gureje, O., Kola, L., & Afolabi, E. (2007). Epidemiology of major depressive disorder in elderly Nigerians in the Ibadan Study of Ageing: A community-based survey. *Lancet, 370*(9591), 957–964.

Gureje, O., Uwakwe, R., Oladeji, B., Makanjuola, V. O., & Esan, O. (2010). Depression in adult Nigerians: Results from the Nigerian Survey of Mental Health and Well-being. *Journal of Affective Disorders, 120*(1–3), 158–164.

Gurland, B., Cross, P., & Katz, S. (1996). Epidemiological perspectives on opportunities for treatment of depression. *American Journal of Geriatric Psychiatry, 4*(Suppl. 1), S7–S13.

Hagberg, J. M., Ehsani, A. A., & Holloszy, J. O. (1983). Effect of 12 months of intense exercise training on stroke volume in patients with coronary artery disease. *Circulation, 67*(6), 1194–1199.

Haines, M., Norris, M., & Kashy, D. (1996). The effects of depressed mood on academic performance in college students. *Journal of College Student Development, 37*(5), 519–526.

Harman, D. (2003). The free radical theory of aging. *Antioxidants and Redox Signaling, 5*(5), 557–561.

Hawkins, H. L., Kramer, A. F., & Capaldi, D. (1992). Aging, exercise, and attention. *Psychology and Aging, 7*(4), 643–653.

Hawkins, S. A., Cockburn, M. G., Hamilton, A. S., & Mack, T. M. (2004). An estimate of physical activity prevalence in a large population-based cohort. *Medicine & Science in Sports & Exercise, 36*(2), 253–260.

Heart and Stroke Foundation of Canada. (2006). Retrieved on December, 2, 2011 from http://www.heartandstroke.com/site/c.ikIQLcMWJtE/b.3483991/k.34A8/Statistics.htm

Helbostad, J. L., Sletvold, O., & Moe-Nilssen, R. (2004). Home training with and without additional group training in physically frail old people living at home: Effect on health-related quality of life and ambulation. *Clinical Rehabilitation, 18*(5), 498–508.

Hertzog, C., Kramer, A., Wilson, R., & Lindenberger, U. (2008). Enrichment effects on adult cognitive development: Can the functional capacity of older adults be preserved and enhanced? *Psychological Science in the Public Interest, 9*(1), 1–65.

Heun, R., Papassotiropoulos, A., & Ptok, U. (2000). Subthreshold depressive and anxiety disorders in the elderly. *European Psychiatry, 15*(3), 173–182.

Heyn, P., Abreu, B. C., & Ottenbacher, K. J. (2004). The effects of exercise training on elderly persons with cognitive impairment and dementia: A meta-analysis. *Archives of Physical Medicine and Rehabilitation, 85*(10), 1694–1704.

Hillman, C. H., Erickson, K. I., & Kramer, A. F. (2008). Be smart, exercise your heart: Exercise effects on brain and cognition. *Nature Reviews Neuroscience, 9*(1), 58–65.

Hillman, C. H., Weiss, E. P., Hagberg, J. M., & Hatfield, B. D. (2002). The relationship of age and cardiovascular fitness to cognitive and motor processes. *Psychophysiology, 39*(3), 303–312.

Hu, S., Ying, Z., Gomez-Pinilla, F., & Frautschy, S. A. (2009). Exercise can increase small heat shock proteins (sHSP) and pre- and post-synaptic proteins in the hippocampus. *Brain Research, 1249*, 191–201.

Huang, C.-J., Chiu, H.-C., Lee, M.-H., & Wang, S.-Y. (2011). Prevalence and incidence of anxiety disorders in diabetic patients: A national population-based cohort study. *General Hospital Psychiatry, 33*(1), 8–15.

Huffman, J. C., Celano, C. M., & Januzzi, J. L. (2010). The relationship between depression, anxiety, and cardiovascular outcomes in patients with acute coronary syndromes. *Neuropsychiatric Disease and Treatment, 6*, 123–136.

Hutton, D. (2008). *Older people in emergencies: Considerations for action and policy development.* Geneva: World Health Organization.

Isaacs, K. R., Anderson, B. J., Alcantara, A. A., Black, J. E., & Greenough, W. T. (1992). Exercise and the brain: Angiogenesis in the adult rat cerebellum after vigorous physical activity and motor skill learning. *Journal of Cerebral Blood Flow & Metabolism, 12*(1), 110–119.

Jongenelis, K., Pot, A. M., Eisses, A. M. H., Beekman, A. T. F., Kluiter, H., & Ribbe, M. W. (2004). Prevalence and risk indicators of depression in elderly nursing home patients: The AGED study. *Journal of Affective Disorders, 83*(2–3), 135–142.

Joseph, J. (2008). Diet, motor behavior, and cognition. In W. Spirduso, L. Poon, & W. Chodzko-Zajko (Eds.), *Exercise and its mediating effects on cognition* (pp. 119–129). Champaign, IL: Human Kinetics.

Julian, L., & Arnett, P. (2009). Relationships among anxiety, depression, and executive functioning in multiple sclerosis. *Clinical Neuropsychologist, 23*(5), 794–804.

Juneau, M., Roy, N., Nigam, A., Tardif, J. C., & Larivee, L. (2009). Exercise above the ischemic threshold and serum markers of myocardial injury. *Canadian Journal of Cardiology, 25*(10), e338–e341.

Jurca, R., Jackson, A. S., LaMonte, M. J., Morrow, J. R., Jr., Blair, S. N., Wareham, N. J., . . . Laukkanen, R. (2005). Assessing cardiorespiratory fitness without performing exercise testing. *American Journal of Preventive Medicine, 29*(3), 185–193.

Katzmarzyk, P. T., Leon, A. S., Wilmore, J. H., Skinner, J. S., Rao, D. C., Rankinen, T., & Bouchard, C. (2003). Targeting the metabolic syndrome with exercise: Evidence from the HERITAGE Family Study. *Medicine & Science in Sports & Exercise, 35*(10), 1703–1709.

Kemoun, G., Thibaud, M., Roumagne, N., Carette, P., Albinet, C., Toussaint, L., . . . Dugue, B. (2010). Effects of a physical training programme on cognitive function and walking efficiency in elderly persons with dementia. *Dementia and Geriatric Cognitive Disorders, 29*(2), 109–114.

Kessler, R. C., Berglund, P., Demler, O., Jin, R., Merikangas, K. R., & Walters, E. E. (2005). Lifetime prevalence and age-of-onset distributions of DSM-IV disorders in the National Comorbidity Survey Replication. *Archives of General Psychiatry, 62*(6), 593–602.

Khuwaja, A. K., Lalani, S., Dhanani, R., Azam, I. S., Rafique, G., & White, F. (2010). Anxiety and depression among outpatients with type 2 diabetes: A multi-centre study of prevalence and associated factors. *Diabetology & Metabolic Syndrome, 2*, 72.

King, A. C., Castro, C., Wilcox, S., Eyler, A. A., Sallis, J. F., & Brownson, R. C. (2000). Personal and environmental factors associated with physical inactivity among different racial-ethnic groups of U.S. middle-aged and older-aged women. *Health Psychology, 19*(4), 354–364.

King-Kallimanis, B., Gum, A. M., & Kohn, R. (2009). Comorbidity of depressive and anxiety disorders for older Americans in the National Comorbidity Survey-Replication. *American Journal of Geriatric Psychiatry, 17*(9), 782–792.

Klavestrand, J., & Vingard, E. (2009). The relationship between physical activity and health-related quality of life: A systematic review of current evidence. *Scandinavian Journal of Medicine & Science in Sports, 19*(3), 300–312.

Kline, G. M., Porcari, J. P., Hintermeister, R., Freedson, P. S., Ward, A., McCarron, R. F.,...Rippe, J. M. (1987). Estimation of VO2max from a one-mile track walk, gender, age, and body weight. *Medicine & Science in Sports & Exercise, 19*(3), 253–259.

Komulainen, P., Lakka, T. A., Kivipelto, M., Hassinen, M., Helkala, E. L., Haapala, I.,...Rauramaa, R. (2007). Metabolic syndrome and cognitive function: A population-based follow-up study in elderly women. *Dementia and Geriatric Cognitive Disorders, 23*(1), 29–34.

Kramer, A. F., Bherer, L., Colcombe, S. J., Dong, W., & Greenough, W. T. (2004). Environmental influences on cognitive and brain plasticity during aging. *The Journals of Gerontology Series A: Biological Sciences and Medical Sciences, 59*(9), M940–M957.

Kramer, A. F., Erickson, K. I., & Colcombe, S. J. (2006). Exercise, cognition, and the aging brain. *Journal of Applied Physiology, 101*(4), 1237–1242.

Kramer, A. F., Hahn, S., Cohen, N. J., Banich, M. T., McAuley, E., Harrison, C. R.,...Colcombe, A. (1999). Ageing, fitness and neurocognitive function. *Nature, 400*(6743), 418–419.

Kramer, D., Allgaier, A. K., Fejtkova, S., Mergl, R., & Hegerl, U. (2009). Depression in nursing homes: Prevalence, recognition, and treatment. *International Journal of Psychiatry in Medicine, 39*(4), 345–358.

Kriska, A. M. (1997). A collection of physical activity questionnaires for health-related research. *Medicine and Science in Sports and Exercise, 29*(6 Suppl), 3–205.

Lam, L. C., Chau, R. C., Wong, B. M., Fung, A. W., Lui, V. W., Tam, C. C.,...Chan, W. M. (2011). Interim follow-up of a randomized controlled trial comparing Chinese style mind body (Tai Chi) and stretching exercises on cognitive function in subjects at risk of progressive cognitive decline. *International Journal of Geriatric Psychiatry, 26*(7), 733–740.

Landi, F., Abbatecola, A. M., Provinciali, M., Corsonello, A., Bustacchini, S., Manigrasso, L.,...Lattanzio, F. (2010). Moving against frailty: Does physical activity matter? *Biogerontology, 11*(5), 537–545.

Landro, N. I., Stiles, T. C., & Sletvold, H. (2001). Neuropsychological function in nonpsychotic unipolar major depression. *Neuropsychiatry, Neuropsychology, and Behavioral Neurology, 14*(4), 233–240.

Langlois, F., Vu, T. T. M., Chassé, K., Dupuis, G., Kergoat, M. J., & Bherer, L. (2010). *Physical activity intervention for frail older adults: Specific impacts on executive functions, working memory, and quality of life.* Paper presented at the Cognitive Aging Conference, April 15–18, 2010, Atlanta, GA.

Larson, E. B., Wang, L., Bowen, J. D., McCormick, W. C., Teri, L., Crane, P., & Kukull, W. (2006). Exercise is associated with reduced risk for incident dementia among persons 65 years of age and older. *Annals of Internal Medicine, 144*(2), 73–81.

Lauer, R. E., Giordani, B., Boivin, M. J., Halle, N., Glasgow, B., Alessi, N. E.,...& Berent, S. (1994). Effects of depression on memory performance and metamemory in children. *Journal of the American Academy of Child and Adolescent Psychiatry, 33*(5), 679–685.

Lautenschlager, N. T., Cox, K. L., Flicker, L., Foster, J. K., van Bockxmeer, F. M., Xiao, J.,...Almeida, O. P. (2008). Effect of physical activity on cognitive function in older adults at risk for Alzheimer disease: A randomized trial. *JAMA, 300*(9), 1027–1037.

Lekan, D. (2009). Frailty and other emerging concepts in care of the aged. *Southern Online Journal of Nursing Research, 9*(3). Retrieved on December 2, 2011 from http://www.resourcecenter.net/images/SNRS/Files/SOJNR_articles2/Vol09Num03Art04.html.

Lenze, E. J., Mulsant, B. H., Shear, M. K., Schulberg, H. C., Dew, M. A., Begley, A. E.,...Reynolds, C. F. (2000). Comorbid anxiety disorders in depressed elderly patients. *American Journal of Psychiatry, 157*(5), 722–728.

Levin, C. A., Wei, W., Akincigil, A., Lucas, J. A., Bilder, S., & Crystal, S. (2007). Prevalence and treatment of diagnosed depression among elderly nursing home residents in Ohio. *Journal of the American Medical Directors Association, 8*(9), 585–594.

Lima, A. F. B. d. S., & Fleck, M. P. d. A. (2011). Quality of life, diagnosis, and treatment of patients with major depression: A prospective cohort study in primary care. *Revista Brasileira de Psiquiatria.* [online]. ahead of print [cited 2011-12-02], pp. 0–0 . Available from: <http://www.scielo.br/scielo.php?script=sci_arttext&pid=S1516-44462011005000001&lng=en&nrm=iso>. Epub Mar 11, 2011. ISSN 1516-4446. http://dx.doi.org/10.1590/S1516-44462011005000001..

Lista, I., & Sorrentino, G. (2010). Biological mechanisms of physical activity in preventing cognitive decline. *Cellular and Molecular Neurobiology, 30*(4), 493–503.

Lledo, P. M., Alonso, M., & Grubb, M. S. (2006). Adult neurogenesis and functional plasticity in neuronal circuits. *Nature Reviews Neuroscience, 7*(3), 179–193.

Lopez, M. (2008). Exercise and sleep quality. In W. Spirduso, L. Poon, & W. Chodzko-Zajko (Eds.), *Exercise and its mediating effects on cognition* (pp. 131–146). Champaign, IL: Human Kinetics.

Mackenzie, C. S., Reynolds, K., Chou, K. L., Pagura, J., & Sareen, J. (2011). Prevalence and correlates of generalized anxiety disorder in a national sample of older adults. *American Journal of Geriatric Psychiatry, 19*(4), 305–315.

Mailey, E. L., White, S. M., Wojcicki, T. R., Szabo, A. N., Kramer, A. F., & McAuley, E. (2010). Construct validation of a non-exercise measure of cardiorespiratory fitness in older adults. *BMC Public Health, 10,* 59.

Manini, T. M. (2010). Energy expenditure and aging. *Ageing Research Reviews, 9*(1), 1–11.

Martin-Merino, E., Ruigomez, A., Johansson, S., Wallander, M. A., & Garcia-Rodriguez, L. A. (2010). Study of a cohort of patients newly diagnosed with depression in general practice: Prevalence, incidence, comorbidity, and treatment patterns. *Primary Care Companion to the Journal of Clinical Psychiatry, 12*(1), PCC.08m00764.

McAuley, E., & Elavsky, S. (2008). Self-efficacy, physical activity, and cognitive function. In W. Spirduso, L. Poon, & W. Chodzko-Zajko (Eds.), *Exercise and its mediating effects on cognition* (pp. 69–84). Champaign, IL: Human Kinetics.

McAuley, E., Elavsky, S., Jerome, G. J., Konopack, J. F., & Marquez, D. X. (2005). Physical activity–related well-being in older adults: Social cognitive influences. *Psychology and Aging, 20*(2), 295–302.

McAuley, E., Szabo, A. N., Mailey, E. L., Erickson, K. I., Voss, M., White, S. M.,...Kramer, A. F. (2011). Non-exercise estimated cardiorespiratory fitness: Associations with brain structure, cognition, and memory complaints in older adults. *Mental Health and Physical Activity, 4*(1), 5–11

McDougall, F. A., Kvaal, K., Matthews, F. E., Paykel, E., Jones, P. B., Dewey, M. E., & Brayne, C. (2007). Prevalence of depression in older people in England and Wales: The MRC CFA Study. *Psychological Medicine, 37*(12), 1787–1795.

Mead, G. E., Morley, W., Campbell, P., Greig, C. A., McMurdo, M., & Lawlor, D. A. (2009). Exercise for depression. *Cochrane Database of Systematic Reviews, 3*, CD004366.

Meeks, T. W., Vahia, I. V., Lavretsky, H., Kulkarni, G., & Jeste, D. V. (2011). A tune in "a minor" can "b major": A review of epidemiology, illness course, and public health implications of subthreshold depression in older adults. *Journal of Affective Disorders, 129*(1–3), 126–142.

Mehta, K. M., Simonsick, E. M., Penninx, B. W., Schulz, R., Rubin, S. M., Satterfield, S., & Yaffe, K. (2003). Prevalence and correlates of anxiety symptoms in well-functioning older adults: Findings from the Health Aging and Body Composition Study. *Journal of the American Geriatrics Society, 51*(4), 499–504.

Michalak, E. E., Tam, E. M., Manjunath, C. V., Solomons, K., Levitt, A. J., Levitan, R., . . . Lam, R. W. (2004). Generic and health-related quality of life in patients with seasonal and non-seasonal depression. *Psychiatry Research, 128*(3), 245–251.

Milani, R. V., Lavie, C. J., Mehra, M. R., & Ventura, H. O. (2011). Impact of exercise training and depression on survival in heart failure due to coronary heart disease. *American Journal of Cardiology, 107*(1), 64–68.

Modrego, P. J., & Ferrandez, J. (2004). Depression in patients with mild cognitive impairment increases the risk of developing dementia of Alzheimer type: A prospective cohort study. *Archives of Neurology, 61*(8), 1290–1293.

Moholdt, T. T., Amundsen, B. H., Rustad, L. A., Wahba, A., Løvø, K. T., Gullikstad, L. R., . . . Slordahl, S. A. (2009). Aerobic interval training versus continuous moderate exercise after coronary artery bypass surgery: A randomized study of cardiovascular effects and quality of life. *American Heart Journal, 158*(6), 1031–1037.

Muangpaisan, W., Intalapaporn, S., & Assantachai, P. (2008). Neuropsychiatric symptoms in the community-based patients with mild cognitive impairment and the influence of demographic factors. *International Journal of Geriatric Psychiatry, 23*(7), 699–703.

Myers, J., Prakash, M., Froelicher, V., Do, D., Partington, S., & Atwood, J. E. (2002). Exercise capacity and mortality among men referred for exercise testing. *New England Journal of Medicine, 346*(11), 793–801.

Nelson, M. E., Rejeski, W. J., Blair, S. N., Duncan, P. W., Judge, J. O., King, A. C., . . . Castaneda-Sceppa, C. (2007). Physical activity and public health in older adults: Recommendation from the American College of Sports Medicine and the American Heart Association. *Medicine & Science in Sports & Exercise, 39*(8), 1435–1445.

Noël, M., Jobin, J., Marcoux, A., Poirier, P., Dagenais, G., & Bogaty, P. (2007). Can prolonged exercise-induced myocardial ischaemia be innocuous? *European Heart Journal, 28*(13), 1559–1565.

Nuti, A., Ceravolo, R., Piccinni, A., Dell'Agnello, G., Bellini, G., Gambaccini, G., . . . Bonuccelli, U. (2004). Psychiatric comorbidity in a population of Parkinson's disease patients. *European Journal of Neurology, 11*(5), 315–320.

Ostergard, T., Andersen, J. L., Nyholm, B., Lund, S., Nair, K. S., Saltin, B., & Schmitz, O. (2006). Impact of exercise training on insulin sensitivity, physical fitness, and muscle oxidative capacity in first-degree relatives of type 2 diabetic patients. *American Journal of Physiology, Endocrinology and Metabolism, 290*(5), E998–E1005.

Palmer, K., Berger, A. K., Monastero, R., Winblad, B., Backman, L., & Fratiglioni, L. (2007). Predictors of progression from mild cognitive impairment to Alzheimer disease. *Neurology, 68*(19), 1596–1602.

Paluska, S. A., & Schwenk, T. L. (2000). Physical activity and mental health: Current concepts. *Sports Medicine, 29*(3), 167–180.

Parmelee, P. A., Lawton, M. P., & Katz, I. R. (1998). The structure of depression among elderly institution residents: Affective and somatic correlates of physical frailty. *The Journals of Gerontology Series A: Biological Sciences and Medical Sciences, 53*(2), M155–M162.

Pasco, J. A., Williams, L. J., Jacka, F. N., Henry, M. J., Coulson, C. E., Brennan, S. L., . . . Berk, M. (2011). Habitual physical activity and the risk for depressive and anxiety disorders among older men and women. *International Psychogeriatrics, 23*(2), 292–298.

Paterson, D. H., Govindasamy, D., Vidmar, M., Cunningham, D. A., & Koval, J. J. (2004). Longitudinal study of determinants of dependence in an elderly population. *Journal of the American Geriatrics Society, 52*(10), 1632–1638.

Penedo, F. J., & Dahn, J. R. (2005). Exercise and well-being: A review of mental and physical health benefits associated with physical activity. *Current Opinion in Psychiatry, 18*(2), 189–193.

Peterson, M., Giuliani, C., Morey, M., Pieper, C., Evenson, K., Mercer, V., . . . Simonsick, E. M. (2009). Physical activity as a preventative factor for frailty: The Health, Aging, And Body Composition Study. *The Journals of Gerontology Series A: Biological Sciences and Medical Sciences, 64*(1), 61–68.

Phillips, A. C., Batty, G. D., Gale, C. R., Deary, I. J., Osborn, D., MacIntyre, K., . . . Carroll, D. (2009). Generalized anxiety disorder, major depressive disorder, and their comorbidity as predictors of all-cause and cardiovascular mortality: The Vietnam Experience Study. *Psychosomatic Medicine, 71*(4), 395–403.

Preisig, M., Merikangas, K. R., & Angst, J. (2001). Clinical significance and comorbidity of subthreshold depression and anxiety in the community. *Acta Psychiatrica Scandinavica, 104*(2), 96–103.

Preville, M., Boyer, R., Grenier, S., Dube, M., Voyer, P., Punti, R., . . . Brassard, J. (2008). The epidemiology of psychiatric disorders in Quebec's older adult population. *Canadian Journal of Psychiatry, 53*(12), 822–832.

Prina, A. M., Ferri, C. P., Guerra, M., Brayne, C., & Prince, M. (2011). Co-occurrence of anxiety and depression amongst older adults in low- and middle-income countries: Findings from the 10/66 study. *Psychological Medicine, 41*(10), 2047–2056.

Raz, N. (2005). The aging brain observed in vivo: Differential changes and their modifiers. In R. Cabeza, L. Nyberg, & D. C. Park (Eds.), *Cognitive neuroscience of aging* (pp. 19–57). New York: Oxford University Press.

Raz, N., Ghisletta, P., Rodrigue, K. M., Kennedy, K. M., & Lindenberger, U. (2010). Trajectories of brain aging in middle-aged and older adults: Regional and individual differences. *Neuroimage, 51*(2), 501–511.

Reiff, J., Schmidt, N., Riebe, B., Breternitz, R., Aldenhoff, J., Deuschl, G., . . . Witt, K. (2011). Subthreshold depression in Parkinson's disease. *Movement Disorders, 26*(9), 1741–1744.

Rejeski, W. J., & Mihalko, S. L. (2001). Physical activity and quality of life in older adults. *The Journals of Gerontology Series A: Biological Sciences and Medical Sciences, 56*(2), 23–35.

Renaud, M., Bherer, L., & Maquestiaux, F. (2010). A high level of physical fitness is associated with more efficient response preparation in older adults. *Journal of Gerontology: Psychological Sciences, 65*(3), 317–322.

Renaud, M., Maquestiaux, F., Joncas, S., Kergoat, M. J., & Bherer, L. (2010). The effect of three months of aerobic training on response preparation in older adults. *Frontiers in Aging Neuroscience, 2*, 148.

Rethorst, C. D., Wipfli, B. M., & Landers, D. M. (2009). The antidepressive effects of exercise: A meta-analysis of randomized trials. *Sports Medicine, 39*(6), 491–511.

Reuter-Lorenz, P. A., & Park, D. C. (2010). Human neuroscience and the aging mind: A new look at old problems. *The Journals of Gerontology Series B Psychological Sciences and Social Sciences, 65*(4), 405–415.

Riedel-Heller, S. G., Busse, A., & Angermeyer, M. C. (2006). The state of mental health in old-age across the 'old' European Union—a systematic review. *Acta Psychiatrica Scandinavica, 113*(5), 388–401.

Rikli, R. E., & Edwards, D. J. (1991). Effects of a three-year exercise program on motor function and cognitive processing speed in older women. *Research Quarterly for Exercise & Sport, 62*(1), 61–67.

Ritchie, K., Artero, S., Beluche, I., Ancelin, M. L., Mann, A., Dupuy, A. M., . . . Boulenger, J. P. (2004). Prevalence of DSM-IV psychiatric disorder in the French elderly population. *British Journal of Psychiatry, 184*, 147–152.

Rivas-Vazquez, R. A., Saffa-Biller, D., Ruiz, I., Blais, M. A., & Rivas-Vazquez, A. (2004). Current issues in anxiety and depression: Comorbid, mixed, and subthreshold disorders. *Professional Psychology: Research and Practice, 35*(1), 74–83.

Roberts, R. O., Knopman, D. S., Geda, Y. E., Cha, R. H., Roger, V. L., & Petersen, R. C. (2010). Coronary heart disease is associated with non-amnestic mild cognitive impairment. *Neurobiology of Aging, 31*(11), 1894–1902.

Rochat, S., Cumming, R. G., Blyth, F., Creasey, H., Handelsman, D., Le Couteur, D. G., . . . Waite, L. (2010). Frailty and use of health and community services by community-dwelling older men: The Concord Health and Ageing in Men Project. *Age and Ageing, 39*(2), 228–233.

Rockwood, K., Howlett, S. E., MacKnight, C., Beattie, B. L., Bergman, H., Hebert, R., . . . McDowell, I. (2004). Prevalence, attributes, and outcomes of fitness and frailty in community-dwelling older adults: Report from the Canadian Study of Health and Aging. *The Journals of Gerontology Series A: Biological Sciences and Medical Sciences, 59*(12), 1310–1317.

Rockwood, K., Song, X., MacKnight, C., Bergman, H., Hogan, D. B., McDowell, I., & Mitnitski, A. (2005). A global clinical measure of fitness and frailty in elderly people. *Canadian Medical Association Journal, 173*(5), 489–495.

Royall, D. (2008). Diabetes, executive control, functional status, and physical activity. In W. Spirduso, L. Poon, & W. Chodzko-Zajko (Eds.), *Exercise and its mediating effects on cognition* (pp. 183–196). Champaign, IL: Human Kinetics.

Rozzini, L., Chilovi, B. V., Peli, M., Conti, M., Rozzini, R., Trabucchi, M., & Padovani, A. (2009). Anxiety symptoms in mild cognitive impairment. *International Journal of Geriatric Psychiatry, 24*(3), 300–305.

Rutledge, T., Linke, S. E., Krantz, D. S., Johnson, B. D., Bittner, V., Eastwood, J. A., . . . Merz, C. N. (2009). Comorbid depression and anxiety symptoms as predictors of cardiovascular events: Results from the NHLBI-sponsored Women's Ischemia Syndrome Evaluation (WISE) Study. *Psychosomatic Medicine, 71*(9), 958–964.

Sallis, J. F., Greenlee, L., McKenzie, T. L., Broyles, S. L., Zive, M. M., Berry, C. C., . . . Nader, P. R. (2001). Changes and tracking of physical activity across seven years in Mexican-American and European-American mothers. *Women Health, 34*(4), 1–14.

Salmon, P. (2001). Effects of physical exercise on anxiety, depression, and sensitivity to stress: A unifying theory. *Clinical Psychology Review, 21*(1), 33–61.

Samper-Ternent, R., Al Snih, S., Raji, M. A., Markides, K. S., & Ottenbacher, K. J. (2008). Relationship between frailty and cognitive decline in older Mexican Americans. *Journal of the American Geriatrics Society, 56*(10), 1845–1852.

Segura, B., Jurado, M. A., Freixenet, N., Albuin, C., Muniesa, J., & Junque, C. (2009). Mental slowness and executive dysfunctions in patients with metabolic syndrome. *Neuroscience Letters, 462*(1), 49–53.

Sigal, R. J., Kenny, G. P., Boule, N. G., Wells, G. A., Prud'homme, D., Fortier, M., . . . Jaffey, J. (2007). Effects of aerobic training, resistance training, or both on glycemic control in type 2 diabetes: A randomized trial. *Annals of Internal Medicine, 147*(6), 357–369.

Singh, N. A., Clements, K. M., & Singh, M. A. (2001). The efficacy of exercise as a long-term antidepressant in elderly subjects: A randomized, controlled trial. *The Journals of Gerontology Series A: Biological Sciences and Medical Sciences, 56*(8), M497–M504.

Singh-Manoux, A., Britton, A. R., & Marmot, M. (2003). Vascular disease and cognitive function: Evidence from the Whitehall II Study. *Journal of the American Geriatrics Society, 51*(10), 1445–1450.

Smalbrugge, M., Jongenelis, L., Pot, A. M., Beekman, A. T., & Eefsting, J. A. (2005). Comorbidity of depression and anxiety in nursing home patients. *International Journal of Geriatric Psychiatry, 20*(3), 218–226.

Smiley-Oyen, A. L., Lowry, K. A., Francois, S. J., Kohut, M. L., & Ekkekakis, P. (2008). Exercise, fitness, and neurocognitive function in older adults: The "selective improvement" and "cardiovascular fitness" hypotheses. *Annals of Behavioral Medicine, 36*(3), 280–291.

Smith, P. J., Blumenthal, J. A., Hoffman, B. M., Cooper, H., Strauman, T. A., Welsh-Bohmer, K., . . . Sherwood, A. (2010). Aerobic exercise and neurocognitive performance: A meta-analytic review of randomized controlled trials. *Psychosomatic Medicine, 72*(3), 239–252.

Sofi, F., Capalbo, A., Cesari, F., Abbate, R., & Gensini, G. F. (2008). Physical activity during leisure time and primary prevention of coronary heart disease: An updated meta-analysis of cohort studies. *European Journal of Cardiovascular Prevention & Rehabilitation, 15*(3), 247–257.

Sofi, F., Valecchi, D., Bacci, D., Abbate, R., Gensini, G. F., Casini, A., & Macchi, C. (2011). Physical activity and risk of cognitive decline: A meta-analysis of prospective studies. *Journal of Internal Medicine, 269*(1), 107–117.

Solfrizzi, V., Scafato, E., Capurso, C., D'Introno, A., Colacicco, A. M., Frisardi, V., . . . Panza, F. (2009). Metabolic syndrome, mild cognitive impairment, and progression to dementia: The Italian Longitudinal Study on Aging. *Neurobiology of Aging, 32*(11), 1932–1941.

Soneira, C. F., & Scott, T. M. (1996). Severe cardiovascular disease and Alzheimer's disease: Senile plaque formation in cortical areas. *Clinical Anatomy, 9*(2), 118–127.

Sparks, D. L., Hunsaker, J. C., 3rd, Scheff, S. W., Kryscio, R. J., Henson, J. L., & Markesbery, W. R. (1990). Cortical senile plaques in coronary artery disease, aging and Alzheimer's disease. *Neurobiology of Aging, 11*(6), 601–607.

Spirduso, W. W. (1975). Reaction and movement time as a function of age and physical activity level. *Journal of Gerontology, 30*(4), 435–440.

Spirduso, W., Francis, K., & MacRae, P. (2005). *Physical dimensions of aging* (2nd ed.). Champaign, IL: Human Kinetics.

Spirduso, W., Poon, L., & Chodzko-Zajko, W. (2008). Using resources and reserves in an exercise-cognition model. In W. Spirduso, L. Poon, & W. Chodzko-Zajko (Eds.), *Exercise and its mediating effects on cognition* (pp. 3–11). Champaign, IL: Human Kinetics.

Spitzer, R. L., Kroenke, K., Linzer, M., Hahn, S. R., Williams, J. B., deGruy, F. V., 3rd,…Davies, M. (1995). Health-related quality of life in primary care patients with mental disorders: Results from the PRIME-MD 1000 Study. *JAMA, 274*(19), 1511–1517.

Stampfer, M. J. (2006). Cardiovascular disease and Alzheimer's disease: Common links. *Journal of Internal Medicine, 260*(3), 211–223.

Stathokostas, L., Jacob-Johnson, S., Petrella, R. J., & Paterson, D. H. (2004). Longitudinal changes in aerobic power in older men and women. *Journal of Applied Physiology, 97*(2), 781–789.

Statistics Canada. (2008). *Canadian demographics at a glance.* Retrieved on December 2, 2011 from http://www.statcan.gc.ca/.

Steffens, D. C., Skoog, I., Norton, M. C., Hart, A. D., Tschanz, J. T., Plassman, B. L.,…Breitner, J. C. (2000). Prevalence of depression and its treatment in an elderly population: The Cache County Study. *Archives of General Psychiatry, 57*(6), 601–607.

Stein, M. B., & Barrett-Connor, E. (2002). Quality of life in older adults receiving medications for anxiety, depression, or insomnia: Findings from a community-based study. *American Journal of Geriatric Psychiatry, 10*(5), 568–574.

Streiner, D. L., Cairney, J., & Veldhuizen, S. (2006). The epidemiology of psychological problems in the elderly. *Canadian Journal of Psychiatry, 51*(3), 185–191.

Stuss, D. T., Shallice, T., Alexander, M. P., & Picton, T. W. (1995). A multidisciplinary approach to anterior attentional functions. In J. Grafman, K. J. Holyoak, & F. Boller (Ed.s), Structure and functions of the human prefrontal cortex (Annals of the New York Academy of Sciences, Vol. 769 (pp. 191–211). New York: New York Academy of Sciences.

Sulaiman, N., Hamdan, A., Tamim, H., Mahmood, D. A., & Young, D. (2010). The prevalence and correlates of depression and anxiety in a sample of diabetic patients in Sharjah, United Arab Emirates. *BMC Family Practice, 11*, 80.

Tanaka, H., & Cortez-Cooper, M. (2008). Exercise, hypertension, and cognition. In W. Spirduso, L. Poon, & W. Chodzko-Zajko (Eds.), *Exercise and its mediating effects on cognition* (pp. 169–181). Champaign, IL: Human Kinetics.

Teresi, J., Abrams, R., Holmes, D., Ramirez, M., & Eimicke, J. (2001). Prevalence of depression and depression recognition in nursing homes. *Social Psychiatry and Psychiatric Epidemiology, 36*(12), 613–620.

Tintle, N., Bacon, B., Kostyuchenko, S., Gutkovich, Z., & Bromet, E. J. (2011). Depression and its correlates in older adults in Ukraine. *International Journal of Geriatric Psychiatry, 26*(12), 1292–1299

Tolin, D. F., Robison, J. T., Gaztambide, S., & Blank, K. (2005). Anxiety disorders in older Puerto Rican primary care patients. *American Journal of Geriatric Psychiatry, 13*(2), 150–156.

U.S. Department of Health and Human Services. (1999). *Mental health: A report of the Surgeon General.* Rockville, MD: U.S. Department of Health and Human Services, Substance Abuse and Mental Health Services Administration, Center for Mental Health Services, National Institutes of Health, National Institute of Mental Health.

U.S. Department of Health and Human Services. (2000). *Healthy People 2010* (2nd ed.). Washington, DC: U.S. Government Printing Office.

U.S. Department of Health and Human Services. (2008). *Physical activity guidelines for Americans.* Washington, DC: U.S. Government Printing Office. Retrieved on December 2, 2001 from www.health.gov/paguidelines.

van Praag, H., Shubert, T., Zhao, C., & Gage, F. H. (2005). Exercise enhances learning and hippocampal neurogenesis in aged mice. *Journal of Neuroscience, 25*(38), 8680–8685.

Veiel, H. O. (1997). A preliminary profile of neuropsychological deficits associated with major depression. *Journal of Clinical and Experimental Neuropsychology, 19*(4), 587–603.

Vitiello, M. V. (2008). Exercise, sleep, and cognition: Interactions in aging. In W. Spirduso, L. Poon, & W. Chodzko-Zajko (Eds.), *Exercise and its mediating effects on cognition* (pp. 146–165). Champaign, IL: Human Kinetics.

Voelcker-Rehage, C., Godde, B., & Staudinger, U. M. (2010). Physical and motor fitness are both related to cognition in old age. *European Journal of Neuroscience, 31*(1), 167–176.

Vogelzangs, N., Seldenrijk, A., Beekman, A. T. F., van Hout, H. P. J., de Jonge, P., & Penninx, B. W. J. H. (2010). Cardiovascular disease in persons with depressive and anxiety disorders. *Journal of Affective Disorders, 125*(1–3), 241–248.

Voss, M. W., Prakash, R. S., Erickson, K. I., Basak, C., Chaddock, L., Kim, J. S.,…Kramer, A. F. (2010). Plasticity of brain networks in a randomized intervention trial of exercise training in older adults. *Frontiers in Aging Neuroscience, 2*, 1–17.

Wang, C. Y., Haskell, W. L., Farrell, S. W., Lamonte, M. J., Blair, S. N., Curtin, L. R.,…Burt, V. L. (2010). Cardiorespiratory fitness levels among US adults 20–49 years of age: Findings from the 1999–2004 National Health and Nutrition Examination Survey. *American Journal of Epidemiology, 171*(4), 426–435.

Windle, G., Hughes, D., Linck, P., Russell, I., & Woods, B. (2010). Is exercise effective in promoting mental well-being in older age? A systematic review. *Aging and Mental Health, 14*(6), 652–669.

Wipfli, B. M., Rethorst, C. D., & Landers, D. M. (2008). The anxiolytic effects of exercise: A meta-analysis of randomized trials and dose–response analysis. *Journal of Sport & Exercise Psychology, 30*(4), 392–410.

Yaffe, K., Haan, M., Blackwell, T., Cherkasova, E., Whitmer, R. A., & West, N. (2007). Metabolic syndrome and cognitive decline in elderly Latinos: Findings from the Sacramento Area Latino Study of Aging study. *Journal of the American Geriatrics Society, 55*(5), 758–762.

Yazdanyar, A., & Newman, A. B. (2009). The burden of cardiovascular disease in the elderly: Morbidity, mortality, and costs. *Clinics in Geriatric Medicine, 25*(4), 563–577.

Yohannes, A. M., Doherty, P., Bundy, C., & Yalfani, A. (2010). The long-term benefits of cardiac rehabilitation on depression, anxiety, physical activity and quality of life. *Journal of Clinical Nursing, 19*(19–20), 2806–2813.

Yunming, L., Changsheng, C., Haibo, T., Wenjun, C., Shanhong, F., Yan, M.,...Qianzhen, H. (2011). Prevalence and risk factors for depression in older people in Xi'an China: A community-based study. *International Journal of Geriatric Psychiatry*, doi: 10.1002/gps.2685.

Zafon, C. (2007). Oscillations in total body fat content through life: An evolutionary perspective. *Obesity Reviews, 8*(6), 525–530.

Zhu, W., & Chodzko-Zajko, W. (2006). *Measurement issues in aging and physical activity : Proceedings of the 10th Measurement and Evaluation Symposium.* Champaign, IL: Human Kinetics.

Children's Motivation for Involvement in Physical Activity

Robert J. Brustad

Abstract

Understanding children's motivation to engage in physical activity is an important and urgent topic given current knowledge about levels of youth inactivity. An improved understanding of children's motivation to be physically active should drive future intervention strategies and help structure public policies. It is necessary to maintain a broad perspective on the topic, because children's physical activity motivation is affected by biological, social, and developmental factors as well as by the psychological and individual-difference factors that are the primary focus here. This chapter discusses the primary contemporary theoretical perspectives on children's physical activity motivation and highlights differences between the physical activity motivation of adults and children. Four major psychological dimensions of influence on youth physical activity motivation are discussed in depth: young people's perceptions of competence and of autonomy, their affective responses to physical activity, and the nature of the social relationships they experience while engaged in physical activity.

Key Words: motivation, children's physical activity, intrinsic motivation.

Understanding children's motivation to engage in physical activity and exercise is a most timely and important topic. The topic is particularly timely given current knowledge about the extent of physical inactivity among children and adolescents and the associated incidence of overweight and obesity among this important segment of our population. The best current estimates indicate that as few as 49% of boys and 35% of girls ages 6–11 years in the United States engage in the recommended amount of moderate and vigorous daily physical activity (Troiano et al., 2008). Of particular concern is that the greatest increase in obesity levels for any age group over the past decade has been for children ages 6–11 years (Ogden et al., 2006), a finding that lends further credence to the belief that American children are more physically inactive than ever before. Physical inactivity during childhood greatly increases the likelihood of short-term and long-term

health care costs for families, communities, and nations, and many of the long-term costs cannot yet be estimated, because there is little historical precedent for extensive levels of physical inactivity and obesity among youth. In addition, physical activity is essential to psychological well-being and effective social functioning among children and adolescents; thus we should be similarly concerned about those outcomes. Given the extent and nature of the issues associated with physical inactivity, children's physical activity behavior has moved well beyond a topic of academic research interest to one that addresses a serious social issue with important implications for intervention and social policy.

The gravity of the current situation makes understanding children's motivation for physical activity and using such knowledge for the promotion of physical activity absolutely essential. It is important to establish physical activity habits during childhood, because children's physical activity patterns track into adolescence and through adulthood (Malina, 1996; Pate, Baranowski, Dowda, & Trost, 1996). For physical activity to be beneficial for children or adults it needs to be adopted as a lifestyle behavior. Merely increasing physical activity opportunities for children without corresponding concern for increasing children's motivation to be active will not be sufficient to enable sustained physical activity involvement throughout the lifetime. Therefore, our primary focus should be on understanding and enhancing children's intrinsic motivation to do physical activity that contributes to desirable affective experiences and outcomes.

Contrasting Child and Adult Physical Activity Motivation

At the outset of this chapter it is worthwhile to contrast the physical activity motivation of children and adults and understand why separate bodies of knowledge exist for each. An important first consideration involves experience. Children simply have much less experience with physical activity than do adults. However, it is during early exposures to various types of physical activity that children begin to form their feelings about physical activity and their future interests in or attractions to its different forms. In contrast, adults have generally had sufficient experience with various forms of physical activity to have well-established likes and dislikes in relation to the type, intensity, and setting for physical activity.

Second, children's physical activity involvement takes place as they are undergoing extensive developmental change, whereas developmental change processes have much less effect on adults. The childhood and adolescent years are accompanied by enormous cognitive, physical, social, and emotional change and these developmental change experiences have an inherent influence on children's interest and involvement in physical activity.

Third, children's forays into physical activity and sport almost always occur in the presence of important significant others, particularly parents, and these significant others can have great influence in shaping children's emerging beliefs and attitudes toward physical activity. Adults, in contrast, do not typically have significant socialization agents serve as "gatekeepers" and interpreters of their physical activity experiences (Fredricks & Eccles, 2004; Welk & Schaben, 2004).

Fourth, adults and children differ greatly in the purposes of their physical activity. Adult physical activity involvement is much more likely to be goal-directed exercise behavior done to improve health, reduce stress, or lose weight. It is almost inconceivable that children would engage in purposeful exercise with an interest in attaining these health and fitness goals, because children do not necessarily see or value the connection between physical activity involvement and physical health changes in the first place (Brustad, 1991). Children further lack the self-management skills to carry out long-term behavioral change strategies. More importantly, children's interest in and attraction to physical activity are most strongly oriented toward their immediate experiences of the activity, and these outcomes depend primarily on the extent to which they enjoy the physical sensations that accompany the activity (e.g., exertion and sweating) and the quality of the social interaction that they experience while engaged in it (Brustad, 1993, 1996).

It should be evident from these four distinctive characteristics why separate bodies of knowledge are needed for the study of the physical activity motivation of adults and of children. It should also be evident that theoretical perspectives developed to address adult physical activity motivation are not necessarily appropriate for children's physical activity motivation. Furthermore, I will argue that a broad range of influences affect children's physical activity motivation and that an exclusive focus on the psychological characteristics related to motivation in youth could result in the loss of an appropriate "bigger picture" understanding of the biological, social, and developmental factors that affect motivation and subsequent physical activity behavior.

A Broad Perspective on Children's Physical Activity Motivation

From one viewpoint, the study of children's physical activity motivation is essentially a matter of understanding the individual differences among children in their desire to be physically active and the effects of these motivational differences on behavior. However, it is also essential to understand the causes of these individual differences, because identifying and appreciating those causes has important implications for the design and promotion of physical activity opportunities through public places such as schools and recreational centers, through organized youth sport programs, and even through the design of public transportation systems. Although the focus of this chapter is on the intrapersonal and psychological contributors to children's physical activity motivation, we would be remiss if we were to ignore the fact that children's involvement in physical activity or in any free-choice activity is subject to broader forms of influence that cannot be directly labeled as "psychological." Such involvement occurs within a broader social and cultural milieu (Bronfenbrenner & Morris, 1998) and is affected by biological, social, and developmental influences in addition to psychological factors. Focusing too narrowly on psychological contributors alone and losing sight of this bigger picture may result in insufficient intervention approaches of limited potential benefit to youth.

One important biological factor is the genetic predisposition to be physically active. A growing body of knowledge points to a tendency for familial aggregation or familial clustering around physical activity, such that family members share common physical activity levels with other family members in a way that reflects shared genetic characteristics (Seabra, Mendonca, Goring, Thomis, & Maia, 2008). Recent scientific advances have enabled us to gain a better appreciation for the role of genetic influences in shaping physical activity characteristics. In contrast to previous ways of considering "nature" and "nurture," modern developmental scientists are reluctant to view genetic and environmental influences as two independent and unrelated forms of influence.

Children's motivation for physical activity is also greatly affected by the social milieu in which they engage in physical activity. In fact, social forms of influence are important in shaping the physical activity motivation of individuals at all phases of the life span, but the type and nature of social influences varies with a person's age and developmental status (Brustad & Babkes, 2004). This chapter discusses three forms of social influence on the physical activity motivation and behavior of children and adolescents. The first form of influence is the role of significant others in affecting physical activity motivation. Socialization agents such as parents, siblings, and peers are highly important in shaping children's physical activity–related attitudes and behaviors, because children's initial experiences with virtually every form of physical play, from crawling, walking, and running to riding a bike, almost invariably take place in the presence of family members and friends. As children mature they are exposed to more structured forms of physical activity through school-based physical activity programs as well as through community-based recreational programs and organized sport programs. In such circumstances, additional significant adults, including teachers and coaches, are influential. Through each new physical activity experience, children are exposed to the attitudes, beliefs, and opinions communicated by these significant others and which give the activity unique meaning. Children may begin to like or dislike activities (e.g., running, swimming, or tennis), properties of physical activity (e.g., sweating or vigorous physical exertion), or characteristics of the physical activity experience (e.g., goal-based exercise, individual activity, or team sport) in accordance with the climate established by and the belief systems of significant others who have been involved in organizing and structuring the experience. The messages children receive from significant others about their competence in physical activity can also play an important role in their continued motivation.

A second form of social influence pertains to gender. A variety of gender-related factors may influence physical activity motivation and involvement. These factors include gender stereotypes and differences in opportunities available to children as a consequence of their gender. Although physical activity and sports in Western societies conform much less to gender stereotypes than ever before, gender-based images and stereotypes nonetheless continue to have an influence on youngsters' attraction to physical activities and the personal meanings that these activities hold for them (Eccles & Harold, 1991; Guillet, Sarrazin, Fontayne, & Brustad, 2006). Physical maturation does not occur at the same age or at the same rate for males and females, and the resultant interaction of gender and maturational status is likely to affect children's physical activity motivation and subsequent behavior.

A third form of social influence shaping children's physical activity motivation revolves around access to physical activity sites and opportunities. Research indicates that children and adolescents are more motivated to participate in physical activity when they perceive that physical activity opportunities are readily accessible to them. However, a considerable disparity in the accessibility of physical activity opportunities for youth arises as a consequence of familial socioeconomic status, family members' perceptions of neighborhood safety, parental opportunities to provide transportation, and the extent to which opportunities for physical activity are present for children after school (e.g., Beets, Beighle, Erwin, & Huberty, 2009; Duncan, Duncan, Strycker, & Chaumeton, 2002; Franzini et al., 2009; Gomez, Johnson, Selva, & Sallis, 2004). Since enhancing children's physical activity behavior is a primary reason for understanding children's physical activity motivation in the first place, it is imperative that we consider how we can enhance children's physical activity motivation by enabling and facilitating greater access to physical activity opportunities through schools, parks, recreational spaces, and the design of public transportation systems. In addition to these three primary forms of social influence on children's physical activity—significant others, gender, and access—there are other forms of influence, including the media, that have an ongoing effect on children's physical activity. It is important to recognize that social influence is a multifaceted and dynamic influence in rapidly changing Western societies.

A third general category of influence involves developmental change. Developmental change processes are related to physical activity motivation and behavior throughout the life span, but the magnitude and rapidity of this change during childhood and adolescence underscore the importance of closely considering the contribution of developmental change processes to children's physical activity motivation. *Development* refers to those sequential change processes that enable an individual to function more effectively. The physical, cognitive, emotional, and social development of children can each independently affect children's physical activity motivation. One of the most evident forms of developmental influence is the child's rate of physical maturation. An earlier-maturing child and a later-maturing child will differ in their capacity to perform a physical activity, which will in turn likely affect their continued motivation to pursue the activity. With regard to the role of cognitive development, children at younger ages do not have a mature understanding of the causes of performance outcomes or of the independent contributions of effort and ability to those outcomes. Through development change processes, children begin to adopt a more mature understanding of performance outcomes in physical activity that has implications for their continued motivation.

Given the breadth of influences that shape the physical activity motivation of youth, a broad and comprehensive perspective is needed. In the past, there has been a tendency for researchers to discuss and attempt to identify "determinants" of physical activity in youth, but the word *determinants* reflects limitations in the research paradigm that has driven much previous investigation. First, the term is problematic because it implies that single factors operate independently from other factors. It is more appropriate to consider physical activity motivation and

behavior in youth as emerging through the interaction of an array of social, psychological, and developmental influences that occur simultaneously and in concert rather than from the independent effect of any single variable. Second, the word *determinants* conveys the idea that children's physical activity motivation can be explained through a cause-and-effect relationship. This is problematic because the knowledge base has been generated largely from correlational studies rather than from longitudinal studies, so it is not appropriate to infer direct causal relationships between any two variables. A better term for describing seemingly influential variables would be *correlates*, given the complex patterns of relationships that may exist among physical activity related variables (Welk & Schaben, 2004).

The primary focus of this chapter is on the psychological factors that help to explain differences among children in their physical activity motivation. But as highlighted above, this is not to imply that only psychological variables are at play. A narrow and reductionist approach to understanding children's physical activity motivation does not serve us well, and problems with our approach and our terminological choices are at least partly responsible for limitations of our current knowledge base and resultant intervention approaches. Effective physical activity interventions cannot be generated unless we also consider the broader biosocial context within which youth physical activity occurs.

Theoretical Perspectives on Children's Physical Activity Motivation

The psychological and intrapersonal factors that underlie youth physical activity motivation have received considerable recent attention, fueled by concerns related to physical inactivity and obesity in youth. To effectively study motivational processes in any domain, it is necessary to use an appropriate theoretical perspective that provides a clearly defined and well-articulated framework for identifying patterns of influence among the key variables that make up the theory. Theoretical frameworks that have been applied to the study of children's physical activity motivation include Harter's (1978, 1981) competence motivation theory, Bandura's (1986, 2001) social cognitive theory, Ajzen's (1991) theory of planned behavior, Duda's (1992) achievement goal perspective as applied to sport, Eccles and colleagues' expectancy-value theory of achievement choice (Eccles et al., 1983; Eccles, Wigfield, & Schiefele, 1998), and Ryan and Deci's (2000) self-determination theory. Each theory was developed to explain motivational processes under given circumstances or in given contexts, but none was developed specifically for the study of children's physical activity motivation. Considerable overlap exists among the theories, and in order not to lose sight of the primary purpose of this chapter, only three theories will be discussed in further detail: competence motivation theory, expectancy-value theory, and self-determination theory. These theories will be presented and reviewed first, and the most relevant theoretically based research will be discussed in the subsequent section on essential psychological contributors to youth physical activity motivation.

Competence Motivation Theory

The developmental considerations of Harter's (1978, 1981) competence motivation theory make it highly relevant to the study of children's and adolescents' exercise and physical activity motivation, in which it has been a frequently employed conceptual perspective. The origins of Harter's theory can be found in White's (1959) model of "effectance motivation." White proposed that individuals have an inherent desire to have an effect on their environment, which leads them to engage in efforts to master various tasks or activities. Although such a perspective seems quite logical today, White's theory emerged in response to more simplistic stimulus–response explanations of human motivation that accompanied the behaviorist legacy in psychology. From the behaviorist perspective, human motivation was generally considered to be the result of extrinsic and environmental forces acting on the individual rather than a consequence of internally generated drives or motives. In White's conceptualization, "effectance motivation" corresponds to an intrinsically satisfying experience whose expression is not dependent on extrinsic forces or rewards.

Harter's competence motivation theory arose out of a desire to explain why children might have the interest and desire to engage in various types of activities or pursue various challenges or, conversely, to avoid these types of activities and challenges. According to Harter, two fundamental psychological contributors to motivation are perceived competence and perceived control: When children feel that they are competent and perceive that they have sufficient control over their environmental circumstances, they are more likely to want to attempt to master corresponding activities or challenges. As Harter noted, children's perceptions of

competence and control do not emerge in a social vacuum but are shaped by significant others, particularly parents. Parents can strengthen or reinforce children's initial attempts at mastery by encouraging the mastery effort itself as opposed to responding to the quality of the product of these mastery attempts. Thus parents can stimulate efforts at mastery through appropriate encouragement and praise or can squelch such efforts by failing to provide support or encouragement for them. In addition, Harter's theory places great emphasis on the role of children's affective experiences as they engage in mastery efforts. Harter was one of the first modern-day motivational theorists to recognize that positive affect and intrinsic pleasure are important outcomes that typically accompany intrinsic motivation. As such, when children or adolescents have favorable perceptions of their competence and control, they are more likely to select intrinsically motivating and optimally challenging activities that have the potential to result in positive affective outcomes such as enjoyment, pride, pleasure, and satisfaction. Conversely, individuals who lack the requisite perceived competence and control are unlikely to have the intrinsic desire to engage in challenging tasks or activities and may even avidly avoid such activities. Competence motivation theory was intended to explain children's motivational orientations across a broad array of contexts and is certainly suitable for application to the study of children's physical activity motivation and behavior.

Expectancy-Value Theory

A second important theory applicable to the study of children's physical activity motivation is Eccles's expectancy-value model (Eccles, 1993; Eccles et al., 1983, 1998). This theoretical model attempts to explain children's motivation across a variety of achievement-related and free-choice contexts and places emphasis on the effect of parental socialization practices on children's motivational characteristics. Eccles's model has many similarities with Harter's in that within each model, children's perceptions of their competence are considered to be fundamentally important in shaping motivation. Eccles and colleagues use the terms *expectations of success* and *success expectancies* to represent children's beliefs that they have the competence necessary to attain success in a given area of achievement. However, Eccles and colleagues also propose that in addition to differing in perceived competence, children differ in the extent to which they value various activities. A child may perceive that being good at physical activity and sport has more value than being good at music even though the child has similarly favorable perceptions of competence for both activities. Differences in perceptions of task value for different activities may be due to perceptions about activities' attainment value ("being good at sport will open more doors for me than being good at music"), intrinsic value ("physical activity is more interesting than other activities"), utility value ("physical activity will help me live a healthy life"), and costs (in terms of time, loss of other opportunities or economic factors).

Expectancy-value theory is similar to Harter's theory in that parents are considered to be highly important socialization agents whose influence includes shaping children's expectancies of success as well as their perceptions of task value. Eccles and colleagues propose that parents have three primary roles in shaping children's success expectancies and task values, whether in physical activity and sport or in any other activity context (see Fredricks & Eccles, 2004). One important role that parents have involves the parental tendency to provide greater opportunity and encouragement for children in those activities in which parents perceive that the child has the greatest aptitude or potential for success. That is, parents enable and facilitate different types of opportunities for children in accordance with parents' own perceptions of the child's unique abilities. Even within the same family, different children are likely to receive different sets of experiences and opportunities in accordance with their parents' perceptions of their interests and aptitudes. The compilation of opportunities will eventually result in greater actual competence and so contribute to a self-fulfilling prophecy whereby children do very well at the very activity that their parents perceived them as most suited to.

The second important role of parents in expectancy-value theory is as "interpreters" of the achievement outcomes of the child's involvement in a given activity. Since children have limited experience with novel activities, they are prone to look to adults for feedback to help them to interpret the causes of outcomes. The parent may convey the idea that the child was successful or unsuccessful and that the outcome was attributable to natural aptitude or to a lack thereof. This feedback will affect children's own appraisals of their abilities and their expectancies for future success.

Third, through observing their parents' own behaviors children see that their parents are more prone to pursue certain possible areas of interest (e.g., physical activity) than others (e.g., music). These observations allow children to make inferences about the relative task value of each activity choice. This form of social influence has commonalities with Bandura's (1986, 2001) social cognitive theory.

A considerable amount of research has been conducted using expectancy-value theory. The bulk of this research supports the contentions that parental behaviors influence children's success expectancies and perceived task value and that these in turn influence children's own motivation to engage in various activities. Academic research supports the view that parents' perceptions of their children's abilities significantly predict children's own perceived abilities and subject matter interests even when the children's actual abilities are controlled for using standardized test scores (Frome & Eccles, 1998; Parsons, Adler, & Kaczala, 1982). In the youth sport setting, a well-supported component of the model has been the relationship between parental expectancies of their children's abilities and the children's own ability appraisals, in that children and their parents tend to hold very similar perceptions of the children's abilities (Babkes & Weiss, 1999; Bois, Sarrazin, Brustad, Trouilloud, & Cury, 2002; Eccles & Harold, 1991).

Developmental considerations are also relevant to Eccles's theory. These considerations have an important but perhaps underappreciated role in affecting children's success expectancies (Weiss & Amorose, 2008). As a consequence of cognitive development, children become more accurate in appraising their own abilities, because they become more effective at using and interpreting the information they gain through sources such as comparison with peers. However, a common consequence of their greater accuracy is that youngsters show a diminished perception of their expectancies of success with age and development (Fredricks & Eccles, 2002), and so motivation is likely to diminish with age. Eccles and colleagues found that children's beliefs about their competence in sport decreased over three years in a sample of elementary school children and this decrease was considered to be at least partially attributable to cognitive development (Rodriguez, Wigfield, & Eccles, 2003).

Self-Determination Theory

A third contemporary perspective that is relevant to the study of children's physical activity motivation is provided by self-determination theory (Ryan & Deci, 2000). Self-determination theory is a widely used theory of motivation with a primary focus on explaining the variability among people in the type of motivation that they display in various contexts. According to self-determination theory, there are three broad categories of motivation: amotivation, extrinsic motivation, and intrinsic motivation. *Amotivation* refers to a state where a person completely lacks motivation to participate in the activity and thus reflects the condition whereby a person simply does not have motivation to be involved in an area of possible interest, such as physical activity.

Extrinsic motivation is said to be present when individuals do have motivation but their motivation does not arise from personal interest or choice. Within self-determination theory there are four types of extrinsic motivation, which differ in their degree of relative autonomy. Starting from the least autonomous and proceeding to increasingly more autonomous forms of regulation, *external regulation* is present when an individual engages in physical activity solely to receive a reward or to avoid receiving a punishment. External regulation might occur in a physical education class in which grades are used to stimulate motivation. Although an individual might be motivated in such an instance, the motivational expression is not optimal because it is merely the result of an external demand ("I have to"). A second form of extrinsic motivation is *introjected regulation,* whereby the person engages in physical activity to avoid feeling guilty about not being active. For example, individuals may feel that they are letting someone down if they fail to participate, so they maintain their involvement even though the activity is not inherently satisfying or enjoyable to them. A third type of extrinsic motivation is *identified regulation,* in which individuals engage in physical activity because they believe that it will be good for their health in the present or future. Identified regulation reflects a greater sense of personal control over the activity than external or introjected regulation but is still considered to be extrinsic because the motive for participation does not reflect the intrinsic motives of enjoyment and personal challenge satisfaction. The fourth category of extrinsic motivation is *integrated regulation*, in which individuals are motivated to engage in physical activity to maintain consistency with their self-image.

Intrinsic motivation represents a state where individuals are involved of their own free choice. According to self-determination theorists, intrinsic motivation occurs when individuals feel competent and autonomous and have favorable feelings of relatedness with others. When individuals experience these three psychological characteristics—competence, autonomy, and relatedness—they are much more prone to engage in intrinsically motivating activities that are accompanied by positive experiences of enjoyment, interest, and challenge. In turn, the positive affect experienced during the intrinsically motivating experience should propel continued intrinsic motivation.

Our purpose and goal in promoting physical activity for youth should be to foster intrinsic motivation. Many types of extrinsic motivation can be fostered, but extrinsic motives for physical activity are unlikely to be sustained for any length of time. Physical activity will be most beneficial to psychological, social, and physical health when it is a lifestyle behavior rather than a short-term, sporadic, or intermittent activity. When extrinsic motives drive physical activity, continued involvement is dependent on the presence of extrinsic factors; in their absence, physical activity will not be maintained because individuals will no longer choose to pursue their involvement. Although much discussion surrounds the need to increase physical activity among young people, it is essential to recognize that practices that increase physical activity involvement without a corresponding increase in intrinsic motivation and enjoyment are unproductive in the long term.

The three theoretical perspectives on motivation presented here share many commonalities and are much more similar than they are different. Each theory places emphasis on social influence either through parental socialization practices or through the motivational benefits associated with feelings of relatedness. Competence motivation theory underscores the importance of positive affect in driving intrinsic forms of motivation, and self-determination theory similarly emphasizes that intrinsic motivation is accompanied by a desirable emotional state. Perceptions of control or autonomy are central components of both competence motivation theory and self-determination theory, and developmental factors that can affect motivation through childhood and adolescence are likewise addressed by both those theories.

Out of this discussion of contemporary theoretical perspectives, four key psychological variables emerge that are most relevant to our understanding of children's physical activity motivation and will be used to frame our discussion. The first key variable will be labeled *perceived competence* and reflects the perceived competence variable from competence motivation theory and self-determination theory as well as success expectancies from expectancy-value theory. A second key variable is *autonomy/perceived control*, which reflects those feelings of personal control that have been deemed important in competence motivation theory and self-determination theory. A third essential psychological variable pertains to *affective experiences*, which include the positive emotional experiences of enjoyment, fun, pride, satisfaction, pleasure, and interest that are essential to the expression of intrinsic motivation from the standpoint of competence motivation theory and self-determination theory. The fourth key variable will be labeled *social relationships* and refers to the nature and quality of young people's social relationships in the context of physical activity, particularly their relationships with parents and other adults, such as teachers and coaches, as well as with peers. Social relationships are central to motivational processes in all three theories.

Essential Psychological Contributors to Children's Physical Activity Motivation
Perceived Competence

Favorable self-perceptions of competence are widely regarded as essential components of any individual's desire to be physically active, whether child, adolescent or adult. Children's perceptions of their competence have been regarded as fundamental precursors to their physical activity motivation because these perceptions reflect the individual's response to the question of "Am I able?" (Fredricks & Eccles, 2004; Welk, 1999). Extensive research has been conducted on the role of competence-related beliefs in affecting physical activity motivation; our discussion will center on some of the more important and innovative recent studies in this area.

Wang and Biddle (2001) used a cluster analytic procedure to examine the motivational characteristics and physical activity behaviors of 12- to 15-year-old youth, with the expressed purpose of identifying distinct motivational profiles that characterized young people's orientations toward physical activity. Wang and Biddle included key variables from primary motivational theories and identified five distinct clusters or patterns that were reflective of physical activity orientations of subgroups within the larger sample of participants. The two clusters with the most favorable physical activity profiles were labeled the "self-determined" and "highly motivated" groups. Two variables that distinguished these clusters were that these individuals had substantially

higher levels of perceived competence and feelings of relative autonomy for physical activity than individuals in the less physically active subgroups. The "poorly motivated" and "amotivated" clusters had low levels of perceived competence, with the "amotivated" group demonstrating quite low levels of autonomy as well. This research is supportive of the view that differences in perceived competence (and autonomy/perceived control) underlie many of the notable differences that we see among adolescents in their motivation to be physically active as well as in their actual physical activity involvement.

In a unique line of research, Welk and Schnaben (2004) conducted a study with a sample of 18 children, ages 10–12 years, who were participants at a summer fitness camp. The researchers examined differences in physical activity motivation and physical activity that were present even though each child had an equal opportunity to be physically active over the course of the camp day. Since children's physical activity is normally affected by many constraints that are outside of their control, such as limited access to parks and recreational spaces, parental work and transportation demands, and length of their school day, Welk and Schnaben considered it worthwhile to examine the physical activity practices of youth in a social environment where all youth had similar physical activity opportunities. Accelerometers were used to provide an objective measure of daily physical activity. Perceived athletic competence was consistently linked to the individuals' actual physical activity behavior, with correlations ranging from .57 to .69 for each of the three weeks of the study. These findings are important, in that virtually no previous knowledge had existed about the relative strength of predictors of physical activity when children have equal opportunity to be physically active. However, the findings from the study are limited by the relatively low number of participants and the fact that youth were only assessed in one setting.

Welk and Eklund (2005) examined relationships of children's perceptions of competence and physical self-perceptions to their actual fitness levels as measured by the Fitnessgram test (Cooper Institute for Aerobics Research, 1999) as well as by individuals' self-reported physical activity characteristics. Part of the purpose of the study was to validate the Children and Youth Physical Self-Perceptions Profile, which contains distinct self-perception dimensions across the areas of perceived sports competence, physical conditioning, body attractiveness, and physical strength. Participants in the study were 754 children of ages 8–12 years from predominantly middle-class families. Results indicated that favorable self-perceptions along each of the four physical self-perception domains were associated with higher levels of physical activity and physical fitness, supporting the expectation that children distinguish between these physical self-perception dimensions and that their physical self-perceptions are important contributors to physical activity involvement.

Shen, McCaughtry, and Martin (2007) found a significant relationship between perceived competence in physical education classes and the leisure-time physical activity behavior of older children and adolescents. Participants in their study were 653 youngsters ranging in age from 11 to 15 years (M = 12.4 years) enrolled in middle schools in a large inner-city school district. Almost all students were from low to lower-middle socioeconomic backgrounds. The study's findings indicated that perceptions of competence (and autonomy) influenced intentions to participate in physical activity via the mediating influence of attitudes, subjective norms, and behavioral control. Thus children's perceptions of competence were identified as an important precursor to physical activity motivation, although other psychological (attitudes) and social (subjective norms and behavioral control) factors exerted a mediating influence on the expression of motivation. The study's findings also revealed that children's perceptions of physical competence in one physical activity context (physical education classes) contributed to physical activity motivation in another physical activity context (leisure-time physical activity practices).

Perceived physical competence also seems to be an important contributor to positive affective experiences and feelings of fun in physical activity. Recent research by Humbert et al. (2008) used focus group protocols to help identify contributors to positive affective experiences and fun as experienced by youth in physical activity settings. Participants were 160 young people of ages 12–18 years. Age-related trends were apparent in the findings in that many factors contributed to self-reported fun at younger ages but that by grade 7 youngsters reported that having confidence and perceiving that they were competent were essential contributors to "fun." These youth reported that they experienced fun when they felt competent and confident in the activity of interest, felt secure that they would not experience negative forms of social interaction with peers, and felt that they would not be made to feel that they didn't "fit in" or "be made fun of" while engaged in the activity.

Barnett, Morgan, van Beurden, and Beard (2008) conducted an interesting longitudinal investigation of the role of physical competence in physical activity and fitness. These authors initially assessed the motor skill proficiency of 929 Australian children of ages 7.9–11.9 years. Six years later, they were able to contact roughly half of the original sample, who provided follow-up information on their physical activity characteristics. Results indicated that perceived sport competence during adolescence mediated the relationship between childhood motor skill proficiency and physical activity levels during adolescence.

A variable that is highly related to perceived competence is self-efficacy, which constitutes a key component of Bandura's (1986, 2001) social cognitive theory of motivation. Self-efficacy reflects the extent to which individuals believe that they can accomplish a specific task of personal importance and thus reflects both their beliefs about their competence and their feelings of personal control relative to completing the task. In a unique study that used a prospective design, Trost et al. (1997) examined children's physical activity–related beliefs and attitudes during the fifth-grade school year and then collected data about actual physical activity levels during the subsequent year. The researchers were primarily interested in examining how the self-efficacy beliefs of these young people would affect the likelihood that they would engage in moderate-to-vigorous or vigorous physical activity as identified through self-reports. Their results indicated that self-efficacy for overcoming barriers to physical activity was a significant predictor of moderate-to-vigorous and vigorous physical activity for the girls in this sample. For the boys, self-efficacy for overcoming barriers to physical activity was related to the likelihood of their participation in vigorous physical activity.

In their review of intervention studies that were conducted with the intent of enhancing physical activity in youth, Lubans, Foster, and Biddle (2008) found good support for the idea that self-efficacy is an important mediating variable that influences the effectiveness of physical activity interventions on subsequent physical activity behavior. In other words, physical activity interventions are more likely to be successful to the extent that they strengthen participants' physical self-efficacy beliefs, as these in turn affect actual physical activity behavior.

The review presented here constitutes just a brief summary of research on the effect of perceived competence beliefs on physical activity motivation and behavior. This research clearly strongly supports the theoretical expectation that self-related perceptions of competence are important contributors to the physical activity motivation of children and adolescents.

Autonomy/Perceived Control

A second important category of influence on motivation involves children's feelings of autonomy and perceived control over their physical activity involvement. Autonomy, which literally means "regulation by the self," reflects an underlying belief that one has free will and choice (Ryan & Deci, 2006). Autonomy is increasingly recognized as an important contributor to intrinsic motivation (see Ryan & Deci, 2006, for a more extensive review), but the variable of autonomy also is important because of developmental considerations. During later childhood and into adolescence, the desire for autonomy becomes an increasingly salient and important dimension of functioning for most young people (Erikson, 1968); thus autonomy should logically be important to youngsters' motivation in the physical domain as in other domains of life. Simply put, older children and adolescents are unlikely to be highly motivated to participate in any interest area if they have little input or perceive themselves as having little control over their involvement. Autonomy, while regarded as a psychological variable, is one that is strongly shaped by social dimensions and constraints, because the child's perception of autonomy is inherently linked to the amount and types of choices that are encouraged or permitted by significant others such as parents, teachers, and coaches.

A rapidly growing body of knowledge has emerged on the importance of autonomy in sport and physical activity motivation. One of the more important research questions in this area focuses on why children and adolescents desire to persist in or drop out of sport (Partridge, Brustad, & Babkes Stellino, 2008). Research by Coakley and White (1992) indicated that a primary contributor to adolescents' desire to discontinue their sport participation was the feeling that they lacked control over their involvement. Similarly, Raedeke (1997) concluded that feelings of limited control over their involvement were important contributors to adolescents' feelings of entrapment and burnout in competitive sport. In a four-week diary study of 33 female gymnasts with a mean age of 13.0 years, Gagne, Ryan, and Bargmann (2003) found that parent and coach support for autonomy was associated with a more favorable motivational profile, including greater intrinsic motivation. The sport-based research indicates that autonomy support is an essential contributor to intrinsic motivation and that a lack of perceived control or autonomy is associated with amotivation and the desire to discontinue sport participation.

More recently, researchers have begun to examine the role of autonomy perceptions in influencing motivation in the physical education setting and the broader physical activity context in an attempt to build on the existing knowledge base. The physical education environment is a social context that is amenable to autonomy supportive strategies, since most school-age youth receive some form of physical education instruction and one of the primary goals of such instruction should be to stimulate a lifelong interest in maintaining a physically active lifestyle. In addition, physical education instruction commonly introduces youth to novel physical activities, and the skills, knowledge, and attitudes that result from these initial experiences should affect their desire to pursue such activities in their free time. A physical education context can be considered autonomy supportive to the extent that it enables and encourages student choice about the physical activities in which students engage and allows them input and choice about the characteristics or qualities of their activity involvement (e.g., intensity levels, competitive vs. noncompetitive focus, or individual vs. group-based activities). An autonomy supportive environment thus stands at the opposite end of the continuum from a more traditional autocratic or controlling environment.

One of the initial explorations into understanding intrinsic vs. extrinsic motivational orientations in the physical education setting was conducted in England by Goudas, Biddle, Fox, and Underwood (1995). This study contrasted the effects of a direct or command style of teaching (Mosston & Ashworth, 1986) in which the physical education teacher makes all of the decisions with those of a more differentiated or inclusive teaching style that allows student choice. One girls' physical education class was taught track and field activities for a 10 weeks, with each lesson being taught with either the command or the inclusive teaching style. At the end of each lesson, the girls completed measures of intrinsic motivation and task involvement; additional interviews were conducted with eight of the study participants. Results revealed that the inclusive teaching style, in comparison to the command style of teaching, resulted in greater intrinsic motivation and task goal involvement which refers to the tendency to use self-referenced criteria of success rather than social comparison criteria for success. In addition, and irrespective of teaching style during a given lesson, those students with higher levels of competence, autonomy, and task orientation had higher levels of intrinsic motivation at all points during the course.

Hagger, Chatzisarantis, Culverhouse, and Biddle (2003) conducted an important study that examined the role of perceived autonomy support in the physical education context. They proposed a transcontextual model of physical activity according to which perceived autonomy support in the physical education context was anticipated to affect young people's perceptions of control, physical activity intentions, and actual physical activity behavior in leisure-time settings. A sample of 295 male and female adolescents with a mean age of 14.5 years completed instruments assessing key motivational constructs from both self-determination theory and the theory of planned behavior (Ajzen, 1991). Measures specific to autonomy support and motivation in physical education classes were completed first, and leisure-time physical activity intentions were assessed one week and six weeks later. The results indicated that perceived autonomy support in the physical education context was directly linked to greater intrinsically motivated behavior in the physical education setting, which in turn was associated with a more intrinsic motivational orientation in leisure-time settings as well as a more generally favorable sense of personal control over physical activity involvement. More positive attitudes and feelings of behavioral control contributed to stronger intentions to be physically active and to greater actual involvement in physical activity among the participants in this study. A direct effect of perceived autonomy support in physical education was also found on physical activity behavior six weeks later, which supports the belief that the characteristics of the physical education environment are important to the maintenance of desirable physical activity behaviors.

In a similar vein, Pangrazi, Beighle, Vehige, and Vack (2003) examined the effects of an elementary school–based program called PLAY (Promoting Lifestyle Activity for Youth) that was intended to enhance the physical activity practices and lifestyle behaviors of the participants. The program was designed to encourage self-directed and enjoyable physical activities by children and to allow children the opportunity to choose their own level of intensity in various physical activities. Results revealed that children who participated in the intervention group had greater resultant physical activity levels (as determined by pedometer-assessed daily step counts) than those in a control group and that that the benefits of autonomy-promoting and enjoyable physical experiences were particularly noteworthy for the girls in the study.

An expanding body of knowledge is coming from direct tests of self-determination theory in the physical education setting. Two studies representative of this knowledge base were conducted by Ntoumanis (2005) and by Standage, Duda, and Ntoumanis (2005). In the first study, Ntoumanis (2005) examined whether feelings of self-determination predicted more favorable psychological and motivational profiles in physical education settings for British adolescents. He found that students' perceptions of autonomy, competence, and relatedness in physical education classes were related to their feelings of self-determined motivation and to desirable affective, cognitive, and behavioral outcomes, including stronger intentions to participate in optional physical education classes during the following school year.

Standage and colleagues (2005) tested the central hypotheses of self-determination theory with 950 secondary school students in England with a mean age of 12.1 years. It was hypothesized that students' perceptions of autonomy support, competence support, and relatedness support in the physical education setting would predict their feelings of need satisfaction and resultant motivation (intrinsic motivation, extrinsic motivation, or amotivation), which, in turn would explain adaptive or maladaptive outcomes in physical education, such as positive or negative affect, degree of concentration, and interest and task challenge. The results provided support for these expectations: Satisfaction of competence, autonomy, and relatedness needs was significantly associated with students' intrinsic motivation, which in turn was associated with favorable and adaptive outcomes in physical education classes, including positive affect, good concentration, and the preference to attempt challenging tasks These findings were consistent across gender.

More recent research by Cox, Smith, and Williams (2008) examined patterns of relationships between motivational characteristics of students in physical education classes and the students' own leisure-time physical activity behaviors. Participants were sixth- and seventh-grade students from five middle schools. Results of the study revealed that students' perceptions of competence, autonomy, and relatedness, their enjoyment of physical activity, their self-determined motivation in physical education, and the amount of physical activity the students engaged in while in the physical education setting were predictive of their leisure-time physical activity behavior. The researchers concluded that a more adaptive form of motivation, as represented by self-determined motivation, results in the transfer of positive physical activity orientations from the physical education setting to other contexts.

In the previously discussed study by Humbert and colleagues (2008) on sources of physical activity enjoyment in adolescents, students indicated that physical activity would be "more fun" if they were allowed to have more influence and control over the rules and structures of the games that they participated in within the school environment. In this sense, feelings of autonomy not only seem to be associated with cognitions about who has control over physical activity involvement but also appear to directly influence the affective properties of the physical activity experience.

Research in physical education contexts about the importance of autonomy support has yielded some important findings. First, these results highlight the importance of autonomy to young people's physical activity motivation and behavior and strongly suggest that intervention efforts intended to promote physical activity involvement in youth should include strategies that facilitate autonomy. Physical education environments vary in the extent to which they give students choice, and students who have their self-determination needs stymied in physical education settings may never fully develop interests in and enjoyment of physical activity. A second important finding from this research is that autonomy supportive experiences seem to transcend their original physical activity contexts. It is thus important to recognize that when young people perceive autonomy support in the physical education context, these experiences transfer to physical activity attitudes, orientations, and behaviors in the leisure-time setting.

Affective Experiences

It seems intuitive that when individuals have positive affective experiences in physical activity, they are more likely to want to maintain their physical activity involvement. As Dishman and colleagues (2005) have argued, enjoyment is an important proximal influence on physical activity involvement that precedes cognitive appraisals of physical activity. In this way, enjoyment of physical activity (or the lack thereof) has an immediate and powerful gut-level effect on young people's motivation to be involved in physical activity. Whereas children's perceptions of their competence relate directly to the question "Can I do it?" their customary affective responses to physical activity provide an answer to the question, "Do I want to do it?" (Welk, 1999). A variety of positive affective experiences can accompany physical activity, including enjoyment, fun, pride, pleasure, and satisfaction. That most physical activity occurs in public settings also means that there is considerable opportunity for youth to experience negative affect as a consequence of feelings of embarrassment that can result from individuals' perceptions of low competence.

Prospective studies have highlighted the importance of children's physical activity enjoyment for their physical activity involvement at a later date. For instance, Trost et al. (1997) assessed various psychological considerations in relation to physical activity in fifth-grade children and then examined levels of vigorous and moderately vigorous physical activity one year later. Their results indicated that for the girls, enjoyment of school physical education was a predictor of physical activity behavior one year later. In similar research, DiLorenzo, Stucky-Ropp, Vander Wal, & Gotham (1998) interviewed older elementary school children in relation to their orientations toward physical activity and then used the same protocol three years later. Results from this study revealed not only that physical activity enjoyment and physical activity involvement were related in the present, but also that for girls enjoyment of physical activity was a significant longitudinal predictor of physical activity involvement three years later.

To gain a better appreciation for the contribution of affect to children's physical activity motivation, it would seem to be beneficial to first identify those properties or characteristics of physical activity that young people regard as enjoyable as well as those qualities of physical activity that children perceive to be undesirable. Some of the initial research in this area involved inductive efforts using small-group and individual interviews to gain elementary school children's perspectives on factors that contributed to their liking or disliking physical activity (Brustad, 1993). This process resulted in the recognition that there are clear individual differences among children in the properties that attract them to or repel them from physical activity. Four general categories of salient physical activity characteristics were identified using this approach that affect young people's interest (or disinterest) in physical activity involvement. One important dimension relates to the physical sensations that accompany the physical activity experience, including sweating, breathing hard, and exerting oneself. Many youth perceive these symptoms of physical exertion to be enjoyable sensations, but others do not. This dimension of physical exertion was found to extend across two distinct contexts, as children make a distinction between exertion in physical activity in general and exertion in contexts that involve more structured, goal-directed, and vigorous forms of physical activity (e.g., physical education class). A second salient affective characteristic of the physical activity experience relates to youngsters' feelings about the social relationships that they encounter in the physical activity environment. For many children, involvement in physical activity results in positive relationships with peers, whereas for many other children the physical activity experience results in negative experiences due to poor interactions with others. This dimension is important because children are in the process of establishing peer groups and friendships and their experiences in physical activity and sport may have important implications for forming and maintaining these social bonds. A third salient dimension of the physical activity experience involves children's like or dislike of competitive games and activities. For many children, particularly children with low perceived competence, competitive games and activities are unattractive because their skills may compare poorly with those of their peers and a competitive emphasis will further magnify their limitations. Finally, children differ in their attraction to physical activity in relation to their perceptions of the importance of physical activity to their health. Many children develop an attraction to physical activity because they realize it is inherently beneficial to physical health, but this element of attraction is not present for all. Out of this research, the Children's Attraction to Physical Activity (CAPA) scale was developed (Brustad, 1993). The CAPA scale reflects each of these four dimensions of physical activity attraction but contains five subscales in all, because separate subscales refer to the liking of physical exertion dimension of physical activity in general physical activity and in contexts structured specifically for exercise. Recent research supports the validity of this measure of attraction for children as young as six years old (Rose, Larkin, Hands, Howard, & Parker, 2009).

Research indicates that children who have greater perceived competence in physical activity are likely to have a stronger attraction to physical activity. In a study involving elementary school children with a mean age of 10.4 years, Brustad (1993) found through path analysis that children's perceptions of competence contributed substantially to their overall level of attraction to physical activity. Related research conducted by Paxton, Estabrooks, and Dzewaltowski (2004) with children ranging in age from 9 to 14 years revealed that perceived competence predicted attraction to physical activity, which mediated the relationship between perceived competence and physical activity involvement. This research highlights the important roles of perceived competence and attraction to physical activity in explaining physical activity behavior of children and adolescents, suggesting that greater perceived competence will lead to stronger attraction to physical activity, which in turn will result in greater physical activity involvement.

Understanding psychosocial correlates of structured physical activity for girls was the focus of research conducted by Barr-Anderson et al. (2007), who devoted specific attention to the role of affective properties of the experience. These researchers considered structured physical activity to be those forms of sport and physical activity that are formally organized. Participants in their study were 2,791 sixth-grade girls from six geographical locations, who provided self-reports of their structured physical activity and sport involvement. Results indicated that girls who experienced greater enjoyment in their physical education classes were more likely to participate in structured forms of physical activity such as basketball, cheerleading and dance, and swimming.

Intervention research has provided further support for the importance of physical activity enjoyment as a fundamental contributor to physical activity motivation and involvement. A school-based study conducted by Dishman and colleagues (2005) revealed that enjoyment of physical activity and physical activity self-efficacy were predictive of actual physical activity among a sample of female high school students. Dishman et al. developed an intervention program that had the goals of increasing student enjoyment and autonomy in physical activity and that was designed to be sensitive to activity preferences related to gender. This intervention resulted in increased physical activity levels among the students involved in the program, whereas a control group of students that did not receive the intervention showed no such increases.

In a recent study in Australia, researchers sought to increase the physical activity enjoyment of adolescent girls who were from linguistically diverse and predominantly low-income backgrounds (Dudley, Okely, Pearson, & Peat, 2010). This group was targeted because girls from these backgrounds are prone to experience substantial declines in their physical activity involvement as they move into adolescence, and proactive intervention efforts could result in their maintaining a more physically active lifestyle. Through their participation in focus groups, participants had the opportunity to identify the types of physical activities that they found to be enjoyable, and activities such as yoga, Pilates, tennis, aquatic activities, and dance were included in the experimental condition for the subsequent intervention. Students who had been randomly assigned to the intervention group showed positive change in their level of physical activity involvement in comparison with control group members, indicating that self-selected and enjoyable activities contribute to greater physical activity involvement for youth.

In sum, our present body of knowledge indicates that youngsters' experiences of positive affect in physical activity contribute to greater physical activity motivation and involvement. Although these findings are hardly surprising, the consistency with which physical activity attraction and enjoyment have been linked to actual physical activity behavior suggests that concerted efforts should be made to facilitate positive emotional experiences with physical activity and that youth should be given an active role in the design of those experiences.

Social Relationships

Social relationships are important to humans throughout the life span and can have favorable or unfavorable effects on individuals' mental and physical health, on their motivation, and on their behavior (see Baumeister & Leary, 1995 for an extensive review). The nature and quality of individuals' social relationships in the physical activity context during childhood and adolescence may have lasting effects on their physical activity motivation and behavior, because youngsters are establishing dispositions toward physical activity during those early years (Partridge et al., 2008). Relationships with parents, siblings, peers, friends, teachers and coaches can all be influential in that process.

The three primary theoretical orientations addressed in this chapter all place extensive focus on the nature of social relationships. Within both competence motivation theory and self-determination theory, an individual's intrinsic motivation is considered to be in part the by-product of favorable patterns of social relationships—such as positive parental socialization practices or strong feelings of connectedness with others—that stimulate an interest in challenging and enjoyable activities. Expectancy-value theory takes a somewhat different tack but provides a framework from which we can understand how young people are motivated to pursue certain activities as a consequence of the value that those activities hold for them and the competence that they feel in the activities, which result from parental socialization practices. Important social agents in the youth physical activity environment include friends and peers, parents, siblings, and teachers and coaches. This section will focus first on the contribution of parents to youth physical activity motivation and then on the effect of similar others—peers and friends—on young people's motivation.

PARENTAL INFLUENCE

The influence of parents in shaping their children's physical activity involvement seems indisputable. Children almost invariably learn to ride a bike, to throw a ball, and to swim in the presence of their parents. Parents assume many important roles in the socialization process, because they commonly introduce children to various physical activities and sports and they also serve as important physical activity role models. Furthermore, parents serve as "gatekeepers" for their children's physical activity, because children rarely have the autonomy to make independent decisions about whether they can engage in vigorous physical activity or play outside, and the type and level of support that parents give their child in the physical activity context play an important role in enabling the child's involvement. Parents also help children interpret, or "make sense of," their physical activity experiences and thus shape children's understanding of their capacities in physical activity as well as their perceptions of the value of the experience. Although it has been traditional to regard the parent–child socialization process as unidirectional, it is more appropriate to view it as a bidirectional process in which children's aptitudes and interests also shape their parents' physical activity interests and practices through an ongoing and reciprocal process (Brustad, 1992; Dorsch, Smith, & McDonough, 2009).

There is a growing body of knowledge on parental influence on children's physical activity, but little of this research has considered the role of children's motivational characteristics in mediating the process. Research has also been conducted from diverse perspectives, some of which lack a clear theoretical orientation, and this makes straightforward conclusions problematic (for a more thorough review, see Gustafson & Rhodes, 2006). Much of the theoretically based research on parental influence on youth physical activity and sport motivation has been designed according to an expectancy-value theoretical framework. In an initial study on youth sport involvement, Eccles and Harold (1991) used a longitudinal design and found that parents' perceptions of their children's sport competence predicted children's own perceived sport competence and their subsequent motivation to participate in sports, a result that was consistent with the central tenets of expectancy-value theory.

In a study that examined parental influence on youth soccer players' motivation, Babkes and Weiss (1999) examined parental practices and children's perceptions of their competence as well as their enjoyment and intrinsic versus extrinsic motivational orientation in soccer. Participants were 9- to 11-year-old male soccer players in a "select" soccer program, and children completed instruments referring to both their mother's and father's soccer-related beliefs and practices. Results revealed that children who believed that their parents held more favorable beliefs about their competence and who received more frequent and contingent responses to their soccer involvement from their parents had more favorable perceptions of their own soccer competence as well as higher levels of intrinsic motivation to participate in soccer than did their peers who reported less favorable perceptions of parental involvement.

In research that examined different forms of parental influence, Brustad (1996) assessed how various parental physical activity socialization practices contributed to the explanation of differences in children's perceptions of physical competence and their attraction to physical activity. Participants were 107 fourth- through sixth-grade children from families of lower socioeconomic status, a population that has been underrepresented in the knowledge base. Results indicated that parental enjoyment of physical activity and parental encouragement of their children's physical activity were associated with

greater perceived physical competence and attraction to physical activity in the children. Gender differences were also identified: Boys liked the exertional properties of physical activity and exercise significantly more than did girls. Parental modeling of physical activity did not help to explain differences among children in their perceptions of competence in physical activity or in their levels of attraction to physical activity.

In a study conducted in France, researchers found that a relationship existed between mothers' perceptions of their children's physical competence and the children's own perceived competence one year later even after controlling for the children's initial perceived competence and actual ability (Bois, Sarrazin, Brustad, Trouilloud, & Cury, 2002). The changes in the children's perceived competence were thus considered to be largely attributable to parental beliefs. This research provided additional support for the theoretically based expectation that parental beliefs are instrumental in shaping children's physical activity–related self-perceptions.

A body of knowledge regarding parental influence in physical activity also exists that did not come from an expectancy-value theoretical perspective. Anderssen and Wold (1992) obtained self-reported leisure-time physical activity data from 904 Norwegian students with a mean age of 13.3 years. In addition, students' reports on parents' and peers' physical activity and on parental and peer support for physical activity were obtained on a separate occasion. Results indicated that parental and peer physical activity levels and parental and peer physical activity support were each significantly related to the level of physical activity involvement of these young adolescents.

Parents assume many other important roles that affect children's motivation to be physically active and their actual opportunities to be physically active. As a consequence of recent societal trends, one of the most important roles that parents assume is as providers of, or gatekeepers to, children's physical activity experiences. This role is infrequently recognized in the public discourse about children's physical activity and inactivity, but parental safety concerns directly affect children's physical activity opportunities in the outdoors (Carver, Timperio, & Crawford, 2008), where children typically receive a substantial amount of their physical activity (Mackett & Paskins, 2008). It has been argued that in recent years children's physical activity and play have become much more controlled by adults, and more subjected to adult supervision, than ever before (Coakley, 2009). Parental safety concerns have a direct impact on the likelihood of children being allowed to play outdoors in the neighborhood or at nearby parks and recreational centers (Davison, 2009), and children and adolescents in inner-city and higher-crime neighborhoods are particularly affected by safety issues (Gomez et al., 2004). Although conclusive data are difficult to obtain, our best available estimates indicate that children have less free time and less leisure time than they did two decades ago and that this loss of physical activity opportunity comes as a consequence of longer school days and more structured after-school experiences (Sturm, 2005). As an outgrowth of these societal changes, parents would seem to have a highly important role in enabling physical activity experiences in the leisure hours (Brustad, 2010).

Given that opportunities for children to engage in physical activity seem to be eroding in the leisure-time hours, parental support for physical activity can be considered to be more important now than in previous decades. Dzewaltowski, Geller, Rosenkranz, and Karteroliotis (2009) examined children's self-efficacy to be physically active in the after-school hours in relation to the children's own self-efficacy beliefs as well as in relation to the children's proxy efficacy, which refers to the children's confidence in their skills and abilities to get important adults to act in ways that facilitate their physical activity opportunities. In this case, the researchers examined children's proxy efficacy in relation to their parents as well as in relation to the program staff for the structured activities that participants were involved in after school. Results indicated that self-efficacy and proxy efficacy are separate but related constructs. The researchers also found gender differences, with males being more confident that they could be physically active than were females, which is also consistent with previous research (Trost et al., 1996).

PEER INFLUENCE

The quality of children's relationships with their peers is a highly salient and important aspect of their feelings of relatedness in the physical activity context and thus can have important effects on their continued physical activity motivation and behavior. Once children enter their school years, their physical activity involvement takes place in school-based recess and physical education classes, through informal after-school free play and through structured sport and physical activity programs. Although the specific type of physical activity

experience will vary, one commonality across contexts is that physical activity will take place in the presence of peers, offering numerous opportunities for both positive and negative forms of peer interaction. Physical ability is an important contributor to popularity with peers during childhood (Adler, Kless, & Adler, 1992) and thus forms a salient dimension of children's peer relationships. These peer relationships are also important contributors to children's social, moral, and cognitive development (Bukowski & Hoza, 1989; Sullivan, 1953; Weiss & Stuntz, 2004).

Our understanding of peer influence on children's physical activity motivation and behavior has been hindered by some general shortcomings in understanding social forms of influence on youth motivation. As Smith and McDonough (2008) note, the preponderance of research relating to the influence of socialization agents on children's physical activity has centered on parental influence. This tendency has been unfortunate, because it portrays children as passive recipients of socialization experiences rather than as active agents in the process. More importantly, the lack of research on peer influence on youth physical activity motivation tends to undervalue the role that peers have in children's physical activity processes. Whereas parents may be highly influential in introducing children to various forms of physical activity and sport, the meaning of these experiences is strongly influenced by the nature and quality of children's interactions with their peers while they are engaged in them (Smith, 2003).

The nature and extent of peer influence varies with developmental status; peer influence for a seven-year-old and peer influence for a 17-year-old are substantially different. During early childhood (six years of age and younger), children tend to spend a great deal of their leisure time in the presence of other family members and have not yet established extensive or stable friendships or peer social networks. During middle childhood (seven to nine years of age) children typically begin to spend much more time in the presence of their peers. But during later childhood (10 to 12 years of age) peer relationships tend to take on much greater importance. During this period youngsters are more likely to want to associate with particular others who are perceived to share qualities with them, and children are more likely to want to have a "best friend" with whom they can have a more intimate personal relationship characterized by esteem support and the disclosure of personally valued information. As a consequence of cognitive development, children of this age are also better able to use peers as sources of reflected appraisal to better understand themselves. Younger children tend to be highly dependent on adult information sources, including parents and teachers, but a developmental shift occurs in later childhood whereby children tend to prefer peer sources of information; this shift is accompanied by a corresponding increase in the accuracy of their self-evaluations (Horn & Weiss, 1991; Stipek, Recchia, & McClintic, 1992). Thus peers become more important as sources of information during later childhood and through adolescence, and youth also look to their peers to provide them with social and emotional support, identity confirmation, and other forms of personal recognition and validation that cannot necessarily be provided through the family (Harter, 1988).

An appreciation of peer influence requires recognition that peer relationships are multifaceted, reciprocal, and dynamic. The multifaceted nature of peer relationships refers to the fact that peers can assume many different roles and that relationships change in accordance with the social setting (Sheridan, Buhs, & Warnes, 2003; Zarbatany, Ghesquiere, & Mohr, 1992). Peer influence is also reciprocal, and inherently dynamic, because children's peers (in contrast to their parents) have similar levels of status and authority and the nature of the relationship among peers tends to emerge and change over time in response to previous interactions. Bukowski and Hoza (1989) characterized peer influence as revolving around two distinct dimensions, consisting of friendships and peer acceptance. Friendships are close dyadic relationships between two individuals that commonly involve shared enjoyable experiences, self-disclosure, and esteem support. Sport-related friendships provide opportunities for positive experiences including self-esteem enhancement, companionship, and intimacy (Weiss, Smith, & Theebom, 1996). Peer acceptance refers to the larger group of similar others that constitute one's social network. The larger peer group contributes to experiences of acceptance or rejection as the "generalized other." Friendships can have greater influence on children's emotional development, including empathy and social disclosure, than the peer group, whereas feedback from the peer group, by offering a form of reflected appraisal from a third-party perspective, may be more influential in assisting children in gaining an understanding of their capacities.

It has long been recognized that a principal motive that children identify for their participation in organized sport is the affiliation and friendship opportunities available in this context (Weiss & Petlichkoff, 1989). More recent research indicates that the desire to develop friendships and to experience favorable relationships with peers is also an important component of children's and adolescents' physical activity motivation (Humbert et al., 2006; Spink et al., 2006; Wilson, Williams, Evans, Mixon, & Rheaume, 2005).

Children and adolescents are also likely to be motivated to develop their capacities in physical activity and sport because peer acceptance is generally greater for those youth who are physically competent. For example, Evans and Roberts (1987) found that the social status of third- through fifth-grade boys was linked to their physical competence on the playground. Similar findings were obtained in subsequent research by Chase and Dummer (1992) and by Weiss and Duncan (1992). These studies support the expectation that the physical activity context provides opportunities to gain peer acceptance. At the same time, the public, social, and sometimes competitive characteristics surrounding physical activity can also result in peer social rejection (Partridge et al., 2008).

With respect to the role of friendship characteristics, Duncan (1993) found that friendship qualities within the physical activity setting, specifically feelings of companionship and esteem support, were related to middle school children's physical activity participation choices outside the physical education setting. In addition, these friendship qualities were associated with more favorable affective experiences in the physical education setting. In a study that was grounded in Harter's competence motivation theory, Smith (1999) examined the relationships among children's perceptions of their peer relationships (both peer acceptance and friendship), their physical self-worth, the nature of their affective responses toward physical activity, and their physical activity motivation. He predicted that perceptions of favorable relationships with peers involving peer acceptance and quality friendships in physical activity would result in stronger feelings of physical self-worth and more positive affect toward physical activity, which in turn would contribute to greater motivation to engage in physical activity. The proposed model was generally supported, in that more favorable perceptions of peer acceptance contributed to greater physical self-worth for both male and female young adolescents. The findings from this study provide support for the belief that the quality of children's peer relationships in physical activity affects their motivation to engage in physical activity, although it should be noted that this is not a direct effect but one that is mediated by physical self-worth and affect.

In a study that addressed the contribution of peer relationships to adolescents' commitment to talent domains such as sport, music, theater and dance, Patrick and colleagues (1999) conducted semi-structured interviews with 41 adolescents who had been identified as highly talented in one of these domains. The participants reported that the talent activity provided them a context within which to make or sustain friendships and that the development of stronger peer relationships and friendships within their talent domain facilitated their social skills and confidence in relating to peers in general. Favorable relationships with peers and friends in the talent domain also contributed to greater ongoing motivation to maintain their commitment to the talent domain. In a subsequent study, Fredricks et al. (2002) found that positive relationships with peers are important to adolescents' decisions about maintaining their involvement in free-choice talent activities.

One of the more frequently examined forms of friendship influence in the physical activity domain is peer support. Peer support can consist of forms of influence such as encouragement and praise or shared physical activity, and it is an important form of social reinforcement for activity involvement (Smith & McDonough, 2008). Various researchers have found that peer support for physical activity is an important contributor to children's physical activity behavior and involvement (Beets, Vogel, Forlaw, Pitetti, & Cardinal, 2006; Duncan, Duncan, & Stryker, 2005; Voorhees, 2005).

In sum, the nature and quality of social relationships in the physical activity context can greatly influence young people's motivation to engage in physical activity. Social relationships take many forms, and the salience of particular social relationships can change with context as well as with development. Much more remains to be known about social influence, particularly with regard to its role in shaping physical activity motivation over the long term.

Developmental Influences on Motivation

This chapter has focused primary attention on the principal theories applicable to understanding children's physical activity motivation and the essential psychological variables that are most important to our understanding. However, an individual's physical activity motivation is not necessarily stable through childhood and adolescence, as developmental and age-related influences are also likely to affect motivational characteristics. Although developmental influences on physical activity motivation are not the central focus of this chapter, it is imperative that we recognize how psychological and developmental processes can interact to influence youth physical activity motivation.

A primary reason to acknowledge the effect of developmental influences on youth physical activity motivation is that efforts to promote physical activity in youth should be structured in ways that address changes in youth physical activity behavior with age. It is well documented that young people's physical activity involvement generally declines from later childhood through adolescence (Nelson, Neumark-Stzainer, Hannan, Sirard, & Story, 2006; Sallis, 2000) and that this decline is particularly noteworthy for girls (Kimm et al., 2002). The decline in physical activity involvement cannot be attributed to any single factor operating in isolation but is probably better explained by the interaction of psychological, social, and biological factors operating in concert with developmental influences. The purpose of the following discussion is to identify some of the key developmental influences that affect the physical activity motivation and behavior of youth.

One developmental process that is highly relevant to our discussion is age-related change in how children and adolescents form perceptions of their physical competence. We have discussed the central importance of perceived competence to the physical activity motivation of youth. Children generally become more accurate at assessing their competence with development, and these improvements in accuracy are primarily the result of advances in cognitive development in middle and later childhood (Stipek et al., 1992). Two primary reasons why youth become more accurate in assessing their competence are that with age, youngsters use more sources of competence information and become more capable of using and integrating the information provided by these sources (Horn & Weiss, 1991; Ruble & Frey, 1991; Weiss, Ebbeck, & Horn, 1997). To be more specific, children become more capable of using information sources such as social comparison, adult and peer feedback, and their own self-referenced sources of knowledge. Although the accuracy of physical self-assessments generally increases with development, the downside is that these judgments tend to be less favorable than they were previously, as younger children tend to be overly optimistic in estimating their abilities. Given that perceptions of physical competence decline for most youth, it is not surprising that children's physical activity interest and involvement decline during later childhood and through the adolescent years. More comprehensive accounts exist that explain the effects of cognitive developmental processes in sport- and physical activity–related self-perceptions and involvement (see Horn, 2004; Weiss & Williams, 2004).

Another important developmental influence is physical maturation. Rate of biological maturation varies considerably as children move into their middle school years. Evidence suggests that early physical maturation is associated with girls' disengagement from physical activity, and this may be attributable to a reduction in the favorability of their physical self-perceptions as they commence puberty (Davison, Werder, Trost, Baker, & Birch, 2007; Knowles, Niven, Fawkner, & Henrety, 2009). In their investigation of potential causes for girls' disengagement from physical activity around puberty, Davidson and colleagues (2007) examined the influence of pubertal development on global self-worth, enjoyment of physical activity, and moderate-to-vigorous physical activity involvement. The 168 participants in the study were assessed on the relevant variables at age 11 years and again at age 13 years. Results indicated that more advanced pubertal status at age 11 was associated with lower psychological well-being at 13, which resulted in lower physical activity enjoyment and lower moderate-to-vigorous physical activity at age 13. Subsequent research by Knowles and colleagues (2009) showed that early adolescent girls' physical activity levels declined over the 12-month span of the study and that less favorable physical self-perceptions that accompanied development partly explained this change. However, these researchers did not find physical maturation to be directly related to declines in physical activity involvement over the 12 months of the study.

Longitudinal studies can be very enlightening about developmental and age-related influences on physical activity motivation, but relatively little research has been conducted with the same participants across developmental phases. As part of a longitudinal study of growth and development, Thompson, Humbert, and Mirwald (2003) conducted individual semistructured interviews with 16 men and 15 women who had been study participants for the previous 25 years and categorized their physical activity status as active, average activity, or inactive. Using thematic analysis, they found that significant others, size and maturation, and physical ability were key variables differentiating among men in the activity categories. These participants reported that significant others (including parents, friends and peers, siblings, and teachers and coaches) had the greatest impact on their physical activity orientations and involvement, and the significant-others variable was the strongest differentiator among men in the three activity categories. Active friends and friends who were heavily involved in sport were cited as essential influences on the sustained physical activity involvement of male participants. With regard to the influence of physical size and maturational status during childhood and adolescence, later-maturing males reported that their later maturation constituted a barrier to involvement in physical activity or sport during their youth that dissuaded them from physical activity involvement during adulthood. As would be anticipated, greater perceived physical competence during childhood and adolescence explained greater sustained interest and involvement for these men during adulthood.

For the women in the Thompson et al. (2003) study, the three most important themes identified were transitions, body weight and shape concerns, and significant others. These women identified school-based transitions between elementary and secondary school as being particularly important to their motivation for sustained involvement in physical activity; for the inactive group, the changing social dynamic in secondary school contributed a great deal to a reduction in physical activity involvement. With regard to body weight and shape concerns, all the women reported that they used physical activity as a means of controlling their weight; women in the more active classifications reported that this motive, which corresponds to the extrinsic motive of introjected regulation from self-determination theory, was particularly central for their physical activity involvement. The third prominent factor affecting adult physical activity patterns for these women was significant others, although these were not as important to sustained involvement as they were for the men. Findings from this study are important because precious little research has examined how influences on physical activity during childhood and adolescence affect lifestyle physical activity practices during adulthood.

Developmental and age-related change processes constitute an understudied area of interest within the knowledge base on physical activity motivation. Although not the primary focus of this chapter, developmental change processes interact with motivational characteristics to influence physical activity behavior. For the purpose of effectively promoting physical activity in youth, attention should be directed toward aspects of development including cognitive, physical, and social development, as these areas can independently or conjointly influence motivation in the physical activity context.

Conclusions

Great advances have been made in the past decade in our understanding of children's motivation for involvement in physical activity. One of the principal reasons that our knowledge base has advanced so rapidly is that appropriate theoretical perspectives have been applied to the topic of children's motivation. In this regard, competence motivation theory and expectancy-value theory are highly useful because they give explicit attention to the important role played by socialization agents while implicitly recognizing other means by which motivational characteristics emerge in children. Self-determination theory is particularly beneficial because it helps to explain differences in motivation among individuals along a continuum from amotivation to various forms of extrinsic motivation to intrinsic motivation. Attention to such motivational differences and their manifestation in physical activity contexts is useful because efforts to promote physical activity interventions with youth are successful only to the extent that they stimulate intrinsic motivation, so that youth are attracted to physical activity for a lifetime. Other theoretical approaches are valuable and encouraged, but these three theories have been highlighted here because of their obvious relevance to understanding physical activity motivation in youth.

This chapter has proposed that four variables are particularly important correlates of physical activity motivation in youth. In accordance with the terminology of the most relevant theories, these variables have been identified as perceived competence, autonomy/perceived control, affective experiences, and social relationships. Our knowledge base indicates that children have much greater intrinsic motivation to engage in physical activity to the extent that they feel competent in their physical skills, feel that they have autonomy or control over their involvement, experience favorable affective outcomes while engaged in physical activity, and develop and maintain positive social relationships with parents, peers, siblings, teachers, and coaches in the physical activity setting. Physical activity interventions should therefore be structured in relation to the goals of enhancing competence and autonomy, increasing enjoyment, and facilitating positive social relationships. There are innumerable ways that these outcomes can be facilitated in relation to individual characteristics and social contexts. Fortunately, a growing body of intervention research supports the expectation that targeting these four outcomes will result in greater physical activity motivation and engagement among youth.

Although our knowledge base has expanded considerably in both quantity and quality, insufficient attention has been devoted to influences that we could label "nonpsychological." Relatively little research interest has been dedicated to understanding biological, social, and developmental influences. Our understanding will expand greatly as further research directs attention to the interaction of these factors with psychological variables to influence motivation in youth.

Future Directions

The past decade has brought considerable attention to issues concerning children's physical activity behavior, with the greatest impetus for this attention stemming from concerns about children's physical inactivity in Western societies and their corresponding tendency toward obesity and related health risks. It has been heartening to see the rapid expansion of interest, because the topic was clearly understudied in preceding decades. I suggest here a few directions that relate to expanding our knowledge in the coming decade.

Understanding children's physical activity motivation is of inherent interest because of the value that this knowledge has in guiding interventions to promote physical activity. Interest in physical activity promotion extends across numerous areas of study, ranging from the medical sciences to public health and community health to sport and exercise science. At times it is easy to lose sight of what should be the primary purpose of our interventions, which is to promote and enable physically active lifestyles. These are most likely to result when individuals are intrinsically motivated to engage in physical activity. As Smith (2003) commented, quality physical activity experiences result in commitment to active living, and thus we should seek to design physical activity experiences in accordance with our best knowledge about the factors that are likely to enhance children's intrinsic motivation to engage in physical activity. To reiterate a main point of this chapter, it is futile merely to increase youth physical activity (e.g., through more time spent in physical education alone) if these approaches do not simultaneously increase young people's desire to adopt a physically active lifestyle. Thus motivational theory should be at the heart of all intervention research. In addition, more longitudinal research is needed to assess the effectiveness of intervention strategies over time and to improve our understanding of how characteristics of the intervention affect young people's intrinsic motivation to engage in physical activity.

A second important consideration in the design of future research is the need to take a broader and more integrative perspective on youth physical activity motivation. Although our knowledge base about children's physical activity motivation has expanded tremendously in the past decade, our approach to knowledge generation can sometimes be faulted for being too narrow. Our interest in identifying psychological factors that underlie motivation has frequently resulted in a tendency to overlook the social, biological, and developmental contexts within which these psychological characteristics have developed. The best research to emerge in the coming decade will explain how physical activity motivation varies in relation to dimensions of the social context, in accordance with physical development, and in conjunction with other influences that are not inherently psychological. For example, an area of current research interest revolves around how physical activity motivation is affected by access to physical activity opportunities, as provided through parks and recreational sites, after-school programming, and even public transportation systems (e.g., Carver et al., 2008; Davison, 2009; Sturm, 2005). Such research has implications for the design of interventions to facilitate greater access to physical activity among youth. Similarly, much more research is needed to help us understand how physical activity motivation varies with physical maturation status, gender and gender-related social stereotypes, cultural and socioeconomic characteristics, and family structure.

It has been heartening to see the growth of interest in understanding children's physical activity motivation and behavior. The development of a strong knowledge base constitutes the best weapon in our efforts to counteract the tendency for youth to be physically inactive in modern Western societies.

Knowledge produced in the coming decade will be beneficial in counteracting this trend to the extent that it adds to our understanding about the effectiveness of various types of interventions across time and in relation to biological, social, and developmental considerations.

References

Adler, P. A., Kless, S. J., & Adler, P. (1992). Socialization to gender roles: Popularity among elementary school boys and girls. *Sociology of Education, 65*, 169–197.

Ajzen, I. (1991). The theory of planned behavior. *Organizational Behavior and Human Decision Processes, 50*, 179–211.

Anderssen, N., & Wold, B. (1992). Parental and peer influences on leisure-time physical activity in young adolescents. *Research Quarterly for Exercise and Sport, 63*, 341–348.

Babkes, M. L., & Weiss, M. R. (1999). Parental influences on children's cognitive and affective responses to competitive soccer participation. *Pediatric Exercise Science, 11*, 44–62.

Bandura, A. (1986). *Social foundations of thought and action: A social cognitive theory.* Englewood Cliffs, NJ: Prentice Hall.

Bandura, A. (2001). Social cognitive theory: An agentic perspective. *Annual Review of Psychology, 52*, 1–26.

Barnett, M., Morgan, P. J., van Beurden, E., & Beard, J. R. (2008). Perceived sports competence mediates the relationship between childhood motor skill proficiency and adolescent physical activity and fitness: A longitudinal study. *International Journal of Behavioral Nutrition and Physical Activity, 5*, 1–12.

Barr-Anderson, D. J., Young, D. R., Sallis, J. F., Neumark-Sztainer, D. R., Gittelsohn, J., Webber, L.,…Jobe, J. B. (2007). Structured physical activity and psychosocial correlates in middle-school girls. *Preventive Medicine, 44*, 404–409.

Baumeister, R., & Leary, M. (1995). The need to belong: Desire for interpersonal attachments as a fundamental human motivation. *Psychological Bulletin, 117*(3), 497–529.

Beets, M. W., Beighle, A., Erwin, H. E., & Huberty, J. L. (2009). After-school program impact on physical activity and fitness: A meta-analysis. *American Journal of Preventive Medicine, 36*(6), 527-537.

Beets, M. W., Vogel, R., Forlaw, L., Pitetti, K. H., & Cardinal, B. J. (2006). Social support and youth physical activity: The role of provider and type. *American Journal of Health Behavior, 30*, 278–289.

Bois, J. E., Sarrazin, P. G., Brustad, R. J., Trouilloud, D. O., & Cury, F. (2002). Mothers' expectancies and young adolescents' perceived physical competence. *Journal of Early Adolescence, 22*(4), 384–406.

Bronfenbrenner, U., & Morris, P. A. (1998). The ecology of developmental processes. In R. M. Lerner (Ed.), *Handbook of child psychology* (5th ed., Vol. 1, pp. 993–1028). New York: Wiley.

Brustad, R. J. (1991). Children's perspectives on exercise and physical activity: Measurement issues and concerns. *Journal of School Health, 61*, 228–230.

Brustad, R. J. (1992). Integrating socialization influences into the study of children's motivation in sport. *Journal of Sport & Exercise Psychology, 14*, 59–77.

Brustad, R. J. (1993). Who will go out and play? Parental and psychological influences on children's attraction to physical activity. *Pediatric Exercise Science, 5*, 210–223.

Brustad, R. J. (1996). Attraction to physical activity in urban schoolchildren: Parental socialization and gender influences. *Research Quarterly for Exercise and Sport, 67*, 316–323.

Brustad, R. J. (2010). The role of family in promoting physical activity. *President's Council on Physical Fitness and Sports: Research Digest, 10*(3), 1–8.

Brustad, R. J., & Babkes, M. L. (2004). Social influence on the psychological dimensions of adult physical activity involvement. In M. R. Weiss (Ed.), *Developmental sport and exercise psychology: A lifespan perspective* (pp. 313–332). Morgantown, WV: Fitness information Technology.

Bukowski, W. M., & Hoza, B. (1989). Popularity and friendship: Issues in theory, measurement, and outcome. In T. J. Berndt & G. W. Ladd (Eds.), *Peer relationships in child development* (pp. 15–45). New York: Wiley.

Carver, A., Timperio, A., & Crawford, D. (2008). Playing it safe: The influence of neighbourhood safety on children's physical activity—a review. *Health & Place, 14*, 217–227.

Chase, M. A., & Dummer, G. M. (1992). The role of sports as a social status determinant for children. *Research Quarterly for Exercise and Sport, 63*, 418–424.

Coakley, J. J. (2009). *Sports in society: Issues and controversies* (10th ed.). New York: McGraw-Hill.

Coakley, J., & White, A. (1992). Making decisions: Gender and sport participation among British adolescents. *Sociology of Sport Journal, 9*, 20–35.

Cooper Institute for Aerobics Research (1999). *The Fitnessgram test administration manual* (6th ed.). Champaign, IL: Human Kinetics.

Cox, A. E., Smith, A. L., & Williams, L. (2008). Change in physical education motivation and physical activity behavior during middle school. *Journal of Adolescent Health, 43*, 506–513.

Davison, K. K. (2009). School performance, lack of facilities, and safety concerns: Barriers to parents' support of their children's physical activity. *American Journal of Health Promotion, 23*(5), 315–319.

Davison, K. K., Werder, J. L., Trost, S. G., Baker, B. L., & Birch, L. L. (2007). Why are early maturing girls less active? Links between pubertal development, psychological well-being, and physical activity among girls at ages 11 and 13. *Social Science & Medicine, 64*, 2391–2404.

DiLorenzo, T. M., Stucky-Ropp, R. C., Vander Wal, J. S., & Gotham, H. J. (1998). Determinants of exercise among children. II. A longitudinal analysis. *Preventive Medicine, 27*, 470–477.

Dishman, R. K., Motl, R. W., Saunders, R., Felton, G., Ward, D. S., Dowda, M., & Pate, R. (2005). Enjoyment mediates effects of a school-based physical-activity intervention. *Medicine & Science in Sports and Exercise, 37*(3), 478–487.

Dorsch, T. E., Smith, A. L., & McDonough, M. H. (2009). Parents' perceptions of child-to-parent socialization in organized sport. *Journal of Sport & Exercise Psychology, 31*, 444–468.

Duda, J. L. (1992). Sport and exercise motivation: A goal perspective analysis. In G. Roberts (Ed.), *Motivation in sport and exercise* (pp. 57–91). Champaign, IL: Human Kinetics.

Dudley, D. A., Okely, A. D., Pearson, P., & Peat, J. (2010). Engaging adolescent girls from linguistically diverse and low income backgrounds in school sport: A pilot randomised controlled trial. *Journal of Science and Medicine in Sport, 13*(2), 217–224.

Duncan, S. C. (1993). The role of cognitive appraisal and friendship provisions in adolescents' affect and motivation toward activity in physical education. *Research Quarterly for Exercise and Sport, 64*, 314–323.

Duncan, S. C., Duncan, T. E., & Strycker, L. A. (2005). Sources and types of social support in youth physical activity. *Health Psychology, 24*, 3–10.

Duncan, S. C., Duncan, T. E., Strycker, L. A., & Chaumeton, N. R. (2002). Neighborhood physical activity opportunity: A multilevel contextual model. *Research Quarterly for Exercise and Sport, 73*(4), 457–463.

Dzewaltowski, D. A., Geller, K. S., Rosenkranz, R. R., & Karteroliotis, K. (2010). Children's self-efficacy and proxy efficacy for after-school physical activity. *Psychology of Sport and Exercise, 11*(2), 100–106.

Eccles, J. S. (1993). School and family effects on the ontogeny of children's interests, self-perception, and activity choice. In J. Jacobs (Ed.), *Nebraska Symposium on Motivation, 1992* (pp. 145–208). Lincoln: University of Nebraska Press.

Eccles, J. S., Adler, T. F., Futterman, R., Goff, S., Kacazala, C. M., Meece, J. L., & Midgley. C. (1983). Expectations, values and academic behaviors. In J. T. Spence (Ed.), *Achievement and achievement motivation* (pp. 75–146). San Francisco: W. H. Freeman.

Eccles, J. S., & Harold, R. (1991). Gender differences in sport involvement: Applying the Eccles et al. model. *Journal of Applied Sport Psychology, 3*, 7–35.

Eccles, J. S., Wigfield, A. W., & Schiefele, U. (1998). Motivation to succeed. In W. Damon (Ed.), *Handbook of child psychology, Vol. 3: Social, emotional, and personality development* (5th ed., pp. 1017–1095). New York: Wiley.

Erikson, E. H. (1968). *Identity: Youth and crisis.* New York: Norton.

Evans, J. R., & Roberts, G. C. (1987). Physical competence and the development of children's peer relations. *Quest, 39*, 23–25.

Franzini, L., Elliott, M. N., Cuccaro, P., Schuster, M., Gilliland, J., Grunbaum, J. A., ... Tortolero, S. R(2009). Influences of physical and social neighborhood environments on children's physical activity and obesity. *American Journal of Public Health, 99*(2), 271–278.

Fredricks, J. A., Alfeld-Liro, C. J., Hruda, L. Z., Eccles, J. S., Patrick, H., & Ryan, A. M. (2002). A qualitative examination of adolescents' commitment to athletics and the arts. *Journal of Adolescent Research, 17*, 68–97.

Fredricks, J. A., & Eccles, J. S. (2002). Children's competence and value beliefs from childhood through adolescence: Growth trajectories in two male sex-typed domains. *Child Development, 38*, 519–533.

Fredricks, J. A., & Eccles, J. S. (2004). Parental influences on youth involvement in sports. In M. R. Weiss (Ed.), *Developmental sport and exercise psychology: A lifespan perspective* (pp. 145–164). Morgantown, WV: Fitness information Technology.

Frome, P. M., & Eccles, J. S. (1998). Parents' influence on children's achievement-related perceptions. *Journal of Personality and Social Psychology, 74*(2), 435–452.

Gagne, M., Ryan, R. M., & Bargmann, K. (2003). Autonomy support and need satisfaction in the motivation and well-being of gymnasts. *Journal of Applied Sport Psychology, 15*, 372–390.

Gomez, J. E., Johnson, B. A., Selva, M., & Sallis, J. F. (2004). Violent crime and outdoor physical activity among inner-city youth. *Preventive Medicine, 39*, 876–881.

Goudas, M., Biddle, S., Fox, K., & Underwood, M. (1995). It ain't what you do, it's the way that you do it! Teaching style affects children's motivation in track and field lessons. *Sport Psychologist, 9*, 254–264.

Guillet, E., Sarrazin, P., Fontayne, P., & Brustad, R. J. (2006). Understanding female sport attrition in a stereotypical male sport within the framework of Eccles' expectancy-value model. *Psychology of Women Quarterly, 35*, 358–368.

Gustafson, S. L., & Rhodes, R. E. (2006). Parental correlates of physical activity in children and early adolescents. *Sports Medicine, 36*(1), 79–97.

Hagger, M. S., Chatzisarantis, N. L. D., Culverhouse, T., & Biddle, S. J. H. (2003). The processes by which perceived autonomy support in physical education promotes leisure-time physical activity intentions and behavior: A trans-contextual model. *Journal of Educational Psychology, 95*(4), 784–795.

Harter, S. (1978). Effectance motivation reconsidered. *Human Development, 21*, 34–64.

Harter, S. (1981). A model of intrinsic mastery motivation in children: Individual differences and developmental change. In W. A. Collins (Ed.), *Minnesota Symposium on Child Psychology* (Vol. 14, pp. 215–255). Hillsdale, NJ: Erlbaum.

Harter, S. (1988). Causes, correlates and the functional role of global self-worth: A life-span perspective. In J. Kolligan & R. Sternberg (Eds.), *Perceptions of competence and incompetence across the life-span* (pp. 67–98). New Haven, CT: Yale University Press.

Horn, T. S. (2004). Developmental perspectives on self-perceptions in children and adolescents. In M. R. Weiss (Ed.), *Developmental sport and exercise psychology: A lifespan perspective* (pp. 101–143). Morgantown, WV: Fitness Information Technology.

Horn, T. S., & Weiss, M. R. (1991). A developmental analysis of children's self-ability judgments. *Pediatric Exercise Science, 3*, 312–328.

Humbert, M. L., Chad, K. E., Bruner, M. W., Spink, K. S., Muhajarine, N., Anderson, K. D., . . . Gryba, C. R. (2008). Using a naturalistic ecological approach to examine the factors influencing youth physical activity across grades 7 to 12. *Health Education & Behavior, 35*, 158–173.

Humbert, M. L., Chad, K. E., Spink, K. S., Muhajarine, N., Anderson, K. D., Bruner, M. W., . . . Gryba, C. R. (2006). Factors that influence physical activity participation among high- and low-SES youth. *Qualitative Health Research, 16*, 467–483.

Kimm, S. Y. S., Glynn, N. W., Kriska, A. M., Barton, B. A., Kronsberg, S. S., & Daniels, S. R., . (2002). Decline in physical activity in black girls and white girls during adolescence. *New England Journal of Medicine, 347*(10), 709–715.

Knowles, A. M., Niven, A. G., Fawkner, S. G., & Henrety, J. M. (2009). A longitudinal examination of the influence of maturation on physical self-perceptions and the relationship with physical activity in early adolescent girls. *Journal of Adolescence, 32*, 555–566.

Lubans, D. R., Foster, C., & Biddle, S. J. H. (2008). A review of mediators of behavior in interventions to promote physical activity among children and adolescents. *Preventive Medicine, 47*, 463–470.

Mackett, R. L., & Paskins, J. (2008). Children's physical activity: The contribution of playing and walking. *Children & Society, 22*, 345–357.

Malina, R. M. (1996). Tracking of physical activity across the lifespan. *Research Quarterly for Exercise and Sport, 67*(Suppl.), s47–s57.

Mosston, M., & Ashworth, S. (1986). *Teaching physical education* (3rd ed.). Columbus, OH: Merrill.

Nelson, M. C., Neumark-Stzainer, D., Hannan, P. J., Sirard, J. R., & Story, M. (2006). Longitudinal and secular trends in physical activity and sedentary behavior during adolescence. *Pediatrics, 118*(6), 1627–1634.

Ntoumanis, N. (2005). A prospective study of participation in optional school physical education using a self-determination theory framework. *Journal of Educational Psychology, 97*(3), 444–453.

Ogden, C. L., Carroll, M. D., Curtin, L. R., McDowell, M. A., Tabak, C. J., & Flegal, K. M. (2006). Prevalence of overweight and obesity in the United States, 1999–2004. *JAMA, 295*(13), 1549–1555.

Pangrazi, R. P., Beighle, A., Vehige, T., & Vack, C. (2003). Impact of Promoting Lifestyle Activity for Youth (PLAY) on children's physical activity. *Journal of School Health, 73*(8), 317–321.

Parsons, J., Adler, T. F., & Kaczala, C. M. (1982). Socialization of achievement attitudes and beliefs: Parental influences. *Child Development, 53*, 310–321.

Partridge, J. A., Brustad, R. J., & Babkes Stellino, M. (2008). Social influence in sport. In T. S. Horn (Ed.), *Advances in sport psychology* (3rd ed., pp. 270–291). Champaign, IL: Human Kinetics.

Pate, R. R., Baranowski, T., Dowda, M., & Trost, S. G. (1996). Tracking of physical activity and physical fitness across the lifespan. *Medicine & Science in Sports & Exercise, 28*, 82–96.

Patrick, H., Ryan, A. M., Alfeld-Liro, C., Fredricks, J. A., Hruda, L. Z., & Eccles, J. S. (1999). Adolescents' commitment to developing talent: The role of peers in continuing motivation for sports and the arts. *Journal of Youth and Adolescence, 28*(6), 741–763.

Paxton, R. J., Estabrooks, P. A., & Dzewaltowski, D. (2004). Attraction to physical activity mediates the relationship between perceived competence and physical activity in youth. *Research Quarterly for Exercise and Sport, 75*, 107–111.

Raedeke, T. (1997). Is athlete burnout more than just stress? A sport commitment perspective. *Journal of Sport & Exercise Psychology, 19*, 396–417.

Rodriguez, D., Wigfield, A., & Eccles, J. S. (2003). Changing competence perceptions, changing values: Implications for youth sport. *Journal of Applied Sport Psychology, 15*, 67–81.

Rose, E., Larkin, D., Hands, B. P., Howard, B., & Parker, H. (2009). Evidence for the validity of the Children's Attraction to Physical Activity questionnaire (CAPA) with young children. *Journal of Science and Medicine in Sport, 12*, 573–578.

Ruble, D. N., & Frey, K. S. (1991). Changing patterns of comparative behavior as skills are acquired: A functional model of self-evaluation. In J. Suls & T. A. Wills (Eds.), *Social comparison: Contemporary theory and research* (pp. 70–112). Hillsdale, NJ: Erlbaum.

Ryan, R. M., & Deci, E. L. (2000). Self-determination theory and the facilitation of intrinsic motivation, social development, and well-being. *American Psychologist, 55*, 68–78.

Ryan, R. M., & Deci, E. L. (2006). Self-regulation and the problem of human autonomy: Does psychology need choice, self-determination, and will? *Journal of Personality, 74*(6), 1557–1585.

Sallis, J. F. (2000). Age-related decline in physical activity: A study of human and animal studies. *Medicine & Science in Sports & Exercise, 32*, 1598–1600.

Seabra, A. F., Mendonca, D. M., Goring, H. H. H., Thomis, M. A., & Maia, J. A. (2008). Genetic and environmental factors in familial clustering in physical activity. *European Journal of Epidemiology, 23*, 205–211.

Shen, B., McCaughtry, N., & Martin, J. (2007). The influence of self-determination in physical education on leisure-time physical activity behavior. *Research Quarterly for Exercise and Sport, 78*(4), 328–338.

Sheridan, S. M., Buhs, E. S., & Warnes, E. D. (2003). Childhood peer relationships in context. *Journal of School Psychology, 41*, 285–292.

Smith, A. L. (1999). Perceptions of peer relationships and physical activity participation in early adolescence. *Journal of Sport & Exercise Psychology, 21*, 329–350.

Smith, A. L. (2003). Peer relationships in physical activity contexts: A road less traveled in youth sport and exercise psychology research. *Psychology of Sport and Exercise, 4*, 25–39.

Smith, A. L., & McDonough, M. H. (2008). Peers. In A. L. Smith & S. J. H. Biddle (Eds.), *Youth physical activity and sedentary behavior* (pp. 295–320). Champaign, IL: Human Kinetics.

Spink, K. S., Shields, C. A., Chad, K., Odnoken, P., Muhajarine, N., & Humbert, L. (2006). Correlates of structured and unstructured activity among sufficiently active youth and adolescents: A new approach to understanding physical activity. *Pediatric Exercise Science, 18*, 203–215.

Standage, M., Duda, J. L., & Ntoumanis, N. (2005). A test of self-determination theory in school physical education. *British Journal of Educational Psychology, 75*, 411–433.

Stipek, D. J., Recchia, S., & McClintic, S. (1992). Self-evaluation in young children. *Monographs of the Society for Research in Child Development, 5*, 71–84.

Sturm, R. (2005). Childhood obesity—what we can learn from existing data on societal trends, part 1. *Preventing Chronic Disease, 2*(1), 1–12.

Sullivan, H. S. (1953). *The interpersonal theory of psychiatry*. New York: Norton.

Thompson, A. M., Humbert, M. L., & Mirwald, R. L. (2003). A longitudinal study of the impact of childhood and adolescent physical activity experiences on adult physical activity perceptions and behaviors. *Qualitative Health Research, 13*, 358–367.

Troiano, R. P., Berrigan, D., Dodd, K. W., Masse, L. C., Tilert, T., & McDowell, M. (2008). Physical activity in the United States measured by accelerometer. *Medicine & Science in Sports & Exercise, 40*(1), 181–188.

Trost, S. G., Pate, R. R., Dowda, M., Saunders, R., Ward, D. S., & Felton, G. (1996). Gender differences in physical activity and determinants of physical activity in rural fifth grade children. *Journal of School Health, 66*, 145–150.

Trost, S. G., Pate, R. R., Saunders, R., Ward, D. S., Dowda, M., & Felton, G. (1997). A prospective study of the determinants of physical activity in rural fifth-grade children. *Preventive Medicine, 26*, 257–263.

Voorhees, C. C. (2005). The role of peer social network factors and physical activity in adolescent girls. *American Journal of Health Behavior, 29*, 183–190.

Wang, C. K. J., & Biddle, S. J. H. (2001). Young people's motivational profiles in physical activity: A cluster analysis. *Journal of Sport & Exercise Psychology, 23*, 1–22.

Weiss, M. R., & Amorose, A. J. (2008). Motivational orientations and sport behavior. In T. S. Horn (Ed.), *Advances in sport psychology* (3rd ed., pp. 115–155). Champaign, IL: Human Kinetics.

Weiss, M. R., & Duncan, S. C. (1992). The relationship between physical competence and peer acceptance in the context of children's sport participation. *Journal of Sport & Exercise Psychology, 14*, 177–191.

Weiss, M. R., Ebbeck, V., & Horn, T. S. (1997). Children's self-perceptions and sources of physical competence information: A cluster analysis. *Journal of Sport & Exercise Psychology, 19*(1), 52–70.

Weiss, M. R., & Petlichkoff, L. M. (1989). Children's motivation for participation in and withdrawal from sport: Identifying the missing links. *Pediatric Exercise Science, 1*, 195–211.

Weiss, M. R., Smith, A. L., & Theebom, M. (1996). "That's what friends are for": Children's and teenagers' perceptions of peer relationships in the sport domain. *Journal of Sport & Exercise Psychology, 18*, 347–379.

Weiss, M. R., & Stuntz, C. P. (2004). A little friendly competition: Peer relationships and psychosocial development in youth sport and physical activity contexts. In M. R. Weiss (Ed.), *Developmental sport and exercise psychology: A lifespan perspective* (pp. 165–196). Morgantown, WV: Fitness Information Technology.

Weiss, M. R., & Williams, L. (2004). The why of youth sport involvement: A developmental perspective on motivational processes. In M. R. Weiss (Ed.), *Developmental sport and exercise psychology: A lifespan perspective* (pp. 223–268). Morgantown, WV: Fitness Information Technology.

Welk, G. (1999). The youth physical activity promotion model: A conceptual bridge between theory and practice. *Quest, 51*, 5–23.

Welk, G. J., & Eklund, B. (2005). Validation of the Children and Youth Physical Self-Perceptions Profile for young children. *Psychology of Sport and Exercise, 6*, 51–65.

Welk, G. J., & Schaben, J. A. (2004). Psychosocial correlates of physical activity in children—a study of relationships when children have similar opportunities to be active. *Measurement in Physical Education and Exercise Science, 8*(2), 63–81.

White, R. W. (1959). Motivation reconsidered: The concept of competence. *Psychological Review, 66*, 297–333.

Wilson, D. K., Williams, J., Evans, A., Mixon, G., & Rheaume, C. (2005). A qualitative study of gender preferences and motivational factors for physical activity in underserved adolescents. *Journal of Pediatric Psychology, 30*, 293–297.

Zarbatany, L., Ghesquiere, K., & Mohr, K. (1992). A context perspective on early adolescents' friendship expectations. *Journal of Early Adolescence, 12*, 111–126.

Exercise Psychology and Children's Intelligence

Phillip D. Tomporowski, Jack A. Naglieri, *and* Kate Lambourne

Abstract

The consensus among academics regarding the malleability of intelligence has vacillated over the past century. Recent observations of brain plasticity over the life span have spurred interest in the effects of environmental interventions on intelligence and cognitive function. Folk psychology has long promoted a link between children's exercise and physical development and their general intelligence. While it is plausible that exercise benefits children's brain development, our review of published studies fails to support the view that exercise training induces robust global improvements in children's intelligence. A few studies, however, provide evidence that exercise may facilitate specific types of cognitive functioning. Children's executive functions appear particularly sensitive to exercise interventions. At present, the ability to draw general conclusions concerning the exercise–intelligence relation is hindered by a lack of methodologically sound studies.

Key Words: children, adolescents, intelligence, cognition, physical activity, exercise, psychometrics, pediatrics.

Introduction

The rapid, dramatic transformations that occur as children pass through the stages of infancy, childhood, adolescence, and into adulthood have been observed and chronicled for thousands of years and in many ways. The changes that occur in children develop into young adults have inspired artists and scientists alike. Parents have long pondered how the plans they have for their child will impact his or her growth and development, and ultimately influence the kind of person he or she will grow to be. Historically, it has long been accepted that a child's developmental path is the result of a complex interaction among genetic and environmental factors. Early developmental psychologists described how genetically linked maturational factors could predict the emergence of children's physical and mental abilities (Gesell, 1925; Piaget, 1963). Maturation reflects a timetable of events that are genetically

arranged and influenced little by environmental factors. Development, on the other hand, reflects changes in physical or mental processes that may be affected by both maturation and experience.

Several basic assumptions guide research on children's physical and mental development (Gabbard, 2004, pp. 9–13). Central to the present review are four assumptions that provide a plausible rationale for hypothesizing that exercise and physical activity behaviors alter children's mental development and, ultimately, the level of their intelligence. First, human development is assumed to be a holistic process that involves relations among physical, cognitive, and psychosocial factors. Second, development is linked to a child's individual history, culture, and environmental affordances. Third, there are periods of time in development during which experiences may influence the emergence of particular brain systems and neuronal networks. Lastly, brain development and subsequent behavior can be aided by positive environmental experiences. The notion that the human brain displays an element of plasticity, or mutability, has emerged over the past decade. Advances in neurological measurement techniques have enabled considerable research with animals and humans that speaks to the positive role of environmental experiences on brain integrity and function.

In concert with advances in neuropsychological research, health professionals have over the past decade developed guidelines for physical education teachers and practitioners that describe physical activity interventions that purportedly enhance both the bodies and minds of developing children. The goals established by the National Association for Sport and Physical Education (NASPE;2009) are oriented toward guiding children to be physically active across the life span. Effective interventions are sensitive to children's developmental levels and abilities and are designed to improve children's mastery of movement skills; develop their understanding of body awareness, space awareness, and effort; and facilitate their cognitive development. From practitioners' frames of reference, children gain fundamental knowledge about themselves and the world around them through physical activity and skill development. The experiences that children derive from learning motor skills lead them to analyze and apply knowledge to overcome lifespan challenges.

The recent NASPE guidelines echo long-standing assumptions concerning intelligence as a set of behaviors necessary for adapting to ever-changing environmental demands. Early views of human development suggested that the manner in which children face developmental tasks could set or modify the trajectory of their life course (Havighurst, 1972). According to this conceptualization, there are challenges associated with particular stages of development. The tasks of infancy and early childhood include learning to walk, talk, and form concepts, and the tasks of middle childhood include mastery of fundamental skills such as reading, writing, and mathematics. These and many other developmental tasks and challenges arise from several sources; they constitute a basic part of individual growth and reflect the constraints of our society. Some are tasks tied closely to biological maturation, others are associated with social and cultural expectations, and still others are linked to personal goals, values, and aspirations. These challenges are unavoidable, and how an individual is able to meet the demands has historically served as a marker of intelligent behavior.

The benefits of exercise for both body and mind have been touted recently in books (Ratey & Hagerman, 2008) and magazines (Carmichael, 2007) directed toward the general public; likewise, monographs have been published that describe the manner in which interventions such as exercise may reap intellectual benefits for individuals at every point across the life span (Hertzog, Kramer, Wilson, & Lindenberger, 2009). The focus of public policy makers has begun to constrict on exercise and physical activity as cost-effective interventions to stem the rise in obesity as well as to improve children's cognitive and intellectual functions (e.g., International Life Sciences Institute, 2003).

The goal of the present chapter is to review the methods and findings of research studies that have focused on the relation between planned exercise programs and children's intellectual and cognitive function. As addressed in the following sections, there are a number of methodological and theoretical issues that influence our ability to draw clear linkages between exercise and intelligence. The chapter is organized into four sections. In the first, we address the assumption that routine exercise can directly influence neurological development of the central nervous system and that resulting changes will be reflected in children's intellectual function. To that end, we will describe the development of children's nervous systems, with reference to the role of experiential factors that may alter the course of brain development. The second section addresses approaches that have been taken to define and measure the construct of intelligence. In our overviews, we describe the history of intelligence tests, the emergence of the field of psychometrics, and the impact of cognitive psychology on test development. Third, we review studies conducted with children and adolescents. The results obtained from these studies are discussed both in terms of theory and in terms of measurement issues. In the final section, we draw conclusions and provide recommendations concerning the assessment of children's intellectual and cognitive function and the level and types of measurement that may have the best chance of verifying whether or not systematic exercise can influence children's intelligence.

Why Would Exercise Be Expected to Influence Children's Intelligence?

The adult human brain consists of at least 100 billion neurons, and the interwoven structures of the central nervous system interact in an exquisite and extremely complex fashion (Taylor, 2006). The study of normal brain and spinal cord development from the point of conception to adulthood provides some insight into the interrelations that exist between genetic and environmental factors that mold the functioning central nervous system. Recent advances in neurological measurement have helped us to understand the biological sequences that unfold on the basis of biological programming and how the trajectories of cell growth and organization may be altered as the developing person interacts with and adapts to an ever-changing environment (Diamond, 2009; Karmiloff-Smith, 2009).

Developmental neuropsychologists and neurophysiologists have made marked progress in elucidating the sequence of cellular events that leads to the development of the adult brain (Craik & Bialystok, 2007; de Haan & Johnson, 2003; Gogtay et al., 2004; Lebel, Walker, Leemans, Phillips, & Beaulieu, 2008). Following conception, cells begins to divide, and by the fourth week a neural tube is formed, from which the structures of the body arise. Precursor cells give rise to the proliferation of neural cells that will make up the central nervous system. Once neurons reach genetically coded locations, they begin to differentiate and take on specific characteristics. Based on gene expression and chemical signals, neuronal dendrite branching begins, as does the extension of cells' axons toward predetermined targets. The processes of synaptogenesis and myelination, which strengthen connections among neurons, begin during the third trimester of prenatal development and continue throughout the life span. The density of cortical neurons increases rapidly, followed by a pruning period, during which cells are eliminated. While the major areas of the brain and spinal cord are set by the time of birth, networks of cells continue to form and emerge at different times throughout childhood and adolescence and into adulthood (Lebel et al., 2008).

Specific areas of the neocortex are traditionally associated with particular functions—for example, vision with the occipital lobes, reasoning with the frontal lobes, and language with the temporal lobes. The prefrontal cortex, which has been associated with intellectual functions such as problem solving, reasoning, and planning, develops in a nonlinear fashion from infancy to young adulthood (Bunge & Wright, 2007; Diamond, 2000, 2002). In general, frontal-lobe processes develop rapidly through the elementary school years and then at a slower pace during adolescence (Brocki & Bohlin, 2004; Huizinga, 2006). The emergence and development of processes that underlie intelligence and cognition continues throughout childhood and adolescence and even into young adulthood (Casey, Amso, & Davidson, 2006; Posner & Rothbart, 2007).

While the fundamental architecture of the brain may be innately determined, there is a growing consensus that networks of cortical cells can be influenced by environmental factors. Impoverished environments can degrade mental development and hinder the refinement of problem-solving skills, whereas enriched environments in which children experience conditions that stress the importance of complex rules to solve problems are hypothesized to lead to thoughtful and more sophisticated problem-solving skills (Frye, Zelazo, & Burack, 1998; Zelazo & Frye, 1998). Considerable evidence has accrued for the plasticity of the neural networks in developing individuals (Nelson, de Haan, & Thomas, 2006) and adults (Pascual-Leone, Amedi, Fregni, & Merabet, 2005). Of particular interest to the present chapter is the role that movement and physical activity play in promoting neurological or behavioral changes.

Infant Research

Research on infants reveals a protracted interrelation between physical activity and cognitive development (Thelen, 1996; Thelen & Smith, 1994). As infants move, they learn about their environments and how tasks are solved (Adolph, 2008; Sommerville & Decety, 2006). Sensorimotor activation has been shown to influence both reasoning and problem solving (Diamond, 2006; Gallese & Metzinger, 2003; Jackson & Decety, 2004). Motor and cognitive development are interrelated phenomena that emerge over a prolonged period (Diamond, 2000), and environments that restrict action–perception couplings are thought to contribute to developmental delays (Spencer et al., 2006; Stockman, 2004; Thelen, 2004). From an evolutionary perspective, it has been argued that the manner in which the brain evolved to organize and control movement explains the emergence of human cognition (Llinas, 2001). Thus an individual's cognitive abilities may be expected to be deeply rooted in the body's physical interactions with the world (Wilson, 2002).

Play Research

Play is a form of physical activity that has been proposed to serve an important role in normal maturation and in the emergence of children's cognitive abilities (Hughes, 1995; Johnson, Christie, & Yawkey, 1987; Panksepp, Siviy, & Normansell,

1984) and socialization skills (Pellis & Pellis, 2007). Indeed, restrictive environments that limit children's access to time for free play, rough-and-tumble play, and physical activity have been hypothesized to impede the development of socially appropriate behavioral patterns (Diamond, Barnett, Thomas, & Munro, 2007; Panksepp, 1998). Though play and physical activity, children are thought to learn to decide when it is appropriate to act and when an action should be inhibited. Children who are motorically active gain from those experiences and acquire greater behavioral control than children who are less motorically active (Campbell, Eaton, & McKeen, 2002). Play that necessitates effortful mental engagement may be linked to children's ability to control their movements and self-regulate their actions. Environments that elicit children's effortful mental involvement may promote behavioral change via the emergence and use of brain processes needed to regulate actions and to achieve goals.

Animal Research

A rapidly growing literature provides compelling support for the positive effects of regular exercise on brain function in animals (van Praag, 2009; Vaynman & Gomez-Pinilla, 2006; Vaynman, Ying, & Gomez-Pinilla, 2004). Chronic exercise training influences the production of neurotransmitters and neurotrophins (Dishman et al., 2006), and exercise training has been linked to the activation of neuromodulators, particularly the monoamine system (Dishman, 1997). Brain-derived neurotropic factors (BDNF) and other neurotrophins have been evaluated as possible moderators of exercise-induced neurocognitive enhancement and protection, as BDNF plays a key role in neuronal proliferation, differentiation, and survival in the mammalian brain (Barde, 1989; Levi-Montalcini, 1987). The BDNF neurotrophin protects cholinergic neurons in the hippocampus and basal forebrain (Hall, Thomas, & Everitt, 2000). New neurons appear in the dentate gyrus of the adult hippocampus rather soon following the onset of aerobic exercise training (Gage, van Praag, & Kempermann, 2000). Changes observed in the density of dendritic spines on neurons and associated changes in long-term potentiation have led some to hypothesize that exercise-induced production of BDNF may affect learning and declarative memory (Kramer & Erickson, 2007; van Praag, 2009; Vaynman et al., 2004). Chronic exercise is also linked to synaptogenesis and angiogenesis. Synaptogenesis is the formation of new synapses and is known to play a critical role in neurological integrity throughout the life span. Angiogenesis is the development of new capillaries from preexisting vessels. Chronic exercise training leads to increased proliferation of endothelial cells and new capillary formation in active brain areas. Insulin-like growth factor also plays a role in these adaptations, as it modulates vascular endothelial growth factor, which is a protein growth factor and prominent molecule involved in angiogenesis and blood vessel growth (Kramer & Erickson, 2007).

In summary, evidence from several areas of research provides evidence that the pattern of children's neural specialization may be determined in part by physical activity. However, caution is advised with regard to the interpretation of the evidence provided above. While chronic physical activity influences the brain at the cellular, structural, and network levels, so do other interventions. Changes in diet (Molteni, Barnard, Ying, Roberts, & Gomez-Pinilla, 2002; Molteni et al., 2004) and specialized educational programs have also been shown to alter brain functions and favorably affect children's (Rueda, Rothbart, McCandliss, Saccomanno, & Posner, 2005) and adults'(Jaeggi, Buschkuehl, Jonides, & Perrig, 2008; Persson & Reuter-Lorenz, 2008) cognitive performance. Thus questions remain concerning the uniqueness of exercise as an intervention that influences intellectual abilities. Some of these questions may be addressed by evaluating closely the manner in which the constructs of intelligence and cognitive abilities have been defined and by assessing how chronic exercise interventions can be varied in mode, intensity, and duration.

Measuring Intelligence and Cognitive Abilities

The scientific study of intelligence began during the mid-19th century. From the very beginning, two different assumptions about the determinants of intelligence guided the work of researchers and theorists—nature vs. nurture. In England, Sir Francis Galton, who was Charles Darwin's cousin and a man influenced greatly by the theory of the evolution by means of natural selection, held an extreme nativistic view. He was of the opinion that an individual's level of intelligence was determined predominantly by lineage. Notions of inheritance and the passage of characteristics from one generation to the next were at the core of Galton's views of intelligence. He also believed that measurement of sensory acuity would provide reliable indices of intelligence. Over several years, he created a battery of tests that measured characteristics such as muscle strength, reaction time, visual judgments, vision, olfaction, and audition. Galton is credited for undertaking the first large-scale administration of psychological tests. Between 1884 and 1890 over 9,000 individuals performed various mental tests administered as part of the London International Health Exhibition and at the South Kensington Museum. The followers of Galton's views developed more expansive test batteries that included laboratory-based tests of basic mental processes. However, the test battery approach lost credibility in the very early years of the 20th century, primarily because low correlations were observed among individual test items and between test measures and student academic performance. The mental task approach developed by Galton and his followers reemerged in the 1970s as the component process approach (Detterman, 1986; Detterman et al., 1992). The majority of contemporary exercise scientists who study the exercise–cognition relationship employ tests that measure constructs hypothesized to reflect specific cognitive processes (e.g., working memory, executive function, or perception), although these constructs have seldom been contextualized within a larger theory of intelligence.

At about the same time that Galton was developing his nativistic views of intelligence, the French government began an initiative to evaluate how children who lived in Paris benefited from universal education. A commission determined that children should be examined to assess their educability (Foschi & Cicciola, 2006). Children identified as being unable to benefit from school were to be placed in special classes (Wasserman & Tulsky, 2005). Alfred Binet, who was a member of the commission, accepted the charge of developing the test, together with Théodore Simon. Binet held a very strong environmentalist view, believing that intelligence was malleable and influenced greatly by experience and social factors. Binet was aware of Galton's mental test approach and its focus on sensory and motor proficiencies, and viewed them as too restrictive. Binet and Simon selected items believed to assess higher-level mental processes such as reasoning and problem solving. The initial version of the Binet–Simon Scale was introduced in 1905; it consisted of 30 items that were ranked in order of difficulty and scored on a pass/fail basis. Unique to the test was the derivation of age-graded norms, which permitted a child's mental age to be determined. In addition to the measurement

advances, the scale was novel in reflecting Binet's underlying view of intelligence. He conceptualized intelligence in terms of a three-level hierarchy that consisted of lower-order elementary processes (e.g., comprehension and inventiveness) and first-order faculties (e.g., memory, imagery, attention, muscular force, coordination skills, and quick visual judgments) topped by a superordinate factor (general intelligence). Binet's pioneering conceptualization of intelligence and insightful selection and organization of test items contributed substantially to the evolution of intelligence tests that emerged in the early 20th century and continue to influence contemporary tests of intelligence.

This very brief historical overview was designed to introduce some element of the nature–nurture debate that has existed within the academic community for over a century. At the heart of the debate lie assumptions concerning the extent to which environmental interventions (e.g., exercise, physical activity, or educational programs) can influence children's intellectual ability. The consensus of academics and educators has vacillated over the past century, with intelligence being viewed as genetically linked and essentially fixed at some times and being seen as malleable and sensitive to environmental factors at other times.

The Psychometric Movement

The hierarchical view of intelligence proposed by Binet, in which complex mental processes are placed at the top and simpler processes, which are subordinate to higher-level processes, are placed at lower levels, is reflected in many contemporary views and tests. The structure of intelligence is studied by researchers who specialize in psychometrics, an academic field that focuses on the measurement of psychological constructs. Constructs are terms that link psychological attributes (e.g., aggression, timidity, personality traits, intelligence, or working memory) to measurement procedures. Measurement provides the basis for operational definitions, which specify the meaning of a construct by denoting measurement operations (Underwood, 1957). The construct "weight," for instance, is operationally defined in terms of values obtained from a scale. Similarly, the construct of intelligence is operationally defined by psychological measurement procedures. An intelligence scale provides numerical representations of the construct. Defining a given construct via direct observation and measurement clarifies both similarities and differences among constructs. As a result, operational definitions restrict the number of concepts available for use within a particular domain or investigation.

Psychometrists have over the past century explored the structure of human intelligence with increasingly sophisticated quantitative methods of measuring human performance. Building on methods of statistical regression developed in the early 20th century, a family of factor analytic procedures provided the basis for understanding the relationships among variables assumed to measure different types of intelligence. Factor analysis is a statistical procedure that examines patterns of correlations among scores on small tests (sometimes called subtests) that comprise an entire test. For example, intelligence tests are comprised a number of individual subtests (each of which contains enough items to have adequate reliability), which have varying degrees of intercorrelation. Factor analysis provides a way to explore the degree to which performance on individual subtests clusters together to form a "factor." Early research using factor analysis provided evidence of a general factor *g*, which is a reflection of the extent to which all variables in the correlation matrix relate to one another. The total IQ score, developed by William Stern, originally was calculated using mental and chronological age scores and came to be used as the primary index of an individual's level of general intelligence (Stern, 1930).

The analyses of the factor structures of the many intelligence tests (e.g., the Stanford–Binet and Wechsler scales) that have been developed and published since the dissemination of the Binet–Simon Scale have focused on the factors that underlie intelligence as measured by these particular tests and how they are linked together within tests. However, the understanding of a test's factorial structure is often confused with an understanding of intelligence as a psychological construct. Because factor analysis can only help discover the relationships among variables being studied, this statistical technique is limited by the initial selection of variables to include in the analysis. For example, the factor solutions for the four versions of the Wechsler Intelligence Scale for Children (Wechsler, 1941, 1991a, 1991b, 2003) have changed from two to three to four factors because of the introduction of new subtests. Factor analysis provides a useful tool for understanding the *test*; however, the original development of the subtests to be included in an intelligence test should have been based on a theory of intelligence. Unfortunately, the psychometric field has historically attempted to build intelligence theories on IQ tests rather than IQ tests on theories of intelligence.

An influential theory based on factor analysis, initially proposed by Raymond Cattell and John Horn in the 1940s, suggested that intelligence is best explained in terms of two dimensions: crystallized intelligence (gc), which reflects the storage of knowledge and the ability to acquire knowledge, and fluid intelligence (gf), which reflects the ability to reason and act adaptively to novel situations (Cattell, 1943). The theory was modified several times (Horn & Cattell, 1966) and the number of ability factors had increased to nine factors by the 1990s.

The rise of psychometrics led to the development of several intelligence tests that have been used worldwide to measure and characterize the abilities of millions of individuals. There was a consensus among psychologists during the first half of the 20th century that human intelligence was essentially fixed by genetic factors and that it could be reliably measured and summarized in terms of one or a few scores. Intelligence tests were employed in many areas (e.g., the military, business, and education) to select individuals for training opportunities and to identify those who required specific educational services. In the 1960s, a number of influential psychologists and social scientists promoted the view that intelligence was mutable and could be affected in a positive or negative manner by environmental factors (Ramey & Ramey, 2004). The merits of using standardized intelligence tests to measure children's abilities were debated vigorously. Head Start, a national, large-scale intervention study that began in the U.S. in 1965, was conducted to evaluate the impact of improved social and educational services on preschool children who lived in low-income, multirisk communities. While the merits of the Head Start initiative and the program's impact on children's intellectual and academic outcomes continue to be discussed (Zigler & Styfco, 2004), and the notion of IQ as a fixed genetically linked characteristic has been challenged.

Researchers of this era who began to explore the effectiveness of interventions on mental development often focused their work on children or adults with developmental disabilities. It was assumed that individuals who possessed lower levels of mental functioning would benefit more from interventions than individuals without developmental disabilities (Ellis & Cavalier, 1982). This assumption provided the impetus for several of the earliest studies conducted specifically to assess the effects of exercise training on intelligence. These studies are reviewed later in this chapter.

The Cognitive Movement

As discussed above, Galton and those he influenced (e.g., James Cattell) approached the study of intelligence by measuring an individual's performance on tests of basic sensory processes. The results of initial studies, however, indicated that measures of memory and perception did not predict general intellectual functioning. As a result, attempts to understand intelligence in terms of simple mental processing tasks were, for the most part, abandoned in favor of the psychometric approaches.

The study of the component properties of the mind was continued, however, by laboratory-based researchers who developed methods to measure such constructs as memory, attention, and problem solving and who proposed theories to explain how these cognitive processes operated. At about the same time that Galton and Binet were working to develop measures of intelligence, Hermann Ebbinghaus, a German scholar, devised the first techniques to measure human memory and learning in a quantitative fashion. These methods served for decades as the nucleus of research conducted by psychologists who studied verbal learning. Research by verbal learning psychologists provided vital information concerning how specific methodological factors influence the retention of knowledge. Modern cognitive psychology emerged in the 1960s as a method that focused not only on how information is stored but also on how it is processed and manipulated. The information processing model heralded a major shift in the manner in which psychologists viewed the working of the mind.

While many models of information processing have been proposed, all have been guided by a particular set of assumptions. Figure 20.1 shows a simple representative model of information processing(Ackerman & Kyllonen, 1991). The model reflects an interaction among four components of the information processing system.

PROCESSING SPEED

A portion of efficient performance can be explained in terms of the speed at which information is transformed and routed through the processing system. The amount of information that is transmitted from one component to another is limited by the integrity of the neural system and how much data can be transmitted in a short period of time. Basic sensory information obtained from the

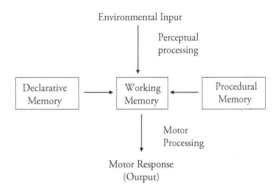

Figure 20.1. A prototypical information processing model. Reproduced with permission from "Trainee Characteristics," by P. L. Ackerman and P. C. Kyllonen,1991, in J. E. Morrison (Ed.), *Training for Performance: Principles of Applied Human Learning* (pp. 193–229), New York: John Wiley & Sons.

environment is organized, transformed into perceptions, and then transferred into working memory. Knowledge gained from past experience and stored in long-term memory is accessed and transferred into working memory. Movement plans developed in working memory are transferred throughout the system and used to initiate action.

BREADTH OF DECLARATIVE KNOWLEDGE

While speed of information processing is important to the execution of efficient performance, it also depends on an individual's store of declarative or factual knowledge. With experience, increasingly sophisticated organizations of facts and rules can be stored; these can be used to solve new problems.

BREADTH OF PROCEDURAL SKILL

The application of factual information to a problem also involves movement and action. Through repeated practice, action patterns become ingrained and are displayed more and more automatically. Unlike factual information, which the individual can describe and define, procedural skills reflect a type of implicit, nonverbal knowledge.

PROCESSING CAPACITY

It is in working memory that information concerning environmental conditions and possible responses is compiled and possible actions are formulated and considered. Because working memory is limited in capacity, the efficiency of the system is tied to the demands placed on it. Two types of processes modify working memory efficiency. Compositional processes collapse long sequences of response productions into shorter sequences. Reducing the number of steps or sequences that are necessary to formulate a response reduces the demand placed on working memory, and as a result responses are produced more efficiently. Proceduralization processes improve working memory efficiency by linking specific environmental conditions to specific responses. Together, these two types of processes reduce the demands placed on working memory and lead to fast and efficient mental processing and skilled performance.

There has been considerable theorizing and research about the components of the information processing model, and a number of laboratory-based tests have been developed to assess them. Indeed, a comprehensive review of the neurocognitive literature by Lezak and her colleagues revealed over 400 tests designed to assess cognitive functions (Lezak, Howieson, & Loring, 2004). Researchers who have focused on the exercise–cognition relationship have tended to select tests that fall into four categories, each of which reflects a component of the information processing model: perception, memory, attention, and executive processes.

PERCEPTUAL TASKS

Human sensory systems provide stimulus information that constitutes the beginning of the transformation of sensation to perception, that is, the change of raw physical energy into something that has meaning. Visual and auditory organs, for example, scan and inspect the outside world. Inspection-time methods (Nettelbeck & Wilson, 1997) and scanning protocols (S. Sternberg, 1969) have been developed that isolate perceptual processes.

SHORT-TERM AND WORKING MEMORY TASKS

Theoretical debate concerning the nature of memory led some researchers to focus on specific aspects of memory processes (J. R. Anderson, 1983; Baddeley, 1986). The construct of working memory evolved from theorizing about the functions of short-term memory. Working memory refers to the temporary storage and manipulation of information necessary for complex tasks such as learning, language comprehension, and reasoning. Subjectively, working memory is analogous to conscious awareness and involves the simultaneous storage and processing of information (Miyake & Shah, 1999). The constraints of working memory are known to limit human performance, and as such it has been a focus of interest for a number of exercise psychologists. Numerous tests of working memory have been developed by cognitive psychologists and clinical neuropsychologists. Evidence for a relation between exercise and working memory is relatively strong, with several studies reporting improved performance, particularly on such tasks as random number generation (Baddeley, Emslie, Kolodny, & Duncan, 1998) and the Paced Auditory Serial Addition Test (Tombaught, 2006).

ATTENTION

Attention is conceptualized as a process that influences the operation of memory systems. It does so in three ways. Focused attention involves selective identification and processing of information. The role of focused attention is to analyze incoming sensory information and to determine what is and what is not relevant. Divided attention involves processing two or more sources of information simultaneously. Short-term memory is limited in the amount of incoming data it can hold and manipulate; as a result, competition for processing takes place. Attention serves to determine the importance of the information that is held and worked on in short-term memory. A trade-off takes place where some information is given more priority than other information. Sustained attention involves vigilance and the maintenance of information in memory, particularly short-term memory stores. Posner's Attentional Network Test (Posner, Sheese, Odludas, & Tang, 2006) has been employed in several studies that examined the effects of acute bouts of exercise on children's attention.

EXECUTIVE PROCESSES

Mental processes that are central to decision making, goal planning, and choice behavior are referred to as "executive" functions (Miyake et al., 2000; Naglieri & Johnson, 2000; Posner & Dahaene, 1994). The construct of executive function has been a focus of interest to cognitive psychologists for decades (Banich, 2009; Monsell & Driver, 2000; Vandierendonck, 2000). While debate concerning the structure of executive function is ongoing, there is a general consensus among researchers that executive function is not a unitary process; rather, it reflects a number of more elemental, underlying processes. Purported component processes include planning, which reflects the ability to use strategies to attain goals; updating, which is closely linked to working memory and the need to monitor its representations; inhibition, which involves the deliberate suppression of a prepotent response; and switching, which requires individuals to disengage the processing operations of an irrelevant task and to engage operations involved in a relevant task. Many of these processes have also been classified as metacognition, which refers to the higher-order thinking that controls thought processes required for problem solving (Borkowski, Carr, & Pressely, 1987; Flavell, 1979). Recently, Etnier and Chang (2009) provided a commentary concerning methods of measuring executive function and their application to research on exercise effects on cognition.

Laboratory-based tests designed to assess the properties of specific components of the information processing model have been valuable for cognitive theory development. Laboratory-based cognitive researchers have conducted a substantial body of research on individual differences in intelligence (See Jensen, 2006).

Impact of Cognitive Psychology on Test Development

The rise in prominence of cognitive psychology and of the assumptions of the information processing model led some behavioral scientists to propose hybrid measurement approaches that combine the methods of classical psychometrics with the component process approach. John Carroll (1976) recognized the merits of merging tests developed by psychometrists that reflected latent processes and the methods used by laboratory-based cognitive psychologists to obtain fine-grained analyses of mental processes. Over the course of three decades of research, he developed a coding scheme for classifying cognitive tasks that reflected both the psychometric assessment of intelligence and research that examined basic information processing (Carroll, 1993). His approach was unique. He employed as a starting point a theory of cognitive processes outlined by Hunt, Frost, and Lunneborg (1973) and linked their processes to corresponding constructs identified via factor analytic methods. On the basis of close evaluation of the measurement properties of a pool of tests assembled by French, Ekstom, and Price (1963), he identified pairs of tests that measured 24 different constructs derived via factor analysis. He then proposed six task coding categories based on cognitive theory: (1) type of stimuli presented, (2) overt response to be made at the end of the task, (3) task structure, (4) operations and strategies, (5) temporal aspects of the operation strategy, and (6) type of memory storage involved. The result of his research was a matrix designed to link tests that measured specific psychometric constructs (e.g., word fluency or speed of closure) with cognitive (e.g., memory search) and memory

(e.g., short- and long-term memory) processes. Carroll's test classification scheme, while underused (see Floyd, 2005), has been used recently by exercise psychologists to categorize cognitive tests for the purpose of meta-analytic evaluation (Etnier, Nowell, Landers, & Sibley, 2006; Lambourne & Tomporowski, 2010).

Influenced by the work of Carroll and other early cognitive scientists, Robert Sternberg (1977, 1985, 2005) developed an influential cognitive theory of intelligence that was designed to expand and extend the definition of intelligence from one tied to scores on abstract items found in traditional intelligence tests to one that reflected peoples' behavior in real-world environments. His triarchic theory attempts to explain human behavior in terms of the interplay among bottom-up basic information processing components, top-down executive processing components, and the selection and execution of behaviors best suited for environmental contexts and challenges faced at a specific point in time. The triarchic theory is hierarchical and consists of three subtheories. The componential subtheory focuses on the processes that lead to the selection, encoding, storage, and combining of information. The experiential subtheory focuses on how individuals are able to use past experiences when confronted with novel tasks or situations and how prior automatization of processes aids problem solving. The contextual subtheory focuses on the extent to which cultural and societal conditions define intelligent behavior. It focuses on the interface between the individual and the external world and how individuals attempt to adapt and shape the environments in which they live. Sternberg proposes that the three subtheories, when taken together, provide a more ecologically representative view of intelligence than more traditional intelligence tests, which are based on the organization of factor loadings rather than on theories of human behavior. The hypotheses derived from the triarchic theory have led to considerable research in many fields (e.g., education, developmental disabilities, giftedness, and individual differences; see R. J. Sternberg, 2005). While the triarchic theory provides a compelling framework for examining conditions that moderate or mediate intelligent behaviors, the model has not been adequately operationalized nor employed by exercise researchers.

Advances in cognitive and neuropsychology have also influenced contemporary theories of intelligence. The Planning, Attention, Simultaneous, Successive (PASS) Theory developed by Jack Naglieri and J. P. Das (Naglieri & Das, 1997, 2005), for example, was based on observations of the Russian physician Alexander Luria (1902–1977). Luria's prescient observations of the functional organization of the central nervous system had a marked impact on researchers interested in normal and atypical mental development (Das, 1999, 2003). Luria identified three functional units of the brain, which he hypothesized to operate in an interrelated fashion. The first unit comprised brain stem structures and their projections to midcortical and cortical areas central to arousal and attention. The second unit included cortical lobes rostral to the central sulcus (parietal, temporal, and occipital) and served to integrate and organize incoming sensory information. The third unit was linked with the prefrontal cortex and was central for processes involved in programming, regulation, and verification of behavior. Luria emphasized that human cognition and behavior was the result of the integration of all three functional units, operating in concert with individual's acquired knowledge and skills.

Naglieri clarified that in PASS the term *cognitive process* describes a foundational neuropsychologically identified ability (Naglieri & Kaufman, 2008). Each PASS process provides a unique kind of function (ability), and the four cognitive processes are needed to meet the multidimensional demands of our complex environment. The variety of cognitive processes affords the capability of achieving the same goal using different types or various combinations of these processes. The PASS cognitive processes underlie all mental and physical activity. The use of PASS cognitive processes (and related factors such as motivation, emotional status, and quality of instruction) greatly influences the acquisition of knowledge, skills, and social competence (Naglieri & Rojahn, 2004).

This neuropsychological conceptualization of brain function provided a theoretical understanding of intelligence which was used to create one of the most recently developed tests of intelligence, the Cognitive Assessment System (CAS; Naglieri & Das, 1997). The CAS was explicitly developed by Naglieri and Das according to the PASS (Planning, Attention, Simultaneous, Successive) theory of intelligence over a 25-year period. This theory-based intelligence test is a nationally standardized instrument designed for children and adolescents 5 through 17 years of age. It differs from traditional intelligence tests in that it emphasizes basic psychological processes and precludes the use of test items that involve academic skills (e.g., vocabulary and

arithmetic). The CAS provides a full-scale standard score and four PASS-scale standard scores (mean of 100 and standard deviation of 15), which are particularly useful for assessing youths' cognitive strengths and weaknesses. The Planning scale assesses the ability to solve goal-directed problems, and as such it provides an index of executive function. The tests that measure planning require the individual to develop and execute a plan, evaluate and monitor the effectiveness of the plan, and to revise or reject the plan as needed. The Attention scale measures the ability to focus attention on relevant task conditions, sustain attention over time, and resist distractions. The Simultaneous scale provides insight into the ability to organize and integrate information into a coherent whole. Lastly, the Successive scale evaluates how well an individual is able to work with series of information based on order and chain-like progressions (Naglieri, 2005). The PASS theory as measured by the CAS has been subjected to considerable experimental examination (for summaries see Naglieri, 2005; Naglieri & Conway, 2009; Naglieri & Das, 2005).

The PASS scales are amenable to profile analysis and have been shown to be useful in identifying individual differences in cognitive ability (Naglieri & Das, 1997). The scales have also been found to be sensitive to educational interventions (Haddad et al., 2003; Iseman & Naglieri, 2011; Naglieri & Gottling, 1995, 1997; Naglieri & Johnson, 2000) and chronic exercise interventions (Davis et al., 2007, in press2011). Naglieri (2005) posits that because the PASS conceptualization of mental ability differs from traditional views of intelligence, which emphasize the role of acquired knowledge (e.g., vocabulary), the CAS provides measures of processing abilities that can better assess the impact of interventions on specific aspects of cognitive function.

Cognitive Test Batteries

Some exercise researchers have conducted studies in which participants perform a battery of cognitive and information processing tests prior to and following exercise training. In these studies, the individual tests that make up the battery are typically selected as measures of specific constructs. A representative study was conducted by Kramer and his colleagues (2002) to assess the effects of aerobic exercise training on older adults' cognitive function. Cognitive tests were selected based on the hypothesis that improvements in aerobic fitness would be associated with selective improvements in cognitive functions that involve executive control processes such as coordination, inhibition, schedule planning, and working memory. The effects of exercise training were evaluated by comparing posttraining changes in the performance of tests or test components hypothesized to reflect executive processing (e.g., switching, working memory, backward digit span, and verbal learning) with changes on tests thought not to require executive processing (e.g., digit–symbol substitution, visual search, spatial attention, the pursuit rotor task, and forward digit span). As predicted, individuals who completed exercise training performed better on cognitive tests than nonexercisers, and the greatest gains were seen on tasks that purportedly measure executive functioning. The test battery approach is limited, however, as conclusions are drawn primarily on the basis of "test counting," that is, the number of tests that show improvements and the number of tests that were not influenced by the intervention.

Several commercially available psychological test batteries have been developed over the past decade. These computer-based test batteries typically include tasks designed for use in laboratory studies of cognition and tasks developed by neuropsychologists. Examples include the Cambridge Neuropsychological Test Automated Battery (CANTAB), HeadMinder, and ImPACT. The CANTAB (Cambridge Cognition, 2011) has been used extensively in psychopharmacological and neuropsychological research, while HeadMinder (Erlanger, Feldman, & Kutner, 2003) and ImPACT (Lovell, Collins, Podell, Powell, & Maroon, 2000) are often used by practitioners in physical rehabilitation and athletic training. There are several advantages to using these test batteries. The tests are designed to be easy to administer, the psychometric properties of the tests that make up the battery have undergone considerable evaluation, and normative data are available. There are, however, limitations. The systems are somewhat expensive, the reliability of some tests has been a concern, and the validity of using the test batteries, particularly with children and older adults, is yet to be fully determined (Broglio, Ferrara, Macciocchi, Baumgartner, & Elliott, 2007; Luciana, 2003; Schatz & Putz, 2006). These test batteries have seldom been used by researchers interested in the relationship of exercise to intelligence and cognition.

Review of Exercise Interventions

We now turn to a review of interventions aimed at using exercise to improve children's cognitive abilities. The studies selected for review were chosen on the basis of their relevance to the hypothesized relation between exercise and children's intelligence, both broadly defined. Studies were limited to published experiments that(a) included an exercise treatment designed to improve specific aspects of participants' physical fitness, (b) targeted participant populations that yield information about mental development, and (c) employed mental tests with acceptable reliability.

Exercise Intervention Studies with Children and Adolescents with Developmental Disabilities

Researchers have had a long-standing interest in how physical activity interventions influence intelligence in individuals with developmental disabilities. The focus on this population is attributable to the view that because of their lower levels of cognitive function, these individuals may evidence greater gains from exercise interventions than individuals without developmental disabilities.

In an early study, Oliver (1958) matched 38 males on age (range = 12–15 years) and IQ scores (mean = 70.1, range = 57–86) and then randomly assigned them to an experimental or control condition. The experimental group completed 10 weeks of exercise conditioning, which consisted of physical education lessons, strength exercises, remedial exercises, and recreational activities performed three hours per day, five days per week. The control group engaged in normal physical education classes three days per week. A battery of physical ability tests (motor educability, athletic achievement, physical fitness, and strength) and mental tests (Terman Merrill IQ, Goodenough test, Raven's matrices, Porteus maze, and Goddard's form board) was administered to each group before and following the intervention. When compared with the control group, the exercise group had significantly greater improvements on the physical tests that measured motor skills, athletic achievement, fitness, and strength. The experimental group also had significantly improved performance on the Terman Merrill IQ, Goodenough test, and Porteus maze test. Of the 19 students in the exercise group, 18 improved their IQ scores, with eight achieving gains of 5 IQ points or more.

Using a similar methodology, Corder (1966) examined the effects of a physical education treatment on the intellectual and physical development of 24 males (age range = 12–16 years; IQ range = 50–80). The participants were matched on age and

IQ and then randomly assigned to an exercise training group, an "officials" group, or a control group. Those assigned to the training group participated in a progressive, physically demanding exercise program that involved activities such as deep knee bends, jumping jacks, push-ups, sit-ups, jumping, sprinting, and running. Each participant assigned to the officials group had the job of rating one of the participants in the training group and recording his running times and number of exercises he performed. This experimental condition was included to explore the effects of the time and attention given to the training group. Children assigned to the control group received regular classroom instruction. The Wechsler Intelligence Scale for Children and the Youth Fitness Test were administered prior to and following treatments. Physical fitness scores improved in the exercise training group but not the officials or control groups. Full-scale IQ scores increased significantly for children in the exercise training condition and in the officials condition. However, the greatest IQ gains were observed in the exercise training group. The authors cited the Hawthorne effect to explain the IQ gain in the officials group and suggested that other factors might have been operating to explain the gain scores in the training group, such as the experience of success and performing tasks that require concentration.

A large study conducted by Rarick, Dobbins, and Broadhead (1976) evaluated the effect of a physical education program on 481 children whose ages ranged between 6 and 13 years; 275 children were classified as educable mentally retarded (IQ range = 50–70), and 206 children were classified as having minimal brain injury. Intact groups of children of each classification were assigned randomly to an individual-oriented physical education program, a group-oriented physical activity program, an attentional control art program, or a regular classroom program. Exercise and art groups met each school day for 35 minutes over 20 weeks of training. In the individual-oriented intervention, children always worked alone, while children in the group-oriented intervention always worked cooperatively with a partner. The primary focus in both training conditions was on improving basic proficiency in movement patterns(e.g., running, jumping, landing, and rolling). Progressively more complex skill training activities were introduced over the course of the program. Similarly, activities such as clay modeling, letter design, and painting in the art training program were made gradually more challenging. Programs were taught by schoolteachers, who received specialized training in instructional methods. Before and following training, children's intelligence was measured (inadequately by today's standards) using the Bender Motor Gestalt Test (a design-copying task) and the Peabody Picture Vocabulary Test (PPVT). Children in the exercise programs and in the art training program showed significantly improved PPVT performance compared with children in the regular treatment condition. Children's PPVT performance did not differ between the exercise and art groups, which suggests that the improvements in intelligence were the result of the Hawthorne effect.

Brown (1967) assessed the effects of an isometric strength training program on the intellectual development of forty 12-year-old males (IQ range = 30–50). The children were assigned randomly to an exercise program or control condition that met daily for six weeks. The exercise program consisted of a series of 12 isometric contractions each held for 10 seconds. An experimenter applied physical resistance during the exercises. Children in the control group interacted socially with a teacher. The exercise program, as compared with the control program, resulted in significant improvements in children's arm, shoulder, abdomen, back, and leg strength as well as significant gains in intelligence as measured by the Stanford–Binet intelligence test.

Exercise Intervention Studies with Adults with Developmental Disabilities

Tomporowski and Ellis (1984) conducted two experiments to determine whether aerobic exercise training would have a positive effect on institutionalized adults with mental retardation. In the first study, 65 participants were matched on IQ (mean = 26, range = 8–44), age (mean = 29 years, range = 17–39), and sex and randomly assigned to an exercise treatment condition that consisted of a progressive program of running and jogging, calisthenics, and circuit training; an attentional control treatment that consisted of a structured educational program emphasizing academics and acquisition of social skills; or a nonintervention control group who received routine care and training. Treatments were provided three hours per day, five days per week. Adults in the exercise condition, compared with the other conditions, evidenced significant improvements in cardiorespiratory capacity as measured via treadmill running. There were no differences in intelligence scores among the three groups as measured by the Stanford–Binet test.

In a systematic replication, Tomporowski and Ellis (1985) increased the intensity of the exercise intervention. Eighty-six subjects were selected from the previous study, matched on sex, age, and intelligence, then randomly assigned to either an experimental or a control group. The experimental group met five days per week for three-hour sessions where they performed circuit training and a group walk/jog program. As each participant adapted to the exercise program, the intensity, duration, or both were gradually increased. The participants in the control group received the normal institutional programs. After the treatment, the cardiorespiratory function of those in the exercise condition improved significantly. However, as in the previous study, Stanford–Binet intelligence test scores did not differ between the groups.

Exercise Intervention Studies with Nondisabled Children and Adolescents

The manner in which exercise might influence the mental functioning of nondisabled youth has been examined in several experiments. An early study conducted by Ismail (1967) involved 142 elementary school children who were matched on IQ (mean = 111) and age (range = 10–12 years) and assigned either to what was described as a well-organized, daily physical education program or to a control group where students performed traditional physical education activities. Children participated in programs throughout an eight-month academic year. Posttreatment IQ scores obtained via the Otis test did not differ between the groups.

Tuckman and Hinkle (1986) assessed the effects of aerobic running exercise on the fitness and mental function of 77 fourth-, fifth-, and sixth-grade students. The treatment condition consisted of three 30-minute running sessions per week for 12 weeks. The fourth- and fifth-grade students also participated in regular physical education classes twice each week. A control group of similar size and age range engaged in regular physical education classes that consisted of sports and occasional jogging. Compared with children in regular physical education classes alone, those who participated in the aerobic running program improved their cardiorespiratory fitness level and also demonstrated higher levels of creativity as measured by the Alternate Uses test. The groups did not differ in performance on the Bender-Gestalt tests of perceptual–motor ability, the Pier–Harris Children's Self-Concept Scale, or teacher responses on the Devereaux Elementary School Behavior Rating Scale.

Hinkle, Tuckman, and Sampson(1993) compared the effects of an aerobic running program with those of traditional physical education on a battery of physical and psychological tests. Eighty-five eighth-grade students were randomly assigned either to an eight-week running program or to regular physical education classes consisting of nonaerobic activities. After the training period, physical fitness of children in the aerobic training condition, when compared with that of children in traditional physical education classes, improved on measures of aerobic capacity (800-meter run), heart rate, systolic blood pressure, and body composition. Aerobic exercise also favorably increased children's creative fluency, creative flexibility, and creative originality as measured by the Figural and Verbal booklets of the Torrance Tests of Creative Thinking.

A unique study conducted by Zervas, Apostolos, and Klissouras (1991) examined the effects of exercise training on children's cognitive response to acute exercise. Nine pairs of monozygotic twins between the ages of 11 and 14 participated in the study. One boy from each pair was randomly assigned to an experimental group and the other to a control group. Another group of eight non-twin boys participated in a second control condition. The experimental group participated in 25 weeks of exercise training that consisted of interval or continuous running on a treadmill. The twins randomized to the control group and the non-twin boys in the second control group participated in regular physical education classes during the 25 weeks. After the treatment period, the twins in the experimental and control group performed a five-minute warm-up on a treadmill followed by a strenuous 20-minute run. The boys in the non-twin control group sat for a period equal to the duration of the exercise bout. A computer-based test of attention was administered prior to and immediately following the exercise bout or rest period. Exercise training did not influence children's cognitive test performance, which was higher following exercise regardless of treatment condition.

Recently, Davis and her associates (2007, 2011) examined the effects of two doses of aerobic exercise on children's cognitive function. Participants were 172 sedentary, overweight (body mass index ≥ 85th percentile) children 7–11 years of age (mean age = 9.3). Children were randomly assigned to a low dose of exercise (20 minutes per day), a highdose of exercise (40 minutes per day), or a control condition. The exercise conditions were equivalent in intensity, differing only in duration. Activities were selected based on their ability to elicit a heart rate greater than 150 beats per minute and included running games, jump rope, and modified basketball and soccer. Analysis of the posttreatment CAS (Naglieri & Das, 1997) scores revealed exercise-related gains on the Planning scale, indicative of selective effects of exercise on executive function. There was a significant linear trend on the Planning scale, suggesting that benefits were related to exercise dose. No significant differences were detected on the other CAS scales.

Interpretation of Empirical Research Findings

Despite the role that games and sport play in societies worldwide, surprisingly few research studies have been conducted that assess the effects of systematic exercise training on children's general intelligence. Results obtained from studies that have employed traditional intelligence tests (e.g., the Stanford–Binet test, Wechsler scales, PPVT, or Otis test) are inconsistent, and close scrutiny of the methods used in studies reporting positive outcomes reveal conditions that cloud interpretation of the exercise–intelligence relation (Brown, 1967; Corder, 1966; Oliver, 1958). Studies in which researchers have employed cognitive test batteries to assess exercise effects provide somewhat more coherent results. The results of a few studies suggest that exercise may exert selective effects on children's cognitive function (Davis et al., 2007, 2011; Hinkle et al., 1993; Tuckman & Hinkle, 1986). The tasks that appear to be influenced most by exercise treatments are those that purportedly measure executive functions (e.g., planning, resistance to distraction, and inhibition). However, it is not readily apparent how predictive changes in performance on specific mental tests are of intelligence or adaptive functioning in real-world situations. Taken together, the available data do not provide compelling support for the view that exercise training induces robust global changes in children's intellectual function, but do suggest that such training may lead to more specific cognitive changes.

We recognize the limitations of our narrative literature review and that alternative, quantitative review methods are available. Indeed, a quantitative review that included a broader sampling of published and unpublished cross-sectional studies and experiments yielded a significant positive overall effect size (0.32), suggesting that physical activity does benefit children's cognitive function (Sibley & Etnier, 2003). The authors of that quantitative review cautioned that the methodological rigor of many studies was questionable.

Our narrative review revealed a number of methodological factors that researchers will need to address before support for a relation between exercise training and intelligence or cognitive function can be established. As in all research, the ability to elucidate a relation between an independent variable (e.g., exercise) and a dependent variable (e.g., intelligence or cognitive function) depends on the precise manipulation of the independent variable, reliable measures of the dependent variable, and research methods that control for the effect of extraneous variables on outcome measures (Tomporowski, 2009). Unfortunately, many of the studies reviewed failed to provide detailed descriptions of the exercise interventions or control group treatments. Further, outcome measures differed considerably among studies. In addition, a number of developmental and maturational factors make it difficult to associate children's physical activity with their intelligence or cognitive function. Below, we examine these issues in some depth and provide suggestions that may aid researchers' attempts to clarify the exercise–intelligence relationship.

EXERCISE METHODOLOGIES

Exercise behavior is complex and can be manipulated in a number of ways. Interventions can be developed to promote specific changes in cardiorespiratory efficiency, muscular strength, muscular endurance, or muscular flexibility. In addition, exercise interventions can differ in modality, intensity, duration, and the social setting in which physical activities are performed.

The concept of specificity of training, which predicts that the body responds to exercise demands in a specific fashion, is a fundamental assumption held by exercise scientists who study training effects on adults (Brooks, Fahey, & White, 1996, p. 414) and children (Rowland, 2005, p. 198). While there are exceptions, the manner in which a child's somatic system and peripheral nervous system respond to the demands of exercise training does not differ qualitatively from that of adults (see Rowland, 2005, Chapter 11). The results of studies conducted with both adults and children show that aerobic training leads to improvements in cardiorespiratory function, anaerobic training leads to improvements in muscle recruitment and speed of muscular contraction, and resistance training leads to increases in strength and power. The magnitude of children's gains in these outcomes, however, may differ from that seen in adults due to differences in maturational factors (e.g., hormone availability). Of interest for the present chapter are explanations concerning how exercise training might alter metabolic processes, structures, or functions in the brain that underlie mental processing and intelligent behavior.

At a basic level, any changes in brain cells that occur in association with exercise training are the result of gene activation that leads to phenotypic expression. To explain adequately the linkage between an exercise stimulus and associated changes in the characteristics of somatic cells (e.g., hypertrophy of muscle), mechanisms that link the repeated contraction of muscles to gene action and link gene action to phenotypic expression need to be identified. As shown in a model developed by Rowland (2005, p. 199) to describe the causal pathway between exercise training and change in somatic systems (Figure 20.2), a mediator is responsible for the link between repetitive muscle contraction and gene action, then another mediator is responsible for phenotypic expression and change in a physiologic function (e.g., increased protein synthesis or augmented neural activity). The results of exercise are specific to the type of training stimulus.

Similar causal pathways have been proposed between exercise training and phenotypic changes of cells in the central nervous system (Dishman

et al., 2006; van Praag, 2009; Vaynman & Gomez-Pinilla, 2006). B. J. Anderson, McCloskey, Tata, and Gorby(2003) hypothesize that the structures and functions of the brain are influenced selectively by the production of physical movement and the sensory feedback derived. Using results from studies conducted with animals, Anderson identified three brain structures that are influenced selectively by exercise: the cerebellum, motor cortex, and hippocampus. Structures within the rodent cerebellum are influenced by exercise training; however, the manner in which the cerebellum responds depends on the type of physical activity performed. Running, for example, which engages large muscles, leads to increased capillary growth in the cerebellum, whereas small-limb actions that are used to climb and maintain balance result in neuronal adaptations and long-lasting structural cerebellar adaptations. The motor cortex plays a fundamental role in both voluntary and reflexive movements. There is a somatotopic mapping of areas of the motor cortex to the skeletal system, and information coming from these areas of the cortex provides basic commands for physical movement. Specific areas of the motor cortex are highly active metabolically during physical activity and the execution of skilled behaviors. Routine running in rats leads to increased tissue volume in the motor cortex, suggesting increases in the number of neuronal synapses in activated cells (B. J. Anderson, Eckburg, & Relucio, 2002). The hippocampus is involved in memory, learning, and movement. Study of cell activation in the hippocampus reveals that the structure plays a role in initiating and coding locomotor movements (Wallace, Hines, & Whishaw, 2002). Hippocampal coding processes, in conjunction with information concerning the spatial location of objects, appear to be responsible for place learning, as numerous studies have found that rats engaged in running training are better than untrained animals in learning and remembering the spatial locations of objects (Vaynman & Gomez-Pinilla, 2006). In humans, the hippocampus plays a pivotal role in relational learning and the encoding of information into long-term memory stores (Erikson et al., 1998).

B. J. Anderson and colleagues' review of the results of animal research led them to propose that exercise selectively influences specific brain structures and processes. The evidence suggests, for example, that aerobic exercise would be expected to affect brain structures and processes differently from anaerobic exercise. Further, physical activity

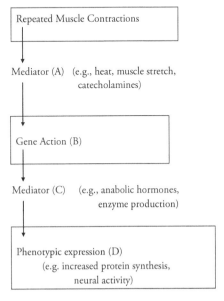

Figure 20.2. A causal pathway between exercise training and changes in somatic systems. Reproduced with permission from *Children's Developmental Physiology*, by T. W. Rowland, 2005, Champaign, IL: Human Kinetics, p. 199.

performed in a complex environment or as part of skilled behavior (e.g., game or sport), would be predicted to affect the brain differently from repetitive activity performed in relative isolation (e.g., treadmill running). While these predictions are based on animal models, if they are accurate, it is all the more important for researchers to examine closely the types of exercise activities employed to study the relationship between exercise and intelligence or cognition.

More recently, a number of experts in exercise psychology, neuropsychology, and motor learning drafted a position statement addressing how exercise might have a neuroprotective effect on the brain (Dishman et al., 2006). They proposed a comprehensive model of possible pathways between exercise and brain structures linked to learning, memory, and adaptive behaviors (see Figure 20.3). Based on that committee's review, exercise should be viewed

as a robust physical stimulus that affects multiple brain structures at the cellular level.

A lack of a detailed description of the exercise intervention employed is common among the studies reviewed above, as well as to most experiments that have assessed effects of chronic exercise treatments on mental function. As a result, it remains unclear whether the results obtained were due exclusively to the types of physical activities performed, the skills that were developed during training, or the social context of the planned exercise programs. Likewise, few studies have provided sufficient information concerning control conditions. Two exceptions to the general rule were the experiments conducted by Corder (1966) and Rarick, Dobbins, and Broadhead (1976), who employed active control group conditions designed to involve the same amount of time and attention as training groups. In both studies, IQ scores increased significantly

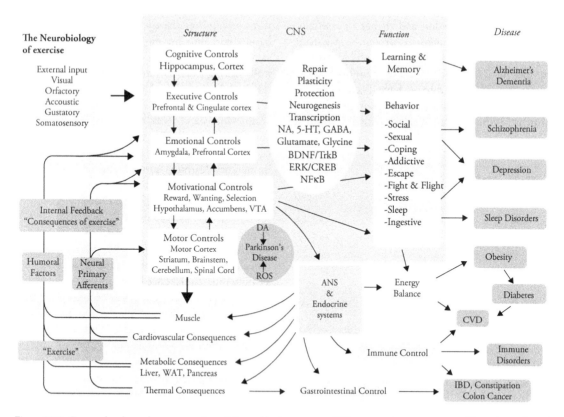

Figure 20.3. Proposed pathways between exercise training and brain structure. ANS, autonomic nervous system; BDNF, brain-derived neurotrophic factor; CNS, central nervous system; CREB, cyclic monophosphate response element–binding protein; CVD, cardiovascular disease; DA, dopamine, ERK, extracellular signal-regulated kinase; 5-HT, 5-hydroxytryptamine; GABA, gamma-aminobutyric acid; IBD, inflammatory bowel disease; NA, noradrenaline; NFκB, nuclear factor kappaB; ROS, reactive oxygen species; TrkB, tyrosine residue kinase receptor-type 2; VTA, ventral tegmental area; WAT, white adipose tissue. Reprinted by permission from "Neurobiology of Exercise," by R. K. Dishman, H.-R. Berthound, F. W. Booth, C. W. Cotman, R. Edgerton, M. R. Fleshner, . . . Zigmond, M. J., 2006, *Obesity, 14*(3), 345–356. Copyright 2006 by Macmillan Publishers Ltd.

for children in both the exercise training condition and the active control condition, suggesting gains due to the Hawthorne effect. Experiments that are designed to separate the effects of exercise training from psychosocial factors are encouraged. Improved research designs that include precise control of the exercise training methods are needed if we are to understand how exercise might modify children's mental functioning.

MEASUREMENT METHODOLOGIES

Psychometrists have created a wide variety of standardized tests that provide global and specific indices of mental abilities (e.g., verbal, quantitative, nonverbal, memory, and reasoning) and cognitive processes (e.g., planning, attention, simultaneous, and successive) (Flanagan & Harrison, 2005; Naglieri & Goldstein, 2009). Most of the studies that have assessed the effects of exercise training on children's mental function have employed tests that essentially measure general intelligence using tests with verbal, nonverbal, quantitative, memory, and speed requirements. It is plausible that exercise training may not influence ability as measured by these general intelligence tests because they do not measure cognitive processes. The only mental tests that do appear to be sensitive to exercise training interventions are those that measure mental processes involved in executive function (e.g., planning on the CAS), which are not measured by tests of general intelligence and underlie flexible, goal-directed behavior(Davis et al., 2007, 2011; Hinkle et al., 1993; Tuckman & Hinkle, 1986).

It may be the case that exercise training in children selectively affects executive processes. This speculation is supported by the results obtained by Davis and her colleagues (2007, 2011), who observed that exercise training resulted in improved performance on the Planning scale of the CAS but not on other subscales. The Planning scale measures strategy generation and application, self-regulation, self-correction, intentionality, and use of knowledge. Future research designed to advance our understanding of the exercise–intelligence relationship will clearly benefit from the selection of appropriate theory-based measures of children's cognitive processing abilities.

Conclusion and Future Directions

The favorable effects of physical activity and exercise on children's physiological functions are well established. The assumption that exercise effects change in children's intelligence, defined in terms of performance on traditional intelligence tests, has yet to be verified, though research indicating effects of exercise on intelligence when it is operationalized with a cognitive processing approach that includes measures of executive function holds promise. The lack of confirmatory data may be due to several factors. First, few well-designed experiments have been conducted to assess the exercise–intelligence relation. Compounding the lack of an adequately sized literature from which to draw conclusions are methodological differences among the published studies. Exercise interventions have varied considerably, with some being based on physical education models and others focusing on skill training, strength, or aerobic programs. Likewise, a wide assortment of measures has been used in these studies, ranging from standardized intelligence tests to laboratory-based component process measures. Evidence from a limited number of studies suggests that chronic exercise training may influence specific aspects of cognitive function and that the relation is strongest when composite measures of mental performance are employed. However, additional theory-based research will be needed to elucidate this hypothesized relation.

Several experiments recently conducted with older adults indicate that routine exercise changes brain structure and function and may offset age-related declines in some cognitive functions. While it is tempting to generalize the results obtained with older adults to children, changes in the brain during older adulthood may differ significantly from changes during early development. It is imperative for researchers to examine closely how maturational factors may influence how exercise may affect brain development and alter mental functioning. There has been a long-standing interest in the cognitive benefits of enriched environments, and considerable data supporting the salutary effects of physical activity have been gathered via animal models. While it remains plausible that exercise benefits children's mental development and intelligence, additional well-designed studies conducted with children and adolescents are warranted.

References

Ackerman, P. L., & Kyllonen, P. C. (1991). Trainee characteristics. In J. E. Morrison (Ed.), *Training for performance: Principles of applied human learning* (pp. 193–229). New York: John Wiley & Sons.

Adolph, K. E. (2008). Learning to move. *Current Directions in Psychological Science, 17*(3), 213–218.

Anderson, B. J., Eckburg, P. B., & Relucio, K. I. (2002). Alterations in the thickness of motor cortical subregions after motor-skill learning and exercise. *Learning and Memory,* *9*, 1–19.

Anderson, B. J., McCloskey, D. P., Tata, D. A., & Gorby, H. E. (2003). Physiological psychology: Biological and behavioral outcomes of exercise. In S. F. Davis (Ed.), *Handbook of research methods in experimental psychology* (pp. 323–345). Malden, MA: Blackwell.

Anderson, J. R. (1983). *The architecture of cognition.* Cambridge, MA: Harvard University Press.

Baddeley, A. D. (1986). *Working memory.* New York: Oxford University Press.

Baddeley, A. D., Emslie, A., Kolodny, J., & Duncan, J. (1998). Random generation and the executive control of working memory. *Quarterly Journal of Experimental Psychology,* *51A*(4), 819–852.

Banich, M. T. (2009). Executive function: The search for an integrated account. *Current Directions in Psychological Science,* *18*(2), 89–94.

Barde, Y. A. (1989). Trophic factors and neuronal survival. *Neuron, 2*, 1525–1534.

Borkowski, J. H., Carr, M., & Pressely, M. (1987). "Spontaneous" strategy use: Perspectives from metacognitive theory. *Intelligence, 11*, 61–75.

Brocki, K. C., & Bohlin, G. (2004). Executive functions in children aged 6 to 13: A dimensional and developmental study. *Developmental Neuropsychology, 26*(2), 571–593.

Broglio, S. P., Ferrara, M. S., Macciocchi, S. N., Baumgartner, T. A., & Elliott, M. D. (2007). Test–retest reliability of computerized concussion assessment programs. *Journal of Athletic Training, 42*(4), 509–514.

Brooks, G. A., Fahey, T. D., & White, T. P. (1996). *Exercise physiology* (2nd ed.). Mountain View, CA: Mayfield.

Brown, B. J. (1967). The effect of an isometric strength program on the intellectual and social development of trainable retarded males. *American Corrective Therapy Journal, 31*, 44–48.

Bunge, S. A., & Wright, S. B. (2007). Neurodevelopmental changes in working memory and cognitive control. *Current Opinion in Neurobiology, 17*, 243–250.

Cambridge Cognition (2011). http://www.cambridgecognition.com

Campbell, D. W., Eaton, W. O., & McKeen, N. A. (2002). Motor activity level and behavioural control in young children. *International Journal of Behavioral Development, 26*(4), 289–296.

Carmichael, M. (2007, March 26). Stronger, faster, smarter. *Newsweek, CXLIX,* 38–55.

Carroll, J. B. (1976). Psychometric tests as cognitive tasks: A new "structure of intellect." In L. B. Resnick (Ed.), *The nature of intelligence* (pp. 27–56). New York: Lawrence Erlbaum.

Carroll, J. B. (1993). *Human cognitive abilities.* Cambridge, UK: Cambridge University Press.

Casey, B. J., Amso, D., & Davidson, M. C. (2006). Learning about learning and development with modern imaging technology. In Y. Munakata & M. H. Johnson (Eds.), *Attention and performance XXI: Processes of change in brain and cognitive development* (pp. 513–533). Oxford: Oxford University Press.

Cattell, R. B. (1943). The measurement of adult intelligence. *Psychological Bulletin, 40*, 153–193.

Corder, W. O. (1966). Effects of physical education on the intellectual, physical, and social development of educable mentally retarded boys. *Exceptional Children, 32*, 357–364.

Craik, F. I., & Bialystok, E. (2007). On structure and process in lifespan cognitive development. In F. I. Craik (Ed.), *Lifespan cognition: Mechanisms of change* (pp. 3–14). Oxford: Oxford University Press.

Das, J. P. (1999). A neo-Lurian approach to assessment and remediation. *Neuropsychology Review, 9*(2), 107–116.

Das, J. P. (2003). A look at intelligence as cognitive neuropsychological processes: Is Luria still relevant? *Japanese Journal of Special Education, 40*, 631–647.

Davis, C. L., Tomporowski, P. D., Boyle, C. A., Waller, J. L., Miller, P. H., Naglieri, J. A., ... Gregoski, M. . (2007). Effects of aerobic exercise on overweight children's cognitive functioning: A randomized controlled trial. *Research Quarterly for Exercise and Sport, 78*(5), 510–519.

Davis, C. L., Tomporowski, P. D., McDowell, J. E., Austin, B. P., Yanasak, N. E., Allison, J. D., ... Miller, P. H. (2011). Exercise improves executive function and academics and alters neural activation in overweight children: A randomized controlled trial. *Health Psychology, 30*(1), 91–98.

deHaan, M., & Johnson, M. H. (2003). Mechanisms and theories of brain development. In M. de Haan & M. H. Johnson (Eds.), *The cognitive neuroscience of development* (pp. 1–18). New York: Psychology Press.

Detterman, D. K. (1986). Human intelligence is a complex system of separate processes. In R. J. Sternberg & D. K. Detterman (Eds.), *What is intelligence? Contemporary viewpoints on its nature and definition* (pp. 57–61). Norwood, NJ: Ablex.

Detterman, D. K., Mayer, J. D., Caruso, D. R., Legree, P. J., Conners, F. A., & Taylor, R. (1992). Assessment of basic cognitive abilities in relation to cognitive deficits. *American Journal on Mental Retardation, 97*, 251–286.

Diamond, A. (2000). Close interrelation of motor development and cognitive development and of the cerebellum and prefrontal cortex. *Child Development, 71*(1), 44–56.

Diamond, A. (2002). Normal development of prefrontal cortex from birth to young adulthood: Cognitive functions, anatomy, and biochemistry. In D. T. Stuss & R. T. Knight (Eds.), *Principles of frontal lobe function* (pp. 466–503). New York: Oxford University Press.

Diamond, A. (2006). Bootstrapping conceptual deduction using physical connection: Rethinking frontal cortex. *Trends in Cognitive Sciences, 10*(5), 212–218.

Diamond, A. (2009). The interplay of biology and environment broadly defined. *Developmental Psychology, 45*(1), 1–8.

Diamond, A., Barnett, W. S., Thomas, J. R., & Munro, S. (2007). Preschool program improves cognitive control. *Science, 318*, 1387–1388.

Dishman, R. K. (1997). Brain monoamines, exercise, and behavioral stress: Animal models. *Medicine & Science in Sports & Exercise, 29*(1), 63–74.

Dishman, R. K., Berthound, H.-R., Booth, F. W., Cotman, C. W., Edgerton, R., Fleshner, M. R., ... Zigmond, M. J. (2006). Neurobiology of exercise. *Obesity, 14*(3), 345–356.

Ellis, N. R., & Cavalier, A. R. (1982). Research perspectives in mental retardation. In E. Zigler & D. Balla (Eds.), *Mental retardation: The developmental-difference controversy.* (pp. 121–154) Hillsdale, NJ: Lawrence Erlbaum.

Erikson, P. S., Perfilieva, E., Bjork-Eriksson, T., Alborn, A. M., Nordberg, C., Perterson, D. A., & Gage, F. H. (1998). Neurogenesis in the adult human hippocampus. *Nature Medicine, 4*, 1313-1317.

Erlanger, D. M., Feldman, D., & Kutner, K. C. (2003). Development and validation of a web-based neuropsychological test protocol for sports-related return-to-play decision-making. *Archives of Clinical Neuropsychology, 18*, 293–316.

Etnier, J. L., & Chang, Y.-K. (2009). The effect of physical activity on executive function: A brief commentary on definitions, measurement issues, and the current state of the literature. *Journal of Sport & Exercise Psychology, 31*, 469–483.

Etnier, J. L., Nowell, P. M., Landers, D. M., & Sibley, B. A. (2006). A meta-regression to examine the relationship between aerobic fitness and cognitive performance. *Brain Research Reviews, 52*, 119–130.

Flanagan, D. P., & Harrison, P. L. (Eds.) (2005). *Contemporary intellectual assessment: Theories, tests, and issues* (2nd ed.). New York: Guilford Press.

Flavell, J. H. (1979). Metacognition and cognitive monitoring: A new area of cognitive-developmental inquiry. *American Psychologist, 34*, 906–911.

Floyd, R. G. (2005). Information-processing approaches to interpretation of contemporary intellectual assessment instruments. In D. P. Flanagan & P. L. Harrison (Eds.), *Contemporary intellectual assessment* (2nd ed., pp. 203–233). New York: Guilford Press.

Foschi, R., & Cicciola, E. (2006). Politics and naturalism in the 20th century psychology of Alfred Binet. *History of Psychology, 9*(4), 267–289.

French, J. W., Ekstrom, R. B., & Price, L. A. (1963). *Manual and kit of reference tests for cognitive factors*. Princeton, NJ: Educational Testing Service.

Frye, D., Zelazo, P. D., & Burack, J. A. (1998). Cognitive complexity and control: I. Theory of mind in typical and atypical development. *Current Directions in Psychological Science, 7*(4), 116–121.

Gabbard, C. P. (2004). *Lifelong motor development* (4th ed.). New York: Pearson.

Gage, F. H., van Praag, H., & Kempermann, G. (2000). Neural consequences of environmental enrichment. *Nature Reviews Neuroscience, 1*(3), 191–198.

Gallese, V., & Metzinger, T. (2003). Motor ontology: The representational reality of goals, action and selves. *Philosophical Psychology, 16*(3), 365–388.

Gesell, A. (1925). *The mental growth of the preschool child*. New York: Macmillan.

Gogtay, N., Giedd, J. N., Lusk, L., Hayashi, K. M., Greenstein, D., Vaituzis, A. C.,...Thompson, P. M. (2004). Dynamic mapping of human cortical development during childhood through early adulthood. *Proceedings of the National Academy of Sciences of the United States of America, 101*, 8174–8179.

Haddad, F. A., Garcia, Y. E., Naglieri, J. A., Grimditch, M., McAndrews, A., & Eubanks, J. (2003). Planning facilitation and reading comprehension: Instructional relevance of the PASS theory. *Journal of Psychoeducational Assessment, 21*, 282–289.

Hall, J. L., Thomas, K. M., & Everitt, B. J. (2000). Rapid and selective induction of BDNF in AD: Expression in the hippocampus during contextual learning. *Nature Neuroscience, 3*, 533–535.

Havighurst, R. J. (1972). *Developmental tasks and education* (3rd ed.). New York: David McKay.

Hertzog, C., Kramer, A. F., Wilson, R. S., & Lindenberger, U. (2009). Enrichment effects on adult cognitive development. *Psychological Science in the Public Interest, 9*(1), 1–65.

Hinkle, J. S., Tuckman, B. W., & Sampson, J. P. (1993). The psychology, physiology, and creativity of middle school aerobic exercisers. *Elementary School Guidance & Counseling, 28*(2), 133–145.

Horn, J. L., & Cattell, R. B. (1966). Refinement and test of the theory of fluid and crystallized general intelligence. *Journal of Educational Psychology, 57*(5), 253–270.

Hughes, F. P. (1995). *Child, play and development*. Boston: Allyn and Bacon.

Huizinga, M. M. (2006). Age-related change in executive function: Developmental trends and a latent variable analysis. *Neuropsychologia, 44*(11), 2017–2036.

Hunt, E. B., Frost, N., & Lunneborg, C. (1973). Individual differences in cognition: A new approach to intelligence. In G. Bower (Ed.), *The psychology of learning and motivation: Advances in research and theory* (Vol. 7, pp. 87–122). New York: Academic Press.

International Life Sciences Institute. (2003). *Childhood obesity—advancing prevention and treatment: An overview for health professionals*. Washington, DC: International Life Sciences Institute.

Iseman, J. S., & Naglieri, J. A. (2011). A cognitive strategy instruction to improve math calculation for children with ADHD: A randomized controlled study. *Journal of Learning Disabilities. 44*, 184–195.

Ismail, A. H. (1967). The effects of a well-organized physical education programme on intellectual performance. *Research in Physical Education, 1*, 31–38.

Jackson, P. L., & Decety, J. (2004). Motor cognition: A new paradigm to study self–other interactions. *Current Opinion in Neurobiology, 14*, 259–263.

Jaeggi, S. M., Buschkuehl, M., Jonides, J., & Perrig, W. (2008). Improving fluid intelligence with training on working memory. *Proceedings of the National Academy of Sciences of the United States of America, 105*, 6829–6833. doi:10.1073/pnas.0801268105

Jensen, A. R. (2006). *Clocking the mind: Mental chronometry and individual differences*. Boston: Elsevier.

Johnson, J. E., Christie, J. F., & Yawkey, T. D. (1987). *Play and early childhood development*. Glenview, IL: Scott, Foresman.

Karmiloff-Smith, A. (2009). Nativism versus neuroconstructivism: Rethinking the study of developmental disorders. *Developmental Psychology, 45*(1), 56–63.

Kramer, A. F., & Erickson, K. I. (2007). Capitalizing on cortical plasticity: Influence of physical activity on cognition and brain function. *Trends in Cognitive Sciences, 11*(8), 342–348.

Kramer, A. F., Hahn, S., McAuley, E., Cohen, N. J., Banich, M. T., & Harrison, C., R. (2002). Exercise, aging, and cognition: Healthy body, healthy mind? In W. A. Rogers & A. D. Fisk (Eds.), *Human factors interventions for the health care of older adults* (pp. 91–120). Mahwah, NJ: Erlbaum.

Lambourne, K., & Tomporowski, P. D. (2010). The effect of acute exercise on cognitive task performance: A meta-regression analysis. *Brain Research Reviews, 1341*, 12–24.

Lebel, C., Walker, L., Leemans, A., Phillips, L., & Beaulieu, C. (2008). Microstructural maturation of the human brain from childhood to adulthood. *NeuroImage, 40*, 1044–1055.

Levi-Montalcini, R. (1987). The nerve growth factor: Thirty-five years later. *Science, 237*, 1154–1162.

Lezak, M. D., Howieson, D. B., & Loring, D. W. (2004). *Neuropsychological assessment* (4th ed.). New York: Oxford University Press.

Llinas, R. (2001). *I of the vortex: From neurons to self*. Cambridge, MA: MIT Press.

Lovell, M. R., Collins, M. W., Podell, K., Powell, J., & Maroon, J. (2000). ImPACT: Immediate Post-Concussion Assessment and Cognitive Testing Software. Pittsburgh, PA: Neuro Health Systems.

Luciana, M. (2003). Practitioner review: Computerized assessment of neuropsychological function in children: Clinical and research applications of the Cambridge Neuropsychological Testing Automated Battery (CANTAB). *Journal of Child Psychology and Psychiatry, 44*(5), 649–663.

Miyake, A., Friedman, N. P., Emerson, M. J., Witzki, A. H., Howerter, A., & Wager, T. D. (2000). The unity and diversity of executive functions and their contributions to complex "frontal lobe" tasks: A latent variable analysis. *Cognitive Psychology, 41*, 49–100.

Miyake, A., & Shah, P. (1999). Toward unified theories of working memory. In A. Miyake & P. Shah (Eds.), *Models of working memory* (pp. 442 481). Cambridge, UK: Cambridge University Press.

Molteni, R., Barnard, R. J., Ying, Z., Roberts, K., & Gomez-Pinilla, F. (2002). A high-fat, refined sugar diet reduces hippocampal brain-derived neurotrophic factor, neuronal plasticity, and learning. *Neuroscience, 112*(4), 803–814.

Molteni, R., Wu, A., Vaynman, S., Ying, Z., Barnard, R. J., & Gomez-Pinilla, F. (2004). Exercise reverses the harmful effects of consumption of a high-fat diet on synaptic and behavioral plasticity associated to the action of brain-derived neurotrophic factor. *Neuroscience, 123*, 429–440.

Monsell, S., & Driver, J. (Eds.). (2000). *Attention and performance XVIII: Control of cognitive processes*. Cambridge, MA: MIT Press.

Naglieri, J. A. (2005). The Cognitive Assessment System. In D. P. Flanagan & P. L. Harrison (Eds.), *Contemporary intellectual assessment: Theories, tests, and issues* (2nd ed., pp. 441–460). New York: Guilford Press.

Naglieri, J. A., & Conway, C. (2009). The Cognitive Assessment System. In J. A. Naglieri & S. Goldstein (Eds.), *A practitioner's guide to assessment of intelligence and achievement* (pp. 3–10). New York: Wiley.

Naglieri, J. A., & Das, J. P. (1997). *Cognitive Assessment System*. Itasca, IL: Riverside.

Naglieri, J. A., & Das, J. P. (2005). Planning, attention, simultaneous, successive (PASS) theory. In D. P. Flanagan & P. L. Harrison (Eds.), *Contemporary intellectual assessment: Theories, tests, and issues* (2nd ed., pp. 120–135). New York: Guilford Press.

Naglieri, J. A., & Goldstein, S. (Eds.) (2009). *A practitioner's guide to assessment of intelligence and achievement*. New York: Wiley.

Naglieri, J. A., & Gottling, S. H. (1995). A cognitive education approach to math instruction for the learning disabled: An individual study. *Psychological Reports, 76*, 1343–1354.

Naglieri, J. A., & Gottling, S. H. (1997). Mathematics instruction and PASS cognitive processes: An intervention study. *Journal of Learning Disabilities, 30*, 513–520.

Naglieri, J. A., & Johnson, D. (2000). Effectiveness of a cognitive strategy intervention to improve math calculation based on the PASS theory. *Journal of Learning Disabilities, 33*, 591–597.

Naglieri, J. A., & Kaufman, A. S. (2008). IDEIA 2004 and specific learning disabilities: What role does intelligence play? In E. Grigorenko (Ed.), *Educating individuals with disabilities: IDEIA 2004 and beyond* (pp. 165–195). New York: Springer.

Naglieri, J. A., & Rojahn, J. R. (2004). Validity of the PASS Theory and CAS: Correlations with achievement. *Journal of Educational Psychology, 96*, 174–181

National Association for Sport and Physical Education. (2009). *National standards and guidelines for physical education teacher education* (3rd ed.). Reston, VA: National Association for Sport and Physical Education.

Nelson, C. A., de Haan, E. H. F., & Thomas, K., M. (2006). *Neuroscience of cognitive development*. Hoboken, NJ: John Wiley & Sons.

Nettelbeck, T., & Wilson, C. (1997). Speed of information processing and cognition. In W. E. MacLean, Jr. (Ed.), *Ellis' handbook of mental deficiency, psychological theory and research* (pp. 245–274). Mahwah, NJ: Lawrence Erlbaum.

Oliver, J. N. (1958). The effect of physical conditioning exercises and activities on the mental characteristics of educationally sub-normal boys. *British Journal of Educational Psychology, 28*, 155–165.

Panksepp, J. (1998). A critical analysis of ADHD, psychostimulants, and intolerance of child impassivity: A national tragedy in the making? *Current Directions in Psychological Sciences, 7*, 91–98.

Panksepp, J., Siviy, S., & Normansell, L. A. (1984). The biology of play: Theoretical and methodological perspectives. *Neuroscience and Biobehavioral Reviews, 8*, 465–492.

Pascual-Leone, A., Amedi, A., Fregni, F., & Merabet, L. B. (2005). The plastic human brain cortex. *Annual Review of Neuroscience, 28*, 377–401.

Pellis, S. M., & Pellis, V. C. (2007). Rough-and-tumble play and the development of the social brain. *Current Directions in Psychological Science, 16*(2), 95–98.

Persson, J., & Reuter-Lorenz, P. (2008). Gaining control: Training executive function and far transfer of the ability to resolve interference. *Psychological Science, 19*(9), 881–888.

Piaget, J. (1963). *The origins of intelligence in children* (M. Cook, Trans.). New York: W. W. Norton.

Posner, M. I., & Dahaene, S. (1994). Attentional networks. *Trends in Neurosciences, 17*, 75–79.

Posner, M. I., & Rothbart, M. K. (2007). *Educating the human brain*. Washington, DC: American Psychological Association.

Posner, M. I., Sheese, B. E., Odludas, Y., & Tang, Y. Y. (2006). Analyzing and shaping human attentional networks. *Neural Networks, 19*, 1422–1429.

Ramey, C. T., & Ramey, S. H. (2004). Early educational interventions and intelligence. In E. Zigler & S. J. Styfco (Eds.), *The Head Start debate* (pp. 3–17). Baltimore, MD: Paul H. Brooks.

Rarick, G. L., Dobbins, D. A., & Broadhead, G. D. (1976). *The motor domain and its correlates in educationally handicapped children*. Englewood Cliffs, NJ: Prentice Hall.

Ratey, J. J., & Hagerman, E. (2008). *Spark: The revolutionary new science of exercise and the brain*. New York: Little, Brown.

Rowland, T. W. (2005). *Children's developmental physiology*. Champaign, IL: Human Kinetics.

Rueda, M. R., Rothbart, M. K., McCandliss, B. D., Saccomanno, L., & Posner, M. I. (2005). Training, maturation, and genetic influences on the development of executive attention. *Proceedings of the National Academy of Sciences of the United States of America, 102*(41), 14931–14936.

Schatz, P., & Putz, B. O. (2006). Cross-validation of measures used for computer-based assessment of concussion. *Applied Neuropsychology, 13*(3), 151–159.

Sibley, B. A., & Etnier, J. L. (2003). The relationship between physical activity and cognition in children: A meta-analysis. *Pediatric Exercise Science, 15*, 243–256.

Sommerville, J. A., & Decety, J. (2006). Weaving the fabric of social interaction: Articulating developmental psychology and cognitive neuroscience in the domain of motor cognition. *Psychonomic Bulletin & Review, 13*(2), 179–200.

Spencer, J. P., Clearfield, M., Corbetta, D., Ulrich, B., Buchanan, P., & Schoner, G. (2006). Moving toward a grand theory of development: In memory of Ester Thelen. *Child Development, 77*(6), 1521–1538.

Stern, W. (1930). *Psychology of early childhood up to the sixth year of age.* New York: Holt.

Sternberg, R. J. (1977). *Intelligence, information processing, and analogical reasoning: The componential analysis of human abilities.* Hillsdale, NJ: Erlbaum.

Sternberg, R. J. (1985). *Beyond IQ: A triarchic theory of human intelligence.* Cambridge, UK: Cambridge University Press.

Sternberg, R. J. (2005). The triarchic theory of successful intelligence. In D. P. Flanagan & P. L. Harrison (Eds.), *Contemporary intellectual assessment: Theories, tests, and issues* (2nd ed., pp. 103–135). New York: Guilford Press.

Sternberg, S. (1969). Memory-scanning: Mental processes revealed by reaction time experiments. *American Scientist, 57*, 421–457.

Stockman, I. J. (2004). A theoretical framework for clinical intervention with pervasive developmental disorders. In I. J. Stockman (Ed.), *Movement and action in learning and development: Clinical implications for pervasive developmental disorders* (pp. 21–31). New York: Elsevier.

Taylor, M. J. (2006). Neural bases of cognitive development. In E. Bialystok & F. I. Craik (Eds.), *Lifespan cognition: Mechanisms of change* (pp. 15–26). Oxford: Oxford University Press.

Thelen, E. (1996). Motor development. *American Psychologist, 50*(2), 79–95.

Thelen, E. (2004). The central role of action in typical and atypical development: A dynamical systems perspective. In I. J. Stockman (Ed.), *Movement and action in learning and development: Clinical implications for pervasive developmental disorders* (pp. 49–74). New York: Elsevier.

Thelen, E., & Smith, L. B. (1994). *A dynamic systems approach to the development of cognition and action.* Cambridge, MA: MIT Press.

Tombaught, T. N. (2006). A comprehensive review of the Paced Auditory Serial Addition Task (PASAT). *Archives of Clinical Neuropsychology, 21*, 53–76.

Tomporowski, P. D. (2009). Methodological issues: Research approaches, research design, and task selection. In T. McMorris, P. D. Tomporowski, & M. Audiffren (Eds.), *Exercise and cognitive function* (pp. 91–112). Chichester, UK: John Wiley & Sons.

Tomporowski, P. D., & Ellis, N. R. (1984). Effects of exercise on the physical fitness, intelligence and adaptive behavior of institutionalized mentally retarded adults. *Applied Research in Mental Retardation, 5*, 329–337.

Tomporowski, P. D., & Ellis, N. R. (1985). The effects of exercise training on the health, intelligence, and adaptive behavior of institutionalized mentally retarded adults: A systematic replication. *Applied Research in Mental Retardation, 6*, 456–473.

Tuckman, B. W., & Hinkle, J. S. (1986). An experimental study of the physical and psychological effects of aerobic exercise on schoolchildren. *Health Psychology, 5*(3), 197–207.

Underwood, B. J. (1957). *Psychological research.* New York: Appleton-Century-Crofts.

Vandierendonck, A. (2000). Executive functions and task switching. *Psychologica Belgica, 40*(4), 211–226.

vanPraag, H. (2009). Exercise and the brain: Something to chew on. *Trends in Neurosciences, 32*(5), 283–290.

Vaynman, S., & Gomez-Pinilla, F. (2006). Revenge of the "sit": How lifestyle impacts neuronal and cognitive health through molecular systems that interface energy metabolism with neuronal plasticity. *Journal of Neuroscience Research, 84*, 699–715.

Vaynman, S., Ying, Z., & Gomez-Pinilla, F. (2004). Hippocampal BDNF mediates the efficacy of exercise on synaptic plasticity and cognition. *European Journal of Neuroscience, 20*, 2580–2590.

Wallace, D. G., Hines, D. J., & Whishaw, I. Q. (2002). Quantification of a single exploratory trip reveals hippocampal formation mediated dead reckoning. *Journal of Neuroscience Methods, 113*(2), 131–145.

Wasserman, J. D., & Tulsky, D. S. (2005). A history of intelligence assessment. In D. P. Flanagan & P. L. Harrison (Eds.), *Contemporary intellectual assessment: Theories, tests, and issues* (2nd ed., pp. 3–22). New York: Guilford Press.

Wechsler, D. (1941). *The Wechsler Intelligence Scale for Children.* New York: The Psychological Corporation.

Wechsler, D. (1991a). *Manual for the Wechsler Intelligence Scale for Children* (3rd ed.). New York: The Psychological Corporation.

Wechsler, D. (1991b). *Manual for the Wechsler Intelligence Scale for Children—Revised.* New York: The Psychological Corporation.

Wechsler, D. (2003). *Manual for the Wechsler Intelligence Scale for Children* (4th ed.). New York: The Psychological Corporation.

Wilson, M. (2002). Six views of embodied cognition. *Psychonomic Bulletin & Review, 9*(4), 625–636.

Zelazo, P. D., & Frye, D. (1998). Cognitive complexity and control: II. The development of executive function in children. *Current Directions in Psychological Science, 7*(4), 121–126.

Zervas, Y., Apostolos, D., & Klissouras, V. (1991). Influence of physical exertion on mental performance with reference to training. *Perceptual and Motor Skills, 72*, 1215–1221.

Zigler, E., & Styfco, S. J. (Eds.) (2004). *The Head Start debate.* Baltimore, MD: Paul H. Brooks.

Cancer Patients

Amy E. Speed-Andrews *and* Kerry S. Courneya

Abstract

The National Cancer Institute estimates there are over 11 million cancer survivors in the U.S. Side effects of cancer and its treatment can undermine quality of life and increase risk of developing secondary cancers and other chronic diseases. Many chronic and late effects of cancer treatments align themselves with the known benefits of physical activity in other medical and nonmedical populations. The purpose of this chapter is to provide an overview of current research on physical activity (PA) in cancer survivors. We divide the chapter into (1) PA studies focusing on health outcomes and (2) behavior change. Accumulating evidence suggests that PA can improve supportive care health outcomes and promote short-term behavior change in select groups of cancer survivors. Many important research questions remain.

Key Words: physical activity, cancer, survivor, quality of life, supportive care, health outcomes, behavior change.

Cancer is a global problem. Worldwide, cancer causes more deaths than AIDS, tuberculosis, and malaria combined (American Cancer Society [ACS], 2007). Cancer is the second leading cause of death in the U.S., surpassed only by heart disease (ACS, 2009a). It is anticipated that in 2009, 562,340 individuals in the U.S. will die from cancer, equating to more than 1,500 cancer deaths per day (ACS, 2009a). Lung cancer is the leading cause of death by cancer in both men (28.3%) and women (26.3%), followed by colorectal and prostate cancers for men, and breast and colorectal cancer for women (ACS, 2009a). Approximately 1.5 million new cases of cancer were expected to be diagnosed in 2009, and this figure was anticipated to increase in subsequent years as a result of a growing and aging population (ACS, 2009a). Anyone can develop cancer. In the U.S., the probability that one will develop some form of cancer in one's lifetime is 1 in 2 for men and 1 in 3 for women (ACS, 2009a). The risk of

diagnosis increases as individuals age, with 77% of cases diagnosed in individuals who are 55 and older (ACS, 2009a).

Nevertheless, improvements in cancer detection and treatment have resulted in improvements in survival rates. The five-year relative survival rate for all cancers increased from 50% in 1975–1977 to 66% to 1996–2004. The National Coalition for Cancer Survivorship (1994–2004) defines *cancer survivor* as "any individual that has been diagnosed with cancer, from the time of discovery and for the balance of life." The National Cancer Institute estimates that there are more than 11 million cancer survivors in the U.S., more than three times the number in 1970 (ACS, 2009a). As the survivor population continues to grow, it is increasingly important to address the unique health needs of cancer survivors. A growing body of evidence suggests that physical activity (PA) can improve supportive care health outcomes and promote short-term behavior change in select groups of cancer survivors.

The purpose of this chapter is to provide an overview of the latest research on PA in cancer survivors. We divide the chapter into two main sections (1) on research examining health outcomes and (2) research examining behavior change. The first section presents an overview of cancer, cancer treatment, and its side effects. We present research examining the impact of PA on health outcomes post cancer diagnosis, including treatment, survivorship, and end-of-life phases of the cancer trajectory. We discuss issues relating to maintenance of the intervention effects and selection of appropriate outcome variables. In the second section, we discuss issues relating to motivation and PA behavior change in cancer survivors within the framework of the major theoretical models predominantly adopted for research with cancer survivors. Additional subsections discuss the determinants of PA behavior and adherence to PA interventions in cancer survivors, motives and barriers to adherence, and preferences for PA programs. We summarize systematic reviews where available and present recent important studies not included in those systematic reviews. Finally, we summarize the main conclusions for each section and present recommendations for further study.

Cancer

Cancer is a catchall term used to describe a group of diseases characterized by uncontrolled growth and spread of abnormal cells that can occur in any tissue or organ in the body. When abnormal cells accumulate, they develop into a tumor or neoplasm (new growth). Tumors can be *benign* (noncancerous) and generally considered nonthreatening, or they can be *malignant* (ACS, 2009a). In comparison with normal cells, cancer cells rapidly grow and divide. Malignant tumors have the unique capacity to spread and invade the surrounding healthy body tissue and organs, disrupting their normal function and ultimately resulting in death if the spread is not controlled. There are over 200 different types of cancer (ACS, 2009a), which can vary dramatically based on pathology, prognosis, treatment, side effects, and demographic and behavioral profiles.

The extent to which cancer has spread is denoted by its stage. A cancer's stage is based on the primary tumor's size at the time of diagnosis and whether or not it has spread to other areas of the body (ACS, 2009a). The "TNM" system establishes disease stage based on extent of the primary tumor (T), regional lymph node involvement (N), and presence or absence of distant metastases, that is, the spread of cancer from one part of the body to another (M). If cancer cells are present only in the layer of cells in which they developed and have not spread, the stage is defined as *in situ* (ACS, 2009a). Once these three factors have been established, a stage of I, II, III or IV is generally assigned, with stage I indicating early or localized disease and stage IV indicating advanced or metastatic disease (ACS, 2009a).

Cancer can be caused by external (e.g., environment and lifestyle behaviors) and internal (e.g., genetics and hormones) factors. These factors can work individually or in conjunction to increase risk for cancer or initiate and promote the growth and spread of the disease (ACS, 2009a). Only about 5% of cancers are hereditary, while evidence suggests that about one-third of the cancer deaths estimated to occur in 2009 were related to preventable lifestyle factors, including overweight/obesity, physical inactivity, and poor diet (ACS, 2009a).

Cancer Treatment and Side effects

The most common treatments for cancer are surgery, radiation therapy (RT), chemotherapy (CT), and hormone therapy. Cancer surgery is the foundation of cancer treatment. The primary purpose is to cure cancer by removing it. A secondary purpose of surgery is to determine the stage of the cancer. Surgery is often combined with other treatments, commonly RT and CT. RT is one of the most common treatments for cancer and may be used as the primary treatment for some cancers (e.g., lung) or in conjunction with surgery and CT (e.g., breast cancer). In this method, high-energy particles or waves are targeted to destroy or damage cancer cells in specific areas of the body. RT works by breaking a strand of DNA inside the cancer cell, which prevents the cancer cell from growing and dividing. RT is a local treatment, affecting primarily the part of the body being treated. Common acute side effects associated with RT are skin irritation in the local area being treated and fatigue. The experience of these side effects and their severity will depend on the treatment dose, part of the body being treated, and general health. RT to the chest area may affect the lungs or heart, and radiation to the abdomen or pelvis can lead to bladder problems, bowel problems, or both (ACS, 2009c).

CT is the use of chemicals (or drugs) to treat disease. CT may be delivered prior to surgery to shrink tumors (neoadjuvant therapy), after surgery to destroy remaining cancer cells (adjuvant therapy), and in the end-of-life stage to slow progress of cancer (palliative therapy). CT drugs are designed to kill fast-growing cells. In contrast to RT, CT is a systemic treatment, and drugs travel throughout the entire body. The advantage of this method is that CT can destroy cancer cells that have metastasized or spread to distal parts of the body. A disadvantage is that CT destroys or damages not only cancer cells but healthy cells as well. CT typically consists of combinations of different drugs, with the exact combination, dose, and scheduling depending on the stage of disease, the goal of CT, and individual factors such as age and existing comorbidities. Side effects often differ depending on these factors. Damage to healthy cells is the main cause of common side effects of CT. Fast-growing cells such as hair follicles, cells in the mouth and digestive tract, and blood-forming cells in the bone marrow are most affected by CT. Thus common CT side effects include hair loss, an altered state of taste, nausea, vomiting, and loss of appetite, anemia, fatigue, and a suppressed immune system. Certain types of CT drugs can also result in loss of lean muscle mass and weight gain. Other types of CT can result in decrements in lean body mass in conjunction with extreme weight loss (cachexia). CT can also damage cells in the heart, kidney, bladder, lungs, and nervous system and increase risk for secondary cancers and other chronic disease (ACS, 2009b).

Hormone therapy is used to reduce or block the action of hormones such as estrogen or testosterone that facilitate the growth of certain cancers. Although this treatment is generally not as toxic as CT, it can still result in significant side effects. Sometimes hormone therapy can be administered over prolonged periods, and it can induce early menopause in some women. Androgen ablation therapy is commonly used as a primary treatment for prostate cancer. Continuous androgen ablation is associated with significant morbidity including fatigue, weight gain, loss of lean body mass, and decline in physical and emotional well-being (Pirl et al., 2002).

Commonly, the approach to treating cancer is multimodal, and oncologists prescribe combinations of different treatment methods. Therefore, cancer survivors cope with multiple side effects on multiple occasions over a prolonged period. Side effects can be acute (occurring during or shortly after treatment and generally disappearing on cessation of treatment), chronic (enduring or frequently occurring), or late (taking months or years to develop). Compared with persons without a history of cancer, cancer survivors are at greater risk of

developing secondary cancers and other diseases and conditions, such as heart disease, diabetes, osteoporosis, and functional decline, which may be directly attributable to cancer treatment, genetics, lifestyle factors, or a combination thereof (ACS, 2007).

Treatment for cancer can also result in significant psychological morbidity, including anxiety and depression (Deimling, Kahana, Bowman, & Shaefer, 2002). Cancer survivors face the shock of diagnosis, the burden of treatment, the loss of good health, uncertainty about the future, and the threat of dying. Depression occurs in response to perceived loss, while anxiety usually results from a real or perceived threat. Rates of depression and anxiety are higher in cancer patients than in the general population (Nordin, Berglund, Glimelius, & Sjoden, 2001; Somerset, Stout, Miller, & Musselman, 2004). Body image can be affected in survivors for whom surgery or other treatments have caused scarring, weight loss, weight gain, alopecia, or loss of a body part or function. Self-esteem may be impaired in survivors who feel that they have lost independence and control over their health and life. Moreover, cancer and its experience can have a detrimental impact on family and relationships, employment, and finances (ACS, 2009b).

Improved cancer treatments have resulted in prolonged survival and better control of disease- and treatment-related complications. Nevertheless, complete recovery of participation in life activities after cancer treatment may take years, particularly when symptoms are long enduring. Hence there is an increasing need for strategies to manage treatment side effects and improve quality of life (QoL) (ACS, 2008). Improved survival rates have generated interest in behavioral strategies that might improve QoL and reduce the risk of recurrence, morbidity, and mortality in cancer survivors.

One lifestyle factor that has generated interest in recent years is PA. The primary purpose of PA interventions is not to treat or cure cancer but rather to manage the symptoms and side effects of the disease, reduce morbidity and mortality, and improve overall QoL. Many chronic and late effects of cancer treatments align themselves with the known benefits of PA in other medical and nonmedical populations. Improvements in adjuvant therapies have led to many cancer survivors being willing and able to participate in PA interventions both during and immediately following treatment (Courneya, 2009). A growing number of trials have assessed the effects of participation in structured exercise programs for cancer survivors.

Physical Activity in Cancer Survivors

Initial interest in PA from a cancer perspective was for primary prevention. Cancer prevention is the most studied and reviewed cancer control outcome (Courneya & Friedenreich, 2007), and there is now a general consensus that PA is associated with reduced risk for developing several cancers, including breast (Monninkhof et al., 2007), colon (Samad et al., 2005), potentially endometrial (Friedenreich et al., 2007), and lung (Tardon et al., 2005).

Early research on PA following a cancer diagnosis centered on rehabilitation following surgery or treatment (Courneya, 2009). More recently, a new research perspective has focused on the benefits of PA in survivorship—in particular, from a supportive care standpoint; the role of PA in improving overall QoL (Courneya, 2009). Supportive care end points are those that are primarily indicators of the quality of a cancer survivor's life and include health measures such as generic and disease-specific QoL, happiness, patient-rated physical and psychosocial functioning, well-being, fatigue, and other symptoms and side effects. Other end points gaining interest include behavioral end points, biopsychosocial mechanisms, and clinical disease end points. Behavioral indicators for PA can include type, volume, intensity, and frequency of PA necessary to bring about change in QoL or disease prognosis. Biopsychosocial end points refer to causal mechanisms (i.e., mediators) that bring about change in supportive care, disease, or behavior end points. In PA research, these mechanisms may include biological markers, health-related fitness, and psychosocial variables (e.g., attitude towards PA and self-efficacy). Clinical disease end points are primarily concerned with the quantitative aspects of expected life, including disease-free survival, recurrence, cancer-specific morbidity and mortality, and overall mortality.

Research studies on PA in cancer survivors can be organized in many ways, including (a) the cancer survivor group being studied, (b) the primary end point of interest and, (c) the timing of the intervention. Early studies focused on heterogeneous groups of cancer survivors on and off treatment. Given the clinical heterogeneity of cancer and its treatments, more recently studies have emerged that focus on one cancer group, most often breast cancer. Similarly, researchers hypothesize PA may play a different role at different phases on the cancer continuum. Systematic reviews have emerged focusing on different phases of the cancer experience, particular symptoms experienced by cancer survivors, or both. In 2007, Courneya and Friedenreich proposed the Physical Activity and Cancer Control (PACC) framework as a method to organize PA research by different stages of the cancer experience (see Figure 21.1).

The PACC framework proposes six cancer-related phases: two prediagnosis (prescreening and screening), and four post diagnosis (pretreatment, treatment, survivorship, and end of life). Prescreening encompasses the entire period prior to cancer screening, whereas screening spans the time from a given test to the results of that test. Pretreatment includes the time after a definitive cancer diagnosis until treatment is initiated. The treatment phase encompasses the time from initiation of primary cancer treatments such as CT, RT, hormone therapy, or a combination to their completion. Survivorship encompasses the period following first diagnosis and treatment and prior to the development of cancer recurrence or death (Hewitt, Greenfield, & Stovell, 2006). In this framework, "end of life" is incorporated as a distinct time period based on the Institute of Medicine's cancer control continuum. Based on these six phases, Courneya and Friedenreich (2007)

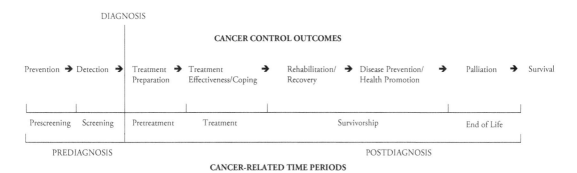

Figure 21.1. The Physical Activity and Cancer Control (PACC) framework. Reproduced with permission from "Physical Activity and Cancer Control," by K. S. Courneya and C. M. Friedenreich, 2007, *Seminars in Oncology Nursing, 23*, 242–252.

propose eight cancer control objectives. In prediagnosis, these are prevention and detection, followed by treatment preparation/coping treatment effectiveness/coping during treatment, recovery/rehabilitation, and disease prevention/health promotion during the survivorship phase, and palliation and survival at the end of life. In the next section, we organize PA research examining health outcomes by the PACC time periods after cancer diagnosis: treatment, survivorship, and end of life. We present evidence for biopsychosocial mechanisms where available and include subsections pertaining to maintenance of the intervention effects and selection of appropriate outcome variables.

Effects of Physical Activity on Supportive Care Outcomes in Cancer Survivors

Supportive care research examines health outcomes that are primarily indicators of the quality of a cancer survivor's life, including generic and disease-specific QoL, happiness, patient-rated physical and psychosocial functioning, well-being, fatigue, and other cancer-related symptoms and side effects.

Treatment

According to the PACC framework (Courneya & Friedenreich, 2007), PA may benefit cancer survivors during treatment in several ways, including (a) managing treatment-related side effects, (e.g., maintaining physical function, preventing muscle loss and weight gain, and improving mood, self-esteem, and overall QoL), (b) facilitating compliance with treatments, and (c) potentiating the efficacy of treatments. The majority of research has focused on management of treatment-related side effects, which will be the primary focus of this subsection.

Several recent systematic reviews on PA in cancer survivors have divided studies into the treatment and survivorship phases. In one of the first meta-analyses to examine the separate effects of PA during and after treatment, Conn, Hafdahl, Porock, McDaniel, and Neilson (2006) reviewed 24 published and six unpublished studies, 13 of which were single-arm, uncontrolled trials. They reported a medium standardized effect size for physical function, with smaller standardized effect sizes for body composition, mood, QoL, and fatigue. With the exception of physical function, the pattern of effects suggested benefits that were more favorable when interventions were delivered after treatment.

Schwartz (2008) reviewed 34 studies examining the effects of exercise during treatment and 38 that examined exercise after treatment. In this review, the literature consistently demonstrated a positive association of PA during treatment with improved QoL, cardiorespiratory fitness, muscle strength, flexibility, anxiety, pain, depression, fatigue, and anthropometric measures of body weight, body fat, and other health-related biomarkers (Schwartz, 2008). In contrast to Conn et al.'s (2006) review, Schwartz (2008) reported that the effect of exercise following treatment did not appear to be as strong as those during treatment, likely because Schwartz included observational studies and uncontrolled trials.

Speck, Courneya, Mass, Duval, and Schmitz (2010) conducted the most recent systematic quantitative review, which included 79 randomized controlled trials (RCTs) of PA interventions in cancer survivors. Outcomes were reported independently for interventions conducted during (39%) and post cancer treatment (61%). The majority of studies reviewed were for breast cancer survivors (84%). Findings from this review indicated quantitative evidence for a large effect of PA interventions post treatment on upper- and lower-body strength and moderate effects on fatigue and breast cancer–specific concerns. During treatment, a small-to-moderate positive effect of PA during treatment was seen for aerobic fitness, muscular strength, anxiety, and self-esteem. A novel aspect of this updated review was evidence that PA interventions significantly reduced fatigue post treatment. A previous review had reported quantitative null findings for the effect of PA on fatigue, both during and post treatment (Schmitz et al., 2005).

Although the majority of studies included in the reviews discussed above involved early-stage breast cancer survivors, the reviews did not separate findings by cancer site. Several systematic reviews and meta-analyses have focused exclusively on a specific cancer group, mainly breast cancer survivors. McNeely et al. (2006) reviewed 14 RCTs examining PA interventions during and post treatment in 717 women diagnosed with breast cancer. Overall, PA interventions had significant positive and meaningful effects on QoL, cardiorespiratory fitness, objective physical functioning, and fatigue. Similar to what was found in the updated review by Speck et al. (2010), the improvement in fatigue was statistically significant in only the two studies conducted post treatment. No significant change in body weight or body mass index (BMI) was reported in any study however, when studies assessed body composition with dual x-ray absorptiometry, favorable changes were reported for lean body mass and bone density (McNeely et al., 2006).

Markes and Resch (2006) reviewed nine RCTs investigating PA interventions in 492 women with stage I, II, and III breast cancer receiving adjuvant treatment. They concluded that exercise can significantly improve cardiorespiratory fitness, with corresponding improvements in activities of daily living. However, owing to a lack of studies there was insufficient evidence for other supportive care outcomes including fatigue, anxiety, depression, immune function, strength, and weight gain. The authors noted considerable heterogeneity between trials for treatment regimens, mode of exercise, and duration of study, which may have resulted in mixed results. Similarly, Speck et al. (2010) reported inconclusive findings for over 60 outcomes examined in their systematic review as a result of insufficient research.

Bicego et al. (2009) conducted a systematic review of nine RCTs examining the effects of exercise on QoL in women living with breast cancer. This review focused exclusively on structured exercise programs lasting a minimum of four weeks and their impact on QoL in women with all stages of breast cancer. Overall, the authors concluded that there is strong evidence that exercise positively influences QoL in women living with breast cancer. Bicego et al. stated that exercise improves mood and QoL by increasing overall health through socialization, goal setting, participation, decreased body weight, and decreased fatigue. This review did not differentiate findings based on treatment status, therefore it is not possible to draw any conclusions concerning whether improvements in QoL were greater during or post treatment.

The growing body of research examining PA interventions in breast cancer survivors has enabled reviews to focus exclusively on specific side effects of the cancer experience. Cancer-related fatigue is defined as a constant, subjective sensation of exhaustion associated with cancer or its treatment that impairs normal functioning and is out of proportion to recent activity. It is often not alleviated with rest (Mock et al., 2007) and is strongly associated with poor QoL and psychological outcomes (Mock et al., 2001). Severe fatigue can result from muscular deconditioning caused by both the disease and treatment but can also be triggered by a sedentary lifestyle (Lucia, Earnest, and Perez, 2003). Recently, Cramp & Daniel (2008) completed a meta-analysis of 28 RCTs that involved 2,083 participants investigating the effect of PA on cancer-related fatigue. Overall findings from the review indicated that PA can be beneficial for individuals with cancer-related fatigue both during and after treatment.

Breast cancer is the most widely studied cancer with respect to PA interventions both during and post treatment. Therefore the evidence for a positive effect of PA in reviews that include all cancers is largely restricted to breast cancer and must be extrapolated with caution. Cancer is a generalized term for many pathologically different diseases with heterogeneous treatment regimes. There is a need to increase the evidence for PA interventions for other cancers.

In the first systematic review of PA in prostate cancer survivors, Thorsen, Courneya, Stevinson, and Fossa (2008) reviewed nine studies examining outcomes of PA interventions, including four RCTs, two single-arm trials, and three observational studies. Most studies were conducted with prostate cancer survivors during treatment, in particular androgen deprivation therapy. Despite the limited number of studies and small sample sizes, preliminary findings suggested that PA interventions, especially resistance training, have beneficial effects on health outcomes in prostate cancer survivors. Promising effects of PA were indicated for muscular fitness, physical functioning, fatigue, and health-related QoL.

Liu, Chinapow, Huijgens, and van Mechelen (2009) reviewed 10 PA intervention studies in 194 patients with hematological cancers (e.g., lymphoma, leukemia, or myeloma) treated with stem cell transplantation. These 10 trials included 159 adults and 35 children. Three studies were RCTs, one was a nonrandomized controlled trial, and six were uncontrolled trials. Despite heterogeneity and modest methodological quality, encouraging findings were reported for improvement in body composition (lean body weight), muscle strength, aerobic capacity, and fatigue. Overall, the authors concluded that PA interventions are safe and feasible for this population, but better-quality studies are needed with larger samples, appropriate control groups, and validated outcome measures.

Several recent large, randomized PA trials with breast, prostate, and lymphoma cancers warrant mention. The largest study of PA during cancer treatment to date is the Supervised Trial of Aerobic versus Resistance Training (START), a multicenter trial comparing aerobic exercise training (AET) and resistance exercise training (RET) to usual care (UC) in 242 breast cancer patients receiving adjuvant CT (Courneya, Segal, Mackey, et al., 2007). The trial demonstrated that AET was superior to UC for improving self-esteem, aerobic fitness, and percentage body fat, whereas RET was superior to

UC for improving self-esteem, lower- and upper-body muscular strength, lean body mass, and CT completion rate. With respect to this latter finding, Courneya, Segal, Mackey, et al. (2007) reported that breast cancer patients engaging in RET completed a higher relative dose intensity of CT than the UC group. This finding was unexpected and warrants replication.

In a novel study, Cadmus et al. (2009) compared the effects of PA in two RCTs with breast cancer survivors, one conducted during treatment and one after treatment. Both interventions were six-month trials examining the impact of moderate-to-vigorous sports or recreational PA versus UC on QoL and psychosocial and physical functioning. The methodological similarities between the two studies enabled a comparison of the intervention at two points in the survivorship trajectory. The IMPACT (Increasing or Maintaining PA during Cancer Treatment) trial examined a home-based intervention in 50 newly diagnosed survivors versus usual care, whereas the YES (Yale Exercise and Survivorship) study examined a combined supervised and home-based intervention versus usual care in 75 posttreatment survivors. Contrary to what was anticipated, Cadmus et al. (2009) found that QoL remained consistent between baseline and six months posttest, and PA did not improve QoL in either study. However, baseline QoL was similar on most measures for newly diagnosed survivors undergoing treatment and survivors on average 3.5 years (range 1 to 10) post treatment . The authors suggested that the results might be due to the high level of functioning of participants reported at baseline. Concomitantly, the percentage of participants receiving a combination of CT and RT in either group or study was relatively low in comparison with other PA studies with breast cancer survivors. It is possible that the study failed to show an effect of exercise in improving QoL outcomes or psychosocial functioning because participants were functioning well enough at the time of enrollment, leaving little room for improvement at posttest. In a secondary analysis, the authors reported that exercise was associated with improved social functioning among posttreatment survivors with low social functioning at baseline. Cadmus et al. suggested that future research may benefit from targeting specifically survivors who are experiencing psychosocial impairment or reduced QoL.

In the first trial to compare AET and RET in prostate cancer survivors, Segal et al. (2009) reported findings from a RCT where 121 prostate cancer patients receiving RT with or without androgen deprivation therapy were randomized to receive AET, RET, or UC. The findings indicated that both resistance and aerobic exercise mitigated fatigue over the short term (12 weeks). However, resistance exercise also resulted in longer-term improvements in fatigue (24 weeks), improved QoL, aerobic fitness, upper- and lower-body strength, and triglyceride levels, and mitigated increases in body fat; Aerobic training also improved fitness.

Courneya, Sellar, Stevinson, McNeely, Peddle, et al. (2009) conducted the first RCT to examine PA in adult lymphoma patients, called the Healthy Exercise for Lymphoma Patients (HELP) trial. In this RCT, 122 lymphoma patients were randomized to UC or supervised AET for 12 weeks. Findings post intervention indicated that aerobic exercise was superior to UC for patient-rated physical function, overall QoL, fatigue, happiness, depression, general health, cardiovascular fitness, and lean body mass. In contrast to results from systematic reviews with breast cancer survivors suggesting larger effects in the postadjuvant setting (Conn et al., 2006; McNeely et al., 2006; Speck et al., 2010), improvements in the HELP trial were similar in patients off treatment or receiving CT.

Adamson et al. (2009) assessed the effect of a group exercise intervention as an adjunct to conventional care on fatigue, physical capacity, general well-being, PA, and QoL in 279 patients undergoing adjuvant CT for advanced cancer. Participants were randomized to one of three conditions: (a) a supervised multimodal exercise program consisting of high-intensity cardiovascular training and resistance training, (b) relaxation training and massage in addition to UC, or (c) UC. Post intervention, the exercise group showed significant improvement on the primary outcome variable, fatigue, and on variables of vitality, physical functioning, role physical and role emotional (problems with work or other daily activities due to physical or emotional health; Ware, Kosinski & Keller, 1994), and mental health. Moreover, objective assessments indicated improvements in aerobic capacity and muscular strength. However, no significant effect was seen on global health status or QoL, and symptoms scales did not show improvements. Failure of the intervention to significantly improve QoL may have been due to high QoL scores at baseline. Similarly, 50–70% of the sample scored in the lowest quartile on six of the symptoms scales, suggesting a possible floor effect. Conversely, the effect of the intervention on fatigue was large. Fatigue was the most frequently reported symptom at baseline, with 65% of participants reporting fatigue at levels greater than that of the general population (Klee et al., 1997).

In summary, the Adamson et al. (2009) study provides preliminary evidence that a supervised multimodal exercise intervention including high- and low-intensity components was feasible and could safely be used in cancer patients receiving adjuvant CT for advanced disease. Adherence to the program was 70.8% and recruitment 53%, which is comparable to figures for other exercise interventions including cancer patients with a lesser disease burden. Moreover, both muscle strength and overall fitness improved during a short period and within the same time range as exercise interventions that recruited patients with lesser burden of disease. Future studies may benefit from comparing the components of the multimodal program to determine the extent to which the program as a whole or independent parts contributed to the improvement in outcome variables.

Overall, meta-analyses and systematic reviews suggest that PA may produce larger and more consistent effects on psychosocial and physical supportive care outcomes during the posttreatment phase of breast cancer survivorship than during treatment. Courneya, Segal, Mackey, et al. (2007) suggested that the small effect of PA on these outcomes may emerge once the psychosocial distress and treatment effects associated with treatment are over. In contrast, the HELP trial found no difference in outcomes between participants on or off treatment (Courneya, Sellar, Stevinson, McNeely, Peddle, et al., 2009). There is a need for further RCTs comparing the benefits of PA in various cancer groups on and off treatment.

Survivorship

In the PACC framework, the cancer control categories spanning the survivorship phase post treatment include shorter-term recovery/rehabilitation and longer-term disease prevention/health promotion. The goal of PA interventions post treatment is to potentiate recovery from the acute and late-appearing effects of treatment, optimize QoL and physical functioning, reduce the risk of recurrence and morbidity, and improve overall survival (Courneya & Friedenreich, 2007). The focus of this next subsection is on the recovery/rehabilitation cancer control category.

Over 50% of cancer survivors indicate a preference for beginning PA programs immediately or soon after treatments rather than during (Jones &

Courneya, 2002; Karvinen et al., 2006; Karvinen, Courneya, Venner, et al., 2007; Vallance et al., 2006). A cancer diagnosis has been referred to as a "teachable moment" where survivors are likely to be motivated to make lifestyle changes to improve their health (Demark-Wahnefried et al., 2005). This phase therefore represents an important time for intervention. Several meta-analyses reviewed earlier compared the effects of PA interventions during the survivorship period with those during the treatment period (Conn et al., 2006; McNeely et al., 2006; Speck et al., 2010). Since the publication of those reviews, several studies have explicitly targeted the survivorship phase and reported beneficial effects of PA on supportive care outcomes.

One of the earliest studies to target the early survivorship phase was the Rehabilitation Exercise for Health after Breast Cancer (REHAB) trial (Courneya et al., 2003). The REHAB trial was an RCT designed to determine the effects of a 15-week exercise training program on cardiovascular fitness and QoL in 53 postmenopausal breast cancer survivors during the early survivorship phase. In light of a 98% adherence rate, significant intervention effects were reported for peak oxygen consumption, peak power output, QoL, fatigue, happiness, and self-esteem.

The Weight Training for Breast Cancer Survivors study examined the effects of twice weekly weight training on supportive care outcomes in 86 breast cancer survivors 4–36 months post treatment (Ohira, Schmitz, Ahmed, & Yee, 2006). The results indicated that weight training had beneficial effects on physical and psychosocial QoL scores, and improvements were associated with increases in lean body mass and upper-body strength. There were no changes in depression scores in this study. Daley et al. (2007) compared the effects of eight weeks of either aerobic exercise or flexibility exercise to UC in 108 breast cancer survivors 12–36 months post treatment. The authors reported beneficial postintervention effects of exercise for QoL, fatigue, self-worth, aerobic fitness, and (in contrast with Ohira et al., 2006) depression.

To date, the studies included in the majority of systematic reviews and meta-analyses have employed predominantly aerobic-type activity both during and post treatment. Speck et al. (2010) reported that 80% of RCTs included in their review were aerobic and or combined aerobic and resistance training protocols. Likewise, in a recent evaluation of PA RCTs in breast cancer survivors, aerobic exercise was the primary modality (60%), followed by some combination of resistance and aerobic PA (White, McAuley, Estabrooks, & Courneya, 2009). Recently there has been an emergence of systematic reviews examining the benefits of other modalities of PA in cancer survivors, predominantly during the posttreatment phase.

De Backer, Schep, Backx, Vreugdenhil, and Kuipers (2009) conducted a recent systematic review of research using resistance training in the posttreatment phase. The final review included 24 studies: 10 randomized control trials, four controlled clinical trials, and 10 uncontrolled trials. Similar to the previous reviews, the majority of studies involved breast (54%) and prostate (13%) cancer survivors; six studies involved heterogeneous groups of cancer survivors. Overall, positive findings were reported for cardiopulmonary function (peak oxygen uptake) and muscular strength. The majority of studies (71%) reported significant improvements in muscle strength and endurance after training. Four studies examined changes in the immune system and found no effect of training, and three studies found no detrimental change in lymphedema. In general, there were no positive effects of training on body composition, with the exception that two studies using dual x-ray absorptiometry reported a significant increase in lean mass and a significant decrease in fat mass. No findings were reported relating to psychosocial outcomes or QoL. A limitation reported by De Backer et al. (2009) is that most studies used mixed aerobic/resistance training protocols, and only four studies focused exclusively on resistance training. Therefore, it is not clear whether the positive changes observed were due to the aerobic or the resistance component or a combination of both. Nevertheless, this review provides support for the feasibility and potential benefits of resistance training for fitness and strength for cancer survivors. Future research is needed to examine the impact of resistance training on psychosocial and QoL parameters.

Two reviews have focused on yoga interventions for cancer survivors (Bower, Woolery, Sternlieb, & Garet, 2005; Smith & Pukall, 2008). Yoga is a low-impact, gentle form of PA that incorporates physical postures (asanas), breathing techniques (pranayama), and relaxation/meditation to integrate and bring balance to the body, mind, and spirit. Yoga interventions for cancer survivors use gentle or restorative postures, typically emphasizing the relaxation component of yoga practice. This relaxation response is an important component of the yoga method; yoga can also include active and dynamic postures to increase strength, flexibility, stability, and balance. Bower et al. (2005) identified nine studies that examined the effects of yoga on psychological and somatic symptoms in predominantly breast cancer survivors. Overall, the review indicated that yoga resulted in modest improvements in sleep quality, mood, stress, cancer-related distress, cancer-related symptoms, and overall QoL.

Recently, Smith and Pukall (2008) conducted an evidence-based systematic review to examine the impact of yoga on psychological adjustment in cancer survivors. Participants were primarily posttreatment (85%). The review included 10 intervention studies, six of which were RCTs and four of which were uncontrolled trials. Overall, positive improvements were reported for sleep, QoL, and levels of stress in both RCTs and uncontrolled trials. However, Smith & Pukall concluded that despite promising evidence for the benefits of yoga, variability across studies in both cancer populations and interventions limits the extent to which this mode of PA can currently be deemed effective for managing psychological symptoms associated with cancer.

Since the publication of these reviews, two recent studies, including findings from our own lab, have supported the beneficial role of yoga for cancer survivors (Danhauer et al., 2009; Speed-Andrews, Stevinson, Belanger, Mirus, & Courneya, 2010). In a small RCT, Danhauer et al. (2009) examined the feasibility of a 10-week restorative yoga program in women with breast cancer. The majority of participants had completed primary treatment for breast cancer (66%). Overall, women participating in the yoga arm reported enjoyment and satisfaction with the activity. Women in the yoga arm reported a significant improvement in fatigue from baseline to post intervention, and favorable improvements were observed for mental health, depression, positive affect, and spirituality in comparison with the control group. Women who reported higher negative affect and lower emotional well-being at baseline derived the greatest benefit from participation in the yoga intervention.

Recently, our group conducted a single-arm pilot study to evaluate the impact of Iyengar yoga on QoL and psychosocial functioning in a select sample of breast cancer survivors (Speed-Andrews et al., 2010). The Iyengar yoga system includes a modified approach for individuals who are stiff, immobile, injured, or ill, using props and supports to adapt postures to the age and fitness levels of participants and permitting modifications on the basis of individual needs. Twenty-four posttreatment breast cancer survivors completed a questionnaire measuring generic and disease-specific QoL and psychosocial functioning before the 12-week classes. Postprogram questionnaires were completed by 17 (71%) participants, who attended an average of 78.9% of the Iyengar yoga sessions. Several indicators of generic QoL improved significantly, including mental health, vitality, role emotional, and bodily pain. Other improvements in QoL and psychosocial functioning were meaningful but were not statistically significant. Findings were further substantiated by participants' positive evaluations of the program's benefits and motivational value.

Although preliminary evidence suggests some psychological and physical benefits from yoga in cancer survivors, the data are still very limited. Preliminary findings suggest yoga can improve QoL in early breast cancer survivors, but few studies have focused on other cancer survivor groups. There is a need to examine whether yoga is beneficial across different groups of cancer survivors at different phases of the cancer trajectory. Yoga is considered a light-intensity PA because of its relatively modest energy requirement (Ainsworth et al., 2000). Consequently, yoga may be a more tolerable and desirable type of PA for cancer survivors who are older, have advanced disease or compromised function, or otherwise prefer a lighter-intensity PA. RCTs comparing yoga with UC or other PA interventions in breast cancer survivors are warranted.

There is some preliminary evidence to support the benefits of exercise for a diverse range of malignancies. Several observational studies using cross-sectional designs have examined the association between PA and QoL in understudied cancer survivor groups. These studies have reported positive associations between PA and QoL in survivors of multiple myeloma (Jones, Courneya, Vallance, et al., 2004), non-Hodgkin's lymphoma (Belizzi et al., 2009; Vallance, Courneya, Jones, & Reiman, 2005), and brain (Jones, Guill, et al., 2006), ovarian (Stevinson et al., 2007), endometrial (Courneya, Karvinen, et al., 2005), bladder (Karvinen, Courneya, North, et al., 2007), colorectal (Lynch, Cerin, Owen, Hawkes, & Aitken, 2008; Peddle, Au, & Courneya, 2008), and lung (Jones et al., 2008) cancer. RCTs are now needed to provide support for the beneficial role of PA in supportive care outcomes across this diverse range of understudied cancer populations.

End of Life

Despite the improvements in treatment and survival, approximately two-thirds of individuals diagnosed with cancer are not cured of the disease, and about half will eventually die from it (Stjernsward, 2007). The cancer control category at the end-of-life phase is palliation. PA research thus far has focused predominantly on palliation. Based on the number of cancer deaths per year and a growing and aging population, the demand for palliative care is likely to dramatically increase in coming years (World Health Organization, 2003). The goal of palliative cancer care is to help advanced cancer patients maximize their QoL by management of cancer-related symptoms (World Health Organization, 2003). The ability to maintain physical independence and perform self-care activities can have a profound impact on QoL. It stands to reason that supportive care interventions that maintain a patient's mobility for as long as possible have the potential to maintain QoL in advanced cancer patients (Jordhoy, 2007).

Evidence for the benefits of PA in alleviating cancer- and treatment-related side effects stems predominantly from studies with early-stage cancer patients. The difference in symptom burden between advanced-stage and early-stage cancer survivors precludes generalizing the benefits from PA to all individuals living with a cancer diagnosis. There is preliminary evidence that select advanced cancer patients are willing and able to participate in PA interventions (Lowe, Watanabe, Baracos, & Courneya, 2009; Oldervoll et al., 2005). In a pilot study, Oldervoll et al. (2005) reported that 63% of cancer patients with advanced incurable disease and clinician-estimated survival between 3 and 12 months were willing to participate in a structured PA intervention. Likewise, a recent pilot survey by Lowe, Watanabe, et al. (2009) found that 92% of participants would be interested and able to participate in a PA program. In this study there was a strong association between higher patient-reported walking or PA and higher QoL, providing a strong rationale for the development of PA programs as a supportive care intervention for palliative cancer patients.

Lowe, Watanabe, and Courneya (2009) reported the first systematic review of PA as a supportive care intervention in palliative cancer patients. They found six studies (largely pilot and case studies) focusing on feasibility issues such as recruitment and adherence, emphasizing the emerging status of this field. The sole RCT (Headley, Ownby, & John, 2004) showed a statistically significant slower rate of decline in total well-being and total fatigue in the treatment versus the control group, and the two single-arm trials demonstrated trends of improvement in QoL, fatigue, and physical function (Oldervoll et al., 2006; Porock, Kristjanson, Tinnelly, Duke, & Blight, 2000). The three case studies likewise showed improvement in selected outcomes.

Overall, there is preliminary evidence that at least some advanced cancer patients are willing and able to participate in PA interventions and that such interventions can benefit QoL. However, the dearth of evidence and heterogeneity between studies preclude definitive conclusions about the efficacy of PA as a supportive care intervention in palliation.

Mediators and Moderators

Several biopsychosocial mechanisms may explain the supportive care benefits in cancer survivors that result from PA training during and post treatment. PA might improve any of a wide variety of mechanisms thought to underlie improved coping and adjustment to cancer, such as physical fitness, self-efficacy, or social interaction. These factors may in turn reduce many of the common symptoms and side effects associated with cancer and its treatments (e.g., fatigue or pain) that affect the ability to perform activities of daily living, leisure activities, and interactions with others and ultimately affect distress, anxiety, and overall QoL.

Mechanisms are commonly referred to as mediators in the social psychology literature. A mediator has been described as an intervening causal variable that is on the pathway between the intervention and behavior (Bauman, Sallis, Dzewaltowski, & Owen, 2002). According to the framework outlined by Baron and Kenny (1986), a variable functions as a mediator when it meets the following three criteria: (1) The independent variable (e.g., PA intervention) significantly accounts for variation in the hypothesized mediator (e.g., physical fitness); (2) the hypothesized mediator accounts for variation in the dependent variable (e.g., QoL), and (3) when both the independent variable and the hypothesized mediator are regressed on the dependent variable, a previously significant relationship between the independent variable and dependent variable is significantly attenuated or no longer exists (Baron & Kenny, 1986). Determining how PA interventions affect various supportive care end points such as QoL (e.g., by decreasing body weight, increasing aerobic capacity, or improving self-esteem) provides an opportunity to clarify how interventions exert their effect, yet few studies have

directly examined mediation in any phase of cancer survivorship.

In one of the few trials to directly test statistical mediation, Courneya et al. (2003) examined potential mechanisms of improvement in supportive care end points in breast cancer survivors. In the REHAB trial, analysis indicated that changes in peak oxygen consumption mediated the effects of PA on cancer-specific QoL and the trial outcome index (an indicator of physical and functional well-being), suggesting that aerobic fitness mediated the effects of the intervention on QoL in this study. Changes in self-esteem, however, were independent of changes in fitness. Similarly, in the HELP trial (Courneya, Sellar, Stevinson, McNeely, Peddle, et al., 2009), improvements in cardiovascular fitness mediated the improvements in patient-rated physical functioning but not psychosocial functioning. Improvements in psychosocial functioning in both studies were suggested by the authors to potentially be results of other aspects of the interventions, such as social interaction or distraction from treatments.

Identification of variables that moderate the effect of PA on supportive care end points is also of importance in research with cancer survivors. A moderator is a factor that can affect the direction and strength of the relationship between the PA intervention and the supportive care end points, equivalent to a statistical interaction (Baron & Kenny, 1986). Within the PA field, it is apparent that one intervention does not fit all groups of cancer survivors at all stages of the cancer experience. Cancer type and modality, duration, and side effects of treatments are likely to influence PA and QoL in cancer survivors during and after treatment and potentially moderate the impact of PA interventions.

Examination of medical and demographic variables as possible moderators of supportive care and behavioral end points can provide insight into characteristics of the population within different cancer groups that may benefit most from different interventions. The START trial (Courneya, Segal, Mackey, et al., 2007) demonstrated that exercise training improved self-esteem, aerobic fitness, muscular strength, lean body mass, body fat levels, and CT completion rate. However, the benefits were most pronounced for women who preferred RET, were unmarried, were under age 50, received non-taxane CT, and presented with more advanced disease (Courneya, McKenzie, Mackey, et al., 2008). In contrast, in the HELP trial, the results were not affected by disease type (Hodgkin's vs. non-Hodgkin's lymphoma) or treatment status (Courneya, Sellar, Stevinson, McNeely, Friedenreich, et al., 2009). However, in this latter study, marital status, general health, and BMI moderated the effects of aerobic training on QoL, with greater improvements for unmarried than married participants, participants in poor or fair health than those in excellent health, and normal weight or obese than overweight participants. Moreover, better outcomes for body composition were observed for participants with advanced disease than for those with early or no disease, and for participants in good health than those in very good to excellent health. We direct the reader to the original research article (Courneya, Sellar, Stevinson, McNeely, Friedenreich, et al., 2009) for a full discussion of these findings.

Maintenance of Change in Supportive Care Outcomes

Few studies have reported whether any of the benefits derived from exercise during treatment are preserved into the posttreatment and longer-term survivorship phases. In one of the few trials to report follow-up of outcomes beyond the immediate postintervention period, Mutrie et al. (2007) reported six-month follow-up data from 201 breast cancer patients receiving CT, RT, or a combination who received either 12 weeks of combined aerobic and resistance exercise or UC. Data indicated that significant postintervention effects on aerobic fitness, shoulder mobility, breast cancer–specific symptoms, depression, and positive mood were largely maintained at six-month follow-up.

At six months, 83.1% of participants in the START trial completed a questionnaire assessing QoL, self-esteem, fatigue, anxiety, depression, and exercise behavior (Courneya, Segal, Gelmon, et al., 2007). The RET group reported greater self-esteem and the AET group lower anxiety in comparison with the UC group. At baseline only 26% of participants were meeting aerobic exercise guidelines and 8% were meeting resistance guidelines, whereas at six-month follow-up almost 60% reported meeting at least one exercise guideline and 20% reported meeting both. Moreover, participants who reported both aerobic and resistance exercise during follow-up reported better functioning on most outcomes, including statistically significant improvements in QoL and fatigue. The results suggest that PA during CT may have longer-term benefits for PA behavior, psychosocial functioning, QoL, and fatigue. In the HELP trial, six-month follow-up indicated that AET was still superior to UC for overall QoL, happiness, and depression (Courneya, Sellar, Stevinson, McNeely, Peddle, et al., 2009). Public health exercise guidelines were being met by 63.6% in the AET group and 40% in the UC group at six-month follow-up.

Finally, in the posttreatment phase, although Daley et al. (2007) reported beneficial postintervention effects for QoL, fatigue, self-worth, aerobic fitness, and depression following eight weeks of aerobic exercise training, only the effect on depression was maintained at six-month follow-up.

Selection of Outcome Variables

As research on the effects of exercise during cancer survivorship grows, an important consideration is the careful selection and measurement of relevant supportive care outcome variables (e.g., fatigue, anxiety, physical function, and QoL). Careful selection of measures will enable appropriate evaluation of the intervention's effectiveness and facilitate comparisons among studies and advancement of knowledge. Moreover, measuring a large number of outcome variables and carrying out multiple subgroup analyses raises the possibility that significant results are due to chance (Bland & Altman, 1995). Outcomes should be selected that are likely to be responsive to the intervention and that are important to the particular cancer survivor population—for example, measuring the effect of PA on fatigue with fatigued patients (Speck et al., 2010). The most responsive or important outcomes likely vary by patient population (e.g., disease type, stage, or treatment) and exercise intervention type (e.g., aerobic, resistance, or yoga), setting (e.g., home based or supervised), and volume (e.g., intensity or frequency), highlighting the importance of identifying potential moderators and mediators of PA and QoL in cancer survivors.

Bennett, Winters-Stone, and Nail (2006) proposed a conceptual model to improve measurement of physical functioning outcomes in studies of cancer survivors (see Figure 21.2). We propose that the main concepts of the model can also be applied to the selection and measurement of supportive care health outcomes in general. The central tenets of the model are that outcomes should be selected that are of importance to the population of survivors being measured, and their selection should therefore take into consideration age, demographic, medical, and health behaviors. Working within a conceptual framework will help determine the efficacy of interventions for groups of cancer survivors and ultimately enable adoption of PA programs into

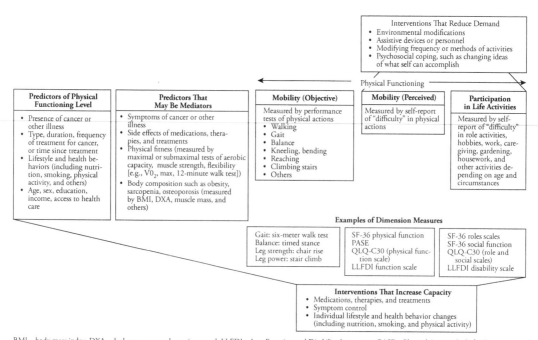

BMI—body mass index; DXA—dual-energy x-ray absorptiometry; L LLFDI—Late Function and Disability Instrument; PASE—Physical Activity Scale for the Elderly; QLQ-C30—European Organization for Research and Treatment of Cancer Quality of Life Questionnaire-Core 30; SF-36—Medical Outcomes Study Short Form-36; V0₂ max—maximal oxygen consumption

Figure 21.2. Conceptual model of physical functioning in cancer survivors. Reproduced with permission from "Conceptualizing and Measuring Physical Functioning in Cancer Survivorship Studies," by J. A. Bennett, K. Winters-Stone, and L. Nail, 2006, *Oncology Nursing Forum, 33*(1), 41–49.

clinical practice guidelines for type, dose, and timing of exercise programs for cancer survivors.

An issue related to selection of outcome variables is recruitment of participants who would benefit from improvement in the outcomes. A potential flaw in PA outcome interventions in cancer survivors thus far is a failure to recruit on a needs-based approach (Speck et al., 2010). In other words, participants are not recruited for PA intervention studies based on their need for improvement in the targeted outcome (e.g., poor QoL or lack of motivation). Several studies discussed have been limited by participants' already high levels of functioning on primary outcomes at baseline, resulting in little room for improvement from participating in exercise programs and underestimation of the intervention effects for a specific outcome (Speck et al., 2010).

In their review of RCTs, Speck et al. (2010) reported that overall, PA interventions had a beneficial effect on fatigue however, the effect size for fatigue was highly variable (0.06 to 2.26) across studies. A possible explanation offered by the authors is that PA interventions have not targeted cancer survivors on a needs-based approach. In support of this, a review of fatigue interventions for cancer survivors indicated that no studies reviewed included eligibility criteria related to the outcome, thus it was possible that many participants were not experiencing fatigue at the time of recruitment, thereby limiting the possibility for improvement (Jacobson, Donovan, Vadaparampil, & Small, 2007). Similarly, several studies reviewed in this chapter indicated that participants scored highly on QoL and other supportive care outcome variables at baseline.

Without careful selection of relevant outcomes, an intervention may be deemed ineffective when in fact it might have been effective if measuring an outcome of relevance to the population (Bennett et al. 2006). More studies are needed that focus on survivors in the greatest need of improvement for the health outcomes of interest.

Conclusions and Future Directions for Supportive Care Outcomes Research

Systematic reviews and meta-analyses and several large RCTs demonstrate that short-term interventions can increase PA and result in corresponding improvements in QoL during treatment and survivorship. The evidence suggests that the effect of PA interventions on supportive care end points in cancer survivors is larger in the survivorship phase than during treatment. As well, there is preliminary evidence that at least some advanced cancer patients are willing and able to participate in PA interventions and that such interventions can have a positive impact on QoL. Results from cross-sectional studies emphasize the need for feasibility studies to examine the benefits of PA interventions on QoL in understudied cancer survivor groups, and preliminary evidence supports a role for modalities of PA other than aerobic exercise in improving supportive care end points. There is a need for further RCTs comparing the benefits of PA in various cancer groups on and off treatment with different modes of PA. Few studies have directly examined mediation, therefore the mechanisms responsible for improving supportive care outcomes have yet to be clarified. These mechanisms likely differ by cancer group and time point in the cancer trajectory.

Supportive care outcome research has focused almost exclusively on efficacy trials. The RE-AIM (Reach, Efficacy/effectiveness, Adoption, Implementation, and Maintenance) framework (Glasgow, 2002) has been applied to PA interventions in the general healthy population and provides an evaluation of the intervention's internal validity (efficacy) and external validity (effectiveness). Efficacy trials determine whether an exercise program does more good than harm under optimal conditions (Flay, 1986). Optimal conditions to maximize the internal validity of the study would include randomization to either the intervention or a standard-care control condition and a supervised exercise protocol with expert staff. Effectiveness trials, on the other hand, examine whether an exercise program does more good than harm when delivered in real-life settings (Flay, 1986)—for instance, the extent to which the benefits of exercise programs are maintained across different settings when implemented by lay health care workers and whether they are generalizable across race, socioeconomic status, or disease stage (White et al., 2009).

White et al. (2009) evaluated the internal and external validity of 25 RCTs with breast cancer survivors within the RE-AIM framework. The majority of studies (60%) were conducted post treatment. They concluded that although there is evidence to suggest that PA improves health outcomes during treatment and survivorship, research to date has focused almost exclusively on the efficacy of such programs (i.e., internal validity) as opposed to their effectiveness (i.e., external validity) and generalizability in real-world practice. In their evaluation, no studies considered the representativeness of participants with respect to eligible nonparticipants or the general population, despite 53.8% of the studies reporting that fewer than half of the eligible women participated. Cancer survivors who elect to participate in exercise interventions are likely different from those who do not (Moyer, Knapp-Oliver, Sohl, Schneider, & Floyd, 2009). Future research is needed that compares participants with eligible nonparticipants. White et al. (2009) suggest that strict inclusion criteria may result in samples of breast cancer survivors who deviate from typical breast cancer survivors. To date, participants have been primarily white, well-educated, urban-dwelling, early-stage breast cancer survivors. Similarly, in a systematic review of 25 years of research, comprising 488 projects, Moyer et al. (2009) reported that fewer than 5% of participants were in the palliative phase of the cancer trajectory. There is a need for PA trials to target specific subgroups of survivors, including specific racial or ethnic groups, those with lower levels of education, rural dwellers, and those diagnosed with later-stage cancer.

Of the supportive care outcome studies reviewed, very few report on maintenance of the interventions' effects. Therefore whether the benefits achieved at posttest are sustainable is uncertain and warrants further research. A consideration here is that conducting research with ill populations means that some participants will be lost because of morbidity or death (Rawl et al., 2002). In addition, physical deterioration resulting from advancing illness may affect psychosocial outcomes (Moyer et al., 2009). In their review, White et al. (2009) report that only 16% of studies assessed maintenance of the interventions' main effects six months post completion, and no studies reported follow-up data concerning the status of exercise programs (i.e., if they are still in existence), cost of maintenance, or the potential for these interventions to be sustained in typical practice. Therefore, the extent to which these programs can be translated into practice warrants further study. There is enough evidence to date from efficacy trials in breast cancer survivors to begin to translate PA programs into effectiveness trials and examine their value in real-life settings.

Careful selection of outcome variables is of importance and warrants recruitment on a needs-based approach of participants who stand to benefit from improvement in the selected outcomes. In addition, there is a need to recruit participants with varied demographic and medical profiles who are representative of the population of cancer survivors at large. Research to date has focused almost exclusively on the efficacy of such programs; there is a need to examine their effectiveness and generalizability in real-world practice. Overall, the persistent evidence for the association between PA and QoL provides a strong rationale for developing effective methods to promote PA behavior in cancer populations.

Physical Activity Motivation and Behavior Change in Cancer Survivors

Exercise motivation and behavior change is a major challenge for health professionals, and even more so for cancer survivors, who often face symptoms and side effects from treatment that present unique barriers to exercise participation and adherence. Given the preliminary positive findings concerning the benefits of exercise in cancer survivors, research has begun to examine the determinants (i.e., correlates) of exercise in cancer survivors and strategies to promote exercise in this population (Courneya, Karvinen, & Vallance, 2007). In this next section, we discuss issues relating to motivation and PA behavior change in cancer survivors. We review the research on PA prevalence, determinants, motives and barriers, preferences, and behavior change interventions in cancer survivors.

Physical Activity Prevalence

PA prevalence estimates require some accepted PA guideline for cancer survivors. To date there are few evidence-based cancer-specific guidelines for exercise. During survivorship, most cancer survivors are generally recommended to follow the public health exercise guidelines from the American College of Sports Medicine and the U.S. Centers for Disease Control, which suggest 150 minutes of moderate or 60 minutes of vigorous activity per week (Haskell et al., 2007). Although the activity dose required for survivors to incur benefits is unknown, this recommendation represents the minimal dose required for health benefits in the general healthy population (Kesaniemi et al., 2001). To date, the prevalence of PA in cancer survivors has generally been assessed based on whether or not they are meeting public health guidelines. Using this benchmark, few cancer survivors, either on or off treatment, are meeting the minimum guidelines recommended to render improvements in health (Courneya, Segal, Mackey, et al., 2007).

Population-based studies in North America have shown that as many as 70% of cancer survivors are not meeting PA recommendations (Blanchard, Courneya, & Stein, 2008; Coups & Ostroff, 2005; Courneya, Katzmarzyk, & Bacon, 2008). Blanchard et al. (2008) found that in a nationally (U.S.) representative sample of six major cancer groups, the majority of cancer survivors were not meeting recommendations for PA, and prevalence estimates were below PA levels of the general population (see Figure 21.3) (U.S. Department of Health and Human Services, 2005). Similarly, in a population-based survey of Canadian cancer survivors, Courneya, Katzmarzyk, and Bacon (2008) found that fewer than 22% of these survivors were physically active, with the lowest PA rates being reported by female colorectal cancer survivors (13.8%), breast cancer survivors (16.6%), female melanoma survivors (19.1%), and male colorectal cancer survivors (20.1%). A recent cross-sectional study reported that fewer than 30% of lung cancer survivors were meeting national PA guidelines (Coups et al., 2009).

Research indicates that cancer patients significantly reduce their activity levels during treatment and do not return to prediagnosis levels after treatment completion (Courneya & Friedenreich, 1997b, 1997c). This pattern appears to hold relatively consistent across various cancer groups (Courneya, Stevinson, & Vallance, 2007; Irwin et al., 2004). Irwin et al. (2004) reported that for breast cancer survivors, time spent being physically active decreased at a rate of 2 hours per week from prediagnosis to off-treatment time points; older age and higher BMI were associated with greater levels of physical inactivity. Harrison, Hayes, and Newman (2009) explored the levels and patterns of PA levels in 511 Australian women 6, 12, and 18 months post breast cancer diagnosis. Although more than 80% of women in this study reported engaging in some PA between 6 and 18 months following breast cancer diagnosis, only 20–30% reported engaging in any vigorous PA, and only 45% were meeting guidelines for sufficient PA. Overall, there was a lack of change between 6 and 18 months post diagnosis. However, there was substantial individual variability, with approximately 40% of participants changing their activity levels (half increasing and half decreasing) over time. Higher levels of PA at baseline predicted lower levels of PA compared with themselves at 18 months, and absence of treatment-related complications

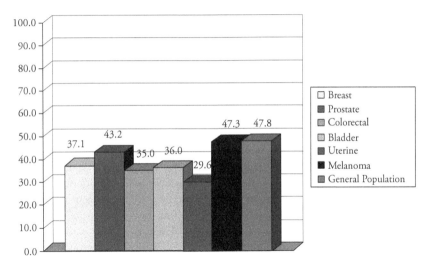

Figure 21.3. Physical activity prevalence rates (%) in cancer survivors. Reproduced with permission: "Cancer Survivors' Adherence to Lifestyle Behavior Recommendations and Associations with Health Related Quality of Life: Results from the American Cancer Society's SCS-II," by C. M. Blanchard, K. S. Courneya, and K. Stein, 2008, *Journal of Clinical Oncology, 26*(13), 2198–2204.

was positively associated with increased PA over time. Vallance et al. (2005) reported significant declines in exercise in non-Hodgkin's lymphoma patients from before to after diagnosis: 33.8% reported meeting guidelines prediagnosis, whereas only 6.5% and 23.7% reported meeting guidelines while on and off treatment respectively. It is well known that the general population overestimates when asked to self-report PA, and therefore it is likely that prevalence rates of PA in cancer survivors are lower than indicated (Courneya, Karvinen, & Vallance, 2007).

Determinants of Physical Activity

Understanding the factors that influence PA is a basic research concern and is crucial to developing and evaluating strategies to increase adoption and maintenance of PA (Bauman et al., 2002). Demographic, medical, social cognitive, physical environment, and exercise characteristics are all likely important determinants of PA in cancer survivors. Increasingly, research into the antecedents of PA behavior in cancer survivors has adopted a theoretical model to guide inquiry. This next subsection provides an overview of the factors related to PA behavior in cancer survivors, with a specific focus on the major theoretical models that have been applied in the exercise domain. Theories can significantly contribute to the knowledge base for guiding the development of new interventions, by informing the interventions and determining the

appropriate constructs to target to bring around change in the primary outcome variables. In a review article, Pinto and Floyd (2008) identified 21 theoretically based RCTs applied to health promotion interventions in cancer survivors, including trials promoting PA in cancer survivors but excluding studies promoting yoga or Tai Chi. For PA interventions, the theories predominantly used included the theory of planned behavior (TPB), the transtheoretical model (TTM), and social cognitive theory (SCT).

The theory that has garnered the most research attention in the exercise and cancer domain is the TPB (Ajzen, 1991). The TPB is a comprehensive model of intentional behavior that has been well validated in the exercise domain (Courneya, 2004). The TPB proposes that a person's intention to perform a behavior is a central determinant of that behavior. Intention in turn is determined by three conceptually independent variables: attitude, subjective norm, and perceived behavioral control (PBC). Attitude is reflected in a positive or negative evaluation of performing the behavior, whereas subjective norm is intended to reflect the perceived social pressure that individuals may feel to perform or not to perform the behavior. Finally, PBC indicates the perceived ease or difficulty of performing the behavior and may have both direct and indirect effects on behavior. Recent research supports the reconceptualization of the major constructs of the theory into a two-component model that divides attitudes into instrumental (i.e., benefits) and affective (i.e., enjoyment) components, norms into injunctive and descriptive components, and PBC into perceived control and self-efficacy components (Ajzen, 2002).

The TPB has been used to explain PA behavior in several cancer survivor groups, including breast (Courneya, Blanchard, & Laing, 2001), colorectal (Courneya & Friedenreich, 1997a), prostate (Blanchard, Courneya, Rodgers, & Murnaghan, 2002), endometrial (Karvinen, Courneya, Campbell, et al., 2007), ovarian (Stevinson, Tonkin, et al., 2009), and bladder cancer (Karvinen et al., 2009) and multiple myeloma (Jones, Courneya, et al., 2006). Research has indicated that intentions are often the strongest predictors of PA behavior in cancer survivors (Courneya et al., 2001; Courneya, Keats, & Turner, 2000), and several studies have also examined the determinants of PA intentions in cancer survivors (Courneya, Vallance, Jones, & Reiman, 2005; Jones et al., 2007). These studies provide support for the usefulness of the TPB in explaining PA behavior and intention in cancer survivors. However, the findings also suggest that the relative importance of the TPB components varies by the cancer survivor group studied. We summarize findings here from a select sample of recent research applying the TPB to understanding PA behavior and intentions in cancer survivors.

In a population based, cross-sectional mailed survey, Stevinson, Tonkin, et al. (2009) investigated the determinants of PA in ovarian cancer survivors. For this cancer group, variables associated with meeting guidelines were younger age, higher education and income, being employed, lower BMI, absence of arthritis, longer time since diagnosis, earlier disease stage, and being disease free. The TPB explained 36% of the variance in PA behavior, with intention being the sole independent correlate.

In one of the few prospective studies to examine PA determinants in cancer survivors, Karvinen et al. (2009) reported that in bladder cancer survivors, intention, PBC, and planning explained 20.9% of the variance in exercise behavior, and PBC, affective attitude, and descriptive norm explained 39.1% of the variance in exercise intention. Moreover, adjuvant therapy, invasive disease, and age were negatively associated with PA, and these effects were mediated by the TPB. Survivors who received adjuvant therapy and with more invasive disease reported less positive affective attitude, suggesting PA is less enjoyable for this group. Survivors with invasive disease also reported lower instrumental attitude,

suggesting they perceived fewer health benefits from PA. For older survivors (≥65 years), PBC was the most important predictor of PA behavior, whereas for those under 65 intention was more important. In addition, instrumental attitude and PBC were more important for intention in older survivors, whereas affective attitude and PBC were more important for intention in younger survivors. This suggests that older adults may be more influenced by the health benefits of PA, while younger survivors may find enjoyment more important. This study is the first to examine the independent contribution of descriptive and injunctive norms, and the results suggest that descriptive norm is the more important component in this cancer group. Karvinen et al. (2009) suggested that interventions that target increasing PA in the lives of important others may be an effective strategy in this group of cancer survivors.

In a cross-sectional study, Courneya, Vallance, et al. (2005) examined the demographic, medical, and social cognitive correlates within a TPB framework of PA intentions in 399 non-Hodgkin's lymphoma survivors. The TPB explained 55% of the variance in exercise intentions, with PBC, affective attitude, and subjective norm accounting for the majority of variance.

Jones et al. (2007) applied the TPB to understand determinants of PA intention in patients diagnosed with primary brain cancer. They found that instrumental attitude, affective attitude, subjective norm, and PBC combined to explain 32% of the variance in PA intentions, with affective attitude and PBC being the most important predictors of PA intentions in this cancer group. The authors suggested that PA interventions promoting enjoyment and confidence to participate in an exercise program may be particularly effective in this cancer group. In general, medical and demographic variables did not significantly modify the relationship between the TPB and intentions. However, male and overweight/obese patients considered the health benefits of exercise to be more important than their female and normal-weight counterparts, suggesting that gender and weight status may influence the PA beliefs of brain cancer survivors. In addition, past PA behavior modified the effect of TPB variables on PA intentions, with higher PA levels over the cancer trajectory being associated with positive PA beliefs.

Bandura's (1986, 1997) SCT has also been examined as a theoretical model for understanding PA behavior in cancer survivors. A central tenet of the theory is the concept of reciprocal determinism, wherein behavior is viewed as a function of the interaction between the person (e.g., beliefs or knowledge), behavior (e.g., past experience), and environment (e.g., physical or social) (Glanz, Lewis, & Rimer, 1997). Self-efficacy, considered one of the key organizing constructs within SCT, is a person's confidence in their ability to perform a specific behavior and overcome barriers to performing that behavior (Bandura, 1986). Self-efficacy has been found to be important in the early stages of PA adoption, and individuals with greater self-efficacy are more likely to adhere to a PA program (McAuley, 1992). Another important construct in SCT is outcome expectation, which refers to the expected likelihood of an outcome or consequence of behavior. Outcome expectations can be incentives when the anticipated outcomes are positive or deterrents when the anticipated outcomes are negative. Other important constructs from this theory include social support and self-regulation (e.g., monitoring and goal setting) of PA behavior.

Using SCT constructs, Rogers et al. (2004) explored PA knowledge, attitudes, and behaviors among breast cancer patients undergoing adjuvant therapy. This was the first published study to apply SCT to PA behavior among breast cancer patients during treatment. The study was qualitative, with each of 12 breast cancer patients attending one of three focus group sessions. Focus group questions were based on the SCT constructs of self-efficacy, environment, behavioral capability, expectations, expectancies, self-control and performance, observational learning, and reinforcement. Rogers et al. reported that most women generally felt confident in their ability to be physically active during treatment. Participants felt that PA was more beneficial than harmful during treatment, with the two most important benefits identified as reduced fatigue and the potential for improved survival. Conversely, the most frequently voiced obstacle to PA was fatigue; a lack of time for exercise was expressed by half of the participants. Walking was the type of exercise felt to be most enjoyable, with yoga being the second most popular. Participants consistently expressed the desire for education and guidance by knowledgeable staff during an exercise program. Rogers et al. concluded that SCT may be a useful framework for future design of larger intervention studies to promote PA behavior among breast cancer patients during treatment.

In a recent study, Coups et al. (2009) examined medical and demographic factors and SCT constructs as correlates of PA among 175 lung cancer survivors. SCT explained 38% of the variance in moderate-to-strenuous PA, which is comparable to the variance explained by the TPB in other cancer groups. Self-efficacy and outcome expectancies were independently associated with moderate-to-strenuous PA. In addition, SCT explained 19% of the variance in leisurely walking. Higher self-efficacy was associated with greater leisure walking, with outcome expectancies and social support from friends approaching significance. Social support from friends was not significantly associated with self-efficacy, suggesting an independent influence of social support from friends on leisurely walking. Additionally, older survivors and survivors with lower levels of education reported engaging in less PA than younger survivors with more years of education. This finding is consistent with research on general adult populations (Trost et al., 2002). The only medical factor associated with moderate-to-strenuous PA was preoperative pulmonary function. Participants with poor pulmonary function reported less engagement in PA, suggesting that this subgroup of cancer survivors is at increased risk of physical inactivity.

In their recent review, Pinto and Floyd (2008) observed that although several interventions have been based on SCT, research predominantly focused on self-efficacy. Similar to the research on determinants of PA intentions, one recent cross-sectional study examined predictors of self-efficacy for exercise in two groups of cancer survivors. Perkins, Baum, Carmack-Taylor, and Basen-Entquist (2009) examined how variables relating to cancer and its treatment relate to self-efficacy for PA in two separate samples of cancer survivors participating in an RCT; breast cancer survivors post treatment, and prostate cancer survivors receiving continuous androgen ablation therapy. In this sample of breast and prostate cancer survivors, several components of health-related QoL were associated with self-efficacy for PA, whereas actual health conditions such as diabetes and arthritis were not, suggesting that subjective perceptions of health-related QoL have a greater influence on self-efficacy for PA than actual health status. For breast cancer survivors, health-related QoL indicators of vitality, bodily pain, and mental health accounted for 21% of the variance in self-efficacy for PA. For prostate cancer survivors, vitality, bodily pain, and education accounted for 16% of the variance in self-efficacy for PA. Men with no college education had lower self-efficacy than those with a bachelor's degree. According to SCT (Bandura, 1997), self-efficacy for a behavior is developed from four sources: mastery experiences (e.g., performance accomplishments), vicarious experience (e.g., observing others or modeling), verbal persuasion (e.g. positive feedback or encouragement), and physiological and affective states (e.g., perceived exertion). Perkins et al. (2009) suggested that perceptions of physiological and affective states may be particularly important in cancer survivors, who often experience physical and emotional side effects during and following treatment. In support of this suggestion, Rogers et al. (2004) found that self-efficacy for PA was lowest when breast cancer survivors felt nauseated and tired during treatment.

The TTM proposes six stages that reflect individuals' temporal progression in changing behavior: precontemplation, contemplation, preparation, action, maintenance, and termination (Prochaska & DiClemente, 1983). In precontemplation, the person is not performing the behavior and has no intention to in the foreseeable future. In the contemplation stage, the person has formed the intention to change in the distant future (within six months). In preparation, the person intends to take action in the immediate future (within one month), has a detailed plan for taking action, and may have taken some small steps toward behavior change. The action stage has been achieved when behavior has been initiated at the target level recommended for that behavior (e.g., exercising 150 minutes per week at at least a moderate intensity). Once this level has been managed for six months the person is considered to be in the maintenance stage. Termination is reached when the risk of returning to the previously unhealthy behavior is zero. In addition, self-efficacy and decisional balance are key constructs of the TTM (DiClemente et al., 1991). Much as in SCT, self-efficacy reflects a person's confidence in performing the health behavior. Decisional balance reflects the benefits and costs (i.e., pros and cons) of behavior change. Cognitive and behavioral processes, another element of the TTM, consist of strategies and techniques that people use to change their behavior and are more or less important as individuals progress through the stages of behavior change. Few studies have examined all constructs at the same time. The most popular construct examined in PA behavior research is the stages of change.

Rhodes, Courneya, and Bobick (2001) examined exercise patterns and prevalence rates during treatment in a sample of 175 breast cancer survivors using the stage construct. Participants were asked to report their stage of change during treatment and their current stage of change. During treatment, 24% of breast cancer survivors were in precontemplation, 10% in contemplation, 47% in preparation, and only 19% in action or maintenance, suggesting that almost a quarter of breast cancer survivors did not even think about exercise during treatment.

Another theory, which has been applied to a lesser extent but nonetheless has demonstrated some utility in explaining PA behavior in cancer survivors, is self-determination theory (SDT; Deci & Ryan, 1985). According to this theory, people have fundamental psychological needs for autonomy, relatedness, and competence. Autonomy is concerned with how autonomous or controlled individuals perceive their choice to be, relatedness refers to the extent to which they feel connected to others in their immediate environment, and competence refers to their ability to interact effectively within their environment. In this theory, motives or regulations are located along a self-determining continuum ranging from strongly controlled by external forces (extrinsic motivation) to entirely autonomous and fully self-determined (intrinsic motivation). The continuum describes the relationship between behavioral regulations and motivational consequences. Extrinsic regulation is the most controlled form and involves the person's behaving in response to a threat or demand. Adjacent to this is introjected regulation, which relates to situations in which individuals engage in behavior to avoid feeling guilty or experiencing negative emotions or to sustain their self-worth (Wilson, Rodgers, Blanchard, & Gessell, 2003). Identified regulation occurs when individuals engage in a behavior they may not particularly enjoy because they recognize its value. Intrinsic motivation is the most autonomous form of motivation, where an individual acts because the sheer enjoyment and pleasure of the behavior itself. Research has indicated that more autonomous forms of regulation can predict moderate-to-vigorous PA (Wilson & Rodgers, 2002) and are positively associated with physical fitness and a positive attitude toward exercise (Wilson, Rodgers, Fraser, & Murray, 2004).

In one of the first studies to apply the SDT to understanding PA in cancer survivors, Wilson, Blanchard, Nehl, and Baker (2006) examined the contribution of autonomous and controlled motives to predicting moderate and vigorous PA (MVPA) and PA outcome expectations in a sample of adult cancer survivors and a noncancer cohort. Findings indicated that in both cancer survivors and the noncancer cohort, autonomous motives independently predicted outcome expectations, whereas both autonomous and controlled motives predicted MVPA, suggesting that cancer status did not moderate the influence of the motives. The results provide support for SDT in that autonomous PA motives predicted more time spent engaging in MVPA and expected benefits from engaging in MVPA.

Similarly, Milne et al. (2008) applied the SDT constructs of autonomy support and competence and the motivation continuum to understand PA motivation and behavior in breast cancer survivors post treatment. In support of the theory's assumptions, participants meeting guidelines for PA (31%) reported significantly greater identified regulation, intrinsic motivation, autonomy support, and competence, and significantly lower extrinsic motivation and amotivation (lacking intention to act), than participants not meeting guidelines. Moreover, variables of competence and autonomy support were positively associated with intrinsic motivation and PA and negatively associated with amotivation and extrinsic motivation. With respect to demographic and medical variables, women with no lymphedema, higher income, and lower BMI were more likely to report meeting guidelines for PA. The authors concluded that SDT may be a useful model for understanding PA motivation in breast cancer survivors. In particular, the findings suggest that future investigations should examine methods to foster a autonomy supportive climate as an effective way to increase PA.

A study by Peddle, Plotnikoff, Wild, Au, and Courneya (2008) explored the medical, demographic, and SDT correlates of PA in a large, population-based random sample of 414 posttreatment colorectal cancer survivors. In this study, SDT and education explained 28% of the variance in PA behavior, with identified regulation, introjected regulation, and education making significant independent contributions. Survivors with less education were significantly less likely to meet PA guidelines. Education remained a significant predictor of PA even after controlling for SDT variables, suggesting that survivors with low education levels could be at risk for physical inactivity. Interestingly, introjected regulation, which is rooted in guilt and compliance, was associated with PA behavior. Although this construct may initiate behavior change, it is not associated with long-term adherence (Peddle, Plotnikoff, et al. 2008). Overall, the study found support for the use of SDT as a model to help understand the social cognitive determinants of PA in this sample of colorectal cancer survivors.

Applications of theoretical models to examine PA behavior in various cancer populations indicate that we can explain on average between 30% and 40% of variance in PA behavior. This suggests that other factors must account for the remaining variance and highlights the importance of examining social cognitive variables in conjunction with medical and demographic variables. Moreover, ecological models have yet to be applied to examine PA behavior in cancer survivors, despite their increase in popularity in the study of PA behavior in general. The primary focus of ecological models is to explain how environments and behaviors affect each other. In particular, they examine the influence on behavior of multiple levels of the social and physical environment, including intrapersonal, interpersonal, institutional, community, and policy levels. It is likely that the levels of influence within ecological models as applied to cancer survivors would be unique to those populations and would differ in importance for survivors at different phases of the cancer trajectory. Ecological influences for cancer patients might include relationships with caregivers at the interpersonal level, care provided by hospitals or cancer centers at the institutional level, support groups and services at the community level, and plans to help long-term survivors at the policy level. An advantage of working within ecological models is that researchers can examine both individual-level and aggregate-level influences on PA behavior, which then enables multiple levels for intervention (Sallis & Owen, 1997). Researchers and practitioners should explore social ecological models when examining correlates of PA behavior in cancer survivors.

It is evident that there are a vast number of diverse and complex variables associated with PA behavior in cancer survivors that seem to vary depending on cancer type and treatment status. Determinant studies are predominantly cross-sectional in design, which limits our ability to define causal relationships of medical, demographic, and theoretical variables to meeting PA guidelines. There is a need to examine causal relationships within theoretically grounded interventions in cancer survivors. Within the PA field, much as in the outcomes research, it is apparent that one behavior change intervention does not fit all groups of cancer survivors at all stages of the cancer experience. A key issue therefore is to find out what types of interventions work for different groups. Identification of possible moderator variables (e.g., medical, demographic, environmental, and social cognitive variables) can aid in this process.

Research has also begun to examine demographic, medical, and social cognitive determinants of adherence to PA interventions in cancer survivors. Courneya et al. (2004) applied the TPB to examine the predictors of exercise adherence in the Colorectal Cancer and Home Based Physical Exercise (CAN-HOPE) trial, a RCT designed to compare the effects of a home-based exercise program on QoL and physical fitness in 102 colorectal cancer survivors. In this study, adherence to the intervention was 76%. The strongest predictors of adherence in the intervention group were exercise stage, employment status, treatment protocol, and PBC. In the intervention group, participants receiving multimodal adjuvant therapy (RT and CT) adhered less than participants receiving only one treatment modality. The authors suggested stratifying based on treatment regime and offering greater support to those receiving multimodal treatments.

Adherence to the START trial was 70%. Courneya, Segal, et al. (2008) found that TPB variables did not predict adherence for breast cancer survivors, rather adherence was predicted by higher cardiovascular fitness, lower body fat, more advanced disease stage, higher education, less depression, and being a nonsmoker. Recently, Courneya et al. (2010) examined predictors of adherence to supervised exercise in lymphoma patients participating in the HELP trial. Overall adherence to the trial was 77.8%, and adherence was predicted by past exercise history, past treatment regime, employment status, and weight. Higher adherence was achieved by participants who did not receive RT, were previous exercisers or previously sedentary compared with those who were insufficiently active (doing some exercise but not regularly), and were a healthy weight. Full-time employment status was a significant negative predictor of adherence, suggesting that cancer patients who are not working may be better able to adhere to supportive self-help strategies. In line with the START trial, motivational variables did not predict adherence however, participants scoring extremely high on the motivation scale in the HELP trial achieved an 85% adherence rate, compared with 66% for participants scoring the lowest. While overall adherence in this trial was higher than for START, all participants in the START trial were concurrently receiving CT, whereas only 44% were in the HELP trial. Adherence rate was 71% for HELP participants undergoing CT and 83% for those off treatment. Failure of motivational variables to predict adherence in the START and HELP trials was thought most likely to be due to ceiling effects

and to reflect a motivational bias for cancer patients willing to participate in exercise studies. In support of this supposition, comparison with a cross-sectional study of lymphoma survivors in Alberta, Canada (Courneya, Vallance, et al., 2005), indicated that HELP participants scored significantly higher on all motivational variables. These results suggest that consideration should be given to medical, demographic, and motivational variables when designing behavioral support interventions in this patient population.

In one of the few behavior change studies to examine predictors of exercise adherence, Pinto, Rabin, and Dunsiger (2009) reported that the best predictor of adherence among breast cancer survivors in a 12-week home-based program was self-efficacy. The Moving Forward study was a RCT telephone-based counseling intervention based on the TTM and SCT (Pinto, Frierson, Rabin, Trunzo, & Marcus, 2005). The mean adherence rate for this trial was 79.94%, which compares favorably with other home-based and supervised trials with breast cancer patients. Three adherence outcomes were measured; minutes of exercise per week, number of steps taken during planned exercise week, and whether participants met their goal. Findings indicated that from week 1 to week 12 participants significantly increased their minutes per week and total steps during the planned exercise week. Baseline self-efficacy was found to be the only variable to predict each adherence outcome. Demographic and medical variables were not significant predictors of any adherence measure, possibly due to the relatively homogenous sample. Decisional balance did not predict adherence or stage of change. The authors noted that stage distribution was restricted in this trial, as women in the action and maintenance phases reported high levels of exercise at screening and therefore were excluded from participation (Pinto et al., 2009).

Motives and Barriers

Early research with cancer patients suggests that while some barriers are common to all populations, cancer survivors also encounter barriers unique to their cancer experience and treatments. Early studies with breast and colorectal cancer survivors reported that the main barriers reported for exercise participation included side effects and symptoms from the cancer experience such as pain, nausea, and fatigue (Courneya & Friedenreich, 1997a; Courneya & Friedenreich, 1999). Likewise, the main benefits reported for PA were related to participant's cancer experience, such as taking their minds off cancer and treatment and recovering from cancer and treatment.

Recent cross-sectional and prospective studies with larger and less studied cancer groups similarly indicate that the main benefits and barriers reported for regular PA participation are related to the cancer experience. In a cross-sectional study of non-Hodgkin's lymphoma survivors (Courneya, Vallance, et al., 2005), the seven most frequent behavioral beliefs reported were similar to those commonly reported by healthy populations, including positive mental attitude, increased muscular strength and tone, and increased energy. On the other hand, the most frequent barriers to exercise were unique to cancer survivors, such as being too weak, pain, and nausea.

In the first prospective study, Courneya, Friedenreich, et al. (2005) examined barriers to weekly exercise in 69 colorectal cancer survivors. The most common barriers in this study were lacking time or being too busy, nonspecific treatment side effects, and fatigue. Participants receiving adjuvant therapy (CT, RT, or both) were more likely to report treatment side effects than those who received surgery alone, suggesting that the reported barriers and motives can differ depending on treatment status.

The START trial was the first study to prospectively examine barriers to exercise in breast cancer patients receiving CT (Courneya, McKenzie, Reid, et al., 2008). Participants in the AET and RET intervention groups attended on average 70.2% of their supervised sessions and provided reasons for missing 89.5% of their missed sessions. The 2,090 reasons given represented 36 barriers, falling into three higher-order themes: (a) disease- or treatment-related barriers (e.g., sickness, fatigue, pain, infection, or CT day; 53% of barriers), (b) life-related barriers (e.g., vacation, family sickness, or weather; 34%), and (c) motivation (e.g., lack of time, home exercise, lost interest, miscommunication, or forgetting; 13%). Demographic and medical variables did not predict the types of exercise barriers reported. The findings suggest that behavioral support programs need to focus on strategies to maintain exercise in the face of difficult treatment side effects.

Preferences

It is likely that exercise and programming preferences of cancer survivors influence their motivation to commence and adhere to a PA program. In the START trial, participants were randomized to RET, AET, or UC. Courneya, Segal, Mackey, et al. (2007) assessed participant preferences prior to randomization and found that 23% had no preference, 41% preferred RET, and 36% preferred AET. Participants stating a preference for RET had improved QoL only when assigned to that condition, whereas those with no preference had improved QoL when assigned to AET but not when assigned to RET (Courneya, Reid, et al., 2008). Because preferences for one type of intervention versus another seem to have important effects, more input from cancer patients in the planning stage is essential and will ensure that researchers are developing appropriate interventions for cancer patients and delivering them in the most acceptable way.

An early study with a mixed group of cancer survivors reported walking (81%), and moderate-intensity PA (56%) as preferable and indicated a preference for PA programs before treatment compared with during or after treatment (Jones & Courneya, 2002). As in the previous study, the majority of participants indicated a preference for walking (55%) compared with other modalities of exercise and moderate-intensity PA (62%) compared with light or strenuous PA. In contrast to the previous study, the preferred start time for the exercise program was three months post treatment (56%) compared to before treatment A cross-sectional sample of 386 endometrial cancer survivors reported being interested (76.9%) and able to participate (81.7%) in exercise and also indicated walking (76.9%), moderate-intensity PA (61.1%), and starting three to six months post treatment (39.3%) as preferable (Karvinen et al., 2006). Ovarian cancer survivors also reported a preference for home-based walking programs after treatment (Stevinson, Capstick, et al., 2009). A recent pilot survey of 50 palliative cancer patients indicated that 92% of participants would be interested and able to participate in a PA program (Lowe, Watanabe, et al., 2009). The majority of participants preferred to be physically active alone (54%), expressed preference for a home-based program (84%), and reported that they were most interested in a walking program (72%).

The majority of findings thus far are for participants recruited from urban settings. In a novel study, Rogers et al. (2009) examined preferences for PA in a sample of rural breast cancer survivors who had completed primary treatment. Rural populations warrant consideration as they tend to be more sedentary than urban dwellers (Trost et al., 2002) and rank poorly on health indicators (Ricketts, 2000). In this study, only 19% of participants met guidelines for PA (Rogers et al., 2009). Preferences for PA programs included home-based (63%), unsupervised (47%), and moderate-intensity programs that were primarily walking, (65%). Counselling time preference indicated by participants was post treatment (36%), while the preferred format was face-to-face counseling (47%), and the preferred source an exercise specialist (40%). Higher self-efficacy was associated with the selection of face-to-face counseling, and participants with less education and less interest were more likely to lack a preference for delivery. Additionally, participants reporting less PA, more comorbidities, lower task self-efficacy, and greater perceived barriers were more likely to prefer lower-intensity PA. Participants reporting greater levels of social support preferred to exercise with friends and family, and those reporting lower support levels preferred to exercise alone. Exercising outdoors was preferred by those with a higher environment score, and exercising at home by those with a lower score. These findings support consideration of medical, demographic, social cognitive, and environmental influences on PA programming preferences among rural cancer survivors.

Although certain preferences are the same across cancer groups, such as mode and intensity, the preferred timing of the intervention varies. The findings discussed above suggest the need to examine variations in preferences by cancer group and treatment status.

Behavior Change Interventions

More recently, researchers have attempted to test PA behavior change interventions in cancer survivors. In a randomized trial, Demark-Wahnefried et al. (2007) examined the effects of the first diet and exercise intervention for cancer survivors delivered exclusively via mailed print materials on diet and PA behavior change, and QoL. FRESH START was based on SCT and the TTM and used print materials tailored to the intervention participant's demographic characteristics, cancer coping style, stage of change, and barriers to change. A total of 306 breast cancer patients and 237 prostate cancer patients diagnosed with early-stage cancer within the previous nine months were recruited and randomized to receive either 10 months of the mailed FRESH START print materials or a 10-month program of publicly available materials on diet and PA. Findings indicated that the intervention group achieved significantly greater improvements in dietary behavior, total weekly minutes of PA, and all other outcomes with the exception of general QoL.

In a secondary analysis, Mosher et al. (2008) examined data from 519 participants who completed the one-year follow-up assessment to determine whether self-efficacy was a possible mediator of the intervention's effect on diet and exercise behavior. Although the results indicated that self-efficacy mediated the effect on dietary outcomes, it did not mediate the effect on exercise. However, a positive relationship between self-efficacy for exercise and exercise duration was observed at follow-up, and examination of the baseline data suggested that participants reported high levels of self-efficacy for exercise prior to the intervention, which might have precluded any additional change (Mosher et al., 2008). A limitation of this study is that a comprehensive examination of all SCT variables was not conducted. Subsequent investigations should examine the contribution of social support, self-regulatory strategies, and outcome expectancies.

In one of the earliest studies to examine theoretical mediators of PA behavior in cancer patients, Jones, Courneya, Fairey, and Mackey (2004) examined the effects of oncologists' recommendations to exercise in newly diagnosed breast cancer survivors attending their first adjuvant therapy consultation.. During the initial consultation, 450 breast cancer patients were randomized to receive (a) an oncologist's recommendation, (b) an oncologist's recommendation plus referral to an exercise specialist, or (c) no recommendation. Participants in either of the two recommendation groups reported significantly more exercise during the six-week follow-up and greater subjective norm, suggesting this time point (i.e., immediately following diagnosis and preceding treatment) may represent an important teachable moment. Moreover, in a follow-up paper, Jones, Courneya, Fairey, and Mackey (2005) examined the impact of the intervention on social cognitive constructs from the TPB (Ajzen, 1991) and reported that subjective norm and PBC increased at six-week follow-up. Moreover, PBC mediated the impact of the oncologist's recommendation on self-reported PA.

Project Leading the Way in Exercise and Diet (LEAD) was developed to determine whether older (≥65 years) breast and prostate cancer survivors assigned to a six-month diet and exercise intervention experienced improvements in diet and exercise behavior and physical function in comparison with a control group (Demark-Wahnefried et al., 2006). The treatment arm received telephone counseling and tailored print materials aimed at increasing exercise and improving diet, whereas the control arm received general health counseling and materials. The materials targeted constructs drawn from SCT and were tailored to the individual's stage of change. Although the intervention resulted in significant changes in overall diet at a six-month posttest, there was no change in PA. Nevertheless, a statistically significant increase in self-efficacy for PA was observed in the intervention group. The authors suggested that lack of sensitivity of the PA instrument (CHAMPS) to detect modest change in activity levels might have been responsible for the null finding for PA. Alternatively, low accrual may have resulted in inadequate power to detect a significant difference. In the first study to evaluate the efficacy of a lifestyle approach for improving exercise behavior and QoL in cancer patients, Carmack-Taylor et al. (2006) developed Active for Life, an adaptation of Project Active for use with prostate cancer patients on androgen ablation therapy. Project ACTIVE was a study conducted by Dunn, Marcus, Kampert, Garcia, Kohl, and Blair (1999) to compare a lifestyle intervention with a supervised structured intervention to increase physical activity and cardiorespiratory fitness in 235 sedentary, healthy adults.

Patients were randomly assigned to one of three study conditions: (a) a lifestyle program targeting self-efficacy and cognitive behavioral skills for adopting and maintaining regular PA, (b) educational support, incorporating facilitated discussion and expert talks on side effects of prostate cancer treatment, or (c) standard care. The education-only support condition was included to control for facilitator support inherent in PA programs. The lifestyle and educational conditions were equivalent in group size, composition, duration, meeting frequency, and time spent with a health educator. Standard-care participants did not attend group meetings but received one mailing of educational material and information about community resources. Results indicated no improvements in energy expenditure or days engaging in 30 minutes of moderate-intensity PA however, lifestyle participants reported a greater increase in stage of change at both six and 12 months compared with the other two conditions. Results indicated no significant improvements in social support or any QoL measure for any of the three conditions at six or 12 months. Likewise, there were no significant differences on measures of body composition or endurance at six or 12 months. Nevertheless, six-month data indicated that participants in the lifestyle program used significantly more cognitive and behavioral processes

of change for PA than those in the other conditions, had significantly higher pros for PA, and showed a trend for higher self-efficacy. At 12 months, lifestyle participants continued to show similar results for cognitive and behavioral processes of change however, the result for pros was no longer significant, and self-efficacy remained nonsignificant.

Overall, the lifestyle approach was not efficacious in improving QoL of prostate cancer patients receiving androgen ablation therapy. However, the lack of significant findings for QoL may be accounted for by the fact that participants reported relatively low levels of distress and pain at baseline, leaving little room for improvement. In a later report, secondary moderator analyses indicated that both the lifestyle and educational programs benefited patients with lower psychosocial functioning at baseline (Carmack-Taylor, Demoor, Basen-Entquist, Smith, and Dunn, 2007). Patients with lower mental health and social support scores had significant improvements in QoL compared with standard care. For those with higher pain, the educational support program resulted in significant improvements compared with the other two conditions. Moreover, 12-month findings indicated lasting effects of body pain.

RCTs examining exercise for cancer patients typically use no-treatment or wait-list control conditions, which do not control for the effects of support, particularly on psychological factors, from a professional or a group. The Carmack-Taylor et al. (2006, 2007) results indicate the importance of PA studies employing control conditions that consider the attention and support provided by health educators and group members. The findings suggest that participation in any group may be better than no group for improving psychosocial parameters in prostate cancer survivors. Without an educational support control condition, the moderator analyses would have shown only that those patients with psychosocial functioning limitations benefited more from the lifestyle program than no program. Research is needed that compares PA with other accepted supportive care interventions such as group support, particularly when examining outcomes such as QoL or emotional well-being.

The Activity Promotion (ACTION) trial (Vallance, Courneya, Plotnikoff, Yasui, & Mackey, 2007) was a RCT based on the TPB that was designed to compare the effects on PA and health-related QoL of breast cancer–specific print materials, a step pedometer, or their combination with those of a standard PA recommendation. At three months post intervention, breast cancer–specific print materials and pedometers were effective in increasing PA and health-related QoL in breast cancer survivors. Specifically, moderate- to vigorous-intensity PA increased by about 40–60 minutes per week in the intervention group compared with controls, and brisk walking increased by 60–90 minutes per week. The combined group also reported significantly better health-related QoL and reduced fatigue compared with the control group. Secondary analysis of intervention groups indicated positive changes in the TPB constructs, instrumental attitude, intention and planning, and several behavioral and control beliefs compared with the control group. Intention and planning were found to partially mediate the effect of the intervention on PA, and several salient beliefs about living longer, reducing risk of cancer recurrence, having no support, family responsibilities, and PA not fitting one's routine mediated the effects of the TPB intervention on intentions at a 12-week posttest (Vallance, Courneya, Plotnikoff, & Mackey, 2008). Analyzing data at the belief level allows researchers to identify components of the intervention materials that were effective at causing behavior change.

The ACTION trial is one of the few studies to report whether the behavior change observed immediately post intervention was maintained at six-month follow-up. Vallance, Courneya, Plotnikoff, Dinu, and Mackey (2008) reported only a small decline in the magnitude of the effect of the intervention during the six-month follow-up period. Although the difference was no longer significant at six months, the intervention groups were still engaging in substantially more PA and brisk walking than they reported at baseline, and they reported 30–60 minutes more of PA and 35–50 minutes more of brisk walking per week than the control group. However, no statistically significant or meaningful differences were found between groups on health-related QoL or fatigue at the six-month follow-up.

The ACTION study provides partial support for the mediating capacity of the TPB and some evidence that the TPB is a reasonable framework on which to base PA behavior change interventions in breast cancer survivors. Further evaluative inquiry is needed to establish stronger support for the use of the TPB for developing, implementing, and evaluating behavior change interventions in other cancer survivor groups.

To date, the interventions in efficacy studies have been delivered by research staff or health care providers. A pilot study conducted by Pinto, Rabin, Abdow, and Papandonatos (2008) examined the feasibility of disseminating a PA intervention program to breast cancer survivors over the telephone by trained community volunteers, also breast cancer survivors. The intervention was based on the Moving Forward trial (Pinto et al., 2005) and consisted of PA counseling matched to the participant's stage of change. In the earlier study, Pinto et al. (2005) had found that the intervention increased PA and vigor, improved fitness, and reduced fatigue among breast cancer survivors when delivered by research staff. Moreover, the intervention participants were more likely than a control group to progress in stages of motivational readiness for PA and to significantly increase their use of behavioral processes; however, the TTM constructs were not mediators of the intervention's effect on exercise behavior. In the later, single-group study, Pinto et al. (2008) reported that the intervention was feasible, with a mean of 10.7 calls delivered out of a possible 12, and was evaluated positively by both participants and volunteers. At 12 weeks there were significant increases in participants' self-reported PA, fatigue, QoL, and vigor, and effects were maintained at 24 weeks. Accelerometer data demonstrated an increase in PA at 12 weeks, but at 24 weeks the effect was no longer significant. This pilot study demonstrated that it was feasible for trained volunteers to deliver a theory-based PA intervention to breast cancer survivors and that an intervention delivered in this manner results in positive effects on survivors PA behavior and psychological outcomes. In the absence of a control group, the findings warrant replication.

Like supportive care research examining health outcomes, the majority of behavior change interventions have been limited to a few cancer survivor groups, predominantly breast cancer survivors. One exception is a study by von Gruenigen et al. (2008) that assessed the feasibility of a lifestyle intervention program for promoting weight loss and increased PA in obese endometrial cancer survivors. Early-stage (stage I to II) endometrial cancer survivors were randomized to a six-month lifestyle program or a UC condition. The lifestyle group received group and individual counseling for six months. At 12 months, the lifestyle group had lost 3.5 kg, compared with a 1.4-kg gain in the control group. Moreover, women in the lifestyle group demonstrated significant improvements in PA compared with UC participants. Weight loss was maintained six months after completion of the intervention. This study demonstrates the feasibility of conducting a weight loss intervention in obese endometrial cancer survivors. Future research efforts should seek to replicate these findings with a larger sample size to determine if there are population characteristics of individuals who benefit more from lifestyle interventions.

Conclusions and Future Directions for Behavior Change Research

Exercise motivation and behavior change is a major challenge for cancer survivors, who often face symptoms and side effects from treatment that present unique barriers to exercise participation and adherence. Prevalence rates for PA indicate that the majority of cancer survivors are not meeting general recommendations for PA. A growing body of research has examined the medical, demographic, and social cognitive determinants (i.e., correlates) of PA in cancer survivors. Research indicates that there are a plethora of demographic, medical, and social cognitive variables associated with PA behavior in cancer survivors and that these appear to vary by cancer group and treatment status.

Increasingly, research into the antecedents of PA behavior in cancer survivors has adopted a theoretical model to guide inquiry. The main theoretical models applied to examine PA behavior in cancer populations explain at best 30–40% of variance in PA behavior. This suggests that other factors must account for the remaining variance; consideration should be given to medical, demographic, and motivational variables when designing behavioral support interventions in this patient population. Few studies have conducted comprehensive examinations of the theoretical models rather, a common approach is to select a few key constructs and examine their independent influences on PA behavior. Subsequent investigations should examine the independent and aggregate contribution of each construct within a given theoretical model. Ecological models have yet to be applied to examine PA behavior in cancer survivors. Research suggests that investigators should consider the influence from both the social and physical environment when designing PA behavior change interventions for different groups of survivors.

Low response rates have been noted in cross-sectional determinants research with cancer survivors, with the percentage of eligible participants completing surveys ranging from 51% in ovarian cancer survivors (Stevinson, Tonkin, et al., 2009) to 82% in rural breast cancer survivors (Rogers et al., 2009). Therefore, it is not clear to what extent we can generalize the findings from determinants research to the general population of cancer survivors.

A main benefit of determinants research is that it enables identifying possible mediators of behavior change. Despite growing recognition of the importance of theory in guiding the development of PA interventions in cancer survivors, the majority of research focuses on the impact of interventions on PA behavior change without examining the underlying theoretical mechanisms along the causal pathway. Only a few studies have assessed change in the theoretical variables due to the intervention and in turn, whether change in the theoretical variables mediates change in PA behavior. Studies to date provide partial support for the mediating capacity of the TPB and SCT, and there is some evidence from determinants research that the TTM and SDT are reasonable frameworks on which to base PA behavior change interventions in breast cancer survivors. More frequent testing of mediators could show how interventions affect behavioral end points and overall QoL. It is prudent to identify components of an intervention that contributed to change in the primary outcomes (Pinto & Floyd, 2008).

The extent to which survivors adhere to a PA intervention program is of importance because it identifies the determinants of PA in survivors who are trying to exercise. In this context, motivational variables do not appear to play a key role in exercise adherence, most likely because of ceiling effects on these variables. Rather, medical and demographic variables seem to be important. Concomitantly, few studies have included long-term follow-up of behavior change. Research is needed to examine whether behavior change observed post intervention is sustained and the mechanisms contributing to maintenance of behavior change.

It is apparent that one behavior change intervention does not fit all groups of cancer survivors at all stages of the cancer experience. A key issue therefore is to find out what types of PA behavior change interventions work for different groups. Identification of possible moderator variables (e.g., medical, demographic, environmental, and social cognitive variables) can aid in this process. Moreover, cancer survivors participating in PA behavior change research have been relatively homogenous and predominantly posttreatment. Participants may be functioning relatively well on various QoL indicators at baseline, which may also account for the lack of change in these variables with change in PA behavior. There is a need for PA behavior change trials to target more demographically diverse groups of survivors across a variety of cancer groups and stages.

Similarly, PA interventions require a certain degree of commitment and involvement from participants, so there is likely selection bias for more motivated participants (Moyer et al., 2009). Several studies discussed above acknowledged high baseline values for motivational variables in PA interventions (Courneya, Segal, et al., 2008; Courneya et al., 2010in press). It is therefore not clear to what extent we can extend our findings to the general cancer population. Identifying preferences for and barriers to PA programs among less motivated eligible participants may help in designing effective methods to enhance recruitment to PA interventions. Although certain PA preferences are the same across cancer groups, such as mode and intensity, the preferred timing of the intervention varies. These findings suggest the need to further examine variations in preferences by cancer group and treatment status. Similarly, studies examining the determinants of PA suggest that barriers to PA can hinder the adoption and maintenance of regular exercise participation. Identifying unique barriers to PA participation in cancer survivors may lead to the development of effective behavioral support interventions to improve adherence and achieve better outcomes. More input from cancer patients in the planning stage is essential and will ensure that researchers are developing interventions appropriate for cancer patients and delivering them in the most acceptable way.

Despite evidence to suggest PA programs are feasible and beneficial for cancer survivors, many important questions remain, including the optimal doses of PA necessary to bring about change in QoL in different groups of survivors, the mechanisms responsible for PA behavior change, and whether changes in behavior and improvements to overall QoL from such programs are sustainable.

Acknowledgment

Kerry S. Courneya is supported by the Canada Research Chairs Program.

References

*Entries marked with asterisks are recommended for further reading.

American Cancer Society (2007). *Global cancer facts and figures.* Atlanta, GA: American Cancer Society.

American Cancer Society (2008). *Cancer facts and figures.* Atlanta, GA: American Cancer Society.

American Cancer Society (2009a). *Cancer facts and figures 2009.* Atlanta, GA: American Cancer Society.

American Cancer Society (2009b). *Understanding chemotherapy: A guide for patients and families.* Atlanta, GA: American Cancer Society.

American Cancer Society (2009c). *Understanding radiation therapy: A guide for patients and families.* Atlanta, GA: American Cancer Society.

Adamson, L., Quist, M., Anderson, C., Moller, T., Herrstedt, J., Kronborg, D.,...Rørth, M. (2009). Effect of a multimodal high intensity exercise intervention in cancer patients undergoing chemotherapy: Randomized controlled trial. *BMJ, 339,* b3410.

Ainsworth, B. E., Haskill, W. L., Whitt, M. C., Irwin, M. L., Swartz, A. M., Strath, S. J.,...Leon, A. S.(2000). Compendium of physical activities: An update of activity codes and Met intensities. *Medicine & Science in Sports & Exercise, 32*(9 Suppl.), S498–S504.

Ajzen, I. (1991). The theory of planned behavior. *Organizational Behavior and Human Decision Processes, 50,* 179–211.

Ajzen, I. (2002). Perceived behavioral control, self-efficacy, locus of control, and the theory of planned behavior. *Journal of Applied Social Psychology, 32,* 665–683.

Bandura, A. (1986). *Social foundations of thought and action: A social-cognitive theory.* Englewood Cliffs, NJ: Prentice Hall.

Bandura, A. (1997). *Self-efficacy: The exercise of control.* New York: W. H. Freeman.

Baron, R. M., & Kenny, D. A. (1986). The moderator–mediator variable distinction in social psychological research: Conceptual, strategic and statistical considerations. *Journal of Personality and Social Psychology, 51,* 1173–1182.

Bauman, A. E., Sallis, J. F., Dzewaltowski, D. A., & Owen, N. (2002). Toward a better understanding of the influences on physical activity: The role of determinants, correlates, causal variables, mediators, moderators, and confounders. *American Journal of Preventive Medicine, 23,* 5–14.

Belizzi, K. M., Rowland, J. H., Arora, N. J., Hamilton, A. S., Miller, M. F., & Aziz, N. M. (2009). Physical activity and quality of life in adult survivors of non-Hodgkin's lymphoma. *Journal of Clinical Oncology, 27,* 960–966.

*Bennett, J. A., Winters-Stone, K., & Nail, L. (2006). Conceptualizing and measuring physical functioning in cancer survivorship studies. *Oncology Nursing Forum, 33*(1), 41–49.

Bicego, D., Brown, K., Ruddick, M., Storey, D., Wong, C., & Harris, S. R. (2009). Effects of exercise on quality of life in women living with breast cancer: A systematic review. *Breast Journal, 15*(1), 45–51.

Blanchard, C. M., Courneya, K. S., Rodgers, W. M., & Murnaghan, D. M. (2002). Determinants of exercise intention and behavior in survivors of breast and prostate cancer: An application of the theory of planned behavior. *Cancer Nursing, 25,* 88–95.

Blanchard, C. M., Courneya, K. S., & Stein, K. (2008). Cancer survivors' adherence to lifestyle behavior recommendations and associations with health related quality of life: Results from the American Cancer Society's SCS-II. *Journal of Clinical Oncology, 26*(13), 2198–2204.

Bland, J. M., & Altman, D. G. (1995). Comparing methods of measurement: Why plotting difference against standard method is misleading. *Lancet, 346*(8982), 1085–1087.

Bower, J. E., Woolery, A., Sternlieb, B., & Garet, D. (2005). Yoga for cancer patients and survivors. *Cancer Control, 12*(3), 165–171.

Cadmus, L. A., Salovey, P., Yu, H., Chung, G., Kasl, S., & Irwin, M. L. (2009). Exercise and quality of life during and after treatment for breast cancer: Results of two randomized controlled trials. *Psycho-oncology, 18,* 343–352.

Carmack-Taylor, C. L., Demoor, C., Basen-Entquist, K., Smith, M. A., & Dunn, A. L. (2007). Moderator analyses of participants in the Active for Life after Cancer trial: Implications for physical activity group intervention studies. *Annals of Behavioral Medicine, 33*, 99–104.

Carmack-Taylor, C. L., Demoor, C., Smith, M. A., Dunn, A. L., Basen-Entquist, K., Nielson, I.,...Gritz, E. R. (2006). Active for Life after Cancer: A randomized trial examining a life-style physical activity program for prostate cancer survivors. *Psycho-oncology, 15*, 847–862.

*Conn, V. S., Hafdahl, A. R., Porock, D. C., McDaniel, R., & Neilson, P. J. (2006). A meta-analysis of exercise interventions among people treated for cancer. *Supportive Care in Cancer, 14*, 699–712.

Coups, E. J., & Ostroff, J. S. (2005). A population based estimate of the prevalence of behavioral risk factors among adult cancer survivors and noncancer controls. *Preventive Medicine, 40*, 702–711.

Coups, E. J., Park, B. J., Feinstein, M. B., Steingart, R. M., Egleston, B. L., & Wilson, D. J. (2009). Correlates of physical activity among lung cancer survivors. *Psycho-oncology, 18*, 395–404.

Courneya, K. S. (2004). Antecedent correlates and theories of exercise behavior. In T. S. Morris & J. Summers Eds.), *Sport psychology: Theories, applications, and issues, 2nd Edition* (pp. 492–512.). Milton, Queensland: John Wiley & Sons Australia, Ltd.

*Courneya, K. S. (2009). Physical activity in cancer survivors: A field in motion. *Psycho-oncology, 18*, 337–342.

Courneya, K. S., Blanchard, C. M., & Laing, D. M. (2001). Exercise adherence in breast cancer survivors training for a dragon boat race competition: A preliminary investigation. *Psycho-oncology, 10*(5), 444–452.

Courneya, K. S., & Friedenreich, C. M. (1997a). Determinants of exercise during colorectal cancer treatment: An application of the theory of planned behavior. *Oncology Nursing Forum, 24*(10), 1715–1723.

Courneya, K. S., & Friedenreich, C. M. (1997b). Relationship between exercise during treatment and current quality of life among survivors of breast cancer. *Journal of Psychosocial Oncology, 15*(3/4), 35–57.

Courneya, K. S., & Friedenreich, C. M. (1997c). Relationship between exercise pattern across the cancer experience and current quality of life in colorectal cancer survivors. *Journal of Alternative and Complementary Medicine, 3*(3), 215–226.

Courneya, K. S., & Friedenreich, C. M. (1999). Utility of the theory of planned behavior for understanding exercise during breast cancer treatment. *Psycho-oncology, 8*(2), 112–122.

*Courneya, K. S., & Friedenreich, C. M. (2007). Physical activity and cancer control. *Seminars in Oncology Nursing, 23*, 242–252.

Courneya, K., Friedenreich, C., Quinney, H., Fields, A., Jones, L., & Fairey, A. (2004). Predictors of adherence and contamination in a randomized trial of exercise in colorectal cancer survivors: An application of the theory of planned behavior and the five factor model of personality. *Annals of Behavioral Medicine, 24*(4), 257–268.

Courneya, K. S., Friedenreich, C. M., Quinney, H. A., Fields, A. L., Jones, L. W., Vallance, J. K., & Fairey, A. S. (2005). A longitudinal study of exercise barriers in colorectal cancer survivors participating in a randomized controlled trial. *Annals of Behavioral Medicine, 29*, 147–153.

Courneya, K. S., Karvinen, K. H., Campbell, K. L., Pearcey, R. G., Dundas, G., Capstick, V., & Tonkin, K. S. (2005). Associations among exercise, body weight, and quality of life in a population based sample of endometrial cancer survivors. *Gynecological Oncology, 97*, 422–430.

Courneya, K. S., Karvinen, K. H., & Vallance, J. K. H. (Eds.). (2007). *Exercise motivation and behavior change.* New York, NY: Springer-Verlag.

Courneya, K. S., Katzmarzyk, P. T., & Bacon, E. (2008). Physical activity and obesity in Canadian cancer survivors: Population-based estimates from the 2005 Canadian Community Health Survey. *Cancer, 112*(11), 2475–2482.

Courneya, K. S., Keats, M. R., & Turner, A. R. (2000). Social cognitive determinants of hospital based exercise in cancer patients following high dose chemotherapy and bone marrow transplantation. *International Journal of Behavioral Medicine, 7*(3), 189–203.

Courneya, K. S., Mackey, J. R., Bell. G. J., Jones, L. W., Field, C. J., & Fairey, A. S. (2003). Randomized controlled trial of exercise training in postmenopausal breast cancer survivors: Cardiopulmonary and quality of life outcomes. *Journal of Clinical Oncology, 21*, 1660–1668.

Courneya, K. S., McKenzie, D. C., Mackey, J. R., Gelmon, K., Reid, R. D., Friedenreich, C. M.,...Segal, R. J.(2008). Moderators of the effects of exercise training in breast cancer patients receiving chemotherapy: A randomized controlled trial. *Cancer, 112*, 1845–1853.

Courneya, K. S., McKenzie, D. C., Reid, R. D., Mackey, J. R., Gelmon, K., Friedenreich, C. M.,...Segal, R. J. Author, A. A. (2008). Barriers to supervised exercise training in a randomized controlled trial of breast cancer patients receiving chemotherapy. *Annals of Behavioral Medicine, 35*(1), 116–122.

Courneya, K. S., Reid, R. D., Friedenreich, C. M., Gelmon, K., Proulx, C., Vallance, J. K.,...Segal, R. J. (2008). Understanding breast cancer patients' preferences for two types of exercise during chemotherapy in an unblinded randomized controlled trial. *International Journal of Nutrition and Physical Activity, 52*(5), 1–9.

Courneya, K. S., Segal, R. J., Gelmon, K., Reid, R. D., Mackey, J. R., Friedenreich, C. M.,...McKenzie, D. C..(2007). Six-month follow up of patient rated outcomes in a randomized controlled trial of exercise training during breast cancer chemotherapy. *Cancer Epidemiology, Biomarkers & Prevention, 16*(12), 2572–2577.

Courneya, K. S., Segal, R. J., Gelmon, K., Reid, R. D., Mackey, J. R., Friedenreich, C. M.,...McKenzie DC. (2008). Predictors of supervised exercise adherence during breast cancer chemotherapy. *Medicine & Science in Sports & Exercise, 40*(6), 1180–1187.

Courneya, K. S., Segal, R. J., Mackey, J. R., Gelmon, K., Friedenreich, C. M., Ladha, A. B.,...McKenzie, D. C. (2007). Effects of aerobic and resistance exercise in breast cancer patients receiving adjuvant chemotherapy: A multicenter randomized controlled trial. *Journal of Clinical Oncology, 25*, 4396–4404.

*Courneya, K. S., Sellar, C. M., Stevinson, C., McNeely, M. L., Friedenreich, C. M., Peddle, C. J.,...Reiman T. (2009). Moderator effects in a randomized controlled trial of exercise training in lymphoma patients. *Cancer Epidemiology, Biomarkers & Prevention, 18*(10), 2600–2607.

Courneya, K. S., Sellar, C. M., Stevinson, C., McNeely, M. L., Peddle, C. J., Friedenreich, C. M.,...Reiman T (2009). Randomized controlled trial of the effects of aerobic exercise on physical functioning and quality of life in lymphoma patients. *Journal of Clinical Oncology, 27*, 1–9.

Courneya, K. S., Stevinson, C., McNeely, M. L., Sellar, C. M., Peddle, C. J., Friedenreich, C. M.,...Reiman T. (2010). Predictors for supervised exercise in lymphoma patients participating in a randomized controlled trial. *Annals of Behavioral Medicine, 40*, 30–39

Courneya, K. S., Stevinson, C., & Vallance, J. K. (2007). Exercise and psychosocial aspects of cancer recovery. In G. T. R. C. Eklund (Ed.), *Handbook of sport psychology* (3rd ed.). New York: Wiley.

Courneya, K. S., Vallance, J. K., Jones, L. W., & Reiman, T. (2005). Correlates of exercise intentions in non-Hodgkin's lymphoma survivors: An application of the theory of planned behavior. *Journal of Sport and Exercise Psychology, 27*, 335–349.

Cramp, F., & Daniel, J. (2008). Exercise for the management of cancer-related fatigue in adults. *Cochrane Database of Systematic Reviews, 16*(2), 1–57.

Daley, A. J., Crank, H., Saxton, J. M., Mutrie, N., Coleman, R., & Roalfe, A. (2007). Randomized trial of exercise therapy in women treated for breast cancer. *Journal of Clinical Oncology, 25*, 1713–1721.

Danhauer, S. C., Mihalko, S. L., Russell, G. B., Campbell, C. R., Felder, L., Daley, K., & Levine, E. A. (2009). Restorative yoga for women with breast cancer: Findings from a randomized pilot study. *Psycho-oncology, 18*, 360–368.

De Backer, C., Schep, G., Backx, F. J., Vreugdenhil, G., & Kuipers, H. (2009). Resistance training in cancer survivors: A systematic review. *International Journal of Sports Medicine, 30*(10), 703–712.

Deci, E. L., & Ryan, R. M. (1985). *Intrinsic motivation and self-determination in human behavior.* New York: Plenum.

Deimling, G. T., Kahana, B., Bowman, K. F., & Shaefer, M. L. (2002). Cancer survivorship and psychological distress in later life. *Psycho-oncology, 11*(6), 479–494.

Demark-Wahnefried, W., Azziz, N., Rowland, J., & Pinto, B. M.(2005). Riding the crest of the teachable moment: Promoting long term health after the diagnosis of cancer. *Journal of Clinical Oncology, 23*, 5814–5830.

Demark-Wahnefried, W., Clipp, E. C., Lipkus, I. M., Lobach, D., Snyder, D. C., Sloane, R.,...Kraus, W. E(2007). Main outcomes of the Fresh Start trial: A sequentially tailored, diet and exercise mailed print intervention among breast and prostate cancer survivors. *Journal of Clinical Oncology, 25*, 2709–2718.

Demark-Wahnefried, W., Clipp, E. C., Morey, M. C., Pieper, C. F., Sloane, R., Snyder, D. C., & Cohen, H. J. (2006). Lifestyle intervention development study to improve physical function in older adults with cancer: Outcomes from Project LEAD. *Journal of Clinical Oncology, 24*, 3465–3473.

DiClemente, C. C., Prochaska, J. O., Fairhurst, S. K., Velicer, W. F., Velasquez, M. M., & Rossi, J. S. (1991). The process of smoking cessation: An analysis of precontemplation, contemplation, and preparation stages of change. *Journal of Consulting and Clinical Psychology, 59*(2), 295–304.

Dunn, A. L., Garcia, M. E., Marcus, B. H., Kampert, J. B., Kohl, H. W., III, & Blair, S. N. (1998). Six-month physical activity and fitness changes in Project Active, a randomized trial. Medicine and Science in Sports and Exercise, 30(7), 1076-1083.

Flay, B. (1986). Efficacy and effectiveness trials (and other phases of research) in the development of health promotion programs. *Preventive Medicine, 15*, 451–474.

Friedenreich, C. M., Cust, A., Lahmann, P. H., Steingdorf, K., Boutron-Ruault, M. C., Clavel-Chapelon, F., & Riboli, E. (2007). Physical activity and risk of endometrial cancer: The European Prospective Investigation into Cancer and Nutrition. *International Journal of Cancer, 121*(2), 347–355.

Glanz, K., Lewis, F. M., & Rimer, B. K. (Eds.) (1997). *Health behavior and health education: Theory, research and practice.* San Francisco, CA: Jossey-Bass.

Glasgow, R. E. (2002). Evaluation of theory-based interventions: The RE-AIM model. In K. Glanz, B. K. Rimer, & F. M. Lewis (Eds.), *Health behavior and health education: Theory, research, and practice (*3rd ed., pp. 531–544*).* San Francisco, CA: Jossey-Bass.

Harrison, S., Hayes, S. C., & Newman, B. (2009). Level of physical activity and characteristics associated with change following breast cancer diagnosis and treatment. *Psycho-oncology, 18*, 387–394.

Haskell, W. L., Lee, I. M., Pate, R. R., Powell, K. E., Blair, S. N., Franklin, B. A.,...Bauman, A. (2007). Physical activity and public health: Updated recommendations from the American College of Sports Medicine and the American Heart Association. *Medicine & Science in Sports & Exercise, 39*, 1423–1434.

Headley, J. A., Ownby, K. K., & John, L. D. (2004). The effect of seated exercise on fatigue and quality of life in women with advanced breast cancer. *Oncology Nursing Forum, 31*, 977–983.

*Hewitt, M., Greenfield, S., & Stovell, E. (2006). *From cancer patient to cancer survivor: Lost in transition.* Washington, DC: The National Academies Press.

Irwin, M. L., McTiernan, A., Bernstein, L., Gilliland, F. D., Baumgartner, R., Baumgartner, K., & Ballard-Barbash, R. (2004). Physical activity levels among breast cancer survivors. *Medicine & Science in Sports & Exercise, 36*(9), 1484–1491.

Jacobson, P. B., Donovan, K. A., Vadaparampil, S. T., & Small, B. J. (2007). Systematic review and meta-analysis of psychological and activity based interventions for cancer related fatigue. *Health Psychology, 26*, 660–667.

Jones, L. W., & Courneya, K. S. (2002). Exercise counselling and programming preferences of cancer survivors. *Cancer Practice, 10*, 208–215.

Jones, L. W., Courneya, K. S., Fairey, A. S., & Mackey, J. R. (2004). Effects of an oncologist's recommendation to exercise on self-reported exercise behavior in newly diagnosed breast cancer survivors: A single-blind, randomized controlled trial. *Annals of Behavioral Medicine, 28*, 105–113.

Jones, L. W., Courneya, K. S., Fairey, A. S., & Mackey, J. R. (2005). Does the theory of planned behavior mediate the effects of an oncologist's recommendation to exercise in newly diagnosed breast cancer patients? Results from a randomized controlled trial. *Health Psychology, 24*(2), 189–197.

Jones, L. W., Courneya, K. S., Vallance, J. K., Ladha, A. B., Mant, M. J., Belch, A. R.,...Reiman, T. (2004). Association between exercise and quality of life in multiple myeloma cancer survivors. *Supportive Care in Cancer, 12*, 780–788.

Jones, L. W., Courneya, K. S., Vallance, J. K., Ladha, A. B., Mant, M. J., Belch, A. R., & Reiman, T.(2006). Understanding the determinants of exercise intentions in multiple myeloma cancer survivors: An application of the theory of planned behavior. *Cancer Nursing, 29*(3), 167–175.

Jones, L. W., Eves, N. D., Peterson, B. L., Garst, J., Crawford, J., West, M. J., . . . Douglas, P. S. (2008). Safety and feasibility of aerobic training on cardiopulmonary function and quality of life in postsurgical nonsmall cell lung cancer patients. *Cancer, 113*(12), 3430–3438.

Jones, L. W., Guill, B., Keir, S. T., Carter, K, Friedman, H. S., Bigner, D. D., & Reardon, D. A. (2006). Patterns of exercise across the cancer trajectory in brain cancer patients. *Cancer, 106*, 2224–2232.

Jones, L. W., Guill, B., Keir, S. T., Carter, K., Friedman, H. S., Bigner, D. D., . . . Reardon, D. A. (2007). Using the theory of planned behavior to understand the determinants of exercise intention in patients diagnosed with primary brain cancer. *Psycho-oncology, 16*, 232–240.

Jordhoy, M. S. (2007). Assessing physical function: A systematic review of quality of life measures developed for use in palliative care. *Palliative Medicine, 21*, 673–682.

Karvinen, K. H., Courneya, K. S., Campbell, K. L., Pearcey, R. G., Dundas, G., Capstick, V., & Tonkin, K. S.(2007). Correlates of exercise motivation and behavior in a population-based sample of endometrial cancer survivors: An application of the theory of planned behavior. *International Journal of Behavior, Nutrition and Physical Activity, 4*, 21.

Karvinen, K. H., Courneya, K. S., Campbell, K. L., Pearcy, R. G., Dundas, G., Capstick, V., & Tonkin, K. S. (2006). Exercise preferences of endometrial cancer survivors: A population based study. *Cancer Nursing, 29*(4), 259–265.

Karvinen, K. H., Courneya, K. S., North, S., & Venner, P. (2007). Associations between exercise and quality of life in bladder cancer survivors: A population based study. *Cancer Epidemiology, Biomarkers & Prevention, 16*, 984–990.

Karvinen, K. H., Courneya, K. S., Plotnikoff, R. C., Spence, J. C., Venner, P. M., & North, S. (2009). A prospective study of the determinants of exercise in bladder cancer survivors using the theory of planned behavior. *Supportive Care in Cancer, 17*, 171–179.

Karvinen, K. H., Courneya, K. S., Venner, P., & North, S. (2007). Exercise programming and counselling preferences in bladder cancer survivors: A population based study. *Journal of Cancer Survivorship: Research and Practice, 1*, 27–34.

Kesaniemi, Y. K., Danforth, E., Jensen, M. D., Kopelman, P. G., Lefebvre, P., & Reeder, B. A. (2001). Dose–response issues concerning physical activity and health: An evidence-based symposium. *Medicine & Science in Sports & Exercise, 33*(6 Suppl.), S351–S358.

Klee, M., Groenvold, M., & Machin, D. (1997). Quality of life of Danish women: Population-based norms of the EORTC QLQ-C30. *Quality of Life Research, 6*, 27–34.

Liu, R. D. K. S., Chinapow, M. J. M., Huijgens, P. C., & van Mechelen, W. (2009). Physical activity exercise interventions in haematological cancer patients, feasible to conduct but effectiveness to be established: A systematic literature review. *Cancer Treatments Reviews, 35*(2), 185–192.

Lowe, S. S., Watanabe, S. M., Baracos, V. E., & Courneya, K. S. (2009). Physical activity interests and preferences in palliative cancer patients. *Supportive Care in Cancer, 18*(11), 1469–1475.

Lowe, S. S., Watanabe, S. M., & Courneya, K. S. (2009). Physical activity as a supportive care intervention in palliative cancer

patients: A systematic review. *Journal of Supportive Oncology, 7*, 1–8.

Lucia, A., Earnest, C., & Perez, M. (2003). Cancer related fatigue: Can exercise physiology assist oncologists? *Lancet Oncology, 4*(10), 616–625.

Lynch, B. M., Cerin, E., Owen, N., Hawkes, A. L., & Aitken, J. F. (2008). Prospective relationships of physical activity with quality of life among colorectal cancer survivors. *Journal of Clinical Oncology, 26*, 4480–4487.

Markes, M., & Resch, B. T. (2006). Exercise for women receiving adjuvant therapy for breast cancer. *Cochrane Database of Systematic Reviews,* Oct 18;(4), CD005001.

McAuley, E. (1992). The role of efficacy cognitions in the prediction of exercise behavior in middle-aged adults. *Journal of Behavioral Medicine, 15*(1), 65–87.

McNeely, M. L., Campbell, K. L., Rowe, B. H., Klassen, T. P., Mackey, J. R., & Courneya, K. S. (2006). Effects of exercise on breast cancer patients and survivors: A systematic review and meta-analysis. *Canadian Medical Association Journal, 175*(1), 34–41.

Milne, H. M., Walkman, K. E., Guilfoyle, A., Gordon, S., & Courneya, K. S.(2008). Self-determination theory and physical activity among breast cancer survivors. *Journal of Sport and Exercise Psychology, 30*, 23–38.

Mock, V., Abernathy, A. M., Atkinson, A., Barsevick, A., Cella, D., Cimprich, B., & Stahl, C. (2007). *The NCCN cancer-related fatigue clinical practice guidelines* (Version 3.2007). Retrieved November 1, 2009, from http://www.nccn.org/professionals/physician_gls.PDF/fatigue.pdf

Mock, V., Pickett, M., Ropka, M. E., Muscari, L. E., Stewart, K. J., Rhodes, V. A., . . . McCorkle, R.(2001). Fatigue and quality of life outcomes of exercise during cancer treatment. *Cancer Practice, 9*, 119–127.

Monninkhof, W. M., Elias, S. G., Vlems, F. A., van der Tweel, I., Schuit, A. J., Voskuil, D. W., & van Leeuwen, F. E.; TFPAC. (2007). Physical activity and breast cancer: A systematic review. *Epidemiology, 18*(1), 137–157.

Mosher, C. E., Fuemmeler, B. F., Sloane, R., Kraus, W. E., Lobach, D. F., Snyder, D. C., & Demark-Wahnefried, W.(2008). Change in self-efficacy partially mediates the effects of the FRESH START intervention on cancer survivors' dietary outcomes. *Psycho-oncology, 17*, 1014–1023.

Moyer, A., Knapp-Oliver, S. K., Sohl, S. J., Schneider, S., & Floyd, A. H. L. (2009). Lessons to be learned from 25 years of research investigating psychosocial interventions for cancer patients. *Cancer Journal, 15*, 345–351.

Mutrie, N., Campbell, A., Whyte, F., McConnachie, A., Emslie, C., Lee, L., . . . Ritchie, D. (2007). Benefits of supervised group exercise programme for women being treated for early stage breast cancer: Pragmatic randomized controlled trial. *BMJ, 334*, 517–523.

National Coalition for Cancer Survivorship. (1994–2004). *Glossary* (Vol. 2009). Retrieved November 1, 2009 from http://canceradvocacy.org/resources/glossary.aspxtop

Nordin, K., Berglund, G., Glimelius, B., & Sjoden, P. O. (2001). Predicting anxiety and depression among cancer patients: A clinical model. *European Journal of Cancer Care, 37*(3), 376–384.

Ohira, T., Schmitz, K. H., Ahmed, R. L., & Yee, D. (2006). Effects of weight training on quality of life in recent cancer survivors: The Weight Training of Breast Cancer Survivors (WTBS) study. *Cancer, 106*, 2076–2083.

Oldervoll, L. M., Loge, J. H., Paltiel, H., Asp, M. B., Vidvei, U., Hjermstad, M. J., & Kaasa, S. (2005). Are palliative cancer patients willing and able to participate in a physical exercise program? *Palliative & Supportive Care, 3*, 281–287.

Oldervoll, L. M., Loge, J. H., Paltiel, H., Asp, M. B., Vidvei, U., Wiken, A. N., ... Kaasa, S. (2006). The effect of a physical exercise program in palliative care: A phase II study. *Journal of Pain and Symptom Management., 31*, 421–430.

Peddle, C. J., Au, H. J., & Courneya, K. S. (2008). Associations between exercise, quality of life, and fatigue in colorectal cancer survivors. *Disease of the Colon and Rectum, 51*, 1242–1248.

Peddle, C. J., Plotnikoff, R. C., Wild, T. C., Au, H. J., & Courneya, K. S. (2008). Medical, demographic, and psychosocial correlates of exercise in colorectal cancer survivors: An application of self-determination theory. *Supportive Care in Cancer, 16*, 9–17.

Perkins, H. Y., Baum, G. P., Carmack-Taylor, C. L., & Basen-Entquist, K. M. (2009). Effects of treatment factors, comorbidities and health related quality of life on self-efficacy for physical activity in cancer survivors. *Psycho-oncology, 18*, 405–411.

*Pinto, B., & Floyd, A. (2008). Theories underlying health promotion interventions among cancer survivors. *Seminars in Oncology Nursing, 24*(3), 153–163.

Pinto, B. M., Frierson, G. M., Rabin, C., Trunzo, J. J., & Marcus, B. H. (2005). Home based physical activity intervention for breast cancer patients. *Journal of Clinical Oncology, 23*, 3577–3587.

Pinto, B. M., Rabin, C., Abdow, A., & Papandonatos, G. D. (2008). A pilot study on disseminating physical activity promotion among cancer survivors: A brief report. *Psycho-oncology, 17*, 517–521.

Pinto, B. M., Rabin, C., & Dunsiger, S. (2009). Home based exercise among cancer survivors: Adherence and its predictors. *Psycho-oncology, 18*, 369–376.

Pirl, W. F., Siegel, G. I., & Goode, M. J., & Smith, M. R. (2002). Depression in men receiving androgen deprivation therapy for prostate cancer: A pilot study. *Psycho-oncology, 168*, 109–116.

Porock, D., Kristjanson, L. J., Tinnelly, K., Duke, T., & Blight, J. (2000). An exercise intervention for advanced cancer patients experiencing fatigue: A pilot study. *Journal of Palliative Care, 16*, 30–36.

Prochaska, J. O., & DiClemente, C. C. (1983). The stages and processes of self-change in smoking: Toward an integrative model of change. *Journal of Consulting and Clinical Psychology, 51*, 390–395.

Rawl, S. M., Given, B. A., Given, C. W., Champion, V. L., Kozachik, S. L., Kozachik, S. L., ... Williams, S. D. (2002). Intervention to improve psychological functioning for newly diagnosed patients with cancer. *Oncology Nursing Forum, 29*, 967–975.

Rhodes, R. E., Courneya, K. S., & Bobick, T. M. (2001). Personality and exercise participation across the breast cancer experience. *Psycho-oncology, 10*(5), 380–388.

Ricketts, T. C. (2000). The changing nature of rural health care. *Annual Review of Public Health, 21*, 639–657.

Rogers, L. Q., Markwell, S. J., Verhulst, S., McAuley, E., & Courneya, K. S. (2009). Rural breast cancer survivors: Exercise preferences and their determinants. *Psycho-oncology, 18*, 412–421.

Rogers, L. Q., Matevey, C., Hopkins-Price, P., Shah, P., Dunningham, G., & Courneya, K. S. (2004). Exploring social cognitive theory constructs for promoting exercise among breast cancer patients. *Cancer Nursing, 27*(6), 462–473.

Sallis, J. F., & Owen, N. (1997). Ecological models. In Glanz, K., F. M., Lewis, & B. K. Rymer (Eds.), *Health behavior and health education: Theory, research and practice* (2nd ed. pp. 403–424). San Francisco, CA: Jossey-Bass.

Samad, A. K., Taylor, R. S., Marshall, T., & Chapman, M. A. (2005). A meta-analysis of the association of physical activity with reduced risk of colon cancer. *Colorectal Disease, 7*(3), 204–213.

Schmitz, K., Holtzman, J., Courneya, K., Masse, L., Duval, S., & Kane, R. (2005). Controlled physical activity trials in cancer survivors: A systematic review and meta-analysis. *Cancer Epidemiology, Biomarkers & Prevention, 14*, 1588–1595.

Schwartz, A. L. (2008). Physical activity. *Seminars in Oncology Nursing, 24*(3), 164–170.

Segal, R. J., Reid, R. D., Courneya, K. S., Segal, R. J., Kenny, G. P., Prud'Homme, D. G., ... Slovinec D'Angelo, M. E. (2009). Randomized controlled trial of resistance and aerobic training in men receiving radiation therapy for prostate cancer. *Journal of Clinical Oncology, 27*, 344–351.

Smith, K. B., & Pukall, C. F. (2008). An evidence-based review of yoga as a complementary intervention for patients with cancer. *Psycho-oncology, 18*(5), 465–475.

Somerset, W., Stout, S. C., Miller, A. H., & Musselman, D. (2004). Breast cancer and depression. *Oncology, 18*(8), 1021–1048.

*Speck, R. M., Courneya, K. S., Mass, L. C., Duval, S., & Schmitz, K. H. (2010). An update of controlled physical activity trials in cancer survivors: A systematic review and meta-analysis. *Journal of Cancer Survivorship, 4*(2), 87–100

Speed-Andrews, A. E., Stevinson, C., Belanger, L. J., Mirus, J. J., & Courneya, K. S. (2010). Pilot evaluation of an Iyengar yoga program for breast cancer survivors. *Cancer Nursing, 33*(5), 369–381.

Stevinson, C., Faught, W., Steed, H., Tonkin, K., Ladha, A. B., Vallance, J. K., ... Courneya, K. S. (2007). Associations between physical activity and quality of life in ovarian cancer survivors. *Gynecologic Oncology, 106*, 244–250.

Stevinson, C., Tonkin, K., Capstick, V., Schepansky, A., Ladha, A. B., Vallance, J. K., Faught, W., Steed, H., & Courneya, K. S. (2009). A population based study of the determinants of physical activity behavior and intentions in ovarian cancer survivors. *Journal of Physical Activity and Health, 6*(3), 339–346.

Stevinson, C., Capstick, V., Schepansky, A., Tonkin, K., Vallance, J. K., Ladha, A. B., Steed, H., Faught, W., & Courneya, K. S. (2009). Physical activity preferences of ovarian cancer survivors. *Psycho-oncology, 18*, 422–428.

Stjernsward, J. (2007). Palliative care: The public health strategy. *Journal of Public Health Policy, 28*, 42–55.

Tardon, A., Lee, W. J., Delgado-Rodriguez, M., Dosemeci, M., Albanes, D., Hoover, R., & Blair, A. (2005). Leisure-time physical activity and lung cancer: A meta-analysis. *Cancer Causes and Control, 16*(4), 389–397.

Thorsen, L., Courneya, K. S., Stevinson, C., & Fossa, S. D. (2008). A systematic review of physical activity in prostate cancer survivors: Outcomes, prevalence, and determinants. *Supportive Care in Cancer, 16*, 987–997.

Trost, S. G., Owen, N., Baumen, A. E., Sallis, J. F., & Brown, W. (2002). Correlates of adults' participation in physical activity: Review and update. *Medicine & Science in Sports & Exercise, 34*, 1996–2001.

U.S. Department of Health and Human Services. (2005). *Centers for Disease Control and Prevention: Behavioral Risk Factor Surveillance System survey data*. Atlanta, GA: U.S. Department of Health and Human Services.

Vallance, J. K., Courneya, K. S., Jones, L. W., & Reiman, A. R. (2005). Differences in quality of life between non-Hodgkin's lymphoma survivors meeting and not meeting public health exercise guidelines. *Psycho-oncology, 14*, 979–991.

Vallance, J. K., Courneya, K. S., Jones, L. W., & Reiman T. (2006). Exercise preferences among a population based sample of non-Hodgkin's lymphoma survivors. *European Journal of Cancer Care, 15*, 34–43.

Vallance, J. K., Courneya, K. S., Plotnikoff, R. C., Dinu, I., & Mackey, J. R. (2008). Maintenance of physical activity in breast cancer survivors after a randomized trial. *Medicine & Science in Sports & Exercise, 40*(1), 173–180.

Vallance, J. K., Courneya, K. S., Plotnikoff, R. C., & Mackey, J. R. (2008). Analyzing theoretical mechanisms of physical activity behavior change in breast cancer survivors: Results from the Activity Promotion (ACTION) trial. *Annals of Behavioral Medicine, 35*(2), 150–158.

Vallance, J. K., Courneya, K. S., Plotnikoff, R. C., Yasui, Y., & Mackey, J. R. (2007). Randomized controlled trial of the effects of print materials and step pedometers on physical activity and quality of life in breast cancer survivors. *Journal of Clinical Oncology, 25*, 2352–2359.

von Gruenigen, V. E., Courneya, K. S., Gibbons, H. E., Kavanagh, M. B., Waggoner, S. E., & Lerner, E. (2008). Feasibility and effectiveness of a lifestyle intervention program in obese endometrial cancer patients: A randomized trial. *Gynecologic Oncology, 109*, 19–26.

Ware, J. E., Kosinski, M., & Keller, S. D. (1994). *SF-36 physical and mental health summary scales: A user's manual*. Boston, MA: The Health Institute, New England Medical Center.

*White, S. M., McAuley, E., Estabrooks, P. A., & Courneya, K. S. (2009). Translating physical activity interventions for breast cancer survivors into practice: An evaluation of randomized controlled trials. *Annals of Behavioral Medicine, 37*(1), 10–19.

Wilson, P. M., Blanchard, C. M., Nehl, E., & Baker, F. (2006). Predicting physical activity and outcome expectations in cancer survivors: An application of self-determination theory. *Psycho-oncology, 15*, 567–578.

Wilson, P. M., & Rodgers, W. M. (2002). The relationship between exercise motives and self-esteem in female exercise participants: An application of self-determination research. *Journal of Applied Biobehavioral Research, 7*(1), 30–43.

Wilson, P. M., Rodgers, W. M., Blanchard, C. M., & Gessell, J. (2003). The relationship between psychological needs, self-determined motivation, exercise attitudes, and physical fitness. *Journal of Applied Social Psychology, 33*, 2373–2392.

Wilson, P. M., Rodgers, W. M., Fraser, S. N., & Murray, T. C. (2004). Relationships between exercise regulations and motivational consequences in university students. *Research Quarterly in Exercise and Sport, 75*(1), 81–91.

World Health Organization (2003). *Palliative care*. Retrieved November 1, 2009, from http://www.who.int/cancer/palliative/en/

PART 6

Exercise Psychology: On the Horizon and into the Future

Psychology of Resistance Exercise

Daniel B. Hollander *and* Robert R. Kraemer

Abstract

Resistance exercise has been identified as an important mode of physical activity to maintain and enhance health. Research has been developing regarding psychological alterations during and after resistance exercise. The purpose of this chapter is to briefly highlight the physical health benefits of resistance exercise and then review research in five domains. First it reviews the relationship between resistance exercise and the sensation of effort. Second, it summarizes research that investigates resistance exercise and affect changes. Third, it discusses research regarding resistance exercise and its effects on self-perception. Fourth, it reviews research on the use of "psyching" strategies prior to maximal and submaximal performance of resistance exercise. The chapter concludes with a discussion of the role of expectation in resistance exercise performance.

Key Words: rating of perceived exertion, pain, anxiety, affect, self-concept, self-esteem, muscle dysmorphia, psyching strategies, deception and ambiguous feedback.

Introduction

Recognized as a critical component of physical culture since the Chou dynasty (3600 BCE) and depicted on Greek sculptures, resistance exercise (RE) has shown benefits to physical functioning for centuries (Webster, 1976). A large number of investigations have demonstrated the positive effects of RE on human physiology (Pollock et al., 2000; Stone, Fleck, Triplett, & Kraemer, 1991; M. A. Williams et al., 2007). However, there have been fewer investigations of the psychology of RE. Consequently, the aim of this chapter will be to briefly review the health benefits of RE and then examine (1) the sensations produced by RE, (2) the relationships between RE and affect/mood (3) the impact of RE on self-concept, self-esteem, and body image, (4) the effects of psychological strategies on strength, and (5) the role of expectation in RE performance. For additional supporting information we direct the reader to the most recent

relevant reviews. Furthermore, we have created tables to permit comparison of study details while the text focuses on exemplary studies.

While searching for information to include in the chapter, we used all relevant databases, including pubmed, medline, psycinfo, eric, sportdiscus, and ebsco, using as key terms *health, effort sense, pain, RPE, exertion, sensations, psychological interventions, placebo, expectancy, body image, self-esteem, self-concept, resistance exercise, resistance training, strength training, weight training, weightlifting,* and *anaerobic.* Articles were identified in specific categories with regard to sample population, methodology, type of RE training employed, and results. Finally, summary sections were developed to guide future research.

The benefits of RE are universally recognized, both clinically and scientifically; RE has been recommended as an effective form of training for disease prevention and health promotion by the

American Heart Association, American College of Sports Medicine, American Geriatrics Society, U.S. Surgeon General's report, British Academy of Sports and Exercise Science, Canadian Society of Exercise Physiology, and American Association of Cardiovascular and Pulmonary Rehabilitation (M. A. Williams et al., 2007). Research has concluded that RE improves physical functioning, reduces falls in the elderly, decreases pain in patients with chronic lower back pain, improves glucose tolerance and insulin sensitivity, increases bone mineral density, increases basal metabolic rate, and improves quality of life (M. A. Williams et al., 2007; M. A. Williams & Stewart, 2009).

A large variety of resistance exercises and training protocols exist. To appreciate the benefits of RE it is critical to understand the distinct characteristics of the numerous types of muscle contraction. In brief, RE can be categorized based on type of contraction employed. The major categories include isometric, isokinetic, and dynamic constant external resistance. Isometric RE refers to exercise that is performed with increased muscle tension and little to no range of movement of the joint. Isokinetic RE refers to RE that is performed through a range of movement at a given speed. Dynamic constant external resistance refers to RE that is performed with free weights or machines that does not vary resistance across the range of movement. Concentric RE refers to dynamic constant external RE that involves the active shortening of the muscle, whereas eccentric RE refers to a form that involves the active lengthening of the muscle. Furthermore, factors such as the speed of movement and type of equipment become important aspects in describing protocols used in this line of research (see W. J. Kraemer & Ratamess, 2004, for a review of RE variables and prescription). Moreover, programming variables such as number of sets and repetitions, work-to-rest ratios, percentage of maximal effort employed, and duration of the intervention are critically important when interpreting results from studies examining the psychology of RE. For example, the type of RE has been shown to be an important determinant of physical exertion, and this in turn can greatly impact perceptions of RE.

Exertional Responses to RE

Borg (1998) noted that the early aerobic exercise studies on effort sense focused on two major components of an individual rating of perceived exertion (RPE): (1) sensation of pressure, force, strain, fatigue, and aches from the somatosensory system, and (2) exertion originating in the chest and cardiopulmonary system. Ekblom and Goldberg (1971) redefined these as *local* and *central* factors. Researchers noted that sensations were generally ranked on one of three continua: general fatigue, leg fatigue (in cycling tasks), and task aversion (emotional response) (Weiser & Stamper, 1977). Physiological state during RE is largely perceived from sensations arising from peripheral working muscles. Thus it is often thought that perception of effort during RE may be more related to peripheral sensations than central fatigue (Weir, Beck, Cramer, & Housh, 2006). While RE clearly has an effect on heart rate and respiratory rate, it is a smaller effect than that from aerobic exercise.

Work RPE in RE has investigated effects of RE variables, pain response (produced in the periphery), caffeine supplementation, muscle contraction types, and chronic training alterations on effort sense. Of the RE studies reviewed that assessed effort sense, more than half assessed RPE using the category ratio-10 (CR-10) scale or similar scales that adhere to a 0–10+ rating for the participants, rather than the conventional 6–20 Borg scale (Borg, 1998). Using a 0–10 scale aids assessment because fatigue onset is rapid in RE and a 0–10 scale is less challenging to interpret and report than a 6–20 scale. RPE may be based on whole-body or active muscle ratings of effort. Generally, active muscle RPE is slightly higher than the whole-body effort rating (Robertson et al., 2003). RPE has also been assessed after an entire session, known as the session RPE method. This method rates perceived exertion via recall of effort for the entire session once the session has ended. Whether it has been assessed using a session method, CR-10 scaling, or 6–20 scaling, as the intensity of RE work increases, so too does RPE (Gearhart et al., 2002; Lagally, Robertson, Gallagher, Gearhart, & Goss, 2002).

The overwhelming majority of investigations have sampled men. Most studies have sampled undergraduate populations, though one study sampled postmenopausal women and another adolescents (see Table 22.1). The latter two investigations are examples of research that has broadened research on exertion to new populations. Several studies have measured RPE and pain concurrently, while other studies have attempted to manipulate RPE nutritionally (Utter et al., 2005), with pharmacological aids (Cook & O'Connor, 2000; Hudson, Green, Bishop, & Richardson,

Table 22.1. Exertional Responses to RE

Study	Sample[a]	Psychological measure[b]	Training type[c]	Results[d]
RE variables that affect perceived exertion				
W. J. Kraemer et al., 1987	9 Bodybuilders, 8 powerlifters	11	DCER	RPE was related to changes in lactate
W. J. Kraemer et al., 1993	8 M UG	11	DCER	↓ RPE for the subsequent set for longer rest periods
R. R. Kraemer et al., 1996	7 M UG	11	DCER	↑ Lactate and RPE associated during low-volume RE
Suminski et al., 1997	8 M UG	2	DCER	RPE and lactate associated
Pincivero et al., 1999	14 M UG	2	ISOK	↔ RPE between rest intervals
Pincivero et al., 1999	17 M UG	2	ISOM	RPE compared to EMG recordings was underestimated in the vastusmedialis
Gearhart et al., 2002	10 M, 10 W UG	12	DCER	↑ RPE related to ↑ intensity
Lagally et al., 2002	20 W UG	11, 12	DCER	↑ Lactate, EMG activity, and RPE with ↑ intensity
Allman & Rice, 2003	M UG, M elderly	9	ISOK	↔ RPE
Robertson et al., 2003	20 M, 20 W UG	3, 12	ISOK	Active muscle and OMNI-RES ratings were associated
Day et al., 2004	9 M, 10 W UG	13	DCER	↑ RPE with ↑ intensity
Lagally et al., 2004	14 W UG, 14 weightlifters	11, 12	DCER	↑ RPE and EMG with ↑ intensity
Sweet et al., 2004	10 M, 10 W UG	13	DCER	≠ Session and mean RPE for low-intensity exercise
Woods et al., 2004	15 M, 15 W UG	9	DCER	↔ RPE between intervals
Duncan, Al-Nakeeb, & Scurr, 2006	10 M, 10 W UG	2, 11, 12	DCER	↑ active muscle RPE compared to overall RPE
Hutchinson & Tenenbaum, 2006	35 UG	11	ISOM	↑ RPE with ↑ intensity
Spreuwenberg et al., 2006	9 M UG	2	DCER	↔ RPE for squat as well as for whole-body workout

(Continued)

Table 22.1. (Continued)

Study	Sample[a]	Psychological measure[b]	Training type[c]	Results[d]
RE variables that affect perceived exertion				
Falvo, Schilling, Bloomer, Smith, & Creasy, 2007	31 M UG	11, 15	DCER	↓ RPE, fatigue, & soreness for single bout of RE than for multiple bouts of eccentric contractions
Simão, Farinatti, Polito, Viveiros, & Fleck, 2007	23 W UG	9	DCER	↑ RPE for later exercises
Singh et al., 2007	15 M UG	11, 13	DCER	↔ Session and regular RPE
McGuigan et al., 2008	61 Children	9, 13	DCER	↓ Session RPE than OMNI RPE immediately post exercise
Robertson et al, 2008	70 Children	8	ISOK	OMNI-RES accurate in prediction of 1-RM
Bellezza et al., 2009	11 M, 18 W UG	3, 11	DCER	↔ RPE between order of exercises
Lagally, Cordero, Good, Brown, & McCaw, 2009	10 M, 10 W UG	8	FRE	ACSM recommendations met using RPE
Wickwire et al., 2009	11 M, 9 W UG	9	DCER	↑ RPE for traditional RE than for superslow protocol
RE, pain, and perceived exertion				
Cook et al., 2000	12 M UG	2, 4, 6, 11, 16	ISOM	↔ Between pain and RPE
Pincivero Bachmeier, & Coelho, 2001	15 M, 15 W UG	9	ISOK	RPE fit both a linear and a quadratic trend
O'Connor, Poudevigne, & Pasley, 2002	21 M, 21 W UG	11	ISOK	Intensity and RPE were related; F rated eccentric exercise as less effortful than M
Hollander et al., 2003	8 M UG	1, 2, 14	DCER	↔ RPE and pain for concentric and eccentric muscle contractions
Hollander et al., 2008	7 M UG	1, 5, 8	DCER	↔ RPE and pain for concentric and eccentric muscle contractions
Robertson et al., 2009	Children	7, 8	ISOK	Children could distinguish between hurt and RPE
Hollander et al., 2010	7 M UG	1, 5, 8	DCER	↔ RPE for 30% of 1-RM with partial occlusion and 70% with no occlusion
RE, caffeine, and perceived exertion				
Green et al., 2007	UG	2	DCER	↑ Number of repetitions in caffeine trial, ↔ RPE with placebo and caffeine

Table 22.1. (Continued)

Study	Sample[a]	Psychological measure[b]	Training type[c]	Results[d]
RE, caffeine, and perceived exertion				
Astorino et al., 2008	22 M UG	11	DCER	↔ RPE with placebo and caffeine
Hudson et al., 2008	15 M UG	10, 11	DCER	↔ RPE with caffeine but ↑ total repetitions
Duncan et al., 2009	15 M UG	11, 12	DCER	↓ RPE in perceived caffeine trial, ↑ active muscle RPE in all conditions
RE, muscle actions, and perceived exertion				
Hollander et al., 2003	8 M UG	1, 2, 14	DCER	≠ RPE and pain for bout of concentric and eccentric muscle contraction
Yarrow et al., 2007	22 M UG	11	DCER with enhanced eccentric contractions	↑ RPE after eccentrically enhanced sets of bench press and squat
Hollander et al., 2008	7 M UG	1, 5, 8	DCER	↔ RPE and pain for concentric and 20% higher eccentric load
Miller et al., 2009	31 W UG	3, 11	DCER	↓ RPE in eccentric contractions
RE training adaptation of perceived exertion				
K. Pierce et al.,1993	23 M UG	12	DCER	↓ RPE and HR at end of 8 weeks
Gearhart et al., 2008	22 M, 27 W elderly	9	DCER	↑ Work done to arrive at RPEs of 4 and 6 after training

[a]M = men; UG = undergraduate college students; W = women.
[b]1 =CR-10 pain (0–10 scale); 2 = CR-10 RPE (0–10 scale); 3=Felt Arousal Scale; 4=McGill Pain Questionnaire; 5=McGill Pain Questionnaire, Short Form; 6= Multiple Affect Adjective Checklist; 7= OMNI Muscle Hurt Scale (0–10);8= OMNI Res (0–10 scale);9= OMNI RPE; 10 = Perceived Pain Index; 11= Rating of Perceived Exertion (6–20 scale); 12= RPE, active muscle (6–20 or 0–10); 13= session RPE; 14= State Anxiety Inventory; 15= Visual Analog Scale for Soreness.
[c]Mode of RE employed in the study. DCER = dynamic constant external resistance (traditional free weight or machine training); FRE = functional resistance exercise;,ISOK = isokinetic resistance machines such as Cybex or Biodyne; ISOM = isometric work.
[d]ACSM = American College of Sports Medicine; EMG = electromyograph; RPE = rating of perceived exertion. ↑, increase or higher; ↓, decrease or lower; ↔, no effect or not significantly different; ≠, not equal.

2008), or partial vascular occlusion (Hollander et al., 2010). Four studies employed the session RPE method (Day, McGuigan, Brice, & Foster, 2004; McGuigan et al., 2008; Singh, Foster, Tod, & McGuigan, 2007; Sweet, Foster, McGuigan, & Brice, 2004). Overall, the dominant research designs have been descriptive and correlational, with few studies employing quasi-experimental or experimental designs.

RE Variables That Affect Perceived Exertion

Manipulation of numerous RE variables (volume, intensity, rest intervals, and upper- vs. lower-body movements) alters RPE. These results have been studied in college-age men (Gearhart et al., 2002) and women (Lagally et al., 2002), older men and women (Gearhart, Lagally, Riechman, Andrews, & Robertson, 2008), and competitive powerlifters and bodybuilders (W. J. Kraemer, Noble, Clark, &

Culver, 1987). For example, W. J. Kraemer and colleagues (1996) demonstrated that RPE rose along with lactate level as successive sets were performed. These findings suggested that volume of work or onset of fatigue was partially responsible for the rise in RPE. Gearhart and colleagues (2002) compared effort sense using seven exercises (bench press, leg press, latissimus dorsi pull-down, triceps press, biceps curl, shoulder press, and calf raise) at either 5 repetitions at 90% of a one-repetition maximum (1-RM, the greatest weight that can be lifted with one maximal effort) or 15 repetitions at 30% of a 1-RM. The higher-intensity protocol was perceived as more difficult, despite requiring a similar amount of relative work. Lagally and colleagues (2002) noted that for a biceps curl at intensities of 30%, 60%, and 90% of a 1-RM, both overall body and active muscle RPE ratings increased as workload (intensity) increased. These findings were further validated in a subsequent study that demonstrated that increases in neural activity recorded with an electromyograph (EMG) paralleled the perception of change in effort during RE (Lagally, McCaw, Young, Medema, & Thomas, 2004).

W. J. Kraemer and colleagues (1993) demonstrated that in addition to RE intensity, rest intervals were also important to the RPE response. Employing three sets at a 10-repetition maximum (~ 75% of 1-RM) for 10 stations, they determined that longer rest periods resulted in significantly lower RPEs during six RE movements. Woods, Bridge, Nelson, Risse, and Pincivero (2004), however, reported that rest intervals of 1, 2, and 3 minutes did not affect RPE across three sets of 10 repetitions of isokinetic knee extensions at 70% of a 10-RM (load (or ~50 % of 1-RM). The discrepant results may possibly be explained by differences in the loads and volumes as well as the type of muscle contraction between these two studies. Thus, degree of load as well as recovery from the previous set seemed to be important factors in perceived effort.

Speed of contraction may be an important variable as well. Wickwire, McLester, Green, and Crews (2009) compared a traditional machine protocol (2-second concentric muscle contraction, 4-second eccentric muscle contraction at 65% of 1-RM to failure) with a superslow protocol (10-second concentric, 5-second eccentric at 40% of 1-RM to failure). Using elbow flexion and knee extension exercises, they determined that the traditional weight training protocol elicited a higher RPE. Another finding has been that larger, multijoint movements elicit lower RPEs than smaller-muscle, single-joint movements

at the 1-RM load (Hollander et al., 2008). Thus speed of contraction and muscle mass recruitment may affect RPE.

RE, Pain, and Perceived Exertion

There are discrepant data regarding the relationship between RPE and pain in RE studies. For instance, Cook and O'Connor (2000) assessed the relationship between RPE and pain during an isometric handgrip task using a fatiguing ramped protocol and found low correlations ($r = -0.02$ to 0.25) between RPE and pain across codeine (analgesic), naltrexone (analgesia blocked), and placebo conditions and within a wide range of work intensities. Other studies have demonstrated that pain and RPE showed moderate-to-high correlations ($r = 0.59–0.85$) when participants assessed concentric and eccentric work at intensities of 65% of a 1-RM (Hollander et al., 2003) as well as eccentric contractions at 85% of a concentric 1-RM (Hollander et al., 2008). O'Connor and colleagues (1998) examined three different eccentric contractions and found a moderate relationship between RPE and pain from 12 to 72 hours post exercise.

One explanation for these equivocal results is that different forms of muscle contractions (isometric, concentric/eccentric, eccentric contractions only, and isokinetic) were employed. Furthermore, it could be that at low workload intensities, pain and RPE are easily discerned, but as the physiologic noise (i.e., increased heart rate, increased pressor response, and increased lactate) becomes greater, sensations become less distinguishable (Borg, 1998). The plausibility of this argument is supported by Lagally and colleagues (2004), who noted that during RE, RPE may have a "breakaway" point beyond which physiological measures are not linearly related to increases in effort sense. Hollander and colleagues (2010) further supported this concept by comparing low-intensity (30% of a 1-RM) RE with partial vascular occlusion, which enhances sensations of exertion and pain, with moderate-intensity (70% of a 1-RM) RE and no occlusion. Specifically, when participants did three successive sets of biceps curls or calf raises, they gave an RPE of "6" in the low-intensity, partial occlusion condition at the same repetition or an earlier repetition than they did in the moderate-intensity, no-occlusion condition. These findings were mirrored in CR-10 pain ratings. Moreover, partial occlusion at 30% of 1-RM elicited similar anaerobic hormonal responses to no occlusion at 70% of 10-RM (Reeves et al., 2006). These results suggest that the changes in blood flow may parallel perceptual changes.

RE, Caffeine, and Perceived Exertion

The relation between administration of caffeine (a stimulant) and RPE has been investigated in a series of studies (Astorino, Rohmann, & Firth, 2008; Duncan, Lyons, & Hankey, 2009; Green et al., 2007; Hudson et al., 2008). These studies have demonstrated mixed results. No significant effects of caffeine on effort ratings were noted in studies by Astorino et al. (2008) and Green et al. (2007) that employed caffeine during RE. Both studies employed undergraduate samples and administered caffeine at 6 mg per kilogram of body weight. Astorino and colleagues (2008) examined 22 resistance-trained men who performed three sets at 60% of a 1-RM to failure on the bench press and the leg press exercises. Caffeine and placebo conditions were randomized in a double-blind design. The group that was administered a caffeine supplement increased their performance by 11% and 12% on the bench press and leg press, respectively, compared with the placebo condition, but these differences were not statistically significant. Green and colleagues (2007) examined peak heart rates, RPE, and number of repetitions in 3 sets of bench press and leg press to failure, in a caffeine (6 mg per kilogram of body weight) or placebo condition. Green et al. (2007) employed a double-blinded experiment with 17 subjects found no significant differences in the bench press condition but did find an enhanced performance (12.5 vs. 9.9 reps) in the caffeine trial. Additionally, peak heart rates were higher in the caffeine trial (158.5 vs 151.8) than the placebo group. However, RPE was not significantly different between the trials. In both the Astorino et al. (2008) and that of Green et al. (2007), RPE was not statistically different between the placebo and caffeine trials. Nonetheless, the results were intriguing. The tendency toward better performance with no change in RPE suggests that caffeine may alter effort sense to benefit performance.

Hudson and colleagues (2008) compared the effects of caffeine and aspirin on the performance of four sets of a 12-repetition maximum load to failure. Results showed that individuals who ingested caffeine performed more repetitions in the first set in leg extensions and arm curls than did those in the aspirin condition. Also, the aspirin condition was associated with significantly higher ratings of perceived pain and RPE in the first set of the exercises. The authors hypothesized that caffeine may reduce pain by blocking pronociceptive adenosine receptors. Greater adenosine concentrations in the blood during higher-intensity exercise may facilitate adenosine signaling on the sensory nerve endings; by blocking adenosine receptors, caffeine would interrupt this signaling, resulting in reduced pain.

In a recent study, Duncan and colleagues (2009) examined the effects of perceived caffeine ingestion on performance. Fifteen undergraduates were randomized to perceived caffeine (participants were instructed that they would receive a 250 ml solution consisting of 3 mg per kilogram of body weight solution of caffeine), placebo (participants were instructed that they would receive 250 ml solution with no caffeine), and control conditions. The subjects performed repetitions to failure of a single-leg leg extension at a 60% of 1-RM load. Participants in the perceived caffeine group completed two more repetitions on average than those in the other groups, and their RPE was lower as well. The results of this deception study mimicked those of the caffeine supplement studies. This deception research suggests that in some circumstances, caffeine's effects may be psychosomatic or expectancy related.

RE, Muscle Actions, and Perceived Exertion

Some research has investigated the impact of muscle-shortening (concentric) versus muscle-lengthening (eccentric) contractions on RPE (Hollander et al., 2003, 2008; Miller et al., 2009; Yarrow et al., 2007). Both Hollander and colleagues (2003) and Miller and colleagues (2009) determined that at an absolute load, eccentric muscle contractions were rated lower on the RPE scale than concentric muscle contractions during RE. The authors hypothesized that this represented not only a perceptual difference but also an "underloading" of the eccentric portion of the lift due to mechanical advantage and gravity. On follow-up, Hollander and colleagues (2008) determined that when eccentric contractions were loaded 20% more than concentric contractions, the RPE values were not statistically different. While previous research had supported the notion that eccentric and concentric contractions might elicit different trends in physiological stress (Bigland-Ritchie, 1981; Bigland-Ritchie, Donovan, & Roussos, 1981; Bigland-Ritchie & Woods, 1976, 1984), most work had been conducted using isokinetic RE (Hortobágyi & Katch, 1990). Contemporary RE machines employed in later studies made the application of results more functionally relevant to healthy and athletic individuals.

RE Training Adaptation of Perceived Exertion

Two studies have demonstrated that chronic adaptations result in lower RPE at the same absolute workload. Gearhart and colleagues (2008) demonstrated this in older adults (≥64 years), after 12 weeks of RE, whereas K. Pierce, Rozenek, and Stone (1993) reported lower RPE in 23 undergraduate men after eight weeks. While the specific duration of training required for reduced RPE at the same workload has not been carefully titrated to determine the actual rate of adaptation, these early investigations reveal that there is a pattern of reduction in effort sense across training time. The perceptual alteration may be due to integrated adaptations of more efficient movement patterns and sensation habituation.

Summary of Research on RE and Perceived Exertion

Research has demonstrated the following regarding RPE responses to acute RE: (1) RE variables of volume, intensity, and speed of contraction affect RPE. (2) Pain and RPE appear to be unrelated at low RE intensities but are related at higher intensities of RE. (3) Preliminary work suggests that caffeine as well as the perception of ingesting caffeine may reduce the RPE response. (4) Perceptions of effort are greater in concentric movements than eccentric movements at absolute workloads, although this effect is greatly diminished when 20% greater loading is used for eccentric muscle actions. (5) After 8–12 weeks of RE training, effort sense ratings are lower at the same absolute workloads.

Future studies should investigate the speed of perceptual adaptation to training loads, potential gender differences in RPE during RE, and the potential influence of physical and mental health on RPE during RE. In addition, future research should make clear whether reported RPEs reflect effort based on immediate sensory signaling during exercise or perceptions of exertion after exercise has ceased. Many past studies have not made this distinction.

Future investigations should include assessment of central factors and peripheral factors to determine which changes most closely align with changes in RPE and pain. Moreover, careful consideration should be given to volume of RE performed, intensity and duration parameters should be clearly defined, and dose–response issues should be addressed. Finally, the term *pain* is perhaps too

broad to reflect the nuances of sensations experienced within RE. With high intensities of RE, it could be that discomfort is actually experienced along with stinging, burning, stabbing, throbbing, and muscle ache (Hollander et al., 2008; Robertson et al., 2009). These terms may more accurately describe the perceived sensations of RE.

RE and Affect

Affect (anxiety, mood, depression, and well-being) is altered during and after RE (for a brief review, see Focht & Arent, 2007). Many investigations of the effect of RE on mood have measured anxiety, several studies have measured depression, and a few studies have measured affect concurrently with self-concept, self-awareness, or self-esteem. A number of studies have employed a state anxiety measure, while at least five studies have employed the Profile of Mood States (POMS) (see Table 22.2). The majority of studies in this area have used undergraduate student samples, while two studies assessed affect in elderly participants. Only a handful of investigations examined mood or affect changes over time. Studies regarding affect and RE have primarily been descriptive and correlational.

RE Variables, Anxiety, and Affect

During acute bouts of RE, anxiety is only minimally reduced or even slightly elevated (Focht and Arent, 2007). However, during recovery, anxiety seems to drop to a lower level than baseline within 120–180 minutes post RE. Tharion, Harman, Kraemer, and Rauch (1991) investigated the effect of RE intensity and rest periods on mood using a 5- or 10-repetition maximum load to failure with rest intervals of 1 or 3 minutes. Overall mood disturbances (as measured by the POMS) were greater with the higher workload and shorter rest period. Bartholomew and Linder (1998) also demonstrated that exercise intensity (load) is a major factor in determining anxiety responses to RE. In a study employing 20 undergraduates, anxiety scores were not altered in response to RE at 75–85% of a 1-RM but were reduced in response to 40–50% of a 1-RM RE.

To examine the dose–response relationship of RE to affect, Arent, Landers, Matt, and Etnier (2005) employed RE protocols of 40%, 70%, and 100% of a 1-RM in 31 undergraduate men and women. The moderate-intensity (70% of a 1-RM) protocol yielded the most positive affective response, despite initiating a hypothalamic-pituitary-adrenal axis stress response (as determined by salivary cortisol

Table 22.2. RE and Affect

Study	Sample[a]	Psychological measure[b]	Training type[c]	Results[d]
RE variables, anxiety, and affect				
Tharion et al., 1991	18 UG	13	DCER	↑ Mood disturbance with ↑ workload and ↓ rest periods
McGowan et al., 1993	10 M, 10 W	13	DCER	↔ Mood and beta-endorphin
O'Connor, Bryant, Veltri, &Gebhardt, 1993	14 W	19	DCER	↓ State anxiety 90–120 min post RE
Raglin et al., 1993	15 M, 11 W	19	DCER	↓ State anxiety after 20 and 60 min of RE
Koltyn,Raglin, O'Connor, & Morgan, 1995	25 UG, 25 controls	4, 19	DCER	↔ State anxiety but ↑ body awareness
Garvin, Koltyn, & Morgan, 1997	30 M UG	19	DCER	↔ State anxiety to 50 min of RE
Bartholomew & Linder, 1998	20 UG	19	DCER	↑ State anxiety for moderate intensity for M but not F
Focht&Koltyn, 1999	84 UG	13, 19	DCER	↓ State anxiety 180 min post exercise at 50% of 1-RM
Focht et al., 2000	54 W UG	4, 19	DCER	↓ State anxiety after 120–180 for all conditions
Bartholomew, Moore, Todd, Todd, & Elrod, 2001	54 UG	5	DCER	↑ Revitalization when workload was low
Focht, 2002	19 W UG	15, 19	DCER	↓ State anxiety in the highest-anxiety individuals
Hale et al., 2002	12W 4 M UG	19	DCER	↓ State anxiety at 10 and 60 min post exercise regardless of order of aerobic or RE training
Annesi, Westcott, & Gann ,2004	17 elderly W	11, 13	DCER	↓ Total mood disturbance, depression, and fatigue; ↑ physical self-concept
Annesi, Westcott, Loud, & Powers , 2004	39 elderly W	5, 13, 21	DCER	↑ Positive feelings post exercise for dissociation group
Arent et al., 2005	31 M & W UG	1, 11, 15, 19	DCER	↑ Mood with moderate RE
Bellezza et al., 2009	11 M, 18 W UG	7, 15	DCER	↑ Positive affect when moving from small- to large-muscle-group exercises

(Continued)

Table 22.2. (Continued)

Study	Sample[a]	Psychological measure[b]	Training type[c]	Results[d]
RE variables, anxiety, and affect				
Herring & O'Connor, 2009	14 adults	13	DCER	↑ Vigor in the 70% of a 1-RM trial (performing 3 different leg exercises for 4 sets X 10 reps.) as compared to the Placebo/Control trial.
Miller et al., 2009	31 W UG	7, 15	DCER	↑ Pleasantness 60 min post RE
Bibeau et al., 2010	58 M, 46 W UG	6, 12, 19	DCER	↑ Anxiety immediately after (5 min.) RE in a high intensity (80-85% of 1-RM)-short rest (30 sec. between sets) vs control group, ↑ positive affect in long rest (90 sec. between sets), ↓ intensity (50-55% of 1-RM) RE vs control group.
RE and positive affect				
Bartholomew, 1999	40 M UG	13	DCER	↑ Anxiety upon onset of RE but ↓ anxiety and ↑ positive mood 30 min post RE
Levinger et al., 2008	22 M 23 W Adults with obesity	14, 17, 20	DCER	↑ Psychological well-being without ↑ psychological distress in W
RE training studies and affect				
Doyne et al., 1987	40 W	3, 8, 10	DCER	↓ Depression in both groups
Norvell & Belles, 1993	43 law enforcement officers	9	Circuit training	↓ Depression, anxiety, and hostility after 4 months
Auchus & Kaslow, 1994	5 W with schizophrenia	16	DCER	↔ Symptoms and depression
Sarsan et al., 2006	60 W adults with obesity	3	DCER	↔ Psychological changes after RE
Bartholomew et al., 2008	135 UG	2, 18	DCER	↑ Strength gains for individuals with low life stress

[a] M = men; UG = undergraduate college students; W=women.
[b] 1 = Activation Deactivation Checklist; 2=Adolescent Perceived Events Scale; 3=Beck Depression Inventory; 4=Body Awareness Scale; 5=Exercise Induced Feeling State Inventory; 6=Exercise Self-Efficacy Scale; 7=Felt Arousal Scale; 8=Hamilton's Rating Scale of Depression;9= Hopkins Symptom Checklist-90; 10= Lubin's Depression Adjective Checklist; 11=Physical Self-Concept Scale; 12= Positive Affect Negative Affect Scale; 13=Profile of Mood States; 14= Quality of Life Scale; 15=Rating of Perceived Exertion; 16= Self-Rated Depression Scale; 17=Short Form 36 for Health And Well-Being;18= Social Support Inventory; 19= State Anxiety Inventory; 20= Subjective Experiences of Exercise Scale; 21= Tennessee Self-ConceptScale-2.
[c] Mode of RE employed in the study. DCER = dynamic constant external resistance (traditional free weight or machine training).
[d] ↑, increase; ↓, decrease; ↔, no effect or not significantly different.

measures). Moreover, the highest-intensity protocol seemed to lead to the greatest adverse mood response. A relationship between high intensity and negative mood is an often identified theme in this line of research. Bellezza, Hall, Miller, and Bixby (2009) demonstrated that varying the order of exercise can alter affect. Specifically, they showed that moving from small to large muscle groups led to more positive affect than moving from large to small muscle groups. However, without direct testing of theories to explain RE–mood relationships, with two exceptions (Arent et al., 2005; Miller et al., 2009) research in this area appears to remain in the descriptive stages and mediating variables are still being uncovered.

A number of studies have attempted to quantify the effect of RE on state anxiety (Focht & Koltyn, 1999; Focht, Koltyn, & Bouchard, 2000; Hale, Koch, & Raglin, 2002; Raglin, Turner, & Eksten, 1993). State anxiety has demonstrated the classic delayed anxiolytic effect, with minimal changes in state anxiety immediately post RE (Bartholomew, 1999; Bibeau, Moore, Mitchell, Vargas-Tonsing, & Bartholomew, 2010) and more pronounced anxiety reductions 60 minutes post RE (Raglin et al., 1993), 120 minutes post RE (Focht & Koltyn, 1999), and 180 minutes post RE (Focht et al., 2000). State anxiety was clearly reduced in these latter studies. Focht (2002) demonstrated that pre-RE baseline anxiety scores had an effect on the degree of anxiety change during RE. The participants who were most anxious had the greatest anxiety reductions during exercise at a self-selected intensity. These findings suggest that in research examining anxiety responses to pre-scribed or self-selected RE, baseline anxiety should be assessed, because its level may affect post-RE anxiety.

RE and Positive Affect

At least 2 studies have examined positive affect and RE. Bartholomew (1999) manipulated pre-exercise mood in a sample of undergraduate students using positive, negative, and neutral/placebo imagery with a counterbalanced protocol. In the experimental RE condition, imagery-induced anxiety and anger dropped below baseline within 30 minutes post RE. Moreover, positive affect was significantly higher for the RE group. The conclusion was that RE served as a distraction from pre-exercise mood and significantly increased positive affect. Levinger and colleagues (2008) demonstrated that after 12 weeks of RE, a sample of obese adults experienced increased ratings of positive well-being without increases in psychological distress or fatigue. Thus preliminary studies suggest that RE can have a positive effect on mood and can enhance positive emotions.

RE Training Studies and Affect

Little is known about the effect of chronic RE training on mood. Most training studies have ranged in time of intervention from approximately eight weeks (Auchus & Kaslow, 1994) to 12 months (Doyne et al., 1987). Participants in these studies have included undergraduate students (Annesi, Westcott, Loud, & Powers, 2004), elderly women (65–66 years old) (Annesi, Westcott, & Gann, 2004), and a small sample of patients with schizophrenia (Auchus & Kaslow, 1994). Studies have found evidence for improved mood across time, particularly with regard to vigor. For instance, Doyne and colleagues (1987) compared the effects of aerobic and strength training on mood in a group of 40 women. Across 12 months, both aerobic and strength training groups demonstrated reductions in depression. It could not be determined whether this result was related to decreased stress or increased self-efficacy. Along these lines, Bartholomew, Stults-Kolehmainen, Elrod, and Todd (2008) examined 135 college students who rated high and low in life stress. Participants underwent a 12-week, RE program and were assessed on physical performance parameters. Individuals high in life stress (a negative affective state) had roughly 2.5–3.0% smaller strength gains as well as 2.5% and 1.21% lower circumferences of the arms and thighs, respectively, than low-stress individuals. However, patients with schizophrenia showed no changes in depression or schizophrenic symptoms of across eight weeks of RE training (Auchus and Kaslow, 1994). Finally, Norvell and Belles (1993) demonstrated that mood was improved in law enforcement officers participating in a circuit training regimen for four months. Those who maintained the circuit training workouts demonstrated decreased physical symptoms of stress, decreased anxiety, depression, and hostility; and greater job satisfaction than a wait-list control group. Moreover, those who dropped out experienced greater depression, hostility, and anxiety than participants who maintained their attendance.

Summary of Research on RE and Affect

Collectively, studies on RE and affect indicate that (1) intensity and order of exercise affect affective response; (2) little change is seen in anxiety immediately following RE, but at 60–120 minutes post exercise, anxiety is typically reduced; (3) baseline level of anxiety affects the anxiolytic effect of RE; (4) RE training enhances positive mood; and (5) RE can reduce depression and anxiety after 12 weeks of training. A limitation in this line of research has been the lack of diversity of the instrumentation used to assess affect. The measure of mood that has dominated this research is the POMS, which unfortunately contains five negative measures of mood and one positive measure. More balanced measures of affect, such as the Positive and Negative Affect Scale (which has equal numbers of positive and negative mood descriptors), have not been consistently employed. Additionally, behavioral or physiological measures have not been used, with one exception (Arent et al., 2005). In general, studies have been descriptive, and little is known about the mediating effects of physiological and sociological variables, baseline mood, personality, and appropriateness of psychometric scaling to capture the most relevant data.

RE and Perceptions of Self

RE research has often focused on the impact of RE on body image, self-esteem, and self-efficacy (see Table 22.3). Most studies in this line of research have measured body image, self-esteem, or self-concept; about a third of the studies have measured body cathexis (a measure of body satisfaction); and the remainder of the studies have measured muscle dysmorphia or drive for bulk. This last group of studies has examined bodybuilders (Fuchs & Zaichkowsky, 1983; Lantz, Rhea, & Cornelius, 2002), college students (Tucker, 1982a, 1983), and athletes including powerlifters (Lantz et al., 2002), football players, and recreational weight lifters (Baghurst & Lirgg, 2009; Wojtowicz & von Ranson, 2006).

Self-esteem/self-concept alterations (changes in perceptions of self-competence or self-efficacy) are one of the most immediate effects of RE. It could be that feedback about a successful or unsuccessful lift is instant and thus efficacy and satisfaction with the performance are immediate and transparent. It might also be that individuals who engage in RE do so to compensate for low self-esteem or self-confidence and thus suffer from social phobias or anxiety about

Table 22.3. RE and Self-Concept

Study	Sample[a]	Psychological measure[b]	Results[a,c]
RE and self-concept			
Darden, 1972	145 Ath	1, 4	≠ Team and individual sports on self and body cathexis
Tucker, 1982a	113 M UG	4, 16, 36	↑ Self-confidence and satisfaction was observed in individuals who trained with weights more often/longer period of time.
Tucker, 1982b	105 M UG	16	↑ Positive scores on physical self, personal self in trained group
Fuchs & Zaichkowsky, 1983	31 BB	16, 27	↑ Emotional health for BB compared with regular population
Tucker, 1983	142 UG	4, 16, 36	↑ Strength was significant predictor of body satisfaction
Tucker, 1987	241 M UG	4, 11, 16, 36,	↑ Body cathexis after strength training
Ford, Puckett, Blessing, & Tucker, 1989	88 W, 20 Con UG	4, 30	↔ Between groups in self- and body concept
Ford, Puckett, Reeve, &Lafavi, 1991	78 M UG	4, 30	↑ Self- and body concept
Tucker & Maxwell, 1992	60 W, 92 Con UG	4, 24	Five variables accounted for 61.5% in body cathexis
Tucker &Mortell, 1994	60 W UG	4	↑ Body image for lifters
Koltyn et al., 1995	50 UG	4, 35	↑ Body awareness

Table 22.3. (Continued)

Study	Sample[a]	Psychological measure[b]	Results[a,c]
RE and self-concept			
P. A. Williams & Cash, 2001	12 M, 27 W, 39 Con UG	20, 25, 32	↓ Social Physique Anxiety Scale (SPA), ↑ body image, and body satisfaction with training
Van Vorst, Buckworth, & Mattern, 2002	159 UG	15, 25	↑ Self-concept for individuals in the preparation stage
Depcik& Williams, 2004	W UG	8	After 13 weeks, 41% of group was not body image disturbed
Edwards, Edwards, &Basson, 2004	60 Ath, 27 health club members, 111 Con UG	25, 27	↑ Psychological well-being for Ath and health club members
Martin Ginis, Eng, Arbour, Hartman, & Phillips, 2005	28 M, 16 W UG	11, 20, 32	↑ Body image with physical changes
Anshel&Seipel, 2009	23M 42 W UG	21,32	↑ Adherence with self-monitoring to RE
RE and muscle dysmorphia			
Parrott et al., 1994	21 BB	9, 17	↑ Aggression for BB during the on-steroid periods
Blouin& Goldfield, 1995	43 BB, 96 Ath	1, 2, 10, 12, 14, 28	↑ Drive to enlarge body parts, ↑ perfectionism, and ↓ self-efficacy for BB
Schwerin, Corcoran, Fisher, & Patterson, 1996	35 AAS &150 UG	31, 32, 39	↓ Social Physique Anxiety or SPA and ↑ upper body esteem for AAS users
Schwerin et al., 1997	185 AAS, Control (Con)	18, 19, 20, 11	AAS use was predicted by the Body Dissatisfaction Index and age
Olivardia et al., 2000	24 M MD, 30 RWL	19	↑ reporting of body dissatisfaction, AAS use anabolic steroid use, and mood disorders for individuals with Muscle dysmorphia levels of body vs RWL
Ung et al., 2000	1 UG	33	Fear of muscle loss and compulsive training were associated with disturbed body image
Choi et al., 2002	24 M MD, 30 Con	20, 25, 32	↓ Body image and happiness for individuals with MD
Lantz et al., 2002	100 BB, 68 powerlifters	22	↑ MD, diet behavior, and pharmacological use for BB
Kanayama et al., 2003	48 AAS, 45 Con	19	↑ Illicit drug use, ↓ body esteem, and ↑ antisocial traits for AAS users

(Continued)

Table 22.3. (Continued)

Study	Sample[a]	Psychological measure[b]	Results[a,c]
RE and muscle dysmorphia			
Hallsworth, Wade, & Tiggemann, 2005	31 BB, 17 Olympic weight lifters, 35 Con	2, 5, 11, 14	↑ Self-objectification and body dissatisfaction for BB
Harne& Bixby, 2005	100 UG	3	↑ Barriers in the non-strength-trained group
Pickett, Lewis, & Cash, 2005	40 BB, 40 RWL, 40 Con	8, 33	↑ Body image and positive appearance for BB and RWL
Goldfield, Blouin, & Woodside, 2006	74 BB	1, 2, 10, 12, 14, 28	↑ Use of binging behaviors for college M BB
Henry, Anshel, & Michael, 2006	72 W UG	8	↑ Body image scores for circuit training compared with aerobic training
Hildebrandt, Schlundt, Langenbucher, & Chung, 2006	237 M RWL	Eight measures of 5	MD positively related to body image dissatisfaction, psychopathology, and drug abuse
Wojtowicz & von Ranson, 2006	53 M, 51W UG	11, 35	Drive for Muscularity Scale helped identify concerns BI
Kuennen & Waldron, 2007	49 M RWL	21, 22, 23, 28	↑ Muscle Dysmorphia Index was associated with perfectionism, self-esteem, and duration of lift
Litt & Dodge, 2008	161 M UG	11	Higher pretest scores on muscularitybehavior predicted performance enhancement use
Wolke & Sapouna, 2008	100 M BB	22 and several clinical scales	↑ MD and childhood bullying/ victimization predicted psychopathology and ↓ self-esteemE
Baghurst & Lirgg, 2009	66 Ath, 115 RWL, & 112 BB	6	↑ Body Dysmorphia Index, dietary behavior, and supplement use in BB
Goldfield, 2009	20 BB, 25 RWL	1, 2, 10, 12, 14, 28	↑ Body dissatisfaction and bulimia in AAS users and college W BB
Vassallo & Olrich, 2010	39 AAS	19	↑ Confidence while using and for return to AAS use by AAS users

[a] AAS = anabolic steroid users; Ath = athletes; BB = bodybuilders; Con = controls; M = men; MD = individuals with muscle dysmorphia; RWL = recreational weight lifters; UG = undergraduate college students; W = women.

[b] 1 = Anabolic Steroids Questionnaire; 2 = Beck Depression Inventory; 3 = Benefits and Barriers to Exercise Scale; 4 = Body Cathexis Scale; 5 =Body Dissatisfaction; 6 = Body Dysmorphia Index ; 8 = Body Self-Image Questionnaire; 9 = Buss Durke Inventory for Hostility and Aggression; 10 = Drive for Bulk Scale; 11 = Drive for Muscularity Scale;12 = Drive for Thinness Scale; 13 =Eating Attitudes Test; 14 = Eating Disorders Inventory; 15 = Exercise stage of change; 16 =Eysenck Personality Inventory; 17 = Feeling State Scale; 18 = General Well-Being; 19 = Interview; 20 = Multidimensional Body Self-Relations Questionnaire; 21 = Multidimensional Perfectionism Scale; 22 =Muscle DysmorphiaIndex; 23 = Narcissistic Personality Inventory; 24 = Physical Self-Description Questionnaire; 25 = Physical Self-Efficacy Scale; 26 = Profile of Mood States; 27 = Psychological Well-Being; 28 = Rosenberg Self-Esteem Scale; 29 = Self-Cathexis Scale; 30 = Self Concept Scale; 31 = Social Anxiety Scale; 32 = Social Physique Anxiety Scale; 33 = Social Self-Esteem; 34 = State Anxiety Inventory; 35 = Swansee Muscular Attitudes Questionnaire; 36 = Tennessee Self-Concept Scale; 37 = Texas Social Behavior Inventory; 38 = Tinker's Somatotype Scale; 39 = Upper Body Esteem Scale

[c] ↑, increase; ↓, decrease; ↔, no effect or not significantly different; ≠, not equal.

their appearance (social physique anxiety). A review of this literature shows that one series of studies has assessed the impact of RE on self-esteem/self-concept in nonathletes, while another has assessed self-esteem/self-concept, social physique anxiety, and muscle dysmorphia of anabolic androgenic steroid (AAS) users and athletes in power sports.

A multitude of measures of self-esteem/self-concept and body image have been used to assess the psychological effect of RE on perceptions of self. A few studies will be highlighted below to demonstrate general findings. One review by Reel and colleagues (2007) demonstrated a greater positive effect size (0.64) for RE than aerobic training (0.40). Most studies in that review addressed body image while some addressed self-esteem and self-concept. It appears that RE and aerobic exercise have similar effects on self-esteem.

RE and Self-Concept

RE has been associated with improved self-esteem, self-concept, and body cathexis. Tucker (1982b), employing the Tennessee Self-Concept Scale and the Body Cathexis Scale, reported that weight lifters had higher scores than an aged matched control group on satisfaction for their physical self, personal self, and identity. In a subsequent study, Tucker (1982a) sampled 113 college weight-trained males and determined that the longer individuals had been training, the better their self-confidence and satisfaction with their body. Additionally, these individuals demonstrated greater social impulsivity than their non-weight training counterparts. But the effects of RE did not appear to last beyond 24–36 weeks post weight training. Tucker and Maxwell (1992) assessed the effect of RE on 60 women across an academic semester. Individuals who had the greatest improvements in general well-being demonstrated lower pretest scores on the General Well-Being scale, reported lower parental income, and demonstrated superior loss of body weight and smaller skinfolds after the 15 weeks of RE training. Body cathexis after training was affected by five variables, which included greater body weight at the onset of the study, greater decreases in skinfold measures after the 15-week intervention, and a lower body cathexis score before the study began.

RE and Muscle Dysmorphia

Early studies investigating bodybuilders suggested that despite an unusual preoccupation with muscularity, these athletes had mood and personality traits similar to those of the general population (Fuchs & Zaichkowsky, 1983). Later work suggested that the drive for muscularity by bodybuilders was related to an obsession with meeting a body image "void," which came to be called "bigorexia" (Pope, Gruber, Choi, Olivardia, & Phillips, 1997) or muscle dysmorphia (a distortion of perception, generally such that individuals perceive themselves as lacking size). Pope and colleagues (1997) suggested that this could be a subclinical form of body dysmorphia, a more chronic clinical psychopathology. Development of scales to measure this phenomenon ensued (Lantz, Rhea, & Mayhew, 2001). Research has demonstrated that men who suffer from muscle dysmorphia reported greater shame, embarrassment, and impairment of social and occupational functioning than healthy participants who do RE, as well as greater use of AASs, body dissatisfaction, and mood disorders (Olivardia, Pope, & Hudson, 2000). These findings were corroborated by Choi, Pope, and Olivardia (2002) and Lantz and colleagues (2002). A case study about a Chinese bodybuilder with muscle dysmorphia demonstrated cross-cultural trends (Ung, Fones, & Ang, 2000). This individual reported a morbid fear of weight and muscle loss, mood disturbance, compulsive training behaviors, forced eating, and disturbed body image. Treatment with antidepressive agents and cognitive psychotherapy reduced his preoccupation with muscularity.

Some support has been garnered for the hypotheses that taking AASs increases aggression and that low self-esteem and childhood bullying and victimization predict the prevalence of psychopathology and AAS use (Parrott, Choi, & Davies, 1994; Wolke & Sapouna, 2008). Other research determined that individuals most at risk for taking AASs had low self-esteem, high body dissatisfaction, and high antisocial personality traits (Kanayama, Pope, Cohane, & Hudson, 2003).

Summary of Research on RE and Self-Concept

Research has demonstrated that individuals who engage in RE tend to have improved body image and body satisfaction. However, if RE has been used to cope with low self-esteem, a potential negative consequence is high body dissatisfaction and a tendency to cope by using AASs. The studies on AAS users have described a link between low self-esteem, childhood bullying, and perceptions of one's own small or lean physical size as potential predictors of AAS use. Moreover, in some but not all studies, AAS users have reported greater antisocial behavior and more impulsivity and aggressiveness. This line of research has not addressed the time line for onset of muscle dysmorphia and which treatments are most effective.

RE and "Psyching" Strategies

Twenty studies have examined the relation between RE and "psyching" (mental preparation or arousal matching/increasing) strategies to elicit maximal or submaximal lifting. The majority of these studies employed undergraduate students and athletes (see Table 22.4). A brief review of psyching strategies has been published by Tod, Iredale, and Gill (2003). Most studies have been done without the guidance of a conceptual framework or guiding theory (Tod, Iredale, McGuigan, Strange, & Gill, 2005), with some exceptions (Murphy, Woolfolk, & Budney, 1988; Perkins, Wilson, & Kerr, 2001; Wilkes & Summers, 1984). The standard methodology for this group of studies has been to have participants use preselected psyching strategies prior to a maximal or submaximal lift, although some studies have included self-selected strategies (Brody, Hatfield, Spalding, Frazer, & Caherty, 2000; McGuigan, Ghiagiarelli, & Tod, 2005; Tod et al., 2005). These techniques have included imagery,

Table 22.4. RE and Psyching Strategies

Study	Sample[a]	Psychological measure[b]	Training type[c]	Results[d]
RE and psyching strategies				
Shelton & Mahoney, 1978	Weight lifters		ISOM	↑ Performance for attentional focus compared with other groups
Gould, Weinberg, & Jackson, 1980	45 M, 45W UG	1, 9	ISOK	Prep arousal worked best in both experiments
Weinberg et al., 1980	10 M, 10 W UG	1, 9	ISOK, balance training	↑ Strength, ↔ balance for psyching strategy
Weinberg et al., 1981	40 M, 40 W UG		ISOK	↑ Performance in psych-up condition
Caudill & Weinberg, 1983	30 M, 30 WUG		DCER	↑ Performance in preparatory arousal, attentional focus, and imagery conditions compared with quiet rest condition
Wilkes & Summers, 1984	60 M UG	1, 8	ISOK	↑ Attention predicted strength change
Weinberg, Jackson, & Seaborne, 1985	24 M UG	4	CALES	↑ Performance during imagery, preparatory arousal, and psych-up conditions
Tynes & McFatter, 1987	36 UG recreational weight lifters		DCER	↑ Performance in preparatory arousal, self-efficacy, attentional focus, and imagery conditions than in a distraction protocol
Brody et al., 2000	15 M UG	3	ISOM	↔ Effects of psyching strategies
Theodorakis, Weinberg, Natsis, Douma, & Kazakas, 2000	54 high school students, 63 UG		ISOK, CALES	↑ Sit-ups in all groups

Table 22.4. (Continued)

Study	Sample[a]	Psychological measure[b]	Training type[c]	Results[d]
RE and psyching strategies				
Tod et al., 2005	12 M, 8 W UG		ISOK	Self-selected psych strategy performed better than distraction placebo
RE and imagery				
Murphy et al., 1988	24 M UG	2, 4, 10	ISOM	↔ Strength for anger and fear imagery
Lee,1990	52 M, 142 W UG	6	CALES	↑ Performance during task-relevant imagery condition
Elko &Ostrow, 1992	30 UG, 30 elderly adults	4, 7, 8	ISOM	↑ Grip strength in older adults using imagery
E. F. Pierce et al., 1993	7 Athletes		DCER	↓ Muscular strength in relaxation condition
Bakker &Boschker, 1996	22 M, 17 W UG	5	DCER	↑ EMG activity during imagery
Perkins et al., 2001	22 M, 8 W athletes	Multiple scales	ISOM	↑ Handgrip scores during paratelic script condition

[a] M = men; UG = undergraduate college students; W = women.
[b] 1 = Activation Deactivation Checklist; 2 = Autonomic Perceptions Questionnaire;3= CR-10 RPE (0–10 scale);4= Competitive State Anxiety Scale-2; 5 = Mental Imagery Questionnaire; 6= Profile of Mood States; 7= Rating of Perceived Exertion; 8= State Anxiety Inventory; 9= State Trait Anxiety Inventory; 10= Tellegen-Atkinson Absorption Scale.
[c] Mode of RE employed in the study. CALES = calesthenics such as sit-ups, push-ups, or jumping jacks; DCER = dynamic external constant resistance (traditional free weight or machine training); ISOK = isokinetic resistance machines such as Cybex or Biodyne; ISOM = isometric work.
[d] ↑, increase; ↓, decrease; ↔, no effect or not significantly different.

preperformance arousal, attentional focus, relaxation, and enhanced self-efficacy; studies have often used distraction controls (e.g., counting backward, mental arithmetic, or focusing on task-irrelevant cues). At least one study attempted to determine whether the duration of a psyching-up strategy has an impact on strength performance and found no significant effect (Caudill & Weinberg, 1983). In most studies, preparatory arousal or attentional focus on the strength task has led to enhanced strength performance, (Weinberg, Gould, & Jackson, 1980; Weinberg & Jackson, 1981; Weinberg, Jackson, Gould, & Yukelson, 1981), whereas relaxation has hindered performance (E. F. Pierce, McGowan, Eastman, Aaron, & Lynn, 1993).

RE and Imagery

To test Oxendine's emotion hypothesis that relaxation and arousal alter strength (Oxendine, 1970), Murphy and colleagues (1988) tested 24 college-age men on a handgrip task under a fear-and-anger imagery condition and a relaxation imagery condition. Relaxation was found to hinder strength performance, but fear and anger were not found to enhance performance. The authors surmised that a more complex model for testing preperformance psyching strategies was in order. Perkins and colleagues (2001) employed Apter's reversal theory (Apter, 2007) to frame their inquiry. Specifically, the goal of the study was to test the notion that according to reversal theory, positive, high-arousal, pleasant imagery scripts would enhance strength performance while high-arousal, goal-directed scripts specific to an athlete's sport would elicit anxiety and could hinder strength. Thirty elite athletes were asked to squeeze a dynamometer after reading two scripts that were specific to their respective sports and that would evoke either a paratelic focus (a playful attitude toward performance) or a telic focus (a goal-directed, serious focus). While measures of psychophysiological outcomes (heart rate, respiratory sinus arrhythmia, and skin conductance) yielded no consistent results, individuals not only showed greater strength in the paratelic condition but also reported more excitement than when they completed the telic script condition. While reading the telic script, participants reported higher levels of anxiety than those who read the paratelic script. This suggests that highly motivated individuals may benefit from paratelic self-talk or imagery scripts when needing to regulate anxiety or attempting to elicit maximal strength.

Summary of Research on RE and Psyching Strategies

Studies investigating the merits of psyching strategies and imagery for RE performance have demonstrated that (1) preperformance arousal manipulation and attentional focus can enhance strength; (2) duration of a psyching strategy is not a major factor in enhancing strength; (3) relaxation strategies prior to RE do not enhance strength, and (4) positive self-talk and imagery may enhance strength. Future research could investigate whether preferred psyching strategies produce optimal performance. Moreover, reproduction of psyching strategies and maximal physical strength could be examined through biofeedback or training approaches that would allow the athlete to develop a performance-enhancing mental skill in a laboratory setting and gradually transfer it to competitive settings. It is possible that an effective psyching strategy for one skill will not have a similar impact on a different skill or the same skill in a different context. Investigators are challenged to address these potential nuances with appropriate research designs and methodology.

RE and Deception/Ambiguity

Among the more interesting lines of inquiry in research on the psychology of RE are the placebo/deception studies that have emerged as tests of expectancy and placebo effects. Specifically, researchers in this area have attempted to determine the extent to which strength and performance are due to expectations, self-deception, or self-handicapping. Some of the studies in this category have examined college students (Kalasountas, Reed, & Fitzpatrick, 2007; Nelson & Furst, 1972; Ness & Patton, 1979; Proske et al., 2004), while others have

involved powerlifters (Maganaris, Collins, & Sharp, 2000), Olympic weight lifters (Mahoney, 1995), or other athletes (Ariel & Saville, 1972) (see Table 22.5). Most studies have used a quasi-experimental or experimental research design; one study has employed a double-blind methodology (Mahoney, 1995). Beedie and Foad (2009) have published a general review of placebo studies in sport. For this review RE studies have been classified based on whether the protocol used deceptive or ambiguous (unknown weight) feedback.

RE and Deception/Placebo

Ariel and Saville (1972) compared the impact of training and placebo on the expectancy outcome of steroid administration in a group of athletes. Performance was examined on the bench press, squat, seated military press, and leg press. Across the 11-week experiment (seven weeks of pre-placebo training and four weeks of training under the placebo condition), all participants gained strength, with greater gains in the placebo condition. In all exercises, with the exception of the seated press, strength improved an average of 19.26 pounds in the placebo condition. Thus the expectancy outcome of the steroid administration had some effect.

Maganaris and colleagues (2000) employed an AA/AB design in a group of 11 powerlifting athletes. During week one, experienced powerlifters were maximally tested on the squat, bench press, and dead lift. One week later, they performed another maximal attempt after taking what they perceived to be a rapid-acting AAS pill. On the third week, the athletes were retested. Prior to the lift on the last testing session of the last week, half of the athletes were told that the supplements were a placebo and not an AAS. As expected, the athletes that were not privy to the deception maintained their mean performance increase of over 10 kg (~24 pounds per lift) compared with the first week. However, participants in the placebo-informed group, who had experienced a 10.56-kg increase from the first week to the second week, showed only a 1.17-kg (2.58-pound) increase after learning of the deception on the third week. The expectancy effect improved performance in the deception group by an impressive 4.1% (as calculated from changes from percent change in strength from baseline across all three lifts) Maganaris et al. mentioned that they were unsure of the duration or "shelf life" of the effect.

Table 22.5. RE and Deception/Ambiguity

Study	Sample[a]	Training type[b]	Results[c]
RE and deception/placebo			
Ariel &Saville, 1972	6 Weight LiftersL	DCER	↑ Performance by 9.5% with placebo
Nelson &Furst, 1972	32 M UG	Arm wrestling	Those deceived won in all but 2 cases
Maganaris et al., 2000	11 Powerlifters	Powerlifting	↑ Performance in participants who perceived they had taken anabolic androgenic steroids; ↓ after deception was revealed
Kalasountas et al., 2007	42 UG	DCER	↑ Performance in placebo groups; ↓ performance after deception was revealed
RE and Ambiguity			
Ness & Patton, 1979	48 M UG	DCER	↑ Performance when weight was unknown and expected to be heavier
Jones & Hunter, 1983	4 M, 6 W UG	ISOM	↑ Force with opposite arm when weight was unknown
Wells, Collins, & Hale,1993	24 UG	DCER	When load was altered, strain scores changed to match performance
Mahoney, 1995	24 Olympic weight lifters	Weightlifting	↑ Performance under ambiguous condition for most athletes

[a] M = men; UG = undergraduate college students; W = women.
[b] Mode of RE employed in the study. DCER = dynamic external constant resistance (traditional free weight or machine training); ISOM = isometric work.
[c] ↑, increase; ↓, decrease.

RE and Ambiguity

Studies by Ness and Patton (1979) as well as Jones and Hunter (1983) have demonstrated that when participants performed in ambiguous conditions—that is, when they did not know the weight they were lifting—they overestimated the necessary force or expectations of heavier attempts led to increases in performance. The quantification of the degree of overcorrection at that time was unknown. A later study by Mahoney (1995) would provide some insight into this issue. Mahoney determined the effects of unambiguous versus ambiguous visual feedback (i.e., knowing how much was placed on a bar versus being unsure) with elite Olympic weight lifters using a double-blind study methodology. Neither the experimenters nor the participants knew which weight plates had been altered until the experiment was finished. Twenty-four lifters performed the snatch lift. Fifteen of the lifters performed better in the ambiguous condition, and the five lifters who set new personal records averaged an increase of 20.7 pounds. Athletes who reported greater difficulties exceeding their past maximum performances and those who expected to lift more showed better performance under ambiguous conditions.

Summary of Research on RE and Deception/Ambiguity

Studies suggest that deception/placebo can alter performance even in elite performers, and the effect appears to be related to expectation of outcome. In ambiguous conditions, improvements in strength ranged from no effect to increases in athletic samples of up to 9.5% (Ariel & Saville, 1972). Future studies should determine how long the expectancy effect persists and what characteristics most predispose an individual to the placebo effect.

Conclusions

Effort sense is affected by the intensity, volume, and speed of contraction of RE. RPE has been related to pain at higher RE intensities. Caffeine blunts perceptual responses, and even expectancy of a caffeine effect can alter RPE. Concentric muscle actions have elicited higher RPEs than eccentric muscle actions at the same absolute workload, and the chronic training effect of RE results in a lower relative RPE after 8–12 weeks of training.

An acute bout of RE does not appear to reduce anxiety immediately; instead the delayed anxiolytic response becomes salient 60–180 minutes post exercise. RE does have some positive effects on psychological well-being while not increasing psychological distress. Similarly, there appears to be fairly positive chronic adaptation of mood (depression).

RE seems to positively affect self-esteem and body image. However, individuals with muscle dysmorphia use RE for reasons other than health or fitness.

Psychological intervention to enhance performance of RE seems to be most effective when arousal is high and attention toward performance is clear but not too intense. Imagery has had marginal success in enhancing performance of RE. Expectations of performance can affect RE performance.

Whether studying sensation, affect, expectancy, optimal psychological strategies, or self-perceptions, much more work is needed to elucidate how RE affects psychological functioning and health. Research on RE has been fruitful in advancing our knowledge of this psychologically potent mode of physical activity. Future investigations will provide greater understanding of the mental health benefits of RE and of motivational strategies that can enhance RE performance.

Acknowledgments

The authors would like to thank several individuals for their contribution to the completion of this chapter. We thank the editor of this text, Dr. Edmund Acevedo, and fellow colleagues Drs. Robert D. Chetlin and Alan S. Kornspan for providing conceptual and content feedback. We are grateful to the graduate assistants (Alyssa Hargett, Virginia Lewis, Dustin R. Smith, and Brittany G. Lawrence) who helped with the literature searches, organization of the tables, and article copying. The final acknowledgment should most appropriately be given to our families (Jenny, Conrad, Owen, Ginger, Ryan, Bradley, and Kyle) for supporting us throughout this endeavor.

References

Allman, B. L., & Rice, C. L. (2003). Perceived exertion is elevated in old age during an isometric fatigue task. *European Journal of Applied Physiology, 89*(2), 191–197.

Annesi, J. J., Westcott, W. L., Loud, R. L., & Powers, L. (2004). Effects of association and dissociation formats on resistance exercise–induced emotion change and physical self-concept in older women. *Journal of Mental Health & Aging, 10*(2), 87–98.

Annesi, J. J., Westcott, W. W., & Gann, S. (2004). Preliminary evaluation of a 10-wk resistance and cardiovascular exercise protocol on physiological and psychological measures for a sample of older women. *Perceptual and Motor Skills, 98*(1), 163–170.

Anshel, M. H., & Seipel, S. J. (2009). Self-monitoring and selected measures of aerobic and strength fitness and short-term exercise adherence. *Journal of Sport Behavior, 32,* 125–151.

Apter, M. J. (2007) *Reversal Theory: The Dynamics of Motivation, Emotion and Personality,* 2nd. Edition. Oxford, England: Oneworld Publications.

Arent, S. M., Landers, D. M., Matt, K. S., & Etnier, J. L. (2005). Dose–response and mechanistic issues in the resistance training and affect relationship. *Journal of Sport & Exercise Psychology, 27*(1), 271–288.

Ariel, G., & Saville, W. (*1972*). Anabolic steroids: The physiological effects of placebos. *Medicine and Science in Sports, 4*(2), 124–126.

Astorino, T., Rohmann, R., & Firth, K. (2008). Effect of caffeine ingestion on one-repetition maximum muscular strength. *European Journal of Applied Physiology, 102*(2), 127–132.

Auchus, M. P., & Kaslow, N. J. (1994). Weight lifting therapy: A preliminary report. *Psychosocial Rehabilitation Journal, 18*(2), 99–102.

Baghurst, T., & Lirgg, C. (2009). Characteristics of muscle dysmorphia in male football, weight training, and competitive natural and non-natural bodybuilding samples. *Body Image, 6*(3), 221–227.

Bakker, F. C., & Boschker, M. S. J. (1996). Changes in muscular activity while imagining weight lifting using stimulus or response propositions. *Journal of Sport & Exercise Psychology, 18*(3), 313–324.

Bartholomew, J. B. (1999). The effect of resistance exercise on manipulated preexercise mood states for male exercisers. *Journal of Sport & Exercise Psychology, 21*(1), 39–51.

Bartholomew, J. B., & Linder, D. E. (1998). State anxiety following resistance exercise: The role of gender and exercise intensity. *Journal of Behavioral Medicine, 21*(2), 205–219.

Bartholomew, J. B., Moore, J., Todd, J., Todd, T., & Elrod, C. C. (2001). Psychological states following resistance exercise of different workloads. *Journal of Applied Sport Psychology, 13*(4), 399–410.

Bartholomew, J. B., Stults-Kolehmainen, M. A., Elrod, C. C., & Todd, J. S. (2008). Strength gains after resiatnce training: The effect of stressful, negative life events. *Journal of Strength & Conditioning Research, 22*(4), 1215–1221.

Beedie, C. J., & Foad, A. J. (2009). The placebo effect in sports performance. *Sports Medicine, 39*(4), 313–329.

Bellezza, P. A., Hall, E. E., Miller, P. C., & Bixby, W. R. (2009). The influence of exercise order on blood lactate, perceptual, and affective responses. *Journal of Strength & Conditioning Research, 23*(1), 203–208.

Bibeau, W., Moore, J. B., Mitchell, N. G., Vargas-Tonsing, T., & Bartholomew, J. B. (2010). Effects of acute resistance training of different intensities and rest periods on anxiety and affect. *Journal of Strength & Conditioning Research, 24*(8), 2184–2191.

Bigland-Ritchie, B. (1981). EMG and fatigue of human voluntary and stimulated contractions. *Ciba Foundation Symposium, 82*, 130–156.

Bigland-Ritchie, B., Donovan, E. F., & Roussos, C. S. (1981). Conduction velocity and EMG power spectrum changes in fatigue of sustained maximal efforts. *Journal of Applied Physiology: Respiratory, Environmental and Exercise Physiology, 51*(5), 1300–1305.

Bigland-Ritchie, B., & Woods, J. J. (1976). Integrated electromyogram and oxygen uptake during positive and negative work. *Journal of Physiology, 260*(2), 267–277.

Bigland-Ritchie, B., & Woods, J. J. (1984). Changes in muscle contractile properties and neural control during human muscular fatigue. *Muscle & Nerve, 7*(9), 691–699.

Borg, G. (1998). *Borg's perceived exertion and pain scales.* Champaign, IL: Human Kinetics.

Blouin, A. G., & Goldfield, G. S. (1995). Body image and steroid use in male bodybuilders. *International Journal of Eating Disorders, 18*, 159–165.

Brody, E. B., Hatfield, B. D., Spalding, T. W., Frazer, M. B., & Caherty, F. J. (2000). The effect of a psyching strategy on neuromuscular activation and force production in strength-trained men. *Research Quarterly for Exercise & Sport, 71*(2), 162–170.

Caudill, D., & Weinberg, R. S. (1983). The effects of varying the length of the psych-up interval on motor performance. *Journal of Sport Behavior, 6*(2), 86–91.

Choi, P. Y. L., Pope, H. G., Jr., & Olivardia, R. (2002). Muscle dysmorphia: A new syndrome in weightlifters. *British Journal of Sports Medicine, 36*(5), 375.

Cook, D. B., & O'Connor, P. J. (2000). Muscle pain perception and sympathetic nerve activity to exercise during opioid modulation. *American Journal of Physiology, 279*(5), R1565.

Darden, E. (1972). Comparison of body image and self-concept variables among various sport groups. *Research Quarterly, 43*(1), 7–15.

Day, M. L., McGuigan, M. R., Brice, G., & Foster, C. (2004). Monitoring resistance exercise intensity during resistance training using the session RPE scale. *Journal of Strength & Conditioning Research, 18*(2), 353–358.

Depcik, E., & Williliams, L. (2004). Weight training and body satisfaction of body-image-disturbed college women. *Journal of Applied Sport Psychology, 16*(3), 287–299.

Doyne, E. J., Ossip-Klein, D. J., Bowman, E. D., Osborn, K. M., McDougall-Wilson, I. B., & Neimeyer, R. A. (1987). Running versus weight lifting in the treatment of depression. *Journal of Consulting and Clinical Psychology, 55*(5), 748–754.

Duncan, M., Al-Nakeeb, Y., & Scurr, J. (2006). Perceived exertion is related to muscle activity during leg extension exercise. *Research in Sports Medicine, 14*(3), 179–189.

Duncan, M. J., Lyons, M., & Hankey, J. (2009). Placebo effects of caffeine on short-term resistance exercise to failure. *International Journal of Sports Performance & Physiology, 4*(2), 244–253.

Edwards, D. J., Edwards, S. D., & Basson, C. J. (2004). Psychological well-being and physical self-esteem in sport and exercise. *International Journal of Mental Health Promotion, 6*(1), 25–32.

Ekblom, B., & Goldberg, A. N. (1971). The influence of physical training and other factors on the subjective rating of perceived exertion. *Acta Physiologica Scandinavica, 83*, 399–406.

Elko, K., & Ostrow, A. C. (1992). The effects of three mental preparation strategies on strength performance of young and older adults. *Journal of Sport Behavior, 15*(1), 34–41.

Falvo, M. J., Schilling, B. K., Bloomer, R. J., Smith, W. A., & Creasy, A. C. (2007). Efficacy of prior eccentric exercise in attenuating impaired exercise performance after muscle injury in resistance trained men. *Journal of Strength & Conditioning Research, 21*(4), 1053–1060.

Focht, B. C. (2002). Pre-exercise anxiety and the anxiolytic responses to acute bouts of self-selected and prescribed intensity resistance exercise. *Journal of Sports Medicine and Physical Fitness, 42*(2), 217–223.

Focht, B. C., & Arent, S. M. (2007). *Psychological responses to acute resistance exercise: Current status, contemporary considerations, and future research directions.* Gottingen: Cuvillier Verlag.

Focht, B. C., & Koltyn, K. F. (1999). Influences of resistance exercise of different intensities on state anxiety and blood pressure. *Medicine & Science in Sports & Exercise, 31*(3), 456–463.

Focht, B. C., Koltyn, K. F., & Bouchard, L. J. (2000). State anxiety and blood pressure responses following different resistance exercise sessions. *International Journal of Sport Psychology, 31*(3), 376–390.

Ford, H. T., Puckett, J. R., Blessing, D. L., & Tucker, L. A. (1989). Effects of selected physical activities on health-related fitness and psychological well-being. *Psychological Reports, 64*(1), 203–208.

Ford, H. T., Puckett, J. R., Reeve, T. G., & Lafavi, R. G. (1991). Effects of selected physical activities on global self-concept and body-cathexis scores. *Psychological Reports, 68*(32), 1339–1343.

Fuchs, C. Z., & Zaichkowsky, L. D. (1983). Psychological characteristics of male and female bodybuilders: The iceberg profile. *Journal of Sport Behavior, 6*(3), 136–145.

Garvin, A. W., Koltyn, K. F., & Morgan, W. P. (1997). Influence of acute physical activity and relaxation on state anxiety and blood lactate in untrained college males. *International Journal of Sports Medicine, 18*(6), 470–476.

Gearhart, R. F., Goss, F. L., Lagally, K. M., Jakicic, J. M., Gallagher, J., Gallagher, K. I., & Robertson, R. J. (2002). Ratings of perceived exertion in active muscle during high-intensity and low-intensity resistance exercise. *Journal of Strength & Conditioning Research, 16*(1), 87–91.

Gearhart, R. F., Lagally, K. M., Riechman, S. E., Andrews, R. D., & Robertson, R. J. (2008). RPE at relative intensities after 12 weeks of resistance-exercise training by older adults. *Perceptual and Motor Skills, 106*(3), 893–903.

Goldfield, G. S. (2009). Body image, disordered eating and anabolic steroid use in female bodybuilders. *Eating Disorders, 17*(3), 200–210.

Goldfield, G. S., Blouin, A. G., & Woodside, D. B. (2006). Body image, binge eating, and bulimia nervosa in male bodybuilders. *Canadian Journal of Psychiatry, 51*(3), 160–168.

Gould, D., Weinberg, R., & Jackson, A. (1980). Mental preparation strategies, cognitions, and strength performance. *Journal of Sport Psychology, 2*(4), 329–339.

Green, J. M., Wickwire, P. J., McLester, J. R., Gendle, S., Hudson, G., Pritchett, R. C., & Laurent, C. M. (2007). Effects of caffeine on repetitions to failure and ratings of perceived exertion during resistance training. *International Journal of Sports Physiology & Performance, 2*(3), 250–259.

Hale, B. S., Koch, K. R., & Raglin, J. S. (2002). State anxiety responses to 60 minutes of cross training. *British Journal of Sports Medicine, 36*(2), 105–107.

Hallsworth, L., Wade, T., & Tiggemann, M. (2005). Individual differences in male body-image: An examination of self-objectification in recreational body builders. *British Journal of Health Psychology, 10*(3), 453–465.

Harne, A. J., & Bixby, W. R. (2005). The benefits of and barriers to strength training among college-age women. *Journal of Sport Behavior, 28*(2), 151–166.

Henry, R. N., Anshel, M. A., & Michael, T. (2006). Effects of aerobic and circuit training on fitness and body image among women. *Journal of Sport Behavior, 29*(4), 281–303.

Herring, M. P., & O'Connor, P. J. (2009). The effect of acute resistance exercise on feelings of energy and fatigue. *Journal of Sports Sciences, 27*(7), 701–709.

Hildebrandt, T., Schlundt, D., Langenbucher, J., & Chung, T. (2006). Presence of muscle dysmorphia symptomology among male weightlifters. *Comprehensive Psychiatry, 47*(2), 127–135.

Hollander, D. B., Durand, R. J., Trynicki, J. L., Larock, D., Castracane, V. D., Hebert, E. P., & Kraemer, R. R. (2003). RPE, pain, and physiological adjustment to concentric and eccentric contractions. *Medicine & Science in Sports & Exercise, 35*(6), 1017–1025.

Hollander, D. B., Kilpatrick, M. W., Ramadan, Z. G., Reeves, G. V., Francois, M. F., Blakeney, A., & Kraemer, R. R. (2008). Load rather than contraction types influences rate of perceived exertion and pain. *Journal of Strength & Conditioning Research, 22*(4), 1184–1193.

Hollander, D. B., Reeves, G. V., Clavier, J. D., Francois, M. R., Thomas, C., & Kraemer, R. R. (2010). Partial occlusion during resistance exercise alters effort sense and pain. *Journal of Strength & Conditioning Research, 24*(1), 235–243.

Hortobágyi, T., & Katch, F. I. (1990). Eccentric and concentric torque–velocity relationships during arm flexion and extension: Influence of strength level. *European Journal of Applied Physiology And Occupational Physiology, 60*(5), 395–401.

Hudson, G. M., Green, J. M., Bishop, P. A., & Richardson, M. T. (2008). Effects of caffeine and aspirin on light resistance training performance, perceived exertion, and pain perception. *Journal of Strength & Conditioning Research, 22*(6), 1950–1957.

Hutchinson, J. C., & Tenenbaum, G. (2006). Perceived effort—can it be considered gestalt? *Psychology of Sport & Exercise, 7*(5), 463–476.

Jones, L. A., & Hunter, I. W. (1983). Perceived force in fatiguing isometric contractions. *Perception & Psychophysics, 33*(4), 369–374.

Kalasountas, V., Reed, J., & Fitzpatrick, J. (2007). The effect of placebo-induced changes in expectancies on maximal force production in college students. *Journal of Applied Sport Psychology, 19*(1), 116–124.

Kanayama, G., Pope, H. G., Cohane, G., & Hudson, J. I. (2003). Risk factors for anabolic-androgenic steroid use among weightlifters: A case-control study. *Drug and Alcohol Dependence, 71*(1), 77–86.

Koltyn, K. F., Raglin, J. S., O'Connor, P. J., Morgan, W. P. (1995). Influence of weight training on state anxiety, body awareness and blood pressure. *International Journal of Sports Medicine, 16*(4), 266–269.

Kraemer, R. R., Acevedo, E. O., Dzewaltowski, D., Kilgore, J. L., Kraemer, G. R., & Castracane, V. D. (1996). Effects of low-volume resistive exercise on beta-endorphin and cortisol concentrations. *International Journal of Sports Medicine, 17*(1), 12–16.

Kraemer, W. J., Dziados, J. E., Marchitelli, L. J., Gordon, S. E., Harman, E. A., Mello, R., . . . Triplett, N. T. (1993). Effects of different heavy-resistance exercise protocols on plasma beta-endorphin concentrations. *Journal of Applied Physiology, 74*(1), 450–459.

Kraemer, W. J., Noble, B. J., Clark, M. J., & Culver, B. W. (1987). Physiologic responses to heavy-resistance exercise with very short rest periods. *International Journal of Sports Medicine, 8*(4), 247–252.

Kraemer, W. J., & Ratamess, N. (2004). Fundamentals of resistance training: Progression and exercise prescription. *Medicine & Science in Sports & Exercise, 36*(4), 674–688.

Kuennen, M. R., & Waldron, J. J. (2007). Relationships between specific personality traits, fat free mass indices, and the muscle dysmorphia inventory. *Journal of Sport Behavior, 30*(4), 453–470.

Lagally, K. M., Cordero, J., Good, J., Brown, D. D., & McCaw, S. T. (2009). Physiologic and metabolic responses to a continuous functional resistance exercise workout. *Journal of Strength & Conditioning Research, 23*(2), 373–379.

Lagally, K. M., McCaw, S. T., Young, G. T., Medema, H. C., & Thomas, D. Q. (2004). Ratings of perceived exertion and muscle activity during the bench press exercise in recreational and novice lifters. *Journal of Strength & Conditioning Research, 18*(2), 359–364.

Lagally, K. M., Robertson, R. J., Gallagher, K. I., Gearhart, R., & Goss, F. L. (2002). Ratings of perceived exertion during low- and high-intensity resistance exercise by young adults. *Perceptual and Motor Skills, 94*(3 Pt. 1), 723–731.

Lantz, C. D., Rhea, D. J., & Cornelius, A. E. (2002). Muscle dysmorphia in elite-level power lifters and bodybuilders: A test of differences within a conceptual model. *Journal of Strength & Conditioning Research, 16*(4), 649–655.

Lantz, C. D., Rhea, D. J., & Mayhew, J. L. (2001). The drive for size: A psycho-behavioral model of muscle dysmorphia. *International Sports Journal, 5*(1), 71–86.

Lee, C. (1990). Psyching up for a muscular endurance task: Effects of image content on performance and mood state. *Journal of Sport & Exercise Psychology, 12*(1), 66–73.

Levinger, I., Goodman, C., Matthews, V., Hare, D. L., Jerums, G., Garnham, A., & Selig, S. (2008). BDNF, metabolic risk factors, and resistance training in middle-aged individuals. *Medicine & Science in Sports & Exercise, 40*(3), 535–541.

Litt, D., & Dodge, T. (2008). A longitudinal investigation of the Drive for Muscularity Scale: Predicting use of performance enhancing substances and weightlifting among males. *Body Image, 5*(4), 346–351.

Maganaris, C. N., Collins, D., & Sharp, M. (2000). Expectancy effects and strength training: Do steroids make a difference? *Sport Psychologist, 14*(3), 272–278.

Mahoney, M. J. (1995). Ambiguity and peak performance: An experimental study with Olympic weightlifters. *International Journal of Sport Psychology, 26*(3), 327–336.

Martin Ginis, K. A., Eng, J. J., Arbour, K. P., Hartman, J. W., & Phillips, S. M. (2005). Mind over muscle? Sex differences in the relationship between body image change and subjective and objective physical changes following a 12-week strength-training program. *Body Image, 2*(4), 363–372.

McGowan, R. W., Pierce, E. F., Eastman, N., Tripathi, H. L., Dewey, T., & Olson, K. (1993). Beta-endorphins and mood states during resistance exercise. *Perceptual and Motor Skills, 76*(2), 376–378.

McGuigan, M. R., Al Dayel, A., Tod, D., Foster, C., Newton, R. U., & Pettigrew, S. (2008). Use of session rating of perceived exertion for monitoring resistance exercise in children who are overweight or obese. *Pediatric Exercise Science, 20*(3), 333–341.

McGuigan, M. R., Ghiagiarelli, J., & Tod, D. (2005). Maximal strength and cortisol responses to psyching-up during the squat exercise. *Journal of Sports Sciences, 23*(7), 687–692.

Miller, P. C., Hall, E. E., Chmelo, E. A., Morrison, J. M., DeWitt, R. E., & Kostura, C. M. (2009). The influence of muscle action on heart rate, RPE, and affective responses after upper-body resistance exercise. *Journal of Strength & Conditioning Research, 23*(2), 366–372.

Murphy, S. M., Woolfolk, R. L., & Budney, A. J. (1988). The effects of emotive imagery on strength performance. *Journal of Sport & Exercise Psychology, 10*(3), 334–345.

Nelson, L. R., & Furst, M. L. (1972). An objective study of the effects of expectation on competitive performance. *Journal of Psychology: Interdisciplinary and Applied, 81*(1), 69–72.

Ness, R. G., & Patton, R. W. (1979). The effect of beliefs on maximum weight-lifting performance. *Cognitive Therapy and Research, 3*(2), 205–211.

Norvell, N., & Belles, D. (1993). Psychological and physical benefits of circuit weight training in law enforcement personnel. *Journal of Consulting and Clinical Psychology, 61*(3), 520–527.

O'Connor, P. J., Bryant, C. X., Veltri, J. P., & Gebhardt, S. M. (1993). State anxiety and ambulatory blood pressure following resistance exercise in females. *Medicine & Science in Sports & Exercise, 25*(4), 516–521.

O'Connor, P. J. & Cook, D. B. (1998). Anxiety and systolic blood pressure reductions following acute exercise is not mediated by muscle contraction type. *International Journal of Sports Medicine, 19*, 188–192.

O'Connor, P. J., Poudevigne, M. S., & Pasley, J. D. (2002). Perceived exertion responses to novel elbow flexor eccentric action in women and men. *Medicine & Science in Sports & Exercise, 34*(5), 862–868.

Olivardia, R., Pope, H. G., & Hudson, J. I. (2000). Muscle dysmorphia in male weightlifters: A case-control study. *American Journal of Psychiatry, 157*(8), 1291–1296.

Oxendine, J. B. (1970). Emotional arousal and motor performance. *Quest, 13*, 23–32.

Parrott, A. C., Choi, P. Y., & Davies, M. (1994). Anabolic steroid use by amateur athletes: Effects upon psychological mood states. *Journal of Sports Medicine and Physical Fitness, 34*(3), 292–298.

Perkins, D., Wilson, G. V., & Kerr, J. H. (2001). The effects of elevated arousal and mood on maximal strength performance in athletes. *Journal of Applied Sport Psychology, 13*(3), 239–259.

Pickett, T. C., Lewis, R. J., & Cash, T. F. (2005). Men, muscles, and body image: Comparisons of competitive bodybuilders, weight trainers, and athletically active controls. *British Journal of Sports Medicine, 39*(4), 217–222.

Pierce, E. F., McGowan, R. W., Eastman, N. W., Aaron, J. G., & Lynn, T. D. (1993). Effects of progressive relaxation on maximal muscle strength and power. *Journal of Strength & Conditioning Research, 7*(4), 216–218.

Pierce, K., Rozenek, R., & Stone, M. H. (1993). Effects of high volume weight training on lactate, heart rate, and perceived exertion. *Journal of Strength & Conditioning Research, 7*(4), 211–215.

Pincivero, D. M., Bachmeier, B., & Coelho, A. J. (2001). The effects of joint angle and reliability on knee proprioception. *Medicine & Science in Sports & Exercise, 33*(10), 1708–1712.

Pincivero, D. M., Gear, W. S., Moyna, N. M., & Robertson, R. J. (1999). The effects of rest interval on quadriceps torque and perceived exertion in healthy males. *Journal of Sports Medicine and Physical Fitness, 39*(4), 294–299.

Pincivero, D. M., Lephart, S. M., Moyna, N. M., Karunakara, R. G., & Robertson, R. J. (1999). Neuromuscular activation and RPE in the quadriceps at low and high isometric intensities. *Electromyography and Clinical Neurophysiology, 39*(1), 43–48.

Pollock, M. L., Franklin, B. A., Balady, G. J., Chaitman, B. L., Fleg, J. L., Fletcher, B.,...Bazzarre, T. (2000). AHA Science Advisory. Resistance exercise in individuals with and without cardiovascular disease: Benefits, rationale, safety, and prescription. An advisory from the Committee on Exercise, Rehabilitation, and Prevention, Council on Clinical Cardiology, American Heart Association; position paper endorsed by the American College of Sports Medicine. *Circulation, 101*(7), 828–833.

Pope, H. G., Gruber, A. J., Choi, P., Olivardia, R., & Phillips, K. A. (1997). Muscle dysmorphia: An underrecognized form of body dysmorphic disorder. *Psychosomatics, 38*(6), 548–557.

Proske, U., Gregory, J. E., Morgan, D. L., Percival, P., Weerakkody, N. S., & Canny, B. J. (2004). Force matching errors following eccentric exercise. *Human Movement Science, 23*(3/4), 365–378.

Raglin, J. S., Turner, P. E., & Eksten, F. (1993). State anxiety and blood pressure following 30 min of leg ergometry or weight training. *Medicine & Science in Sports & Exercise, 25*(9), 1044–1048.

Reel, J. J., Greenleaf, C., Baker, W. K., Aragon, S., Bishop, D., Cachaper, C.,...Hattie, J. (2007). Relations of body concerns and exercise behavior: A meta-analysis. *Psychological Reports, 101*(3), 927–942.

Reeves, G. V., Kraemer, R. R., Hollander, D. B., Clavier, J., Thomas, C., Francois, M., & Castracane, V. D. (2006). Comparison of hormone responses following light resistance exercise with partial vascular occlusion and moderately difficult resistance exercise without occlusion. *Journal of Applied Physiology, 101*(6), 1616–1622.

Robertson, R. J., Goss, F. G., Aaron, D. J., Gairola, A., Kowallis, R. A., Liu, Y., Randall, C., Tessmer, K. A., Schnorr, T., Schroeder, A., & White, B. (2008). One repetition maximum prediction models for children using the OMNI RPE scale. *Journal of Strength & Conditioning Research, 22*(1), 196–201.

Robertson, R. J., Goss, F. L., Aaron, D. J., Nagle, E. F., Gallagher, M., Jr., Kane, I. R.,...Hunt, S. E. (2009). Concurrent muscle hurt and perceived exertion of children during resistance exercise. *Medicine & Science in Sports & Exercise, 41*(5), 1146–1154.

Robertson, R. J., Goss, F. L., Rutkowski, J., Lenz, B., Dixon, C., Timmer, J.,...Andreacci, J. (2003). Concurrent validation of the OMNI perceived exertion scale for resistance exercise. *Medicine & Science in Sports & Exercise, 35*(2), 333–341.

Sarsan, A., Ardiç, F., Ozgen, M., Topuz, O., & Sermez, Y. (2006). The effects of aerobic and resistance exercises in obese women. *Clinical Rehabilitation, 20*(9), 773–782.

Schwerin, M. J., Corcoran, K. J., Fisher, L., & Patterson, D. (1996). Social physique anxiety, body esteem, and social anxiety in bodybuilders and self-reported anabolic steroid users. *Addictive Behaviors, 21*(1), 1–8.

Schwerin, M. J., Corcoran, K. J., LaFleur, B. J., Fisher, L., Patterson, D., & Olrich, T. (1997). Psychological predictors of anabolic steriod use: An exploratory study. *Journal of Child & Adolescent Substance Abuse, 6*(2), 57–68.

Shelton, T. O., & Mahoney, M. J. (1978). The content and effect of 'psyching-up' strategies in weight lifters. *Cognitive Therapy and Research, 2*(3), 275–284.

Simão, R., Farinatti, P. D. T. V., Polito, M. D., Viveiros, L., & Fleck, S. J. (2007). Influence of exercise order on the number of repetitions performed and perceived exertion during resistance exercise in women. *Journal of Strength & Conditioning Research, 21*(1), 23–28.

Singh, F., Foster, C., Tod, D., & McGuigan, M. R. (2007). Monitoring different types of resistance training using session rating of perceived exertion. *International Journal of Sports Physiology and Performance, 2*(1), 34–45.

Spreuwenberg, L. P. B., Kraemer, W. J., Spiering, B. A., Volek, J. S., Hatfield, D. L., Silvestre, R, & Fleck. S. J. (2006). Influence of exercise order in a resistance-training exercise session. *Journal of Strength & Conditioning Research, 20*(1), 141–144.

Suminski, R. R., Robertson, R. J., Arslanian, S., Dasilva, S. G., Kang, J. G., Utter, A. C.,...Metz K. F. (1997). The perception of effort during resistance exercise. *Journal of Strength & Conditioning Research, 11*(4): 261–265.

Stone, M. H., Fleck, S. J., Triplett, N. T., & Kraemer, W. J. (1991). Health- and performance-related potential of resistance training. *Sports Medicine, 11*(4), 210–231.

Sweet, T. W., Foster, C., McGuigan, M. R., & Brice, G. (2004). Quantitation of resistance training using the session rating of perceived exertion method. *Journal of Strength & Conditioning Research, 18*(4), 796–802.

Tharion, W. J., Harman, E. A., Kraemer, W. J., & Rauch, T. M. (1991). Effects of different weight training routines on mood states. *Journal of Applied Sport Science Research, 5*(2), 60–65.

Theodorakis, Y., Weinberg, R., Natsis, P., Douma, I., & Kazakas, P. (2000). The effects of motivational versus instructional self-talk on improving motor performance. *Sport Psychologist, 14*(3), 253–271.

Tod, D. A., Iredale, F., & Gill, N. (2003). 'Psyching-up' and muscular force production. *Sports Medicine, 33*(1), 47–58.

Tod, D. A., Iredale, K. F., McGuigan, M. R., Strange, D. E. O., & Gill, N. (2005). Psyching-up enhances force production during the bench press exercise. *Journal of Strength & Conditioning Research, 19*(3), 599–603.

Tucker, L. A. (1982a). Effects of a weight training program on self concepts of college males. *Perceptual and Motor Skills, 54*(3 Pt. 2), 1055–1061.

Tucker, L. A. (1982b). Relationship between perceived somatotype and body cathexis of college males. *Psychological Reports, 50*(31), 983–989.

Tucker, L. A. (1983). Effect of weight training on self-concept: A profile of those influenced most. *Research Quarterly for Exercise & Sport, 54*(4), 389–397.

Tucker, L. A. (1987). Effect of weight training on body attitudes: Who benefits most? *Journal of Sports Medicine & Physical Fitness, 27*(1), 70–78.

Tucker, L. A., & Maxwell, K. (1992). Effects of weight training on the emotional well-being and body image of females:

Predictors of greatest benefit. *American Journal of Health Promotion, 6*(5), 338–371.

Tucker, L. A., & Mortell, R. (1994). Comparison of the effects of walking and weight-training programs on body image in middle-aged women: An experimental study. *American Journal of Health Promotion, 8*, 34–42.

Tynes, L. L., & McFatter, R. M. (1987). The efficacy of 'psyching' strategies on a weight-lifting task. *Cognitive Therapy and Research, 11*(3), 327–336.

Ung, E. K., Fones, C. S. L., & Ang, A. W. K. (2000). Muscle dysmorphia in a young Chinese male. *Annals of the Academy of Medicine of Singapore, 29*(1), 135–137.

Utter, A. C., Kang, J., Nieman, D. C., Brown, V. A., Dumke, C. L., McAnulty, S. R., & McAnulty, L. S. (2005). Carbohydrate supplementation and perceived exertion during resistance exercise. *Journal of Strength & Conditioning Research, 19*(4), 939–943.

Van Vorst, J. G., Buckworth, J., & Mattern, C. (2002). Physical self-concept and strength changes in college weight training classes. *Research Quarterly for Exercise & Sport, 73*(1), 113–117.

Vassallo, M. J., & Olrich, T. W. (2010). Confidence by injection: Male users of anabolic steroids speak of increases in perceived confidence through anabolic steroid use. *International Journal of Sport & Exercise Psychology, 8*(1), 70–80.

Webster, D. (1976). *The iron game: An illustrated history of weight-lifting., Irvine, Scotland*: John Geddes Printers.

Weinberg, R. S., Gould, D., & Jackson, A. (1980). Cognition and motor performance: Effect of psyching-up strategies on three motor tasks. *Cognitive Therapy and Research, 4*(2), 239–245.

Weinberg, R. S., & Jackson, A. (1981). Effect of psyching-up strategies on motor performance. *TAHPERD Journal, 49*(3), 16–17.

Weinberg, R. S., Jackson, A., Gould, D., & Yukelson, D. (1981). Effect of preexisting and manipulated self-efficacy on a competitive muscular endurance task. *Journal of Sport Psychology, 3*(4), 345–354.

Weinberg, R. S., Jackson, A., & Seaborne, T. (1985). The effects of specific vs nonspecific mental preparation strategies on strength and endurance performance. *Journal of Sport Behavior, 8*, 175–180.

Weir, J. P., Beck, T. W., Cramer, J. T., & Housh, T. J. (2006). Is fatigue all in your head? A critical review of the central governor model. *British Journal of Sports Medicine, 40*(7), 573–586.

Weiser, P. C., & Stamper, D. A. (1977). Psychophysiological interactions leading to increased effort, leg fatigue, and respiratory distress during prolonged strenuous bicycle riding. In G. Borg (Ed.), *Physical work and effort* (pp. 401–416). New York: Permagon Press.

Wells, C. M., Collins, D., & Hale, B. D. (1993). The self-efficacy–performance link in maximum strength performance. *Journal of Sports Sciences, 11*(2), 167–175.

Wickwire, P. J., McLester, J. R., Green, J. M., & Crews, T. R. (2009). Acute heart rate, blood pressure, and RPE responses during super slow vs. traditional machine resistance training protocols using small muscle group exercises. *Journal of Strength & Conditioning Research, 23*(1), 72–79.

Wilkes, R. L., & Summers, J. J. (1984). Cognitions, mediating variables, and strength performance. *Journal of Sport Psychology, 6*(3), 351–359.

Williams, M. A., Haskell, W. L., Ades, P. A., Amsterdam, E. A., Bittner, V., Franklin, B. A.,...Stewart, K. J. (2007).

Resistance exercise in individuals with and without cardiovascular disease: 2007 update. A scientific statement from the American Heart Association Council on Clinical Cardiology and Council on Nutrition, Physical Activity, and Metabolism. *Circulation, 116*(5), 572–584.

Williams, M. A., & Stewart, K. J. (2009). Impact of strength and resistance training on cardiovascular disease risk factors and outcomes in older adults. *Clinics in Geriatric Medicine, 25*(4), 703–714.

Williams, P. A., & Cash, T. F. (2001). Effects of a circuit weight training program on the body images of college students. *International Journal of Eating Disorders, 30*(1), 75–82.

Wojtowicz, A. E., & von Ranson, K. M. (2006). Psychometric evaluation of two scales examining muscularity concerns in men and women. *Psychology of Men & Masculinity, 7*(1), 56–66.

Wolke, D., & Sapouna, M. (2008). Big men feeling small: Childhood bullying experience, muscle dysmorphia and other mental health problems in bodybuilders. *Psychology of Sport & Exercise, 9*(5), 595–604.

Woods, S., Bridge, T., Nelson, D., Risse, K., & Pincivero, D. M. (2004). The effects of rest interval length on ratings of perceived exertion during dynamic knee extension exercise. *Journal of Strength and Conditioning Research, 18*(3), 540–545.

Yarrow, J. F., Borsa, P. A., Borst, S. E., Sitren, H. S., Stevens, B. R., & White, L. J. (2007). Neuroendocrine responses to an acute bout of eccentric-enhanced resistance exercise. *Medicine & Science in Sports & Exercise, 39*(6), 941–947.

Tai Chi as an Alternative Mode of Exercise Activity for Older Adults

Fuzhong Li

Abstract

There is strong research evidence that regular participation in physical activity is associated with a variety of health benefits in older adults. While there are many mainstream exercise modalities (e.g., resistance, endurance, stretching, and balance), Tai Chi, an alternative exercise modality, is receiving increasing attention. The volume of empirical research on Tai Chi has steadily increased over the past two decades, with findings showing its positive impact in preventing and treating chronic illnesses and functional loss and enhancing overall functioning and quality of life. These results have implications for public health promotion to ameliorate illness and disability in the aging population. This chapter is intended to summarize the current research on Tai Chi (with a focus on a small group of rigorous studies), discuss findings with respect to their practical implications, and highlight future research directions.

Key Words: health, older adults, physical activity, Tai Chi.

The projected increase in the population aged 65 and over across the world (United Nations, 2007) has significant ramifications due to increases in the number of people with age-related disabilities, including adding significant strain on healthcare costs and undermining the quality of life of the aging population at large. The public health concern is that with advancing age come progressive declines in physical and mental capacity in older adults. To preserve normal physiological function and physical independence, it is crucial that older adults avoid a sedentary lifestyle by engaging in regular exercise and physical activity. Compelling evidence from a large number of epidemiological and intervention studies shows the benefits of exercise for older adults in preventing or delaying many diseases and disabilities (Chodzko-Zajko et al., 2009; Nelson et al., 2007). While numerous types of exercise or physical activity have been recommended for older adults (National Institute on Aging, 2010), one that has been increasing in interest and popularity in both scientific research and community-wide adoption is Tai Chi.

Tai Chi

Tai Chi, or more formally, Tai Ji Quan, consists of a series of individual postures that are linked together in a continuous movement sequence, with variations for long or short routines. Each of the movements is derived from either imitation of the movements of animals or self-defense postures used in combat. A sequence of Tai Chi movements is generally performed under conscious, controlled mental focus, making it a moving meditation exercise. Although there are inherent intricacies associated with this ancient exercise that are largely unexplored by the scientific community, Tai Chi essentially is an integrated exercise involving deliberate movements, meditation, and qi ("chee," or energy) synchronized to create a dynamic, continuous reciprocity of what ancient philosophers called yin and yang states. Conceptually, the states consist of opposite but complementary forces of nature (e.g., male/female, active/passive, static/moving, forceful/yielding, tension/relaxation) that need to be "in balance" for optimal functioning. The resulting equilibrium of these counterforces is believed to bring about sustained health and well-being, leading to prolonged life.

Traditionally, there are multiple styles or schools of Tai Chi (e.g., Chen, Yang, Sun, and Wu), with Chen being historically considered the original (People's Sports, 1996). However, the Yang school of Tai Chi (Liang & Wu, 1996; Yang, 1991) is the most popular, especially as a result of the development of a simplified 24-form routine (China Sports, 1980) with an easy-to-difficult progression; even, slow tempo; and low-to-moderate intensity, which make it amenable to people of all ages, especially older adults (F. Li, Fisher, Harmer, & Shirai, 2003). For centuries Tai Chi, regardless of style, has been practiced as combative, with self-defense applications, but it continues to evolve from a martial art to a competitive demonstration sport to, on a broader scale, a health-enhancing, artful exercise practiced by individuals of all ages to maintain health and prevent disease. Thanks in part to accumulating evidence of its therapeutic value to overall health and well-being (J. X. Li, Hong, & Chan, 2001; Wolf, Coogler, & Xu, 1997), Tai Chi is drawing greater interest in the domains of public health and clinical practice.

Empirical Research

As in any field of medical treatment, early research with Tai Chi focused primarily on exploring its physical and mental health benefits using nonexperimental design paradigms. The resultant outcomes, although preliminary in nature, laid the foundations for studies with more scientific rigor, particularly randomized controlled trials (RCTs). Evidence established through RCTs has indicated the effectiveness and therapeutic value of Tai Chi practice as an exercise modality for maintaining optimal physical and psychological function. The majority of research conducted to date has applied the Yang school of Tai Chi (China Sports, 1980; People's Sports, 1996), with variation in the number of forms implemented (Liang & Wu, 1996; Yang, 1991). Although specific rationales in many studies are often not fully described, one reason for using Yang style may be that its characteristics, such as

gentleness, slowness, and easiness, make it amenable to elderly, frail, or disabled populations.

In what follows, a selective review of RCT studies or those that involve at least a comparison group for Tai Chi is provided. The review focuses on several geriatric syndromes deemed clinically important with respect to functional capacity, chronic disease and condition management, life independence, and well-being.

Muscular Strength

The repetitive movements of Tai Chi practice engage practitioners in a continuous, symmetrical body weight shift between the dominant leg and the nondominant leg, which exerts a training effect on major lower-extremity muscle groups, such as the tibialis anterior (dorsal flexion), quadriceps femoris (knee extensor), and hamstring (knee flexor) muscles. There is evidence from both controlled and noncontrolled studies (Christou, Yang, & Rosengren, 2003; Lan, Lai, Chen, & Wong, 1998; Wu, Zhao, Zhou, & Wei, 2002) for this effect of weight-bearing activity on muscular strength, although findings have been equivocal (Woo, Hong, Lau, & Lynn, 2007).

In a nonrandomized study, Christou et al. (2003) showed that in comparison to a no-exercise control, a 20-week program of three hours a week of Tai Chi (Chen style) improved knee extensor strength and force control in older adults (mean age = 71.9±1.8 years). Similarly, in a prospective nonrandomized controlled study, Lan et al. (1998) examined muscle strength of the knee in a cohort of long-term Tai Chi practitioners and sedentary controls over a 12-month period and observed significant increases in both knee extensor (18%) and flexor (15%) values in the Tai Chi group compared with the control group. However, in a 12-month Hong Kong–based RCT reported by Woo et al. (2007), there was no difference in the strength measure (quadriceps femoris) between Tai Chi and control conditions. The authors indicated that the intensity of the Tai Chi training may not have been sufficiently high to produce observable improvements in strength.

Tai Chi has been shown to help older adults maintain exercise gains. Wolfson et al. (1996) reported that in a sample of older adults (mean age = 79±5 years), six months of Tai Chi (Yang style) training following a three-month balance training intervention preserved lower-extremity strength gains developed during the intervention phase.

Functional Balance

With controlled and continuous movements, the transition between weight-bearing and non-weight-bearing stances, and large body (center of mass) displacement during the motion, Tai Chi practice imposes a great challenge to practitioners' balance mechanisms. Most noticeably, Tai Chi practice often requires that one control for the limits of stability (with respect to the base of support), especially when the center of mass exceeds the base of support. Therefore, Tai Chi is viewed as an appropriate exercise for training postural stability and balance. This hypothesis has been evaluated in a number of empirical studies (Hain, Fuller, Weil, & Kotsias, 1999; W. W. N. Tsang & Hui-Chan, 2003; Tse & Bailey, 1992).

In a RCT, F. Li, Harmer, et al. (2005) examined the efficacy of a six-month intervention of Tai Chi three times a week in improving functional balance in older persons (mean age = 77±5 years). At the end of the intervention, Tai Chi participants showed significant improvements in several important clinical measures of functional balance, including the Berg Balance Scale, Dynamic Gait Index, Functional Reach, and single-leg standing, compared with control participants who had done stretching exercises, who showed no significant change in these outcomes. Intervention gains in these measures were maintained at a six-month postintervention follow-up.

There is also some evidence that improved functional balance from Tai Chi training reduces fall frequency. F. Li, Fisher, Harmer, and McAuley (2004) followed a cohort of older adults who completed a six-month training and found that Tai Chi participants, who showed improvements in measures of functional balance (Berg Balance Scale, Dynamic Gait Index, and Functional Reach) during the intervention, also had a significantly reduced risk of falls during the six-month postintervention period compared with participants in a control condition.

Few studies have investigated potential underlying mechanisms of the observed functional benefits, such as better balance, of Tai Chi training. Hass et al. (2004) examined whether Tai Chi (Yang style) training improved postural control by altering the center of pressure during gait initiation—an important indicator of balance dysfunction. These authors showed that older adults (mean age = 79.6±5 years), after a 48-week intervention of intense Tai Chi training, significantly improved the magnitude by which they shifted their center of pressure backward, which helps to generate the forward momentum needed to initiate gait. In addition, Tai Chi training improved the smoothness of movements,

possibly as a result of enhanced coordination from the training. In combination, these findings suggest that Tai Chi may improve postural control.

Bone Health

Tai Chi movements are performed in a semi-squat (lowered center of gravity) position that stresses lower-extremity muscles. Although of low-to-moderate impact, the emphasis of constant weight-shift makes Tai Chi a bone-loading activity. While muscle action on bone has been shown to promote bone health, evidence concerning the influence of Tai Chi training on bone structure is limited and the results are equivocal.

Chan et al. (2004) tested the hypothesis that Tai Chi may retard bone loss in a sample of early postmenopausal women (mean age = 54.0±3.5 years) in Hong Kong. Participants were randomized into a Tai Chi group, which practiced 45 minutes a day, five days a week, for 12 months or a sedentary control group. Main outcome measures of bone mineral density (BMD) were taken at the lumbar spine and proximal femur, using dual-energy x-ray absorptiometry (DXA), and in the distal tibia, using multislice peripheral quantitative computed tomography (pQCT). At the end of the trial, BMD measurements revealed a general bone loss in both Tai Chi and control participants at all measured skeletal sites, but with a slower rate for those in the Tai Chi group. Although the DXA findings were equivocal, the pQCT data indicated a significant retardation of bone loss in the distal tibia in the Tai Chi group compared with the controls.

The prediction that Tai Chi helps retard bone loss was partially supported in a more recent Hong Kong–based study (Woo et al., 2007) involving a sample of community-dwelling older adults (mean age = 69±3 years). Specifically, Woo et al. evaluated the effects of Tai Chi (Yang style), in comparison with a resistance training program and a control group, on BMD (total hip, femoral neck, total spine, and intertrochanteric area). The authors found that after 12 months of training three times a week, female participants in both the Tai Chi and resistance training groups had significantly less loss for total hip BMD only compared with those in the control group. In men, however, there was no difference in percentage change in BMD between the three treatment groups.

Reduced Fear of Falling

There is a strong association between falls and fear of falling, and because of this, several Tai Chi studies have included a measure of fear of falling. Sattin, Easley, Wolf, Chen, and Kutner (2005) examined whether an intense Tai Chi exercise program (Wolf et al., 2003) could reduce fear of falling better than a wellness education (control) program in older adults who had fallen previously and met criteria for transitioning to frailty. These authors reported that after 12 months of intervention confidence about not falling was significantly greater in the Tai Chi group than in the control group, with the differences increasing over the trial period.

Similarly, the study by F. Li, Fisher, Harmer, et al. (2005) showed that among other health outcomes, a six-month Tai Chi intervention significantly reduced fear of falling in adults aged 70 and over. Specifically, Tai Chi participants had a 55% reduction in fear of falling as operationalized by the Survey of Activities and Fear of Falling in the Elderly (Lachman et al., 1998), compared with a 13% reduction for those assigned to a stretching control condition. This was the first Tai Chi–based study that employed a measure of fear of falling that includes broader activities such as activities of daily living and instrumental activities of daily living as well as social and exercise activities.

Preventing Falls and Reducing Risk of Falling

If Tai Chi training can improve lower-extremity strength, balance, and gait and possibly maintain bone integrity, it is reasonable to speculate on its impact in preventing falls, a significant public health problem among older adults (Centers for Disease Control and Prevention, 2010). Three RCTs designed to address this question have been conducted in the United States. Wolf et al. (1996) compared the efficacy of two methods of exercise in reducing frequency of falls. Older adult participants (mean age = 76±5years) were randomized to 15 weeks' participation in one of three groups (Tai Chi, computerized balance training, or a control). The computerized balance training and control groups attended sessions once a week, but the Tai Chi (Yang style) participants attended twice-weekly sessions. Results showed that compared with the control group, the Tai Chi participants experienced a significant reduction (approximately 47%) in falls.

In a RCT extension of this work, Wolf and colleagues (2003) examined whether Tai Chi exercise could benefit older individuals who were less robust (i.e., transitioning to frailty). Participants (mean age = 81±6years) took part for 48 weeks in either a Tai Chi (Yang style—practiced two sessions per week,

starting at 60 minutes and progressing to 90 minutes over the course of the study) or exercise control (wellness education) condition. Results showed that after excluding the first three months of training data (because of significant between-group variation), a 46% reduction in falls was observed in the Tai Chi group compared with the exercise control group.

A later study by F. Li, Harmer, et al. (2005) confirmed the findings reported by Wolf and his colleagues. In a sample of adults aged 70 years and older (mean age = 77±5 years) Li and colleagues found that at the end of a six-month intervention there had been significantly fewer falls (38 vs. 73) and lower proportions of fallers (28% vs. 46%) and injurious falls (7% vs. 18%) in the Tai Chi condition compared with a stretching control group. After adjustment for baseline covariates, the risk of multiple falls in the Tai Chi group was 55% lower than that in the controls (risk ratio = 0.45, 95% confidence interval, 0.30–0.70).

In a study conducted in Australia, Voukelatos, Cumming, Lord, and Rissel (2007) reported that a program of Tai Chi (a mixture of several styles including Yang) delivered for one hour a week to relatively healthy community-dwelling adults aged 60 and older (mean age = 69±7 years) reduced the fall incidence rate by 28% after 16 weeks and 33% after 24 weeks. On the basis of their findings, the authors concluded that participation in once-per-week Tai Chi classes for 16 weeks can prevent falls in relatively healthy community-dwelling older adults.

Not all trials conducted to date provide conclusive support for the efficacy of Tai Chi in reducing frequency of falls or risk of falling in older adults. For example, in a study in the Netherlands, Logghe et al. (2009) found that a 13-week training program of Tai Chi for one hour a week failed to produce a difference in risk of falling between Tai Chi participants and controls. Similarly, although Woo et al. (2007) used a higher frequency and greater duration of training (three times per week for 12 months) in their Hong Kong study, they also did not show any significant differences in number of falls between the Tai Chi and control groups.

Physical Functioning

In a six-month RCT involving a sample of community-dwelling older adults (mean age = 73±5 years), F. Li, Harmer, et al. (2001) found that Tai Chi training improved self-reported physical function, in areas ranging from daily activities (e.g., walking) to moderate-to-vigorous activities (e.g., running), by 65%. A reanalysis of the study outcomes showed that Tai Chi participants with lower levels of physical function at baseline benefited more from the Tai Chi training than those with higher baseline physical function scores (F. Li, Fisher, Harmer, & McAuley, 2002). In contrast, Kutner, Barnhart, Wolf, McNeely, and Xu (1997) found at a four-month postintervention follow-up evaluation that there was no significant improvement in self-reported physical function among participants who completed a 15-week Tai Chi training program. To overcome weaknesses associated with self-report, F. Li, Fisher, Harmer, et al. (2004) used clinical measures of physical function in a six-month sleep quality trial (participants mean age = 75±8 years). They reported that Tai Chi participants showed better scores on measures including single-leg standing, timed chair rise, and 50-foot walk than those who were assigned to a low-impact physical activity control condition.

Blood Pressure and Lipid Profile

Young, Appel, Jee, and Miller (1999) compared the effects of aerobic exercise and Tai Chi in a sample of older adults (mean age = 67±5 years) with blood pressure levels ranging from prehypertension (120–139 mm Hg systolic, 80–89 mm Hg diastolic) to stage 1 hypertension (140–159 mm Hg systolic, 90–99 mm Hg diastolic). These researchers found that although both blood pressure values decreased significantly over 12 weeks of training in both intervention groups, the magnitudes of the improvements did not differ between the groups for either systolic pressure (-8.4±1.6 mm Hg and -7.0±1.6 mm Hg in the aerobic exercise and Tai Chi groups, respectively) or diastolic pressure (-3.2±1.0 mm Hg and -2.4±1.0 mm Hg in the aerobic exercise and Tai Chi groups, respectively). These results indicate that Tai Chi may have a health impact similar to that of moderate-intensity aerobic exercise. Wolf et al. (1996) observed a reduction in systolic blood pressure (by 13 mm Hg) during a 12-minute walk following Tai Chi participation.

In a RCT that involved a sample of middle-aged adults (mean age = 51±13 years) in Taiwan, Tsai et al. (2003) showed that a 12-week Tai Chi (Yang style) program was beneficial for lowering blood pressure and improving lipid profiles. Specifically, in comparison with the control group, Tai Chi participants showed significantly greater decreases in systolic and diastolic blood pressure (by 15.6 mm Hg and 8.8 mm Hg, respectively) and total serum cholesterol level (by 15.2 mg/dL). High-density lipoprotein cholesterol increased by 4.7 mg/dL in the Tai Chi group compared with those in the control group.

Immunity

In a RCT of community-dwelling healthy older adults (mean age = 70±6years), Irwin, Olmstead, and Oxman (2007) showed that a 25-week Tai Chi training program of 40-minute classes, three times weekly, significantly increased participants' immunity to varicella-zoster virus compared with those in a health education control. After 16 weeks, participants in both groups received a single injection of Varivax, the chicken pox vaccine. Nine weeks later, the investigators assessed each participant's level of varicella immunity, comparing it with immunity at the start of the study. They found that Tai Chi alone increased participants' immunity to varicella, and Tai Chi combined with the vaccine produced an approximately 40% higher level of immunity than the vaccine alone. These findings suggest that Tai Chi training may help protect older adults from the varicella virus, which causes both chicken pox and shingles.

Qualify of Sleep

F. Li, Fisher, Harmer, et al. (2004) showed that Tai Chi three times weekly for six months significantly improved self-reported sleep quality in a sample of older adults (mean age = 75±8 years) who had sleep complaints. Participants reported improvements in five of the Pittsburgh Sleep Quality Index (PSQI) subscale scores, with particular improvements in sleep latency (reduced by about 18 minutes per night) and sleep duration (increased by about 48 minutes per night). The results also provided preliminary evidence linking Tai Chi to decreased daytime sleepiness.

These findings were supported in a trial that compared Tai Chi with a no-treatment control. Irwin, Olmstead, and Motivala (2008) reported that in comparison with controls, participants (mean age = 70±6 years) in a 16-week Tai Chi program showed significant improvements in PSQI global scores and in subscale scores for sleep efficiency, duration, and disturbance.

Self-Efficacy

Tai Chi is performed in a self-controlled, rhythmic manner, with frequent transitioning from a wide base of support to a narrow base. Over time, this may help develop confidence in controlling one's balance. In a RCT, F. Li, McAuley, Harmer, Duncan, and Chaumeton (2001) examined the effects of Tai Chi training on perceptions of movement efficacy in a sample of community-dwelling older adults (mean age = 73±5 years). At the end of six months of practice, Tai Chi participants registered significant improvements in movement efficacy. Subsequent analysis showed that participants' changes in efficacy were associated with greater attendance at practice sessions and that improvements in movement self-efficacy as a function of Tai Chi were related to increased levels of perceived physical capability (F. Li, McAuley, Harmer, Fisher, et al., 2001). The findings suggest that Tai Chi can enhance self-efficacy and that the changes in self-efficacy may improve exercise adherence and physical functioning.

F. Li, Fisher, Harmer, and McAuley (2005) explored whether self-efficacy mediates change in fear of falling in a secondary analysis. Participants (mean age = 77±5 years) were involved in either a Tai Chi or a stretching exercise control intervention three times per week for six consecutive months. Results supported the mediational hypothesis in that Tai Chi participants, who evidenced improvement in falls self-efficacy over the intervention, also reported greater reductions in fear of falling than those in the stretching control condition. The authors concluded that Tai Chi may be used to enhance older adults' confidence in their balance, which may in turn reduce their fear of falling.

Sense of Well-Being, Esteem, and Perception of Benefits

Traditionally, Tai Chi has also been thought to enhance overall mental well-being, and there is increasing research to support this view. F. Li and his colleagues provided a series of reports from a single, six-month RCT study that examined the extent to which Tai Chi (Yang style) training enhanced elderly individuals' multidimensional psychological well-being. Older adults (mean age = 73±5 years) were randomly assigned to two hours a week of either a control condition or Tai Chi. Results indicated that compared with those in the control condition, Tai Chi participants showed higher levels of health perceptions, life satisfaction, positive affect, and well-being and lower levels of depression, negative affect, and psychological distress (F. Li, Duncan, et al., 2001). Similarly, Tai Chi participants showed not only higher levels of general self-esteem and domain-specific physical self-worth but also subdomain-specific esteem of body attractiveness, physical strength, and physical condition (F. Li, McAuley, Harmer, Duncan, & Chaumeton, 2002).

Participation in Tai Chi also is reported to result in better perceptions of benefits. For example, Kutner et al. (1997) conducted an exit interview four months postintervention on a group of older adult participants (mean age not known) who completed a 15-week Tai Chi program and found that in comparison with a control group, the Tai Chi participants reported significant improvements in confidence in their balance and movement and greater benefits and positive effects on their normal physical activity and lives.

Chronic Disease Populations
HEART DISEASE

In a RCT, Yeh et al. (2004) examined the effects of a 12-week Tai Chi (Yang style) program on quality of life and exercise capacity in patients with chronic stable heart failure and left ventricular ejection fraction less than 40%. At 12 weeks, patients in the Tai Chi group showed improved quality-of-life scores, increased distance walked in six minutes, and decreased (improved) serum B-type natriuretic peptide levels compared with patients in the control group. The authors concluded that Tai Chi may be a beneficial adjunct treatment that enhances quality of life and functional capacity in patients with chronic heart failure. In a subsequent 12-week trial, the investigators from the same research group (Yeh et al., 2011) showed again that Tai Chi exercise improved self-reported quality of life, exercise self-efficacy, and mood measures among patients with chronic systolic heart failure.

DIABETES

T. Tsang, Orr, Lam, Comino, and Singh (2008) examined whether Tai Chi could improve glucose homeostasis and insulin resistance in older adult patients with type 2 diabetes. Patients were randomized into a Tai Chi program (a mixture of Sun and Yang styles) or a sham-exercise control for twice-a-week practices for 16 weeks. The trial results showed that Tai Chi training did not improve glucose homeostasis or insulin sensitivity measured 72 hours after the last bout of exercise. The authors concluded that higher-intensity Tai Chi training may be required to elicit changes in body composition associated with metabolic benefits in type 2 diabetes.

OSTEOARTHRITIS

The slow and fluid movements of Tai Chi, coupled with deep diaphragmatic breathing and an emphasis on body–mind connection, may also have a positive effect on chronic diseases related to the musculoskeletal system. A few RCTs have provided evidence of the potential of Tai Chi in the management of lower-extremity osteoarthritis. For example, Wang et al. (2009) examined the effectiveness of a twice weekly, 12-week Tai Chi (Yang style) program on pain in a sample of patients with knee osteoarthritis (mean age = 65±8 years). Their results showed that in comparison with participants assigned to an attention control, Tai Chi participants reported significant reductions in their pain level as indexed by the Western Ontario and McMaster Universities Osteoarthritis Index. A similar 12-week trial conducted in Korea produced some evidence of the efficacy of a Sun-style Tai Chi program in reducing arthritic symptoms in older women with osteoarthritis (Song, Lee, Lam, & Bae, 2003). Results from the two trials also indicated improvements in physical function as a result of Tai Chi training.

Physical limitations experienced by patients with osteoarthritis often lead to a diminished sense of personal capability and self-efficacy. In a RCT, Hartman et al. (2000) examined whether Tai Chi (Yang style) could improve self-efficacy in managing pain, physical function, and other arthritis symptoms in older adults with osteoarthritis (mean age = 68±7 years). After a 12-week intervention, the authors found that in comparison with a control group, Tai Chi participants had improved confidence in managing arthritis symptoms.

FIBROMYALGIA

In a 12-week RCT, Wang and her colleagues (Wang, Schmid, Rones et al., 2010) examined whether Tai Chi could improve musculoskeletal pain in patients with fibromyalgia (mean age = 50±12 years). Patients were randomized to either a Tai Chi group (practicing a set of 10 forms from the classic Yang style) or a control group consisting of wellness education and stretching. At completion of the study, compared to those in the control group, Tai Chi participants showed a clinically significant reduction (–18.4 points) in the overall severity of fibromyalgia, as indicated by a significant decrease in the total Fibromyalgia Impact Questionnaire score (–27.8 points in Tai Chi vs. –9.4 points in control). Significant improvements were also observed among Tai Chi participants in the measures of physical and mental components of the 36-item Health Survey. The authors concluded that Tai Chi may be used as part of multidisciplinary therapies for patients with fibromyalgia.

PARKINSON'S DISEASE

In a preliminary study, Hackney and Earhart (2008) examined the effects of Tai Chi (Yang style) on balance, gait, and mobility in people with Parkinson's disease. The Tai Chi group participated in 20 one-hour training sessions over 10–13 weeks. Compared with those in the control condition, Tai Chi participants showed improved scores on the Berg Balance Scale, Unified Parkinson's Disease Rating Scale, Timed Up&Go, tandem stance test, six-minute walk, and backward walking. The authors concluded that Tai Chi is an appropriate, safe, and effective form of exercise for patients with mild to moderately severe Parkinson's disease.

On the basis of their prior work (Li et al., 2007), F. Li and his colleagues (Li et al., 2012) conducted an RCT examining whether a tailored Tai Chi program could improve postural stability in patients with Parkinson's disease. The investigators randomly assigned 195 patients (mean age = 69±9 years), who were classified as stages 1 through 4 on the Hoehn–Yahr staging scale (Hoehn & Yahr, 1967), to one of three groups: Tai Chi, resistance training, or stretching control. These patients participated in 60-minute group-based exercise sessions twice weekly for 24 weeks. The study included primary outcomes of the Limits of Stability test (maximum excursion, directional control), secondary outcomes of gait and knee strength, Functional Reach, Timed Up&Go, motor scores of the Unified Parkinson's Disease Rating Scale (Fahn, Elton, & members of the UPDRS Development Committee, 1987), and number of falls. At completion of the study, the authors showed that the Tai Chi group performed consistently better than the stretching and resistance groups in the primary outcome measures. Tai Chi participants also scored better than the stretching group in all secondary outcomes and outperformed the resistance group in stride length and Functional Reach. Tai Chi training was shown to reduce the incidence of falls compared to stretching but not to resistance. The 6-month Tai Chi training effects were sustained at 3-month postintervention follow-up. The investigators concluded that Tai Chi training may be used to reduce balance impairments in patients with mild-to-moderate Parkinson's disease, with additional health benefits of improved physical functioning and reduced falls.

Future Research

There has been a significant increase in the volume of research on Tai Chi over the past two decades. Although knowledge regarding the health benefits of Tai Chi practice has improved from the early anecdotal reports to studies grounded on more rigorous scientific approaches, the considerable variation in the results currently available affects the extent to which claims of benefits can be confidently stated. There is a significant need for continued research, and the field will benefit from further investigation in a number of areas. In what follows, several of these needs are highlighted to stimulate future efforts.

First, more clinical RCTs designed with appropriate scientific rigor are needed. As noted in several major reviews of current work (Harmer & Li, 2008; Wang, Collet, & Lau, 2004; Wayne et al., 2004), significant study design weaknesses include a lack of randomization for intervention assignment, failure to mask (blind) study assessors, inadequately developed training protocols, lack of details on the qualifications of instructors, poorly defined intervention conditions, small sample sizes, underpowered end points, and high dropout rates. RCTs are needed to allow researchers to make multiple functional, medical, behavioral, and biomechanical measurements in a more rigorous fashion; study outcome efficacy and mechanisms of action; and draw valid causal inferences.

There is a need to address dose–response questions, particularly in regard to what constitutes optimal Tai Chi training to achieve desirable health benefits. Relevant program variables include intensity, duration, and frequency, none of which has been examined in previous RCTs. With respect to duration and frequency, training schedules in completed RCTs vary widely, although most have used 60-minute sessions one to three times per week for 12 to 48 weeks. Regarding intensity, in a RCT by Wolf et al. (2003), the investigators used two sessions a week starting at 60 minutes each and progressing to 90 minutes over the course of 48 weeks. No trend analysis on the time intervals, however, was performed to determine whether the incremental approach influenced the outcomes differentially across the two training intervals. Future studies should address the influence of these training variables on health outcomes by considering a RCT with a within-group design or a factorial design within a RCT that involves comparisons of Tai Chi training doses.

Additionally, there is a need to conduct intervention follow-up evaluations, which would be both clinically important and relevant to identifying sustained training effects, if any, or the maintenance of training effects. For example, F. Li, Harmer, et al. (2005) showed that although participants in both Tai Chi and low-impact exercise control groups showed significant reductions in functional measures from the end of a six-month intervention to follow-up six months postintervention, the Tai Chi group showed significantly slower deterioration in these measures than the control group. Importantly, however, Tai Chi participants who showed improvements in measures of functional balance at the intervention end point had a significantly reduced risk of falls during the six-month postintervention period compared with the control group.

The extent to which the experience and qualifications of a Tai Chi instructor affect research outcomes is unclear. Although there is a spectrum of opinions on what constitutes a qualified instructor, as noted by several investigators (Wolf et al., 1996; Wu, 2002), qualifications matter as they may affect the quality of the intervention and whether fidelity is maintained and, hence, the efficacy of the intervention outcomes. With differences in Tai Chi styles, length of forms within and between styles, and different philosophies and practice/training emphases among the styles, it is quite conceivable that variation in qualifications among instructors introduces a significant covariate that has not often been attended to in RCTs. To date, there has been no evaluation of the potential impact of instructor quality on intervention delivery and outcomes.

There is a pressing need to explore the mechanism(s) underlying observed changes in clinical outcomes as a result of Tai Chi training. Research to date has largely involved Tai Chi as a therapeutic modality with end points of interest focused on improving clinical outcomes. However, a balance is needed between establishing the efficacy of Tai Chi training on health outcomes and understanding the mechanisms (physiological, biomechanical, social, or psychological) that underlie the Tai Chi–health relationship. Identifying mechanisms is vital for guiding decisions that will shape the design and evaluation of future intervention studies. For example, although Tai Chi has been shown to reduce falls, the training mechanism(s) responsible remains largely unexplored. In one study, F. Li et al. (2004) showed that improvements in balance may be responsible for reductions in falls following Tai Chi training. However, other mechanisms may be operating concomitantly to produce this effect. Clearly, a mechanistic approach is needed to fully understand how to produce meaningful changes in clinical outcomes.

It is important to demonstrate that an evidence-based preventive intervention is not only beneficial but cost-effective. This information is vital for policy makers and public health practitioners as they determine the economic feasibility of offering a program to improve population health outcomes. In general, Tai Chi has been shown to be a low-cost exercise administratively (F. Li et al., 2001; F. Li, Harmer, Glasgow, et al., 2008). In a cost–benefit analysis, Wilson and Datta (2001) showed that Tai Chi was cost saving both in direct benefits alone (hip fracture costs averted) and in direct plus indirect benefits, with a total net cost savings of $1,274.43 per person per year. Their analyses also indicated that a Tai Chi intervention could avert approximately 50 falls per 100 participants annually; that approximately 200 patient-years of Tai Chi exposure would prevent 1 hip fracture, at a savings of $17,268 per hip fracture averted; and that 800 patient-years of Tai Chi exposure would prevent 1 death. Although the Wilson and Datta (2001) data speak to the potential impact versus cost of Tai Chi for nursing home residents, they need to be viewed critically because the efficacy of Tai Chi in reducing falls for this frail institutionalized population has not been established with RCTs. At a minimum, this information will be useful for future large-scale dissemination efforts in broader community settings as well as for promoting evidence-based behavioral medicine in clinical practice.

There is clearly a need to evaluate the efficacy of Tai Chi specifically for clinical subpopulations and geriatric-specific chronic diseases and conditions, such as heart disease, diabetes mellitus, depression, and osteoporosis. The paucity of empirical trials in this area is evident. Similarly, although Tai Chi training has been shown to improve balance and postural control, no studies have targeted patients with vestibular disease (Wayne et al., 2004). On the positive side, the current research has provided impetus for further investigation in these areas.

Finally, relatively little is known about whether successful, evidence-based interventions can make the transition to mainstream use (i.e., be configured for community or clinical practice). RCTs are conducted under predefined study control conditions with specific inclusion/exclusion criteria. Consequently, whether efficacious programs derived from rigidly controlled trials can be directly applied and disseminated in the diverse circumstances of public health practice to reach broader, community-based service providers remains to be determined. Similarly, the uptake of evidence-based clinical practices continues to lag well behind the accumulation of scientific knowledge, and the identification and implementation of best practices has received scant attention. Thus, there is a need for broader dissemination once Tai Chi training has been shown effective for particular disease conditions. Some initial efforts in the areas of promoting general health (Jones, Dean, & Scudds, 2005) and falls prevention (F. Li, Harmer, Glasgow, et al., 2008; F. Li, Harmer, Mack, et al., 2008) have shown promising outcomes in terms of feasibility, uptake, program fidelity, effectiveness, and program sustainability.

Implications

From the perspective of public health promotion, Tai Chi has several inherent benefits: It does not require special equipment, clothing, or footwear and can take place almost anywhere. These unique features are likely to appeal to and are well suited for older adult populations. Moreover, a specific Tai Chi routine can be modified to accommodate the functional level of participants, including individuals in wheelchairs or those with restricted levels of physical activity. There are at least two research-based, simplified Yang-style programs that have been evaluated and shown to be effective in improving strength and balance, reducing the risk of falls, and promoting overall physical functioning and well-being in older adults (Li et al., 2005, Li, Harmer, Glasgow, et al. 2008; Wolf et al., 1996). These modified programs are safe, appropriate, and sufficiently flexible to allow communities of older adults to perform to their potential.

Although studies have varied significantly in design, outcome measures, and Tai Chi styles and forms implemented, findings with public health and clinical implications relating to improved balance and reduced risk of falls are clearly supported. However, evidence is lacking or insufficient for specific disease treatment; therefore, it would be premature to derive any clinically meaningful implications. With this in mind, the following provides a summary of practical implications derived from the current research inquiry.

Findings from existing Tai Chi research preclude any conclusive recommendations in regard to appropriate training frequency, duration, and intensity. However, given that Tai Chi is generally considered a low- to moderate-impact exercise, decisions on proper training parameters should depend on the health outcome under scrutiny. For example, it may take significantly less time or effort to observe a treatment effect on psychologically based end-point measures (e.g., mental health or well-being) than to detect meaningful change in physiologically or physically based end-point measures (e.g., strength, gait, reductions in falls).

From the perspective of physical rehabilitation, the effectiveness of Tai Chi for improving lower-extremity strength, balance, and gait suggests that exercises need not be performed at high intensity for therapeutic benefits. For example, Tai Chi, as a low- to moderate-intensity exercise, may be beneficial as a stand-alone exercise regimen or an add-on for community-dwelling older adults to improve balance (F. Li, Harmer, Fisher, et al., 2005; Wolf et al., 1996; Wolfson et al., 1996). Although the optimal duration and frequency remain to be determined, studies that have shown improvements in balance-related parameters suggest a regimen of twice weekly practice for 16 weeks. Although Tai Chi training improves balance in older adults, whether it will specifically benefit a clinical patient population with vestibulopathic disease by remediating impaired postural control remains uncertain (Wayne et al., 2004).

There is good evidence that Tai Chi can reduce fear of falling, fall frequency, and risk of falling for community-dwelling older adults (F. Li, Fisher, Harmer, & McAuley, 2004; Li, Harmer, Fisher et al., 2005; Sattin et al., 2005; Voukelatos et al., 2007; Wolf et al., 1996, 2003). However, there are important caveats. First, efficacy of falls reduction has been established primarily in community-dwelling older adults. There is no compelling evidence that the same outcomes would occur in institutionalized frail elders. Second, the intervention data from these efficacy studies clearly indicate that at least three months of training are needed before a meaningful reduction in frequency of falls can be achieved. Despite these considerations, Tai Chi is recommended as a falls prevention exercise for the older adult population by the American Geriatrics Society, British Geriatrics Society, and American Academy of Orthopaedic Surgeons (American Geriatrics Society, British Geriatrics Society, and American Academy of Orthopaedic Surgeons Panel on Falls Prevention, 2001), American College of Sports Medicine (Chodzko-Zajko et al., 2009), and the Centers for Disease Control and Prevention (2010).

With health spending on chronic conditions rising among older adults, particularly Medicare patients, there is an increasing need for making evidence-based preventive programs available in the community (Thorpe, Ogden, & Galactionova,

2010). Tai Chi has much potential in this regard, and there are preliminary indications that disseminating a Tai Chi program in a broad community context is both receptive and feasible. In falls prevention, for example, F. Li and colleagues (F. Li, Harmer, Glasgow, et al., 2008; F. Li, Harmer, Mack, et al., 2008) built on a prior RCT (F. Li, Harmer, et al., 2005) to evaluate whether their evidence-based *Tai Chi: Moving for Better Balance* program could be translated and implemented in a local community setting. Within the RE-AIM framework (Glasgow & Emmons, 2007), the outcomes of the dissemination project showed promising results in terms of adoption by community activity centers, reach into the older adult target population, feasibility of program implementation, and fidelity, as well as sustainability. At this writing, the program has been adopted by the departments of health in several U.S. states, including Oregon, Colorado, California, Connecticut, Florida, Maryland, New Mexico, and New York, and in numerous local communities across the country.

F. Li and his colleagues are currently extending the dissemination work to involve health care providers (physicians, physical therapists, and nurse practitioners) in referring their patients into a Tai Chi program. If this research-to-practice effort proves to be successful in terms of uptake among clinical practitioners and effective in reducing frequency of falls and maintaining or improving physical function, the project will have far-reaching implications for clinical or service delivery agencies that wish to implement falls prevention programs.

Summary and Conclusions

Tai Chi has a history going back more than 300 years (China Sports, 1980) and is practiced by millions worldwide. It is gradually being recognized as a viable alternative exercise modality for people of all ages. Accumulating evidence, obtained primarily on the basis of RCTs, suggests that Tai Chi may be efficacious as a behavioral medicine approach for the prevention and rehabilitation of chronic diseases and dysfunctional mental and physical conditions commonly associated with advancing age. Although a number of issues of methodological and clinical importance have yet to be critically examined, it is time to promote Tai Chi as an exercise regimen for maintaining routine physical functioning, delaying disabilities, and consequently improving independence and quality of life for the older adult population across broad community settings.

Acknowledgment

The work is supported by a grant from the Centers for Disease Control and Prevention, National Center for Injury Prevention and Control (1-R18 CE001723).

References

American Geriatrics Society, British Geriatrics Society, and American Academy of Orthopaedic Surgeons Panel on Falls Prevention. (2001). Guideline for the prevention of falls in older persons. *Journal of the American Geriatrics Society, 49,* 664–672.

Centers for Disease Control and Prevention. (2010). *Falls among older adults: An overview.* Retrieved on February 25, 2010, from http://www.cdc.gov/HomeandRecreationalSafety/Falls/adultfalls.html

Chan, K., Qin, L., Lau, M., Woo, J., Au, S., Choy, W.,...Lee, S. (2004). A randomized, prospective study of the effects of Tai Chi Chun exercise on bone mineral density in post-menopausal women. *Archives of Physical Medicine and Rehabilitation, 85*(5), 717–722.

China Sports. (1980). *Simplified "Taijiquan."* Beijing: Foreign Language Printing House.

Chodzdo-Zajko, W. J., Proctor, D. N., Fiatarone Singh, M. A., Minson, C. T., Nigg, C. R., Salem, G. J., & Skinner, J. S. (2009). Exercise and physical activity for older adults. *Medicine & Science in Sports & Exercise, 41,* 1510–1530.

Christou, E. A., Yang, Y., & Rosengren, K. S. (2003). Taiji training improves knee extensor strength and force control in older adults. *Journal of Gerontology: Biological Sciences and Medical Sciences, 58*(8), 763–766.

Fahn, S., Elton, R. I., Members of the UPDRS Development Committee (1987). Unified Parkinson's Disease Rating Scale. In: S. Fahn, C. D. Marsden, D. B. Calne, M. Goldstein, editors. *Recent developments in Parkinson's disease* (pp. 153–163, vol. 2). Florham Park, NJ: Macmillan Health Care Information.

Glasgow, R. E., & Emmons, K. M. (2007). How can we increase translation of research into practice? Types of evidence needed. *Annual Review of Public Health, 28,* 413–433.

Hackney, M. E., & Earhart, G. M. (2008). Tai Chi improves balance and mobility in people with Parkinson disease. *Gait & Posture, 28*(3), 456–460.

Hain, T. C., Fuller, L., Weil, L., & Kotsias, J. (1999). Effects of T'ai Chi on balance. *Archives of Otolaryngology—Head and Neck Surgery, 125*(11), 1191–1195.

Harmer, P., & Li, F. (2008). Tai Chi and falls prevention in older people. In Y. Hong (Ed.), *Tai Chi Chuan: State of the art in international research* (pp. 124–134). Basel, Switzerland: Karger.

Hartman, C. A., Manos, T. M., Winter, C., Hartman, D., Li, B., & Smith, J. C. (2000). Effects of T'ai Chi training on function and quality of life indicators in older adults with osteoarthritis. *Journal of the American Geriatrics Society, 48,* 1553–1559.

Hass, C. J., Gregor, R. J., Waddell, D. E., Oliver, A., Smith, D. S., Fleming, R. P., & Wolf, S. L. (2004). The influence of Tai Chi training on the center of pressure trajectory during gait initiation in older adults. *Archives of Physical Medicine and Rehabilitation, 85,* 1953–1958.

Hoehn, M., & Yahr, M. (1967). Parkinsonism, onset, progression and mortality. *Neurology, 17,* 427–442.

Irwin, M. R., Olmstead, R., & Motivala, S. J. (2008). Improving sleep quality in older adults with moderate sleep complaints: A randomized controlled trial of Tai Chi Chih. *Sleep, 31,* 1001–1008.

Irwin, M. R., Olmstead, R., & Oxman, M. N. (2007). Augmenting immune responses to varicella zoster virus in older adults: A randomized, controlled trial of Tai Chi. *Journal of the American Geriatrics Society, 55,* 511–517.

Jones, A. Y., Dean, E., & Scudds, R. J. (2005). Effectiveness of a community-based Tai Chi program and implications for public health initiatives. *Archives of Physical Medicine and Rehabilitation, 86,* 619–625.

Kutner, N. G., Barnhart, H., Wolf, S. L., McNeely, E., & Xu, T. (1997). Self-report benefits of Tai Chi practice by older adults. *Journal of Gerontology: Psychological Sciences, 52,* 242–246.

Lachman, M., Howland, J., Tennstedt, S., Jette, A., Assmann, S., & Peterson, W. (1998). Fear of falling and activity restriction: The Survey of Activities and Fear of Falling in the Elderly (SAFE). *Journal of Gerontology B: Psychological Sciences, 53*(1), P43–P50.

Lan, C., Lai, J.-S., Chen, S.-Y., & Wong, M.-K. (1998). 12-Month Tai Chi training in the elderly: Its effect on health fitness. *Medicine & Science in Sports & Exercise, 30,* 345–351.

Li, F., Duncan, T. E., Duncan, S. C., McAuley, E., Chaumeton, N. R., & Harmer, P. (2001). Enhancing the psychological well-being of elderly individuals through Tai Chi exercise: A latent growth curve analysis. *Structural Equation Modeling: A Multidisciplinary Journal, 8,* 53–83.

Li, F., Fisher, K. J., Harmer, P., & McAuley, E. (2002). Delineating the impact of Tai Chi training on physical function among the elderly: Modeling the moderating effects of unobserved class trajectories. *American Journal of Preventive Medicine, 23,* 92–97.

Li, F., Fisher, K. J., Harmer, P., Irbe, D., Tearse, R. G., & Weimer, C. (2004). Tai Chi and self-rated quality of sleep and daytime sleepiness in older adults: A randomized controlled trial. *Journal of the American Geriatrics Society, 52,* 892–900.

Li, F., Fisher, K. J., Harmer, P., & McAuley, E. (2004). Tai Chi: Improving functional balance and predicting subsequent falls in older persons. *Medicine & Science in Sports & Exercise, 36*(12), 2046–2052.

Li, F., Fisher, K. J., Harmer, P., & McAuley, E. (2005). Falls self-efficacy as a mediator of fear of falling in an exercise intervention for older adults. *Journal of Gerontology: Psychological Sciences, 60*(1), P34–P40.

Li, F., Fisher, K. J., Harmer, P., & Shirai, M. (2003). A simpler 8-form easy Tai Chi for elderly persons. *Journal of Aging and Physical Activity, 11,* 217–229.

Li, F., Harmer, P., Fisher, K. J., McAuley, E., Chaumeton, N., Eckstrom, E., & Wilson, N. L. (2005). Tai Chi and fall reductions in older adults: A randomized controlled trial. *Journal of Gerontology: Biological Science and Medical Sciences, 60*(2), 187–194.

Li, F., Harmer, P., Fisher, K. J., Xu, J., Fitzgerald, K., & Vongjaturapat, N. (2007). Tai Chi-based exercise for older adults with Parkinson's disease: A pilot program evaluation. *Journal of Aging and Physical Activity, 15,* 139–151.

Li, F., Harmer, P., Fitzgerald, K, Eckstrom, E., Stock., Galver, J., Maddalozzo, G., & Batya, S. S. (2012). Tai Chi postural stability in patients with Parkinson's disease patients. *New England Journal of Medicine, 366,* 511–519.

Li, F., Harmer, P., Glasgow, R., Mack, K. A., Sleet, D., Fisher, K. J., …Tompkins, Y. (2008). Translation of an effective Tai Chi intervention into a community-based falls prevention program. *American Journal of Public Health*, 98(7), 1195–1198.

Li, F., Harmer, P., Mack, K. A., Sleet, D., Fisher, K. J., Kohn, M. A.,…Tompkins, Y. (2008). Tai Chi: Moving for Better Balance: Development of a community-based falls prevention program. *Journal of Physical Activity & Health*, 5, 445–455.

Li, F., Harmer, P., McAuley, E., Duncan, T. E., Duncan, S. C., Chaumeton, N. R., & Fisher, J. (2001). An evaluation of the effects of Tai Chi exercise on physical function among older persons: A randomized controlled trial. *Annals of Behavioral Medicine*, 2, 89–101.

Li, F., McAuley, E., Harmer, P., Duncan, T. E., & Chaumeton, N. R. (2001). Tai Chi influences on self-efficacy and exercise behavior in older adults. *Journal of Aging and Physical Activity*, 9, 161–171.

Li, F., McAuley, E., Harmer, P., Duncan, T. E., & Chaumeton, N. R. (2002). Tai Chi as a means to enhance self-esteem: A randomized controlled trial. *Journal of Applied Gerontology*, 21, 70–89.

Li, F., McAuley, E., Harmer, P., Fisher, J., Duncan, T. E., & Duncan, S. C. (2001). Tai Chi, self-efficacy, and physical function in the elderly. *Prevention Science*, 2(4), 229–239.

Li, J. X., Hong, Y., & Chan, K. M. (2001). Tai Chi: Physiological characteristics and beneficial effects on health. *British Journal of Sports Medicine*, 35, 148–156.

Liang, S.-Y., & Wu, W.-C. (1996). *Tai Chi Chuan: 24 & 48 postures with martial applications*. Roslindale, MA: YMAA Publication Center.

Logghe, I. H. J., Zeeuwe, P. E. M., Verhagen A. P., Wijnen-Sponselee, R. M. T., Willemsen, S. P., Bierma-Zeinstra, S. M. A., …Koes, B. W. (2009). Lack of effect of Tai Chi Chuan in preventing falls in elderly people living at home: A randomized clinical trial. *Journal of the American Geriatrics Society*, 57, 70–75.

National Institute on Aging (2010). *Exercise and physical activity: Your everyday guide from the National Institute on Aging*. Retrieved on February 15, 2010, from http://www.nia.nih.gov/HealthInformation/Publications/ExerciseGuide/

Nelson, M. E., Rejeski, W. J., Blair, S. N., Duncan, P. W., Judge J. O., King A. C.,…Castaneda-Sceppa, C. (2007). Physical activity and public health in older adults: Recommendation from the American College of Sports Medicine and the American Heart Association. *Medicine & Science in Sports & Exercise*, 39, 1435–1445.

People's Sports. (1996). *Tai Chi Chuan: Collected works*. Beijing: People's Sports Publications.

Sattin, R. W., Easley, K. A., Wolf, S. L., Chen, Y., & Kutner, M. H. (2005). Reduction in fear of falling through intense Tai Chi exercise training in older, transitionally frail adults. *Journal of the American Geriatrics Society*, 53, 1168–1178.

Song, R., Lee, E. O., Lam, P., & Bae, S. C. (2003). Effects of Tai Chi exercise on pain, balance, muscle strength, and perceived difficulties in physical functioning in older women with osteoarthritis: A randomized clinical trial. *Journal of Rheumatology*, 30, 2039–2044.

Thorpe, K. E., Ogden, L. L., & Galactionova, K. (2010). Chronic conditions account for rise in Medicare spending from 1987 to 2006. *Health Affairs*, 29, 718–724.

Tsai, J.-C., Wang, W.-H., Chan, P., Lin, L.-J., Wang C.-H., Tomlinson, B.,…Liu, J. C. (2003). The beneficial effects of Tai Chi Chuan on blood pressure and lipid profile and anxiety status in a randomized controlled trial. *Journal of Alternative and Complementary Medicine*, 9, 747–754.

Tsang, T., Orr, R., Lam, P., Comino, E., & Singh, M. F. (2008). Effects of Tai Chi on glucose homeostasis and insulin sensitivity in older adults with type 2 diabetes: A randomised double-blind sham-exercise-controlled trial. *Age and Ageing*, 37, 64–71.

Tsang, W. W. N., & Hui-Chan, C. W. Y. (2003). Effects of Tai Chi on joint proprioception and stability limits in elderly subjects. *Medicine & Science in Sports & Exercise*, 35, 1962–1971.

Tse, S. K., & Bailey, D. M. (1992). T'ai Chi and postural control in the well elderly. *American Journal of Occupational Therapy*, 46, 295–300.

United Nations. (2007). *World population prospects: The 2006 revision. Highlights* (Working Paper No. ESA/P/WP.202). New York: United Nations Department of Economic and Social Affairs, Population Division. Also available at http://www.un.org/esa/population/publications/wpp2006/WPP2006_Highlights_rev.pdf

Voukelatos, A., Cumming, R. G., Lord, S. R., & Rissel, C. (2007). A randomized, controlled trial of Tai Chi for the prevention of falls: The Central Sydney Tai Chi Trial. *Journal of the American Geriatrics Society*, 55, 1185–1191.

Wang, C., Collet, J. P., & Lau, J. (2004). The effects of Tai Chi on health outcomes in patients with chronic conditions: A systematic review. *Archives of Internal Medicine*, 164, 493–501.

Wang, C., Schmid, C. H., Hibberd, P. L., Kalish, R., Roubenoff, R., Rones, R., & McAlindon, T. (2009). Tai Chi is effective in treating knee osteoarthritis: A randomized controlled trial. *Arthritis & Rheumatism*, 61, 1545–1553.

Wang, C, Schmid, C. H., Rones, B. S., Kalish, R., Yinh, J., Goldenberg, D. L.,…McAlindon, T. (2010). A randomized trial of Tai Chi for fibromyalgia. *New England Journal of Medicine*, 363, 743–754.

Wayne, P. M., Krebs, D. E., Wolf, S. L., Gill-Body, K. M., Scarborough, D. M., McGibbon, C. A.,…Parker, S. W. (2004). Can Tai Chi improve vestibulopathic postural control? *Archives of Physical Medicine and Rehabilitation*, 85, 142–152.

Wilson, C. J., & Datta, S. K. (2001). Tai Chi for the prevention of fractures in a nursing home population: An economic analysis. *Journal of Clinical Outcomes Management*, 8, 19–27.

Wolf, S. L., Barnhart, H. X., Kutner, N. G., McNeely, E., Coogler, C., Xu, T., & the Atlanta FICSIT Group (1996). Reducing frailty and falls in older persons: An investigation of Tai Chi and computerized balance training. *Journal of the American Geriatrics Society*, 44, 489–497.

Wolf, S. L., Coogler, C., & Xu, T. (1997). Exploring the basis for Tai Chi Chuan as a therapeutic exercise approach. *Archives of Physical Medicine and Rehabilitation*, 78, 886–892.

Wolf, S. L., Sattin, R. W., Kutner, M., O'Grady, M., Greenspan, A. I., & Gregor, R. J. (2003). Intense Tai Chi exercise training and fall occurrences in older, transitionally frail adults: A randomized, controlled trial. *Journal of the American Geriatrics Society*, 51, 1693–1701.

Wolfson, L., Whipple, R., Derby, C., Judge, J., King, M., Amerman, P.,…Smyers, D. (1996). Balance and strength training in older adults: Intervention gains and Tai Chi maintenance. *Journal of the American Geriatrics Society*, 44, 498–506.

Woo, J., Hong, A., Lau, E., & Lynn, H. (2007). A randomized controlled trial of Tai Chi and resistance exercise on bone health, muscle strength and balance in community-living elderly people. *Age and Ageing, 36,* 262–268.

Wu, G. (2002). Evaluation of the effectiveness of Tai Chi for improving balance and preventing falls in the older population—a review. *Journal of American Geriatrics Society, 50,* 746–754.

Wu, G., Zhao, F., Zhou, X, & Wei, L. (2002). Improvement of isokinetic knee extensor strength and reduction of postural sway in the elderly from long-term Tai Chi exercise. *Archives of Physical Medicine and Rehabilitation, 83,* 1364–1369.

Yang, Z. (1991). *Yang style Taijiquan* (2nd ed.). Beijing: Morning Glory.

Yeh, G. Y., McCarthy, E. P., Wayne, P. M., Stevenson, L. W., Wood, M. J., Forman, D., . . . Phillips, R. S. (2011). Tai Chi exercise in patients with chronic heart failure: A randomized clinical trial. *Archives of Internal Medicine, 171*(8), 750–757.

Yeh, G. Y., Wood, J. M., Lorell, B., H., Stevenson, L. W., Eisenberg, D. M., Wayne, P. M., . . . Phillips, R. S. (2004). Effects of Tai Chi mind–body movement therapy on functional status and exercise capacity in patients with chronic heart failure: A randomized controlled trial. *American Journal of Medicine, 117,* 541–548.

Young, D. R., Appel, L. J., Jee, S. H., & Miller, E. R. (1999). The effects of aerobic exercise and T'ai Chi on blood pressure in older people: Results of a randomized trial. *Journal of the American Geriatrics Society, 47,* 277–284.

INDEX

A

ACC. *See* anterior cingulated cortex

ACSM. *See* American College of Sports Medicine

ACTH. *See* adrenocorticotrophic hormone

Action for Health in Diabetes Trial, 107

action stage, in TTM, 284

action theory, for personality and physical theory, 206

ACTivity PromoTION (ACTION) trial, 452–453

acute exercise, 41
  anxiety levels and, 43
  body image and, as research topic, 67
  cognition and, 77–82. *See also* cognitive-energetic model
  catecholamines and, 82
  CBF and, 81–82
  central fatigue hypothesis for, 79
  duration as influence on, 78
  inverted-U hypothesis for, 78–79
  mechanisms for, 81–82
  serotonin and, 82
  theoretical basis for, 78–81
  transient hypofrontality hypothesis for, 79–80, 80

AD. *See* Alzheimer's disease

ADAPT. *See* Arthritis, Diet, and Activity Promotion Trial

adaptive immunity, 137
  function of, 176

adenosine triphosphate (ATP), 146–147

adolescents
  with disabilities, physical activity for, 338–339
    barriers to, 344–346
    community disapproval for, 345
    competence and, 338, 350
    enjoyment levels for, 350–351
    environmental barriers to, 345–346
    feelings of normalcy from, 338
    independence and, 338
    individual self-perceptions for, 338

institutional barriers to, 345
institutional predictors for, 351
pain as barrier to, 344–345
parents as barrier to, 345
peer disapproval, 345
among peers, 338–339
PE personnel disapproval, 345
physical construction barriers to, 345–346
predictors for, 350–351
reciprocity and, among peers, 339
self-efficacy from, 350
in social environments, 338–339
type of disability as barrier to, 344
intelligence and exercise in, 410–412
  interventions for, 419–425
  measurement for, 425
  methodologies for, 422–425
  NAPSE guidelines for, 410
  research findings for, 422–425
physical activity for, 26
  with disabilities, 338–339
  recommendation guidelines for, in U.S., 29
sedentary behavior among, 26
self-efficacy for, 393

adrenocorticotrophic hormone (ACTH), 131, 175

adults
  with disabilities, physical activity for, 339–343
    barriers to, 346–349
    competence and, 339
    economic costs of, 348
    enjoyment levels for, 339–340
    environmental barriers to, 348–349
    exercise interventions for, with developmental disabilities, 420–421
    family influence on, 342–343
    fatigue from, 347
    fear as factor in, 347
    fitness facility personnel disapproval, 348

health care personnel and, 348, 353
illness and, 347
individual self-perceptions for, 339–341
injury and, 347
institutional barriers to, 348–349
lack of knowledge and, 347
lack of opportunity for, 349
neighborhood topography as barrier, 349
pain from, 347
parental influence on, 343
predictors for, 351–353
prior experience as predictor for, 351–352
QoL for, 340–341
relationship complexity and, 341–342
self-concept for, 352
self-efficacy from, 339, 352
siblings as influence on, 343
social barriers to, 348
in social environments, 341–343
social interactions and, 342
time constraints for, 347–348
TPB for, 352–353
TRA for, 353
by type of disability, 346–347
physical activity recommendation guidelines for, in U.S., 28, 253–254

aerobic exercise
  anxiety levels and, 42–43
  guidelines for, 5
  mental health benefits from, 5
  for older adults, 369
    cognitive impairment and, 374–375

affect
  core, 322–323
  in decision research, 301
  in exercise psychology, 247–248. *See also* dual-mode theory

event related potentials (ERPs), 78–79
evolution, physical activity and, 10
executive processes, for intelligence,
    416–417
exercise. *See also* acute exercise; aerobic
        exercise; anaerobic exercise;
        chronic exercise; exercise
        psychology; psychosocial
        influences, on exercise;
        resistance exercise
    ACSM guidelines for, 5
    AHA guidelines for, 5
    anxiety and, 41–45
        academic literature on, 41–42
        with acute exercise, 43
        with aerobic exercise, 42–43
        anaerobic exercise and, 44, 44–45,
            45
        change mechanisms for, 50–51
        with chronic exercise, 43
        consensus statements for, 52
        distraction/time-out hypothesis
            for, 51
        dose-response approaches to,
            44–45, 50
        future research applications with,
            51–52
        pharmacotherapy compared to, 44
        practical recommendations for, 51
        preventive effects for, evidence
            of, 42
        research on, 41–42
        thermogenic hypothesis for, 51
        traditional treatment therapies
            versus, 43–44
        treatment therapies with, 45–51
    anxiolytic effects of, 40, 44
    assessment measures for, 5–6
    BDNF expression with, 136
    body image and
        by age, 64–65
        baseline body image with, 63
        body composition and, 60–61
        cardiovascular fitness and, 61
        characteristics of exercise, 65–66
        dose-response approach in, 69–70
        for eating disorder therapy, 69
        environmental influences on, 67
        by ethnicity, 65
        exerciser characteristics, 63–65
        experience level, with exercise, 63
        focus on body function over
            appearance in, 71
        by gender, 63–64
        gender-role orientation and, 64
        mechanisms for, 57–60, 58–59
        meta-analytic studies for, 56–57
        moderators for, 63, 59–71
        multiple dimensions of,
            measurement criteria for,
            71–72
        objective improvements to, 60–62
        perceived improvements from, 62

recommendations for, 70–72
self-efficacy improvements from, 62
strength fitness and, 61
study design theories for, 70–71
among women, 62
brain structure after, 369, 370,
    411–412
    angiogenesis, 369, 412
    animal studies on, 412
    infant research on, 411
    neurogenesis from, 369
    play research on, 411–412
    synaptogenesis from, 369, 412
definition of, 4, 360
dependency, 6
FITT principles of, 65
health risks from, 6
HRQL influenced by, 100–108
    appropriateness of interpretation
        for, 111–112
    with cancer, 98, 101–104
    with COPD, 98, 104
    future research for, 111
    gender and, 108
    mediators for, 108
    moderators for, 108
    for multiple sclerosis, 98, 109
    with obesity, 98, 106–108
    with osteoarthritis, 98, 100–101
    social and behavioural
        characteristics for, 112–113
intelligence and, in children, 419–425
intention and, 225
kinesiophobia and, 308
methodological parameters for, 5–7
muscle pain and, 149–153
    as analgesic intervention, 156–158
    BKN and, 146, 151
    cardiorespiratory increases as
        analgesic, 158
    definition of, 144
    distraction as analgesic, 158
    DOMS and, 144, 149–151
    during exercise, 151–153
    5-HT serotonin and, 146
    gate-control theory for, 148–149,
        158
    gender and, 155–156
    H^+ ions in, 145–146
    noxious chemicals and, 145–146
    opioid mechanisms during, 158
    performance influenced by,
        161–162
    possible mechanisms for, 152
    proton ions in, 145–146
    repeated-bout effect from,
        156–157
    by type of exercise, 157–158
neuroticism levels influenced by,
    42, 48
overuse injuries from, 6
for panic disorder, 48
physical activity compared to, 4–5

PMT for, 289–290
positive psychology and, 123–125
    BPS intervention for, 124
    hedonic adaptation theory for,
        123
    SDT for, 123–124
    set point theory for, 123
    strengths-based approach to,
        124–125
psychophysiological stress responses
        during
    HPA activity, 133
    with physical activity, 133–136
    SNS activity, 133
    in SCT, 281–282
    SDT and, 123–124
        physical activity with, 287–288
    self-efficacy from, 62
    TPB and, 229–235
        advantages of, 230
        comparison studies for, 229–230
        control beliefs in, 229
        dual route models in, 231
        explicit processes in, 232
        flexibility of, 230–231
        implementation strategies in, 232
        implicit processes in, 231–232
        integrated approaches to,
            232–235
        intention in, 230–231, 232
        limitations of, 230, 231
        perceived control in, 229
        planning strategies for, 232
        SCT and, 227
        SDT and, 233, 233–234
        social beliefs in, 229
        in social psychology, 230
        subjective norms in, 229
        testing limitations of, 231
    tranquilizer effects of, 44
exercise dependency, 6
exercise psychology
    affect in, 247–248. *See also* dual-mode
            theory
        as anticipated, 247
        associations for, 247
        attitudes for, 247
        as behavioral motivator, 309–311
        enjoyment in, 310–311
        parameters of, 247
        reason in conflict with, 323–324
        reassessment of, 311–314
        theories for, 244–245
    affective processes in, 247–248
        as anticipated, 247
        associations for, 247
        attitudes for, 247
        as behavioral motivator, 309–311
        enjoyment in, 310–311
        parameters of, 247
        reassessment of, 311–314
        in theories for, 244–245
    dominant paradigm in, 298

estrogen role in, 155–156
during exercise, 155–156
thresholds, 155
tolerance levels, 155
negative body image among, 56
environmental influences on
exercise for, 67
exercise interventions for, 63–64
physical fitness and, 62
during pregnancy, 68–69
SPA, 61, 62
osteoporosis in, physical activity
and, 24

pain tolerance levels for, 155
personality and physical activity for,
213–214
physical fitness for, 62
psychological stress for, cardiorespiratory
adaptations to, 171
SPA among, 62
exercise environment and, 61
work, physical activity and. *See*
occupational studies
working memory
aging and, 367
intelligence and, 416

World Health Organization (WHO)
aging demographic predictions, 359
HRQL definition of, 99
WTBS study. *See* Weight Training
for Breast Cancer
Survivors study

Y
yoga, after cancer, 438–439
Young, Paul T., 307

Z
Zajonc, Robert, 300